G. KELLY C/N
9B

a **LANGE** clinical manual

Practical Oncology

GW00697528

DO NOT

REMOVE

FROM

WARD

a **LANGE** clinical manual

Practical Oncology

First Edition

Edited by

Robert B. Cameron, MD
Department of Surgery
University of California, Los Angeles, School of Medicine
Los Angeles, California

APPLETON & LANGE
Norwalk, Connecticut

ISBN   0-8385-1326-3

9 780838 513262   90000

Notice: The authors and the publisher of this volume have taken care to make certain that the doses of drugs and schedules of treatment are correct and compatible with the standards generally accepted at the time of publication. Nevertheless, as new information becomes available, changes in treatment and in the use of drugs become necessary. The reader is advised to carefully consult the instruction and information material included in the package insert of each drug or therapeutic agent before administration. This advice is especially important when using new or infrequently used drugs. The publisher disclaims any liability, loss, injury, or damage incurred as a consequence, directly or indirectly, of the use and application of any of the contents of this volume.

Copyright © 1994 by Appleton & Lange
Simon & Schuster Business and Professional Group

All rights reserved. This book, or any parts thereof, may not be used or reproduced in any manner without written permission. For information, address Appleton & Lange, 25 Van Zant Street, East Norwalk, Connecticut 06855.

94 95 96 97 98 / 10 9 8 7 6 5 4 3 2

Prentice Hall International (UK) Limited, *London*
Prentice Hall of Australia Pty. Limited, *Sydney*
Prentice Hall Canada, Inc., *Toronto*
Prentice Hall Hispanaoamericana, S.A., *Mexico*
Prentice Hall of India Private Limited, *New Delhi*
Prentice Hall of Japan, Inc., *Tokyo*
Simon & Schuster Asia Pte. Ltd., *Singapore*
Editoria Prentice Hall do Brasil Ltda., *Rio de Janeiro*
Prentice Hall, *Englewood Cliffs, New Jersey*

ISSN: 1072-1495

Acquisitions Editor: Shelley Reinhardt

PRINTED IN THE UNITED STATES OF AMERICA

This book is dedicated to Dianne and Brian, for their understanding, patience, and encouragement during the long and arduous task of preparing this text; to my mother for her steadfast love and support throughout my life; and to the memory of A. Malcolm Cameron and A. Bruce Cameron, both of whom experienced cancer's capricious and virulent nature.

ASSOCIATE EDITORS

Leonard Gomella, MD
Assistant Professor, Department of Urology, Jefferson Medical College of Thomas Jefferson University, Philadelphia, Pennsylvania.

James Heaps, MD
Clinical Assistant Professor, Department of Obstetrics and Gynecology, University of California, Los Angeles, School of Medicine, Los Angeles, California.

Howard L. Parnes, MD
Assistant Professor of Medicine and Oncology, University of Maryland, School of Medicine, Baltimore, Maryland.

CONSULTING EDITORS

Robert E. Bellet, MD
Clinical Associate Professor of Medicine; Head, Clinical Services; Associate Director of Clinical Oncology, Jefferson Medical College of Thomas Jefferson University, Philadelphia, Pennsylvania.

Gary E. Fishbein, MD
Clinical Assistant Professor of Medicine, Division of Neoplastic Diseases, Jefferson Medical College of Thomas Jefferson University, Philadelphia, Pennsylvania.

James Mulé, PhD
Senior Investigator, Surgery Branch, National Cancer Institute, National Institutes of Health, Bethesda, Maryland.

Steven Paikin, MD
Associate Professor, Division of Gastroenterology, Department of Medicine, Jefferson Medical College of Thomas Jefferson University, Philadelphia, Pennsylvania.

Lewis J. Rose, MD
Clinical Assistant Professor of Medicine, Division of Neoplastic Diseases, Jefferson Medical College of Thomas Jefferson University, Philadelphia, Pennsylvania.

Contents

Contributors

Mindy S. Bohrer, MD
Assistant Clinical Professor of Medicine, Tufts University School of Medicine; Department of Oncology/Hematology, Lawrence Memorial Hospital, Medford, Massachusetts.

James K. Bredenkamp, MD
Head and Neck Associates of Orange County, Laguna Hills, California.

Robert B. Cameron, MD
Chief Resident, Department of Surgery, University of California, Los Angeles, School of Medicine, Los Angeles, California.

Gregory Chow, MD
Chief Resident, Department of Orthopedic Surgery, University of California, Los Angeles, School of Medicine, Los Angeles, California.

Steven D. Colquhoun, MD
Clinical Instructor, Department of Surgery, University of California, Los Angeles, School of Medicine, Los Angeles, California.

Cynthia A. Corporan, MD
Fellow in Pediatric Surgical Oncology, MD Anderson Cancer Center, Houston, Texas.

Jeffrey Eckardt, MD
Professor of Orthopedic Surgery and Orthopedic Oncology, University of California, Los Angeles, School of Medicine, Los Angeles, California.

Mark F. Ellison, MD
The Urology Clinic, Georgia Lithotripsy Center, Athens, Georgia.

Fawzy I. Fawzy, MD
Professor and Deputy Chair, Department of Psychiatry and Biobehavioral Sciences, University of California, Los Angeles, School of Medicine, Los Angeles, California.

R. Bruce Filmer, MD
Chief, Department of Urology, Alfred I. DuPont Institute, Wilmington, Delaware.

Beth Fisher, MD
Charlottesville, Virginia

Jeffrey M. Fowler, MD
Assistant Professor, Department of Obstetrics and Gynecology, Division of Gynecologic Oncology, University of Minnesota Medical School, Minneapolis, Minnesota.

Leonard Gomella, MD
Assistant Professor, Department of Urology, Jefferson Medical College of Thomas Jefferson University, Philadelphia, Pennsylvania.

Michael Grasso, MD
Assistant Professor, Department of Urology, Loma Linda University School of Medicine, Loma Linda, California.

James Heaps, MD
Clinical Assistant Professor, Department of Obstetrics and Gynecology, University of California, Los Angeles, School of Medicine, Los Angeles, California.

Carl B. Heilman, MD
Chief Resident, Department of Neurosurgery, Tufts New England Medical Center, Boston, Massachusetts.

Thomas J. Howard, MD
Assistant Professor of Surgery, Indiana University Medical Center, Indianapolis, Indiana.

Christian Jensen, MD
Assistant Professor, Division of Urology, University of Utah School of Medicine, Salt Lake City, Utah.

Nora C. Ku, MD
Assistant Clinical Professor, Division of Hematology/Oncology, University of California, Irvine, College of Medicine, Irvine, California.

J. Michael Lahey, MD
Visiting Assistant Professor, Department of Ophthalmology, University of California, Los Angeles, School of Medicine, Los Angeles, California.

Matthew J. Lando, MD
Department of Otolaryngology–Head and Neck Surgery, Kaiser Permanente Medical Group, Hayward, California.

Robert S. Lavey, MD, MPH
Assistant Professor, Department of Radiation Oncology and Biomedical Physics, University of California, Los Angeles, School of Medicine, Los Angeles, California.

Alan T. Lefor, MD
Assistant Professor of Surgery and Oncology, Department of Surgery, University of Maryland School of Medicine, Baltimore, Maryland.

Joe K. McIntosh, MD
Assistant Professor of Surgery, Department of Pediatric Surgery, State University of New York Health Science Center at Brooklyn, College of Medicine, Brooklyn, New York.

Carlin J. McLaughlin, DO
Regional Internal Medicine Associates, Langhorne, Pennsylvania.

Jeffrey Miller, MD
Clinical Associate in Hematology/Oncology, University of Maryland School of Medicine, Baltimore, Maryland.

F.J. Montz, MD
Assistant Professor, Department of Obstetrics and Gynecology, University of California, Los Angeles, School of Medicine, Los Angeles, California.

Laila I. Muderspach, MD
Assistant Professor, Department of Obstetrics and Gynecology, Division of Gyneco-
logic Oncology, University of Southern California School of Medicine, Los Angeles,
California.

Barbara Natterson, MD
Resident, Department of Psychiatry, University of California, Los Angeles, School
of Medicine, Los Angeles, California.

Richard G. Nord, MD
Attending Physician, Youngstown Urologic Associates, Youngstown, Ohio.

Howard L. Parnes, MD
Assistant Professor of Medicine and Oncology, University of Maryland School of
Medicine, Baltimore, Maryland.

Joseph C. Poen, MD
Department of Radiation Oncology, University of California, Los Angeles, School of
Medicine, Los Angeles, California.

Cecilia Marina C. Prela, PharmD
United States Food and Drug Administration, Rockville, Maryland.

Patrick Roth, MD
Chief Resident, Department of Neurosurgery, Tufts New England Medical Center,
Boston, Massachusetts.

Victor Santana, MD
Associate Professor, Department of Pediatrics, University of Tennessee College of
Medicine; Associate Member, St. Jude Children's Research Hospital, Memphis,
Tennessee.

Stephen Saris, MD
Associate Professor, Department of Neurosurgery, Tufts New England Medical
Center, Boston, Massachusetts.

Edward Shlasko, MD
Assistant Professor of Surgery, Department of Pediatric Surgery, State University
of New York Health Science Center at Brooklyn, College of Medicine, Brooklyn,
New York.

James Stephanelli, MD
Chief Resident, Department of Urology, Jefferson Medical College of Thomas Jefferson University, Philadelphia, Pennsylvania.

Stephen Strup, MD
Chief Resident, Department of Urology, Jefferson Medical College of Thomas Jefferson University, Philadelphia, Pennsylvania.

Andres Taleisnik, MD
Resident, Department of Surgery, University of California, Los Angeles, School of
Medicine, Los Angeles, California.

Terence P. Wade, MD
Assistant Professor of Surgery, St. Louis University School of Medicine, St. Louis,
Missouri.

David E. Weissman, MD
Department of Medicine, Medical College of Wisconsin, Milwaukee County Medical
Complex, Milwaukee, Wisconsin.

Jan Wong, MD
Associate Clinical Professor of Surgery, Division of Surgical Oncology, University
of California, Los Angeles, School of Medicine, Los Angeles, California.

Preface

PURPOSE

In contradistinction to other oncology manuals, this text was conceived as a multidisciplinary synopsis of the art and science of oncology. It is the culmination of the work of over 40 authors from the specialties of medical, surgical, and radiation oncology. The authors have distilled the knowledge in their own area of special interest into concise, yet exhaustive, chapters on nearly every aspect of the practice of oncology from basic principles to each specific malignancy. The goal of the authors and editor is to provide a book that serves as both a portable textbook and a practical guide to the care of oncology patients. I hope that the contents will prove useful to medical and nursing students, interns, residents, oncology fellows, and practicing oncologists, alike.

ORGANIZATION AND SCOPE

The manual is divided into 4 major sections. The first segment discusses general principles of oncology. This includes basic information on medical, surgical, and radiation oncology as well as material on specific problems encountered by oncology patients. The second part of the manual outlines the details involved in each individual adult malignancy, from presentation and diagnosis through therapy and follow-up. The third major portion of the book addresses pediatric oncology in a similar fashion. Finally, an extensive appendix is included that summarizes pharmacologic data on chemotherapeutic agents and combination chemotherapy regimens.

OTHER USEFUL FEATURES

- The convenient outline format and selective use of boldface type afford quick, easy access to key aspects of patient assessment and management.
- Basic summaries of the appropriate pathophysiologic processes are provided if important for the understanding of the rationale behind the approach to diagnosis and therapy.
- Thorough descriptions of the appropriate surgical considerations and procedures are given.
- Extensive appendices cover nearly all chemotherapeutic agents, their indications, their uses in combination regimens, their dosages, and their toxicities.
- References are provided at the end of each chapter, listing only the most up-to-date clinical studies and reviews.

Although oncology is not an exact science, every attempt has been made to provide information that is generally accepted as exemplifying the standard of medical care. Where ambiguity or controversy exists, the authors have tried to objectively discuss available data so that intelligent decisions may be made regarding the care and treatment of the oncologic patient. Like all Lange manuals, feedback from the reader is vital to the success and future evolution of this book, and therefore, comments regarding this text are both welcomed and encouraged.

Robert B. Cameron, MD
July 1, 1993

1 Introduction to the Cancer Patient

Robert B. Cameron, MD

THE MAGNITUDE OF THE PROBLEM

In the United States, cancer is the **second leading cause of death** (23% of all deaths) after heart disease (34% of all deaths). Estimates indicate that in 1993, approximately **1,170,000 people will be diagnosed with cancer and 526,000 will die** from cancer-related illnesses. These figures do not include the more than 600,000 people who will develop nonmelanoma skin cancer. One of every 3 people living in the United States today will eventually battle a life-threatening malignancy. Unfortunately, the situation is not improving. With the exception of stomach and uterine cancers, which have declined 60% and 63%, respectively, over the last 30 years, the incidence of most cancers has remained unchanged, and the number of lung cancer cases has increased more than 160%. The estimated site- and sex-specific cancer incidences and deaths for 1992 are shown in Figure 1–1. Together, 4 malignancies— **lung, colorectal, breast, and prostate**—account for **55% of all new cancers and 54% of all cancer deaths**. The economic impact of cancer is staggering. In 1985 the overall cancer-related medical costs in the United States were estimated to exceed **$71.5 billion**.

PATIENT EVALUATION

I. **Performance status.** Although not formally included in cancer staging (see p 3, **V**), the patient's functional status often determines what therapeutic interventions he or she will tolerate. Appendix A provides 3 common scales of performance status.

II. **Medical history and physical examination.** A thorough medical history, including family history and pertinent cancer risk factors, must be obtained from all patients who have suspected neoplasms. In addition, a detailed physical examination that includes common metastatic sites is necessary.

III. **Nutritional status.** Many cancer patients, especially those with advanced disease, suffer from **cancer cachexia**. The severity of their malnutrition is determined by a number of factors, including the degree of (1) tumor- or chemotherapy-induced **anorexia**, (2) tumor-induced **increase in metabolism**, (3) tumor-induced **functional impairment of the gastrointestinal (GI) tract**, and (4) **fasting** required by diagnostic tests. The evaluation of the cancer patient requires a **complete nutritional assessment** and, if necessary, formulation of a **plan for nutritional therapy** that may include dietary changes, enteral feedings (through nasogastric, gastrostomy, or jejunostomy tubes), or parenteral nutrition (either peripheral or central).

IV. **Common diagnostic tests and procedures.** The following tests and procedures are often performed for specific reasons during the evaluation:

   A. **Blood tests**

   1. **Complete blood count.** Low hemoglobin levels may indicate external blood loss (eg, gastrointestinal and urologic), anemia (often associated with chronic diseases), or chemotherapy- or radiation-induced myelosuppression, whereas high hemoglobin levels (erythrocytosis) are characteristic of certain neoplasms such as hepatocellular carcinoma. In addition, many cancer patients have thrombocytosis; however, thrombocytopenia and leukopenia, along with anemia, are signs of significant myelosuppression.

   2. **Hepatic transaminases.** Elevated serum glutamic oxaloacetic transaminase (SGOT) and glutamic pyruvic transaminase (SGPT) levels may indicate the presence of hepatic metastases, coexisting acute or chronic liver disease, or toxicity induced by a chemotherapeutic agent such as fluorouracil, cisplatin, or methotrexate.

   3. **Alkaline phosphatase.** The serum enzyme alkaline phosphatase is a sensitive

1993 ESTIMATED CANCER INCIDENCE by SITE and SEX[1]

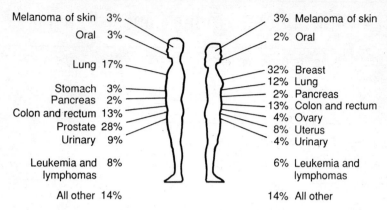

Melanoma of skin	3%			3%	Melanoma of skin
Oral	3%			2%	Oral
Lung	17%			32%	Breast
				12%	Lung
Stomach	3%			2%	Pancreas
Pancreas	2%			13%	Colon and rectum
Colon and rectum	13%			4%	Ovary
Prostate	28%			8%	Uterus
Urinary	9%			4%	Urinary
Leukemia and lymphomas	8%			6%	Leukemia and lymphomas
All other	14%			14%	All other

[1]Excluding nonmelanoma skin cancer and carcinoma in situ

1993 ESTIMATED CANCER DEATHS by SITE and SEX

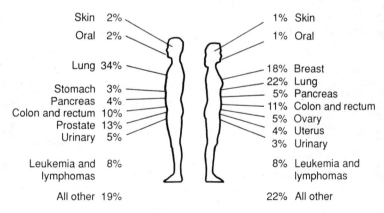

Skin	2%			1%	Skin
Oral	2%			1%	Oral
Lung	34%			18%	Breast
				22%	Lung
Stomach	3%			5%	Pancreas
Pancreas	4%			11%	Colon and rectum
Colon and rectum	10%			5%	Ovary
Prostate	13%			4%	Uterus
Urinary	5%			3%	Urinary
Leukemia and lymphomas	8%			8%	Leukemia and lymphomas
All other	19%			22%	All other

Figure 1–1. *Reproduced from Boring CC, Squires BA, Tong T. Cancer Statistics, 1993. 1993;43:9. With permission from JB Lippincott and the American Cancer Society.*

indicator of both hepatic and bony metastases. Hepatic metastases are associated with elevations in the heat-stable alkaline phosphatase fraction, whereas bony metastases are accompanied by an increased heat-labile fraction. Benign biliary diseases such as gallstones in the common bile duct also raise serum levels of this enzyme.
4. **5′-Nucleotidase.** Because elevated 5′-nucleotidase levels are associated with liver metastases, serum levels of this enzyme can be substituted for heat fractionation of alkaline phosphatase. Normal nucleotidase levels occur with bony metastases.
5. **Gammaglutamyl transpeptidase (GGTP).** Levels of GGTP can be used to evaluate the origin of elevated alkaline phosphatase levels in a manner identical to that of 5′-nucleotidase.

6. **Blood urea nitrogen (BUN) and creatinine.** Measurements of BUN and creatinine provide an estimate of renal function that may determine whether a kidney lesion is resectable or whether a planned chemotherapy regimen must be altered to avoid agents with potential renal toxicity (eg, cisplatin, methotrexate).

7. **Albumin.** Measurement of serum albumin, combined with prealbumin, transferrin, ferritin, and total iron-binding capacity, can be used to evaluate a patient's nutritional status.

B. **Urine tests.** Routine chemical and microscopic analysis of a random-voided urine specimen may demonstrate **hematuria** caused by primary urologic neoplasms or chemotherapy-induced hemorrhagic cystitis (see Chapter 12), **pyuria** indicating a urinary tract infection often found in immunocompromised cancer patients, or **calculi** associated with rapid chemotherapy-induced cytolysis.

C. **Imaging studies**
   1. **Chest x-ray.** The chest x-ray is a simple and inexpensive screening test for lung and rib metastases, mediastinal masses, and coexisting pulmonary disease. In early asymptomatic esophageal carcinoma, a **thickened posterior tracheal stripe (> 4.5 mm)** may be observed on a lateral chest x-ray.
   2. **Computed tomography (CT).** CT is often the best method of documenting both the anatomic location and extent of primary neoplasms. In addition, CT is frequently the most sensitive method of detecting the existence of distant metastases.
   3. **Magnetic resonance imaging (MRI).** MRI yields information similar to that obtained with CT scans. In some instances, however, T2 and spin inversion (IR) windows provide better delineation of normal and malignant tissue.
   4. **Ultrasound.** Masses previously detected by MRI and CT scans can be evaluated by ultrasound to distinguish **solid from cystic lesions**. In addition, ultrasonography is a relatively inexpensive screening tool for **hepatic** and **renal** abnormalities, including **liver masses, biliary dilation, ascites, renal masses and cysts, hydronephrosis, and abdominal fluid collections**.
   5. **Technetium-99m bone scan.** Bony pain or increased levels of heat-labile alkaline phosphatase are strong indications for using a technetium-99m bone scan to localize possible bony metastases. To exclude the presence of malignancy, plain x-ray films of any abnormality should be obtained.
      Note: Multiple myeloma produces pure lytic lesions that are not imaged by a bone scan. A skeletal series (plain x-rays) is indicated for this disease.

V. **Staging**
   A. **Goals of cancer staging.** Cancer staging is the practice of categorizing patients into groups according to the extent of their disease. The goals of cancer staging are to (1) provide information about the **prognosis**, (2) guide the **planning** of appropriate therapy, (3) help **evaluate** and compare different treatments, particularly those developed at different medical centers, and (4) obtain information about the **basic biology** of cancer.
   B. **The TNM staging system.** Because different organizations frequently propose separate staging systems, cancer staging has been hindered by a lack of uniformity. In 1987, however, the **American Joint Committee on Cancer and the Union Internationale Contre le Cancer** developed a uniform **TNM staging system** for most cancers.
      1. **Components.** The TNM tumor-staging system describes the extent of disease on the basis of four components:
         a. **T.** The size and extent of the primary tumor.
         b. **N.** The status of lymph node metastases.
         c. **M.** The presence or absence of distant metastases.
         d. **G.** The histopathologic grade of the tumor.
      2. **General rules**
         a. **Pathology.** Histology must be confirmed.
         b. **Classification.** Four types of classification are possible: (1) **clinical,** which is based on all available information except that obtained from pathologic examination, (2) **pathologic,** which is based on complete pathologic examination of the tumor, (3) **re-treatment,** which applies after a disease-free interval if histologic confirmation of recurrence is documented and additional definitive treatment is planned, and (4) **autopsy,** which is performed if the patient dies.
         c. **Stage assignment.** Once assigned, the tumor stage cannot be changed.
         d. **Category assignment.** If doubt about the correct TNM category exists, the tumor should be assigned to the lower category.

  e. **Multiple tumors.** If multiple primary tumors are present, the stage is assigned according to the most advanced tumor and the existence of multiple tumors is indicated: eg, T3(m).

TREATMENT EVALUATION

I. **Types of clinical trials**
   A. **Phase I.** Phase I studies explore the **dose-schedule** of the treatment and document **toxicity**.
   B. **Phase II.** Phase II studies attempt to **identify tumor types** that may respond to the therapy.
   C. **Phase III.** Phase III studies determine the efficacy and morbidity of the treatment relative to the natural history of the disease and the standard therapies previously used.
II. **Definition of response.** To avoid confusion, the definition of clinical responses must be uniform. The generally accepted definitions of the various responses are listed below:
   A. **Complete.** A complete response is defined as the disappearance of all detectable disease.
   B. **Partial.** A response cannot be categorized as partial unless the **sum of the products of the greatest perpendicular diameters** of all measurable lesions has decreased by **at least 50%**, no new areas of tumor have appeared, and no single area of known tumor has progressed.
   C. **Minimal.** The criteria for a minimal response are similar to those for a partial response, excluding the 50% reduction requirement.
   D. **Stable.** Stable disease is defined as an absence of response and progression of the disease.
   E. **Progression.** Disease progression is defined as cancer-related death, appearance of new lesions, or an increase of **at least 25%** in the sum of the greatest perpendicular diameters of all measurable lesions.

2 Principles of Surgical Oncology

Robert B. Cameron, MD

Surgery is the oldest form of cancer therapy. In addition, surgical biopsy plays a key role in the diagnosis of most malignancies. Although the development of newer therapeutic modalities, including chemotherapy, radiation therapy, and immunotherapy, has led to decreased use of radical surgical procedures, surgery remains the only potentially curative treatment for many cancer patients.

ROLES OF SURGERY IN CANCER TREATMENT

I. **Prevention.** There are numerous well-documented cases in which mild cellular abnormalities progress to invasive malignancy. When cellular abnormalities are encountered, **prophylactic surgery** can prevent the development of what otherwise would become a life-threatening disease. Several types of cancer that can arise from cellular abnormalities and may be prevented by early prophylactic surgery are discussed below.

   A. **Cervical carcinoma.** Extensive studies have proved that cervical carcinoma often begins as mild cellular atypia, progresses over a period of years to carcinoma in situ, then develops into frankly invasive cancer. The Papanicolaou (Pap) test has been responsible for a dramatic **70% decline** in the incidence of invasive cervical cancer over the past 40 years. Now, early detection of dysplasia and carcinoma in situ and prompt surgical treatment can prevent the development of invasive cancer.

   B. **Squamous cell carcinoma of the mouth.** Constant irritation from tobacco and alcohol can cause degeneration of the oral mucosa that progresses from normal squamous epithelium to dysplasia to carcinoma in situ and, finally, to invasive carcinoma. The **leukoplakia (whitish plaques)** associated with dysplasia often can be detected early by primary care physicians and dentists and then removed by surgeons, thus eliminating the risk of cancer.

   C. **Gastroesophageal carcinoma.** Peptic-induced columnar metaplasia of the distal esophagus **(Barrett's esophagus)** has been associated with the development of dysplasia and carcinoma. Serial endoscopies with multiple biopsies can be used to monitor patients for severe dysplasia. If dysplasia or carcinoma in situ develops, an esophagogastrectomy can be performed to abort the development of invasive carcinoma.

   D. **Bladder carcinoma.** Bladder carcinoma often begins as a superficial lesion that eventually evolves into invasive carcinoma. With the aid of cystoscopy, such lesions can be removed before they become true invasive cancers. Even if superficially invasive cancer is found, an early cystectomy can cure the patient.

   E. **Testicular carcinoma.** The association between **cryptorchidism** and the subsequent development of testicular carcinoma has long been appreciated. When cryptorchidism is detected, a simple surgical procedure, **orchiopexy,** can correct the problem and minimize any increased risk of testicular carcinoma.

   F. **Breast carcinoma.** Because breast cancer has a strong genetic component, the incidence among women with a significant family history of breast cancer (premenopausal bilateral breast cancer in the mother, sister, or both) approaches **4% per year.** Some women in this high-risk group prefer to have a **prophylactic mastectomy** to eliminate the risk of developing the disease.

   G. **Colon carcinoma.** Certain colonic diseases such as **familial polyposis and ulcerative colitis** are known to increase the risk of colon cancer. Patients with these conditions should be monitored closely and a **prophylactic proctocolectomy or total abdominal colectomy** with a mucosal proctectomy and an ileo-anal pull-through procedure should be considered to eliminate the risk of colon cancer.

II. **Diagnosis.** In many cases of malignancy, surgeons are asked to perform a biopsy to help determine a diagnosis. Because all subsequent treatment hinges on the histologic appearance of the tissue, a biopsy is an essential part of treatment planning. Some common biopsy techniques are described below.

A. Fine needle aspiration biopsy. A 22-gauge needle can be percutaneously placed almost anywhere in the body, including the brain. Tumor cells aspirated through the needle can be identified by an experienced cytologist. Although the track of the needle is theoretically contaminated with malignant cells during the biopsy and should be surgically excised during the definitive surgery, in practice fine needle track metastases are rarely a clinical problem.

B. Core needle biopsy. A needle specifically designed to excise a core of tissue with recognizable architecture (eg, Tru-Cut) can be used to diagnose a high percentage of cases without resorting to an open biopsy (see **C** below). However, masses in certain locations, such as those near large vascular structures and deep-seated lesions of the central nervous system (CNS), are not amenable to this procedure. Because needle track metastases are more likely after core needle biopsies than after fine needle aspirations, the needle should be placed in a manner that enables the surgeon to remove the track easily during a subsequent definitive surgical procedure.

C. Open biopsy. In many instances, a piece of tissue must be removed to confirm a suspected diagnosis of malignancy. Two types of open biopsy are generally used.

  1. Excisional biopsy. In this type of biopsy, the entire abnormality is excised. Thus, the pathologist has the entire lesion with which to make the diagnosis. This type of open biopsy is usually appropriate for small (< 2 cm) superficial lesions.

  2. Incisional biopsy. Occasionally, an abnormality is so large or is situated in such a precarious place that excisional biopsy should not be attempted. In this situation, an incision is made into the lesion and a wedge of tissue large enough for an accurate diagnosis is removed. This procedure occasionally requires a frozen section of the tissue to confirm that an adequate amount of tissue has been obtained.

D. Incisions. Selecting the most appropriate type and orientation of the biopsy incision requires a thorough understanding of not only the anatomy but also the subsequent surgical procedures that may be required. Before performing any of the specific biopsies listed below, the optimal orientation of the surgical incision must be intelligently planned.

  1. Breast biopsy. Three types of incisions are used in biopsies for breast cancer: **curvilinear, transverse, and radial.** Traditionally, a curvilinear incision that could be completely encompassed within a modified radical mastectomy was recommended. When segmental mastectomy (lumpectomy) and axillary dissection, followed by radiation therapy, were adopted as an acceptable treatment regimen, this recommendation was modified slightly. **Curvilinear and transverse incisions are still preferred.** These incisions are placed best directly **over the mass** to avoid creating skin flaps, and they do not necessarily have to be within the scope of a mastectomy incision. If skin or superficial tissue is to be removed, particularly in the lower half of the breast, radial incisions are preferred and curvilinear, and transverse incisions should be avoided because they result in an unacceptable degree of breast distortion. Conversely, because radial incisions yield cosmetically inferior results, they should not be used in the upper half of the breast. The biopsy incision should not be incorporated into the longitudinal or transverse incision used for an axillary dissection. Incorporating it produces a contour defect, which should be avoided. Drains should not be used, and the skin should be closed with a fine (4-0 or 5-0) absorbable subcuticular suture.

  2. Soft-tissue biopsy of the extremities

    a. Masses smaller than 2 cm in diameter. When the mass is small, an excisional biopsy can be performed safely by using a **longitudinal** incision placed directly over the mass. Transverse incisions should be avoided because, if re-excision of the area is required, they increase the difficulty and compromise the cosmetic result of any subsequent re-excision.

    b. Masses larger than 2 cm in diameter. Larger masses require an **incisional** biopsy, again using a **longitudinal** incision. With an accurate diagnosis, the mass can subsequently be excised completely, along with appropriate margins.

III. Staging. The surgeon is often responsible for determining the extent of a patient's disease. This staging is commonly determined during definitive resection of the primary lesion. Several procedures in the surgeon's arsenal are specifically designed to stage a variety of cancers.

A. Mediastinoscopy and mediastinotomy. Pathologic assessment of mediastinal nodes is sometimes crucially important for determining the most appropriate treatment for patients with lung cancer. A biopsy of these nodes can be performed either by means of substernal mediastinoscopy or, more directly, by means of parasternal mediastinotomy (also called a Chamberlain procedure).

B. Laparotomy. Exploring the abdominal cavity with biopsy of all the appropriate organs and lymph nodes is a common procedure for evaluating Hodgkin's disease, ovarian carcinoma, and testicular carcinoma.

  1. Hodgkin's disease. Use of an exploratory laparotomy with (singular)-splenectomy, liver biopsies (three left and right needle biopsies and a right wedge biopsy), and lymph node biopsies (right and left para-aortic and iliac nodes) has altered the clinical staging and treatment in as many as 35% of patients with Hodgkin's disease.

  2. Ovarian carcinoma. A thorough staging laparotomy is an essential part of treating ovarian cancer. In addition to removing the primary lesion (see Chapter 46), this procedure includes the following:

  a. Collection of ascites (if present).

  b. Washings of the pelvis and, if no ascites is present, both pericolic gutters and subdiaphragmatic areas.

  c. Omentectomy, including supracolic omentum if it is involved.

  d. Strip biopsies (1×3 cm) of both pericolic gutters and right diaphragmatic peritoneum.

  e. Biopsy of any liver lesions.

  f. Resection of all gross disease if possible, including resection of the bowel if necessary.

  g. Biopsies of pelvic and para-aortic nodes if no other gross lesions larger than 2 cm are present.

The results of this staging and cytoreductive laparotomy correlate directly with length of survival.

  3. Testicular carcinoma. Although laparotomy and **retroperitoneal lymphadenectomy** are performed less commonly today because combination chemotherapy is so successful, they remain the most accurate methods of staging nonseminomatous testicular carcinoma. Furthermore, overall survival of patients with pathologic Stage I disease now approaches 100% after retroperitoneal lymphadenectomy. In patients with advanced disease who respond to initial chemotherapy, this treatment can determine the extent of the response and, by removing residual disease, improve the prognosis.

IV. Treatment. Surgical treatment of cancer can be divided into treatment of the primary lesion and treatment of metastatic foci.

A. Primary lesions. Adequate surgical treatment of a specific malignancy is defined as the procedure that will cure the primary disease in the vast majority of, if not all, patients with a minimum degree of morbidity. Surgical therapy usually involves complete removal of the primary lesion plus a rim of surrounding normal tissue. Regional lymph nodes also are frequently removed either to determine the likelihood of systemic disease (eg, in breast cancer patients) or to cure patients whose tumors may have only regional spread (eg, in patients with melanoma). Surgical procedures usually must be individualized to meet the needs of a particular patient, and the precise surgical procedure indicated may change over time as information about the nature and spread of the malignancy increases and as new therapeutic modalities are developed. For example, breast cancer, which formerly was almost always treated by radical mastectomy, is currently often treated by modified radical mastectomy or, in many cases, by lymphectomy and axillary dissection. Similarly, bony and soft tissue sarcomas of the extremities, which formerly were treated by amputation, are often treated adequately with limb-sparing surgery. Thus, surgical oncology is an evolving, dynamic specialty.

B. Metastatic lesions. In the past, surgery rarely was used to remove metastatic cancer. With more experience in the resection of selected metastatic lesions, however, surgeons discovered that 25–30% of patients with malignancies such as **bony and soft tissue sarcomas** who otherwise would succumb to their disease can be cured by aggressive resection of distant (pulmonary) metastases at the time of diagnosis. Furthermore, among patients who have been disease-free for a long interval (usually more than 1 year) after treatment for certain primary cancers, resection of distant metastases (eg, liver or lung) has prolonged the survival of and even cured as many as 32%. Therefore, resection of distant metastases is indicated in selected situations and should be attempted.

V. **Palliation.** Many operations are performed each year for the sole purpose of improving the patient's quality of life. Indications for palliative procedures include hemorrhage, obstruction, perforation of a hollow viscus, painful masses, and extreme anxiety. For instance, even in the face of metastatic disease, resection of gastrointestinal tumors–esophageal, gastric, and colorectal–provides important palliation from the effects of a painful obstructive mass. In addition, complete resection of primary tumors of the CNS provides significant palliation. Metastatic disease does not signal termination of the surgeon's involvement in the care of cancer patients; rather it invites a new effort to provide patients with the best quality of life that surgery can offer.

SPECIAL SURGICAL PROBLEMS: VASCULAR ACCESS

Many cancer patients need frequent catheterization for phlebotomy and chemotherapy and, occasionally, for administration of fluid. Because sites for simple intravenous catheterization are quickly exhausted and more dependable vascular access is then required, surgeons are regularly called on to provide adequate vascular access in medical and surgical patients. Vascular access can be accomplished by venous or arterial catheterization, depending on the therapeutic requirements.

I. **Venous catheterization**

A. **Percutaneous catheters.** Soft, cuffed catheters made of polyurethane and silicone elastomers (Hickman, Broviac) have been developed for percutaneous placement into a central vein.

1. **Placement.** The catheter can be placed into the superior or inferior vena cava either through percutaneous subclavian, internal jugular, or femoral approaches or through a cephalic, external jugular, or saphenous vein cutdown.

2. **Maintenance.** Patency can be maintained by flushing the catheter with 5 mL of heparinized saline (100 U/mL) every month and after each use. If a rare episode of catheter thrombosis occurs, patency can be re-established by infusing 0.5 mL of streptokinase (5000 U/mL).

3. **Disadvantages.** The major disadvantages of percutaneous catheters are that they require constant and diligent care and constant changes of dressings by the patient.

B. **Implantable catheters.** Completely implantable catheters (Port-A-Cath, Mediport) have been developed to relieve patients of the encumbrances of daily catheter care and, potentially, to reduce the incidence of catheter sepsis. Implantable catheters and percutaneous catheters are inserted and maintained in the same way; however, in the case of implantable catheters, instead of creating a cutaneous exit site, a small metal port containing a silicon rubber septum is implanted in a subcutaneous pocket. When access is needed, a special needle **(Huber needle)** that punctures but does not tear the rubber septum of the port is used to pierce the skin and port.

II. **Arterial catheterization.** Although the arterial route is used less often than the venous route, it is often used to treat a variety of **hepatic metastases.** This type of application requires a **hepatic angiogram** to assess the vascular anatomy, followed by major surgery to implant a subcutaneous pump (Infusaid) and to place the tip of the catheter in the hepatic artery through the **gastroduodenal artery.** Cholecystectomy is required to prevent chemotherapy-induced chemical cholecystitis. Maintenance of a patent catheter requires weekly flushing with 5 mL of heparinized saline (100 U/mL).

REFERENCES

Margolese R et al. The technique of segmental mastectomy (lumpectomy) and axillary dissection: a syllabus from the National Surgical Adjuvant Breast Project workshops. *Surgery* 1987;**102**:828.

Marx AB, Landmann J, Harder FH: Surgery for vascular access. *Curr Probl Surg* 1990;**27**(1):7.

3 Principles of Chemotherapy

Carlin J. McLaughlin, DO

BIOLOGY OF THE NEOPLASTIC CELL

I. **Systemic nature of cancer.** Because of the systemic nature of metastatic neoplasms, a systemic approach to treatment (ie, chemotherapy) is often required.

II. **Tumor growth**

   A. **Selective toxicity.** No unique biochemical differences exist between malignant cells and rapidly proliferating normal cells such as those in gastrointestinal epithelium, bone marrow, and skin. Consequently, chemotherapy affects both neoplastic and normal tissues, producing therapeutic and toxic effects, respectively. However, levels of cellular enzymes and rates of reaction differ slightly in malignant and normal cells, and these small **quantitative differences** account for the selective antitumor toxicity mediated by administration of chemotherapeutic agents.

   B. **Growth fraction and control.** Malignant cells are associated with the elimination of normal regulatory mechanisms that control cell growth, including **contact inhibition** (inhibition of growth upon cell-to-cell contact) and **programmed cell death** (planned cell senescence after a preset number of cell divisions). Neoplastic growth is governed by **Gompertian kinetics**—the tumor doubling time increases and the fraction of dividing cells (growth fraction) decreases exponentially with increasing tumor mass. The maximal growth fraction occurs at approximately 37% of **largest tumor size.** Large tumors that have relatively small growth fractions are less susceptible to the effects of chemotherapy than are small tumors that have relatively large growth fractions. The effect of chemotherapy follows the rule of first-order kinetics: in other words, the fraction of cells killed relative to the total number of cells is constant. With each exposure, the maximum reduction of viable tumor cells is 2–5 logs (100–100,000 times). Therefore, the fact that tumor burdens often approach 10^{10}–10^{12} cells clearly indicates that repeated high-dose chemotherapy is essential for a successful outcome. Chemotherapy fails only if insufficient drug is administered or if the tumor possesses either inherent or acquired drug resistance.

III. **Cell cycle.** The cell cycle, relative time intervals, and sites of action of the various classes of antineoplastic agents are depicted in Figure 3–1.

CHEMOTHERAPEUTIC AGENTS

Appendix B contains a complete list of chemotherapeutic agents. In addition, classification of the different agents by their mechanism of action and cell-cycle specificity have been used extensively and are reviewed below.

I. **Cell cycle specificity.** The cell cycle consists of **4 phases.** The initial phase is gap$_1$, or **G$_1$ phase**, which is highly variable in length. The next phase is that of rapid DNA synthesis, or **S phase,** followed by another gap (**G$_2$ phase**), during which RNA and protein are made. The final phase, **M phase,** is that of cell division (mitosis), a process that is entirely dependent on microtubule function. Chemotherapy agents often act during a specific phase of the cell cycle and consequently are grouped into the following categories (Table 3–1).

   A. **Cell cycle-nonspecific agents.** These agents are effective against cells in any phase of replication, including those in **G$_1$ phase**, and are useful in tumors with low proliferative activity.

   B. **Cell cycle-specific agents**

      1. **S phase-specific agents.** Chemicals that block purine and pyrimidine synthesis as well as disrupt normal DNA proliferation affect cells in S phase when intense DNA replication occurs. Since this phase is relatively short, frequent or continuous administration is required so that adequate drug levels are present when the cell enters this phase. In addition, tumors with slow replication rates

9

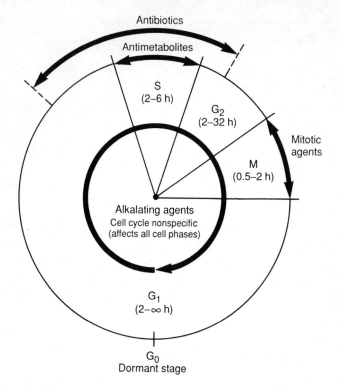

Figure 3–1. Phases of the cell cycle, relative time intervals, and sites of action of the various classes of antineoplastic agents.

(minimum number of cells in S phase) generally are not susceptible to these agents.

2. **M phase-specific agents.** Microtubular inhibitors interfere with mitosis and block cell division in M phase.

3. **Other.** Some agents block cell replication at several sites (eg, G_2 phase, etc.) and can act as both cell cycle-specific and cell cycle-nonspecific agents.

II. **Mechanism of action.** Common classifications of chemotherapy agents involve the mechanism of antitumor action. This method of categorizing chemotherapeutic agents is important, since chemicals with different modes of action may be rationally combined to increase antitumor effects. A summary is presented below and includes the following categories (Table 3–2).

A. **Alkylating agents.** These chemicals bind DNA nucleotides, thus preventing accurate genetic transcription and translation.

B. **Antimetabolites.** These agents block purine and pyrimidine synthesis as well as disrupt normal DNA proliferation.

C. **Mitotic inhibitors.** These standard nomenclature-vinca alkaloid derivatives block cell division by interfering with microtubular assembly.

D. **Antibiotics.** Antibiotic agents intercalate between DNA base pairs and disrupt normal function.

CHEMOTHERAPY DOSE CONSIDERATIONS

I. **Dose-response relationship.** Intuitively, a dose-response relationship should govern the administration of chemotherapeutic agents, with higher doses producing greater response rates in sensitive tumors. Yet, this has been difficult to document clinically despite some reports of improved response rates with higher doses in some tumors.

II. **Relative dose intensity (RDI).** The RDI (mg/m²/week) represents the potency of ther-

TABLE 3–1. CELL CYCLE SPECIFICITY OF CHEMOTHERAPEUTIC AGENTS

Nonspecific	Cell Cycle Specific			
	G_1 Phase Specific	S Phase Specific	G_2 Phase Specific	M Phase Specific
Busulfan	Asparaginase	Cytosine arabino-	Bleomycin	Vinblastine
Carboplatin		side (ARA-C)	Etoposide (VP-16)	Vincristine
Carmustine		Floxuridine		
Chlorambucil		(FUdR)		
Cisplatin		Fluorouracil		
Cyclophosphamide		Hydroxyurea		
Dacarbazine		Mercaptopurine		
(DTIC)				
Dactinomycin		Methotrexate		
Daunorubicin		Thioguanine		
Doxorubicin				
Hexamethyl-				
melamine (thio-				
tepa)				
Ifosfamide				
Lomustine (CCNU)				
Mechlorethamine				
(nitrogen mustard)				
Melphalan (phen-				
ylalanine mus-				
tard)				
Mitomycin-C				
Mitotane				
Mitoxantrone				
Pipobroman				
Plicamycin				
(mithramycin)				
Procarbazine				
Streptozotocin				
Uracil mustard				

apy and may be related to the resulting response rate. RDI can be reported for one drug or for a combination of drugs with a weighted average.

COMBINATION CHEMOTHERAPY

Combinations of chemotherapeutic agents have been tried with the expectation of improved results. Common chemotherapeutic combinations are listed in Appendices C1 and C2. The rationale for combination chemotherapy is based on the following principles.

    I. **Additive activity.** Each drug has demonstrated activity as a single agent, ideally with confirmed reports of complete responses. When they are combined, the antitumor effects are additive, yielding a higher response rate than with any single agent.

    II. **Nonoverlapping toxicity.** Each drug possesses toxicities that are not greatly enhanced by the addition of the other drugs. Consequently, the optimal relative dose intensity (drug dose and frequency of administration) of the individual drugs can be maintained without significantly increasing the risk of life-threatening side effects.

PHARMACOKINETICS

The antineoplastic effects of chemotherapeutic agents are dependent on a number of factors that influence the tumor's exposure over time to a concentration of drug. While dosage is the most important element in the concentration over time ($C \times T$) relationship, other determinants include (1) **route of administration** (absorption), (2) **volume of distribution** (transport and drug interactions), (3) **metabolism** (transformation to active metabolite), and (4) **excretion** (elimination).

TABLE 3–2. MECHANISMS OF ACTION OF CHEMOTHERAPEUTIC AGENTS

Alkylating Agents	Anti-metabolites	Mitotic Inhibitors	Antibiotics	Miscellaneous Agents
Busulfan	Cytosine arabin-oside (ARA-C)	Etoposide (VP–16)	Bleomycin	Asparaginase
Carboplatin	Floxuridine (FUdR)	Teniposide	Dactinomycin	Hydroxyurea
Carmustine (BCNU)	Fluorouracil	Vinblastine	Daunorubicin	Mitotane
Chlorambucil	Mercaptopurine	Vincristine	Doxorubicin	Procarbazine
Cisplatin	Methotrexate	Vindesine	Mitomycin-C	
Cyclophosphamide	Thioguanine		Mitoxantrone	
Dacarbazine (DTIC)			Plicamycin	
Hexamethylmela-mine (thiotepa)			(mithramycin)	
Ifosfamide				
Lomustine (CCNU)				
Mechlorethamine (nitrogen mustard)				
Melphalan (phen-ylalanine mustard)				
Pipobroman				
Methyl-CCNU				
Streptozotocin				
Uracil mustard				

DRUG RESISTANCE

Inherent or acquired drug resistance of tumor cells is a major cause of chemotherapy failure. The development of drug resistance is directly proportional to both the total number of tumor cells present and the rate of mutation. Three basic types of drug resistance exist: (1) cytotoxic resistance, (2) biochemical resistance, and (3) pleiotropic drug resistance, or so-called multiple drug resistance (MDR).

   I. **Cytotoxic resistance.** Tumor cells that remain in the G_1 phase of the cell cycle, and therefore are not undergoing active mitosis, are resistant to chemotherapeutic agents. This is called "cytotoxic drug resistance." Strategies to overcome this form of drug resistance, including continuous infusion chemotherapy, are currently being evaluated.

  II. **Biochemical drug resistance.** Multiple mechanisms (listed below) may prevent active drugs from functioning at the target site within the tumor cell. To counter these phenomena, synergistic drug combinations (ie, fluorouracil and one of the following: leucovorin, allopurinol, thymidine, melphalan, or methotrexate) recently have been utilized to decrease the development of this biochemical drug resistance.

   A. Defects in drug transport.
   B. Defects in drug activation.
   C. Increased drug inactivation.
   D. Improved DNA repair.
   E. Target-site gene amplification.
   F. Increased competing biochemical pathways.
   G. Chemical change in target structure.
   H. Increased competing substrates.

 III. **Multiple-drug resistance (MDR).** Tumor cells that exhibit drug resistance to disparate classes of cytotoxic drugs with different mechanisms of action, such as antibiotics, vinca alkaloids, podophyllotoxins (etoposide), and dactinomycin demonstrate the characteristic of multiple-drug resistance. This phenomenon may result from mutations in any one of several "MDR genes" and is associated with the following biochemical changes.

   A. **Increased activity of 170 Kd surface glycoprotein.** This membrane protein serves as an **energy- and calcium-dependent intracellular-to-extracellular drug pump.** In experimental models, this drug resistance can be reversed by calcium channel blockers, quinidine, quinine, tricyclic antidepressants and phenothiazines, and efforts are currently underway to clinically reverse the MDR phenomenon with calcium channel blockers and quinidine.

B. **Abnormal topoisomerase activity.** A proposed mechanism of MDR involves abnormal topoisomerase activity. Normally, topoisomerase is required for DNA replication and creation of secondary and tertiary structure in the nucleus, and changes in this activity may alter tumor cell susceptibility to the antitumor effects of chemotherapeutic agents.

ADMINISTRATION OF CHEMOTHERAPY

I. **Requirements.** To guarantee the patient a reasonable likelihood of therapeutic benefit, the following criteria must be satisfied before instituting any cytotoxic therapy.
  A. **Established diagnosis.** A histologic diagnosis must be firmly established and the stage of the malignancy carefully ascertained. This information is crucial in determining the natural history of the disease, tumor responsiveness, and appropriate therapeutic goals (cure or palliation).
  B. **Adequate patient health.** The patient's health status and **ability to tolerate the planned therapy** should be critically evaluated in light of his or her age, performance status (see Appendix A), and hepatic, renal, cardiac, and pulmonary function.
  C. **Disease markers present.** Except for accepted standard adjuvant therapy, chemotherapy should be administered only in the presence of **objective measures of tumor response** (eg, decrease in tumor size, tumor antigen levels, or paraprotein levels).
  D. **Supportive services available.** Laboratory and radiologic support must be available to monitor patients for potential life-threatening side effects as well as tumor response. When complications of therapy are detected, treatment must be instituted promptly to avoid significant morbidity. It is the ability to maximize the therapeutic benefit while minimizing morbidity that defines successful administration of chemotherapy.
II. **Indications.** Chemotherapy should only be administered to cancer patients with one of the following goals in mind.
  A. **Cure.** Some malignancies are curable with chemotherapy alone or in combination with other therapeutic modalities (ie, surgery, radiation therapy). Examples of diseases amenable to cure with chemotherapy include acute lymphocytic or myelocytic leukemia, Hodgkin's disease, non-Hodgkin's lymphomas, ovarian cancer, testicular cancer, and pediatric solid tumors. In addition, adjuvant chemotherapy may cure patients with breast cancer and bladder carcinoma as well as those with osteogenic and soft tissue sarcomas.
  B. **Palliation.** Chemotherapy may afford significant relief of symptoms and, in some circumstances, prolongation of survival in the following malignancies: chronic lymphocytic and myelocytic leukemia, hairy cell leukemia, multiple myeloma, chronic lymphomas, Kaposi's sarcoma, mycosis fungoides, carcinoid malignancies, esophageal cancer, colon cancer, small cell and non-small cell lung cancer, prostate cancer, bladder cancer, malignant melanoma, endometrial cancer, and adrenal neoplasms.
III. **Contraindications.** For some tumors, chemotherapy has no proven curative or palliative role. In such circumstances, unproven drug regimens should not be offered outside of an approved clinical trial. Examples of malignancies in this category include thyroid cancer, islet cell cancers, renal cell carcinoma, cervical cancer, pancreatic cancer, nonsmall cell lung cancer, hepatocellular carcinoma, biliary neoplasms, and gliomas.

TOXICITY

The side effects of chemotherapeutic agents are numerous and, at times, life-threatening. Intensive chemotherapy regimens are associated with **mortality rates as high as 2–10% and morbidity rates of 50–100%.** A complete list of common side effects associated with various chemotherapeutic agents is given in Appendix D. Briefly, the toxicities can be categorized as follows.
I. **Local and dermal side effects** include alopecia, photosensitivity, phlebitis, tissue necrosis, and local infiltration of chemotherapeutic agents (see Chapter 18).
II. **Myelosuppression** is the **most dangerous side effect** of chemotherapeutic agents.
  A. **Etiology.** The pattern and duration of the myelosuppressive effect varies, depending on the drug. In addition, the effects may be cumulative. Certain alkylating agents, such as **mitomycin-C, busulfan, chlorambucil, and the nitrosoureas are particularly toxic,** rarely leading to stem cell depletion and irreversible myelosuppression. **Drugs that are generally minimally myelotoxic include**

bleomycin, vincristine, and methotrexate (with leucovorin rescue). As a rule, standard doses of most agents can be given every 3–4 weeks. A nadir white blood count obtained 7–10 days after drug administration aids in the grading of toxicity and in dose modifications.

B. Diagnosis. Myelosuppression is diagnosed on the basis of complete blood counts and is graded according to the scale outlined in Appendix F (Toxicity Grading).

C. Therapy. Until recently, the complications of myelosuppression were treated by **supportive therapy** alone. However, a new era of specific therapy with **myeloid growth factors** has dawned with the recent approval of recombinant human granulocyte colony-stimulating factor (G-CSF) (Filgrastim, Neupogen) for prevention of febrile neutropenia and of recombinant human granulocyte-macrophage colony-stimulating factor (GM-CSF) (Sargramostim, Prokine, Leukine) for autologous bone marrow transplantation.

III. Infectious side effects

A. Etiology. Infections in patients receiving chemotherapy are related to the severity and duration of neutropenia and to alterations in the integrity of infection barriers, such as mucous membranes and skin. Infectious organisms associated with granulocytopenic defects include enteric gram-negative bacteria, gram-positive bacteria (*Staphylococcus epidermidis, Staphylococcus aureus,* and diptheroids), viruses (herpes simplex and zoster), and fungi (*Candida* and *Aspergillus* species). Fungal infections occur more commonly after induction therapy for acute leukemia.

B. Diagnosis. Although **fever in a neutropenic patient** is sufficient evidence to suspect an occult infection and begin antibiotic therapy, cultures are necessary to confirm the presence of infection. **Culture-confirmed infections occur in only 40%** of all febrile neutropenic episodes.

C. Therapy. The mainstay of therapy consists of the **administration of broad-spectrum antibiotics** until the granulocytopenia and fever resolve. As mentioned above, therapy with G-CSF for febrile neutropenia and GM-CSF for bone marrow transplantation may dramatically alter the treatment of this complication.

IV. Cardiac side effects. Daunorubicin and doxorubicin possess significant cardiac toxicity, as outlined in Chapter 10.

V. Pulmonary side effects. Although methotrexate, mitomycin-C, procarbazine, and cytosine arabinoside may all produce pulmonary fibrosis, the most common etiologic agent is bleomycin, as discussed in Chapter 9.

VI. Hepatic side effects. Transient hepatic dysfunction as manifested by transaminase and alkaline phosphatase elevations is relatively common; however, cholangitis, hepatic necrosis, and hepatic veno-occlusive disease can also occur. Chemotherapy-induced hepatic toxicity is more extensively discussed in Chapter 13.

VII. Gastrointestinal side effects

A. Stomatitis and other types of mucositis

1. **Etiology.** Inflammation of the oral mucosa from cytotoxic damage occurs most commonly with **antimetabolites,** such as methotrexate, fluorouracil, and cytosine arabinoside. Continuous infusion antimetabolite therapy produces a greater incidence of stomatitis and other types of mucositis than that observed with intermittent therapy.

2. **Diagnosis. Pain (odynophagia) and erythema** in the context of recent chemotherapy should raise the suspicion of stomatitis and other types of mucositis. **Tumor infiltration and superinfection must be excluded,** however.

3. **Treatment.** Treatment is aimed at symptomatic relief with **topical anesthetics, such as 2% viscous lidocaine,** 5-mL gargle every hour. In addition, **prophylactic antifungal agents** (nystatin, 500,000 units swished in the mouth and swallowed every 6 hours) and, in some cases, antiviral medications (eg, acyclovir, 200 mg 5 times daily) are recommended to neutralize the increased risk of infection due to the breakdown of the normal oral mucosal barrier.

B. Nausea and vomiting

1. **Etiology.** The emetigenic potential of different chemotherapeutic agents varies widely (Table 3–3). Receptors in the chemoreceptor trigger zone of the fourth ventricle, cortex, and gastrointestinal tract are thought to be responsible for inducing emesis.

2. **Diagnosis.** Symptoms of nausea and vomiting **temporally related to the administration of chemotherapy** are diagnostic of chemotherapy-induced emesis. However, **gastrointestinal obstruction must be excluded,** especially if abdominal distention or obstipation is present.

3. **Therapy.** Treatment includes the use of **antiemetic drugs** (Table 3–4). **Ondansetron, a new serotonin S-3 receptor blocking agent,** has shown

TABLE 3–3. EMETIGENIC POTENTIAL OF CHEMOTHERAPEUTIC AGENTS

Highly Emetigenic	Modestly Emetigenic	Minimally Emetigenic
Cisplatin	Carboplatin	Chlorambucil
Dacarbazine (DTIC)	Carmustine (BCNU)	Fluorouracil
Dactinomycin	Cyclophosphamide	Hydroxyurea
Nitrogen mustard	Cytosine arabinoside (ARA-C)	Melphalan (phenylalanine
Procarbazine	Daunorubicin	mustard)
Streptozotocin	Doxorubicin	Vincristine
	Etoposide (VP-16)	
	Ifosfamide	
	Lomustine (CCNU)	
	Methyl-CCNU	
	Mitoxantrone	
	Vinblastine	

promise in significantly reducing emesis associated with cisplatin and other highly emetigenic drugs.

C. **Diarrhea**
   1. **Etiology.** Diarrhea frequently accompanies stomatitis. A denuded mucosal membrane results in the development of isotonic diarrhea. Diarrhea associated with the **combination of fluorouracil and leucovorin** can be particularly serious, and **high-dose cytosine arabinoside** (induction therapy for acute leukemia) may produce a syndrome of profound diarrhea and abdominal pain mimicking an acute surgical emergency. In patients receiving chemotherapy, the risk of **pseudomembranous colitis from *Clostridium difficile* infection** is also increased due to the frequent administration of broad-spectrum antibiotics.
   2. **Diagnosis.** Diarrhea **temporally related to the administration of chemotherapy** is most likely not infectious in origin. If an infection is suspected, however, a stool specimen should be examined for the presence of white blood

TABLE 3–4. ANTIEMETIC THERAPY FOR CHEMOTHERAPY-ASSOCIATED NAUSEA/EMESIS

Drug	Dosage	Route
Histamine antagonists		
Hydroxyzine (Atarax)	50–100 mg every 6 h	IV/PO
Diphenhydramine (Benadryl)	10–50 mg every 6 h	IV/IM/PO
Muscarine antagonists		
Scopolamine (Transderm-Scop)	0.5 mg every 3 days (apply 4 h before needed)	Transdermal
Dopamine antagonists		
Metoclopramide (Reglan)	1–2 mg/kg every 3 h	IV/IM/PO
Droperidol (Inapsine)	0.5–2.5 mg/2.5–10 mg every 4 h	IV/IM
Haloperidol (Haldol)	0.5–5.0 mg every 4 h	IM/PO
Prochlorperazine (Compazine)	2.5–10 mg/5–10 mg/5–10mg/25 mg every 4 h	Slow IV/IM/PO/PR
Chlorpromazine (Thorazine)	2–25 mg/25–50 mg/10–25 mg/50–100 mg every 4 h	Slow IV/IM/PO/PR
Thiethylperazine (Torecan)	2 mg/10 mg every 8 h	IM/PO
Trimethobenzamide (Tigan)	200 mg/250 mg/200 mg	IM/PO/PR
Corticosteroids		
Methylprednisolone (Solu-Medrol)	250–500 mg every 6 h	IV
Dexamethasone (Decadron)	4–25 mg every 6 h	IV/PO
Benzodiazepines		
Lorazepam (Ativan)	1–2 mg/1–4 mg/1–2 mg /1–2 mg every 4 h	IV/IM/PO/SL
Cannabinoids		
Dronabinol (Delta-9-tetrahydrocannabinol)	5–15 mg/m^2 every 4 h	PO
Nabilone (Cesamet)	1–2 mg every 8 h	PO
Serotonin antagonists		
Ondansetron (GR C-507/75)	0.15 mg/kg before and every 4 h × 2 after therapy	IV/PO

cells, enteric pathogens (eg, *Salmonella, Shigella*), ova and parasites, and *C difficile* toxin.

   3. **Therapy.**

      a. **In the absence of infection,** treatment is mainly supportive with anti-diarrheal drugs such as Kaopectate (kaolin and pectin), 30 mL after each loose stool; loperamide, 4 mg initially, followed by 2 mg after each loose stool to a maximum of 8 mg daily; or diphenoxylate (with atropine), 5 mg every 6 hours.

      b. **Patients with severe diarrhea associated with antimetabolite chemotherapy** occasionally require hospitalization for intravenous fluids.

      c. **For the diarrheal syndrome related to high-dose cytosine arabinoside therapy,** complete bowel rest with central venous hyperalimentation and careful observation is usually all that is required.

      d. **For diarrhea associated with pseudomembranous colitis and *C difficile*** infection, therapy consists of oral vancomycin or metronidazole, 500 mg every 6 hours.

  D. **Constipation**

    1. **Etiology.** Constipation is a side effect usually seen in patients with neurogenic gastrointestinal atony who are being treated with vinca alkaloids. In general, doses of these drugs should be reduced in diabetics and those over the age of 65 to avoid symptomatic constipation. In severe cases of constipation, ileus may result.

    2. **Diagnosis.** A vinca alkaloid-associated decrease in stool frequency or difficulty in evacuation in the absence of mechanical intestinal obstruction is sufficient to diagnose chemotherapy-induced constipation.

    3. **Therapy.** Treatment includes hydration, stool softeners (docusate sodium, 100 mg twice daily), laxatives (milk of magnesia, 30 mL daily), enemas, and cathartics.

VIII. Allergic reactions. Acute allergic reactions occasionally occur with chemotherapeutic agents, most commonly etoposide and teniposide. Acute pulmonary reactions have classically occurred with **methotrexate,** resulting in steroid-responsive pulmonary infiltrates. **Bleomycin** can cause anaphylaxis, skin reaction, fever, chills, and pulmonary fibrosis on a more chronic basis. Other side effects associated with chemotherapeutic agents are listed in Appendix D.

  IX. Cystitis. This occurs primarily with 2 agents, **cyclophosphamide** and **ifosfamide** (see Chapter 12).

   X. Neurotoxicity

    A. **Etiology.** The vinca alkaloids **vincristine sulfate** and **vinblastine sulfate** as well as **fluorouracil** and **cytosine arabinoside** have been implicated in the development of peripheral, central, and visceral neuropathies. Other agents with similar mechanisms of action also may not be tolerated due to overlapping toxicity.

    B. **Diagnosis**

      1. **Vinca alkaloid-induced neuropathy** is suggested by absent reflexes, constipation, and ileus. Rarely, cranial nerve abnormalities may be seen. Severe muscle cramping has been reported with high doses (> 0.2 mg/kg) of vinblastine used in the treatment of testicular cancer.

      2. Cerebellar toxicity is a characteristic result of **constant infusion or high doses of fluorouracil and cytosine arabinoside.**

      3. **Asparaginase** may cause encephalopathy by inhibiting protein synthesis and increasing ammonia levels.

    C. **Therapy.** The sole treatment of neurologic toxicity is discontinuation of the offending chemotherapeutic agent.

DOSE MODIFICATION

Dose modifications are complex and are based on the degree of organ dysfunction. A guide to dose modifications for most chemotherapeutic agents is given in Appendix E.

REFERENCES

DeVita VT: The relationship between tumorous mass and resistance to treatment of cancer. *Cancer* 1983;**51**:1209.

Goldie JH: Scientific basis for adjuvant and primary (neoadjuvant) chemotherapy. *Semin Oncol* 1987;**14**:1.

4   Principles of Radiation Oncology

Robert S. Lavey, MD, MPH, and Joseph C. Poen, MD

Ionizing radiation has been used in cancer therapy since 1896 and currently plays a role in the management of almost all types of cancer. Nearly **60%** of all cancer patients in the United States undergo radiation therapy sometime during the course of their disease **(50% for cure and 50% for palliation).**

BIOLOGY OF RADIATION-INDUCED CELL DAMAGE

A **1-cm³** tumor contains **10 million viable cells.** To eradicate such a tumor, each cell must be made incapable of reproduction (sterilized).

I. **Goal. The goal of radiation therapy is to sterilize a targeted tumor completely while preserving the integrity of surrounding normal structures.**

II. **Mechanism.** Radiation generates highly reactive free radical molecules that irreparably alter the cell's DNA structure, thereby rendering the cell incapable of proliferation.

III. **Clinical response.** A cell that has been sterilized by radiation may appear to be histologically normal and remain physiologically active but be unable to reproduce. Actual cell death may not occur until the time of cell division, when the cell attempts to replicate faulty DNA. Therefore, the time course of clinical response in any tissue, normal or malignant, is determined by the rate of tissue turnover. Rapidly proliferating normal tissues (eg, bone marrow and gastrointestinal mucosa) and neoplasms (eg, small-cell lung cancer and lymphoma) generally exhibit cell loss within days or weeks after the first dose of radiation; however, normal tissues (eg, nerves and hepatocytes) and tumors with slow turnover rates (well-differentiated prostatic carcinoma) may not manifest cell loss for months to years. The rate of response is characteristic of the cell population but not of the eventual outcome. Biopsies obtained after radiation therapy may demonstrate that tumor cells are present, but serial examinations (clinical, chemical, or radiologic) are required to determine whether they are capable of reproduction.

IV. **Radiosensitivity and radioresistance.** A unit dose of ionizing radiation causes a similar degree of DNA damage in most cell types. No tissue is intrinsically resistant to radiation injury. For most tumors, a dose of **200 centigray (cGy)** will reduce the number of reproductively viable cells by **50%,** resulting in a **cumulative 1-log decrease in malignant cells every 3 or 4 doses.** The goal is to deliver enough radiation to sterilize **every** malignant cell. With few exceptions, the number of malignant cells is the major factor in successful tumor control. **Some neoplasms are mistakenly characterized as "radioresistant" because they either have a slow clinical response time or are located at sites that do not permit adequate irradiation without excessive damage to normal tissues.**

V. **Modification of responses to irradiation.** Extrinsic factors can modify the degree of cellular radiosensitivity.

   A. **Oxygen.** Cellular oxygen stabilizes radiation-induced **free radical molecules,** thereby increasing their chance of binding to the DNA of the cell. Under hypoxic conditions, 2–3 times more radiation is required to produce the same effect as that produced under well-oxygenated conditions. Although the clinical consequences of tumor cell hypoxia are unknown, local tumor cell hypoxia resulting from abnormal tumor vascularity has been proposed as a major factor in cases of radiation failure. Methods designed to increase tumor oxygenation—including therapy with hyperbaric oxygen, oxygen-carrying perfluorocarbons, and red-blood cell transfusion—are being tested clinically. However, all these maneuvers should be viewed as experimental.

   B. **Radiosensitizers and radioprotectors.** Several agents that preferentially increase sterilization of malignant cells or reduce radiation damage to normal cells are currently being evaluated. To date, however, none have gained widespread acceptance or approval by the Federal Drug Administration in standard radiation therapy.

   1. Radiosensitizers can enhance radiation-induced malignant cell damage by (1) stabilizing free radicals (eg, **2-nitroimidazole compounds**), (2) synchronizing cells in G_1 phase **(hydroxyurea),** (3) incorporating thymidine analogs into DNA **(bromodeoxyuridine),** and (4) depleting the supply of intracellular free radical-scavenging thiol compounds **(L-BSO).**

   2. Conversely, radioprotectors that increase the level of intracellular thiol (eg, **WR-2721**) may be useful in minimizing normal tissue injury.

  C. Cytotoxic chemotherapy. The chemotherapeutic agents **cisplatin** and **fluorouracil** are often used concomitantly with radiation therapy to increase tumor cell sterilization. These agents are termed "radiosensitizers," although their exact mechanism is unknown. Acute and chronic radiation toxicity may be increased by the simultaneous administration of chemotherapy and radiation. Because of this enhanced toxicity, the doses of radiation, chemotherapy, or both may need to be modified. In addition, certain chemotherapeutic agents (eg, doxorubicin) should not be given during radiation therapy.

TYPES OF RADIATION

Two methods of administering radiation exist—teletherapy and brachytherapy. **Teletherapy** uses an external radiation source and beam that is directed toward the tumor area. In contrast, **brachytherapy** uses an internal radiation source that is placed adjacent to or within the tumor itself.

  I. Teletherapy, or "external beam radiotherapy" is delivered using **gamma-rays, x-rays,** or **electrons,** and in specialized centers, **neutrons, protons,** or **alpha particles.** Each variation exhibits unique physical and biological characteristics that may be advantageous in certain settings.

   A. Gamma rays delivered by cobalt equipment is the oldest and simplest method of modern high-energy (megavoltage) radiation therapy, and in many centers it remains the preferred technique for treatment of tumors situated in superficial areas of the body such as the extremities, breasts, and head and neck. Radioactive cobalt undergoes nuclear decay, producing photons with **energies of 1.17 and 1.33 million electron volts (MEV).** The maximum dose of these gamma rays is delivered **0.5 cm beneath the skin surface.**

   B. X-rays are produced in a linear accelerator by focusing a beam of high-speed electrons onto a high-density metal target (usually tungsten). The kinetic energy transferred to the metal results in the release of photons. X-rays and gamma rays are both photon beams, differing only in the way they are produced.

    1. Megavoltage equipment. Megavoltage (linear accelerators) in clinical use produce photons with a **maximum energy of 4–25 MEV.** The depth of tissue penetration is directly proportional to the mean energy of the photon beam (about one-third of the maximum photon energy). Megavoltage equipment deposits less energy near the skin surface than cobalt machines. The greatest energy deposition occurs at **1–6 cm beneath the surface,** making these machines ideal for **treatment of tumors within deep body cavities such as the thorax, abdomen, and pelvis.**

    2. Orthovoltage equipment. Orthovoltage x-ray machines produce photons with energies of **0.1–0.4 MEV,** lower than either cobalt or megavoltage equipment. These photons deposit most of their energy **at or within millimeters of the skin surface,** making orthovoltage x-rays suitable for the **treatment of superficial tumors of the skin and subcutaneous tissues.** Before the development of higher energy (megavoltage) machines, orthovoltage equipment was the mainstay of external-beam radiation therapy, and at high doses its use produced a sunburn-like skin reaction and subcutaneous fibrosis.

   C. Electrons. By eliminating the metal target used in linear accelerators, high-speed electrons can be used for radiation therapy. Because the dose of radiation delivered by electrons diminishes rapidly with tissue depth, treatment with electrons is desirable for tumors that are situated within a few centimeters of the skin surface or that overlie radiation-sensitive normal tissues (eg, spinal cord). The energy of the electron beam is chosen according to the desired depth of tissue penetration. Electrons also are combined with photon irradiation to deliver a homogeneous dose of radiation to a desired tissue depth. In addition, some radiation centers are investigating a single high-dose intraoperative electron treatment for unresectable abdominal tumors. Direct surgical exposure of the tumor reduces the dose of radiation delivered to normal tissues, thereby reducing the toxicity of treatment. However, special facilities, which are not yet widely available, are required to deliver the radiation.

D. Heavy Particles. A few specialized centers use expensive cyclotrons to treat selected patients with neutrons, protons, pions, and alpha (helium nuclei) particles. Clinical trials are underway to establish their role in the treatment of cancer.

1. **Neutrons** are heavy, electrically neutral particles. Neutron-induced damage is influenced less by hypoxia and DNA repair processes than is photon- or electron-mediated injury. Neutrons may be advantageous in the treatment of **large, slow-growing tumors** such as unresectable salivary gland neoplasms and well-differentiated prostate carcinoma.

2. **Protons and alpha particles** are positively charged nuclear particles that deliver their radiation dose at a defined tissue depth to small noninfiltrating tumors situated in highly radiation-sensitive tissues such as chordomas and uveal melanomas, which may be treated best with this modality.

II. **Brachytherapy** involves the placement of radioactive sources directly into a malignancy such as a tongue or prostate tumor **(interstitial therapy)** or into a body cavity adjacent to the tumor **(intracavitary insertion).** Brachytherapy is often combined with teletherapy to provide an extra **"boost"** dose to accessible tumor. This approach takes advantage of the exponential decrease in radiation dose with increasing distance from a radioactive source to deliver a high dose of radiation to the tumor site while minimizing the radiation exposure of the surrounding normal tissues. Commonly used radioactive materials are chosen on the basis of specific characteristics such as half-life and photon energy.

A. Cesium^{137} decays by **beta emission** to barium^{137} with a **half-life of 30 years,** emitting a powerful gamma ray of 0.66 MEV. Cesium^{137} is often used in temporary intracavitary implants for large **cervical, uterine,** and **vaginal cancers.**

B. Iridium^{192} decays by **beta emission** to platinum^{192} with a **half-life of 74 days,** producing gamma rays with an average energy of 0.34 MEV. Iridium^{192} is commonly implanted in the lip, tongue, breast, and other sites to deliver about 2000 cGy to the tumor over a period of 2–3 days.

C. Iodine^{125} decays by **electron capture** to telurium^{125} with a **half-life of 60 days.** It emits an extremely low-energy gamma ray of 0.028 MEV, limiting its dose range to a tiny volume. This is advantageous in the treatment of tumors situated in vital structures such as the brain.

D. Gold^{198} decays by **beta emission** to mercury^{198} with a **half-life of 2.7 days,** emitting a 0.41 MEV gamma ray. This short half-life is ideal for permanent implantation in areas that are difficult to treat, such as the pulmonary bronchi.

FIELDS, DOSES, & FRACTIONATION

The likelihood of tumor control is **directly related to the radiation dose and inversely proportional to the number of tumor cells.** The major factor limiting the radiation dose is the tolerance of the normal tissues in the irradiated volume. Because radiation is delivered locally, complications depend on tumor location. For example, diarrhea is associated with intestinal irradiation, alopecia with scalp irradiation, and odynophagia with throat or esophageal irradiation. **Treatment volume, dose distribution,** and **dose fractionation** must be carefully controlled and monitored to deliver sufficient therapy while avoiding serious toxicity to normal tissue.

I. **Radiation treatment fields.** Radiation treatment fields (ports) are designed to encompass the entire tumor volume while excluding as much normal tissue as possible. A **"simulation"** session is required to individualize the size, shape, and location of the field or fields before radiation therapy begins. For potentially curative treatment, all areas of gross and suspected microscopic tumor and regional lymphatics must be included in the fields. With palliative radiation therapy, the irradiated volume may be limited to tumor sites producing symptoms to minimize the side effects of treatment.

A. Single-field therapy. A single field frequently is indicated for **superficial tumors** (eg, basal cell carcinoma, Kaposi's sarcoma), **superficial lymphatic regions** (cervical and supraclavicular nodes), and **anatomic areas that do not require a deeply penetrating beam** (eg, the hand or spinal cord). By using a single treatment field, the maximum dose is delivered at or near the body surface.

B. Multiple-field therapy. For large or deeply situated tumors, **2–4 treatment fields** that converge on the tumor from different directions are used to **increase both the dose homogeneity within the tumor and the tumor to normal tissue dose ratio.** In general, the addition of more fields decreases the maximum dose of radiation given to areas of normal tissue in exchange for increasing the total volume of normal tissue irradiated.

C. **Arc (rotating beam) therapy** extends the multiple field concept to an extreme by centering the tumor at a point around which the radiation machine rotates during treatment. This, in effect, creates an infinite number of radiation ports.

D. **Stereotactic radiation therapy** is used to localize the radiation dose precisely to a small area, particularly in the brain. The patient's head is immobilized in a stereotactic metal frame attached to the treatment table. A single large dose of radiation is given via multiple fields to a small intracranial target. This procedure is gaining acceptance for the treatment of cranial arteriovenous malformations and small cerebral tumors.

E. **Shrinking-field therapy.** The radiation dose required for tumor eradication is directly related to the number of malignant cells in an area. The **shrinking field** technique reduces the size of the fields after a moderate radiation dose has been delivered to the initial volume to include only the areas with the greatest concentration of tumor cells.

II. **Radiation doses.** The standard unit of radiation, replacing the rad, is the **gray (Gy)**. One gray equals 100 rad or cGy, which is the energy required to deliver 1 joule of energy to 1 kilogram of tissue. For most malignancies, the total dose used over a complete course of therapy is **30–50 Gy for palliation, 45–50 Gy for eradication of subclinical disease,** and **60–70 Gy for elimination of clinically apparent disease.** Lower doses may be appropriate for unusually radiosensitive cancers such as **leukemia, lymphoma,** and **seminoma.** The effective dose required to achieve a desired result depends on the following factors: **daily radiation dose, therapeutic goal** (curative or palliative), **tumor cell type and radiosensitivity, tumor size, tolerance of the surrounding normal tissues, future therapeutic plans** (chemotherapy, surgical resection, or both), and the **patient's general physical condition.**

III. **Fractionation.** Division of external-beam therapy into small daily doses over a prolonged period increases the therapeutic ratio. Dose fractionation increases the therapeutic ratio by allowing normal cells to repair DNA damage, by redistributing malignant cells into more radiosensitive cell-cycle phases, and by increasing oxygenation of hypoxic tumor cells. Clinically, dose fractionation permits an effective dose of external-beam radiation to be delivered to the tumor while maintaining acceptable injury to normal tissue.

A. **Conventional fractionation** has been empirically derived. Typically, **180–200 Gy/d is given 5 times per week for 5–8 weeks** (total dose of 50–70 cGy).

B. **Altered fractionation.** Altered fractionation schemes are commonly used in a variety of situations.

1. **Hypofractionation (250–300 cGy)** delivers a reduced number (10–15) of larger than conventional fractions (total dose of 30–39 Gy). This approach is generally used for palliative treatment in patients with metastatic disease. Hypofractionation is designed to minimize the conventional toxicity of treatment. The likelihood of long-term tumor control, however, is diminished.

2. **Hyperfractionation** delivers an increased number of smaller than conventional fractions twice a day over 5–7 weeks (total dose of 60–84 Gy). This aggressive treatment attempts to improve tumor control rates without increasing toxicity and is commonly used in lung and head and neck malignancies.

3. **Accelerated fractionation** shortens the course of radiation therapy to 1.5–5 weeks by giving 2 or 3 treatments per day separated by 6–8 hours. This approach is advocated for rapidly proliferating tumors such as carcinomas of the head and neck and uterine cervix. However, tumor cell repopulation is decreased. Because the time for DNA repair and repopulation of normal tissues also is shortened, acute toxicity limits the total dose that can be given. Accelerated fractionation is often combined with hyperfractionation (150–180 cGy 2–3 times a day) to balance normal tissue tolerance with therapeutic efficacy.

TOXICITIES

The time course and severity of normal tissue reactions are highly dependent on **total dose, dose fractionation, treatment volume,** and **energy of radiation.** Because radiation, unlike chemotherapy, is a local treatment, side effects are limited to the tissues that are situated within the radiation fields. The following is a guide to the management of frequently encountered radiation toxicities.

I. **Skin toxicity.** With megavoltage radiation, serious skin reactions are minimized. However, **late subcutaneous fibrosis** can develop, especially with **doses exceeding 65**

Gy. An acute skin reaction commonly does become evident during the third week of therapy, increasing until the completion of treatment. The associated **erythema, desquamation, and pruritus** completely resolve within 3 weeks after therapy ends. During therapy, topical corticosteroids or moisturizing creams applied several times daily afford symptomatic palliation and promote healing. With current methods of radiation therapy, radiation-induced skin ulceration or necrosis is **rare.**

II. **Oral cavity and mandibular toxicity.** Radiation doses over **20 Gy** to the major salivary glands produce **decreased salivation and xerostomia.** The degree of permanent salivary and taste impairment is proportional to the **total radiation dose, proportion of the glands irradiated, and age of the patient.** Xerostomia may be partially relieved by frequent hydration and synthetic saliva preparations. Because xerostomia predisposes to the development of dental caries, extractions and other necessary oral surgery should be performed before treatment is initiated. In addition, fluoride treatments should be given regularly after irradiation to minimize the formation of caries. It is essential for good oral hygiene to be maintained throughout the patient's life to prevent tooth decay and mandibular osteonecrosis. Dental surgery should be avoided permanently after irradiation of the oral cavity.

III. **Hematologic toxicity** is manifested primarily as **myelosuppression.** The volume of marrow irradiated and total radiation dose determine the severity of hematologic toxicity. In adults, **40% of active marrow is located in the pelvis, 25% is in the vertebral column, and 20% is in the ribs and skull.** Extensive irradiation of these sites, particularly in patients with underlying bone marrow disease, can cause marked myelosuppression. Radiation therapy to areas other than these sites, even at high doses, will not significantly impact on peripheral blood counts or bone marrow reserve. Bone marrow **injury is reversible after fractionated radiation doses as large as 25 Gy.** Occasionally, **transfusions** are required to support the patient during the recovery period.

IV. **Gastrointestinal toxicity**

A. **Acute complications. Nausea, vomiting, and diarrhea** commonly occur 2–6 hours after abdominal or pelvic irradiation and may begin on the first day of treatment. The incidence and severity of these side effects increases with the fraction size and treatment volume.

1. Nausea may be prevented by oral administration of prochlorperazine (10 mg) or promethazine (25 mg) 1 hour before treatment.
2. A low-residue diet and administration of an anticholinergic agent such as loperamide as needed are useful for controlling diarrhea.
3. Occasionally, a reduction in fraction size or a break in treatment is required to control the acute symptoms.

B. **Chronic diarrhea, obstruction caused by bowel adhesions, and fistula formation** are uncommon (< 1%) but serious complications of intestinal irradiation. **Progressive odynophagia** caused by pharyngeal or esophageal irradiation commonly occurs during the treatment course but resolves 1 to 2 weeks after cessation of therapy.

1. **Alcohol and tobacco consumption, which exacerbate odynophagia,** should be avoided. Odynophagia may limit the patient's diet to **soft or liquid (nonacidic) foods.** Liquid nutritional supplements are often useful for maintenance of adequate oral nutrition, and, in severe cases, a temporary nasogastric feeding tube may be helpful.
2. **Oral administration of nonsteroidal anti-inflammatory drugs or narcotic analgesics and a mouthwash of viscous xylocaine** usually diminishes the symptoms of **mucositis.** Opportunistic *Candida* infection may exacerbate the mucositis and should be treated with **ketoconazole, fluconazole,** or **nystatin.**

REFERENCES

Moss WT, Cox JD (editors): *Radiation Oncology: Rationale, Technique, Results,* 6th ed. St. Louis, MO: CV Mosby; 1989:1–57, 83–172.

Peres CA, Brady LW (editors): *Principles and Practice of Radiation Oncology.* Philadelphia, PA: JB Lippincott; 1987:1–43.

Suit HD, Muneyasu U: Radiation biology of radiation therapy. In: Wang CC (editor), *Clinical Radiation Oncology.* Littleton, MA: PSG Publishing; 1988:7–55.

5 Principles of Immunotherapy

Robert B. Cameron, MD

THE IMMUNE SYSTEM

Lymphocytes, antigen presenting cells (eg, macrophages, dendritic cells), **and specialized epithelial cells** of the spleen and thymus constitute the human immune system. These cells interact with foreign antigens and with each other to mediate both the **humoral** and the **cellular** arms of the immune response. The primary goal of immunotherapy is to recruit the host's natural defense mechanism, the immune system, to combat the invading malignancy.

I. **Lymphocytes.** Lymphocytes are a heterogeneous group of cells found in the bone marrow, spleen, lymph nodes, tonsils, thymus, intestines (Peyer's patches), and blood. Several subsets of lymphocytes exist.

   A. **B lymphocytes.** Bone marrow-derived CD19+ B cells are the precursors to **immunoglobulin (Ig)** secreting or **plasma** cells. In response to soluble or cellular antigens and dependent on **"help"** provided by **T cells** in the form of soluble or membrane-bound growth factors), specific antibodies are elaborated. Structural differences in the heavy chains result in 5 classes of Ig: **IgA**, a dimer present in **secretions), IgD**, a B cell **membrane** receptor; **IgE**, mast cell and basophil allergic responses; **IgG**, 75% of circulating Ig; and **IgM**, a monomer as a B cell membrane receptor and a pentamer as the initial Ig formed in the immune response.

   B. **T lymphocytes.** T or thymus-dependent CD3+ lymphocytes include CD3+, CD4+ **helper** (T_h) cells that provide B or T cell **cognate** help (direct cell contact) or **factor-dependent** help (cytokine release); CD3+, CD8+ **suppressor** (T_s) cells that **inhibit** T_h cells; and CD3+, CD8+ cytotoxic (T_c) cells that mediate cytotoxicity.

   C. **Null cells.** Null cells are devoid of the usual mature T and B cell markers and include CD3- CD16+ **natural killer (NK) cells** and E-rosette-, CD3-, CD11- **lymphokine (interleukin-2)-activated killer (LAK) cells** that mediate nonspecific, contact-dependent cytotoxicity.

II. **Antigen-presenting cells (APC). The primary APCs are the monocyte-macrophages**. These phagocytic cells may bear Fc and complement (C3) receptors as well as Class II major histocompatibility complex (MHC) antigens. In addition, when "activated" by lipopolysaccharide, muramyl dipeptide, or interferon-gamma, macrophages may bind to and directly lyse viable tumor cells. They also may secrete a variety of chemotactic and cytotoxic **factors**, such as collagenase, elastase, protease, lipase, ribonuclease, glycosidase, complement components, superoxide, prostaglandins, leukotrienes, and cytokines (interleukin-1, tumor necrosis factor-alpha, and macrophage colony-stimulating factor).

TUMOR IMMUNOLOGY

The concept of immunotherapy rests entirely on the assumption that tumor cells possess immunologically reactive surface antigens that do not exist on normal cells. The following data support this premise:

I. **Clinical information.** Certain malignancies (renal cell carcinoma and malignant melanoma) may undergo **spontaneous regression**, presumably due to immune surveillance.

II. **Monoclonal antibodies.** Specific **oncofetal** (eg, carcinoembryonic antigen, alphafetoprotein) and **tumor-associated antigens** (17–1A, L6, and B72.3 [adenocarcinoma] and 48.7, 9.2.27, 96.5, and Mel-1 [melanoma] have been demonstrated by monoclonal antibodies.

III. **Specific cytotoxic lymphocytes.** Although "nonspecific" in their tumor target lysis pattern, LAK cells specifically lyse tumor cells but not fresh normal cells, presumably because of an as yet undefined cell surface antigenic change. In addition, recent data demonstrate **specific** cytotoxic T lymphocyte lysis of autologous, but not allogeneic, tumor targets by **tumor-infiltrating lymphocytes**. The latter finding suggests the existence of tumor-associated antigens that are either unique to each individual malignancy or more universal but uniquely recognized in the context of the proper autologous Class I MHC antigens.

ACTIVE IMMUNOTHERAPY

Active immunotherapy consists of the administration of substances designed to provoke an antitumor response by the tumor-bearing host's own immune cells.

  I. In vivo induced immunity. This involves administration of immunomodulatory agents directly to the tumor-bearing host.

    A. Nonspecific immunotherapy. This type of treatment produces antitumor reactivity that does not depend on a unique tumor-associated antigen.

      1. Bacillus Calmette-Guerin (BCG). Intralesional BCG may eliminate up to **70–90% of cutaneous tumor nodules in breast cancer and melanoma**, and intrapleural administration of BCG has been reported to delay the recurrence of lung cancer. In addition, intravesicle instillation produces **70% complete responses in patients with superficial bladder cancer**. Macrophage destruction of tumor cells as **innocent bystanders** during a vigorous immune reaction to BCG represents the most likely mechanism, yet **systemic** immunity rarely occurs.

      2. *Corynebacterium parvum*. Although active in animals,*C. parvum* has no documented efficacy in humans.

      3. Cytokines. With recent genetic advances, a myriad of cytokines with potential antitumor activity have become available.

        a. Interferons (IFN). Since their discovery in 1957, 3 major interferons have been described. All inhibit tumor growth, promote partial reversal of the malignant phenotype, enhance expression of cell surface molecules (including beta-2-microglobulin, Fc receptors, tumor antigens, and histocompatibility antigens), augment NK activity, modulate B cell function, inhibit T cell suppressor activity, and activate macrophages. The side effects mimic a **flulike illness** with anorexia, weight loss, fatigue, lethargy, and disorientation.

          (1) Interferon-alpha (IFN-alpha). IFN-alpha is produced primarily by **leukocytes** after **viral (Class I) stimulation**. Multiple species encoded by **15 different genes** exist, and IFN-alpha shares a cell surface receptor with IFN-beta. IFN-alpha is most active against **hairy cell leukemia and chronic myelogenous leukemia**, but it also has some activity against lymphoma, myeloma, Kaposi's sarcoma, renal cell carcinoma, melanoma, ovarian carcinoma, and glioma.

          (2) Interferon-beta (IFN-beta). Although only **2 genes in fibroblasts** encode for this **Class I IFN**, nearly all other properties of this cytokine are identical to those of IFN-alpha. Clinical experience with IFN-beta, however, has been extremely limited.

          (3) Interferon-gamma (IFN-gamma). IFN-gamma, or **immune interferon**, is produced by T lymphocytes on antigenic stimulation (**Type II interferon**). Only a **single gene** encodes for IFN-gamma, and it has its own cell surface receptor. To date, clinical trials using IFN-gamma have been disappointing.

        b. Interleukin-1 (IL-1). IL-1, or **lymphocyte-activating factor**, is produced primarily by macrophages but also by NK cells, lymphocytes, and endothelial cells. Two forms, IL-1-alpha and IL-1-beta, exist and mediate pyogenic responses; release of cytokines from T cells; neutrophil, macrophage, and lymphocyte chemotaxis; growth of fibroblasts and endothelial cells; activation of NK cells; differentiation of B cells; and proliferation of hematopoietic stem cells. Together with granulocyte colony-stimulating factor, IL-1 may play a role in **bone marrow protection and recovery from radiation- or chemotherapy-induced leukopenia**.

        c. Interleukin-2 (IL-2). Produced by activated T cells, IL-2 induces LAK and T cell growth, cytotoxicity, and lymphokine production. **High doses (eg, 100,000 units/kg/8 h) may produce objective regression of advanced tumors in as many as 15% of patients, particularly those with melanoma and renal cell carcinoma**. However, substantial reversible IL-2 toxicities (as a result of lymphoid organ infiltration and a vascular leak syndrome) frequently occur and include (1) flulike symptoms such as chills (49%), nausea and vomiting (75%), and diarrhea (70%); (2) hepatic dysfunction manifested by hyperbilirubinemia or elevated liver enzymes (85%); (3) renal dysfunction with oliguria (38%) and elevated creatinine (79%);

(4) pulmonary dysfunction, ie, bronchospasm (1%), pleural effusions (3%), and respiratory insufficiency occasionally requiring intubation (14%); (5) cardiac toxicity, including hypotension requiring pressors (66%), arrhythmias (9%), and myocardial infarction (1%); (6) bone marrow depression manifested as anemia requiring transfusion (66%) and thrombocytopenia (78%); (7) central nervous system toxicity with disorientation (28%), somnolence (14%), and coma (4%); (8) edema and weight gain greater than 5% of body weight (64%); (9) sepsis (10%); (10) and death (1%).

d. **Interleukin-4 (IL-4).** IL-4, also known as **B cell growth factor (BCGF)**, is produced by activated T cells and serves as a growth factor for both T and B cells. Preliminary data suggest that IL-4, in combination with IL-2, may generate **more specific cytotoxic tumor-infiltrating lymphocytes** than those induced with IL-2 alone.

e. **Interleukin-6 (IL-6).** IL-6, previously referred to as **interferon-beta-2** and **B cell stimulatory factor-2 (BSF-2)**, is manufactured by monocytes, fibroblasts, and certain tumors. It induces fibroblast expression of Class I MHC antigens, hepatic production of acute phase proteins, and T cell proliferation. However, potential antitumor activity has not been confirmed in humans.

f. **Tumor necrosis factor (TNF).** TNF-alpha (**cachectin**) is produced by macrophages, endothelial cells, and T cells, while TNF-beta (**lymphotoxin**) is made exclusively by T cells. Both induce fever, cachexia, endothelial cell changes, and neutrophil chemotaxis. Clinical trials in humans, however, have failed to demonstrate the impressive antitumor activity originally observed in animals.

g. **Colony stimulating factors (CSF).** The CSFs are required growth factors in the normal proliferation and differentiation of bone marrow elements.

    (1) Granulocyte CSF (G-CSF). G-CSF induces the differentiation of **granulocytes** (ie, neutrophils and eosinophils) and some monocytes. Studies in mice, primates, and humans demonstrate that G-CSF **reduces the period of neutropenia** following radiation therapy or chemotherapy.

    (2) Granulocyte-macrophage CSF (GM-CSF). Although theoretically more potent than for G-CSF **macrophages** stimulation, GM-CSF has not proved to be substantially different clinically from G-CSF.

    (3) Macrophage CSF (M-CSF). M-CSF stimulates the production of **monocytes and macrophages**; however, its role, if any, in the immunotherapy of human tumors is not yet defined.

    (4) Other compounds. Although **levamisole** was recently proved effective in the adjuvant treatment of colorectal carcinoma, other derivatives of bacteria cell walls (**trehalose dimycolate, muramyl dipeptide**), and the drug **flavone acetic acid (FAA)** have not met with success.

B. **Specific immunotherapy.** Specific immunotherapy, directly or indirectly, mediates antitumor activity that depends on a unique tumor-associated antigen. **Tumor vaccines** that provide permanent and systemic immunity have been a long-time goal of immunotherapists. Most protocols use viable or inactivated **autologous or allogeneic tumor cells** (antigens) and **an adjuvant** to augment immunogenicity. **Xenogenization** (alteration of the surface antigenic structure to increase immunogenicity) with viruses, radiation (eg, ultraviolet light), heat, and chemicals also is used. Although a recent clinical study using 3 weekly vaccinations with irradiated tumor cells and BCG documented **active immunity** (as measured by delayed-type hypersensitivity responses) in **67% of patients with colorectal carcinoma** and fewer recurrences and deaths than in the control group (Hoover et al, 1985), most trials do not report successful immunization or prolonged survival.

II. **Ex vivo induced immunity (adoptive immunotherapy).** This form of **active** immunotherapy results from in vitro exposure of the tumor-bearing host's tissues to immunologically active substances, resulting in immune activity that may be adoptively transferred back to the host.

A. **Nonspecific immunotherapy. Lymphokine-activated killer cells,** originally described in 1980, are primarily CD3⁻, CD16⁺ lymphocytes that are capable of lysing fresh tumor cells and NK-resistant targets (but not fresh normal cells) in short-term lytic assays after in vitro exposure to IL-2 for 3–6 days. Recent clinical trials of LAK cells (administered with IL-2) in patients with advanced cancer report a **7.8% complete and 25% overall response rate** in patients with a variety of tumors. The response rates were as high as **35% (25 of 72 patients) with renal cell carcinoma and 60% (3 of 5 patients) with non-Hodgkin's lymphomas** (Rosenberg et al, 1987). Response rates in patients given IL-2 alone were 3.5% complete and 17% overall.

B. **Specific immunotherapy. Tumor-infiltrating lymphocytes (TIL)** are an example of specific immune cells. These lymphocytes, grown from tumor cell suspensions incubated in IL-2, differ from LAK cells in that their cytotoxicity is often specific for the tumor from which they were derived. TIL have been cultured from a variety of human tumors and have been characterized as cytotoxic CD3+ T cells that variably express CD4, CD8, and CD25 (IL-2 receptor) antigens. In 2 recent studies, **objective responses were reported in as many as 60% of patients** treated with as many as 7.5×10^{11} cells (Kradin et al, 1987; Rosenberg et al, 1988). The toxicity reported was essentially identical to that observed with IL-2 alone. However, combinations of TIL and other therapies (eg, radiation therapy, chemotherapy) and the transduction into TIL of genes coding for various cytokines (eg, IL-2, TNF-alpha) may increase the therapeutic efficacy of TIL and simultaneously decrease the associated toxicity.

PASSIVE IMMUNOTHERAPY

Immunity created by the transfer of exogenous reagents to a tumor-bearing host is termed **passive immunity**.

I. **Monoclonal antibodies (MoAb).** Although MoAbs have not been the panacea that they once were thought to be, they may prove to be beneficial in both the imaging and treatment of cancer. MoAbs may mediate tumor cell destruction by producing antibody-dependent cellular cytotoxicity, by increasing effector cell binding to tumor, by blocking receptors for autocrine growth factors, by activating complement, and by exerting an innocent bystander effect during a host anti-MoAb reaction. Generally, most MoAbs are generated from murine sources and do not function well with human effector cells. However, with new genetic techniques, it may be possible to increase the efficacy of these antibodies by constructing both **heteroconjugates** (2 different linked antibodies) and **chimeric antibodies** (a murine antigen-binding region and a human effector cell-binding area).

A. **Cancer imaging.** The use of specific MoAbs labeled with iodine-125 or 131, indium-111, or technetium-99m can **detect 50–100% of metastatic tumor sites**, depending on their size and location, the blood flow to the area, and the antigen-antibody combination used. However, even with maximal binding, no more than **0.0047% of the injected dose is bound per gram of tissue**, making detection of small foci of disease extremely difficult.

B. **Cancer therapy.** Most trials involving MoAb administration as antitumor therapy have failed to demonstrate any efficacy. An exception is **B cell lymphoma, which may respond in 50%** of patients to infusion of anti-idiotype antibodies (antibodies directed against antigenic determinants on the variable regions of immunoglobulins). Generally, problems with MoAbs are that (1) antibody doses are limited; (2) antibodies are frequently given without conjugates (eg, ricin,[131]I, doxorubicin), cytokines (eg, IFN-gamma), or effector cells (eg, LAK); (3) tumor antigens are variable and change with time; (4) antibodies bind to soluble antigen released by the tumor; (5) antibodies cannot gain access to the tumor because of limitations in blood supply; and (6) blocking anti-Fc receptor **human antimouse antibodies** develop in **90–100%** of patients.

II. **Other agents.** Active investigation to identify substances that remove or neutralize tumor growth factors, angiogenic factors, and other tumor factors is continuing.

REFERENCES

Hoover HC et al: Prospectively randomized trial of adjuvant active specific immunotherapy for human colorectal cancer. *Cancer* 1985;**55**:1236.

Kradin RL et al: Tumor-derived interleukin-2 dependent lymphocytes in adoptive immunotherapy of lung cancer. *Cancer Immunol Immunother* 1987;**24**:76–85.

Ortaldo JR, Longo DL: Human natural lymphocyte effector cells: definition, analysis of activity, and clinical effectiveness. *JNCI* 1988;**80**:999–1010.

Rosenberg SA et al. A progress report on the treatment of 157 patients with advanced cancer using lymphokine-activated killer cells and interleukin-2 or high-dose interleukin-2 alone. *N Engl J Med* 1987;**316**:889–897.

Rosenberg SA et al: Use of tumor-infiltrating lymphocytes and interleukin-2 in the immunotherapy of patients with metastatic melanoma: a preliminary report. *N Engl J Med* 1988;**319**:1676–1680.

Topalian SL, Rosenberg SA: Tumor-infiltrating lymphocytes (TIL): evidence for specific immune reactions against growing cancers in mouse and man. DeVita V, Hellman S, Rosenberg SA (editors), *Important Advances in Oncology.* Philadelphia, PA: JB Lippincott; 1990.

6　Bone Marrow Transplantation

Carlin J. McLaughlin, DO and Nora C. Ku, MD

Bone marrow transplantation (BMT) may be used for a wide variety of benign as well as malignant diseases. Both allogeneic and autologous transplantation have proved to be curative in cancers that were previously uniformly fatal. In cancer therapy, BMT affords the opportunity to exploit doses of chemotherapy and irradiation that normally produce excessive hematologic toxicity.

TYPES OF BONE MARROW TRANSPLANTATION

I. **Autologous BMT.** The reinfusion of bone marrow or peripheral blood stem cells that are harvested **from the same patient** prior to ablative chemotherapy or radiation therapy (or both) is termed autologous BMT. This type of transplantation permits administration of chemotherapeutic agents at levels previously associated with fatal bone marrow aplasia and, at the same time, avoids histocompatibility problems that arise with allogeneic BMT (see **III,** below). Autologous BMT is **most useful in patients with disease-free bone marrow and responsive malignancies who are** *not* **candidates for allogeneic or syngeneic BMT** because of age or absence of a suitable bone marrow donor.

II. **Syngeneic BMT.** Syngeneic transplantation utilizes bone marrow **from a human leukocyte antigen (HLA)-identical twin** and is limited to patients with twin siblings who are free of significant genetic diseases. Although syngeneic BMT averts the morbidity and mortality related to HLA incompatibility—ie, graft-versus-host disease (GVHD)—that occurs with allogeneic BMT, it is associated with a **higher relapse rate resulting from a weaker graft-versus-tumor response** (see **III,** below).

III. **Allogeneic BMT.** Although HLA-mismatched BMT is sometimes attempted, standard allogeneic BMT employs HLA-compatible bone marrow **from a related or unrelated donor.** This form of BMT is associated with a **higher morbidity than syngeneic or autologous BMT.** However, in the treatment of leukemia, it yields an **overall survival comparable to syngeneic BMT.** This stems from an immunologically mediated graft-versus-tumor effect that does not occur with syngeneic BMT and that accompanies mild to moderate chronic GVHD (see p 31).

USES OF BONE MARROW TRANSPLANTATION

Although BMT has been used to treat benign disorders such as severe combined immunodeficiency, aplastic anemia, and thalassemia major, BMT has been much more extensively employed to treat the following malignancies.

I. Hematologic malignancies

A. **Acute lymphocytic leukemia (ALL).** Because **70%** of patients with low-risk ALL (see Chapter 63) are cured with conventional chemotherapy, **BMT should not be considered prior to relapse.** However, patients with high-risk ALL may be evaluated for BMT once remission is achieved, but only within the context of an approved clinical trial.

B. **Acute nonlymphocytic leukemia (ANLL).** For selected patients (with HLA-compatible donors), superior survival may be achieved with allogenic BMT following induction chemotherapy than with standard maintenance chemotherapy. The most appropriate time for BMT is controversial, but once relapse occurs, allogeneic BMT offers the only hope for long-term, disease-free survival.

C. **Chronic myelogenous leukemia (CML).** After undergoing BMT during the first year of the chronic phase of this disease, 70–80% of patients less than 30 years old and 50–60% of those 30 years or older are cured. In addition, 15–20% of patients who are in the otherwise uniformly fatal blast phase may be cured by syngeneic or allogeneic BMT. The lower cure rate for patients over 30 years of age is due to higher treatment-related mortality and an increased rate of relapse.

D. **Chronic lymphocytic leukemia (CLL).** CLL usually occurs in older patients, and **BMT is generally not indicated.** However, BMT remains an alternative for young CLL patients because results with standard chemotherapy are poor.

E. **Hodgkin's disease.** Patients who have **failed standard chemotherapy** may be candidates for autologous BMT, which has yielded high response rates and some durable complete remissions in preliminary clinical trials.

F. **Non-Hodgkin's lymphoma.** High overall response rates and a 30% 3-year disease-free survival in patients who have failed standard chemotherapy have prompted investigational use of autologous BMT as consolidation therapy in high-risk patients with intermediate- or high-grade lymphoma. Contaminating neoplastic cells in autologous bone marrow may be purged with monoclonal antibodies or avoided by harvesting peripheral blood stem cells (see Transplantation Procedure, p 28).

G. **Multiple myeloma.** Several patients with relapsing or refractory multiple myeloma have been treated with high doses of alkylating agents, radiation therapy, and autologous BMT using cryopreserved bone marrow or peripheral blood stem cells. Unfortunately, remissions have been short-lived, with most patients dying of malignant disease.

II. **Solid tumors.** BMT (usually autologous) has been tested in virtually every solid malignancy; however, the results have been difficult to interpret because of patient selection bias and inappropriate or absent control groups. Currently, BMT is under investigation as a form of therapy for the following solid cancers:

A. **Neuroblastoma.** Recently, a combination of multiagent chemotherapy and autologous BMT has been shown to improve overall survival from 22% to 53% at 40 months.

B. **Testicular carcinoma.** Complete and durable remissions have been obtained in 12% of heavily pretreated patients who have failed conventional and salvage chemotherapy. However, the toxicity is considerable (21% mortality). Currently, trials are in progress comparing autologous BMT to standard therapy (vincristine, bleomycin, and cisplatin) in the initial treatment of testicular carcinoma.

C. **Breast cancer.** In a number of uncontrolled trials, high initial response rates have been documented in patients with advanced or refractory disease who undergo autologous BMT. Unfortunately, after 3 years, the survival rates are similar to those for patients treated with chemotherapy alone. Currently, clinical trials are evaluating the role of adjuvant autologous BMT in the treatment of high-risk patients with breast cancer.

D. **Ewing's sarcoma.** Preliminary results in otherwise unresponsive patients with Ewing's sarcoma who are treated with intensive chemotherapy using cyclophosphamide (200 mg/kg over 4 days), etoposide, busulfan, and cisplatin, followed by autologous BMT, are encouraging but inconclusive.

E. **Malignant melanoma.** High-dose combination chemotherapy, together with autologous BMT, for metastatic disease produces better response rates, but overall survival remains unchanged.

PATIENT SELECTION

Selection requirements differ depending on the indication for BMT and type of transplant planned. In general, the most stringent criteria are employed for patients undergoing allogeneic BMT for hematologic cancers (eg, leukemia).

I. **Autologous BMT.** Patients undergoing autologous transplantation for leukemia, lymphoma, or solid tumors should be in **excellent physical condition;** however, age requirements generally are less restrictive than with allogeneic BMT because of the absence of GVHD and its associated morbidity. **Responsive disease** is an important criterion, as patients with refractory disease respond poorly.

II. **Allogeneic BMT.** The ideal patient to receive allogeneic BMT is **less than 30 years of age** and has **no underlying cardiopulmonary disease.** Patients 30–49 years old may be considered for allogeneic BMT if they are in good physical condition; however, their survival is usually lower due to transplant-associated morbidity from GVHD.

DONOR SELECTION

Generally, bone marrow donors for allogeneic BMT are **siblings with identical HLAs.** These antigens, which constitute the major histocompatibility complex in humans, are encoded by genes located on chromosome 6. Class I antigens (A, B, and C) are defined serologically, whereas Class II antigens (D, DR, SB, MB, and MT) are defined by mixed lymphocyte cultures. Since 2 haplotypes are inherited (1 from each parent), the probability that 2 siblings carry identical major histocompatibility antigens is 25%. If a compatible sibling is not available, a search of the extended family and bone marrow donor registries may be conducted for an HLA-matched donor. If a complete match is not available, a 1- or 2-antigen mismatched donor may be considered, although the risks of GVHD and rejection increase with the degree of mismatch. The chance of finding an HLA-matched, unrelated donor in a registry is between 1 in 1000 and 1 in 100,000.

MYELOABLATIVE THERAPY (CONDITIONING)

Two important goals of conditioning are (1) **cytoreduction** to make space for the transplanted bone marrow and (2) **immunosuppression** to reduce the chance of rejection. Myeloablative therapy typically utilizes cytotoxic agents with or without total body irradiation. Representative conditioning regimens are provided in Table 6–1.

   I. **Chemotherapy.** Cytotoxic agents used in BMT conditioning are selected for their prominent myelosuppression; other toxicities usually are minimal. **Cyclophosphamide** is used most widely and may be administered alone or with other agents such as **cytosine arabinoside, etoposide, carmustine, thiotepa,** and **mitoxantrone.**
   II. **Total body irradiation (TBI).** In some conditioning regimens, TBI (500–1575 cGy over 2.5–7 days) is given in addition to chemotherapy.

TRANSPLANTATION PROCEDURE

   I. **Bone marrow harvest.** Although few complications follow bone marrow donation, the donor should be healthy because collection requires general or regional anesthesia. During the harvesting procedure, **400–1000 mL of bone marrow containing at least $1–5 \times 10^7$ cells/kg (syngeneic or autologous BMT) or $1–5 \times 10^8$ cells/kg (allogeneic BMT)** are aspirated from the anterior and posterior iliac crests and, if necessary, the sternum. Bone and tissue debris are removed by filtration through mesh or by centrifugation. Neoplastic cells, if present, can be purged (see **III,** below); then the stem cells are reinfused (after completion of myeloablative therapy) or else frozen (cryopreserved) for later use (see **II,** below). Recently, **stems cells isolated from peripheral blood** have been used successfully in autologous BMT and may represent an alternative source of pluripotent stem cells.
   II. **Cryopreservation.** To preserve bone marrow for more than 24 hours, the **cells must be mixed with 5–10% dimethylsulfoxide with or without 4% human albumin, 6% hydroxyethyl starch, and polyvinyl pyrolidone** in order to prevent formation of lethal intracellular ice crystals. The marrow is diluted to a concentration of $4–5 \times 10^7$ **cells/mL,** cooled using a controlled-rate freezer to $-194\ ^\circ C$, and then stored in liquid nitrogen until the patient is ready for transplantation.
   III. **Purging procedures**
   A. **Positive selection schemes.** Positive selection using **fluorescence-activated cell sorting** is limited by a slow rate of cell separation.
   B. **Negative selection schemes**
   1. **Physical methods.** Counterflow **elutriation** and **immunoabsorption** are examples.
   2. **Biochemical methods. Phototherapy, cytotoxic drugs** (4-hydroxyperoxy-cyclo-phosphamide, etoposide, vincristine, and methylprednisolone), and **bone marrow culture** are typical biochemical methods of bone marrow purging.
   3. **Immunologic methods.** Purging with **cytotoxic cells** (eg, lymphokine-activated killer cells) and **cytokines** (interleukin-2, interferons) as well as comple-

TABLE 6–1. COMMON CONDITIONING REGIMENS FOR BONE MARROW TRANSPLANTATION

Institution	Chemotherapy[1]	Radiation Therapy
Johns Hopkins University	CY 60 mg/kg/d × 2 days	1200 cGy over 4 days
M.D. Anderson Hospital	CY 4.5–6.0 g/m², BCNU 300 mg/m², etoposide 600 mg/m²	None

[1]CY = Cyclophosphamide; BCNU = carmustine.

ment, antibody, toxin, rosette, and magnetic bead mediated separations have been used.

POSTTRANSPLANT IMMUNOSUPPRESSION

Although immunosuppression is not required after autologous or syngeneic BMT, it is **essential after allogeneic BMT to prevent or minimize GVHD.** The immunosuppression is usually maintained for up to 1 year, although prolonged treatment may be necessary to control chronic GVHD. During this period of intense immunosuppression, the patient is highly susceptible to opportunistic infections.

  I. **Cyclosporin A (CsA).** (1–3 mg/kg/d) is a fungal metabolite that primarily inhibits helper T lymphocytes but also affects B cell function. At a molecular level, CsA **interferes with early T cell activation** by altering lymphokine gene transcription. Since CsA has **no myelosuppressive activity,** it is an ideal immunosuppressive agent for BMT. **Side effects** may be severe, however, and include nephrotoxicity, hepatotoxicity, hypertension, and central nervous system effects (tremors, altered mentation, and seizures). The dose should be individualized based on serum creatinine and cyclosporin blood levels as measured by radioimmunoassay or high-pressure liquid chromatography.

 II. **Corticosteroids directly suppress lymphocytes, particularly B cells,** reducing immunoglobulin and complement levels and tissue reactivity to antigen-antibody interactions. **Methylprednisolone** and **prednisone** (0.5 mg/kg) are used most commonly, whereas higher doses (pulse doses) are used during flares of GVHD.

III. **Cytotoxic agents.** Low doses of cytotoxic agents, such as **cyclophosphamide** and **methotrexate,** may be used for additional immunosuppression. These agents **inhibit lymphocyte expansion** and are most beneficial in BMT using a HLA-mismatched or unrelated donor. Methotrexate also reduces hemolysis in BMT patients with an ABO blood group mismatched donor.

IV. **Other agents**
   A. **FK-506.** Like CsA, **FK-506** (another fungal by-product) **inhibits T cell function by regulating cytokine gene expression.** Preliminary data indicate that FK-506 is more potent than CsA, and clinical trials evaluating its use in bone marrow and solid organ transplantation are in progress.
   B. **Monoclonal antibodies.** Complement-mediated depletion of donor bone marrow T cells, using anti-CD3 or campath 1 monoclonal antibodies before infusion, reduces the incidence and severity of GVHD. More recently, selective depletion of the CD8$^+$ T "cytotoxic/suppressor" cell subset has had a similar effect. However, the incidence of graft failure increases with depletion of donor T cells.

SUPPORTIVE CARE

During the immediate post-BMT period, patients require intensive support, often including **blood products** and **antimicrobial therapy,** until the donor bone marrow engrafts and the initial period of pancytopenia resolves.

  I. **Antimicrobials.** If an infection is suspected, empiric antimicrobial therapy must be initiated immediately and continued until any existing neutropenia and fever completely resolve.
   A. **Antibiotics.** Appropriate management of suspected or documented infections in BMT recipients includes the administration of **broad-spectrum antibiotics** once initial culture specimens (eg, blood, urine, sputum) are obtained. Potent cytocidal antibiotics that are devoid of nephrotoxicity are ideal, and therefore the combination of a **third-generation cephalosporin** (eg, ceftazidime, ceftizoxime) and a **semi-synthetic antipseudomonal penicillin** (eg, piperacillin, mezlocillin) is recommended. Therapy may be adjusted if cultures reveal a specific organism.
   B. **Antifungal agents.** Because of profound immunosuppression and widespread use of broad-spectrum antibiotics, BMT patients are extremely susceptible to fungal infections, particularly with *Candida* species. Although **amphotericin B** (0.6 mg/kg/d, adjusting for renal function) remains the standard antifungal agent for suspected systemic fungal infections, the new drug **fluconazole** (200 mg initially followed by 100 mg daily), which may be given intravenously or orally without significant nephrotoxicity, may also be effective, particularly with oropharyngeal and esophageal candidiasis.
   C. **Intravenous immune globulin** (500 mg/kg/wk for 14 weeks) has been shown to decrease the risk of GVHD as well as systemic infection.

 II. **Blood products** (erythrocyte and platelet transfusions) are often required during recovery from BMT (usually 3–4 weeks) as well as intermittently for weeks to months. Platelet counts, in particular, rebound more slowly than other blood components. All blood products should be irradiated with 1500–2000 cGy to reduce the incidence of HLA sensitization and to prevent transfusion-associated GVHD. In addition, blood products that are seronegative for cytomegalovirus should be given to seronegative patients.

  A. **Red blood cells.** In general, the hemoglobin level should be maintained **above 8.5 mg/dL**. If both the recipient and donor blood types are ABO compatible, then that ABO type should be used for transfusions; however, if the donor and recipient are ABO incompatible, **O-negative** blood should be transfused.

  B. **Platelets.** Platelet counts of **20,000/μL or higher** should be maintained with platelet transfusions, since the incidence of **life-threatening hemorrhage** increases dramatically below these levels. In general, **random donor platelets** pooled from 4 to 10 random donors of varying HLA types should be utilized. If platelet sensitization occurs (ie, platelet count does not increase with transfusion), single-donor or HLA-matched platelets obtained by apheresis may be necessary to overcome documented platelet resistance.

III. **Colony-stimulating factors (CSF).** Recently, **granulocyte-macrophage CSF (sargramostim, Prokine, Leukine)**, 5 μg/kg/d, SC or IV) was approved for use in patients undergoing BMT after clinical trials established that it shortens the period of BMT-associated neutropenia by 7 days.

SPECIFIC COMPLICATIONS

The complications of BMT depend on the type of myeloablative regimen used (high-dose chemotherapy alone vs chemotherapy plus irradiation), the type of BMT (syngeneic vs allogeneic vs autologous), and the method of posttransplant immunosuppression, if any. In all cases, the doses of chemotherapy and radiation therapy employed are sufficient to cause **fatal bone marrow aplasia** if not rescued by the infusion of viable stem cells. As a result, the nonhematologic toxicities are more severe than those seen with conventional doses of chemotherapy and become the limiting factors in dose selection. The significantly greater early morbidity and mortality for allogeneic BMT (25–30%) compared with autologous and syngeneic BMT (10%) are largely the result of the development of **acute GVHD**.

  I. **Early complications (occurring less than 100 days after BMT).** Acute complications may be classified into infectious and noninfectious problems.

  A. **Infectious complications.** Infections comprise a major source of morbidity following BMT and are related to the duration and severity of treatment-induced neutropenia.

  1. **Bacterial infections.** In the acute posttransplant phase, bacterial pathogens predominate. **Gram-positive bacterial infections** have become prevalent because of the proliferation of indwelling venous catheters and should be treated with vancomycin (1 gm every 12 hrs) until the antimicrobial susceptibility is known; however, **gram-negative bacterial infections** are also common.

  2. **Fungal infections.** Systemic fungal infections (*Candida albicans* and *Aspergillus flavus*) frequently complicate the acute posttransplant period. Intravenous antifungal therapy (**amphotericin B**, 0.5–0.6 mg/kg/d intravenous) is routinely initiated if defervescence does not occur promptly in a febrile patient receiving appropriately selected broad-spectrum antibiotics.

  3. **Viral infections**

  a. Primary or secondary (reactivation) **herpes simplex** infections are extremely common in BMT patients and are treated with intravenous **acyclovir** (500 mg/m^2 intravenously every 8 hours) and intravenous CMV immunoglobulin (500 mg/kg).

  b. **Cytomegalovirus (CMV)** infection is associated with high morbidity and mortality rates but may be managed successfully with **ganciclovir** (5 mg/kg intravenously every 12 hours) and **intravenous CMV immunoglobulin** (500 mg/kg).

  B. **Noninfectious complications**

  1. **Mucositis,** particularly stomatitis, is an almost ubiquitous complication of high-dose chemotherapy and radiotherapy. **Painful oral ulcerations as well as potential airway obstruction** may occur. **Management** includes meticulous oral care, narcotic analgesia, and the prompt recognition and treatment of fungal or viral infection.

  2. **Subacute (occurring 30–100 days after BMT) nonbacterial interstitial pneumonia** is a major threat to BMT patients. **Almost 20% of allogeneic BMT patients** develop this complication, which is associated with a high mortality rate.

3. **Hemorrhagic cystitis.** Myeloablative regimens that utilize high-dose **cyclo-phosphamide** therapy may produce significant cystitis. Aggressive measures should be instituted to prevent this serious complication (see Chapter 12).
4. **Veno-occlusive disease of the liver occurs in 20–30% of patients** undergoing high-dose chemotherapy. It is characterized pathologically by nonthrombotic occlusion of the small hepatic blood vessels. **Right upper quadrant pain, jaundice, hepatomegaly,** and **ascites** are its clinical manifestations. **Mortality ranges from 5–50%,** depending on the severity of the syndrome as assessed by clinical and laboratory abnormalities. Treatment consists of supportive care (eg, sodium restriction, use of plasma volume expanders and avoidance of diuretics and prostaglandin inhibitors).
5. **Acute graft-versus-host disease.** Acute GVHD results from the engraftment of donor allogeneic T lymphocytes that recognize disparate HLA and non-HLA host antigens, initiating a cytotoxic response directed against host tissues. Acute GVHD characteristically presents as **erythroderma, voluminous diarrhea,** and **immune-mediated hepatitis.** The extent of HLA disparity correlates with the incidence of acute GVHD, with 35–50% of HLA-matched and nearly all unrelated transplant recipients developing signs or symptoms of GVHD or both. Prevention and management involve **immunosuppression with CsA, corticosteroids, and methotrexate.** In patients treated with high-dose chemotherapy and autologous BMT, GVHD can be a complication of using **non-irradiated** blood products.

II. **Chronic complications (more than 100 days after BMT).** Chronic problems, like early complications, can be classified as infectious or noninfectious.
  A. **Infectious complications**
    1. **Bacterial infections.** Sinopulmonary infections (eg, sinusitis, pneumonia), particularly with **encapsulated organisms and *Pneumocystis carinii*,** are major causes of long-term morbidity and mortality in BMT patients. In patients with chronic GVHD, **prophylaxis with trimethoprim-sulfamethoxazole (Bactrim, Septra) or penicillin** should be considered.
    2. **Viral infections.** Disseminated **varicella zoster** infections in the late post-transplant phase are associated with significant morbidity and mortality, and antiviral therapy (**acyclovir,** 10 mg/kg intravenously every 8 hours) should be instituted promptly.
  B. **Noninfectious complications**
    1. **Pulmonary complications.** Recently, pulmonary problems have been recognized as an increasing source of morbidity and mortality in the late posttransplant phase. **Obstructive lung disease** affects 10% of patients with chronic GVHD and may be associated with obliterative bronchiolitis.
    2. **Chronic graft-versus-host disease.** Chronic GVHD develops in up to 35% of patients who receive allogenic BMT and may occur de novo or as a progression of acute GVHD. The risk of developing chronic GVHD is greater in patients who (1) are more than 30 years old, (2) have manifested acute GVHD, and (3) have received buffy coat transfusions to enhance bone marrow engraftment. Chronic GVHD is a **multisystem autoimmune disease resembling scleroderma. It involves all mucosal surfaces as well as the skin, lungs, liver, and eyes.** It also causes **profound immunodeficiency.** However, in some cancers (particularly leukemia), a **beneficial graft-versus-tumor (GVT) response** occurs that may decrease the tumor relapse rate.
    3. **Ocular complications.** Frequently, **cataracts** are observed in BMT patients receiving total body irradiation as part of the myeloablative regimen.
    4. **Endocrine complications.** Commonly, **infertility and hypothyroidism** occur in patients treated with total body irradiation, and it is therefore important to counsel patients regarding fertility issues before proceeding with BMT.
    5. **Secondary malignancies.** The use of **alkylating agents and total body irradiation** is associated with a fivefold to sixfold increased risk of developing a second (usually hematologic) malignancy.

REFERENCES

Anderson KC, Weinstein HJ: Transfusion-associated graft-versus-host disease. *N Engl J Med* 1990;**323**:315.

Ash RC et al: Successful allogeneic transplantation of T-cell-depleted bone marrow from closely HLA-matched unrelated donors. *N Engl J Med* 1990;**322**:485.

Barlogie R et al: Autologous bone marrow transplantation (ABMT) in multiple myeloma (MM). *Proc Am Soc Clin Oncol* 1990;**9**:287.

Barrett J, McCarthy D: Bone marrow transplantation for genetic disorders. *Blood Rev* 1990;**4**:116.

Cheson BD et al: Autologous bone marrow transplantation: Current status and future directions. *Ann Intern Med* 1989;**110**:51.

Gulati S, Yahalow J, Portlock C: Autologous bone marrow transplantation. *Curr Probl Cancer* 1991;**15**(1):5.

Jagannath S et al: High-dose cyclophosphamide, carmustine, and etoposide and autologous bone marrow transplantation for relapsed Hodgkin's disease. *Ann Intern Med* 1986;**104**:163.

Philip T et al: High-dose therapy and autologous bone marrow transplantation after failure of conventional chemotherapy in adults with intermediate-grade or high-grade non-Hodgkin's lymphoma. *N Engl J Med* 1987;**316**:1493.

Press OW, Schaller RT, Thomas ED: Bone marrow transplant complications. Pages 399–424 in: *Complications of Organ Transplantation,* Toledo-Pereyra LH (editor). Marcel Dekker, 1987.

Ramsay NKC, Kersey JH: Indications for marrow transplantation in acute lymphoblastic leukemia. *Blood* 1990;**75**:815.

Sullivan KM: Acute and chronic graft-versus-host disease in man. *Int J Cell Cloning* 1986;**4** (Sup 1):42.

Sullivan KM: Current status of bone marrow transplantation. *BMT Proc* 1989;**21**(sup 1):41.

Sullivan KM et al: Chronic graft-versus-host disease in 52 patients: Adverse natural course and successful treatment with combination immunosuppression. *Blood* 1981;**57**:267.

Sullivan KM et al: Late complications after marrow transplantation. *Semin Hematol* 1984;**21**(1):53.

Takvorian T et al: Prolonged disease-free survival after autologous bone marrow transplantation in patients with non-Hodgkin's lymphoma with a poor prognosis. *N Engl J Med* 1987;**316**:1499.

Thomas ED, Clift RA, Storb R: Indications for marrow transplantation. *Annu Rev Med* 1984;**35**:1.

7 Principles of Pain Management

David E. Weissman, MD

Pain occurs in up to 70% of cancer patients during the course of their illness. Although over 90% of cases of cancer pain can be well controlled using available techniques, it is often undertreated because of inadequate education of health professionals; excessive and unwarranted physician and public concern about opiate-induced respiratory depression, tolerance, and psychological dependence; and excessive physician concern about regulatory scrutiny.

ETIOLOGY OF CANCER PAIN

Pain commonly occurs as a result of direct tumor involvement of bone, nerves, soft tissue, and viscera, especially in patients with cancer of the breast, prostate, lung, or kidney, melanoma, and myeloma. In addition, pain commonly occurs as a result of cancer treatment, such as post-thoracotomy pain, pain from radiation-induced mucositis, or pain accompanying chemotherapy-induced peripheral neuropathy.

TYPES OF CANCER PAIN

I. **Somatic pain and visceral pain** arise from stimulation of **nociceptive afferent nerves** in skin, soft tissue, or bone (somatic pain) or in the viscera (visceral pain), respectively. Somatic pain is often described as **dull or aching** and is well localized, while visceral pain is **poorly localized,** often being referred to dermatomes distant from the source of pain. Examples include bone metastases; liver metastases with capsular distention; biliary, bowel, or ureteral obstruction; and mucositis. Somatic and visceral pain can usually be well controlled with antineoplastic treatment, conventional analgesics (eg, aspirin, acetaminophen, NSAIDs, opiates), or both.

II. **Neuropathic pain,** also referred to as **"deafferentation pain,"** results from injury to peripheral nerves and is described as a **sharp, burning, or shooting pain associated with paresthesias and dysesthesias.** Examples include metastatic brachial plexopathy and dermatomal herpes zoster. Response to conventional analgesics is often poor, but **anticonvulsants and antidepressants** as well as **anesthetic, neurosurgical, and non-drug therapies** may be helpful.

PAIN ASSESSMENT

I. **Doctor–patient relationship.** Successful pain management is enhanced by a strong doctor–patient relationship. Since pain is a subjective phenomenon that cannot be validated by diagnostic tests or procedures, the physician should accept the pain as "real" and convey that sentiment to the patient prior to instituting therapy. Taking time to sit, listen, and reassure the patient will greatly improve the chances for a good analgesic outcome. Placebos should be avoided, as they instill mistrust between doctor and patient, and the results are usually uninterpretable.

II. **Pain history.** It is important to document the quality, location, and duration of the pain and to investigate its effect on activities of daily living such as sleeping, eating, movement, and emotions. Asking patients to quantitate their pain using a verbal or written 0–10 scale is frequently useful.

III. **Analgesic history.** Important aspects of an analgesic history include what drug and non-drug treatments have been attempted, the response to such treatments, and the observed side effects. In additon, the time to maximal effect and duration of analgesia should be documented. Finally, the physician should determine whether analgesics are taken around-the-clock or only for severe pain.

IV. **Diagnostic evaluation.** A complete assessment of pain includes a thorough physical examination and review of pertinent laboratory and radiologic studies to establish the cause of the pain. Common signs and symptoms accompanying acute pain, such as tachycardia, diaphoresis, and facial grimacing, are frequently absent in chronic cancer pain syndromes. Analgesics should be provided as needed to complete the diagnostic evaluation. Re-evaluation of the pain and the patient's response to analgesics must be performed frequently.

ANTINEOPLASTIC TREATMENT

All cancer patients with pain should be evaluated for the potential application of antineoplastic therapy. A decline or total withdrawal of analgesic medication is a common measure of the efficacy of antineoplastic therapy.

   I. **Radiation therapy** is an effective analgesic modality, especially when treating tumor pain at discrete anatomic sites. Partial or total analgesia is achieved in almost 80% of patients following completion of radiation therapy. The analgesic response is generally superior if treatment is begun soon after the onset of pain rather than waiting until severe pain develops. **Common indications** for radiation therapy are:

      A. Painful bone or soft tissue metastases.

      B. Epidural spinal cord compression.

      C. Retroperitoneal adenopathy causing nerve compression.

   II. **Chemotherapy and hormonal therapy.** Usually, antineoplastic drugs are administered as systemic therapy rather than being directed at discrete, localized tumor. A significant antitumor and analgesic response is most likely to be observed in Hodgkin's or non-Hodgkin's lymphoma, leukemia, breast or prostate cancer, germ cell tumors, and small cell lung cancer. Patients with a good performance status (see Appendix A) who have received little or no prior antineoplastic therapy are most likely to experience a good antitumor and analgesic response. The **time to onset of analgesia** depends on the speed of the antitumor effect; times ranging between 3 and 14 days following multi-agent chemotherapy for leukemias and lymphomas to 1–6 weeks following the initiation of hormonal therapy for breast and prostate cancer are typical.

DRUG THERAPY

   I. **General principles.** Analgesic medications are the **mainstay** of cancer pain management. The initial choice of analgesic should be based on the severity of the patient's pain. Oral administration ought to be attempted whenever possible, avoiding intramuscular injections. Furthermore, for continuous pain, medications should be ordered around-the-clock rather than "as needed," and additional medication should be provided for breakthrough pain. Side effects should be anticipated.

   II. **Non-opiate analgesics**

      A. **Aspirin and nonsteroidal anti-inflammatory drugs (NSAIDs)** have analgesic, antipyretic, and anti-inflammatory activity; side effects include gastrointestinal irritation, renal insufficiency, and prolongation of the bleeding time, limiting their usefulness in neutropenic and thrombocytopenic patients. NSAIDs are particularly useful in the treatment of pain from bony metastases and may be synergistic with opiates.

      B. **Acetaminophen** has analgesic and antipyretic activity. **Hepatic toxicity** may occur following ingestion of large doses of the drug and is the dose-limiting factor when prescribing acetaminophen–opiate combination products.

   III. **Opiate analgesics**

      A. **Morphine agonists.** Morphine, hydromorphone, oxymorphone, methadone, levorphanol, oxycodone, codeine, meperidine, fentanyl, and propoxyphene all share a common mechanism of analgesic action. However, they differ in their relative analgesic potency, duration of activity, and amount of absorption following oral administration. Most of the morphine agonists can be interchanged to produce equianalgesia after calculating an equipotent dose. There is no ceiling dose when using a morphine agonist (except codeine or propoxyphene), and there is no standard opiate dose for an individual patient or pain syndrome. Table 7–1 summarizes the equipotent doses of most commonly used opiate compounds.

        1. **Morphine** is the drug of choice for severe cancer pain. **Immediate-release oral or parenteral morphine** has analgesic activity for 3–4 hours, and **sustained-release morphine preparations** produce analgesia for 8–12 hours. Under conditions of chronic opiate use, 30 mg of oral morphine is equipotent to 10 mg of parenteral morphine; 60 mg orally is equipotent to 10 mg of parenteral morphine in patients not receiving chronic opiates.

        2. **Hydromorphone** has a duration of activity of 3–4 hours, and 1.5–2 mg of pa-

TABLE 7–1. EQUIPOTENT DOSES OF OPIATE ANALGESICS

Medication	Parenteral (mg)	Oral (mg)
Morphine	10	60/30[1]
Hydromorphone (Dilaudid)	1.5–2	7.5
Methadone	10	20
Levorphanol (Levo-Dromoran)	2	4
Oxymorphone (Numorphan)	1	10[2]
Oxycodone (Percocet, Percodan, Roxicet, Roxicodone, Roxiprin, Tylox)	—	30
Meperidine (Demerol, Mepergan)	75	300
Codeine	130	200

[1]30 mg of oral morphine is equipotent to 10 mg of parenteral morphine when used chronically.
[2]Rectal preparations only.

renteral or 7.5 mg of oral hydromorphone is equipotent to 10 mg of parenteral morphine.

3. **Methadone** has analgesic activity for 4–6 hours but a **plasma half-life of 1–2 days.** With rapid dose escalation, methadone may accumulate and cause excessive sedation, especially in the elderly or patients with renal or hepatic dysfunction. Methadone's long plasma half-life makes rapid dose adjustments impractical; **dosages should not be increased more frequently than every 2–3 days.** Two milligrams of parenteral or 20 mg of oral methadone is equipotent to 10 mg of parenteral morphine.

4. **Levorphanol** provides analgesic activity for 4–6 hours and has a **plasma half-life of 12–16 hours.** Therefore, it should be used with the **same precautions as for methadone.** Ten milligrams of parenteral or 4 mg of oral levorphanol is equipotent to 10 mg of parenteral morphine.

5. **Oxymorphone** is a short-acting opiate similar to morphine. One milligram of parenteral or 10 mg of rectal oxymorphone is equipotent to 10 mg of parenteral morphine.

6. **Oxycodone** has a 3- to 4-hour duration of activity, and although it is usually administered as a fixed-dose oral product combined with aspirin or acetaminophen, it may also be given alone. Thirty milligrams of oral oxycodone is equipotent to 10 mg of parenteral morphine.

7. **Meperidine** is a **poor choice** for chronic cancer pain. Repeated administration leads to neurotoxicity due to accumulation of the **toxic metabolite normeperidine,** especially in patients with impaired renal function. In addition, meperidine is often administered by the intramuscular route, creating unnecessary pain in patients requiring analgesics over a prolonged period. Seventy-five milligrams of parenteral or 300 mg of oral meperidine is equipotent to 10 mg of parenteral morphine.

8. **Codeine** is substantially less potent than morphine but has a similar duration of activity (3–4 hours). Although it is often administered as a fixed-dose combination product with aspirin or acetaminophen, it also may be given alone. Two hundred milligrams of oral codeine is equipotent to 10 mg of parenteral morphine.

9. **Propoxyphene** is substantially less potent than morphine but has a similar duration of activity (3–4 hours). However, propoxyphene should not be administered on a long-term basis due to accumulation of the **toxic metabolite norpropoxyphene.**

10. **Fentanyl** is a very potent, short-acting opiate available for parenteral or transdermal (patch) administration. The transdermal product provides up to 72 hours of continuous analgesia although after initial administration, steady-state blood levels are not achieved for up to 24 hours. The dose of transdermal drug should not be increased more frequently than every 72 hours. After patch removal, fentanyl will continue to be absorbed into the blood for up to 24 hours.

B. **Morphine agonist-antagonists.** Medications in this class include **pentazocine, nalbuphine,** and **butorphanol.** These drugs **are usually not indicated** for chronic cancer pain management, since they can cause **psychotomimetic effects** following repeated administration and can induce **opiate withdrawal** if administered to a patient receiving a morphine agonist. **Buprenorphine** is an opiate 30 times more potent than morphine and is classified as a partial agonist, although at standard doses (0.3–0.6 mg intramuscularly or intravenously every 6 hours) it has pharmacologic activity similar to that of morphine. Significantly, buprenorphine dissociates from the opiate receptor more slowly than morphine, creating **respiratory depression** that may be difficult to reverse with naloxone.

C. **Routes of administration**

1. **Oral.** The oral route should be utilized whenever possible, since most opiates are now available in both tablet and liquid preparations. Liquid preparations are especially useful for patients with feeding tubes. With this route, drug levels will peak between **30 and 90 minutes** after administration.

2. **Rectal.** Morphine, hydromorphone, and oxymorphone are available for rectal administration. The dose of most opiates administered rectally is equivalent to the oral dose. Rectal administration should be avoided in neutropenic patients, however.

3. **Intravenous.** Opioids given intravenously as boluses have the **most rapid onset of analgesia** but a **greater risk of acute respiratory depression** than orally or rectally administered opiates. The duration of analgesia following a bolus dose of an intravenous opiate is shorter than with oral or rectal administration, and tolerance frequently develops more quickly with intravenous administration.

4. **Subcutaneous.** All parenterally available opiates may be administered subcutaneously. This is a useful route for patients who cannot take oral medication and in whom intravenous access is not feasible or desirable. Dosing of subcutaneous injections or infusions is the same as with intramuscular or intravenous dosing, and the medications may be given as a repeated intermittent bolus or by continuous infusion.

5. **Intramuscular.** This is the **least desirable route** for chronic opiate administration because of **injection-related pain** and **erratic absorption.** Neutropenic and thrombocytopenic patients should not receive any intramuscular injections.

6. **Spinal.** Opioids can be administered into the epidural or intrathecal space through indwelling catheters as either intermittent boluses or continuous infusions. This route of administration may cause a higher incidence of **pruritus** and **urine retention** than with oral or parenteral administration.

7. **Continuous infusion.** Opioids may be given as continuous infusions by the intravenous, subcutaneous, or spinal route. Although any parenteral opiate may be used for intravenous or subcutaneous infusion, morphine or hydromorphone is most commonly chosen. The starting hourly rate of administration is calculated by totaling the current 24-hour opiate dose, converting this to an equipotent dose of the desired opiate, and dividing by 24. For example, a patient receiving 40 mg of oral morphine every 4 hours would begin at 3.3 mg/h of intravenous morphine (40 mg/dose × 6 doses/d × 1 mg intravenous morphine/ 3 mg oral morphine × $\frac{1}{24}$ = 3.3 mg/h). A bolus dose equivalent to the hourly infusion rate is given before starting the infusion and before each dose escalation. The bolus should not exceed 30 mg of morphine and must be administered at a rate not exceeding 2 mg of morphine per minute. Subcutaneous opiate infusions are useful for home pain care. A 25- or 27-gauge butterfly needle changed every 3–7 days may be used. The drug and concentration (mg/mL) should be chosen so that infusions are administered at a rate of less than 2 mL/h.

8. **Transdermal.** This route is a good alternative for patients unable to take oral medication.

D. **Beginning opiate therapy**

1. **Mild pain.** Treatment should be **initiated with nonopiate analgesics** such as acetaminophen, 650 mg every 4 hours, or aspirin, 650 mg every 4 hours. An NSAID such as ibuprofen, 400–800 mg 3–4 times daily, naproxen, 250–500 mg 2–3 times daily, or choline magnesium trisalicylate, 1500 mg twice daily, may also be tried. **If the pain is due to bony metastases, a trial of NSAIDs** rather than acetaminophen is recommended.

2. **Moderate pain.** When acetaminophen, aspirin, and NSAIDs are not adequate, a moderate-strength opiate analgesic such as **codeine** or **oxycodone** can be tried. Although codeine and oxycodone may be prescribed as single preparations, they are commonly given as combination products containing aspirin or

acetaminophen. When given in this formulation, the toxicities of aspirin and acetaminophen are the dose-limiting factors.

3. **Severe pain.**
   a. For severe pain, **short-acting, strong oral opiate analgesics,** either alone or in combination with a nonopiate analgesic, should be used. If other opiates are already in use, begin with an equipotent dose of a strong opiate; otherwise, start at the lower end of the recommended dosage range. **Morphine** is the drug of choice for severe pain and can be administered at a dose of 15–30 mg every 3–4 hours and increased in increments of 25–50% every 8–12 hours until adequate analgesia is obtained. Alternatively, **hydromorphone** may be started at a dose of 2–4 mg every 3–4 hours. Once adequate analgesia is obtained with short-acting preparations, an equipotent dose of a longer-acting drug may be substituted.
   b. Alternatively, severe pain may be treated with **long-acting morphine preparations.** These are available as specially formulated pills and should not be broken or crushed. They can be administered every 8–12 hours and, if necessary, upward dose titration can occur every 24 hours until adequate analgesia is obtained. During this time, patients should receive a supply of a short-acting opiate such as morphine, hydromorphone, or oxycodone to use for breakthrough pain.

E. **Opiate side effects**
   1. **Constipation.** Constipation is best treated by increasing regular exercise, encouraging oral fluid intake, administration of daily stool softeners and bulk-forming agents, and judicious use of laxatives. One bowel movement every other day is a reasonable goal.
   2. **Nausea.** Tolerance to opiate-induced nausea usually develops after repeated administration. If needed, patients should be provided with antiemetics such as prochlorperazine (10–25 mg), haloperidol (1–2 mg), or metoclopramide (10 mg).
   3. **Respiratory difficulties.** Because of the rapid development of tolerance, respiratory depression is an **uncommon problem** in patients receiving chronic opiates, especially by the oral or rectal route. **Risk factors** for respiratory depression include rapid intravenous administration, rapid dose escalation (especially with methadone and levorphanol), and hepatic or renal insufficiency. Significant respiratory depression can be treated in an emergent manner by the prompt administration of 1 ampule of **naloxone** (Narcan) or, if time permits, a single 0.4-mg ampule of naloxone can be diluted in 10 mL of saline and slowly infused until respirations increase but with continued analgesia. Comatose patients should be intubated to prevent **aspiration** from naloxone-induced salivation and bronchospasm. In addition, naloxone may precipitate **seizures** in patients receiving meperidine, and in standard doses, it may not reverse buprenorphine-induced respiratory depression.
   4. **Sedation.** Opiates may cause sedation by direct depression of the central nervous system. With chronic use, most patients develop tolerance to opiate-induced sedation. If sedation becomes a continuing problem, lower doses of shorter-acting drugs given more frequently or a continuous opiate infusion may improve this side effect. In addition, low doses of **amphetamines** such as dextroamphetamine (2.5–5 mg) or methylphenidate (2.5–5 mg) administered early in the day may be used in carefully selected patients with refractory sedation. However, amphetamines must be used cautiously in the elderly and in patients with underlying cardiovascular disease.
   5. **Miscellaneous.** Opiate administration may lead to acute urine retention, orthostatic hypotension, delirium, hallucinations, pruritis, or the syndrome of inappropriate antidiuretic hormone secretion (SIADH).

F. **Opiate tolerance and dependence**
   1. **Tolerance** is a normal response to chronic opiate therapy and **should be anticipated and accepted,** especially in patients receiving intravenous or spinal opiates. However, increasing complaints of pain more often indicate **cancer progression** rather than opiate tolerance. Tolerance is marked by a decrease in the duration of analgesic activity and is best treated by escalating the opiate dose.
   2. **Physical dependence** is defined as the development of opiate withdrawal symptoms when opiates are discontinued or when opiate antagonists are administered. This normal pharmacologic response to chronic opiate therapy should be anticipated in patients who receive opiate antagonists or who are acutely withdrawn from opiates.

3. **Psychological dependence (addiction)** is defined as a behavioral condition characterized by an overwhelming involvement in the acquisition and use of a drug. This occurs very rarely in patients who receive opiates for pain control, and patients and their families should be counseled about this fact.

G. **Regulatory, licensing, and prescribing information.** Opiate analgesics are controlled substances in the United States. Physicians who wish to prescribe, administer, or dispense opiates must register with the **Drug Enforcement Administration (DEA)** and hold a valid state medical license. Regulations vary between states regarding specific limitations on opiate prescriptions including quantity, number of refills, telephone prescriptions, and whether patients receiving chronic opiates must be reported to a state regulatory agency.

IV. **Adjuvant drugs**

A. **Antidepressants.** The most commonly used drug in this class is **amitriptyline.** Doses between 25 and 75 mg are given at bedtime for neuropathic pain syndromes. The analgesic effect appears to be unrelated to the antidepressant effect. Lower doses than those needed for full antidepressant activity are generally effective. Although amitriptyline has been the standard antidepressant prescribed for neuropathic pain, other antidepressants, such as **desipramine** (10–50 mg) and **doxepin** (10–75 mg), may be tried due to advantages in side effect profiles. In general, a trial of an antidepressant is attempted prior to anticonvulsants for control of neuropathic pain.

B. **Anticonvulsants.** Carbamazepine and phenytoin have been used successfully to treat neuropathic pain syndromes. **Carbamazepine** is begun at 100 mg twice daily and slowly increased to 400–800 mg/d; plasma levels are closely monitored. **Phenytoin** is initiated at 3–5 mg/kg/d and escalated according to plasma levels and clinical toxicity.

C. **Corticosteroids** may be administered for pain caused by nerve compression or bony involvement. Positive side effects include **mild euphoria, increased appetite,** and **improved sense of well being.** Dose recommendations are empiric; 4–16 mg of **dexamethasone** or 20–80 mg of **prednisone** per day may be given. The duration and dose of corticosteroid therapy should be kept to a minimum to avoid the serious side effects of **adrenal and immunologic suppression.**

ANESTHETIC AND NEUROSURGICAL PROCEDURES

Patients with pain that is not well controlled by antineoplastic or drug therapy may be candidates for anesthetic or neurosurgical procedures. Neurodestructive procedures, such as surgery, radiofrequency, and neurolytic drugs, are indicated only for very select patients and should not be attempted unless patients have failed all other analgesic modalities.

I. **Trigger point injections.** Intramuscular injections of **saline or a local anesthetic** are used for localized musculoskeletal pain reproduced by direct palpation.

II. **Peripheral nerve blocks** are used for somatic pain syndromes occurring in a limited, discrete anatomic area. Examples include **intercostal nerve blocks** for rib pain or **gasserian ganglion blocks** for craniofacial pain.

III. **Autonomic nerve blocks.** Autonomic nerve blockade may be used to treat localized pain syndromes including mid-upper abdominal pain from pancreatic cancer **(celiac plexus block)** and urogenital pain caused by lumbar plexus metastases **(lumbar plexus block).**

IV. **Spinal infusions and blocks.** Infusions of opiates or local anesthetics (or both) into the epidural or intrathecal space is effective for difficult lower body pain syndromes. Alternatively, neurolytic agents can be infused into the epidural or intrathecal space for more permanent analgesia, but this is associated with a **significant risk of major sensory, motor, and autonomic nerve damage.**

V. **Rhizotomy.** Interruption of a single nerve root is most commonly performed for **craniofacial pain** such as that mediated by metastatic tumor invading the trigeminal or glossopharyngeal nerve.

VI. **Dorsal root entry zone (DREZ) Disruption.** Patients with unilateral neuropathic pain, such as a brachial or lumbar plexopathy, may benefit from **surgical disruption of the spinal cord dorsal root entry zone.**

VII. **Cordotomy.** Patients with lower body somatic pain that is refractory to all other treatments may respond to **unilateral** or **bilateral** cordotomy. This procedure involves disruption of the spinothalamic tract within the spinal cord. It may be accomplished as a percutaneous procedure using radiofrequency or surgically as an open procedure.

VIII. **Chemical hypophysectomy. Alcohol** injected directly into the pituitary gland may provide analgesia for patients with severe, diffuse pain unrelieved by other measures.

IX. **Neurostimulatory approaches.** Peripheral nerve stimulation with **transcutaneous electrical nerve stimulation (TENS)** may be attempted in any patient with focal pain amenable to the application of a stimulating electrode. Direct implantation of stimulating electrodes in peripheral nerves, spinal cord, or brain is rarely used in cancer patients, and only for refractory neuropathic pain syndromes.

BEHAVIORAL TECHNIQUES

Behavioral techniques may be helpful in patients with episodic pain or pain related to specific activities and in patients for whom maintenance of self-control plays an important role in pain management. Specific modalities include biofeedback, hypnosis, guided imagery, relaxation training, and individual or group psychotherapy.

REFERENCES

Appropriate management of pain in primary care practice: Proceedings of a symposium. *Am J Med* 1984;**77**(3A):1.

Cleeland CS: Nonpharmacologic management of cancer pain. *J Pain Symptom Management* 1987;**2**:S23.

Foley KM: Medical progress: The treatment of cancer pain. *N Engl J Med* 1985;**313**:84.

Lipton S: Neurodestructive procedures in the management of cancer pain. *J Pain Symptom Management* 1987;**2**:219.

Payne R, Foley KM (editors): Cancer pain. *Med Clin North Am* 1987;**71**:153.

Portenoy RK: Continuous infusion of opiate drugs in the treatment of cancer pain: Guidelines for use. *J Pain Symptom Management* 1986;**1**:223.

Weissman DE et al: *Handbook of Cancer Pain Management.* Wisconsin Cancer Pain Initiative, 1988.

8 Psychological Care of the Cancer Patient

Fawzy I. Fawzy, MD, and Barbara Natterson, MD

Today, cancer patients live longer and lead more physically active lives than in the past. The overall 5-year survival rate for all cancers now exceeds 50%, with more than 3 million cancer victims living longer than 5 years and many living much longer. As a result, the psychosocial needs of cancer patients have expanded beyond mere help with "death and dying" and now include support with multiple stressors encountered during various phases of the disease. Caring for the emotional and psychological needs of cancer patients and their families remains a critical but often difficult task for the health care team. This chapter gives guidelines for the psychosocial care of cancer patients. In addition, adaptive and maladaptive psychological responses are described that may manifest in each phase of the disease process. Emphasis is placed on recognizing (1) **adaptive psychological symptoms** that should be supported by the physician, (2) **maladaptive psychological manifestations** that may be successfully treated by the primary care physician, and (3) **severe syndromes** that require psychiatric referral.

CANCER PHASES

I. **Prediagnostic phase.** For some patients, even the possibility of cancer may be devastating psychologically by raising a variety of anxieties and concerns, including fear of pain, disfigurement, isolation, and death. Individual responses to the prospect of cancer differ markedly.
   A. **Adaptive responses.** Many patients present with real symptoms and the fear of cancer. These patients should be given calm professional reassurance that the proper tests and treatment will be performed.
   B. **Maladaptive responses**
      1. **Hypervigilance.** Overly vigilant patients interpret any change in body function as a sign of cancer.
      2. **Inappropriate preoccupation.** These individuals spuriously believe that they have cancer despite negative test results and reassurances to the contrary. Patients exhibiting both inappropriate preoccupations and hypervigilance require repeated assurances that they are, in fact, cancer free. However, if their behavior interferes with everyday functioning, psychiatric referral is indicated.
      3. **Spurious symptoms.** Patients who develop symptoms of cancer in the absence of disease require psychiatric referral.
      4. **Denial.** Individuals whose response is one of denial **ignore worrisome symptoms,** resulting in a delay in diagnosis. Patients suffering from excessive denial rarely visit their doctors and, when seen, require strong reassurance that they will receive the best medical care and that prompt diagnosis and treatment affords the best prognosis.

II. **Diagnostic phase.** Once the diagnosis of cancer is confirmed, the physician (ideally, the primary care physician who has an established relationship with the patient and is familiar with the patient's personal coping patterns) must inform the patient. Discussion should be conducted in private, be unhurried and honest, convey realistic hope, and reassure the patient that the physician will continue to stand by him or her. The presence of a supportive family member is helpful and should be encouraged by the physician. Information should be presented at the patient's level of understanding and, if necessary, disclosed during several visits. Frequently, repetition is necessary because anxiety often blocks full comprehension and assimilation of all information. Once the diagnosis has been communicated, the patient may exhibit the following psychological responses.
   A. **Adaptive responses**
      1. **Shock/disbelief.** This common initial response may be so severe that the details of a treatment plan cannot be discussed until a later date. The physician

must be especially supportive at this time, and additional appointments should be scheduled as needed.

2. **Immediate and partial denial.** This is a normal protective mechanism and should not be discouraged.

3. **Anger.** The patient should be encouraged to ventilate any hostility that may be felt toward the physician, family, friends, or a religious deity. It is imperative that the physician not interpret anger as a personal attack.

4. **Anxiety.** Emotional support and reassurance may alleviate much of the expected anxiety and apprehension.

5. **Depression.** A mild depression (sadness-grief) should be expected, but a more severe clinical depression requires intervention.

B. **Maladaptive responses**

1. **Excessive denial.** Persistent denial that interferes with the patient's therapy despite repeated discussions between the patient and the primary care physician requires psychiatric referral.

2. **Despair and depression.** Clinical depression may occur at any time after the diagnosis of cancer. Neurovegetative symptoms (eg, anorexia, anhedonia, sleep disturbance) and psychological symptoms (eg, hopelessness, decreased concentration, excessive guilt) suggest a major depression. In addition, the patient may fatalistically refuse treatment if he or she views death as inevitable. In these cases, early psychiatric referral is essential.

3. **Seeking alternative therapy.** The use of experimental therapies that "may not help but do not hurt" in conjunction with standard medical treatment should not be discouraged. However, when a patient's hunt for "quick cures" interferes with the delivery of conventional therapy, psychiatric consultation should be considered.

III. **Initial treatment phase.** Each of the various cancer treatment modalities provides specific psychological challenges.

A. **Surgery.** Most patients perceive surgery as the therapy with the greatest curative potential. However, because of its invasiveness, it raises many fears as well as expectations.

1. **Adaptive responses**

a. **Fear.** Preoperatively, patients often express fears of surgical pain and death. Anxiety generated by the loss of control and vulnerability that occurs while under anesthesia also is common. Patients must be encouraged to voice their feelings, and any misconceptions should be dispelled by repeated explanations and reassurances.

b. **Grief reactions to changes in body image.** Certain site-specific psychological responses to surgery are common. Mastectomy, for example, commonly interferes with femininity, sexuality, and self-esteem. Similarly, colostomy and genitourinary surgery may adversely affect body image and sexuality. Because of its conspicuous nature, disfiguring head and neck surgery also may be detrimental. A realistic appraisal of the results of disfiguring surgery and reconstructive options (such as plastic surgery and new, less bulky prostheses) should be discussed.

2. **Maladaptive responses**

a. **Avoidance.** Some patients use numerous excuses to postpone or cancel surgery because of excessive fear of surgical procedures. When identified, these patients benefit from psychiatric intervention.

b. **Seeking alternative therapy.** In psychologically predisposed patients, extreme fear and concern may be manifested as a pathologic preoccupation with finding an alternative to surgery. The surgeon and the oncologic team should maintain vigilance for such behavior because timely psychiatric referral may help attenuate the patient's distress, thereby allowing smooth perioperative care.

c. **Postoperative reactive depression.** Postoperative symptoms of depression (see II.B.2, above) are common but, if excessive, may require psychiatric treatment.

d. **Severe, prolonged postoperative grief reaction.** A severe grief reaction that produces symptoms identical to a major depression (see II.B.2, above) requires psychiatric intervention.

B. **Radiation Therapy.** The goal of irradiation (ie, cure, palliation, local tumor control) must be compassionately but clearly explained to the patient.

1. **Adaptive responses**

a. **Fear of machines and side effects.** Anxiety and fear of radiation are common. An explanation of the fundamental principles of radiation therapy helps correct any misconceptions. A detailed discussion of possible side effects and available therapy to control them also helps alleviate the patient's fears.

    b. Fear of abandonment. To alleviate the patient's fear of being abandoned by the primary care physician and of fragmentation of care during this phase of treatment, regular contact with the primary care physician is imperative.

  2. Maladaptive responses. If the fear of radiation therapy is severe, psychotic-like responses, including frank delusions and hallucinations, may occur and compel psychiatric referral. Some patients even refuse therapy.

C. Chemotherapy. At times, the fear of chemotherapy and its side effects may exceed the fear of cancer itself. Clear, accurate information about contemporary chemotherapeutic regimens acts to defuse the horror stories originating from the use of high-dose alkylating agents in the 1950s and 1960s.

  1. Adaptive responses

    a. Anticipatory anxiety. Anticipation as well as the actual experience of chemotherapeutic side effects (eg, nausea, vomiting, alopecia) may lead to anxiety and depression. Relaxation techniques, including hypnosis, biofeedback, and muscle relaxation, increase the patient's psychological participation in chemotherapy and help reduce discomfort. In addition, medications (eg, 0.5 mg of lorazepam 3 times per day) reduce anxiety levels and the memory of unpleasant events.

    b. Changes in body image. Although alopecia is a major concern, careful patient preparation, including clinics that demonstrate head coverings, makeup, and skin care products, markedly reduce the trauma of hair loss.

    c. Altruism. Organ donation (if desired) should be encouraged and applauded because it fosters the feeling that some benefit may arise from a difficult situation.

  2. Maladaptive responses

    a. Delirium/organic brain syndrome. Many chemotherapeutic agents and associated medications produce disorientation, hallucinations, and delusional experiences. This iatrogenic organic brain syndrome may be exacerbated by other medical conditions such as infection, fever, and polypharmacy. Supportive measures (reassurance and full explanation to the patient of what is occurring), dosage reduction, discontinuation of the offending agent, and psychotropic agents (1 mg of haldol, as needed) may be necessary, depending on the severity of symptoms. Psychiatric consultation is advised.

    b. Isolation-induced psychotic disturbance. Many patients with neutropenia are placed in reverse isolation. The decrease or absence of human physical contact may lead to feelings of isolation, depression, or even psychosis. The additional emotional needs of the cancer patient during this period must be addressed to avoid severe disturbances requiring psychiatric consultation.

IV. Recurrence. The psychological stress of recurrent cancer is similar to that encountered at the time of initial diagnosis (see p 40, **II**); however, the situation may be more difficult because of the failure of curative therapy. It is imperative that the changing treatment goals be discussed with the patient and that realistic hope be maintained. The physician must be aware that with each successive treatment plan, the patient may go through this adaptive response cycle several times, each time with more difficulty adjusting to the situation. The patient may cope well the first, second, and even the third time but may eventually require professional help.

V. Terminal phase. Most patients are aware of the irreversible and progressive nature of their disease when it reaches the terminal stage, regardless of whether their situation has been discussed or explained to them. Several particular areas of fear and concern that these patients experience may necessitate early psychiatric referral for supportive psychotherapy and, at times, medication to attenuate the emotional distress.

A. Fear of abandonment. Frequently, patients are concerned that once deemed "terminal," they will lose the care and attention of the health care team. Unfortunately, studies have shown that health care providers often devote significantly less time to terminally ill patients. Steps should be taken to sustain the high level of care, and the patient must be reassured that the physician and health care team will remain committed to continued support. As the patient approaches death, the physician's active and supportive listening facilitates acceptance.

B. Fear of loss of composure and bodily dignity. The physical and mental impairment associated with the dying process generates tremendous fear and anxiety in the cancer patient. Although cancer and its treatment may be dehumanizing, one must remember that the right to die with dignity (of even comatose patients) is important.

C. **Fear of pain.** During the terminal stages of therapy, adequate analgesia is a paramount goal. Some physicians overlook the importance of pain control, confusing compulsory narcotic habituation in cancer patients with recreational addiction in normal individuals (see, also, Chapter 7).

D. **Fear of leaving unfinished business.** These concerns may include both practical and psychological matters and often vary with the developmental stage of a patient's life. Young parents, for example, are consumed with apprehension about their small children, whereas other patients are preoccupied with financial and unresolved family matters.

CARE OF THE FAMILY

Faced with a family member's diagnosis of cancer, families must develop new coping strategies and adapt to new demands. Among other roles, family members suddenly become medical caregivers, psychological supporters, transportation providers, and financial managers. With the significance placed on the cancer patient's care, the psychological needs of other family members may be overlooked. Individual family members respond differently, depending on a variety of factors, including their relationship to the patient, their previous experiences with illness and cancer, and their prior psychological state.

I. **Spouse.** The cancer patient's spouse often hides feelings of helplessness and fear in an effort to appear optimistic and reassuring. In fact, studies suggest that shared involvement in decision making by both patient and spouse results in improved adjustment. Spouse support groups are emerging at many medical centers and are an excellent resource.

II. **Parents.** The death of a child invariably results in a high level of stress on the surviving parents. Because family disintegration, substance abuse, and serious psychopathology are common among parents of a dying patient, early psychiatric referral is recommended even in the absence of overt psychiatric symptoms.

III. **Children.** Preschool and school-age children often act out their emotional distress, which is manifested by school and behavioral problems. Care must be exercised to explain to children at their own level what is happening to their parent. Older children and adolescents often experience role reversal as they become caregivers to their own sick parent. Again, acting out through school and behavioral difficulties may signal profound emotional distress that warrants psychiatric attention.

RESOURCES FOR THE CANCER PATIENT

Once a physician has accepted the responsibility of helping the cancer patient adjust psychologically to the new realities of life and death, a number of resources exist that both the patient and physician can call on.

I. **Self-help groups.** These therapeutic groups, established by experienced cancer patients for newly diagnosed patients, provide the opportunity to express fears and discover how others are coping with cancer.

II. **Other individual cancer patients.** Patients who have previously undergone surgery are an especially good psychosocial resource for patients who are about to experience radical surgery, particularly surgery involving colostomy, laryngectomy, or mastectomy. Through physical survival and attainment of normal function, patients who have undergone a procedure give hope to other patients who are confronting the same or a similar procedure.

III. **Oncology nurses.** These specially trained professionals are invaluable to physicians and patients. They often become deeply involved in their patients' lives and serve as invaluable resources for many community psychosocial organizations.

IV. **Medical social workers.** Social workers are an excellent and frequently underutilized source of support and information for cancer patients and their families. They regularly serve as liaisons between members of the health care team and community-based support groups.

V. **Clergy** can be extremely supportive and helpful to patients and their families.

VI. **Community services.** The American Cancer Society, the Wellness Community, Reach for Recovery, and Vital Options (for young adults, 20–40 years of age) are examples of indispensible community support groups that serve cancer victims.

PRINCIPLES OF CANCER CARE

The following are major rules that physicians should follow in caring for cancer patients:

I. **Rule 1.** Provide the time and the atmosphere for patients and their families to express their feelings and to ask questions throughout the course of the disease.

II. **Rule 2.** Reassure patients that they will not be abandoned and that the best possible medical care, including adequate pain control, will be provided.

III. **Rule 3.** Include patients and their families in all phases of decision making, including treatment planning.

IV. **Rule 4.** Use all available resources to provide emotional support for patients, their families, and the physician.

REFERENCES

Fawzy FI, Fawzy NW: Psychosocial aspects of cancer. In: Nixon D (editor), *Diagnosis and Management of Cancer.* Addison-Wesley, 1982: 111–123.

Fawzy FI et al: Psychosocial management of cancer. *Psychiatric Med* 1983;**1**(2):165.

Holland JC, Rowland JH (editors): *Handbook of Psychooncology: Psychological Care of the Patient with Cancer.* Oxford University Press, 1989.

9 Pulmonary Problems & Emergencies

Jeffrey Miller, MD, and Howard L. Parnes, MD

Cancer patients may develop multiple pulmonary problems that potentially can lead to respiratory failure and death. Common pulmonary complications are discussed below.

AIRWAY OBSTRUCTION

  I. **Etiology.** Airway obstruction in cancer patients is a **rare oncologic emergency** caused by (1) primary tracheal neoplasms, (2) head and neck cancers, (3) bronchogenic carcinoma, or (4) tracheal invasion by esophageal, thyroid, or lung cancer.
 II. **Presentation.** Patients with impending airway obstruction present with **dyspnea, cough,** and **hemoptysis.**
III. **Diagnosis.** Although occasionally normal, **physical examination** often reveals wheezing, stridor, or both, particularly with forced exhalation. **Chest x-ray studies, plain film x-ray studies of the neck, and computed tomography (CT) scan or magnetic resonance imaging (MRI) of the neck** are helpful in defining the cause and site of the obstruction. Generally, **bronchoscopy** is indicated and may be both diagnostic and therapeutic (see **IV,** below).
 IV. **Therapy.** The treatment and prognosis of airway obstruction depend on the site of obstruction, etiology, and stage of the underlying neoplasm. **Treatment options** include tracheostomy (for high lesions), surgical resection (rarely indicated), laser bronchoscopy, phototherapy, external beam irradiation, and brachytherapy (with radioisotope-coated wire). **Adjuvant therapy** consists of antibiotics to eliminate infection and corticosteroids to decrease local inflammation and edema.

HEMOPTYSIS

  I. **Etiology.** Common causes of hemoptysis include the following conditions.
   A. **Infection.** This is the most common cause of hemoptysis and includes **bacterial, mycobacterial, viral,** and **fungal** processes, all of which may be either diffuse (pneumonia) or focal (abscess). Mycobacterial (eg, tuberculosis) and fungal (eg, aspergilloma) infections are associated with massive hemoptysis.
   B. **Inflammation.** Irritation and inflammation due to bronchitis, bronchiectasis, and Goodpasture's syndrome may cause hemoptysis.
   C. **Vascular abnormalities.** A wide variety of vascular abnormalities, such as arteriovenous malformations, pulmonary embolism, and mitral stenosis, may cause hemoptysis.
   D. **Iatrogenic trauma.** This is a frequent cause of hemoptysis. It may result from percutaneous transthoracic needle biopsy of the lung, transbronchial lung biopsy, or surgery.
   E. **Bleeding diatheses.** Coagulation and both quantitative and qualitative platelet abnormalities may be associated with significant hemoptysis.
   F. **Neoplasm.** Bronchogenic carcinoma is a common cause of hemoptysis, particularly in patients more than 40 years of age, and may produce massive hemoptysis. In addition, tracheal and laryngeal cancers may cause hemoptysis.
 II. **Presentation.** Symptoms vary from expectoration of a small amount of blood-tinged sputum to massive bleeding.
III. **Diagnosis.** The diagnosis is confirmed by **microscopic examination and culture of a sputum sample.** In 5% of cases, **massive hemoptysis (> 600 mL of blood in 24 hours)** occurs and is considered a **life-threatening emergency.** To exclude nonmalignant causes, sputum must be examined microscopically for bacteria, acid-fast bacilli, and fungus, and must be cultured. Although the history, symptoms, and chest x-ray findings may suggest the bleeding site, **flexible bronchoscopy** is indicated, and suc-

45

cessfully localizes the bleeding in 85–90% of patients. Rigid bronchoscopy may be necessary in patients with massive hemoptysis.

IV. **Therapy.** Management of the patient with hemoptysis may be divided into nonspecific and specific treatment.
   A. **Nonspecific therapy** includes bed rest, semi-upright positioning, mild sedation, humidified oxygen, intravenous fluids, blood transfusion (as needed), and correction of bleeding diatheses. Because patients with fungal pneumonia and fungal (eg, aspergilloma) cavitary lesions are particularly prone to massive hemoptysis, prophylactic correction of thrombocytopenia and coagulation abnormalities is recommended.
   B. **Specific therapy** includes **bronchoscopic identification of the bleeding site,** if possible, and **airway protection** by placing the ipsilateral thorax in a dependent (lateral decubitus) position to prevent aspiration into the contralateral lung. Massive hemoptysis should be treated by **selective intubation of the normal lung** with either a single- or double-lumen endotracheal tube since massive hemoptysis, if untreated, usually leads to death from asphyxiation, not exsanguination. Definitive therapy involves **surgical resection** of the involved pulmonary segment(s) or lobe(s).

DYSPNEA

I. **Etiology.** The lungs represent the most common site of metastatic cancer. Metastases may occur as pulmonary nodule(s), diffuse lymphatic permeation resulting in interstitial infiltrates **(lymphangitic metastases),** and, rarely, endobronchial lesions. Lymphangitic spread develops from tumor emboli (usually from breast, pancreas, stomach, liver, or prostate cancer) that pass through the pulmonary vessels to fill the perivascular and peribronchial lymphatics, causing fibrosis. Although all 3 forms of metastases may cause shortness of breath, dyspnea is most commonly associated with lymphangitic metastases.

II. **Presentation.** Besides dyspnea, a **nonproductive cough** and **hypoxia** are characteristic.

III. **Diagnosis.** Interstitial pneumonia, chemotherapy-induced lung injury, and pulmonary embolus must be distinguished from lymphangitic pulmonary metastases. **Chest x-rays** usually show varying degrees of bilateral interstitial infiltrates but may be normal. In patients with normal chest x-ray films, further imaging studies may be required to exclude other conditions, such as pulmonary embolus (ventilation-perfusion scan or pulmonary angiogram), or to make the diagnosis (CT scan of the chest). In some patients, **bronchoalveolar lavage, transbronchial biopsy, or open lung biopsy** may be necessary to confirm the diagnosis. **Pulmonary function tests** demonstrate a restrictive ventilatory defect and impaired diffusing capacity.

IV. **Therapy** consists of **oxygen, prednisone,** and **appropriate chemotherapy** directed against the underlying cancer. Although the prognosis varies depending on the underlying malignancy, the **median survival** of patients with lymphangitic metastases is only 1–6 months.

MALIGNANT PLEURAL EFFUSION

I. **Etiology.** Pleural effusions are a common complication in cancer. **Benign effusions** most commonly result from congestive heart failure, hypoalbuminemia, hepatic insufficiency, nephrotic syndrome, or pneumonia. **Malignant effusions may be due to increased capillary permeability from inflammation or damage of the endothelium, or lymphatic obstruction by tumor.**

II. **Presentation.** Patients with pleural effusions commonly present with **dyspnea, cough,** discomfort, and **nonspecific chest pain;** however, 20–25% of patients are **asymptomatic.**

III. **Diagnosis.** It is important to establish the underlying cause of the pleural effusion in order to institute appropriate therapy. A variety of examinations may be helpful in the diagnostic evaluation of patients with pleural effusion.
   A. **Physical examination.** Examination of the chest may reveal characteristic signs of pleural effusions, ie, **distant breath sounds, dullness to percussion,** and **absence of fremitus.** Large effusions may produce a shift of the trachea to the contralateral side.
   B. **Imaging studies.** An **upright posteroanterior chest x-ray** may reveal costophrenic angle blunting (200 mL minimum), and a **lateral decubitus study** may demonstrate a fluid layer (100 mL minimum). **Ultrasonography** may differentiate

between pleural fluid and thickening. **CT scan of the chest** may be required to image small pleural effusions. In addition CT imaging is helpful in delineating pleural anatomy, underlying lung parenchyma, and the mediastinum.

C. **Invasive procedures**
1. **Thoracentesis (diagnostic).** Diagnostic thoracentesis is required to obtain a pleural fluid specimen to determine the cause of the effusion. The specimen should be sent to the laboratory for complete cell count and differential, lactate dehydrogenase level (LDH), protein level, pH, glucose level, gram's stain, bacterial and fungal cultures, mycobacterial (acid-fast) stain and culture, and cytologic examination. Malignant pleural effusions are usually classified as **exudative (total protein > 3.0 g/dL, fluid:serum LDH ratio > 0.6, or fluid:serum protein ratio > 0.5).** Cytologic examination of pleural fluid is critical and verifies the diagnosis in 70–80% of patients with malignant pleural effusion. If it fails to confirm a suspected malignancy, repeat thoracentesis is recommended.
2. **Pleural biopsy.** If multiple cytologic examinations of pleural fluid are nondiagnostic, a pleural biopsy should be performed. A blind needle biopsy of the pleura **increases the diagnostic yield to 90%.** If no diagnosis is made with a blind biopsy, fiberoptic thoracoscopy, with pleural biopsy under direct vision, increases the diagnostic yield to 95%.
3. **Thoracotomy** is rarely necessary.
IV. **Therapy**
A. **Symptomatic treatment**
1. **General.** Routine measures for concomitant reversible airway disease (eg, supplemental oxygen, bronchodilators) should be instituted .
2. **Thoracentesis (therapeutic)** is generally indicated to establish a diagnosis (diagnostic) and may be required to palliate symptoms (therapeutic). Steps should be taken to avoid and treat preventable **complications** such as **bleeding** (correct thrombocytopenia and coagulation defects prior to the procedure), **pneumothorax** (obtain a chest x-ray film before and after the procedure), **vasovagal reaction** (supply adequate physical support) and, **re-expansion pulmonary edema,** a rare complication (remove no more than 1000 mL of fluid at a time).
3. **Tube thoracostomy (chest tube)** is generally indicated for **large or recurrent pleural effusions.** (Loculated effusions may require more than one chest tube.) This procedure should be performed by a surgeon and is usually followed by chemical pleurodosic (coo bclow).
4. **Pleurodesis**
a. **Chemical.** Chemical pleurodesis (sclerosis) may be safely accomplished once the chest tube drainage decreases to less than 200 mL/d. A **sclerosing agent,** such as tetracycline (500–3000 mg/100 mL saline) or bleomycin (60 mg), is sterilely instilled into the thorax. Then the chest tube is clamped, and the patient is placed in 6 positions (supine, prone, left and right lateral decubitus, sitting, and Trendelenburg's) over 2–3 hours (20–30 minutes per position). Subsequently, the chest tube is unclamped and then removed when the drainage falls below 120–150 mL/d. This technique is successful in 50–75% of patients and may be repeated.
b. **Surgical.** Occasionally, **thoracotomy and open mechanical or talc pleurodesis** are required, particularly for difficult loculated effusions. **Pleurectomy** (stripping parietal pleura) is rarely performed because it is associated with significant morbidity (23%) and mortality (9%).
5. **Pleuroperitoneal shunt.** A shunt may be placed from the pleural space to the peritoneal cavity in **patients who have failed pleurodesis.** A one-way pump valve is placed near the middle of the shunt under local anesthesia. This pump valve device allows the patient (or family) to manually empty the pleural cavity. Placement of a pleuroperitoneal shunt is associated with few complications and has a **success rate of 74%.**
B. **Specific treatment.** Once a specific malignancy is diagnosed, effective **antineoplastic therapy** must be instituted. Chemotherapy, radiation therapy and, rarely, surgery are employed, depending on the type of cancer present.

CHEMOTHERAPY-INDUCED LUNG INJURY

I. **Etiology.** Many chemotherapeutic agents cause pulmonary injury (see Appendix D). Frequently the injury is due to chronic pneumonitis with subsequent pulmonary fibrosis, but occasionally it may be caused by a hypersensitivity reaction. The 3 agents associated with the highest risk of inducing a hypersensitivity reaction are **bleomycin,**

mitomycin-C, and **methotrexate.** For bleomycin, an increased risk of lung injury occurs with cumulative doses of more than 450–500 mg. Lower doses may cause pulmonary injury in patients more than 60 years old, with prior or simultaneous radiation therapy to the lung, and patients requiring simultaneous or subsequent oxygen therapy, particularly with an F_{IO_2} of more than 35%.

II. **Presentation.** Clinically, patients complain of **dyspnea, nonproductive cough, fatigue, malaise,** and **low-grade fever** lasting weeks to months.

III. **Diagnosis.** The **physical examination** may be normal or may reveal dry rales or pleural rub. There is no pathognomonic chest x-ray finding, but usually a reticulonodular infiltrate is present either diffusely or at the lung bases. Typically, **pulmonary function tests** demonstrate a decreased diffusing capacity and restrictive ventilatory defect. An **open lung biopsy** may be required to differentiate between chemotherapy-induced lung injury and opportunistic infection, since these two entities are sometimes indistinguishable. **Bronchoalveolar lavage,** a less invasive procedure, is currently considered investigational in this setting.

IV. **Therapy.** The primary treatment for chemotherapy-induced lung injury consists of **stopping the offending agent.** Diffusing capacity measurements before and during treatment, analogous to the use of radionuclide angiography in anthracycline-induced cardiomyopathy (see Chapter 10), has been proposed as a way to avoid clinically apparent lung injury; however, the criteria used in determining toxicity include a combination of clinical, radiographic, and pulmonary function measurements.

RADIATION-INDUCED LUNG INJURY

I. **Etiology.** Radiation-induced lung damage depends on the **volume of lung irradiated and the total radiation dose.** Radiation pneumonitis seldom occurs with doses of less than 2000 cGy but will invariably occur 2–3 months following doses of more than 6000 cGy. **Concomitant chemotherapy** or **steroid withdrawal** (see **IV,** below) during or immediately following radiation therapy, increases the risk of radiation-induced lung damage; however, advanced age and chronic obstructive pulmonary disease do not increase the risk. Almost all symptomatic patients and a few who do not develop acute symptoms subsequently develop progressive pulmonary fibrosis over 6–24 months.

II. **Presentation.** The most common symptoms of radiation pneumonitis are **acute dyspnea, nonproductive cough, fever,** and **leukocytosis.** The patient may have **tachypnea, cyanosis,** and **cor pulmonale** in severe cases.

III. **Diagnosis.** The **physical examination** is usually normal, but occasionally there are moist rales or a pleural friction rub. Although **chest x-ray findings** are variable, a normal chest film is rare. Typically a hazy, "ground-glass" opacification over the irradiated area occurs early, followed by alveolar infiltrates and dense consolidation. **CT scans of the chest** demonstrate abnormalities that conform sharply to the radiation field. **Pulmonary function tests** remain normal until the patient develops clinical evidence of pneumonitis. Subsequently, a restrictive defect develops accompanied by decreased diffusing capacity. Ultimately, **open lung biopsy** may be required to differentiate radiation-induced pneumonitis from lymphangitic metastases and infection.

IV. **Therapy.** The primary goal of treatment is **prevention through radiation dose limitations.** However, if acute radiation-induced pneumonitis develops, **steroids** (prednisone, 1 mg/kg/d for several weeks) are the only therapeutic agents available and are effective only if initiated before fibrosis has developed. Prophylactic use has not proved helpful. After 3–4 weeks, the corticosteroids are slowly tapered to avert a "flare" in pneumonitis.

REFERENCES

Ginsberg SJ, Comis RL: The pulmonary toxicity of antineoplastic agents. *Semin Oncol* 1982;**9**:34.

Rubin P, Casarett GW: *Clinical Radiation Pathology.* Saunders, 1968.

Stover DE: Pulmonary toxicity. In: DeVita VT, Hellman S, Rosenberg SA (editors): *Cancer: Principles and Practice of Oncology,* 3rd ed. Lippincott, 1989:2162–2169.

10 Cardiovascular Problems & Emergencies

Jeffrey Miller, MD, and Howard L. Parnes, MD

PERICARDIAL TAMPONADE

I. **Etiology.** In tamponade, excess pericardial fluid (normal amount = 20–50 mL) interferes with diastolic filling of the heart, leading initially to tachycardia and increased cardiac contractility and eventually to decreased cardiac output and hemodynamic compromise. The quantity of fluid required to cause tamponade varies from less than 200 mL for rapid fluid accumulations to more than 1000 mL for slow fluid collections. Pericardial effusions in cancer patients result from **venous and lymphatic obstruction** secondary to metastatic disease (25–35% of breast and lung cancer patients), **primary pericardial tumors** (sarcoma or mesothelioma), or **direct local tumor extension,** and may precipitate an oncologic emergency.

II. **Presentation.** The symptoms of pericardial effusion/cardiac tamponade depend on the total volume and rate of fluid accumulation as well as underlying cardiac function. Patients may be asymptomatic or complain of **chest pain, dyspnea, anxiety,** and occasionally cough, hoarseness, hiccups, nausea, and abdominal pain.

III. **Diagnosis**

A. **Noninvasive studies.** In the asymptomatic patient, **physical examination** may be normal; however in symptomatic patients, distant heart sounds, increased jugular venous pressure, narrowed arterial pulse pressure, tachycardia, and pulsus paradoxus (> 10 mm Hg drop in systolic blood pressure upon inspiration) are frequently present. **Laboratory tests** generally are not helpful. With fluid accumulations of more than 250 mL, **chest radiograph** may reveal a large, globular cardiac silhouette ("**water bottle**" heart); however, a normal cardiac silhouette does not exclude the possibility of tamponade. **Other radiologic findings** include small unilateral or bilateral pleural effusions, widening of the subcarinal angle, and normal pulmonary vasculature. The **electrocardiogram** often demonstrates sinus tachycardia, nonspecific ST segment and T wave changes, low-voltage QRS complexes, and sometimes QRS electrical alternans. **Two-dimensional echocardiography** represents the most accurate and least invasive method of documenting pericardial effusions and cardiac tamponade. False-positive results are rare but may occur with tumor infiltration or encasement of the heart. **Computed tomography (CT) or magnetic resonance imaging (MRI) of the chest** may be helpful in these instances and may also be useful in further defining the pericardial anatomy.

B. **Invasive studies**

1. **Swan-Ganz right heart catheterization.** Cardiac tamponade is confirmed by **equalization of diastolic pressures** in the right atrium, ventricle, and pulmonary artery. In addition, **rapid, early diastolic elevation of the right atrial pressure to a plateau** that is maintained throughout diastole is highly suggestive of tamponade.

2. **Diagnostic pericardiocentesis.** The precise diagnosis of malignant pericardial effusion requires the demonstration of malignant cells in either the pericardial fluid or tissue. Pericardiocentesis, when performed under ultrasound guidance, is associated with a low complication rate. (Possible complications include arrhythmias, hemorrhage, myocardial or coronary artery laceration, and cardiac arrest.) A pericardial fluid sample should be examined by an experienced cytopathologist for malignant cells, which are identified in 80–90% of patients. Generally, measurement of fluid lactate dehydrogenase (LDH) and protein levels are not helpful, but Gram's and acid-fast stains as well as bacterial and mycobacterial cultures should be performed. Pericardial fluid may be **serous, serosanguineous,** or **hemorrhagic.** Hemorrhagic pericardial fluid

may be distinguished from frank blood resulting from intracardiac aspiration by its ability to form a clear ring around a drop placed on a gauze pad and its inability to form a clot in a red top tube (nonclotting). If the cytopathologic studies are nondiagnostic in a patient with a suspected malignant pericardial effusion, **surgical exploration** may be required for a tissue diagnosis.

IV. **Therapy.** Treatment depends on the histologic type of the malignancy, availability and effectiveness of antitumor therapy, and performance status of the patient (see Appendix A).

A. **Nonspecific treatment.** The following procedures are used in the absence of effective antineoplastic therapy to palliate the symptoms of cardiac tamponade.

1. **Therapeutic pericardiocentesis.** At the time of diagnostic pericardiocentesis, a **pigtail catheter** may be inserted over a needle and left in the pericardial space for 3–5 days. The patient should be given intravenous antibiotics during this period to prevent infection.

2. **Pericardiodesis.** Sclerosis (irritation and subsequent fibrotic obliteration) of the pericardial space with **tetracycline** (500 mg in 25 cc normal saline instilled into a pericardial catheter over 2–3 min) or bleomycin (30 units in 20 cc) until the drainage is less than 1 mL/h. This procedure has no major complications and prevents recurrence for more than 1 month in 75% of patients. **Side effects** include chest pain, fever, and arrhythmias. The chest pain may be ameliorated by the addition of 150 mg of lidocaine (15 mL of 1% solution) to the tetracycline solution.

3. **Surgery.** Failure to establish a definitive diagnosis by cytopathologic examination and to manage symptomatic cardiac tamponade by nonoperative means necessitates one of the following 3 procedures.

a. **Subxiphoid pericardiotomy.** This procedure externally drains the pericardial sac without a thoracotomy and may be accomplished under **local anesthesia.** It is the preferred method of drainage at many centers and has a recurrence rate of 6–12%.

b. **Pericardial window.** This requires thoracotomy (usually left anterolateral) and drains the pericardium into the pleural space. These procedures are associated with a lower complication rate but a higher recurrence rate (5–20%) than pericardiectomy (see below).

c. **Pericardiectomy.** The majority of the pericardium is removed during this procedure, resulting in a very low recurrence rate. However, relatively high morbidity and mortality rates limit its usefulness except for carefully selected patients. Although it is the treatment of choice for **pericardial tamponade secondary to constrictive pericarditis** (see p 51, **IV.B).**

B. **Specific treatment.** Therapy aimed at the underlying malignancy should be promptly instituted, if available.

1. **Chemotherapy.** Systemic therapy with cytotoxic agents may be indicated in patients with **breast cancer, lymphoma,** and **leukemia** but rarely produces immediate relief of tamponade.

2. **Radiotherapy.** Radiation therapy (2000–3000 cGy over 2–3 weeks) is indicated for radiosensitive neoplasms. However, additional measures may be required for immediate palliation of tamponade.

SUPERIOR VENA CAVA SYNDROME

I. **Etiology. Superior vena cava (SVC) syndrome** is a symptom complex that results from partial or complete obstruction of the thin-walled superior vena cava caused by external compression from mediastinal tumor (80–95%), thrombosis (venous access devices) and, less commonly, mediastinal fibrosis or direct tumor invasion. Obstruction leads to **increased venous pressure** in the head, neck, arms, and upper thorax, causing facial and upper extremity edema as well as pleural and pericardial effusions. In severe cases, SVC obstruction represents an oncologic emergency due to **tracheal, laryngeal, and cerebral edema** that results in irreversible brain damage and death. The types of cancer that most commonly cause SVC syndrome are **small cell lung cancer** and **non-Hodgkin's lymphoma.** Hodgkin's disease commonly involves the mediastinum, but rarely causes SVC obstruction.

II. **Presentation.** Patients complain of **positional dyspnea** (worse when supine), **facial and upper extremity swelling,** cough, headache, nausea, dizziness, visual change, hoarseness, and dysphagia.

III. **Diagnosis.** The medical **history** is often suggestive, while **physical examination** may reveal tachypnea, neck vein distention, and facial and upper extremity edema, as well as dilated superficial veins of the abdomen, upper chest, and back (collaterals from chronic obstruction). Conjunctival edema and dilated retinal veins may also be present, while Horner's syndrome, laryngeal stridor, altered mental status, syncope, and seizures rarely develop. **Chest x-ray studies** may demonstrate superior mediastinal widening (64%) or hilar mass (12%). **CT scan of the chest** (with contrast) and **technetium-99m or standard venography** confirm the diagnosis but are not required. The presence of pain in the upper middle back should raise the suspicion of impending spinal cord compression. **Special tests and procedures directed at identifying the underlying malignancy** include sputum cytology, lymph node or bone marrow biopsy, bronchoscopy, percutaneous needle biopsy of masses, mediastinoscopy, and (rarely) thoracotomy.

IV. **Therapy.** Rarely, signs and symptoms of increased intracranial pressure or laryngeal edema necessitate the initiation of specific therapy prior to establishment of a histologic diagnosis; however, this should be avoided if possible, since the resulting tumor fibrosis makes subsequent histologic interpretation difficult or even impossible.

   A. **Nonspecific treatment.** Supportive treatment should be initiated immediately and includes head elevation, oxygen supplementation, corticosteroids (prednisone, 1 mg/kg/d), and judicial use of diuretics. Administration of anticoagulants should be avoided (except with thrombosis due to indwelling venous catheters), since invasive diagnostic procedures are frequently required, as discussed in the preceding section on diagnosis.

   B. **Specific treatment.** Once the histologic diagnosis is known, specific therapy (radiation and/or chemotherapy) directed at the underlying tumor is instituted. **Chemotherapy must be given through lower extremity veins,** since administration in upper extremity vessels is more likely to cause extravasation because of the increased venous pressure. **Palliation is excellent,** but the overall prognosis is determined by the underlying malignancy. Generally, patients with non-Hodgkin's lymphoma do better than those with small cell carcinoma.

RADIATION-INDUCED CARDITIS

I. **Etiology.** The incidence of radiation-induced acute or chronic carditis (pericarditis) increases with the dose of radiation and the volume of heart tissue irradiated. Nearly 5% of patients with Hodgkin's disease who have received more than 4000 cGy of mantle-field irradiation develop radiation-induced pericarditis.

II. **Presentation.** Common presenting complaints are identical to those described for pericardial tamponade (see p 49, **II**). Acute pericarditis usually occurs within 12 months of irradiation but may not appear for several years.

III. **Diagnosis.** The diagnosis is suggested by the characteristic symptoms in a patient who has undergone mediastinal irradiation. Histologic confirmation is not required; however, other processes that may produce a similar clinical picture, such as pericardial tamponade (see p 49, **III**), must be excluded.

IV. **Therapy**

   A. **Acute disease.** Most patients are successfully treated with **nonsteroidal anti-inflammatory drugs (NSAIDs), corticosteroids,** and **antipyretics.**

   B. **Chronic disease.** Chronic pericarditis may be treated symptomatically; however, patients with symptomatic constrictive pericarditis may rarely require **pericardiectomy** (see p 50, **3.c**). Myocarditis infrequently leads to cardiomyopathy or coronary arteritis.

ANTHRACYCLINE-INDUCED CARDIOMYOPATHY

I. **Etiology.** Anthracycline antitumor antibiotics **(doxorubicin and daunorubicin)** cause irreversible cardiomyopathy that is either dose dependent or dose independent.

   A. **Dose-dependent toxicity.** Dose-dependent cardiomyopathy rarely occurs with cumulative doxorubicin doses of less than 450 mg/m^2 but develops in **> 15% of patients receiving more than 600 mg/m^2.** Since it is irreversible, prevention is imperative, and therefore detection of subclinical disease is mandatory (see **IV,** below). **Risk factors** for the development of anthracycline-induced cardiomyopathy include large cumulative doses, concurrent or prior mediastinal irradiation, preexisting heart disease or hypertension, advanced age, and administration of intermittent boluses rather than continuous administration.

   B. **Dose-independent toxicity (arrhythmias).** This rare process is reversible, usually within 24–48 hours after discontinuation of the drug.

II. **Presentation.** Typically, anthracycline toxicity manifests with **symptoms of conges-**

tive heart failure (eg, dyspnea, fatigue), but conduction disturbances, arrhythmias, and myocarditis or pericarditis also occur.

III. **Diagnosis. Monitoring of baseline and sequential cardiac function** is done to detect subclinical cardiomyopathy before overt symptoms develop. **Radionuclide angiography** or **multiple gated acquisition (MUGA)** scans are used most frequently to determine the left ventricular ejection fraction (LVEF) both at rest and after exercise. A **resting LVEF of less than 45% or an increase of less than 5% with exercise indicates significant disease** and mandates discontinuation of anthracyclines or further evaluation with biopsy. **Endomyocardial biopsy is the "gold standard"** for detecting subclinical anthracycline toxicity. Histopathologic grading of anthracycline damage closely correlates with the development of clinical toxicity and may be used to gauge the safety of continued anthracycline therapy.

IV. **Therapy.** No effective therapy exists for established anthracycline cardiomyopathy other than **standard therapy for congestive heart failure;** therefore, recent research has been directed toward the development of **anthracycline analogs** that have similar antitumor efficacy but reduced cardiotoxicity. In addition, clinical trials evaluating **cardioprotective agents, such as ICRF-187,** currently are being conducted.

PARANEOPLASTIC SYNDROMES

Nonbacterial thrombotic endocarditis (NBTE) is characterized by the presence of sterile verrucous fibrin or platelet thrombi on the left-sided heart valves.

I. **Etiology.** NBTE may occur with any malignancy but is most common in **adenocarcinomas** of the lung (7%), prostate (3%), pancreas (3%), ovary, and stomach.

II. **Presentation.** Patients present with signs and symptoms of either **emboli** to the brain (focal or diffuse findings), peripheral vessels, and visceral organs or **bleeding** in the skin, brain, urinary tract, gastrointestinal tract, and respiratory tract. In addition, they may develop acute **peripheral arterial insufficiency.**

III. **Diagnosis.** Although the manifestations of bacterial endocarditis are typically absent and patients are afebrile, **blood cultures** must be obtained to exclude subacute bacterial endocarditis. **Physical examination** identifies a systolic heart murmur in less than 33% of patients. Most valvular lesions are less than 2 mm, and therefore **echocardiography** frequently gives false-negative results. **Cerebral angiography** may demonstrate multiple arterial occlusions, definitively establishing the diagnosis in patients with no other signs of thromboembolism.

IV. **Therapy.** Treatment is **directed primarily at the underlying neoplasm.** Although no data on platelet inhibition exists, success with systemic anticoagulation (heparin and coumadin) in preventing emboli has been anecdotally reported.

REFERENCES

Helms SR, Carlson KM: Cardiovascular emergencies. *Semin Oncol* 1989;**16**(6):463.

Pass H: Treatment of malignant pleural and pericardial effusions. In DeVita VT, Hellman S, Rosenberg SA (editors): *Cancer: Principles and Practice of Oncology,* 3rd ed. Philadelphia: Lippincott, 1989; 2317–2327.

Schwartz RG et al: Congestive heart failure and left ventricular dysfunction complicating doxorubicin therapy: Seven-year experience using radionuclide angiocardiography. *Am J Med* 1978; **65**:823.

Speyer JL: Protective effect of the bispiperayinedione ICRF-187 against doxorubicin-induced cardiac toxicity in women with advanced breast cancer. *N Engl J Med* 1988;**319:**745.

Torti FM, Lum BL: Cardiac toxicity. In DeVita VT, Hellman S, Rosenberg SA (editors): *Cancer: Principles and Practice of Oncology,* 3rd ed. Philadelphia: Lippincott, 1989; 2153–2162.

Yahalom J: Superior vena cava syndrome. In DeVita VT, Hellman S, Rosenberg SA (editors): *Cancer: Principles and Practice of Oncology,* 3rd ed. Philadelphia: Lippincott, 1989; 1971–1977.

11 Neurologic Problems & Emergencies

Patrick Roth, MD, and Stephen Saris, MD

INCREASED INTRACRANIAL PRESSURE

I. **Etiology.** The skull is a closed space containing 3 relatively noncompressible substances: blood, brain, and cerebrospinal fluid (CSF). Intracranial masses (metastases or primary brain tumors) displace a small volume of CSF and blood and, with further growth, produce increased intracranial pressure (ICP). As masses expand, intracranial compliance decreases so that subsequent small increases in mass size result in large ICP elevations and acute neurologic deterioration. In general, slowly expanding neoplasms produce fewer symptoms than rapidly enlarging.

II. **Presentation.** The common signs and symptoms of increased ICP are **headaches, nausea,** and **vomiting;** however, if pressure elevation is diffuse, the patient may be asymptomatic. Pressure gradients between different cranial compartments may develop and produce brain herniation syndromes. **Transtentorial temporal lobe (uncal) herniation** usually compresses the ipsilateral brainstem, causing a depressed level of consciousness, ipsilateral dilated pupil, and contralateral hemiplegia. **Tonsillar herniation** is rare but may compress the brainstem, causing a stiff neck, depressed level of consciousness, and finally death. Shift of the anterior cingulate gyrus under the falx cerebri **(subfalcian herniation)** is often asymptomatic. If **posterior fossa lesions block CSF pathways,** hydrocephalus, expansion of the ventricles, and compression of the brain occur, causing headache and depressed level of consciousness.

III. **Diagnosis.** The diagnosis of increased ICP is suggested by the signs and symptoms listed above and by radiologic findings seen on clinical grounds and **computed tomography (CT) scan (with and without intravenous contrast) or magnetic resonance imaging (MRI).** Demonstration of a mass lesion with compression of adjacent brain and displacement of the midline structures is diagnostic. **Lumbar puncture must not be performed** in any patient with suspected or documented intracranial mass lesion accompanied by a mass effect.

IV. **Therapy.** Treatment of increased ICP varies, depending on the mechanism of pressure elevation.

A. **Increased ICP associated with herniation (severe symptoms)**

1. **Head elevation.** Elevation of the head to 30 degrees provides optimal venous return and decreased arterial pressure.

2. **Hyperventilation.** Intubation and hyperventilation is the most rapid method of lowering the ICP. A 1-mm Hg decrease in the P_{CO_2} will produce a 4% decrease in cerebral blood flow. The effects of hyperventilation persist for 48–72 hours, when renal compensation for the respiratory alkalosis occurs. Theoretically, hyperventilation also shunts blood from normal brain to compressed hypoxic brain, since blood vessels in hypoxic areas remain dilated.

3. **Manipulation of serum osmolarity.** Elevation of serum osmolarity reduces ICP by osmotically diminishing the water content of brain cells. This effect most commonly is achieved with **mannitol** (1 g/kg by intravenous push), which is administered until the serum osmolarity reaches 320 mmol/dL. Above this level, significant toxicity may occur. **Furosemide** (10 mg by intravenous push) may also be used to raise serum osmolarity; it has the advantage of avoiding the transient elevation of cerebral blood flow associated with mannitol.

4. **Surgery.** In the presence of a solitary, easily accessible intracranial neoplastic mass with or without evidence of extracranial disease, surgical resection is usually appropriate if the elevated ICP has been controlled.

B. **Increased ICP without herniation (severe symptoms)**

1. **Corticosteroids. Dexamethasone** (10 mg intravenously every 4 hours) may dramatically improve symptoms of increased ICP.

2. **Whole brain irradiation** (3000 cGy over 2 weeks) is sometimes effective in

palliating symptomatic brain metastases once the elevated ICP has been controlled by medical means.

3. **Anticonvulsants. Phenytoin** (15 mg/kg by intravenous infusion at < 50 mg/min to a maximum of 1 g, followed by 300 mg/d) should be administered in all patients with central nervous system (CNS) malignancies to prevent seizures.

C. **Increased ICP associated with hydrocephalus.** Acute symptomatic hydrocephalus is best treated by **CSF diversion.** Most commonly, a ventricular catheter is either placed to drain externally or is tunneled subcutaneously to drain into the peritoneum.

NEOPLASTIC MENINGITIS

I. **Etiology.** Involvement of the leptomeninges with metastatic tumor is termed "neoplastic meningitis." The tumor usually enters the central nervous system (CNS) through the choroid plexus, and once the tumor has seeded the leptomeninges, widespread dissemination throughout the subarachnoid space frequently occurs. **Adenocarcinomas (breast and lung), melanoma,** and **lymphomas** all have a predilection for metastasis to the leptomeninges.

II. **Presentation.** Signs and symptoms of neoplastic meningitis reflect the characteristic widespread involvement of the CNS, with **hydrocephalus, meningismus, diffuse cortical damage,** or all three frequently present. **Headache** and a **change in mental status** are common, and **cranial nerve abnormalities** (most commonly involving cranial nerves VII, III, V, and VI) develop in up to 95% of patients because of involvement of the basal cisterns. **Pain and weakness** (40%) from spinal root involvement (usually lumbar or sacral) also occurs. The propensity of neoplastic cells to "settle" in dependent portions of the CSF space is thought to be responsible for the high incidence of cranial nerve and spinal root involvement.

III. **Diagnosis.** Initially, a **CT scan (with and without contrast) or MRI** of the brain should be obtained to evaluate the size of the ventricles and to exclude concurrent focal masses prior to lumbar puncture, as well as to demonstrate characteristic meningeal enhancement. Subsequently, the presence of malignant cells in the CSF may be confirmed in 50% of patients with initial **lumbar puncture.** Repeated collections (up to 5) in the remaining patients will detect malignant cells in an additional 30%. Other **nonspecific CSF findings** include decreased glucose levels (classically very low), increased protein levels, and the presence of inflammatory cells, either neutrophils or lymphocytes.

IV. **Therapy.** Because of the characteristic diffuse CNS involvement, optimal treatment is directed toward the entire neuraxis.

A. **Radiation therapy.** Although radiation therapy is effective, the required widespread exposure commonly results in unacceptable myelosuppression.

B. **Chemotherapy.** The most effective agents are **methotrexate** and **cytosine arabinoside** administered intrathecally through a ventricular catheter **(Ommaya reservoir).**

SPINAL CORD COMPRESSION

I. **Etiology.** About 5% of all cancer patients experience symptomatic spinal cord metastases. Spinal metastases occur as a result of (1) local tumor extension from vertebral body metastases (90%), (2) contiguous spread from paraspinal tumors through intravertebral foramens (< 10%), and (3) direct metastasis to the epidural space (< 10%). Common tumors involved include (in order of frequency): lung, colon, breast, prostate, and other genitourinary malignancies. The distribution of spinal metastases (10% cervical, 70% thoracic, and 20% lumbosacral) correlates with the proportion of vertebral body mass in each spinal segment.

II. **Presentation.** The most common presenting symptom of spinal metastases is **subacute, relentless, segmental back pain (90%),** and therefore, back pain must be recognized as a possible early symptom of spinal metastasis in cancer patients. The pain may develop into a **radiculopathy, myelopathy,** or **conus medullaris or cauda equina syndrome.**

III. **Diagnosis.** In the presence of epidural metastases, **plain film x-ray findings** such as bony pedicle erosion, vertebral body collapse, and the presence of a paraspinal soft tissue mass may be identified in 85% of patients; however, only 20% of patients with back pain and abnormal findings on **plain x-ray films** have corresponding epidural disease, particularly in the absence of radiculopathy. In the past, myelography was considered the most sensitive diagnostic examination; however, **MRI with gadolinium** is now the "gold standard" imaging test. Cancer patients with back pain and either abnormalities on plain x-ray studies or radicular pain warrant further evaluation with an MRI scan of the spine.

IV. **Therapy**

   A. **General considerations.** Typically, **therapy is most effective if begun prior to the onset of symptoms,** and in the presence of neurologic deterioration, the degree of neurologic recovery is inversely proportional to the extent of the attendant neurologic deficit. The **goals of treatment are palliation of pain, neurologic improvement, and stabilization.** Although corticosteroids are indicated in nearly all patients, surgery (laminectomy or vertebral body resection), radiation therapy, and chemotherapy should be selectively employed based on tumor location, type, and stage; neurologic status; radiation history; and bony stability.

   B. **Corticosteroids** may alleviate pain and stabilize or improve neurologic deficits through a transient, dose-dependent reduction in vasogenic edema. **Dexamethasone** (10 mg intravenously every 4 hours) is routinely employed in the initial therapy for symptomatic spinal metastases.

   C. **Radiation therapy** may reduce the size of epidural metastases (particularly in patients with radiosensitive tumors such as **lymphoma, neuroblastoma, seminoma,** and **Ewing's sarcoma**) and should be initiated as soon as a firm diagnosis is established. (If the diagnosis is in doubt, a biopsy must be performed.) In general, 4000 cGy is delivered over 21–28 days, but the spinal cord toxicity of high-dose radiation therapy (> 4500 cGy in less than 33 days or fields involving > 10 cm of spinal cord) limits its effectiveness in this area.

   D. **Surgery.** Because multiple retrospective studies have failed to demonstrate significant benefit of decompressive laminectomy followed by radiation therapy over irradiation alone in the treatment of spinal cord compression, **decompressive laminectomy** traditionally has been reserved for (1) radioresistant tumors, (2) symptomatic progression despite optimal radiation therapy, (3) tumor that is located mostly posteriorly or posterolaterally, and most commonly, (4) tumors in fields that were previously maximally irradiated. Recently, **tumor resection, with internal stabilization** if necessary, has been advocated for symptomatic spinal cord metastases. Besides permitting resection of all or most of the tumor, this approach provides a definitive diagnosis. Removal of the tumor is accomplished anterolaterally (transthoracic, transabdominal, or anterocervical approaches) or posterolaterally (costotransversectomy or transverse process osteotomy). As experience with this approach has increased, the associated morbidity and mortality have declined. In one study, 80% of patients were ambulatory after therapy, and more than 50% of previously nonambulatory patients were able to walk after treatment.

LUMBAR AND BRACHIAL PLEXOPATHIES

Metastatic cancer may manifest as neurologic symptoms of brachial or lumbosacral plexopathy.

Brachial Plexopathy

   I. **Etiology.** Brachial plexopathy occurs most frequently with **lung and breast cancer.** Lymphatic metastases to the axillary lymph nodes are usually responsible; however, brachial plexopathy may also result from local extension of upper lobe pulmonary lesions. **Malignant brachial plexopathy** may be confused or coexist with **radiation-induced brachial plexopathy,** since radiation portals used in breast and lung cancer often include the brachial plexus.

  II. **Presentation**

   A. **Malignant brachial plexopathy** presents primarily with **pain,** initially involving the **lower brachial plexus trunk** (C8/T1 dermatome distribution), producing **medial hand and arm pain** as well as **hand weakness.** In addition, a concurrent **Horner's syndrome** from stellate ganglion involvement may be present, and some patients also have epidural spread of tumor.

   B. **Radiation-induced brachial plexopathy** more commonly affects the **upper trunk,** since the lower plexus is shielded by the first rib, and produces **upper lateral arm and shoulder weakness and paresthesias** rather than pain. In addition, **ipsilateral arm lymphedema** due to fibrosis is evident with radiation-induced plexopathy. These changes develop 6–12 months following radiation therapy and occur only with doses of more than 6000 cGy.

 III. **Diagnosis.** The diagnosis may be difficult to confirm. **CT- or MRI-guided fine-needle**

      aspiration of cervical masses may provide the necessary information in the hands of an experienced cytopathologist.

IV. **Therapy**
    A. Radiation therapy is most widely used in the treatment of metastatic lesions to the brachial plexus. However, the results have not been encouraging—only 50% of patients obtain pain relief.
    B. Chemotherapy. Occasionally, chemotherapy may be beneficial in reducing pain in patients with chemotherapy-sensitive tumors.

Lumbosacral Plexopathy

  I. **Etiology.** Lumbosacral plexopathy results from direct extension or metastatic spread of intra-abdominal and pelvic tumors, most commonly **colorectal and gynecologic carcinomas,** as well as **sarcomas.** Direct extension frequently involves the upper lumbosacral plexus (L1–L4), while metastatic spread commonly affects the lower portions (L5–S4).
  II. **Presentation.** Common complaints are **lower extremity pain and weakness,** and physical examination may reveal asymmetric reflexes. Nearly 50% of patients have **concurrent spinal metastases,** usually below the level of the conus. Other findings, such as rectal mass, lower extremity edema, and hydronephrosis, implicate the sacral plexus as the cause of the symptoms. Incontinence is more common with cauda equina lesions.
  III. **Diagnosis.** As with brachial lesions, CT- or MRI-guided fine-needle aspiration of documented lumbosacral masses provides the only alternative to open surgical exploration and biopsy.
  IV. **Therapy**
    A. Radiation therapy is used in the treatment of lumbosacral metastatic lesions, with results similar to those of brachial plexus lesions (see **IV.A,** above).
    B. Chemotherapy. (See Brachial Plexopathy, **IV.B,** above).

RADIATION-INDUCED NEUROPATHY

  I. **Etiology.** Although the CNS is theoretically resistant to radiotherapy-induced toxicity because of the low proliferative rate of neurons, possible deleterious effects limit the amount of radiation that may be given. In general, the maximal radiation dose that may be safely administered to the brain is 6000 cGy over 7 weeks. Although the exact maximum tolerated spinal cord dose is debated, most authorities agree that **large radiation fractions, short treatment times, high total doses,** and **long segments of irradiated spinal cord** are associated with greater toxicity. The toxic effects of cranial irradiation may be **acute (< 2 weeks after radiation),** due to peritumoral edema, or **delayed (> 6–24 months after radiation),** due to death or hyperplasia of radiosensitive endothelial cells, oligodendrocyte damage, or immunologically induced damage, producing multiple focal areas of necrosis, demyelination, mineralization, and vascular proliferation in the subcortical white matter.
  II. **Presentation**
    A. Acute symptoms. Headaches, somnolence, and **increased neurologic deficits** are common findings. In children, a period of subacute somnolence and malaise without focal findings, lasting 2 weeks and resolving spontaneously, may occur 6–8 weeks after the end of therapy. With involvement of the spinal cord, electrical, shooting sensations that travel down the back into the extremities when the neck is flexed **(Lhermitte's sign)** characterize subacute transient myelopathy, which occurs 2–4 months following the end of treatment and resolves over several months.
    B. Delayed symptoms. Delayed symptoms start 6–24 months after the end of treatment and are more serious. Patients may present with a **seizure disorder, focal deficit, or more generalized finding (progressive dementia),** which may mimic tumor recurrence. Neuropsychological testing in children has demonstrated deficiencies in the verbal intelligence quotient (IQ), memory, and a variety of other cognitive functions. These effects occur predominately in younger patients, particularly those aged 2–6 years. About 6–12 months after spinal cord irradiation, some patients develop **progressive transverse myelopathy.** This is manifested by **paresthesias and loss of pain and temperature sensation,** which over 6 months progresses to involve all spinal cord elements.
  III. **Diagnosis.** The diagnosis of radiation-induced neuropathy is largely one of exclusion. The presentation is often similar to recurrent or progressive neoplastic disease. **MRI**

may help to exclude recurrence and document a characteristic diffuse or patchy increase in white matter intensity on T_2-weighted images. Definitive diagnosis requires **histologic examination** of the abnormal brain tissue.

    IV. **Therapy**
        A. **Acute symptoms.** Acutely, edema is controlled with **dexamethasone** (2 mg intravenously every 12 hours) administered throughout the course of radiation therapy.
        B. **Delayed symptoms.** There is no therapy for delayed progressive myelopathy, although temporary remissions following high-dose corticosteroids have been reported.

CHEMOTHERAPY-INDUCED NEUROPATHY

    I. **Etiology.** In patients with chemotherapy-induced neuropathy, the type of neuronal damage depends on the mechanism of action of the specific chemotherapeutic agent (see Appendix B).
    II. **Presentation.** Signs and symptoms of chemotherapy-induced neuropathy are summarized in Appendix C. Specific complications are discussed below.
        A. **Alkylating agents.** The **nitrosoureas,** agents often used at high doses and combined with radiation therapy in the treatment of high-grade gliomas, may produce encephalopathy. **Cisplatin** may produce a predominately sensory peripheral neuropathy with loss of position and vibratory sense. Rarely, **nitrogen mustard** produces confusion, lethargy, personality changes, and seizures that occur several days after therapy and last 2 weeks (acute) or that begin 6 months after therapy and continue for 3 months (delayed).
        B. **Antimetabolites.** When administered in high intravenous doses or intrathecally, **methotrexate** may produce aseptic meningitis that begins within hours of administration and lasts up to 3 days. With intrathecal administration of methotrexate, acute myelopathy may rarely occur within 30 minutes of therapy and last 1–24 months (occasionally permanently). Acute seizures may occur but are transient. Leukoencephalopathy is a chronic problem in patients with (1) acute lymphocytic leukemia receiving high-dose intrathecal methotrexate, (2) brain tumors previously treated with radiation therapy or methotrexate, (3) meningeal carcinomatosis, and (4) osteogenic sarcoma. At high doses, fluorouracil produces acute cerebellar symptoms (ataxia, dysarthria, nystagmus, and hypotonia). Rarely, high doses may cause encephalopathy.
        C. **Vinca alkaloids. Vincristine** and **vinblastine** are limited by neurotoxicity, most commonly a dose-related, reversible axonal neuropathy in which symmetric weakness, pain, sensory findings, and gait disturbances are preceded by loss of deep tendon reflexes (in particular, the ankle jerk). Cranial, spinal, and autonomic nerves may be affected by damage to the axonal transport mechanism.
        D. **Other.** Although **asparaginase** has not been shown to cross the blood-brain barrier, it may cause encephalopathy. Some degree of cerebral dysfunction occurs in 20–60% of patients. Subacute encephalopathy related to asparaginase deficiency has also been described.

PARANEOPLASTIC SYNDROMES

Paraneoplastic syndromes are **symptom complexes that occur as a remote, indirect effect of a tumor or its metastases (or both).** On occasion, these syndromes may be the only presenting complaints, and certain syndromes, such as subacute cerebellar degeneration, subacute motor neuropathy, dermatomyositis, Eaton-Lambert syndrome, and dorsal root ganglionitis, are highly associated with underlying cancers and should trigger a full evaluation for cancer. The pathogenesis of most of the neurologic paraneoplastic syndromes is not fully understood, although in many instances an autoimmune mechanism is suspected. Paraneoplastic syndromes that affect the nervous system fall into the following categories.

Cerebral Syndromes

    I. **Dementia.** This common, albeit nonspecific syndrome is **associated with lung cancer** and presents as variably progressive mental deterioration. A rapid variant, **angioendotheliomatosis,** may be caused by proliferation of endothelial cells in response to tumor-secreted angiogenic factors.
    II. **Limbic encephalomyelitis.** This irreversible inflammatory disorder of gray matter affects the brain, brainstem, spinal cord, and dorsal root ganglia in patients with **lung cancer** or **Hodgkin's disease.** Progressive dementia associated with seizures, cranial nerve dysfunction, depression, and a subacute form of poliomyelitis (progressive motor

loss sparing sensation) marks this disease, which causes death in less than 1 year. The pathologic changes include perivascular lymphocytic infiltration, loss of neurons, and the presence of reactive astrocytes, typically in the mesial temporal lobe, cingulate gyrus, brainstem nuclei, inferior olive, substantia nigra, anterior gray horn cells, and dorsal root ganglia.

III. **Optic neuritis.** This autoimmune phenomenon described in patients with **lung cancer** is characterized by unilateral or bilateral scotomas, papilledema, and decreased visual acuity. Pathologically, demyelination and retinal ganglion cell loss occur.

IV. **Progressive multifocal leukoencephalopathy.** This demyelinating disease is caused by a papovavirus in immunosuppressed patients with **leukemia, lymphoma** and, **most commonly, acquired immunodeficiency syndrome (AIDS).** It is characterized by rapidly progressive dementia, dysarthria, aphasia, ataxia, blindness, and death (within 6 months). It affects multiple areas of the neuraxis.

Cerebellar Syndromes

I. **Subacute cerebellar degeneration.** This syndrome is associated with **lung, colorectal, prostate, ovary,** and **cervical cancer** and is characterized by subacute bilateral ataxia, nystagmus, dysarthria, opsoclonus (rapid and chaotic conjugate eye movements), and dementia. Pathologically there is (1) mild atrophy with loss of Purkinje cells, (2) CSF lymphocytosis, and (3) elevated CSF protein levels. A high correlation with underlying malignancies exists; however, treatment of the underlying cancer has little effect on this syndrome.

II. **Myoclonic encephalopathy.** This syndrome occurs in 2–7% of children less than 2 years of age with neuroblastoma (frequently preceding the diagnosis) and typically presents with acute or subacute irritability, ataxia, polymyoclonus, and opsoclonus in previously healthy children < 2 years of age. Often there is partial remission of the disease when the underlying neuroblastoma is successfully treated, but most children have some residual neurologic deficits.

Spinal Cord Syndromes

I. **Subacute necrotizing myelopathy.** Rapidly progressive upper and lower motor neuron, sensory, and autonomic dysfunction to the thoracic spine characterize this syndrome. Pathologically, necrosis of spinal cord gray and white matter over several levels is observed. Most commonly seen in patients with **lung and kidney cancer,** this syndrome precedes the diagnosis of cancer in 50% of cases.

II. **Subacute motor neuropathy.** This syndrome is associated with **lymphoma** (particularly when lymphoma is treated with radiation therapy) and is distinguished by a slowly progressive isolated lower motor neuron dysfunction manifested as weakness. No known treatment exists, but spontaneous recovery has been reported.

III. **Amyotropic lateral sclerosis (ALS).** This symptom complex, which occurs in 10% of cancer patients, consists of spasticity, muscle wasting, and fasciculation caused by upper and lower motor neuron involvement.

Peripheral Neuropathies

I. **Polyneuropathy.** This mixed motor-sensory neuropathy is the **most common of the paraneoplastic syndromes** and is associated with **lung, gastrointestinal, and breast cancer.** It presents with paresthesias, pain, areflexia, muscle wasting, and distal muscle weakness, which may progress to paralysis. Rarely, it is manifested as neuromyotonia or dysautonomia. Pathologic findings include **elevated CSF protein levels.** The process is generally not affected by treatment of the underlying cancer.

II. **Ascending polyneuropathy (Guillain-Barré syndrome).** This syndrome is associated with **Hodgkin's and non-Hodgkin's lymphomas** and is manifested in a manner similar to that described in patients without cancer, ie, symmetric, ascending distal motor neuropathy.

III. **Sensory neuropathy.** Pure sensory neuropathy is a dorsal root ganglionitis that is strongly associated with **thoracic cancers (lung, laryngeal, and esophageal cancer, lymphoma, thymoma)** and, on occasion, is accompanied by encephalomyelitis. All of the sensory modalities appear to be affected. Patients experience the subacute onset of gait disturbances, paresthesias, extremity pain, loss of deep tendon reflexes, and distal sensory and proprioception loss. Pathologically, an autoimmune disorder caused by an anti-myelin IgM kappa antibody has been proposed. Motor nerve conduction is normal, but CSF protein is elevated. Of all the peripheral neuropathies, sensory neuropathy is the most common in patients with cancer and precedes the diagnosis of cancer in more than 50% of cases.

IV. **Autonomic neuropathy.** Axonal and neuronal degeneration accompanied by lympho-cytic infiltration characterizes this disorder. The syndrome is associated with **small cell lung cancer.** It presents as orthostatic hypotension, neurogenic bladder, altered gas-trointestinal peristalsis, and pseudo-obstruction (Ogilvie's syndrome).

Neuromuscular Disorders

I. **Myasthenia gravis.** This syndrome occurs in 30% of patients with **thymoma;** con-versely, 10–20% of patients with myasthenia gravis harbor thymomas. The hallmark of the disorder is fatigability with exercise and a positive edrophonium or Tensilon test. The ocular, respiratory, axial, and limb muscles all may be affected. Most patients may be adequately treated with **anticholinesterase inhibitors (pyridostigmine [Mestinon]), corticosteroids, immunosuppressants, plasmapheresis, and, if nec-essary, thymectomy.**

II. **Myasthenic (Eaton-Lambert) syndrome.** This syndrome, which is similar to myasthe-nia gravis, affects the neuromuscular junction; however, instead of fatigability with re-petitive exercise, the patient's strength increases and the patient has a negative edrophonium or Tensilon test. Patients with myasthenic syndrome commonly present with proximal muscle weakness (thigh and pelvic girdle), pain and, rarely, ptosis and diplopia. Dysarthria, dysphagia, paresthesias, impotence, and dry mouth are common and suggest a more systemic problem, including the cholinergic autonomic system. This syndrome may develop in up to 6% of patients with **small cell lung cancer,** but it may also occur in patients with other cancers. Diagnosis is assisted by **electromyog-raphy:** amplification of the evoked muscle response is seen when 20–50 Hz of electri-cal stimulation is administered to the motor nerve. The syndrome may improve with treatment of the underlying malignancy, but **guanidine** may also be beneficial.

III. **Polymyositis/dermatomyositis.** Up to 34% of patients with this muscular syndrome (70% of men > 50 years old) have underlying cancer. The myopathy generally presents within 1 year of the diagnosis of cancer. The syndrome is characterized by the gradual onset of proximal muscle weakness and pain. The **erythrocyte sedimentation rate** and **muscle enzyme levels** are usually elevated, and **electromyography** reveals brief, small-amplitude muscle action potentials. **Corticosteroids, azathioprine, plas-mapheresis,** and **radiation therapy** may be beneficial.

REFERENCES

Gilber RW et al: Epidural spinal cord compression from metastatic tumor: Diagnosis and treatment. *Ann Neurol* 1978;**3**:40.

Gilbert MR, Grossman SA: Incidence and nature of neurologic problems in patients with solid tu-mors. *Am J Med* 1986;**81**:951.

Goldwin JW: Radiation myelopathy: A review. *Med Pediatr Oncol* 1987;**15**:89.

Hefner JE, Sahn SA: Controlled hyperventilation in patients with intracranial hypertension. *Arch Intern Med* 1983;**143**:765.

Jaeckle KA et al: The natural history of lumbosacral plexopathy in cancer. *Neurology* 1985;**35**:8.

Kori SH et al: Brachial plexus lesions in patients with cancer: 100 cases. *Neurology* 1981;**31**:45.

Kun LE et al: Quality of life in children treated for brain tumors. *J Neurosurg* 1983;**58**:1.

Little JR: Meningeal carcinomatosis. In Wilkins RH, Rengachary SS (editors): *Neurosurgery.* New York: McGraw-Hill, 1985; 610–612.

Martins AN et al: Delayed radiation necrosis of the brain. *J Neurosurg* 1977;**47**:336.

Siegal T: Surgical decompression of anterior and posterior malignant epidural tumors compressing the spinal cord: A prospective study. *Neurosurgery* 1985;**17**:424.

Wilson KV, Masaryk TJ: Neurologic emergencies in the cancer patient. *Semin Oncol* 1989;**16** (6):490.

12 Urologic Problems & Emergencies

Mark F. Ellison, MD, Leonard Gomella, MD,
and Robert B. Cameron, MD

HEMORRHAGIC CYSTITIS

Hemorrhagic cystitis, which has both benign and malignant causes, may account for a significant degree of morbidity and mortality. A stepwise approach to prevention and management may minimize this complication.

I. **Etiology**
   A. **Chemotherapeutic agents.** Acrolein, a metabolite of the alkylating agents **cyclophosphamide** and **ifosfamide,** may damage the bladder epithelium and result in subsequent angiogenesis. The incidence of hemorrhagic cystitis secondary to use of these alkylating agents ranges from 4–40%, and the mortality, from 4–75%. There is no specific dose or temporal relationship to therapy associated with the development of hemorrhagic cystitis; cases have been reported from 1 month to 8 years after therapy and after only 1 intravenous injection of cyclophosphamide.
   B. **Pelvic radiation therapy** with either external beam or brachytherapy carries a 3–12% risk of hemorrhagic cystitis, which increases to 34% with concomitant cyclophosphamide therapy. Damage to vascular endothelium, resulting in ischemia, tissue necrosis, fibrosis, and the subsequent development of telangiectatic vessels, is responsible. Hemorrhagic cystitis may occur from 3 months to 10 years after radiation exposure. The presence of fluid within the bladder may ameliorate both the acute and late toxic effects of radiation therapy.
   C. **Pelvic cancer.** Primary or recurrent pelvic cancer may present with gross hematuria, which may be classified as hemorrhagic cystitis. **Bladder, prostate, and cervical cancers** are the most common causes of hemorrhagic cystitis in this category. Therapy in this case is directed mainly toward the primary neoplastic disease.
   D. **Infections**
      1. **Bacterial cystitis** is not an uncommon cause of hemorrhagic cystitis (gross hematuria); it usually responds to antimicrobial therapy.
      2. **Adenovirus and BK-type human polyomavirus infections** have been associated with hemorrhagic cystitis, particularly in bone marrow transplant recipients and other immunocompromised patients.
   E. **Coagulopathies.** Coagulation disorders such as **hemophilia** and those resulting from **use of anticoagulants** may cause hemorrhagic cystitis. Correction of the underlying coagulation disorder is usually all that is required.
II. **Presentation.** The patient with hemorrhagic cystitis usually presents with **gross hematuria** with or without antecedent irritative voiding symptoms (frequency, urgency, and dysuria).
III. **Diagnosis.** Initial evaluation involves a **history focusing on risk factors** (see I, above) and **physical examination** (inspection for petechiae or ecchymoses, palpation for distended bladder, and rectal and pelvic examination to exclude recurrent or primary pelvic malignancies). Required **laboratory evaluation** includes urinalysis, urine culture, complete blood count and differential, platelet count, prothrombin time, partial thromboplastin time, blood urea nitrogen (BUN), and creatinine. Intravenous pyelography (IVP) should be obtained to rule out upper urinary tract abnormalities and obstruction.
IV. **Therapy**
   A. **Preventive measures.** For patients receiving cyclophosphamide or ifosfamide, prophylactic measures including **intravenous hydration, forced diuresis,** and **frequent voiding** to minimize exposure to acrolein may be appropriate. **Indwelling urinary catheters** and **continuous bladder irrigation** have also been proposed as preventive measures for high-risk patients. Intravesical administration of **N-acetylcysteine** or **2-mercaptoethane sodium sulfonate (mesna),** which detoxify acrolein, may be used to prevent cyclophosphamide- and ifosfamide-induced cysti-

tis. Mesna has been approved by the FDA and does not interfere with antineoplastic effects, which may occur with N-acetylcysteine. Since mesna is rapidly excreted, timing of its administration relative to administration of the alkating agent is important. Recommendations for use with ifosfamide include an intravenous bolus dose of mesna equal to 20% of the ifosfamide dose given 15 minutes prior to as well as 4 and 8 hours after ifosfamide administration.

B. **Initial management.** The mainstays of initial therapy are **intravenous hydration** (and transfusion, if necessary) to maintain brisk urine output, **correction of coagulopathies,** and **discontinuation of any anticoagulants or antiplatelet drugs and inciting factors** (therapy with cyclophosphamide, ifosfamide, or radiation). If a genitourinary infection is suspected, **empiric antibiotics** should be instituted (usually an aminoglycoside together with ampicillin or a third-generation cephalosporin) until confirmed by culture.

C. **Clot management.** Initially, clots should be evacuated with **bladder irrigation using a large caliber urethral catheter (20–24 F).** This allows the vessels to constrict by emptying the bladder completely and collapsing the bladder walls. A pulsatile technique with a catheter-tipped syringe is recommended. If initial irrigation is successful, **continuous bladder irrigation with sterile saline,** using a 3-way foley catheter to prevent further clot formation, should be started and maintained until the hematuria resolves. However, if all clots cannot be removed, **cystoscopy, using a large-caliber rigid cystoscope,** may be necessary. Cystoscopy requires intravenous administration of a sedative or regional or general anesthesia. **Electrocautery** may be used during this procedure to coagulate any bleeding vessels.

D. **Intravesical agents.** For rare refractory cases, a variety of agents may be instilled into the bladder to arrest hemorrhage. These agents should be used after evacuation of all clots but must not be instilled immediately after bladder biopsy because of the high risk of extravasation and systemic absorption.

1. **Aluminum potassium sulfate (Alum), an astringent that precipitates protein on mucosal surfaces, is mixed as a 1% solution (30 g in 3 L sterile water) and instilled as continuous bladder irrigation** (without anesthesia and regardless of the presence of vesicoureteral reflux). Irrigation should continue until 24 hours after all bleeding has stopped. Even though systemic absorption of the agent is low, **serum aluminum levels** should be monitored, particularly in patients with renal insufficiency.

2. **Silver nitrate ($AgNO_3$).** Use of silver nitrate, a cauterizing agent, requires **regional or general anesthesia.** Silver nitrate, 200 mL of a 1.0–9.5% solution, is instilled under gravity drainage from no higher than 15 cm above the symphysis pubis. The catheter is clamped for 15 minutes and then **continuous bladder irrigation with sterile water** (rather than normal saline, which precipitates silver) is performed for 24–48 hours. Even though silver nitrate has been used for upper urinary tract bleeding, **preinstillation cystography** is required to detect vesicoureteral reflux. If present, reflux may be prevented or minimized by using **ureteral or Fogarty balloon catheters,** positioning the patient in a **marked Fowler (reverse Trendelenberg) position** during instillation, and maintaining **brisk diuresis.** Bleeding usually abates within 24–48 hours, although repeat instillations are occasionally necessary.

3. **Formalin.** Irrigation with a 1–10% formalin (3.7% formaldehyde) solution, which hydrolyzes proteins and coagulates tissues, may be utilized. Caution must be exercised in ordering the solution. A 1–2% solution is generally recommended for initial therapy to avoid the complications of anuria, acute tubular necrosis, ureteral and bladder fibrosis, and ureteral obstruction. As with silver nitrate, **anesthesia** and **preinstallation cystography** to exclude vesicoureteral reflux are required. Reflux may be prevented or minimized by the maneuvers described in **2** above. The formalin solution is instilled under gravity drainage from no higher than 15 cm above the symphysis pubis, using a Foley catheter. The catheter is not clamped but is held at this level for 3–4 minutes, preventing excess pressure and extravasation. Then the bladder is drained and the procedure is repeated for a total contact time of 15 minutes. Finally, irrigation with sterile water is performed and continuous saline irrigation instituted. **Repeat treatment** may be used after 24–48 hours, and the concentration may be increased to 4%. Repeat cystography is required before each retreatment since formalin may induce fibrosis and subsequent vesicoureteral reflux.

4. **Other agents.** Recent advances have been reported with intravesical use of **the prostaglandins F_5-alpha, E_2,** and 0.2% carboprost-tromethamine, a prostaglandin F_2-alpha analog available in the United States for the treatment of

cyclophosphamide-induced hemorrhagic cystitis. These agents may be instilled with no anesthesia and have no side effects. Intravesical administration of amicar is of little benefit.

E. **Miscellaneous modes of therapy. Sodium pentosanpolysulfate (Elmiron)** (administered orally) and **hyperbaric oxygen** have been used successfully for the treatment of radiation-induced hemorrhagic cystitis. Effective use of **hyperthermic saline irrigation, cryosurgery,** and **Helmstein intravesical balloon hydrodistention (internal compression) in combination with the use of a gravity suit (external compression)** have been reported. Oral or intravenous **aminocaproic acid (Amicar),** a synthetic inhibitor of fibrinolysis used for prostate bleeding, may be beneficial if disseminated intravascular coagulation (DIC) has been excluded. **Desmopressin** (DDAVP Injection) is a new agent with potential for the treatment of refractory hemorrhagic cystitis. Desmopressin is a vasopressin analog that increases serum levels of factor VIII and von Willebrand's factor.

F. **Surgery.** Surgical measures employed for refractory, life-threatening hemorrhagic cystitis usually involve **urinary diversion with or without cystectomy.** Diversion of urine by use of bilateral ureteral catheters or percutaneous nephrostomy tubes, by cutaneous ureterostomies, or by creation of an intestinal conduit reduces bleeding. In addition, the bladder may be opened and the mucosa treated directly with phenol or 10% formalin. **Angiographic embolization or surgical ligation of the internal iliac (hypogastric) arteries** may also be performed. In general, cystectomy should be avoided because of the high mortality rate associated with the procedure in this setting.

URETERAL OBSTRUCTION

I. **Etiology.** The causes of ureteral obstruction in cancer patients may be classified as benign or malignant.

A. **Benign obstruction.** Ureteral obstruction from radiation-induced retroperitoneal, bladder, or periureteral fibrosis is usually a late sequelum (up to 13 years after radiation treatment) and occurs in 2–3% of patients with **prostate cancer,** 1–5% of patients with **cervical cancer,** and patients with Hodgkin's disease treated with external beam radiation therapy. Surgery alone may lead to ureteral blockage from either direct injury or scarring. Surgical manipulation and devascularization of the ureter often contribute to subsequent fibrosis.

B. **Malignant obstruction.** Malignant ureteral obstruction may be caused by direct invasion of the ureteral wall or by extrinsic compression by tumor or lymphatic metastases. **Cervical, prostate, urothelial, ovarian, uterine,** and **colorectal cancers** are commonly responsible. Distant metastases from breast cancer and periaortic lymph node enlargement from lymphomas are less frequent causes. Generally, malignant ureteral obstruction is associated with a poor prognosis.

II. **Presentation.** Symptoms attributable to ureteral blockage are present in 50–60% of patients. Symptoms associated with azotemia **(weakness, fatigue, decreased mental status, nausea, vomiting)** and **flank or back pain** are the most common presenting symptoms. Elevated serum creatinine and BUN are often present. Hematuria, pyuria, nonspecific voiding symptoms (frequency, dysuria, incontinence), a palpable abdominal mass, and anuria are less common. Fever may be associated with pyelonephritis and sepsis, and fistulas from ureteral obstruction may lead to incontinence, recurrent infections, and abscesses.

III. **Diagnosis.** Ureteral obstruction may be detected at the time of initial cancer diagnosis, during staging procedures, or during routine follow-up studies. Anuria secondary to urethral obstruction or a neurogenic bladder must be excluded by **bladder catheterization. IVP, computed tomography (CT) scan (with or without intravenous contrast),** and **radionuclide renal scans** are common diagnostic tests. Ultrasonography is preferred because it is noninvasive, is readily available, and avoids possible nephrotoxic contrast agents. If clinically indicated, retrograde or antegrade pyelography may be needed to determine the point of obstruction. (Bone scans may incidentally detect ureteral blockage by asymmetric renal uptake.)

IV. **Therapy**

A. **Indications.** Before instituting therapy for malignant ureteral obstruction, consideration must be given to the **histology and stage of the primary neoplasm, previous and possible future treatment options, presence of symptoms (eg, pain, sepsis), quality of life,** and the **socioeconomic impact of prolonging the patient's life.** In general, if a patient's life may be prolonged with minimal pain, normal mentation, few complications, and a significant time (with good quality of life) outside the hospital, then attempts at urinary diversion are appropriate. If the patient has unilateral, asymptomatic obstruction with a normally functioning contralateral kidney, then intervention is seldom indicated unless renal reserve is required for therapy with potentially nephrotoxic chemotherapeutic agents (eg, cisplatin). Furthermore, if bilateral obstruction exists, urinary diversion is usually performed on only the better functioning kidney (as determined by renal scan, cortical thickness, or contrast studies). In debilitated patients, especially those with intractable pain, senility, or severe unrelated medical disease, nonintervention, allowing progressive azotemia and providing for a relatively comfortable demise, may be appropriate.

B. **Techniques of urinary diversion**
  1. **Cystoscopic stent placement.** Urinary diversion for malignant ureteral obstruction usually may be accomplished by means of endoscopic or percutaneous techniques. Initially, cystoscopic stent placement should be attempted using general or regional anesthesia or intravenous administration of a sedative. (Subsequent stent changes are usually accomplished with local anesthesia.) Placement of retrograde ureteral catheters in the presence of extensive local disease involving the trigone may be very difficult because of inability to locate and cannulate the ureteral orifices. Various methods using guidewires and different catheters are available, including types with stents that have a "*J*" configuration at each end ("double *J*" stents) to prevent migration from the renal pelvis and bladder.
  2. **Percutaneous nephrostomy.** If cystoscopic stent placement fails, percutaneous nephrostomy may be performed under local or general anesthesia using ultrasonic or contrast (retrograde or intravenously administered) guidance. A **simple nephrostomy tube** may be placed, or an **indwelling ureteral stent** may be passed antegrade over a guidewire into the bladder, even if the retrograde approach has previously failed. Combination catheters with both distal (internal) and proximal (external) drainage capabilities are available. Ideally, a percutaneous nephrostomy tube is replaced with an indwelling stent, which is more comfortable for the patient and associated with fewer infections. The nephrostomy tube is clamped for 24–48 hours to assure adequate internal drainage before removal, and the internal stents may subsequently be changed cystoscopically without repeat percutaneous procedures.
  3. **Open surgical nephrostomy** is associated with numerous complications. However, if endoscopic and percutaneous techniques fail, open surgical procedures may be considered. Open procedures include **ureterolysis, cutaneous ureterostomy or nephrostomy, ureteral reimplantation into the bladder, creation of an intestinal conduit,** and **transureteroureterostomy** (normal contralateral ureter). Creation of an intestinal conduit using non-irradiated bowel and ureter is the most reliable and least morbid method of palliation. Ureterosigmoidostomy usually is not feasible because of extensive pelvic malignancy or previous pelvic radiation therapy. Rarely, **nephrectomy** may be necessary for patients with symptomatic obstruction and a poorly functioning kidney that cannot be drained by other methods.

C. **Morbidity and mortality.** The primary complications associated with either cystoscopic or percutaneous placement of ureteral stents are **bleeding, infection,** and **obstruction.** Bleeding is almost always minor and self-limited. Although urinary tract infections should be treated with antibiotics, long-term antibiotics are not indicated, since sterilization is impossible and resistant organisms often develop. **Stent incrustations and obstruction** may occur; stent patency should be monitored by means of serum BUN and creatinine levels and cystography, which normally demonstrates reflux of contrast into the renal pelvis. Stent incrustations and obstruction may be minimized by hydration, treatment of infections, and frequent stent changes (every 2–3 months). **Irritative bladder symptoms** may be managed with antispasmodics (eg, propantheline bromide or oxybutynin chloride). After relief of ureteral obstruction, particularly with a solitary kidney or bilateral obstruction, the patient must be monitored for **postobstructive diuresis** requiring fluid replacement. Finally, long-term indwelling catheters may break, complicating their removal and replacement.

RADIATION NEPHRITIS

I. **Etiology.** Radiation nephritis may develop, depending on the cumulative radiation dose and volume of kidney irradiated. It usually occurs with radiation doses of more than 2000 cGy, and the resulting nephritis is classified as **acute** (occurring 6–12 months following radiation) or **chronic** (occurring more than 12 months following radiation).

    II. Presentation. Although patients are often asymptomatic, symptoms of uremia and renal failure **(fatigue, dyspnea, anorexia, nausea, and vomiting)** may be present.

  III. Diagnosis

    A. Acute radiation nephritis. Physical examination often reveals hypertension, which may be severe. Examination of the urinary sediment is nonspecific, with microscopic hematuria, proteinuria (< 2 g/d) and granular casts typically present.

    B. Chronic radiation nephritis. As in the acute form, physical examination frequently demonstrates severe hypertension. In addition, the urinary sediment is usually described as benign or unremarkable.

  IV. Therapy. Treatment is directed at 2 major complications.

    A. Hypertension. The hypertension may be extremely malignant, requiring prompt aggressive therapy. **Nephrectomy** may be necessary in patients with unilateral disease and uncontrolled hypertension.

    B. Renal failure. Management of this problem is symptomatic, following the standard indications for dialysis. In the acute setting, **corticosteroids** are controversial but may provide some benefit; however, they must be tapered slowly to avoid a "flare" of the nephritis.

PARANEOPLASTIC SYNDROMES

The only true renal paraneoplastic syndrome that has been described is the paraneoplastic **nephrotic syndrome, consisting of proteinuria** (> 3.5 g/1.73 m^2/d), hypoalbuminemia, hyperlipidemia, and edema.

    I. Etiology. Although direct tumor infiltration and amyloidosis may cause nephrotic syndrome, true paraneoplastic nephrotic syndrome is the most common type in cancer patients. It is most frequently associated with **Hodgkin's disease** but is also reported in association with **carcinomas.**

   II. Presentation. Symptoms at presentation are related to the underlying malignancy (eg, type B symptoms in patients with Hodgkin's disease) and to the nephrotic syndrome itself (eg, pitting edema, dyspnea).

  III. Diagnosis. In the appropriate setting, proteinuria (> 3.5 g/1.73 m^2/d) is defined as nephrotic proteinuria. Pitting edema, hypoalbuminemia, hyperlipidemia, or all three may be present. Pleural effusions and ascites may also occur. **Kidney biopsy** demonstrates minimal change disease (80%), glomerulonephritis, focal sclerosis, or membranoproliferative glomerulonephritis (in patients with Hodgkin's disease) or membranous glomerulonephritis (in patients with carcinoma). (Five to ten percent of all patients with membranous glomerulonephritis have cancer.)

  IV. Therapy. The primary therapy for all patients is **treatment of the underlying malignancy.** All other therapeutic intervention is directed at palliation of symptoms.

REFERENCES

Bahrassa F, Federico A: Post-treatment ureteral obstruction of uterine cervix. *Int J Radiat Oncol Biol Phys* 1987;**13**:23.

Donahue JA, Frank IN: Intravesical formalin for hemorrhagic cystitis: Analysis of therapy. *J Urol* 1989;**141**:809.

Eyre RC et al: Management of the urinary tract involved by recurrent cancer. *Arch Surg* 1987;**122**:493.

Levine LA, Richie JP: Urological complications of cyclophosphamide. *J Urol* 1989;**141**:1063.

Parsons CL: Successful management of radiation cystitis with sodium pentosanpolysulfate. *J Urol* 1986;**136**:813.

Orlip SA, Fraley EE: Indications for palliative urinary diversion in patients with cancer. *Urol Clin North Am* 1982;**9**:79.

Weiss JP, Neville EC: Hyperbaric oxygen: Primary treatment of radiation-induced hemorrhagic cystitis. *J Urol* 1989;**142**:43.

Zadra JA et al: Nonoperative urinary diversion for malignant ureteral obstruction. *Cancer* 1987;**60**:1353.

13 Gastrointestinal Problems & Emergencies

Alan T. Lefor, MD

OBSTRUCTION

Obstruction of the gastrointestinal tract is one of the most common complications of intra-abdominal malignancies. The symptoms are similar regardless of the site of obstruction. Treatment varies with the level of the lesion.

Esophageal Obstruction
   I. **Etiology.** Intraluminal growth of a **primary malignancy** and **extrinsic compression** of the esophagus by mediastinal tumors are common causes of esophageal obstruction. Rarely, the esophagus is the site of metastatic disease or of strictures or webs.
  II. **Presentation.** Patients with esophageal obstruction typically relate a history of **progressive dysphagia,** first for solid foods and eventually for liquids as well. In the late stages, patients often report regurgitation of undigested food. Pneumonia due to **chronic aspiration** is not uncommon, and patients often physically sense the exact level of the obstruction.
 III. **Diagnosis.** Workup usually includes **esophagoscopy** and **barium swallow esophagraphy. Biopsy** should be obtained at the time of endoscopic examination, but with mediastinal tumors this usually is not diagnostically helpful.
  IV. **Therapy.** Treatment is symptomatic and depends on the nature of the problem and its location. **Totally obstructing esophageal cancer** may be managed by the placement of a proximal nasoesophageal tube for decompression and fluid resuscitation, followed by esophagectomy, esophageal bypass, dilation, laser therapy, intraluminal intubation, cervical esophagostomy ("spit fistula"), radiation therapy, or chemotherapy (or a combination of these). Gastrostomy to maintain adequate nutrition during therapy may be necessary. **Esophageal compression by an** extrinsic lesion necessitates treatment of the primary problem, either with surgery or by radiation therapy.

Gastric Obstruction
   I. **Etiology.** Gastric outlet obstruction in cancer patients may be caused by benign ulcers. It may also be caused by large gastric tumors or extension of pancreatic tumors.
  II. **Presentation.** The classic symptoms of gastric outlet obstruction are **nausea and vomiting.** The vomitus is described as clear, yellow, nonbilious, or all of these and may occasionally be projectile.
 III. **Diagnosis.** The diagnosis is generally made after obtaining a medical history and is easily confirmed with **barium upper gastrointestinal studies or gastroscopy.** At the time of endoscopy, biopsies and brush cytologic specimens are obtained to confirm the presence of malignancy.
  IV. **Therapy.** Relief of obstruction and maintenance of nutrition are the major goals of therapy for obstruction of the stomach. **Prompt nasogastric decompression and fluid resuscitation** are used to stabilize the patient. Malignant obstruction may occur with local or regional disease, and therefore **curative resection** should always be considered. Inoperable gastric outlet obstruction of any cause may, however, be alleviated with **palliative resection, gastroenterostomy, or gastrostomy.** Feeding jejunostomy may be necessary to maintain nutrition in patients with extensive gastric involvement. Peptic ulcer disease may also cause gastric outlet obstruction in cancer patients. Acutely, H_2 blocking agents may obviate surgery, but an ulcer operation may ultimately be required.

Small Bowel Obstruction

I. **Etiology.** Many cases of small bowel obstruction in patients with cancer are due to intra-abdominal tumor implants, which occur most commonly as a result of gastric, ovarian, pancreatic, and colonic carcinomas. Intra-abdominal tumor implants may also occur in patients with malignant melanoma, sarcomas, and lung cancer. Benign causes of obstruction must also be considered in the differential diagnosis. The most common benign causes are adhesions due to previous operations and hernias, both internal and external. Overall, the rate of occurrence of malignant causes of small bowel obstruction in cancer patients is equal to that of benign causes.

II. **Presentation.** Patients usually present with **nausea** and **intractable bilious vomiting.** The vomitus is sometimes described as "feculent." **Abdominal distention** and **obstipation** complete the clinical picture.

III. **Diagnosis.** Small bowel obstruction is usually a clinical diagnosis. **Plain film x-ray studies of the abdomen** (both supine and upright) and **upright x-ray studies of the chest** are important to confirm the diagnosis and to exclude perforation. Occasionally, an enema with water-soluble contrast is necessary to eliminate the possibility of large bowel obstruction. "Thin" or "dilute" upper GI barium studies are obtained by some physicians, although these are not essential and are frequently nondiagnostic.

IV. **Therapy.** The treatment of **complete small bowel obstruction** always consists of nasogastric decompression and adequate fluid resuscitation followed by prompt surgery. **Partial small bowel obstruction,** however, may initially be treated conservatively utilizing intravenous fluids and nasogastric suction for decompression. A long tube (Cantor or Miller-Abbott) may be useful in patients with partial small bowel obstruction and those with early postoperative obstruction. it is helpful to localize the site of obstruction as early as possible by the judicious use of radiographic studies (contrast studies) and endoscopy. Surgery is reserved for patients who do not respond to decompression and bowel rest. While patients with benign causes of small bowel obstruction usually benefit from surgery, those with malignant causes usually do not achieve long-term survival. Furthermore, surgery in patients with carcinomatosis may be extremely hazardous and is associated with a significant risk of enterocutaneous fistulas.

Colonic Obstruction

I. **Etiology.** In cancer patients, colonic obstruction is usually the result of a primary neoplastic process, although secondary involvement from tumor invasion also occurs.

II. **Presentation.** Signs and symptoms of large bowel obstruction are essentially identical to those of small bowel obstruction. **Abdominal distention, obstipation, nausea,** and **intractable feculent emesis** are characteristic, especially in patients with complete obstruction.

III. **Diagnosis.** In patients with the appropriate symptoms, the diagnosis is commonly made by **plain film x-ray studies of the abdomen** (supine and upright) and **upright chest x-ray studies,** which reveal gas in the proximal colon and evidence of small bowel obstruction. The diagnosis is confirmed by **enema with water-soluble contrast or by endoscopy** (which also permits simultaneous biopsy). The use of barium is contraindicated, since it frequently forms concretions and may cause peritonitis and abscesses if perforation exists.

IV. **Therapy.** Early diagnosis and treatment is critical for prevention of potentially fatal complications such as perforation. Therapy should always include **prompt nasogastric decompression** and **fluid resuscitation** followed by **early surgical decompression.** Except for cecal lesions, which may be treated with primary resection and anastomosis, all lesions require some form of **proximal diverting colostomy (loop or end).** Resection of the primary lesion may be performed simultaneously or at a later date, depending on the patient's condition and the extent of the tumor. In seriously ill patients with left-sided lesions, a **right transverse colostomy** may be easily performed under local anesthesia through a transverse incision that divides the rectus muscle. For right-sided lesions, **cecostomy or end-ileostomy** may be performed.

PERFORATION

Perforation may occur at any point in the gastrointestinal tract and may be caused by either benign or malignant processes. Perforation of the gastrointestinal tract in acutely ill patients almost always leads to immediate surgery. In cancer patients this may be particularly disastrous, since many are receiving chemotherapy, corticosteroids, or both. It is important to remember that immunosuppression resulting from chemotherapy or corticosteroids may significantly mask the usual signs and symptoms of gastrointestinal perforation and the resulting peritonitis.

Esophageal Perforation

I. **Etiology.** Perforations of the esophagus are almost always due to **esophageal carcinoma,** since simple mechanical obstruction produces vomiting that provides a rapid means of decompression. Nonneoplastic causes of esophageal perforation include **foreign bodies** (eg, chicken and fish bones) and **Boerhaave's syndrome** secondary to chemotherapy-induced emesis. **Trauma resulting from diagnostic endoscopy** is another common cause of esophageal perforation.

II. **Presentation.** Patients may present with **neck crepitus, chest pain** due to mediastinitis, **cough** (especially while eating) due to tracheoesophageal fistulas, **abdominal or shoulder pain** (or both) due to subdiaphragmatic infection, **pleural effusions** due to intrapleural rupture, or signs and symptoms of **sepsis.**

III. **Diagnosis.** The diagnosis is most often made based on clinical findings and confirmed by a **chest-x-ray** demonstrating neck and mediastinal air or pleural fluid. The level of perforation may be established by **water-soluble contrast esophagraphy,** unless a tracheoesophageal fistula is suspected, in which case barium should be used.

IV. **Therapy.** In most cases, perforation of the esophagus is a life-threatening emergency. After initial **nasogastric decompression** and **fluid resuscitation,** treatment consists of **surgical closure,** proximal or distal diversion (cervical esophagostomy or "spit fistula" and gastrostomy), or both, as well as any therapy necessary for the primary process, eg, esophagectomy for esophageal carcinoma, removal of a foreign body causing esophageal perforation. **Drainage** is performed using chest and mediastinal tubes, and **broad-spectrum antibiotics** should be instituted immediately. Perforations of the proximal cervical esophagus may occasionally be treated with nasogastric decompression, fluid resuscitation, and broad-spectrum antibiotics; however, such perforations are uncommon.

Gastric Perforation

I. **Etiology.** Perforation of the stomach may be caused by malignant processes (eg, gastric carcinoma and lymphoma, especially after chemotherapy) or by benign diseases or invasive procedures (eg, gastric ulcers and gastroscopy).

II. **Presentation.** Although contained perforations may present with moderate abdominal pain, fever, nausea, and vomiting , most perforations freely communicate with the peritoneum and cause **sudden severe abdominal pain, nausea, vomiting,** and **sepsis** (fever, tachycardia, and hypotension).

III. **Diagnosis.** The **hallmark physical finding** is that of a rigid, "board-like" abdomen. **Laboratory findings** may include hyperamylasemia due to peritoneal resorption of leaking salivary and pancreatic amylase, as well as leukocytosis. Perforation of a hollow viscus is confirmed by demonstration of free air under the diaphragm on **upright chest x-ray** although 20% of patients do not have this finding. Injection of air through a nasogastric tube may increase the percentage of patients with radiographically demonstrated subdiaphragmatic air, but this maneuver, is generally not recommended since it can reopen a sealed perforation. The location of the perforation may be demonstrated on an upper gastrointestinal series using **water-soluble contrast,** but this is not always necessary.

IV. **Therapy.** Treatment is similar to that for any acute gastrointestinal process. Initial therapy consists of **nasogastric decompression** and **fluid resuscitation. Broad-spectrum antibiotics** followed by **prompt surgery** are also instituted early. The perforation is either repaired with an omental patch (Graham closure) or excised, depending on the cause and location. If a peptic ulcer is involved, **vagotomy** and **pyloroplasty** may be indicated.

Small Bowel Perforation

I. **Etiology.** Small bowel perforation may result from peptic ulcer disease (duodenum), cancer, blind intestinal loops created by neoplastic obstruction, adhesions, or surgery.

II. **Presentation.** Common signs and symptoms include **abdominal pain, nausea, vomiting,** and **sepsis** (fever, tachycardia, and hypotension).

III. **Diagnosis.** As with gastric perforations, the **hallmark physical finding** is that of a rigid, "boardlike" abdomen reflecting diffuse peritonitis. **Laboratory examination** may also reveal hyperamylasemia and leukocytosis. An **upright chest x-ray** may demonstrate subdiaphragmatic air in up to 75% of cases. Radiographic contrast studies are generally unrevealing except with peptic ulcer disease of the duodenum.

IV. **Therapy.** Surgery is preceded by **nasogastric decompression, fluid resuscitation,** and **broad-spectrum antibiotics.** For duodenal ulcer diatheses, **closure of the perforation** with an omental patch (Graham closure) is recommended. For most other lesions, **resection** of the involved loop of small bowel with primary anastomosis is the treatment of choice.

Colonic Perforation

I. **Etiology.** Malignancies and diverticulitis are responsible for the majority of colonic perforations, although colonoscopy, toxic megacolon, colitis (ischemic or inflammatory), volvulus, and cecal perforation secondary to distal obstruction are other known causes.

II. **Presentation.** Symptoms of colonic perforation include abdominal pain, nausea, vomiting, and sepsis (fever, tachycardia, and hypotension).

III. **Diagnosis.** As with other gastrointestinal perforations, the **pre-eminent physical finding** is that of a rigid, "boardlike" abdomen reflecting diffuse peritonitis. **Laboratory examination** may reveal leukocytosis. **Upright chest x-ray** demonstrate free air under the diaphragm in a majority of cases. Unless distal obstruction exists, the diagnosis is confirmed and the point of obstruction defined by **water-soluble contrast enema.**

IV. **Therapy.** After initial **nasogastric decompression, fluid resuscitation,** and **broad-spectrum antibiotics, surgery** is performed to resect the perforated segment, if possible. Proximal diverting colostomy or ileostomy should be considered a mandatory part of the procedure since primary anastomosis in this setting is extremely hazardous, although right-sided lesions may be excised and an ileotransverse colostomy created if soilage is minimal. The distal colon may either be closed (Hartmann's procedure) or brought out as a separate mucous fistula. Alternatively, the defect may be exteriorized as a loop colostomy. **Intra-abdominal abscesses following surgical procedures** for colonic perforations are common, and aggressive surgical drainage is frequently required.

HEMORRHAGE

Bleeding may occur anywhere in the gastrointestinal tract and may be due to either benign or malignant conditions. Initial therapy is almost always nonoperative. Coagulation abnormalities and platelet deficiencies are corrected and the hemoglobin level is maintained at or above 10 mg/dL. Surgery is considered only if the bleeding is intractable to medical management. **Common arbitrary guidelines for surgical intervention include bleeding requiring more than 6 units of blood in any 24-hour period or a total of 10 units during the entire episode.** Variations from these guidelines depend on the patient's condition and desires.

Esophageal Hemorrhage

I. **Etiology.** Carcinoma, inflammation (esophagitis), ulcerations or erosions (chemotherapy-induced), mucosal lacerations (Mallory-Weiss syndrome), metaplasia (Barrett's mucosa), and varices all may cause esophageal bleeding.

II. **Presentation.** Esophageal bleeding presents as upper gastrointestinal bleeding and is accompanied by **melena, iron-deficiency anemia** and, if brisk bleeding occurs, **hematemesis** and **hematochezia.**

III. **Diagnosis.** A history of melena or hematemesis suggests upper gastrointestinal blood loss. **Nasogastric lavage of the stomach** will produce an aspirate that contains hemoglobin ("coffee grounds" or frank blood). Subsequently, **esophagogastroduodenoscopy** is required to localize the bleeding and pinpoint the cause. In addition, **endoscopic therapy, including sclerotherapy and electrocautery,** may avert the need for surgery. For cases of massive bleeding, endoscopy may not be possible; in these circumstances, **angiography** may be both diagnostic and therapeutic.

IV. **Therapy.** In addition to standard medical management, **tamponade with Sengstaken-Blakemore or Linton tubes, intravenous or intra-arterial vasopressin infusion** (0.4 units/min), and **endoscopic sclerotherapy** may be tried. Because of high operative morbidity and mortality rates, especially in patients with cirrhosis, surgery should be considered only if aggressive nonoperative therapy fails. When indicated, surgery consists of (1) selective portosystemic shunt (distal splenorenal shunt) or esophageal interruption (Sugiura procedure) for variceal bleeding or (2) esophagectomy for nonvariceal bleeding.

Gastric Hemorrhage

I. **Etiology.** Gastric blood loss may be caused by neoplastic (carcinoma; rarely lymphoma) or nonneoplastic conditions (peptic ulcer disease, gastritis, and erosions).

II. **Presentation.** Usually, gastric hemorrhage presents as acute upper gastrointestinal bleeding accompanied by **melena, iron-deficiency anemia,** and **hematemesis.** Rarely, gastric bleeding may cause hematochezia.

III. **Diagnosis.** If the patient has signs and symptoms suggestive of upper gastrointestinal bleeding, a **nasogastric tube** should be placed and the stomach lavaged with room-temperature saline. In patients with gastric hemorrhage, gross blood or "coffee grounds" material is usually obtained. The nasogastric tube is also used to clear clotted blood and decompress the stomach (the presence of blood and gastric distention promotes bleeding). Next, **esophagogastroduodenoscopy** is required to localize and diagnose the source of bleeding. With massive bleeding, **angiography** may be required for localization.

IV. **Therapy.** In most cases, initial treatment consists of **conservative medical management,** including gastric lavage with room-temperature saline to evacuate existing clot, correction of coagulation and platelet abnormalities, and red cell transfusions. If these conservative measures fail, **intravenous infusions of vasopressin, therapeutic endoscopy** (eg, sclerotherapy, electrocautery), and **angiography** may be attempted. **Surgery** is reserved for patients who do not respond to these more conservative measures. Massive bleeding refractory to medical therapy requires surgical intervention. At the time of surgery, benign bleeding ulcers may be oversewn or excised, but malignant sites of bleeding should be excised if possible, even if subtotal gastrectomy is required.

Small Bowel Hemorrhage

I. **Etiology.** Usually, small bowel bleeding originates in the duodenum and is caused by peptic ulcer disease. However, primary small bowel tumors, small bowel metastases, ischemia, and aortoenteric fistulas also may cause gastrointestinal bleeding.

II. **Presentation.** The presentation depends on the site and rate of bleeding. Proximal sites and slow oozing produce **signs and symptoms of upper gastrointestinal bleeding** (melena, iron-deficiency anemia and, with rapid proximal sites, hematemesis), while distal and more rapid hemorrhage presents with **signs and symptoms of lower gastrointestinal bleeding** (hematochezia and iron-deficiency anemia).

III. **Diagnosis.** With the exception of duodenal bleeding, which is easily diagnosed with upper gastrointestinal **endoscopy,** the diagnosis of small bowel bleeding is difficult and imprecise. **Aspiration of gastric contents** may or may not reveal blood, depending on the site. If bleeding is brisk, **angiography** should be performed. **Radiolabeled red blood cell scans** are useful for slower intermittent blood loss.

IV. **Therapy.** Initial therapy involves **conservative medical management.** If this fails and the bleeding has been localized, **surgery** is indicated. Resection or oversewing of duodenal ulcers is usually curative. In addition, the enterotomy is frequently incorporated into a pyloroplasty which, together with a truncal vagotomy, treats the underlying ulcer diathesis. For nonduodenal sites, resection of the involved bowel is simple and curative. If complete excision is not technically feasible, partial excision with fulguration of the remaining bowel to prevent mucocele formation generally may be accomplished.

Colonic Hemorrhage

I. **Etiology.** Although colon cancer frequently causes bleeding, massive hemorrhage due to cancer is unusual. Diverticulosis, angiodysplasia, and inflammatory bowel disease more commonly produce massive lower gastrointestinal bleeding. Hemorrhoids, fissures, perirectal abscesses, polyps, ischemia, and colitis are other disorders associated with colorectal bleeding.

II. **Presentation.** Typically, lower gastrointestinal bleeding presents with **hematochezia,** which is described as either red or purple in hue. **Abdominal pain** is uncommon but may occur because of hyperperistalsis.

III. **Diagnosis.** After an appropriate **history** has been obtained, a simple **rectal examination** usually confirms either gross blood or guaiac-positive fecal matter in the rectal vault. Although contrast studies are occasionally helpful in the diagnosis of underlying diseases, **colonoscopy** is the gold standard for locating the source of colorectal bleeding and confirming the diagnosis (by obtaining a biopsy, if appropriate). If endoscopy is inadequate because of brisk or intermittent bleeding, **angiography or radiolabeled red blood cell scans,** respectively, may be required.

IV. **Therapy.** In the majority of patients, **conservative medical therapy** arrests the bleeding. However, prompt surgical intervention is required if conservative measures fail. Generally, **partial colectomy** is curative, although if diffuse bleeding exists or if the exact site of bleeding is unknown, a **subtotal colectomy** may be necessary.

Hemorrhage From Other Sites
Intrahepatic and intrasplenic hemorrhage may occur secondary to coexisting lesions, such as splenic artery aneurysms and hepatic cysts. Because these entities are rare, they are only mentioned here.

FISTULAS

I. **Etiology.** Fistulas are connections between 2 epithelial surfaces. Gastrointestinal fistulas are generally caused by **malignancies, infection, inflammatory diseases, or surgery.** Connections that may develop include enteroenteric, enterocolic, gastrocolic, enterocutaneous, colocutaneous, biliary-enteric, colovesical, tracheoesophageal, and aortoenteric fistulas.

II. **Presentation.** The signs and symptoms vary, depending on the type and location of the fistula. Sudden coughing while eating and recurrent pneumonia are characteristic of tracheoesophageal fistulas, while sentinel upper gastrointestinal bleeding characterizes aortoenteric fistulas. Pneumaturia and chronic urinary tract infections are associated with colovesical fistulas, and chronic diarrhea is seen with gastrocolic fistulas. Rectovaginal fistulas lead to vaginal discharge, while entero- and colocutaneous fistulas commonly produce feculent drainage, frequently from wounds. Enteroenteric and enterocolic fistulas may, however, be asymptomatic.

III. **Diagnosis.** The most important aspect in the diagnosis is clinical suspicion. Once a fistula is suspected, a simple **radiographic study** using **water-soluble contrast** may be obtained to confirm the presence or absence of a fistula (with tracheoesophageal fistulas, however, **barium contrast** is required). In addition, **cystoscopy** is occasionally necessary to demonstrate colovesical fistulas. Some fistulas cannot be imaged by any study.

IV. **Therapy.** The basic principle in the treatment of fistulas is **proximal diversion** of the gastrointestinal tract. This allows the fistula to close unless a **secondary factor** is present. "FRIEND" (**F**oreign body, **R**adiation, **I**nfection, **E**pithelialization, **N**eoplasm, **D**istal obstruction) is useful for remembering these secondary causes. If a fistula, regardless of the site, persists because of one of these factors, surgery is required to separate the two epithelial surfaces, resect abnormal or damaged tissue, and interpose normal tissue. Because of the inflammation associated with fistulas, the surgical procedure is often difficult and therefore should not be undertaken without careful planning.

ASCITES

I. **Etiology.** Malignant ascites usually results from obstruction of the subdiaphragmatic lymphatic channels; however, in some cases, tumor cell secretion and portal hypertension secondary to advanced hepatic metastatic disease, cirrhosis, or the Budd-Chiari syndrome contribute to the accumulation of fluid.

II. **Presentation.** Ascites typically presents with abdominal distention, anorexia, early satiety, difficulty breathing and ambulating, and fatigue.

III. **Diagnosis.** The presence of ascites is a clinical diagnosis. **Abdominal distention, dullness to percussion,** and a **fluid wave** are sufficient to diagnose ascites. In addition, **abdominal x-ray studies** reveal a "ground glass" appearance. **Abdominal ultrasonography or computed tomography (CT) scan** may be used to confirm the diagnosis, especially if small amounts or loculated fluid is suspected. **Paracentesis** produces fluid with elevated concentrations of total protein (> 40% of serum) and lactate dehydrogenase (> 100% of serum), elevated red blood cell (> 10,000/μL) and white blood cell (> 1000/μL) counts, and in some circumstances, elevated tumor markers (eg, carcinoembryonic antigen, alpha-fetoprotein).

IV. **Therapy**
   A. **Medical therapy.** Although malignant ascites is frequently refractory to medical management, conservative therapy (bed rest, dietary sodium restriction, and loop and aldosterone-inhibiting diuretics such as furosemide or spironolactone at high doses) should be tried.
   B. **Paracentesis.** Repeated paracentesis may be used as a temporizing maneuver; however, the incidence of complications (eg, bleeding, peritonitis, bowel perforation, ascitic leak) is significant, and patient discomfort leads to low acceptance of this procedure.
   C. **Local antineoplastic therapy.** Intraperitoneal chemotherapy, irradiation, and im-

munotherapy have all been attempted without success and currently are not recommended.

D. **Peritoneovenous shunt.** Since 1975, shunts have been used to connect the peritoneal cavity with the vascular system (superior vena cava) for drainage of malignant ascites. A one-way valve, either a disc valve (LeVeen) or a flap valve in a compressible casing to allow manual flushing (Denver), is utilized to allow only unidirectional flow of fluid.

   1. **Contraindications.** A peritoneal shunt may be placed in any patient who has failed medical therapy and do not have one of the following contraindications to shunt placement.
      a. Positive peritoneal cultures.
      b. Coagulopathy.
      c. Thrombocytopenia.
      d. Jaundice (bilirubin > 6 mg/dL).
      e. Congestive heart failure.
      f. Poor medical health.
      g. Short life expectancy (< 4 weeks).
      h. Thick, bloody, or loculated ascites.

   2. **Monitoring.** After shunt placement, central venous pressure, urine output, coagulation time, platelet count, fibrin degradation products, and daily weight must be monitored closely. An increase in fibrin degradation products (caused by delivery of proteinaceous material to the vascular system) is to be expected and indicates good shunt function. Shunt function may also be evaluated with manual compression of the pump (Denver shunt), Doppler studies, or technetium-99m sulfur colloid studies.

   3. **Complications.** While results of peritoneal shunting have generally been favorable, problems may arise. **Occlusion** occurs in 10–50% of patients within 8 weeks. However, pulmonary edema, disseminated intravascular coagulation (DIC), superior vena cava thrombosis, pulmonary embolism, gastrointestinal bleeding from esophageal varices, ascitic leak, and infection—all common after shunt placement in cirrhotic patients—are rare in the treatment of malignant ascites. Tumor dissemination as a result of peritoneal shunts, although theoretically a potential catastrophe, has been shown by autopsy studies to be extremely uncommon.

CHEMOTHERAPY-INDUCED HEPATIC INJURY

Since the liver is the site of metabolism for many drugs, it is not surprising that liver injury may be caused by administration of chemotherapeutic agents. While the spectrum of possible liver injury ranges from mild elevation of liver function tests to fulminant hepatic necrosis, liver damage is a rare complication of chemotherapy.

   I. **Etiology.** A number of chemotherapeutic agents may cause hepatic injury. **Nitrosoureas** (carmustine [BCNU], lomustine [CCNU]) commonly cause transient elevations of serum liver enzymes, alkaline phosphatase, and bilirubin. **Antimetabolites** may lead to cirrhosis, fatty infiltration, hepatitis (methotrexate), or hepatic necrosis (mercaptopurine). **Asparaginase** has been associated with bleeding diatheses caused by altered production of the liver-dependent clotting factors II, VII, IX and X.

  II. **Presentation.** Hepatic injury, if detected early, is usually asymptomatic. Severe injury may be accompanied by **jaundice, right upper quadrant pain** from liver swelling and capsular distention, **anorexia,** and **unusual bleeding.**

 III. **Diagnosis.** Elevations of serum liver enzymes, alkaline phosphatase, bilirubin, and coagulation times in a patient being treated with a potentially toxic chemotherapeutic agent suggests the diagnosis.

  IV. **Therapy.** No specific therapy exists other than to decrease the dose or entirely discontinue administration of the offending chemotherapeutic agent. The decision must be made in light of the degree of hepatic injury and the potential benefits of continued chemotherapy.

RADIATION ENTERITIS

Radiation therapy is used in the treatment of several types of cancer, including cervical, uterine, rectal, ovary, and bladder. Following the standard doses of 4000–6000 cGy, severe gastrointestinal symptoms develop in 2–5% of patients. Although most patients respond well to nonoperative management, up to 40% ultimately require surgery as a direct consequence of radiation therapy. Radiation enteritis may be classified as **acute** or **chronic.**

I. **Etiology.** The pathophysiology of radiation-induced bowel injury is complex and not well understood. Intestinal injury is potentiated by preexisting mesenteric vascular disease and the concomitant administration of chemotherapy. Small bowel is most sensitive to radiation injury, followed by stomach, esophagus, colon, and rectum. Acute injury from the direct toxic effects of radiation on the rapidly dividing epithelial cells usually occurs within a few weeks (after about 4000 cGy). Chronic radiation damage is manifested from 6 months to 20 years following irradiation. Radiation injury appears to be a progressive disease, and the final result depends on tissue sensitivity to radiation, blood supply, mobility, and the scarring that results from the acute injury.

II. **Presentation.** Symptoms of acute radiation enteritis may include **anorexia, diarrhea, nausea, vomiting, crampy abdominal pain,** and **bleeding.** These symptoms usually regress within a few weeks as the bowel heals. The sequelae of chronic injury include obstruction, perforation, abscess formation, fistulization, and even neoplasia.

III. **Diagnosis.** The diagnosis of radiation-induced gastrointestinal injury remains a clinical finding and one of exclusion. Ischemia, obstruction, strangulation, and infection must all be excluded before a diagnosis of radiation enteritis can be made with confidence.

IV. **Therapy.** Therapy for radiation injury generally is nonoperative; however, some patients require operative intervention for certain complications.

    A. **Medical management.** Nonoperative management is usually directed at the relief of symptoms. **Antispasmodics, anticholinergics,** and **opiates** may provide some relief. A low-residue, low-fat, lactose-free diet may also relieve symptoms. By decreasing inflammation, **sulfasalazine** (40–60 mg/kg daily in 3–6 divided doses) has proved beneficial for selected patients. **Steroid enemas** have proved advantageous in patients with proctitis.

    B. **Surgical management.** Although general indications for operation and specific surgical procedures are the same whether or not the gastrointestinal injury resulted from irradiation surgical options must be carefully considered since the postoperative morbidity and ability to heal are strongly affected by previous irradiation. Specifically, the choice between resection, bypass, and diversion is much more complex. While resection and primary anastomosis is occasionally indicated for patients with a single discrete area of radiation injury, the majority of patients have generalized damage requiring bypass rather than resection. The treatment of fistulas is particularly complex. Fistulas resulting from radiation-induced injury rarely close spontaneously, and bypass of the involved segment yields better results than resection. Finally, perforation is best treated by exteriorization of the affected segment, avoiding primary anastomosis.

V. **Prevention.** A number of new approaches are being devised to decrease the incidence of radiation-induced complications. These include (1) **use of absorbable mesh to exclude small bowel from the pelvis** when postoperative irradiation is planned and (2) **increased use of intraoperative radiation therapy (IORT),** which theoretically leads to fewer complications, although recent studies indicate a complication rate similar to that for conventional radiation therapy.

TYPHLITIS

I. **Etiology.** Typhlitis is inflammation of the cecum. The cause of typhlitis is unknown, although the most common underlying diagnosis in these patients is leukemia.

II. **Presentation.** Patients commonly complain of **fever, abdominal pain,** and **tenderness.**

III. **Diagnosis.** The symptoms of fever and abdominal pain in a neutropenic patient is suggestive of typhlitis.

IV. **Therapy.** Surgery should be avoided unless necessary in this population, since the rate of major morbidity is 50% and 30-day mortality is 32%. Specific problems include a high rate of anastomotic leak as well as an increased risk of appendectomy-associated complications. In patients requiring cytotoxic chemotherapy, most are found to have medical problems with surgical diseases occurring in only 5%. Therefore, only a minority of patients with abdominal pain severe enough to prompt consultation actually require surgery. However, localized pain and tenderness increase the probability that surgical intervention is needed.

PARANEOPLASTIC SYNDROMES

A variety of gastrointestinal manifestations of malignancy have been reported. The following paraneoplastic syndromes have been reported to manifest remote gastrointestinal effects that decrease with tumor regression or resection.

Zollinger-Ellison Syndrome

Zollinger-Ellison Syndrome (ZES) occurs in patients with gastrinomas, which most often occur in the endocrine pancreas. Gastrinomas are discussed in detail in Chapter 58.

  I. Etiology. All aspects of the syndrome may be ascribed to **hypersecretion of gastrin** by G cell-like endocrine tumors found in the pancreas, duodenum, and jejunum as well as in ectopic locations such as lymph nodes, liver, stomach, spleen, mesentery, and ovary.

 II. Presentation. Patients with ZES typically complain of **abdominal pain** (85–98%) from a severe ulcer diathesis, **diarrhea** (30–50%) secondary to acid-induced small bowel injury and bile salt precipitation, and occasionally **dysphagia** and **pyrosis.** The syndrome should be suspected in anyone who presents with an ulcer that is (1) associated with diarrhea, (2) recurrent or resistent to therapy, (3) in an unusual location, (4) familial, and (5) severe enough to require an ulcer operation.

III. Diagnosis. Fasting hypergastrinemia (> 1000 pg/mL) is diagnostic of ZES; however, patients with lower levels of gastrin require one or more **collaborating tests** in order to distinguish other causes of hypergastrinemia (retained gastric antrum, antral G-cell hyperfunction or hyperplasia, and gastric outlet obstruction). These tests include basal acid output (> 15 meq/h), secretin stimulation test (> 200 pg/mL increase in gastrin), calcium infusion test (> 395 pg/mL increase in gastrin), and rarely a maximum acid output test (meal test). Currently, the **secretin stimulation test** is preferred due to its simplicity and relative paucity of side effects.

IV. Therapy. Initially, treatment is directed at control of acid hypersecretion with **H$_2$ antagonists** (cimetidine, ranitidine, famotidine), **proton pump antagonists** (omeprazole), and rarely (resistant patients only) **total gastrectomy.** The amount of medication required may be 20 times the normal dose, and should be titrated while measuring acid secretion. The long-term treatment goal is to successfully control the gastrinoma with surgery, chemotherapy, hormonal therapy, and immunotherapy.

Carcinoid Syndrome

The carcinoid syndrome is observed in association with carcinoid tumors (see Chapter 59) and rarely in association with medullary carcinoma of the thyroid, small cell lung carcinoma, pancreatic endocrine tumors, neuroblastoma, and chromaffin tumors.

  I. Etiology. The carcinoid syndrome of diarrhea, cutaneous flushing, wheezing, and fibrotic valvular heart disease is produced by a combination of **vasoactive amines:** 5-hydroxytryptamine (serotonin), 5-hydroxytryptophan, tachykinins (substance K and P, neuropeptide K), histamine, bradykinin, prostaglandins, and adrenocorticotropic hormone (ACTH). These substances are normally metabolized by the liver and lung, preventing the development of symptoms; however, when hepatic metastases occur, the metabolic capacity is overwhelmed or bypassed and carcinoid symptoms may develop.

 II. Presentation. Patients frequently complain of **diarrhea** (70–85%), **facial and neck flushing** (65–95%), **wheezing** (5–25%), **congestive heart failure** (10–50%), **pain** (< 10%), and **pellagra-like skin lesions** (5%). Recent data indicate that only 73% of patients with increased serotonin levels complain of carcinoid symptoms. Thus, elevated serotonin levels and the development of carcinoid symptoms are not closely correlated. The flushing is classified into one of 4 types.

    A. Type I flushing. These flushes are **transient erythematous flushes** of the face and neck, lasting only 1–2 minutes. They are associated with midgut carcinoids and occasionally with foregut carcinoids.

    B. Type II flushing. A **violaceous tinge lasting several minutes** is characteristic of this type of flushing. **Permanent cyanotic coloration, dilated facial veins,** and **telangiectasia** are also present. Like type I flushes, these flushes are associated primarily with midgut carcinoids but are also seen in patients with foregut carcinoid tumors.

    C. Type III flushing. This type of flush is associated with **deep forehead furrowing, profuse lacrimation, permanently injected sclerae,** and sometimes hypotension. They last for hours to days and usually occur in patients with foregut carcinoids.

    D. Type IV flushing. Type IV flushes are **patchy, bright red flushes** of the lower neck and arms. These uncommon flushes are triggered by histamine release from gastric carcinoids.

III. Diagnosis. Measurement of **24-hour urinary serotonin or 5-hydroxyindole acetic acid (5-HIAA)** confirms the diagnosis of carcinoid syndrome. 5-HIAA is more commonly used, is 73% sensitive, and is 100% specific. However, false-positive results occur with certain foods (avocados, bananas, pineapple, kiwi, plantains, walnuts, pecans, and hickory nuts) and medications (acetaminophen, salicylates, guaifenesin, and L-dopa). Measurement of **urinary and platelet serotonin** may be helpful if the urinary 5-HIAA is normal but the clinical index of suspicion is high.

TABLE 13–1. PHARMACOLOGIC THERAPY FOR THE CARCINOID SYNDROME

Group	Drug	Dose	Mechanism/Toxicity	Diarrhea	Flushing
Alpha-adrenergic agonists	Phenoxybenzamine (Dibenzyline)	10–30 mg PO daily	Blocks alpha-adrenergic receptors	—	Improves
	Chlorpromazine (Thorazine)	10–25 mg PO every 8 hours	Blocks acetylcholine, histamine, serotonin, and kinin	—	May improve
Serotonin synthesis inhibitors	Methyldopa (Aldomet)	4–6 g PO daily	Blocks tryptophan decarboxyla and alpha-adrenergic receptors	—	May improve
	Parachlorophenyl alanine	0.5–1.0 g PO every 6 hours	Blocks amino acid hydroxylase	Improves	May improve
Serotonin receptor antagonists	Cyprohepadine (Periactin)	4–10 mg PO every 8 hours	Blocks H_1 receptors/causes somnolence	Improves	—
	Ketanserin	40–160 mg PO daily	Blocks H_1, alpha-adrenergic, and dopamine receptors	Improves	May improve
	Methysergide (Sansert)	2 mg PO every 6–8 hours	Blocks acetylcholine and H_1 receptors	Improves	—
Somatostatin analogues	Octreotide acetate (Sandostatin)	50–150 μg SC every 8–12 hours	Blocks serotonin release/causes gallstones (20%)	Improves	Improves
Calcium channel blockers	Verapamil (Calan, Isoptin)	40–120 mg PO every 6–8 hours	Blocks calcium channels/causes atrioventricular block	Improves	May improve

Adapted, with permission, from Bunn PA, Ridgway ED: Paraneoplastic syndromes. Pages 1928–1931 in: DeVita VT, Hellman S, Rosenberg SA (editors). Cancer: Principles and Practice of Oncology. Lippincott, 1989.

IV. **Therapy.** A variety of agents may be used to palliate the symptoms of carcinoid syndrome (Table 13–1); however, **surgical resection,** if possible, remains the only curative option. **Chemotherapy for metastatic disease** may help improve symptoms, but to date, responses have been disappointing. Radiation therapy is not helpful (see p 484, **IX**).

Malabsorption

Many patients with cancer lose weight because of anorexia and cachexia (see below); however, some patients experience weight loss despite adequate oral intake. These patients may have a malabsorption syndrome.

I. **Etiology.** Although major surgery, radiation therapy, chemotherapy, gastrointestinal lymphoma, and gastric, hepatic, and biliary neoplasms may all exert direct effects on the gastrointestinal tract resulting in malabsorption, carcinomas of the colon, pancreas, lung, and prostate may cause villous atrophy of the small bowel as a "remote" effect of the tumor.

II. **Presentation.** Symptoms generally are those of cachexia from chronic malabsorption, although diarrhea may sometimes occur.

III. **Diagnosis.** A presumptive diagnosis may be made in patients with adequate oral intake and normal thyroid function tests but progressive weight loss. If it is necessary to confirm the diagnosis, small bowel biopsy should be performed; **mucosal flattening and simple villous atrophy** on histologic examination confirm the diagnosis.

IV. **Therapy.** Primary therapy involves treatment of the underlying malignancy; however, **parenteral nutrients, vitamins,** and **calories** may be required.

Anorexia and Cachexia

Many cancer patients develop reversible anorexia, cachexia, asthenia, and inability to maintain normal metabolic homeostasis (ie, caloric expenditure remains high when intake is low) without regard to the site, size, or type of neoplasm present.

I. **Etiology.** Cytokines, particularly **tumor necrosis factor (TNF)-alpha** (also known as cachectin) and **interleukin-1 (IL1)-beta,** have been shown to produce an anorexia/cachexia syndrome in rats. Inhibition of peripheral lipoprotein lipase as well as other effects may be responsible. Altered regulation of hormones (insulin, glucagon, growth hormone, and cortisol) and anorexigenic pituitary polypeptides have also been implicated.

II. **Presentation.** Patients commonly complain of **weight loss, anorexia, taste alterations** (decreased sensitivity to sweet, increased sensitivity to bitter, and aversion to meat), **early satiety, fatigue,** and **loss of energy.**

III. **Diagnosis.** The diagnosis is based on the appropriate symptoms being present in a cancer patient without evidence that they may be explained by toxic effects of therapy or tumor infiltration of organs (liver, bowel).

IV. **Therapy.** Treatment is aimed mainly at the primary tumor, although **increased oral intake** and **parenteral nutrition** may be required.

Hepatopathy

I. **Etiology.** Elevations in liver enzymes as well as decreases in serum levels of hepatic proteins have been reported in patients with malignant schwannoma and renal cell carcinoma without metastases to the liver. This distant effect has been attributed to hepatic amyloid or periportal inflammation. The hepatic abnormalities have reverted to normal upon resection of the primary tumor.

II. **Presentation.** Patients are generally asymptomatic, although low albumin levels may lead to troublesome peripheral edema.

III. **Diagnosis.** A sample of peripheral blood frequently reveals decreased serum albumin and cholesterol levels, prolonged prothrombin time, hyperglobulinemia, or increased serum alkaline phosphatase levels (or all of these). Imaging studies fail to demonstrate hepatic metastases.

IV. **Therapy.** Although fluid restriction (to control edema) and fresh-frozen plasma (to reverse the coagulopathy if significant bleeding develops) may occasionally be required, the only therapy usually needed is treatment of the underlying neoplasm.

REFERENCES

Cromack DT et al: Are complications in intraoperative radiation therapy more frequent than in conventional treatment? *Arch Surg* 1989;**124:**229.

Feldman JM: Carcinoid tumors and the carcinoid syndrome. *Curr Probl Surg* 1989;**26**(12):831.

Glenn J, Funkhouser WK, Schneider PS: Acute illnesses necessitating urgent abdominal surgery in neutropenic cancer patients: Description of 14 cases and review of the literature. *Surgery* 1989;**105:**778.

Gleysteen JJ: Surgical management of malignant ascites. *Surg Rounds* 1984;(June):73.

Lacy JH, Shively EH: Management of malignant ascites. *Surg Gynecol Obstet* 1984;**159:**397.

Russell JC, Welch JP: Operative management of radiation injuries of the intestinal tract. *Am J Surg* 1979;**137:**433.

Souter RG et al: Surgical and pathologic complications associated with peritoneovenous shunts in management of malignant ascites. *Cancer* 1985;**55:**1973.

Yeoh EK, Horwitz M: Radiation enteritis. *Surg Gynecol Obstet* 1987;**165:**373.

14 Hematologic Problems & Emergencies

Jeffrey Miller, MD, and Howard L. Parnes, MD

ERYTHROCYTE ABNORMALITIES

Erythrocytosis

I. **Etiology.** Tumor-associated erythrocytosis (TAE) is a physiologically inappropriate increase in erythrocyte mass that occasionally develops in certain neoplasms, such as 9–20% of cerebellar hemangioblastomas and 1–6% of renal tumors. The incidence of TAE for various tumors is as follows: kidney, 38%; liver, 19%; cerebellum (hemangioblastoma), 15%; uterine, 7%; adrenal, 3%; miscellaneous (lung, ovaries, thymus), 3%. The proposed mechanisms of TAE are **increased erythropoietin** (72% of all cases), **androgens,** and **prostaglandin production.**

II. **Presentation.** Most patients are **asymptomatic;** however, with increasing red blood cell mass, the blood viscosity escalates, leading to complaints of headache, malaise, diaphoresis, pruritus, dizziness, diplopia, blurred vision, paresthesias, facial plethora, and conjunctival congestion. In addition, physical findings of retinal vein engorgement and hypertension are common.

III. **Diagnosis.** The demonstration of a **hematocrit greater than 55% in males and greater than 50% in females in the absence of hypovolemia** is diagnostic of erythrocytosis. The diagnosis of TAE can be made only after excluding other nonmalignant causes (chronic lung disease, cyanotic heart disorders, heavy smoking, hemoglobinopathies, polycythemia vera, exogenous corticosteroid administration, Cushing's disease, hydronephrosis, renal cysts, and high altitudes) with a detailed history and physical examination, arterial P_{O_2} determination, and hemoglobin electrophoresis.

IV. **Therapy.** Although successful treatment of the primary tumor controls the erythrocytosis in more than 97% of patients, **phlebotomy** rarely may be required if the neoplasm cannot be effectively managed with surgery, chemotherapy, or radiation therapy.

Anemia

I. **Etiology.** Anemia is present in 60% of cancer patients. It is often multifactorial in origin. Some patients exhibit an "anemia of chronic disease" characterized by normocytic and normo- or hypochromic indices; normal reticulocyte count; red cell maturation; normal or increased ferritin, and iron stores; decreased serum iron, iron binding capacity, and red cell half-life; and increased erythropoiesis. However, most patients are anemic for one of the following reasons.

    A. **Blood Loss.** Gastrointestinal neoplasms regularly lead to occult blood loss, resulting in a microcytic, hypochromic, iron deficiency anemia. Frequent phlebotomy and surgery may also result in blood loss."

    B. **Myelosuppression.** Both irradiation and chemotherapy may cause myelosuppression and a normocytic, normochromic anemia.

    C. **Malnutrition.** Inadequate nutrition may lead to iron deficiency (microcytic, hypochromic anemia) and vitamin B_{12} or folate deficiency (megaloblastic anemia). Vitamin B_{12} deficiency develops in patients following gastrectomy (loss of intrinsic factor) for gastric cancer.

    D. **Hypersplenism.** The hypersplenism that occurs with hematologic malignancies (eg, myelofibrosis, chronic myelogenous leukemia) may shorten red cell survival and lead to anemia.

    E. **Hemolysis.** About 2–3% of cancer-related anemias are due to hemolysis.

        1. **Autoimmune hemolytic anemia (AHA).** Two types of AHA exist: warm and cold. **Cold-type** AHA is associated with **B cell lymphoproliferative diseases** (lymphoma, chronic lymphocytic leukemia, Waldenström's macroglobulin-

emia), although the monoclonal paraprotein (IgM) produced by the malignant cells does not directly cause the hemolysis. **Warm-type** AHA is particularly characteristic of **chronic lymphocytic leukemia, lymphoma and non-Hodgkin's), angioimmunoblastic lymphadenopathy, and ovarian teratoma.** It also has been reported as a rare occurrence in patients with squamous cell carcinoma, adenocarcinoma and hairy cell leukemia. **The anemia of AHA is often severe, with a mean presenting hemoglobin level of 7.4 g/dL.** Rarely, **immune thrombocytopenia** may occur concomitantly with AHA (Evans's syndrome).

2. **Microangiopathic hemolytic anemia (MAHA)** occurs primarily in patients with **adenocarcinomas,** such as gastric cancer; cancers of the breast, lung, prostate or seminal vesicle, colon, pancreas, or ovary; hepatocellular cancer; cholangiocarcinoma; and adenocarcinoma of unknown primary site. Like AHA, MAHA typically presents with **severe anemia** and a **mean hemoglobin concentration of 7 g/dL.** Rarely, cancer patients with **intraluminal mucin-producing tumor emboli and chemotherapy-induced intimal proliferation** develop MAHA due to excessive shearing forces on erythrocytes. The onset of hemolysis is often abrupt and severe, and may be associated with **disseminated intravascular coagulation (DIC)** in 50–60% of patients.

F. **Renal insufficiency.** Renal failure of any cause is associated with decreased erythropoietin production and normochromic, normocytic anemia.

G. **Bone marrow infiltration.** Although cortical bone metastases are common in cancer, they usually don't cause functional bone marrow impairment. However, bone marrow infiltration in the late stages of prostate and breast cancer may cause anemia.

H. **Red cell aplasia.** Rarely, selective loss of erythropoiesis with or without hypogammaglobulinemia produces severe anemia in patients with thymomas (5%) as well as in patients with adenocarcinoma of the breast, stomach, thyroid, and unknown primary sites, squamous cell carcinoma of the lung and skin, anaplastic and small cell lung cancer, lymphomas, and many leukemias.

II. **Presentation.** Presenting signs and symptoms vary greatly depending on the degree of anemia. Many patients with mild anemia are **asymptomatic,** while patients with moderate reductions in erythrocyte mass may experience **fatigue, weakness, pallor, and palpitations.** In severe cases, **tachycardia, orthostatic hypotension, dyspnea,** and **congestive heart failure** may occur.

III. **Diagnosis.** A **complete blood count** and reticulocyte count should be obtained and the **peripheral blood smear** examined. Anemia is defined as a hemoglobin concentration of less than 14.0 g/dL in males and less than 12.0 g/dL in females. To aid in the differential diagnosis, the anemia is classified as microcytic, normocytic, or macrocytic based on **red cell indices.** Serum iron, total iron binding capacity, ferritin, vitamin B_{12}, and folate levels may be helpful if iron or vitamin deficiency is likely, and serum lactate dehydrogenase level, indirect bilirubin level, and Coombs' tests (direct and indirect) should be ordered if hemolysis is suspected. Schistocytes, nucleated red blood cells, and hyperbilirubinemia strongly suggest MAHA. MAHA is seen in DIC, thrombotic thrombocytopenic purpura, hemolytic uremic syndrome, prosthetic heart valves, and Kasabach-Merritt syndrome.

IV. **Therapy.** For most cancer patients with anemia, **treatment of the underlying malignancy** constitutes primary therapy. **Repletion of iron, vitamin B_{12}, folate, and blood** should be done as necessary. For example, patients with gastric cancer require B_{12} (100 µg intramuscularly once a month). Patients with anemia associated with renal failure often benefit from administration of erythropoietin (Epogen), 50–100 units/kg 3 times weekly. **Splenectomy** may be necessary for patients with hypersplenism or AHA but should be considered only if all other measures fail. Corticosteroids may be helpful in patients with AHA. Some authorities recommend the use of heparin for DIC in acute promyelocytic leukemia.

LEUKOCYTE ABNORMALITIES

Leukocytosis

I. **Etiology.** A leukemoid reaction usually results from **tumor production of colony-stimulation factors (CSF).**

II. **Presentation.** A leukemoid reaction is almost always asymptomatic.

III. **Diagnosis.** An elevated **leukocyte count of more than 20,000/µL in the absence of infection, glucocorticoid administration, and evidence of chronic myelogenous leukemia (CML)** is diagnostic of a leukemoid reaction. The following characteristics mitigate against the diagnosis of CML: (1) leukocyte count of more than 100,000/μL with no immature forms, (2) normal platelet and basophil counts, (3) absence of splenomegaly, (4) elevated leukocyte alkaline phosphatase level, (5) absence of the Philadelphia chromosome, and (6) normal vitamin B_{12} levels.

IV. **Therapy.** No specific therapy is required. Treatment is directed at the underlying malignancy.

Hyperleukocytosis

I. **Etiology.** Extremely high levels of circulating leukocytes (hyperleukocytosis) occur in CML, acute lymphocytic leukemia (ALL), myelogenous leukemia (AML), and chronic lymphocytic leukemia (CLL).

II. **Presentation. Leukostasis** in the microcirculation of the lungs is characterized by pulmonary infiltrates, hypoxia, and the adult respiratory distress syndrome. When the central nervous system is involved, blurred vision, dizziness, ataxia, stupor, papilledema, engorged retinal veins, coma, and sudden death (intracerebral hemorrhage may occur). Because of the large size and rigidity of white blood cells, intravascular leukostasis is more common in patients with CML or AML and is rare in ALL or CLL. In addition, **pseudohypoglycemia, pseudohypoxemia,** and **pseudohyperkalemia** may obscure true laboratory results because of the large number of metabolically active cells present in blood samples. For this reason, all blood should be collected on ice and immediately processed.

III. **Diagnosis.** A leukocyte count of more than 100,000/μL in a patient with AML, CML, ALL or CLL is diagnostic of hyperleukocytosis.

IV. **Therapy.** Prior to initiation of definitive therapy, **nonspecific measures** such as increasing inspired oxygen concentrations, mechanical ventilation, cranial irradiation, and leukapheresis may be necessary. **Specific chemotherapy (hydroxyurea** for myeloid leukemia and **prednisone** for lymphocytic leukemia) is instituted as soon as possible after administration of **allopurinol** and **intravenous hydration** to prevent the tumor lysis syndrome (see p 86). Red blood cell transfusions should be avoided in patients with hyperleukocytosis since this may precipitate symptoms by increasing blood viscosity.

Leukopenia

I. **Etiology. Antineoplastic therapy (chemotherapy, radiation therapy)** is almost always responsible for leukopenia in cancer patients, although sepsis and drugs (eg, cimetidine, sulfonamides, penicillins) may also cause low white blood cell counts. Rarely, malignant bone marrow infiltration may cause leukopenia. Paraneoplastic leukopenia occurs primarily in patients with thymoma, but also in those with T-gamma lymphoproliferative disease and Hodgkin's disease. This syndrome may be mediated by immune complexes and responds to chemotherapy but not to splenectomy.

II. **Presentation.** Most patients receiving chemotherapy and irradiation are monitored closely, and therefore leukopenia is usually discovered in an otherwise **asymptomatic** patient. Fever may be the only sign of infection in patients with leukopenia. Common sites of infection include the mouth, rectum and lungs.

III. **Diagnosis.** A complete blood count reveals an **abnormally low white blood count, usually less than 3000/μL.** However, the risk of infection is most closely related to neutrophils. The incidence of infections significantly increases when the absolute neutrophil count is less than 500/μL. Sepsis and drug-related leukopenia must be excluded.

IV. **Therapy.** Since most leukopenia in cancer patients is related to chemotherapy, radiation therapy, and infection, treatment is **supportive** (antibiotics, colonly stimulating factors). Any patient, regardless of etiology, with an absolute neutrophil count of less than 500/μL and fever should receive empiric antibiotics to prevent septic deaths. For patients with paraneoplastic leukopenia, normal blood counts may be restored by treatment of the underlying malignancy and with G-CSF therapy (neupogen).

PLATELET ABNORMALITIES

Thrombocytosis

I. **Etiology.** Thrombocytosis is commonly observed in patients with solid tumors, occurring in up to one third of patients. It also frequently occurs in patients with iron deficiency, collagen vascular disease, and other inflammatory states. Rarely, thrombocytosis is not associated with malignancy or any other disease process, in which case it is called "**essential thrombocytosis.**"

II. **Presentation.** The majority of patients with thrombocytosis and 20% of patients with essential thrombocytosis are **asymptomatic.** Patients with essential thrombocytosis may, however, present with mucosal hemorrhage (50%; epistaxis, gastrointestinal bleeding); headaches; easy bruising; thrombosis (30%) of the superficial, deep, or hepatic (Budd-Chiari syndrome) veins or carotid, mesenteric, renal, or peripheral arteries; transient ischemic attacks; cerebral infarcts; and intermittent, painful erythema, cyanosis, and gangrene of the digits (erythromelalgia).

III. **Diagnosis.** A **platelet count of more than 400,000/μL in the absence of diseases that cause secondary thrombocytosis,** ie, iron deficiency anemia, hemolysis, acute hemorrhage, acute and chronic inflammatory diseases (eg, rheumatoid arthritis, inflammatory bowel disease), splenectomy, and infection, warrants an evaluation for an underlying malignancy (history and physical exam, stool hemoccult, chest radiograph, complete blood count, serum electrolytes, calcium and liver function tests). Platelet counts in excess of 1,000,000/μL suggest a myeloproliferative disorder (polycythemia rubra vera, CML, myelofibrosis, essential thrombocytosis).

IV. **Therapy.** Most patients with platelet counts of less than 1,000,000/μL do not require specific therapy. For patients with platelet counts of more than 1,000,000/μL or minor thrombotic complications, **aspirin,** 625 mg daily, may be beneficial. Patients with major thrombotic or hemorrhagic sequelae (essential thrombocytosis) must be anticoagulated with **heparin** and subsequently **warfarin** (Coumadin). In emergency situations, the platelet count may be lowered acutely with **plateletpheresis** and chronically with **cytotoxic agents (hydroxyurea).**

Thrombocytopenia

I. **Etiology.** Tumor-associated thrombocytopenia presents as an idiopathic thrombocytopenic purpura (ITP)-like syndrome. Although it occurs in older patients (mean age, 54 years) and no immune mechanism has been documented, ITP-like syndrome follows a course similar to that of classic ITP and is most commonly associated with **Hodgkin's disease** and **CLL.** Other diseases known to produce an ITP-like thrombocytopenia are immunoblastic lymphadenopathy (30% of cases), non-Hodgkin's lymphoma, ALL, immunoblastic sarcoma, epidermoid carcinomas, and carcinomas of the breast, lung, rectum, pancreas, gallbladder, ovary, testis, and prostate. This paraneoplastic thrombocytopenia is rarely responsible for thrombocytopenia in cancer patients. In most cases, thrombocytopenia is secondary to chemotherapy, radiation therapy, malignant bone marrow infiltration, DIC, and thrombotic microangiopahty as well as nonmalignant causes such as drugs (eg, heparin, thiazides, sulfonamides, gold, quinidine), hypersplenism, sepsis, and blood transfusions (posttransfusion purpura).

II. **Presentation.** Patients are often **asymptomatic** despite very low platelet counts (ie, less than 10,000/μL). Symptoms may include **purpura, petechiae,** and **excessive bleeding** after procedures. Rarely, intracranial bleeding may precipitate changes in mental status, coma, and death.

III. **Diagnosis. By definition, thrombocytopenia is a platelet count of less than 150,000/μL;** however, clinical symptoms arise only with platelet counts of less than 50,000/μL. Most patients with the ITP-like syndrome present with platelet counts of less than 30,000/μL, circulating megathrombocytes, increased bone marrow megakaryocytes, normal red cell counts, no evidence of DIC, and an absence of other causes of thrombocytopenia.

IV. **Therapy.** As with many hematologic abnormalities, primary therapy consists of treating the underlying malignancy. In patients with platelet counts of less than 50,000/μL and ITP-like syndrome, a therapeutic effect may be obtained by the administration of **prednisone,** 1 mg/kg/d, and if refractory splenectomy may be performed. In general, platelet transfusion is not indicated in patients with immune thrombocytopenia, however, it may be utilized in emergency situations.

COAGULATION ABNORMALITIES

Disseminated Intravascular Coagulation (DIC)

I. **Etiology.** Tumor-associated **procoagulants and activators of fibrinolysis** trigger acute and chronic DIC and fibrinolysis with abnormalities of coagulation times, clotting factors, platelets, and fibrinogen. Most commonly, DIC is associated with **acute promyelocytic leukemia** and **adenocarcinoma** of the prostate, pancreas, stomach, colon, gallbladder, lung, ovary, and breast. Rarely, primary fibrinolysis may be present without thrombosis.

II. **Presentation.** Chronic DIC is usually asymptomatic, presenting only with laboratory abnormalities. Acute DIC is rare in cancer patients and typically presents with thrombotic or hemorrhagic complications, eg, thrombophlebitis, purpura, hemorrhage from biopsy or venipuncture sites, and rarely intracranial hemorrhage.

III. **Diagnosis.** Table 14–1 summarizes the laboratory findings associated with acute DIC, chronic DIC, and primary fibrinolysis.

IV. **Therapy.** If possible, the primary therapy should be **directed at the underlying malignancy.** The indications for anticoagulation are **controversial.** For acute DIC (often accompanied by severe complications) and symptomatic chronic DIC, **intravenous heparin** (300–600 units/kg/d) may be instituted. **Transfusion of fresh-frozen plasma, cryoprecipitate, and platelets** may be performed as necessary.

Thrombophlebitis

I. **Etiology.** Due to procoagulants released by tumor cells many cancer patients acquire a **hypercoagulable state.** Decreased levels of antithrombin III, protein C, and protein S have also been implicated in this process. This results in an increased incidence of thrombophlebitis which may involve the deep or superficial veins. A specific **syndrome of migratory superficial thrombophlebitis (Trousseau's syndrome)** is associated with **mucin-secreting adenocarcinomas** (lung, pancreas, breast, prostate, and ovary).

II. **Presentation.** Generally, patients present with **pain, swelling,** and **erythema of the involved extremity,** although physical examination accurately diagnoses the disorder in only 50% of patients. The possibility of occult malignancy should be considered in patients with deep venous thrombosis who do not have underlying risk factors (obesity, post-operative, and immobilization).

III. **Diagnosis.** Superficial thrombophlebitis is a clinical diagnosis; however, involvement of the deep venous system must always be excluded. Currently, the diagnosis of deep venous thrombophlebitis may be confirmed in more than 95% of cases with noninvasive techniques, ie, **color Doppler and duplex scanning. Venography** may be required to establish the diagnosis.

IV. **Therapy.** Acutely, deep venous thrombosis requires anticoagulation with **heparin.** The **chronic** treatment of tumor-associated thrombosis does not respond well to warfarin and may require prolonged anticoagulation with subcutaneous heparin.

Thrombotic Microangiopathy

I. **Etiology.** Two syndromes related to the hemolytic-uremic syndrome may occur in cancer patients: **tumor-associated thrombotic microangiopathy (TATM)** and **chemotherapy-associated thrombotic microangiopathy (CATM).** TATM occurs in patients with extensive (usually metastatic) disease and involves intravascular coagulation, hyaline thrombi (primarily in the lung), and endothelial damage. CATM usually develops in patients with minimal disease and is characterized by microthrombi in the kidneys and immune complex formation. TATM arises most commonly in patients with adenocarcinoma of the stomach but may occur in those with carcinoma of the breast, pancreas, colon, lung, prostate, or ovary. CATM typically arises in patients with carcinoma of the stomach, pancreas, colon, liver, or ovary as well as those with epidermoid

TABLE 14–1. LABORATORY FEATURES OF COAGULOPATHIES

Feature	Acute DIC[1]	Chronic DIC[1]	Primary Fibrinolysis
Prothrombin time	Prolonged	Normal	Normal
Partial thromboplastin time	Prolonged	Normal	Normal
Thrombin time	Prolonged	Normal	Normal
Platelet count	Reduced	Elevated	Normal
Fibrinogen	Reduced	Elevated	Reduced
Protamine test	Positive	Positive	Negative
Fibrin degradation products	Elevated	Elevated	Elevated
Fibrinopeptide A	Elevated	Elevated	Elevated
D-dimers	Elevated	Elevated	Elevated

[1]DIC = disseminated intravascular coagulopathy.

cancers that are treated with mitomycin-C or, less commonly, fluorouracil and cisplatin. More than 90% of CATM is due to mitomycin-C.

II. **Presentation.** Both syndromes typically present with thrombocytopenia, microangiopathic hemolytic anemia, coagulation abnormalities suggestive of DIC, renal insufficiency, proteinuria, hematuria, and neurologic symptoms (eg, headache, lethargy, confusion, hemiparesis). CATM often includes hypertension and noncardiogenic pulmonary edema.

III. **Diagnosis.** The diagnosis of TATM and CATM is made on clinical grounds. Characteristic laboratory findings (see **II,** above) in the appropriate clinical setting (see **I,** above) is sufficient to confirm the diagnosis.

IV. **Therapy**
   A. Primary therapy for **TATM** involves **treatment of the underlying malignancy,** if possible. Supportive care includes the administration of fresh frozen plasma (FFP) and **heparinization** if DIC is present. Glucocorticoids and platelet inhibitors have not been helpful.
   B. Primary therapy for **CATM** includes **aggressive plasmapheresis.** Anecdotal improvement with **vincristine** and **staphylococcal protein A immunoperfusion** have been reported, but corticosteroids, heparin, platelet inhibitors, and immunosuppressive agents generally have exhibited no therapeutic value. Plasma transfusion in CATM may precipitate noncardiogenic pulmonary edema and should be used with caution.

V. **Prognosis.** The prognosis for both syndromes is **extremely poor.** Nearly all patients with TATM die of metastatic disease, while more than 80% of patients with CATM succumb to the complications of the syndrome (eg, renal failure).

TRANSFUSION THERAPY

Red Blood Cell Transfusion
   I. **Indications.** The indications for red blood cell transfusions vary with age, coexisting disease (eg, cardiac, renal, cancer) and clinical situation, and therefore the decision to transfuse must be individualized. In general, red blood cell transfusion should be considered in patients with a hemoglobin of less than 10.0.
   II. **Administration.** Blood should be given through an intravenous line containing normal saline and generally requires a 20-gauge or larger intravenous catheter. The transfusion should be given slowly for 15–30 minutes and discontinued if signs or symptoms of **hemolytic transfusion reaction** (low back pain, chest tightness, nausea, vomiting, hypotension, hematuria), **allergic reaction** (pruritus and urticaria), **bacterial contamination** (septic shock), **pulmonary insufficiency,** or **cardiac failure** develop.

Leukocyte Transfusion
   I. **Indications.** Although controversial, the indication for leukocyte transfusion is sepsis in a patient with an **absolute neutrophil count of less than 250/μL** and no prospect of recovery for greater than one week. In addition, no response must have occurred for 72 hours of therapy with appropriate antibiotics.
   II. **Administration.** At least 1×10^{10} granulocytes are required to be effective. Leukocytes should be transfused in a monitored setting. Large increments in peripheral white blood counts should not be expected.

Platelet Transfusion
   I. **Indications.** Platelet transfusion is indicated in (1) patients with platelet counts of 20,000–50,000/μL and active bleeding or impending surgery, (2) patients with platelet counts of less than 30,000/μL and potential bleeding sites (eg, peptic ulcer, brain metastasis, fungating tumor mass), coagulation abnormalities, and platelet dysfunction (most commonly drug induced), and (3) patients with platelet counts of less than 20,000/μL.
   II. **Administration.** In general, 1 unit of single-donor platelets obtained by apheresis contains an equivalent number of platelets as 6–10 units of random-donor platelets (3.5–5.5 x 10^{11} platelets in 300–400 mL of plasma). Platelets may be stored for 5 days; once transfused, they survive for 2–3 days. To determine the efficacy of the transfusion, the corrected count increment is calculated by the following equation: corrected count increment = observed increment (count/uL) × BSA (m^2)/number of platelets transfused × 10^{11}. An increment greater than 7500/uL per unit of platelets with a corrected count increment of greater than 10,000/uL is satisfactory. If the patient has fever, DIC, sepsis, hemorrhage or alloimmunization (due to previous platelet transfusion) a smaller incre-

ment may be seen. A platelet count should be obtained between 10 min and 1 hour after transfusion to determine efficacy.

Plasma Transfusion
   I.   **Indications.** Fresh-frozen plasma transfusion is necessary for **disease states requiring replacement of coagulation factors,** such as liver disease or mild factor IX deficiency, DIC, tumor-associated thrombotic microangiopathy (TATM), and the coagulopathy associated with massive blood transfusion.
   II. **Administration.** Fresh-frozen plasma (250mL/unit) is thawed and given through a 20-gauge or larger intravenous catheter. Each unit may be delivered over 30–60 minutes. Standard precautions for transfusing blood products should be observed.

REFERENCES

Colman RW et al (editors): *Hemostasis and Thrombosis: Basic Principles and Clinical Practice,* 2nd ed. Lippincott, 1987.

Erslev AJ: Clinical manifestations and classification of erythrocyte disorders. In Williams WJ et al (editors): *Hematology,* 4th ed. New York: McGraw-Hill, 1990;423–429.

Murphy S: Primary thrombocytopenia. In Williams WJ (editor): *Hematology,* 4th ed. New York: McGraw-Hill, 1990;232–236.

O'Connell B, Lee EJ, Schiffer CA: The value of a 10 minute post-transfusion platelet counts. *Transfusion* 1988;**28**:66.

Nichols CR, Akard LP. Hematologic problems in patients with cancer and chronic inflammatory disorders. In Hoffman R, Benz EJ, Shatil SJ, Furie B, Cohen HJ, (editors): *Hematology: Basic Principles and Practice.* New York: Churchill Livingston, 1991;1733–1746.

15 Metabolic Problems & Emergencies

Jeffrey Miller, MD, and Howard L. Parnes, MD

HYPERURICEMIA

I. **Etiology.** Elevated serum uric acid levels may be caused by **overproduction of uric acid** in certain malignancies, (ie, chronic myelogenous leukemia, erythroleukemia, multiple myeloma, myeloid metaplasia, and mast cell diseases) as well as by **massive release of uric acid** from cells as they are destroyed during cytotoxic therapy (see Tumor Lysis Syndrome, p 86). Also, certain drugs, such as **diuretics** (furosemide, thiazides, and ethacrynic acid) and **antituberculin medications,** increase serum uric acid levels. If untreated, hyperuricemia leads to hyperuricosuria (> 800 mg/24 h), uric acid nephropathy, and renal failure.

II. **Presentation.** With close monitoring (eg, daily uric acid levels during cytotoxic therapy) and prophylactic measures, most patients experience only mild asymptomatic hyperuricemia. However, if the uric acid level is markedly elevated, then **nephroureterolithiasis, nephrocalcinosis, oliguria,** and **renal insufficiency** may occur.

III. **Diagnosis.** The diagnosis of hyperuricemia is confirmed when the uric acid level is greater than 8.0 mg/dl.

IV. **Therapy.** Ideally, treatment is directed at prevention. Before cytotoxic therapy is initiated a baseline uric acid measurement is obtained and hyperuricemic drugs (eg, thiazide diuretics) are withdrawn. If the uric acid level is more than 9 mg/dL or less if cytotoxic therapy is used in a patient with a high risk tumor (Burkitts, ALL, lymphoblastic lymphoma) therapy is begun with **intravenous hydration** (3000 mL/m²/d), **alkalinization of the urine** with intravenous or oral sodium bicarbonate (50 meq per liter of intravenous fluid) or acetazolamide (500 mg orally or intravenously every 6 hours). Allopurinol, the xanthene oxidase inhibitor, is also started before therapy (600 mg loading followed by 300 mg/day orally). Simultaneously, the doses of drugs such as mercaptopurine and other agents metabolized by xanthine oxidase must be reduced.

HYPOCALCEMIA

I. **Etiology.** Low serum calcium levels in cancer patients may be caused by **hyperphosphatemia** (see Tumor Lysis syndrome, p 86), **widespread or rapidly healing bone metastases** (eg, as a result of breast or prostate cancer), and **rare tumors** (eg, calcifying chondrosarcoma). In addition, persistent hypocalcemia may result from vitamin D deficiency, pseudohypoparathyroidism, pancreatitis, and inhibition of parathormone release and activity secondary to **hypomagnesemia** as a consequence of cisplatin therapy. In general, increased serum calcitonin resulting from medullary carcinoma of the thyroid does not cause hypocalcemia. In patients with bone metastases, hypocalcemia may actually be more common than hypercalcemia.

II. **Presentation.** Nearly all patients are **asymptomatic,** although some may complain of **paresthesias, irritability, lethargy, depression,** and **muscle cramps. Chvostek's sign** (facial twitching with tapping of the facial nerve trunk in front of the ear) and **Trousseau's sign** (carpal spasm with inflation of a brachial blood pressure cuff) may be present. If severe hypocalcemia develops, **papilledema, tetany, laryngospasm,** and **seizures** may occur.

III. **Diagnosis.** Hypocalcemia in (1) the presence of normal dihydroxycholecalciferol (vitamin D), calcium intake, and parathormone levels and (2) the absence of hypomagnesemia is sufficient to confirm the diagnosis.

IV. **Therapy.** No specific therapy is indicated unless troublesome muscle spasms or tetany develop. Acutely, 1 or 2 ampules of **10% calcium gluconate or chloride** (1–2 g/10–20 mL) may be given intravenously over 3 minutes, followed by a calcium infusion (1 ampule/L D_5W at 100 mL/h). For chronic symptoms, **oral calcium supplementation** (15 mg/kg/d) with calcium carbonate (Calci-chew, Nephro-calci, Caltrate), and a **vitamin D analog** (eg, ergocalciferol [vitamin D_2; 50,000 units twice weekly], calcitriol [Rocaltrol; 0.25–2μg/d]) should be instituted. If serum magnesium levels are low, magnesium should be replenished and serum calcium levels should be monitored closely.

HYPOPHOSPHATEMIA

I. **Etiology.** The **administration of glucose** (in total parenteral nutrition, for example) to treat malnutrition is the most common cause of a low serum phosphorous concentration in cancer patients. In addition, hypophosphatemia has been reported in patients with certain cancers that produce a "phosphaturic" substance with resulting severe phosphaturia (multiple myeloma, ossifying mesenchymal tumors and, rarely, lung and prostate cancer), neoplasms associated with hyperparathyroidism (MEN-I and MEN-IIa), and (rarely) rapidly growing tumors (rapid metabolic utilization).

II. **Presentation.** Patients characteristically experience **confusion, irritability, nervousness,** and **weakness.** If severe, hypophosphatemia leads to hemolytic anemia, rhabdomyolysis, leukocyte and platelet dysfunction, and **seizures** due to membrane instability and depleted energy stores.

III. **Diagnosis.** Hypophosphatemia is defined as a **measured serum phosphate concentration of less than 2.5.**

IV. **Therapy.** For **severe hypophosphatemia** (< 1 mg/dL), elemental phosphorus (2.5–5 mg/kg) should be cautiously infused intravenously over 6–8 hours to avoid intramyocardial hypocalcemia. For **mild to moderate hypophosphatemia** (1–2.5 mg/dL), an oral phosphorus preparation (Neutra-Phos or K-Phos; 250–2000 mg/d in divided doses) may be prescribed, provided the serum calcium level is not elevated. In some cases (eg, ossifying mesenchymal tumors), **surgery** is curative.

HYPERKALEMIA

I. **Etiology.** In cancer patients, elevated serum potassium levels are most often due to **exogenous administration, renal insufficiency,** adrenal insufficiency (bilateral adrenal metastases), use of potassium-sparing diuretics (spironolactone [Aldactone]), and the **tumor lysis syndrome** (see p 86).

II. **Presentation. Electrocardiographic changes** (peaked T waves, short QT interval, ST segment depression, and widened QRS complex), **weakness,** paralysis, and increased release of some hormones (aldosterone, epinephrine, insulin, and glucagon) are typical clinical features of hyperkalemia.

III. **Diagnosis. A serum potassium concentration of more than 5.5 mg/dL** is diagnostic. However, in the presence of erythrocytosis (Hct > 50%), leukocytosis (> 50,000/μL), and elevated platelet counts (> 1 million/μL), the serum potassium level may be falsely elevated (**pseudohyperkalemia**) due to cytolysis that occurs with the clotting process after the blood is drawn. In these cases, the **plasma potassium level** should be determined using heparinized blood.

IV. **Therapy.** Specific therapy depends on the degree of hyperkalemia, renal function, and the presence or absence of electrocardiographic abnormalities. **Mild hyperkalemia** (serum potassium level of 5–5.5 mg/dL and no electrocardiographic changes) may require only **intravenous hydration** (half-normal saline) and **furosemide** (Lasix) along with dietary restriction and withdrawal of any exogenous source (potassium supplements and potassium-sparing diuretics). **Moderate hyperkalemia** (serum potassium level 5.5–6.5 mg/dL and no electrocardiographic changes) requires the same measures but with the addition of **cation (sodium-potassium) exchange resins** (sodium polystyrene sulfonate [Kayexalate], 15–30 g in 100 mL of 20% sorbitol orally or 30–50 g in 100 mL of 70% sorbitol rectally, every 6 hours to exchange 1.0 meq potassium per gram). **Severe hyperkalemia** (serum potassium level of 6.5 mg/dL or electrocardiographic changes) mandates close cardiac monitoring in the intensive care unit, administration of **dextrose** and **insulin** (1 ampule of $D_{50}W$ (25 g/50mL) with 5 units of regular insulin (1 unit/5 g dextrose) 1 ampule of **sodium bicarbonate** (50 meq/50 mL) which may be repeated in 10–15 minutes if EKG abnormalities persist. To preserve the myocardium, 1–2 ampules of 10% **calcium gluconate** may be given intravenously over 3 minutes. Since these are only temporary measures Kayexalate should also be administered, but in certain circumstances (oliguria, extreme hyperkalemia) emergent dialysis may be required.

TUMOR LYSIS SYNDROME

  I. **Etiology.** This syndrome of hyperuricemia, hyperkalemia, hyperphosphatemia, and hypocalcemia results from **massive cell death and release of intracellular** uric acid, potassium, and phosphate. The hyperphosphatemia causes hypocalcemia. It occurs primarily during treatment of neoplasms with the following characteristics: (1) large tumor burden, (2) high proliferative rates, and (3) profound sensitivity to therapy. Cancers associated with this syndrome are primarily **lymphoproliferative disorders,** eg, high grade leukemias (acute and blast crisis of CML) and lymphoma (Burkitt's), but has been described with the treatment of **solid tumors** (eg, small cell lung and breast cancer).

 II. **Presentation.** The signs and symptoms of tumor lysis syndrome are **hyperuricemia** (see p 84, **II**), **hyperkalemia** (see p 85, **II**), **hyperphosphatemia** (symptoms of hypocalcemia), and **hypocalcemia** (see p 84, **II**).

III. **Diagnosis.** High-risk patients must be monitored with daily electrolyte, phosphate, and uric acid levels before and during cytotoxic therapy. The diagnosis is confirmed by laboratory values demonstrating increased levels of serum uric acid, potassium, and phosphate and a decreased serum calcium level.

IV. **Therapy.** The principal treatment is **prevention.** Therapy must be instituted prior to the administration of therapy and is directed at correcting the 4 metabolic abnormalities outlined below:

   A. **Hyperuricemia.** (See p 84, **IV**.) Alkalinization should be avoided in patients with hyperphosphatemia to prevent calcium phosphate deposition.

   B. **Hyperkalemia.** (See p 85, **IV**.)

   C. **Hyperphosphatemia.** Elevated serum phosphate levels are treated with intravenous hydration (half-normal saline), dietary restriction, and phosphate binding agents (aluminum hydroxide [Amphojel], 30 mL every 3–4 hours) Phosphate binding agents prevent absorption of oral phosphate and therefore, are only useful in patients who are eating. Extremely high levels (> 20 mg/dL) may require emergent dialysis.

   D. **Hypocalcemia.** (See p 84, **IV**.)

LACTIC ACIDOSIS

  I. **Etiology.** Lactic acidosis associated with cancer (type B) stems from a **simultaneous increase in lactate production and decrease in lactate metabolism,** and differs from lactic acidosis occurring with shock and sepsis (type A). This syndrome occurs most often in patients with **leukemia** and **lymphoma,** but it has been described in patients with solid tumors and extensive hepatic metastases, as well.

 II. **Presentation.** Typically, patients present with signs and symptoms of metabolic acidosis, ie, **tachypnea, weakness, nausea, confusion,** and **somnolence. Tachycardia and hypotension** are also common and, if not corrected, progress to shock and death.

III. **Diagnosis.** The diagnosis is confirmed by **blood gas and serum electrolyte values demonstrating an anion-gap metabolic acidosis that has no other explanation.** Serum lactate levels may be directly measured, although this is not required.

IV. **Therapy.** The primary therapy is **treatment of the underlying malignancy,** since treatment of the acidosis itself, in the absence of antineoplastic therapy, is usually unsuccessful. The utility of sodium bicarbonate infusion is controversial.

ADRENAL INSUFFICIENCY

  I. **Etiology.** Although adrenal metastases are common, **bilateral adrenal metastases** causing adrenal insufficiency (Addison's disease) are rare. Other causes of adrenal insufficiency in cancer patients include **bilateral adrenalectomy,** administration of **agents with adrenal toxicity** (aminoglutethimide, mitotane, metyrapone), as well as rapid tapering of chronic glucocorticoid therapy.

 II. **Presentation.** Although adrenal insufficiency may have an insidious onset, most patients develop several signs and symptoms typical of adrenal crisis, including **weakness, anorexia, weight loss, hyperpigmentation, postural hypotension, hyponatremia, and a hyperkalemic acidosis.**

III. **Diagnosis.** The diagnosis is confirmed by the **cosyntropin (ACTH) stimulation test.** In this test, 0.25 mg of cosyntropin is administered intravenously after securing a baseline plasma cortisol level. An additional cortisol determination is obtained 60 minutes following cosyntropin injection. A cortisol increase of less than 5–7 µg/dL (total < 15 µg/dL) is considered abnormal and mandates corticosteroid replacement therapy.

IV. **Therapy.** For patients with chronic adrenal insufficiency, physiologic replacement of glucocorticoids is achieved with **cortisone acetate** (25 mg orally every morning and 12.5 mg every afternoon), while mineralocorticoid replacement, if necessary, requires **fludrocortisone** (0.05–0.1 mg/d). For acute adrenal insufficiency (adrenal crises) large doses of parenteral glucocorticoids (eg, hydrocortisone, 100 mg intravenously every 8 hours) are needed.

PARANEOPLASTIC SYNDROMES

Hypercalcemia

 I. **Etiology.** Hypercalcemia is the **most common life-threatening metabolic paraneoplastic abnormality.** It occurs in 10–20% of all patients with cancer and in 20–40% with multiple myeloma. Hypercalcemia is most common in patients with lung cancer (because of its higher prevalence), followed by breast cancer. Hypercalcemia is a consequence of (1) **tumors that produce parathormone-like proteins** (squamous carcinoma of the lung, esophagus, pharynx, larynx, genitourinary tract, and anus as well as renal cell carcinoma), (2) **tumors metastatic to bone that produce local humoral factors,** ie, prostaglandins, interleukin-1, tumor necrosis factor, transforming growth factors, platelet-derived growth factor, and colony-stimulating factors (adenocarcinoma of the breast and pancreas as well as lymphoma), (3) **tumors that produce osteoclast-activating factor** (multiple myeloma), and (4) **tumors associated with hyperparathyroidism** (pheochromocytoma, pancreatic islet cell neoplasms, and parathyroid carcinoma). **Decreased renal excretion and increased gastrointestinal absorption of calcium** are rare mechanisms of hypercalcemia.

 II. **Presentation.** Common symptoms include **fatigue, lethargy, confusion, weakness, polyuria, polydipsia, dehydration, anorexia, nausea, constipation, and pruritus.** Depending on the rapidity and extent of the calcium elevation, **electrocardiographic changes** (bradycardia, prolonged PR interval, shortened QT interval, widened T wave), **seizures, stupor,** and **coma** may develop.

 III. **Diagnosis.** The diagnosis of hypercalcemia of malignancy is confirmed by **an elevated total or ionized serum calcium level (total > 10.5 mg/dL).** Because calcium is protein bound, patients with hypoalbuminemia have spuriously low calcium levels. In such patients the severity of the hypocalcemia can be estimated by the formula: corrected calcium (mg/dl) = measured calcium + [4-albumin (gm/dl] × 0.8. Conversely, patients with multiple myeloma may have pseudohypercalcemia since elevated total serum proteins may increase the measured serum calcium erroneously. Before the diagnosis of hypercalcemia of malignancy may be made, **other conditions associated with hypercalcemia** (primary hyperparathyroidism, vitamin D intoxication, use of thiazide diuretics, milk-alkali syndrome, granulomatous diseases, immobilization, and adrenal insufficiency) must be excluded.

 IV. **Therapy.** Ideally, treatment of hypercalcemia is directed at the underlying malignancy; however, frequently the tumor is widely metastatic and refractory to available therapy. Therefore, nonspecific measures are instituted as outlined below.

 A. **General measures.** Initial steps should be taken to discontinue any oral calcium and vitamin D supplementation. In addition, thiazide diuretics, which cause increased renal calcium reabsorption, as well as nonsteroidal anti-inflammatory drugs (NSAIDs) and H_2 receptor antagonists (cimetidine, ranitidine, famotidine), which cause decreased renal blood flow, should be withdrawn. Retinoids (vitamin A) in large doses also may cause hypercalcemia and should be avoided.

 B. **Fluids.** Fluid administration constitutes the backbone of treatment for hypercalcemia. For asymptomatic patients with mild hypercalcemia (< 12.5 mg/dL), **oral fluids** (2–4 L/d above normal) may be sufficient; with more severe hypercalcemia (> 12.5 mg/dL or symptoms present), hospital admission and **intravenous hydration** is indicated. Normal saline is infused at 200–500 mL/h, depending on cardiac and renal function, to reverse dehydration and encourage calcium excretion. **Furosemide** (20–80 mg intravenously every 4–6 hours) should not be used routinely (due to the risk of dehydration) but may be added if symptoms of fluid overload develop. **Serum potassium and magnesium levels must be monitored closely** and repleted as necessary, since significant urinary losses may occur during the forced diuresis. With diuresis alone, 20–30% of patients become normocalcemic.

 C. **Phosphates.** Oral phosphate preparations have very little utility in treating hypercalcemia. Intravenous phosphate, however, rapidly normalizes serum calcium but is reserved for patients with life threatening cardiac arrhythmias because the risk of metastatic calcification is high.

D. **Corticosteroids.** Prednisone (1–2 mg/kg/d orally) or hydrocortisone (100–200 mg intravenously every 8 hours) may lower serum calcium concentrations by inhibiting bone resorption and decreasing gastrointestinal calcium absorption. The most prominent hypocalcemic action of corticosteroids is, however, their antitumor effect in multiple myeloma, leukemia, lymphoma and, in certain circumstances, breast cancer. Nearly 40% of patients with these cancers become normocalcemic following corticosteroid therapy. The success rate of corticosteroids for the treatment of hypercalcemia in patients with other cancers is much lower.

E. **Diphosphonates.** These compounds, including **ethane-1-hydroxydiphosphate (EHDP, etidronate disodium)** and the experimental agents aminohydroxybutylidene biphosphate (AHButBP) and aminohydroxypropylidene diphosphonate (APD), are analogs of pyrophosphate and inhibit bone resorption. EHDP (Didronel), given intravenously (5–7.5 mg/kg/d over 4–6 hours for 3–7 days), normalizes calcium levels in 27% of patients, but if administered orally, EHDP is less effective. Prominent side effects of EHDP consist of renal failure (acute toxicity) and osteomalacia (chronic toxicity).

F. **Calcitonin.** Salmon calcitonin (1 unit subcutaneously as a skin test followed by 200 units subcutaneously every 8–12 hours) may normalize serum calcium concentrations in 30% of patients. However, the effect is modest and brief, decreasing after 48 hours. The use of corticosteroids to prolong the effectiveness of calcitonin is *controversial.*

G. **Plicamycin (Mithracin)** (10–50 µg/kg, but usually 25 µg/kg, intravenously in 1 L of D_5W over 4–6 hours every 2–7 days) is a cytotoxic agent that kills osteoclasts and prevents bone resorption. The onset of action requires 1–2 days and lowers serum calcium to normal in 80% of patients. **Blood chemistries and cell counts must be monitored** for evidence of thrombocytopenia, hypocalcemia, renal and hepatic toxicity, and coagulopathy.

H. **Gallium nitrate.** This agent directly inhibits bone resorption. It is given as a continuous 5-day intravenous infusion (100–200 mg/m^2/d) and normalizes serum calcium levels in 75–85% of patients. The maximal effect may occur several days after the infusion is stopped. Because of the severe renal toxicity of this agent, aggressive hydration during therapy and avoidance of other nephrotoxic drugs (eg, aminoglycosides, NSAIDs) is required.

I. **Prostaglandin inhibitors.** Rarely, tumor production of prostaglandins causes hypercalcemia. This hypercalcemia is amenable to therapy with prostaglandin inhibitors (indomethacin, NSAIDs). The adverse effects of these agents on renal blood flow limit their utility, however. Currently, routine use of these drugs cannot be recommended.

Hypoglycemia

I. **Etiology.** Carcinomas that produce somatomedins with nonsuppressible insulin-like activity (NSILA) are responsible for cancer-related hypoglycemia. Hypoglycemia is commonly associated with **insulinomas** and less frequently with **mesenchymal tumors** (eg, mesothelioma, fibrosarcoma, neurofibrosarcoma, and hemangiopericytoma) hepatoma; adrenal cortical carcinoma; gastrointestinal carcinomas; and, rarely, renal cell carcinoma. Ectopic insulin production (non-islet cell tumors), excessive neoplastic glucose utilization, extensive liver disease (cancer or alcoholism), and insulin receptor proliferation have been proposed as the basis of neoplastic hypoglycemia; however, data supporting these mechanisms is lacking.

II. **Presentation.** The signs and symptoms of hypoglycemia are the same regardless of the etiology— **confusion, headache, fatigue, muscle weakness, aphasia, tremor, personality changes, palpitations, diaphoresis, seizures, and coma**—are related to the degree and rate of glucose depression. These manifestations occur during fasting or after exercise and are relieved by food intake.

III. **Diagnosis.** Once the common nonneoplastic causes of hypoglycemia (exogenous insulin and oral sulfonylurea hypoglycemic agents, adrenal insufficiency, alcoholism, and malnutrition) have been excluded, a carefully monitored 72-hour fast is performed. Over 50% of patients develop hypoglycemia (serum glucose level < 50 mg/dL) within 12 hours and over 95%, within 72 hours. However, in the presence of significant leukocytosis (> 50,000/µL) such as that which occurs in patients with acute leukemia, serum glucose levels may be falsely low (**pseudohypoglycemia**) due to metabolism of the glucose by the leukocytes.

IV. **Therapy.** For patients with mild symptoms, **frequent feedings** may be all that is necessary. With more severe hypoglycemia, **glucose** is initially administered either orally (sugar water or juice in alert patients) or intravenously ($D_{50}W$ 25 g in 50 mL in obtunded patients). In patients with insulinomas unresponsive to dietary management, **diazoxide** (200–600 mg orally) may be instituted to inhibit insulin secretion. **Glucagon, corticosteroids,** and **somatostatin** also have occasionally been used. Definitive treatment, (ie, surgery, radiation therapy, chemotherapy) is directed at the underlying tumor.

Hyperglycemia

I. **Etiology.** Although the most common causes of hyperglycemia in the cancer patient are diabetes mellitus and the exogenous administration of glucose (eg, total parenteral nutrition), rare gastrointestinal endocrine tumors (**glucagonoma** and **somatostatinoma**) as well as **pheochromocytoma** are associated with glucose intolerance.

II. **Presentation.** Patients are generally **asymptomatic;** however, in severe cases, patients may complain of typical diabetic symptoms (**polydipsia, polyphagia, polyuria, blurred vision, and fatigue**).

III. **Diagnosis.** A fasting blood sugar determination of more than 140 mg/dL is abnormal and suggests impaired glucose tolerance.

IV. **Therapy.** Management of hyperglycemia of malignancy is identical to that of diabetes mellitus. **Dietary modification** (caloric and simple sugar restriction) may be all that is required in cases of mild hyperglycemia. For moderate hyperglycemia, **oral hypoglycemic agents** such as glipizide (Glucotrol, 2.5–40 mg/d in divided doses), and glyburide (Micronase, DiaBeta; 1.25–20 mg/d in divided doses) usually provide adequate glucose control. For severe hyperglycemia, **subcutaneous insulin** administration is necessary to prevent diabetic ketoacidosis and nonketotic hyperosmolar coma.

Syndrome of Inappropriate Secretion of Antidiuretic Hormone

I. **Etiology.** Ectopic tumor production of antidiuretic hormone (ADH) or arginine vasopressin (AVP), which is normally produced by the posterior pituitary in response to hypovolemia and hyperosmolality, is responsible for the syndrome of inappropriate secretion of antidiuretic hormone (SIADH). It is characterized by hyponatremia, low serum osmolality, and inappropriate high urine sodium and osmolality. Excessive levels of serum AVP increase water resorption in the kidney, and the resulting hypervolemia triggers the release of atrial natriuretic hormone (ANH), which increases renal sodium excretion, leading to hyponatremia. SIADH occurs almost exclusively in **small cell carcinoma of the lung,** although it has been described in association with malignancies of the gastrointestinal tract, prostate, adrenal cortex, and head and neck, as well as thymomas, lymphomas, and bronchial carcinoids.

II. **Presentation.** Many patients with SIADH are **asymptomatic** and the disorder is discovered incidentally on routine blood electrolyte determinations. However, symptoms may develop depending on the rapidity and severity of the hyponatremia, and include **anorexia, nausea, lethargy, confusion, headache, weakness, seizures, coma,** and even death.

III. **Diagnosis.** The diagnosis of SIADH rests on the demonstration of (1) **hyponatremia (< 135 meq/L)** and normokalemia, (2) **low serum osmolality (< 280 mosm/L),** (3) **high urine sodium (> 20 meq/L) and osmolality (> 200 mosm/L),** (4) **no evidence of hypovolemia,** and (5) **normal cardiac, renal, hepatic, adrenal, and thyroid function.** Before a diagnosis of cancer-related SIADH can be made, other known causes of SIADH must be excluded, such as pulmonary infections, head trauma, intracranial mass lesions or infection, drugs (cyclophosphamide, vincristine, diuretics, narcotics, alcohol), acute intermittent porphyria, adrenal insufficiency, and pain.

IV. **Therapy.** Primary treatment involves **cytotoxic chemotherapy directed at the underlying malignancy** (usually small cell lung cancer); however, additional **supportive measures** may be necessary as outlined below.

A. **Fluid restriction.** Restriction of fluid to 500–1000 mL/d should be instituted immediately in all patients, and this may be adequate in patients with mild hyponatremia (> 130 meq/L). If hydration is required for chemotherapy (eg, cyclophosphamide), the serum sodium must be corrected first and then hydration accomplished with careful monitoring of serum sodium, daily weight, fluid intake, and urine output.

B. **Demeclocycline.** Large doses of demeclocycline (800–1000 mg/d orally) block the effect of AVP on the renal tubule (production of cyclicAMP) and increase free water excretion. This increases serum sodium and, in many patients, decreases the need for fluid restriction.

C. **Hypertonic saline.** In patients with severe symptoms (coma) or a serum sodium concentration of less than 110 meq/L, infusion of 3% saline (1 L every 8–12 hours) is indicated. If the serum sodium concentration is corrected too quickly, cerebral edema and intracranial herniation may occur. Therefore, the serum sodium concentration is corrected slowly, 0.5–1 meq per hour.

Syndrome of Inappropriate Adrenocorticotropic Hormone (Cushing's Syndrome)

I. **Etiology.** Ectopic tumor production of adrenocorticotropic hormone (ACTH), which is normally secreted by the pituitary, is responsible for this syndrome of hypokalemia, hyperglycemia, edema, muscle weakness, and hypertension (Cushing's syndrome). Adrenal overstimulation induces bilateral adrenal hyperplasia and hypercortisolism. Cushing's syndrome ordinarily is associated with **small cell lung cancer** (5.5% of all cases = 50% of cases of ectopic Cushing's syndrome), **bronchial and thymic carcinoids, thymomas,** and **pancreatic islet cell tumors.** Less commonly, it may occur in medullary carcinoma of the thyroid; pheochromocytoma; gastrointestinal and renal carcinoids; ovarian, prostatic, and renal cell carcinoma; rhabdomyosarcoma; and pancreatic cystadenoma. Among all cases of Cushing's syndrome, 68% are of pituitary origin, 17–27% have an adrenal cause, and 5–15% are ectopic.

II. **Presentation.** Typically, ectopic Cushing's syndrome presents with **hypokalemia, alkalosis, hyperglycemia, hypertension, edema,** and **muscle weakness.** Except with indolent tumors, other characteristic features of cortisol excess (central obesity, increased dorsal neck fat ["buffalo hump"], moon facies, abdominal striae, and hirsutism) generally are not prominent.

III. **Diagnosis.** Elevated urinary free cortisol (> 100 μg/d), fasting plasma cortisol (> 10 μg/dL), plasma ACTH concentration (> 200 pg/mL), and 8 AM plasma cortisol (> 5 μg/dL) following "high-dose" dexamethasone suppression (2 mg every 6 hours for 2 days or a single dose of 8 mg at midnight) all suggest an ectopic (extrapituitary) source of ACTH, although in 50% of patients with carcinoids that produce ACTH, cortisol is suppressed by dexamethasone administration. Other conditions that produce weakness (neuromuscular disorders), hypokalemic alkalosis (nasogastric suction, emesis, diuretic use, diarrhea, and gastrointestinal fistulas), hyperglycemia (diabetes mellitus), and edema (nephrotic syndrome, fluid overload, and malnutrition) also must be excluded.

IV. **Therapy.** The primary treatment for ectopic Cushing's syndrome is direct **antitumor therapy** (surgery, radiation, chemotherapy). This is successful in the majority of patients, but some may require **additional measures** to control the hypercortisolism, as outlined below.

   A. **Correction of hypokalemia.** Potassium losses frequently amount to 80–120 meq/d. Replacement of this amount is difficult to achieve in some patients. The potassium supplementation may be reduced by administration of a potassium-sparing diuretic (spironolactone). Unfortunately, however, very high doses are required.

   B. **Inhibition of adrenal glands.** Drugs that lower the effective cortisol concentration (**ketoconazole**) and drugs that decrease adrenal cortisol production (**aminoglutethimide, metyrapone, and mitotane**) may be necessary if attempts at tumor control are unsuccessful. These agents must be administered with great care while the patient is monitored closely for signs and symptoms of **adrenal insufficiency,** which frequently occurs following such therapy. In rare instances, **bilateral adrenalectomy** may be necessary.

REFERENCES

Ebie N, Ryan W, Harris J. Metabolic emergencies in cancer medicine. *Med Clin Nam* 1986;**70**: 1151–1166.

Narins RG, et al: Diagnostic strategies in disorders of fluid, electrolyte, and acid-base homeostasis. *Am J Med* 1982; **72**:496.

Risken RA, Heath DA, Bold AM: Hypercalcemia: A hospital survey. *Q J Med* 1980;**49**:405.

Silverman P, and Distelhorst CW: Metabolic emergencies in clinical oncology. *Semin Oncol* 1989;**16**(6):504.

16 Infectious Problems & Emergencies

Howard L. Parnes, MD, Jeffrey Miller, MD, and Robert Cameron, MD

INFECTIOUS AGENTS

Life threatening infections are common in cancer patients. The major factors contributing to this increased risk are neutropenia, decreased antibody production, deficiencies in cell mediated immunity, disruption of mucosal surfaces, and the use of chronic indwelling catheters. Although bacteria cause the majority of infections in compromised patients, fungal and viral organisms are becoming increasingly important due to the effectiveness of antibacterial therapy, longer periods of neutropenia, and alterations in microbial flora induced by antibiotics.

BACTERIA

Aerobes
I. **Gram-positive.** Although the clinical significance of gram positive organisms decreased significantly following the advent of beta-lactam penicillins, there has been a resurgence in staphylococcal infections over the past decade. This has been attributed to the emergence of antibiotic resistant organisms and the more frequent use of indwelling venous catheters. Currently, *S aureus* and *S epidermidis* are the most common bacterial isolates in cancer patients. These bacteria often require therapy with *vancomycin* because of increasing resistance to beta-lactam penicillins. Other important pathogens include *streptococcus* (alpha-hemolytic species, and *S viridans*) and *Corynebacterium*.

II. **Gram-negative.** Patients with neutropenia are at risk for serious infections due to three common gram negative organisms: *Escherichia coli, Klebsiella pneumoniae,* and *Pseudomonas aeruginosa.* In addition, the use of broad spectrum antibiotics has resulted in the selection of multi-drug resistant bacterial strains, such as *Enterobacter species, Citrobacter species, Acinetobacter species, Serratia marcescens* as well as non-aeruginosa pseudomonads.

Anaerobes
Although anaerobic bacteria rarely cause primary infections, they are frequently isolated in **mixed infections**. *Clostridium* species (*C perfringens, C septicum,* and *C tertium*) and *Bacillus* species are commonly found in mixed infections of the gastrointestinal tract. **Metronidazole and clindamycin** continue to be indicated in the treatment of these mixed infections, although 50% of *C tertium* infections are resistant to these antibiotics and require **vancomycin.**

Mycobacteria
Infections in cancer patients rarely involve *Mycobacterium* species, although catheter infections with *M chelonei* and *M fortuitum* have been documented. **Isoniazid, rifampin, streptomycin, and capreomycin** are effective antibiotics for mycobacterial infections.

FUNGI

Fungal species frequently cause serious infection in immunocompromised patients. Patients with prolonged granulocytopenia and those who have received protracted courses of broad spectrum antibiotics are particularly susceptible to fungal infections. The most common fungal pathogens are *Candida* species, *Aspergillus* species, and *Cryptococcus neoformans*. Although less common, Mucor species can cause pulmonary disease or invasive sinusitis. Empirical therapy with Amphotericin B should be strongly considered in persistently febrile, neutropenic patients due to the high prevalence of fungal infections in this setting. Amphotericin B can be administered over a period of two hours at doses ranging from 0.6 mg/kg/day (*candida* esophagitis) to 1.0–1.5 mg/kg/day (aspergillus infections). Corticosteroids administered intravenously at the start of the infusion help to decrease acute reactions (fever and chills). The administration of normal saline before and after Amphotericin infusion decreases the nephrotoxicity of this drug. Fluconazole is a new, orally administered anti-fungal agent. Fluconazole does not provide coverage against *aspergillus* and *mucor* although it is an excellent drug for the treatment of oral candidiasis. Invasive fungal infections should be treated with Amphotericin B.

VIRUSES

Viruses represent an important cause of morbidity and mortality for the immunocompromised cancer patient. The most significant viral pathogens belong to the herpes group, specifically herpes simplex virus (HSV), varicella zoster virus (VZV) and cytomegalovirus (CMV). Infection due to these pathogens may be either primary or represent reactivation of latent virus. HSV infections in patients with acute leukemia are almost exclusively recurrent infections. Similarly, the majority of CMV infections represent reactivation. Both oral and intravenous acyclovir are effective therapy for acute and chronic HSV infections. Treatment shortens the duration of viral shedding, reduces the clinical symptoms, and speeds healing. Prophylactic therapy with acyclovir in seropositive patients can substantially reduce the morbidity from chemotherapy induced viral reactivation. Doses of 250 mg/m^2 every 12 hours intravenously or 800 mg orally twice daily provide greater than 95% clinical efficacy. High dose intravenous acyclovir may decrease the probability of CMV infection in bone marrow transplant recipients. The early administration of gancyclovir also appears to prevent CMV infections in the transplant setting. For patients with CMV pneumonia, gancyclovir at a dose of 7.5 mg/kg/day coupled with intravenous immune globulin at 500 mg/kg every other day may be of major therapeutic benefit. Foscarnet also has activity against CMV and can be used to treat resistant herpes virus infections.

PARASITES

Although generally uncommon in cancer patients, parasitic infections, particularly with *Pneumocystis carinii*, are important pathogens in patients receiving corticosteroids and in AIDS patients. Infection with this organism typically produces an interstitial pneumonia. Trimethoprim-sulfamethoxazole (Bactrim, Septra) is the best drug for *P carinii* prophylaxis. This drug is given at a dose of 1 double strength tablet BID, 3 times a week. For patients allergic to sulfonamides, pentamidine may be used.

SPECIFIC SITES OF INFECTION

DERMIS

The skin represents the primary barrier to invading organisms. This barrier is frequently disrupted by the effects of surgery, radiation and chemotherapy as well as by the use of intravenous catheters. In addition, the skin is a common site for primary infections in cancer patients. This underscores the importance of good personal hygiene (including hand washing) by both the patient and health care personnel, the use of sterile technique when performing invasive procedures, including venipuncture, and careful physical examination of the skin on a regular basis. Occasionally, the dermis is involved secondarily in patients with systemic infections. Therefore, cutaneous lesions should be aggressively evaluated by aspirate, culture, and biopsy. Examination with Gram's stain (bacteria), potassium hydroxide preparation (fungi), acid fast stain (mycobacteria), Wright-Giemsa stain (Tzanck test for virus), immunofluorescence, and methylene blue stains may be helpful. The following organisms may be isolated from cutaneous lesions:

  I. **Bacteria.** *S aureus* may produce localized cellulitis or disseminated erythematous, sometimes purulent lesions that reveal clusters of gram-positive cocci on aspiration. Systemic *P aeruginosa* infection (vasculitis) occasionally manifests as round, "bull's-eye" lesions with a colorful or necrotic vesicular center (ecthyma gangrenosum), although similar lesions may occur with *Aeromonas hydrophila* and *Enterobacter* infections. *S marcescens, Nocardia,* halophilic *Vibrio,* and *Mycobacterium* infections are rarely manifested as cutaneous lesions.

II. **Fungi.** *Candida tropicalis* and other *candidal infections* may present with coin-like lesions. A multitude of other fungal infections, including *Aspergillus* organisms, *C neoformans, Histoplasma capsulatum, Phycomycetes, Mucor, Petriellidium,* and *Sporothrix schenckii* infections, also periodically have cutaneous manifestations.

III. **Viruses.** Although both CMV and rubella (measles) may produce erythematous rashes, the most important viral pathogens are the herpes viruses, particularly primary and secondary herpes zoster infection.

A. **Primary varicella.** Primary varicella (chickenpox) is caused by the varicella zoster virus (VZV) of the herpesvirus group. Varicella is primarily a disease of childhood with approximately 85% of infections occurring by age 9. Although this disease is benign and self-limited for the general population, there is a high incidence of systemic dissemination (approximately 30%) and bacterial superinfection in previously unexposed (seronegative) adult and pediatric cancer patients. Passive immunization with varicella zoster immune globulin (VZIG) reduces the incidence of pneumonitis and encephalitis and decreases the mortality associated with primary varicella from 7% to 0.5% in immunocompromised patients. It must be administered within 72 hours of exposure to be maximally effective. The current recommended dose is 1 vial/10 kg of body weight with a maximum dose of 5 vials. A single dose is protective for approximately 4 weeks. If VZIG is not available, intravenous gamma globulin may be an acceptable substitute. Isolation of infectious individuals provides the most important method of preventing VZV infection. Furthermore, individuals who have not had chickenpox but who have been exposed to this virus, should not be allowed contact with immunosuppressed patients from 1 week following the initial exposure until at least 3 weeks following the exposure.

B. **Secondary herpes zoster.** Secondary herpes zoster (zoster or shingles) is a more common viral infection among immunosuppressed adults than is primary varicella. This dermatomal cutaneous lesion is cause by reactivation of latent virus in dorsal root ganglia. Patients with Hodgkin's disease and patients who have undergone allogeneic bone marrow transplant are at highest risk for shingles (50% and 30%, respectively). One to three percent of patients with Hodgkin's disease and zoster will have viral dissemination. This most commonly involves the lungs, CNS, and liver and is associated with a mortality rate of 10%. Herpes zoster can cause substantial morbidity due to acute pain, post-herpetic neuralgia, blindness (trigeminal nerve involvement), myelitis, and secondary bacterial infections. Severe pain in the affected dermatome may precede the appearance of skin lesions and mimic an acute abdomen. VZV infection can be differentiated from other causes of vesicular rashes (vaccinia, variola, rickettsial pox, enterovirus) by Tzanck smear (multinucleated giant cells seen by Wright-Giemsa stain) or immunofluorescent staining of cells scraped from the base of a fresh vesicle. Patients undergoing autologous transplantation are also at high risk (approximately 30%) of developing zoster. Patients with non-Hodgkin's lymphoma and solid tumors have a 7–9% risk of developing zoster.

In the setting of bone marrow transplantation, oral acyclovir at a dose of 800 mg bid for a duration of 1 year appears to provide effective prophylaxis against herpes zoster. Intravenous acyclovir at a dose of 500 mg/m^2 of body surface area q8h is indicated for the treatment of herpes zoster infections in immunocompromised patients. Interferon alpha and vidarabine also have demonstrated efficacy in the treatment of this infection. Oral acyclovir is not appropriate therapy for zoster infections in immunocompromised patients due to poor oral bioavailability.

CENTRAL NERVOUS SYSTEM

CNS infections are uncommon in cancer patients but, if they occur, may be catastrophic. Symptoms typical of intracranial infection (fever, headache, dizziness, nuchal rigidity, and mental status changes) may or may not be present. Focal symptoms and seizures are common in patients with **encephalitis.** If a CNS infection is suspected, cerebrospinal fluid (CSF) should be obtained (eg, lumbar puncture, aspiration of Ommaya reservoir) and examined by Gram's (bacteria) and India ink *(C neoformans)* stains, culture (bacterial, mycobacterial, fungal, and viral), cryptococcal antigen determination, and cytologic examination. In addition, measurement of CSF glucose and total protein levels and cell counts may help distinguish **meningitis** from encephalitis (Table 16–1). If increased intracranial pressure is suspected, an intracranial mass lesion must be excluded by computed tomography or magnetic reso-

TABLE 16–1. DISTINGUISHING CLINICAL AND LABORATORY FEATURES OF MENINGITIS AND ENCEPHALITIS

Test	Meningitis	Encephalitis
Diffuse neurologic findings	Yes	Yes
Focal neurologic findings/seizures	Uncommon	Common
CSF glucose level	Low	Normal
CSF protein level	High	High
CSF cell count	Polymorphonuclear pleocytosis	Mononuclear pleocytosis

nance imaging scan prior to CSF sampling. Generally, bacteria and fungi produce meningitis, while viruses and parasites cause encephalitis.

I. **Bacteria.** Although rare in normal patients, *Listeria monocytogenes* (gram-positive rods) is the most common cause of bacterial meningitis in immunosuppressed cancer patients. **Ampicillin** is the drug of choice for this organism. Other bacterial pathogens that may cause meningitis include *P aeruginosa, S aureus, Nocardia* species, and *Mycobacterium tuberculosis*. Gram negative bacteria and fungi are responsible for the majority of brain abscesses in the cancer population.

II. **Fungi.** Approximately one-third of CNS infections in cancer patients are fungal with *cryptococcus neoformans* being the most common organism. Since India ink stain of CSF fluid detects the presence of *C neoformans,* organisms in only 50% of patients, **CSF (or serum) cryptococcal titers** are crucial. Therapy for central nervous system *cryptococcus* is Amphotericin B (0.5 mg/kg/day) and flucytosine (5-FC; 25–37.5 mg/kg orally every 6 hours) for six weeks. In immunosuppressed patients who cannot tolerate 5-FC, amphotericin can be used alone but should be continued for a minimum of 10 weeks. Maintenance therapy with fluconazole (200 mg/day) may be helpful for a long-term suppressive therapy in AIDS patients. Chronic therapy with fluconazole (200 mg/d) is started when the patient is afebrile and cultures are negative. Alternatively, **fluconazole** may be used for acute therapy instead of flucytosine.

III. **Viruses.** Herpesviruses (both HSV and VZV) are the main etiologic agents of viral encephalitis, although encephalitis due to mumps also occurs. Patients with viral encephalitis usually present with characteristic findings (Table 16–1). Although definitive diagnosis requires **brain biopsy,** positive CSF antibody titers and increased convalescent serum antibody titers (compared to acute titers) in the appropriate clinical setting are sufficient to begin therapy with **acyclovir** (500 mg/m^2 every 8 hours).

IV. **Parasites.** The intracellular parasite *Toxoplasma gondii* may present as encephalitis or as a mass lesion with typical CSF findings of encephalitis (Table 16–1). Definitive diagnosis requires demonstration of intracellular parasites on brain biopsy. Effective treatment requires either **pyrimethamine** (100 mg as a single dose, then 25 mg/d) and **sulfadiazine** (4–6 g/d) or **"triple sulfa" therapy** (sulfadiazine, sulfamethazine, and sulfamerazine) for 4–5 weeks.

RESPIRATORY SYSTEM

The upper and lower respiratory tracts are common sites for infection in immunosuppressed cancer patients.

Upper Respiratory Tract

Sinusitis is a common cause of infection in neutropenic patients. In addition, patients with tumors obstructing sinus drainage (eg, nasopharyngeal carcinoma) are at high risk for developing acute or chronic sinusitis. Although patients with sinusitis may present with localized pain, pressure, and purulent drainage, symptoms may be diminished in the neutropenic patient. Although *S pneumoniae* and *H influenza* are the most common causes of sinusitis in the normal host, gram negative organisms and anaerobic bacteria are also frequent pathogens in the neutropenic host (Table 16–2). Fungal infections with *Aspergillus* species and *Mucor* species are important causes of sinusitis in patients with prolonged durations of

TABLE 16–2. ORGANISMS THAT ARE COMMON CAUSES OF UPPER RESPIRATORY TRACT INFECTION

Infection	Organisms
Otitis externa	*Pseudomonas aeruginosa*
Otitis media	*Streptococcus pneumoniae, Hemophilus influenzae*
Sinusitis	*Streptococcus pneumoniae, Hemophilus influenzae, Branhamella catarrhalis*
Epiglottitis	*Hemophilus influenzae*

myelosuppression who have received broad spectrum antibiotics. Amphotericin B is required for the treatment of fungal sinusitis.

Lower Respiratory Tract

The lungs represent an important source of serious infections in the cancer patient. Immunosuppressed cancer patients are susceptible to a wide variety of organisms and may present with a minimum of signs and symptoms since neutrophils are an important component of the inflammatory response. In patients with pulmonary infiltrates detected by chest x-ray studies, empiric, broad spectrum antibiotics should be initiated. If the patient does not have a favorable clinical response, bronchoalveolar lavage or open lung biopsy are indicated. Material obtained by these procedures should be cultured for bacterial, viral, and fungal pathogens. In addition, the specimen should be examined with gram stain (bacteria), acid fast stain (mycobacteria), and methenamine silver stain (P. carinii).

  I. **Bacteria.** Bacterial pneumonia remains a significant problem in cancer patients. A large number of bacterial pathogens are responsible for pulmonary infections in this population. In addition to organisms which commonly cause pneumonia in the non-compromised patient (*Streptococcus pneumoniae, Hemophilus influenzae*), the possibility of other gram positive bacteria, gram negatives and a variety of uncommon organisms must be considered. Infections with *mycobacteria* and *nocardia* are increasing in frequency and are associated with significant mortality. *Legionella, Mycoplasma*, and *Chlamydia* are uncommon causes of diffuse interstitial pneumonitis in the granulocytopenic host.

 II. **Fungi.** Fungal infections are a major cause of mortality in patients with prolonged periods of neutropenia. *Candida* is the most common fungal infection followed by *Aspergillus*. Due to the frequency and seriousness of fungal pneumonia, granulocytopenic patients who develop a new infiltrate on chest radiograph while on antibiotics should receive Amphotericin B empirically. A definitive diagnosis usually requires an invasive procedure to obtain tissue, however, this is not always feasible. Positive blood cultures for *Candida* are unlikely despite the presence of invasive or disseminated infection. Endophthalmitis (white, fluffy retinal lesions) has been associated with disseminated candidiasis. *Aspergillosis* is characterized by blood vessel invasion and causes a necrotizing bronchopneumonia and the potential for life threatening hemoptysis. Dissemination (sinuses, CNS, liver, kidney, skin, heart valves) occurs in up to 30% of patients, however, blood cultures are rarely positive. Additional fungal pathogens include the *Phycomycetes* (*Mucor* and *Rhizopus*), histoplasmosis, *Coccidioides immitis, Cryptococcus neoformans, Torulopsis glabrate, Trichosporon, Fusarium, and Pseudoallecheria boydii*. Amphotericin B is the treatment of choice for invasive fungal disease. It is important to administer adequate saline hydration to minimize nephrotoxicity and patients must be monitored closely for the development of hypokalemia and hypomagnesemia. Fluconazole is a new, oral anti-fungal agent, with activity against *Candida* and *Cryptococcus* but not *Aspergillus*. This drug should not be used alone for the treatment of invasive fungal infections.

III. **Viruses**

   A. **CMV pneumonia** is the most important viral infection of the lower respiratory tract. It occurs within 4 months of bone marrow transplantation in 20% of patients with hematologic malignancies undergoing this procedure and has an 85–90% fatality rate. Diagnosis can be made using centrifugation cultures and monoclonal antibody staining of specimens obtained by bronchoalveolar lavage. The sensitivity and specificity of this approach is nearly 100%. Treatment with acyclovir, gancyclovir, vidarabine, and interferon alpha has been largely unsuccessful. However, gancyclovir in combination with intravenous immunoglobulin has resulted in significant clinical benefit. A clinical response rate of 52% has been reported for this combination therapy. The Memorial Sloan Kettering trial utilized gancyclovir at a dose of 7.5 mg/kg/day plus intravenous gamma globulin at 500 mg/kg every other day for a total treatment course of 20 days. Gancyclovir was continued at a dose of 5 mg/kg/day 3–5 days a week for 20 further doses, while intravenous immunoglobulin was continued at a dose of 500 mg/kg twice a week, for eight further doses. The use of **seronegative blood products** for seronegative bone marrow transplant recipients is the best method of preventing this infection.

   B. **Other Viruses.** Other viral causes of diffuse pneumonia include HSV, VZV, rubella (German measles), influenza, parainfluenza, rhinovirus, adenovirus, and respiratory syncytial virus (RSV). Bronchaleolar lavage or open lung biopsy is required for diagnosis of these less common causes of viral pneumonia. HSV and VZV may be successfully treated with acyclovir (500 mg/m^2 every 8 hours). The diagnosis of these infections may be difficult since positive respiratory cultures may be due to viral shedding from the oral cavity and lavage fluid showing multi-nucleated giant cells is not specific.

IV. **Parasites.** *Pneumocystis carinii* is an important cause of pneumonia in immuno-compromised patients. This infection is most commonly associated with hematologic malignancies, AIDS and in patients receiving corticosteroids. Fever, cough, tachycardia and tachypnea are the characteristic manifestations in non-AIDS patients. The diagnosis is confirmed by observation of **trophozoites** in methenamine silver-stained specimens obtained by BAL or open lung biopsy. The infection is treated with **trimethoprim-sulfamethoxazole** (Bactrim, Septra) (20 mg/kg/d); **pentamidine** (4 mg/kg/d) should be used for sulfonamide-sensitive individuals. Disseminated *Toxoplasma gondii* and *Strongyloides stercoralis* rarely cause pulmonary infections.

CARDIOVASCULAR SYSTEM

Serious infections of the cardiovascular system, albeit uncommon, are increasing in frequency due to the proliferation of indwelling venous catheters.

   I. **Intravenous catheters.** Indwelling venous catheters are associated with significant morbidity, particularly catheter related infections. *Staphylococcus aureus* is the most common pathogen responsible for catheter related infections. However, other gram positive bacteria, gram negative organisms and candida may be involved. Catheter removal is often unnecessary in treating catheter related infections. However, patients with fungemia, infections that extend along the subcutaneous ("tunnel infection") and those with persistently positive blood cultures should have their catheters removed.

   II. **Endocarditis.** Subacute bacterial endocarditis (SBE) in cancer patients is identical to that in immunocompetent patients, presenting with fever, chills, night sweats, weight loss, heart murmur, splinter hemorrhages, Roth's spots, Janeway lesions, splenomegaly, and other characteristic symptoms and signs. Endocarditis in immunosuppressed cancer patients, however, is associated not only with gram-positive bacteria (*Streptococcus viridans, Enterococcus* species, and *S aureus*) but also with gram-negative bacteria (*P aeruginosa*), fungi (*Candida* and *Aspergillus* species), parasites (*Toxoplasma gondii*), and viruses. Viral SBE is much harder to treat successfully, and fungal SBE frequently requires valve replacement. *Streptococcus bovis* is another pathogen that can cause SBE; it is associated with an underlying gastrointestinal malignancy, usually colon cancer.

GASTROINTESTINAL SYSTEM

Infections of the gastrointestinal system are responsible for 20–30% of all infections in cancer patients that lead to sepsis. Opportunistic infections occur frequently. Standard intra-abdominal infections (eg, appendicitis, cholecystitis, diverticulitis) may also occur, but due to immunosuppression, often manifest with atypical symptoms.

Oropharynx

The mouth is an important source of infection for patients receiving chemotherapy. Bacteria, viruses, and fungi are responsible for the majority of these infections. With the wide spread use of broad spectrum antibiotics, fungal overgrowth and invasive fungal infections are increasingly common. *Candida* species are the most common offending organism. Oral candidiasis can be treated with clotrimazole troches (10 mg 5 times daily). For severe infection unresponsive to oral antifungal agents, amphotericin B should be utilized until the granulocyte count has recovered. Fluconazole may be an acceptable alternative for the treatment of oral candidiasis. It is important to culture these lesions for the presence of herpes simplex virus due to the high prevalence of viral reactivation in cancer patients undergoing chemotherapy. Acyclovir (250 mg/m^2 intravenously every 8 hours) is effective therapy for HSV infection.

Esophagus

Esophagitis may have an infectious etiology or may be a sequela of radiation or chemotherapy. Infectious esophagitis can be caused by fungal, viral or bacterial organisms in the granulocytopenic patient. In this setting, *candida* and HSV are the most common causes. In the febrile, granulocytopenic patient with odynophagia, EGD (esophagogastroduodenoscopy) is a valuable diagnostic tool. Invasive fungal infection should be treated with amphotericin B in granulocytopenic patients. Acyclovir provides an effect therapy for HSV esophagitis.

Liver

I. **Bacteria.** Bacterial infections of the liver (hepatic abscesses) may occur via hematogenous seeding. Gram positive, gram negative or anaerobic bacteria may be involved. Percutaneous catheter drainage or surgical drainage may be required in addition to antibiotic therapy.

II. **Fungi.** The diagnosis of hepatosplenic candidiasis should be considered in a patient with persistent fever following recovery of the granulocyte count. Additional characteristic findings include right upper quadrant pain and increased serum alkaline phosphatase. The majority of symptoms occur following bone marrow recovery. Liver biopsy is necessary for confirmation of the diagnosis. Treatment consists of high dose amphotericin therapy (1.0–1.5 mg/kg per day to a total dose of 2.5 gm). The addition of flucytosine may be beneficial.

III. **Virus.** Viral hepatitis is particularly prevalent among patients with hematologic malignancies due to the large number of transfusions that these patients require. Non-A, Non-B (NANB) hepatitis is most frequently caused by hepatitis C and is the most common transfusion related hepatitis. Patients with NANB hepatitis are often anicteric and tend to present with a less severe acute illness than those with hepatitis B infection. The risk of developing chronic hepatitis following NANB infection is approximately 60%. In patients with hematologic malignancies, chronic NANB hepatitis is more likely to progress to cirrhosis than in the non-immunosuppressed patients. Therapy with interferon alpha (2 × 10^6 units subcutaneously 3 × weekly for 6 months) may be beneficial.

Small and Large Intestine

I. **Bacteria.** *Clostridium difficile* infection is an important cause of antibiotic-associated colitis (AAD). The administration of chemotherapy also predisposes patients to infection with this organism. The presence of *C difficile* toxin should be demonstrated in the stool to confirm this diagnosis. Patients with *C difficile* colitis should be isolated to prevent the spread of this infection to other patients. Treatment includes vancomycin (125–250 mg orally 4 times a day) or metronidazole (250 mg orally 4 times daily).

   A. **Traditional pathogens** (ie, *Salmonella, Shigella*, and *Campylobacter* species) that occur in noncancer patients also occur in cancer patients and should be treated with **ciprofloxacin** (500 mg twice daily) for 5–7 days.

   B. **Typhlitis.** Typhlitis or **necrotizing enterocolitis** is an inflammatory condition involving the cecum (see p 72). This infection is most commonly observed in patients with acute leukemia with prolonged periods of granulocytopenia and is associated with a 30–40% mortality rate. It is characterized by right lower quadrant pain, fever and diarrhea. Gram-negative bacteria, particularly *P aeruginosa* are most commonly implicated. In addition to broad spectrum antibiotic therapy, surgical resection of necrotic bowel may be required.

   C. Rarely, *Clostridia* species *(C perfringens, C septicum,* and *C tertium)* are responsible for **fulminant peritonitis** (with abdominal wall ecchymosis and crepitus) in children with ALL. This antibiotic-resistant disorder should be treated with **vancomycin.** Note: AAD, necrotizing enterocolitis, and *Clostridia* peritonitis all occur in the setting of prolonged broad-spectrum antibiotic administration and neutropenia.

II. **Parasites.** Fever, nausea, vomiting, diarrhea and abdominal pain characterize the *hyperinfection syndrome,* a highly lethal disease caused by *Strongyloides stercoralis.* The diagnosis is confirmed by documentation of fecal larvae. In the immunocompromised patient, treatment with thiabendazole (25 mg/kg twice daily for 2–3 weeks) is indicated.

Rectum

Perirectal cellulitis and abscess are common causes of infection in the granulocytopenic patient. For this reason, a careful rectal examination is mandatory in granulocytopenic patients with fever. Gram negative bacteria, group D *streptococci* and anaerobes are common pathogens. In addition to broad spectrum antibiotic therapy, sitz baths and stool softeners are helpful supportive measures. Surgical intervention is rarely necessary. It is often helpful to place the patient with a perirectal abscess on parenteral nutrition to allow bowel rest and permit healing.

GENITOURINARY SYSTEM

Urinary tract infections are relatively uncommon in the granulocytopenic patient. However, this source must be considered in patients with urinary obstruction.

FEBRILE NEUTROPENIA

Fever (temperature greater than 100.4°F or 38°C) in the neutropenic patient (absolute neutrophil count less than 1,000 per mm^3) is associated with significant mortality if left untreated. It has therefore become standard practice to institute empiric broad spectrum antibiotic therapy in this setting.

  I. **Diagnostic workup.** It is important to remember that the classic signs and symptoms of infection may be diminished or absent in the granulocytopenic patient since the granulocyte is responsible for much of the inflammatory response. Keeping this in mind, a thorough history and physical examination should be performed with special attention to the skin, venipuncture sites, intravenous catheters, biopsy sites, mouth and oral pharynx, sinus, lungs, abdomen and anus. Before beginning antibiotics, blood and urine cultures should be obtained. It is important to obtain cultures from a peripheral site in addition to obtaining blood from each lumen of all indwelling catheters. Cultures of skin and mucosal lesions should also be obtained. A chest radiograph and, particularly in patients with acute leukemia, sinus radiographs should be performed.
 II. **Therapy**
   A. **Antibiotics.** Broad spectrum antibiotics should be started immediately after cultures have been obtained. Standard initial antibiotic regimens consist of combinations of antibiotics to provide double coverage against the virulent gram negative pathogens. Such coverage has traditionally included an aminoglycoside and either a beta-lactam penicillin or a third generation cephalosporin. In order to avoid the nephrotoxicity associated with aminoglycosides, double beta-lactam therapy, eg, piperacillin plus ceftazidime may be utilized. Some authors have advocated the use of single agent antibiotic therapy (monotherapy) with either ceftazidime or imipenen. Patients receiving only one antibiotic may require more frequent adjustments in their antibiotic regimen and must be watched particularly closely. There is little data to support the use of empiric vancomycin as part of the initial empiric antibiotic therapy. The duration of antibiotic therapy is dependent upon the patient's clinical course.
   B. **Antifungal Agents.** Although the issue of empiric antifungal therapy is somewhat controversial, most investigators recommend the institution of empiric amphotericin for neutropenic patients with persistent fever despite seven days of broad spectrum antibiotics. Following a test dose of 1 mg given over 1 hour, the dose should be increased to 0.5 mg/kg per day.
   C. **C-Colony stimulating factors (CSF).** Growth factors such as G-CSF at a dose of 5 μg/kg/day subcutaneously have been shown to shorten the period of neutropenia and to decrease the number of febrile episodes requiring hospitalization. Therapy with growth factors has not however, been demonstrated to decrease the incidence of infections or to improve survival. The utility of growth factor therapy to allow the administration of higher doses of chemotherapy is an area of active investigation.

PARANEOPLASTIC FEVER

Nearly 5% of cancer patients are found to have fever stemming solely from their cancer. Cancers associated with paraneoplastic fever include **Hodgkin's disease, renal cell carcinoma, osteogenic sarcoma,** and **myxomas.** The diagnosis is one of exclusion and is suggested by fever that correlates with progressive tumor growth and disappears with successful therapy (surgery, radiation therapy, or chemotherapy). **Endogenous pyrogens** produced by either neoplastic cells or normal cells incorporated in the tumor have been implicated in the pathogenesis of this paraneoplastic syndrome.

REFERENCES

Crawford J et al: Reduction by granulocyte colony-stimulating factor of fever and neutropenia induced by chemotherapy in patients with small-cell lung cancer. *N Engl J Med* 1991;315:164.

Morstyn G et al: Effect of granulocyte colony-stimulating factor on neutropenia induced by cytotoxic chemotherapy. *Lancet* March 26, 1988.

Pizzo PA. Drug therapy: Management of fever in patients with cancer and treatment induced neutropenia. *NEJM* 328:1323, 1993.

Wade JC. Management of infection in patients with acute leukemia. *Hematology/Oncology Clinics of North America* 7:293, 1993.

Rubin M, Walsh TJ, Pizzo PA. Clinical approach to infections in the compromised host. In *Hematologic Malignancies*, pp 1063.

Wade JC. Viral infections among patients with hematologic malignancies. In PH Wiernik, GP Canellos, RA Kyle, CA Shiffer (eds). *Neoplastic Diseases of the Blood, 2nd Ed.* New York: Churchill Livingston, 1991;817–852.

17 Orthopedic Problems & Emergencies

Gregory Chow, MD

BONE METASTASES

Nearly all malignancies can metastasize to bone, and **50–80% of patients with breast, lung, kidney, prostate, gastrointestinal, and thyroid cancers develop bone metastases**. Although bone metastases are generally not life-threatening, they are usually painful, thereby greatly affecting the quality of the cancer patient's life. As cancer therapy and survival have improved the incidence of bone metastases has increased.

- I. **Clinical evaluation.** The possibility of bone metastases must be considered in all cancer patients who complain of **pain in the spine, extremities, ribs, or sternum** or who have recent onset of **ambulatory dysfunction**.
  - A. **Medical history.** Typically, pain is **well localized** and **occurs with activity**. A prior diagnosis of cancer may not have been made, so that the discovery of a metastatic bone lesion may be the **initial diagnostic finding** of occult malignancy, particularly in patients with lung cancer. **Spinal metastases** may cause extremity weakness, paresthesias, and bowel or bladder dysfunction, or all of these symptoms.
  - B. **Physical examination.** Although localized swelling is sometimes noted in a slender patient, **point tenderness on deep palpation** is often present. Limitations in the range of motion (ROM) of all affected joints must be documented and should be compared to the ROM of the contralateral side (remember to check hip and shoulder rotational motions, abduction, and adduction). **Tenderness with joint ROM and exertion should be identified**. Motor strength, sensation, and deep tendon reflexes must be checked.
  - C. **Laboratory tests.** Serum **calcium, phosphorus, and alkaline phosphatase** levels should be measured. They are often elevated in patients with bone metastases.
  - D. **Imaging studies**
    1. **Plain film x-rays.** Good quality conventional x-rays of the affected area **in at least 2 planes** (anteroposterior and lateral) must be obtained (oblique views of the spine also should be included); however, x-rays are often normal because they cannot detect an abnormality until **more than 50% of bone density is lost**.
    2. **Technetium-99m bone scan.** These are the most sensitive and cost-effective tests for documenting bone metastases, although they have a **10% false-positive rate**.
    3. **Other imaging studies.** CT and MRI scans are not routinely indicated unless spinal metastases are present and are associated with neurologic dysfunction. In these circumstances, myelography also should be obtained.
- II. **Management of long bone metastases.** Bone lesions are often discovered incidentally. Purely **osteoblastic lesions**, such as those from prostate cancer, are **often asymptomatic**. Lesions that do not cause pain or systemic effects (ie, hypercalcemia) may be managed by observation alone and do not require specific treatment. Moderately painful lesions often respond to radiation therapy, systemic chemotherapy, hormonal therapy, or all of these. However, severely painful lesions warrant special intervention to preserve function, ease nursing care, and improve the quality of life.
  - A. **Nonoperative management.** Immobilization by **splinting, casting, cast bracing, or bed rest** is essential for pain relief and healing. Because bone exposed to systemic chemotherapy or local irradiation heals slowly, **immobilization periods generally are 2–3 times longer** for pathologic and impending pathologic fractures than for conventional traumatic fractures.
  - B. **Operative management. Rigid internal fixation provides pain relief and eliminates the need for immobilization measures;** however, standard fixation techniques must be modified (eg, augmented with methylmethacrylate) to improve sta-

bility in diseased bone. Periarticular fractures are often treated best by artificial joint replacement.

1. **Selection of surgical candidates.** The following guidelines should be considered in selecting patients for surgical management:
   a. **Life expectancy.** This should be more than 3 weeks.
   b. **Anesthesia.** The patient must be able to tolerate general anesthesia.
   c. **Mental obtundation.** An inability to appreciate pain may negate the need to palliate bone metastases.
   d. **Hematopoietic compromise.** Chemotherapy- or radiation-induced bone marrow suppression that would compromise host immunity during the immediate postoperative period is a contraindication to operation. Local irradiation of surgical wounds (**up to 3500 cGy**) is well tolerated and is *not* a contraindication to surgery

2. **Surgical indications**
   a. **Pathologic fracture.** Most painful pathologic fractures amenable to surgical stabilization should be treated **operatively** regardless of life expectancy.
   b. **Failure of conservative therapy.** Surgery is indicated for any painful, surgically amenable metastasis that is not palliated by irradiation, chemotherapy, or hormonal therapy.
   c. **Impending pathologic fractures.** These should be internally fixed prophylactically to prevent patient distress and inconvenience. No absolute criteria for identifying impending fractures exists; however, guidelines for identifying high-risk lesions are (1) **destruction of more than 50% of the cortex in long bones,** (2) lytic **lesions involving more than 2.5 cm of the cortex,** and (3) painful intramedullary lytic **lesions consisting of more than 50% of the cross-sectional diameter** of the bone.

3. **Surgical technique.** The goals of surgery are to provide **immediate, lasting rigid fixation** for both pain relief and for early patient mobilization. Diseased bone frequently does not heal; therefore, implanted devices must bear stress for an extended period—often for 1–2 years. **Methylmethacrylate cement** is a useful adjunct to fill voids created by tumor resection, improve the strength of fixation, and make postoperative immobilization unnecessary. Nearly **90% of patients achieve excellent pain relief and return of function**. Radiation therapy (3500–4000 cGy) is administered routinely following surgery to control tumor growth. If indicated, chemotherapy also may be instituted 2–3 weeks postoperatively.
   a. **Upper extremity.** A fixation device (either an **intramedullary device such as a Rush rod or an osteosynthesis plate and screws**) appropriate for the location is selected. Intramedullary devices are technically easy to implant; however, they do not provide rigid rotational stability and are known to **loosen or migrate in 5–15% of cases,** causing pain and loss of fixation from impingement of the device on other structures. Methylmethacrylate should be used to improve fixation whenever possible. Proximal lesions that are close to or involve the shoulder joint are best treated by **cemented prosthetic replacement**.
      (1) **Preparation. Lesions are exposed and thoroughly curetted** to remove as much tumor as possible. Normal cortex is preserved, even if only a thin shell remains.
      (2) **Intramedullary devices.** The appropriate size is selected and the **insertion site is exposed**. First, the gaps and intramedullary canal are filled with methylmethacrylate. Then, **while the methylmethacrylate is still soft, the device is inserted.**
      (3) **Osteosynthesis plate and screws. The intramedullary canal is reamed proximally and distally** with curettes. Then, **methylmethacrylate is placed in the void** created by the tumor and pressurized into the canal as far proximally and distally as possible. The **plate is then fixed with screws** using standard technique.
   b. **Lower extremity.** Postoperatively, **pain relief and ambulation are achieved in more than 90% of patients,** thus easing nursing care and facilitating transfer activities such as bed to wheelchair to bathroom and so forth. **Fifty percent of patients who are not ambulatory before surgery can be expected to regain the ability to walk after surgery**. Technical aspects of surgery are similar to those for the upper extremity.
      (1) **Tibial and femoral diaphyses.** Like lesions in the upper extremity, le-

sions of the tibial and femoral diaphyses can be stabilized by **plate and screw or intramedullary fixation**. However, unlike the procedure for the upper extremity, intramedullary devices can be sized exactly to the reamed canal and locked proximally and distally with screws to provide rotational stability. Intramedullary nailing may be accomplished without exposing the tumor site (**closed**). Intramedullary reaming removes most of the tumor focus without spreading tumor cells. Methylmethacrylate may not be necessary but, if used, can be inserted via the canal using a cement delivery gun or be placed directly through the open fracture site. **All devices should be locked with screws** if cortices are compromised by tumor or osteoporosis or if additional rotational stability is needed.

- (2) **Femoral neck and acetabulum.** Lesions in these regions are best treated by **hip arthroplasty**. Isolated femoral neck lesions with intact acetabular cartilage can be treated by **cemented bipolar hemiarthroplasty**. If acetabular cartilage is damaged or if metastases are present in the acetabulum, **cemented total hip arthroplasty** is the treatment of choice. The metastatic lesion(s) may compromise prosthesis fixation and must be completely removed. This may be achieved by excising a femoral neck lesion or by thoroughly curetting the lesion from the acetabulum. Acetabular reconstruction may require a custom prosthesis or mesh reinforcement. **Cemented arthroplasty allows for immediate, pain-free weight bearing** and should provide durability for the remainder of the patient's lifetime.
- (3) **Intertrochanteric femoral lesions.** These metastases may be managed as femoral neck lesions: that is, treated with **prosthetic replacement**. Alternatively, they may be **internally fixed using a compression screw-plate device** supplemented with methylmethacrylate.
- (4) **Subtrochanteric femoral lesions.** Fractures of the subtrochanteric region of the femur generally heal slowly because of poor vascularity and high stress forces in the area. However, pathologic or impending pathologic fractures that are well fixed will allow for **ambulatory function in 65–85% and pain relief in 90% of patients** even though the fracture may not heal.
    - (a) **Zickel intramedullary appliance.** This device, used with or without methylmethacrylate, has proved to be effective in treating subtrochanteric metastatic lesions.
    - (b) **Condylar blade plate and screws.** A 95-degree angled condylar blade plate and screws augmented with methylmethacrylate can be used instead of the Zickel device, although placement is technically more demanding.
    - (c) **Intramedullary nail.** An interlocking intramedullary nail also may be an appropriate alternative for fractures and lesions in this area.

III. **Management of spinal metastases.** The spine is the **site of metastatic disease in up to 70% of all patients**. The majority of cases, however, are **asymptomatic** and require no treatment. Symptomatic involvement of the spine ranges from **minor pain** that resolves spontaneously to **paralysis and irreversible loss of bowel or bladder control or both**. The clinical and radiographic evaluation of patients with spinal metastases is described on p 100, I. Frequently, biopsy is required prior to therapeutic intervention to establish the diagnosis of malignant spinal involvement. Although this may be obtained by radiographically guided needle biopsy; however, more commonly, **surgical biopsy is necessary**. A posterior transpedicular approach is frequently used for surgical biopsy.

- A. **Compression fractures**
    1. **Compression fractures of the thoracic and lumbar spine** are a common and painful complication of spinal metastasis. Although they are painful, the **spine is stable** and neither surgical intervention nor braces are necessary. Irradiation, chemotherapy, and hormonal therapy directed at the tumor, as well as **symptomatic management of the pain**, should be instituted. Pain should resolve within 3–4 weeks if the tumor responds to treatment. **Transcutaneous electric nerve stimulation (TENS)** has been shown to aid in pain relief.
    2. **Cervical compression fractures are often unstable** and require bracing for stability while the tumor is treated.
- B. **Neurologic dysfunction.** CT scan with myelography or MRI scan is essential if neurologic dysfunction is present. **Neurologic dysfunction implies instability of the bony structures**. The anterior elements (ie, the vertebral bodies) are most frequently involved.

C. **Surgical intervention.** Surgery plays an infrequent role in the treatment of spinal metastases. An experienced orthopedic spine surgeon must be involved in making the operative decisions. If surgery is used, pain relief is excellent in **90% of patients**, and **80% of patients who are nonambulatory** because of spinal metastases can be expected to regain ambulatory function. Neurologic complications from surgery are reported to be **extremely rare (< 5% of patients)**.
   1. **Decompressive posterior laminectomy.** This procedure **is usually not indicated** because metastases frequently are anterior and the **posterior elements may be the only bony structures providing stability to the spine**. Patients subjected to this procedure are often bedridden until death occurs.
   2. **Anterior stabilization.** This is the procedure of choice for the surgical treatment of spinal metastases and involves **resection of the tumor and vertebral body, if necessary, as well as anterior instrumentation and stabilization**. Methylmethacrylate should be used to fill spaces left by vertebrectomy.
   3. **Laminectomy with posterior stabilization.** If the posterior elements are involved with tumor or if **life expectancy exceeds 1–2 years, laminectomy with posterior stabilization** is indicated. **Bone grafting** is performed as a second-stage procedure after appropriate irradiation or chemotherapy.

RADIATION-INDUCED ORTHOPEDIC COMPLICATIONS

The biologic effect of radiation on tissue depends on the magnitude of the absorbed dose (see Chapter 4). Superficial surfaces of bone absorb much larger amounts of radiation than the surrounding soft tissues, especially when orthovoltage radiation is used. **The risk to bone is less with megavoltage radiation**; however, most bone changes have been shown to occur when the absorbed dose reaches **4000–10,000 cGy**.

I. **Atrophic changes and osteitis.** These pathologic processes are similar. Ewing first described **"radiation osteitis"** in an irradiated bone with a nonhealing pathologic fracture. Currently, the problem is termed **"radiation osteitis"** only if inflammation can be demonstrated, whereas the term **"radiation bone atrophy"** is reserved for other conditions.
   A. **Severity.** The severity of radiation atrophy ranges from mild through moderate to severe. Mild changes include **diffuse demineralization, cortical thickening, and coarsening of the trabecular pattern**; moderate changes involve problems such as **cystic lesions with a sclerotic rim**; and severe changes involve **complete loss of trabecular bone, often accompanied by osteonecrosis**.
   B. **Incidence.** No good data exists regarding the true incidence of radiation atrophy. Mild-to-moderate changes may be seen in as many as **80% of patients who have received orthovoltage radiation**. Megavoltage radiation is less damaging, resulting in a **20% incidence of mild changes**.
   C. **Clinical manifestations.** Symptoms and radiographic changes associated with irradiation usually occur from **1–3 years after exposure**. Patients may be asymptomatic, may complain of pain, or may present with pathologic fractures. The differential diagnosis must include **metastatic lesions and radiation-induced sarcoma**. Biopsy may be necessary for a definitive diagnosis.
   D. **Management.** Pathologic and impending pathologic fractures should be managed as described above on p 100, **II**.

II. **Radiation-induced sarcoma (RIS).** RIS of bone is **extremely rare**. Its overall incidence in patients who survive 5 years after cancer the diagnosis is **0.035%**. In the past, RIS was often identified in patients who had received radiation to benign bony abnormalities (eg, giant cell tumors). Because of this, irradiating benign lesions is no longer standard practice.
   A. **Diagnostic criteria.** There are strict criteria for a diagnosis of RIS, which are as follows: (1) there must be **radiographic or histologic evidence that the bone was normal** before irradiation, (2) the sarcoma must arise in a region that was **within the irradiated field**, (3) an **asymptomatic period of 5 years** must have passed since radiation ended, and (4) there must be **histological confirmation** of sarcoma.
   B. **Histology. Osteosarcoma** is, by far, the most common histologic type of RIS. Others are malignant fibrous histiocytoma, fibrosarcoma, chondrosarcoma, and spindle cell sarcoma.
   C. **Therapy.** Management must be aggressive and include surgical resection (including amputation, if necessary) and chemotherapy (see p 411, **IX**).
   D. **Prognosis.** The prognosis for these tumors is extremely poor—the **5-year survival rate is 10–20%**.

REFERENCES

Bragg DG et al: The clinical and radiographic aspects of radiation osteitis. *Radiology* 1970;**97:**103–111.

Colyer RA: Surgical stabilization of pathological neoplastic fractures. *Curr Probl Cancer* 1986; **10:**119–168.

Douglass HO, Shukla SK, Mindell E: Treatment of pathological fractures of long bones excluding those due to breast cancer. *J Bone Joint Surg* 1976;**58A:**1055–1060.

Habermann ET, Lopez RA: Metastatic disease of bone and treatment of pathological fractures. *Orthop Clin North Am* 1989;**20:**469–486.

Harrington KD et al: Methylmethacrylate as an adjunct in internal fixation of pathological fractures. *J Bone Joint Surg* 1976;**58A:**1047–1054.

Harrington KD (editor): *Orthopedic Management of Metastatic Bone Disease.* St. Louis, MO: CV Mosby; 1988.

Howland WJ et al: Postirradiation atrophic changes of bone and related complications. *Radiology* 1975;**117:**677–685.

Lewallen RP, Pritchard DJ, Sim FH: Treatment of pathologic fractures or impending fractures of the humerus with Rush rods and methylmethacrylate. *Clin Orthop* 1982;**166:**193–198.

McAfee PC, Zdeblick TA: Tumors of the thoracic and lumbar spine: surgical treatment via the anterior approach. *J Spinal Disorders* 1989;**2:**145–154.

Harrington KD (editor): *Orthopedic Management of Metastatic Bone Disease.* St. Louis, MO: CV Mosby; 1988.

Sim FH (editor): *Diagnosis and Management of Metastatic Bone Disease: A Multi-disciplinary Approach.* New York: Raven Press; 1988.

Smith J: Radiation-induced sarcoma of bone: clinical and radiographic findings in 43 patients irradiated for soft tissue neoplasms. *Clin Radiol* 1982;**33:**205–221.

Tountas AA et al: Postirradiation sarcoma of bone. *Cancer* 1979;**43:**182–187.

Yazawa Y et al: Metastatic bone disease. *Clin Orthop* 1990;**251:**213–219.

Zickel RE, Mouradian WH: Intramedullary fixation of pathological fractures and lesions of the subtrochanteric region of the femur. *J Bone Joint Surg* 1976;**58A:**1061.

18 Dermatologic Problems & Emergencies

Howard L. Pames, MD, Jeffrey Miller, MD, and Robert B. Cameron, MD

COMPLICATIONS OF THERAPY FOR MALIGNANT DISEASE

ALOPECIA

Hair loss (**alopecia**) is the most common and the most visible and psychologically traumatic dermatologic side effect of irradiation and chemotherapy. Severe alopecia almost always occurs as a side effect of **doxorubicin and cyclophosphamide** administration and is frequently observed as a side effect of ifosfamide, 5-fluorouracil, dactinomycin, daunorubicin, bleomycin and vindesine. It is occasionally associated with mechlorethamine, thiotepa, methotrexate, vinblastine, vincristine, etoposide, BCNU and hydroxyurea. Alopecia is rarely observed as a complication of busulfan, chlorambucil, melphalan, cytarabine, deoxycoformycin, mithramycin, mitomycin C, CCNU, L-asparignase, cisplatin, DTIC, hexamethylamine, and procarbazine. Hair in any location, including the scalp, face, axillas, chest, abdomen, pubic area and legs, may be affected. Open discussion of alopecia and abatement methods with the patient and immediate family prior to the institution of therapy may minimize the emotional trauma associated with hair loss.

   I. **Kinetics.** Alopecia is dose-dependent and, except with high doses of radiation, is nearly always reversible. With **chemotherapy-induced alopecia,** hair loss starts 1–2 weeks following administration of adequate doses of cytotoxic agents (> 50 mg/m^2 doxorubicin; > 500 mg/m^2 cyclophosphamide), peaks in 1–2 months, and is followed by hair regeneration. **Radiation-induced alopecia** generally begins after 500 cGy has been administered and peaks in 2 months. Hair regeneration may begin 8–9 weeks following the end of therapy, however, following high dose radiation hair loss is often permanent.

  II. **Prevention of alopecia.** Hair loss may be prevented by decreasing blood flow to the scalp during and immediately after chemotherapy administration. Either of 2 methods of prevention may be used to decrease the delivery of cytotoxic agents to the scalp hair follicles. The first is called the **"tourniquet technique,"** in which a **narrow sphygmomanometer cuff** is inflated to 50 mm Hg above systolic pressure and placed below the hair line. The second method entails **generation of local hypothermia** by the application of a commercial **"ice turban"** maintained at 24 °C. The tourniquet technique may be used for a maximum of 20 minutes, which limits its usefulness because plasma levels of chemotherapeutic agents sufficiently high to produce alopecia are sustained much longer than this. The hypothermia method requires a highly motivated patient and has produced inconsistent results because of various factors affecting drug half-life. Methods to prevent alopecia should not be used for patients undergoing potentially curative chemotherapy, eg, treatment for acute leukemia, because they may provide a sanctuary for tumor cells and put the patient at risk for subsequent relapse in the scalp.

 III. **Palliation of alopecia.** Most patients desire to cover their heads during the period of alopecia. The various methods of head covering (hats, scarves, turbans, and wigs) should be discussed with the patient before initiating therapy. Wigs must be ordered and prepared ahead of time in order to match the original hair color and to guarantee availability when hair loss occurs.

PHOTOSENSITIVITY

Although uncommon, chemotherapy may induce photosensitivity reactions characterized by erythema, edema, blistering, peeling, and hyperpigmentation. Drugs associated with photosensitivity include: 5-FU, vinblastine, DTIC, and 6-thioguanine. 5-FU may result in rapid darkening of the skin following exposure to ultraviolet light. Patients receiving any of these drugs should be advised to limit their exposure to sunlight and to use adequate sunscreens. In addition, **photosensitizers** (eg, hematoporphyrin derivative, dihematoporphyrin ether/ester) used in photodynamic therapy, may cause exquisite, albeit temporary, photosensitivity.

EXTRAVASATION OF CHEMOTHERAPY AGENTS

The most feared acute toxicity of chemotherapy is extravasation of a vesicant agent with resulting tissue necrosis. Local injury varies from mild erythema and pain to severe skin and soft tissue necrosis. Extravasation of doxorubicin for example, may require surgical debridement followed by plastic surgery reconstruction or amputation.

  I. **Etiology.** Relatively little is known about the biochemical mechanisms that result in local tissue damage. Agents such as doxorubicin bind to nucleic acids and remain in the infiltrated tissues causing severe tissue damage. Other drugs such as the vinca alkaloids which do not bind to nucleic acids are able to undergo metabolism and clearance limiting the degree of tissue injury. The major vesicants are doxorubicin, actinomycin-D, daunorubicin, estramustine, mechlorethamine (nitrogen mustard), mitomycin C, vinblastine, vincristine, and vindesine.

 II. **Prevention.** Chemotherapeutic agents should be infused only by experienced personnel, and each infusion **should be given through a side port of an intravenous line at a new intravenous site or through an indwelling central catheter.** The dorsum of the hand and joints should be avoided. In addition, blood return should be checked at regular intervals (every 1–2 minutes) before, during, and immediately after infusion.

III. **Presentation.** Patients may complain of **pain, burning,** and **swelling** at the infusion site; however, a large number of patients with extravasation are asymptomatic.

IV. **Diagnosis.** Extravasation should be suspected if pain, edema, slowing of the infusion, or loss of blood return develops. If extravasation of a chemotherapeutic agent is suspected, it should be assumed to have occurred. The infusion should be stopped, and the patient treated accordingly.

 V. **Therapy.** If extravasation occurs, the drug should be discontinued immediately and aspiration should be attempted before removing the needle. If an antidote is to be administered through the needle, any residual drug remaining in the needle, tubing, and tissues should be aspirated before administering the antidote. If the extravasation occurs at a peripheral site, it may be helpful to elevate the affected extremity and to apply ice. No pressure should be applied, since this may spread the drug into the surrounding area. Local injection of numerous agents has been tried as antidotal therapy but none has proved to be efficacious; agents that have been used include bicarbonate, corticosteroids, propranolol, isoproterenol, acetylcysteine, glutathione, lidocaine, bupivacaine, diphenhydramine, cimetidine, and butylated hydroxytoluene. **If dermal necrosis and ulceration develop, prompt surgical debridement is indicated** and should be followed by skin grafting 2–3 days later. Specific measures for individual drugs are outlined below.

  A. **Anthracyclines.** The application of ice to the affected area may be helpful. Limited data suggest that topical dimethyl sulfoxide (DMSO) may help to prevent ulceration. Some clinical and experimental data suggest that topical **dimethyl sulfoxide (DMSO)** with or without alpha-tocopherol may prevent ulceration in these patients.

  B. **Vinca alkaloids and epipodophyllotoxins.** Tissue toxicity from vinblastine, vincristine, vindesine and etoposide extravasation may be diminished by treatment with hyaluronidase (500–1000 units administered directly into the extravasation site). Therapy with hyaluronidase appears to work by diluting the vesicant drug and promoting the absorption of the offending agent from local tissues.

  C. **Mechlorethamine.** Isotonic **sodium thiosulfate** may act as an alternative substrate for mechlorethamine-mediated alkylation. Injection of 10 mL of 4% thiosulfate into the affected area is recommended in addition to the standard measures (eg, elevation, icing).

  D. **Mitomycin-C.** Like damage from anthracyclines, damage from mitomycin-C may be ameliorated by topical application of **DMSO** with or without alpha-tocopherol.

  E. **Vinca alkaloids.** Experimental evidence suggests that tissue toxicity from vinblastine, vincristine, and vindesine extravasation may be lessened with **hyaluronidase** given in a manner identical to that for etoposide extravasation. (see **B,** above).

MANIFESTATIONS OF OCCULT MALIGNANCY

Familiarity with the cutaneous manifestations of malignancy is important since dermal lesions may be the only presenting sign or symptom of an underlying cancer.

HEREDITARY DISORDERS

Autosomal Dominant Disorders

I. **Bourneville's disease.** This phakomatosis, also known as "tuberous sclerosis," presents with hypopigmented macules, sebaceous adenomas, and subungual fibromas. It is rarely associated with **astrocytomas** and **glioblastomas.**

II. **Cowden's disease.** Acral verrucous papules, facial trichilemmomas, and oral mucosal fibromas characterize this disorder (also called "multiple hamartoma syndrome"), which is associated with **breast and thyroid cancer.**

III. **Gardner's syndrome.** This syndrome of epidermal and sebaceous cysts, dermoid tumors, fibromas, and lipomas is frequently associated with **adenocarcinoma of the colon.**

IV. **Multiple mucosal neuromas.** Head and neck (eyelids, nasal, lips, tongue, and laryngeal) neuromas are often associated with **pheochromocytoma** and **medullary carcinoma of the thyroid** (multiple endocrine neoplasia [MEN], type IIb).

V. **Multiple basal cell neuroma syndrome.** This syndrome is infrequently associated with medulloblastoma and fibrosarcoma of the jaw. The associated dermal manifestations are epidermoid cysts, pits in the palms and soles, and multiple basal cell carcinomas.

VI. **Peutz-Jeghers syndrome.** A low incidence of **gastric, duodenal, small bowel, and colonic carcinomas** is linked to this syndrome, consisting of pigmented macules on the lips, oral mucosa, face, and digits.

VII. **Sturge-Weber syndrome.** This phakomatosis is characterized by facial capillary or cavernous hemangiomas. Neurologic malignancies develop in a minority of patients.

VIII. **Tylosis palmaris et plantaris.** After age 10, this syndrome appears as hyperkeratosis of the palms and soles and is closely associated with the development of **esophageal cancer.**

IX. **Von Hippel–Lindau disease.** This rare phakomatosis (cerebelloretinal hemangioblastoma) produces retinal, cerebellar, and pancreatic angiomas and papilledema. It occurs rarely in conjunction with **neurologic and renal malignancies.**

X. **Von Recklinghausen's disease.** Manifestations of this phakomatosis (also called "neurofibromatosis") include café au lait spots, axillary "freckles," giant nevi, and neurofibromas. Pheochromocytoma is the predominant malignancy associated with this disorder but only occurs in a minority of patients. Other malignancies associated with neurofibromatosis are neurofibrosarcoma, neurilemoma, astrocytoma, and glioma.

Autosomal Recessive Disorders

I. **Ataxia-telangiectasia.** Telangiectasias of the ears, malar area, neck, and antecubital and popliteal fossas characterize this disorder, which is associated with the development of **leukemias** and **lymphomas.**

II. **Bloom's syndrome.** This syndrome of photosensitivity and telangiectasias of sun-exposed skin is often associated with leukemia.

III. **Chédiak-Higashi syndrome.** Recurrent pyoderma, giant melanosomes, and dilution of skin and hair color occur in conjunction with **lymphoma** in this rare disease.

IV. **Fanconi's disease.** This anemia presents with patchy hyperpigmentation and is associated with a high incidence of leukemia.

V. **Werner's syndrome.** Also referred to as **adult progeria,** this syndrome presents as premature aging (eg, graying hair, sclerodermalike skin changes, balding) and leg ulcers. About 10% of patients with this syndrome will develop sarcomas, meningiomas, or other malignancies.

Sex-linked Recessive Disorders

I. **Bruton's sex-linked agammaglobulinemia.** Recurrent dermal infections in this disease are associated with a 5% incidence of **leukemia** and **lymphoma.**

II. **Dyskeratosis congenita. Carcinomas** (and less frequently, **leukemia**) are found in patients with this syndrome of nail loss, hyperkeratosis of the palms and soles, skin atrophy of extensor surfaces, mucosal leukoplakia, and reticulate hyperpigmentation.

III. **Wiskott-Aldrich syndrome.** Nearly 10% of patients with this disorder (recurrent pyoderma, eczematous dermatitis, and petechiae-purpura) develop **leukemia** or **lymphoma.**

NON-HEREDITARY DISORDERS

I. **Alopecia mucinosa.** In patients more than 40 years old, this syndrome of multiple areas of dermal papules with follicular accentuation is highly associated with the presence of **lymphoma.**

II. **Amyloidosis.** Secondary amyloidosis, characterized by macroglossia, purpura, and diffuse yellowish papules or plaques, arises in 10–20% of patients with **multiple myeloma.**

III. **Arsenical keratosis.** Arsenic exposure may cause skin and visceral malignancies after a latency period of 10 years. Multiple discrete, firm corn-like hyperkeratoses appear on the palms and soles. Chronic arsenic exposure is associated with lung cancer.

IV. **Bowen's disease.** Single or multiple sharply defined, brownish red, scaly plaques, resembling eczema and psoriasis, are typical of squamous cell carcinoma in situ (Bowen's disease). **Respiratory, gastrointestinal, and genitourinary tract cancers** frequently develop in patients with this disease after a mean latency period of 8 years.

V. **Dermatitis herpetiformis.** In patients more than 50 years old, this uncommon disorder, characterized by pruritic clusters of vesicles on the scalp, back, buttocks, and extensor surfaces, particularly if unresponsive to sulfapyridine treatment is associated with underlying lymphoma.

VI. **Erythema annulare centrifugum.** This syndrome occurs in association with **prostate cancer** and **multiple myeloma** as well as other malignancies, infections, and disorders. It consists of annular, slowly migrating erythematous lesions.

VII. **Erythema multiforme.** In rare instances, this disorder of symmetric, vivid red skin lesions and "target" ("iris") lesions may occur in association with **lymphomas, leukemias,** and deep-seated **solid tumors** (following radiation therapy).

VIII. **Erythroderma.** This symptom complex is characterized by a generalized erythematous scaling eruption. If severe, (> 17 g/m^2/d), it may lead to negative nitrogen balance, edema, hypoalbuminemia, loss of muscle mass, and dehydration (due to loss of dermal water barrier) and thus become a true **dermatologic emergency.** Although it generally occurs with **lymphomas (in particular, mycosis fungoides)** and **leukemias,** it sometimes arises in patients with **deep-seated solid tumors.**

IX. **Melanosis.** Melanosis, sometimes called the **"slate gray syndrome,"** occurs in association with metastatic **melanoma** and **hepatocellular carcinoma.** Melanin precursors are deposited in tissues (including dermis) and cause the skin to appear gray instead of dark brown. In addition, the **urine turns black** on exposure to oxygen because of oxidation of the excreted precursors.

X. **Paget's disease. Mammary** Paget's disease results from intraductal **breast cancer** that has invaded the epidermis, causing eczematous, weeping, crusted, and scaly lesions. **Extramammary** Paget's disease (similar eczematous lesions on the pubis, perineum, thighs, or genitalia) is a consequence of **adenocarcinoma of the apocrine or eccrine sweat glands, rectum, or urethra.** Both disorders (mammary and extramammary) resemble atopic eczema and contact dermatitis; however, lesions fail to respond to topical corticosteroids. **Biopsy** must be performed for the diagnosis of Paget's disease.

XI. **Pyoderma gangrenosum.** An atypical form of this lesion may be associated with **myelogenous leukemia, multiple myeloma, polycythemia,** or **myeloid metaplasia.** As with the more common form, painful papules, nodules, or bullae progress to central necrosis.

PARANEOPLASTIC SYNDROMES

SYNDROMES WITH ERYTHEMA

Cutaneous Flushing
This paraneoplastic syndrome occurs in association with the **carcinoid syndrome** (see Carcinoid Syndrome, p 73, **II**).

Erythema Gyratum Repens
I. **Etiology.** The pathogenesis of this syndrome, also referred to as **"erythema perstans,"** has not been defined.

II. **Presentation.** Patients present with pruritic, concentric, arcuate, urticarial lesions that look similar to wood grain and that arise in association with **lung, breast,** and **other adenocarcinomas.**

III. **Diagnosis.** Typical dermal lesions in the setting of an appropriate malignancy are sufficient for a tentative diagnosis. Identification of an underlying malignancy confirms the diagnosis.

IV. **Therapy.** Supportive local care and treatment of the occult malignancy (once diagnosed) are the only available forms of therapy.

Exfoliative Dermatitis
   I. **Etiology.** The pathogenesis has not been defined, but this form of erythroderma is most often associated with mycosis fungoides.
   II. **Presentation.** Patients complain of progressive erythema that subsequently develops into scaling.
   III. **Diagnosis.** Characteristic lesions noted in the proper clinical setting are sufficient to make the diagnosis.
   IV. **Therapy.** Supportive local care and treatment of the underyling malignancy are the only available forms of therapy.

Necrolytic Migratory Erythema
This symptom complex occurs with **glucagonomas** (see p 468, **III. B.3**).

SYNDROMES WITH PIGMENTED LESIONS

Acanthosis Nigricans
   I. **Etiology.** The pathogenesis of this syndrome has not been defined. Common malignancies associated with this paraneoplastic syndrome are **gastrointestinal adenocarcinomas (92%)** and, in particular, **stomach cancer (60%).** Benign causes of acanthosis nigricans include: acromegaly, adrenal insufficiency, thyroid disease and diabetes mellitus.
   II. **Presentation.** Distinctive areas of hyperkeratosis and hyperpigmentation occur on the neck, axilla, anogenital region, and intertriginous areas.
   III. **Diagnosis.** In the presence of representative areas, the diagnosis may be by visual inspection made after **exclusion of pseudoacanthosis** of obesity, gigantism, acromegaly, Stein-Leventhal syndrome, and diabetes mellitus as well as **exclusion of benign acanthosis** of childhood.
   IV. **Therapy.** Supportive local care and treatment of the underlying malignancy (once diagnosed) are the only available forms of therapy.

Bazex's Disease
   I. **Etiology.** The pathogenesis of Bazex's disease has not been defined; however, the disease is known to occur in association with **head and neck neoplasms** and **gastrointestinal and lung cancers.**
   II. **Presentation.** Patients (males only) develop distinctive erythema and hyperkeratosis of the palms and soles, with scaling and pruritus.
   III. **Diagnosis.** Typical lesions found in the appropriate setting are diagnostic of this syndrome.
   IV. **Therapy.** Although the response to removal of the underlying tumor is usually good, substantial improvement may be obtained with **etretinate** (Tegison), 0.75–1.5 mg/kg/d in divided doses.

Leser-Trelat Syndrome
   I. **Etiology.** The exact pathogenesis of this syndrome has not been defined, but it is known to occur in association with **non-Hodgkin's lymphoma** and **gastrointestinal adenocarcinoma.**
   II. **Presentation.** Acute proliferation of many seborrheic, wartlike keratoses is characteristic of this disorder.
   III. **Diagnosis.** Infection of multiple slow-growing seborrheic keratoses that are more common than, but appear similar to, rapidly proliferating Leser-Trelat lesions confirms the diagnosis.
   IV. **Therapy.** Supportive local care and treatment of the underlying malignancy (once diagnosed) are the only available forms of therapy.

Sweet's Syndrome
   I. **Etiology.** Although not confirmed, **tumor secretion of interleukin-1 (IL-1)** probably accounts for the cutaneous manifestations of this syndrome. A variety of **hematologic malignancies and solid tumors** are associated with this disorder in 10–15% of cases.
   II. **Presentation.** Fever, neutrophilic dermal infiltrate, multiple painful cutaneous plaques, and neutrophilia are common findings.
   III. **Diagnosis.** The diagnosis is based on documentation of characteristic dermal lesions.
   IV. **Therapy.** The dermal lesions may respond rapidly to administration of **corticosteroids.**

MISCELLANEOUS SYNDROMES

Acquired Ichthyosis
I. **Etiology.** The pathogenesis of this syndrome has not been defined, although a close association with **Hodgkin's disease, multiple myeloma,** and **other lymphomas** exists.
II. **Presentation.** The appearance of generalized dry, cracking skin, rhomboidal scales with flaky edges, epidermal atrophy, and hyperkeratosis of the palms and soles is characteristic of the syndrome.
III. **Diagnosis.** Histopathologic findings of epidermal atrophy and hyperkeratosis in the appropriate setting and in the absence of a family history of similar disorders confirm the diagnosis.
IV. **Therapy.** Supportive local care and treatment of the underlying malignancy are the only available forms of therapy.

Cushing's Syndrome
This well-known symptom complex characterized by a round face, truncal obesity, wasting of the extremities, and atrophic skin with purple striae most often occurs in association with small cell lung cancer. It may also occur in cancers of the thyroid, adrenal gland, pancreas (islet cell) and other sites.

Dermatomyositis
I. **Etiology.** The pathogenesis of this syndrome has not been defined; however, malignant disease has been reported in up to 50% of patients with dermatomyositis. The dermatologic manifestations precede the carcinoma by days to years with an average latency of 6 months.
II. **Presentation.** This disorder is characterized primarily by an inflammatory myopathy with proximal muscle weakness. The cutaneous lesions consist of purplish-pink heliotrope erythema of the face with edema of the eyelids. Erythematous lesions over the knuckles and interphalangeal joints **(Grotton's sign)** are a characteristic late finding.
III. **Diagnosis.** The development of typical findings (clinical picture, characteristic results on electromyography, elevation of serum creatine phosphokinase and aldolase levels, and a positive biopsy) is sufficient to make the diagnosis of dermatomyositis.
IV. **Therapy.** Supportive systemic (aspirin and corticosteroids) and local (physiotherapy) care and treatment of the underlying malignancy (once it is identified) are the only available forms of therapy.

Hypertrichosis Lanuginosa
I. **Etiology.** This rare syndrome has been reported in association with **breast, lung, colorectal, uterine, gallbladder, and bladder carcinoma;** however, the cause has not been determined.
II. **Presentation.** Patients often complain of rapid growth of fine, silky, light (lanugo) hair, primarily over the face and ears.
III. **Diagnosis.** The syndrome may be diagnosed by the striking and characteristic lanugo hair growth. Several other entities (ie, the hereditary form of the disorder called "dog face" or "monkey face," porphyria cutanea tarda, erythropoietic porphyria, phenytoin use, and overproduction of androgens (in females)), must be excluded, however.
IV. **Therapy.** Treatment of the underlying malignancy is the only available form of therapy.

Pachydermoperiostosis
I. **Etiology.** The pathogenesis of this syndrome has not been defined although the acquired form is strongly associated with lung cancer.
II. **Presentation.** The main features are thickening of the skin (forehead, eyelids, ears, and lips) and creation of new skin folds (leonine facies) along with hypertrophic osteoarthropathy.
III. **Diagnosis.** The presence of hypertrophic pulmonary osteoarthropathy and the patient's appearance is diagnostic. A familial form (not associated with malignancy) may be seen in patients less than 40 years of age.
IV. **Therapy.** Treatment of the occult malignancy (once diagnosed) is the only successful mode of therapy.

Porphyria Cutanea Tarda
This syndrome occurs rarely in patients with **hepatocellular carcinoma** (see p 259, **III.B.1**).

Pruritus
   I. **Etiology.** The pathogenesis of this syndrome has not been defined, but it is known to occur with **lymphomas (particularly Hodgkin's disease), mycosis fungoides,** and **carcinoma of the breast, lung, colon, prostate, and stomach.**
   II. **Presentation.** Patients generally complain of intense, unremitting pruritus.
   III. **Diagnosis.** This paraneoplastic syndrome remains a **diagnosis of exclusion.** Non-malignant causes of pruritus, such as xerosis (dry skin), must be excluded.
   IV. **Therapy.** Treatment is primarily directed at the underlying malignancy.

Systemic Nodular Panniculitis
This paraneoplastic syndrome occurs in patients with **pancreatic carcinoma** (see p 249, **III.B.1**).

REFERENCES

Braverman I. Cancer. In Braverman I. *Skin Signs of Systemic Disease, 2nd ed.* Philadelphia: Saunders, 1981;1–108.

Bunn PA, Ridgway EC. Paraneoplastic syndromes. In DeVita, VT, Hellman S, and Rosenberg SA, (editors): *Cancer: Principles and Practice of Oncology, 3rd ed.* Philadelphia: Lippincott, 1989;1896–1940.

Callen JP. Skin signs of internal malignancy. In Callen et al (editors): *Dermatological Signs of Internal Disease.* Philadelphia: Saunders, 1988;99–109.

DeSpain JD. Dermatologic toxicity. In Perry MC (editor): *The Chemotherapy Source Book.* Baltimore: Williams and Wilkins, 1991.

Dewys WD, Killen JY. The paraneoplastic syndromes. In *Clinical Oncology for Medical Students and Physicians,* 6th ed. Atlanta: American Cancer Society, 1983;112–118.

Haynes HA: Cutaneous manifestations of internal malignancy. In Isselbacher KJ, Adams RD, Braunwald E, et al (editors): *Harrison's Principles of Internal Medicine,* 11th ed. New York: McGraw Hill, 1987;1588–1592.

Higgins EM, DuVivier AW. Cutaneous manifestations of malignant disease. *British Journal of Hospital Medicine,* 1992;**48;**552–561.

Worret WI. Skin signs and internal malignancies. *International Journal of Dermatology,* 1993;**32;** 1–5.

19 Reproductive Problems & Emergencies

F.J. Montz, MD

Cancer and cancer therapy may affect 3 areas of the reproductive system: (1) production of sex hormones, (2) fertility, and (3) sexual function. Although fertility and sex hormone production are intimately related, cancer patients, who often are elderly, are more commonly affected by the physiologic and psychological impact of cancer and cancer therapy on sex hormone production than by changes in fertility. In addition, even though sexual function, fertility, and sex hormone production are interdependent, it is possible to maintain satisfying coital and orgasmic function despite altered fertility and sex hormone production.

PROBLEMS WITH SEX HORMONE PRODUCTION

In both sexes, the gonads (ovaries and testes) are the primary site of sex hormone production; however, extragonadal tissues (eg, adrenal glands, tumors) also produce small but occasionally clinically significant amounts of these hormones. Although gynecomastia in males and hirsutism in females may occur secondary to neoplastic overproduction of sex hormones, the primary problem encountered in cancer patients is one of decreased sex hormone production.

  I. **Etiology.** Deficient production of sex hormones usually follows physical removal of gonadal tissue (surgical castration) or damage to gonadal tissue mediated by radiation therapy, chemotherapy, or both (functional castration).
   A. **Surgical castration.** Orchiectomy and oophorectomy immediately and irreversibly remove the primary site of sex hormone production; however, removal of a single gonad has little impact on the serum levels of sex hormones (assuming that the remaining gonad is functional). **Oophorectomy** is used primarily in the treatment of cancer of the ovary, uterus (corpus and cervix), and breast, whereas **orchiectomy** is used in the therapy of testicular, prostatic, and male breast carcinoma.
   B. **Functional castration**
    1. **Chemotherapy-induced dysfunction.** The risk of chemotherapy-induced gonadal dysfunction varies with sex, age, the agent or agents administered, and dose.
     a. **Sex.** In general, males are more sensitive than females to the effects of cytotoxic agents. For instance, 80% of males but only 40–50% of females develop gonadal failure following MOPP chemotherapy (mechlorethamine, Oncovin, procarbazine, and prednisone) for Hodgkin's disease.
     b. **Age.** Age is also important. Prepubertal testes and ovaries are resistant to chemotherapy-induced dysfunction. After the onset of puberty, however, testes become markedly sensitive to chemotherapeutic agents, and ovaries gradually grow increasingly susceptible to cytotoxic damage (only 20% of females less than 20 years old and more than 50% of females past 40 years old develop permanent amenorrhea).
     c. **Cytotoxic agents.** Gonadal failure occurs most commonly with alkylating agents. Nearly 60% of menstruating females develop complete ovarian failure following therapy with a single alkylating agent. **Cyclophosphamide, phenylalanine mustard, busulfan,** and **nitrogen mustard** are known to cause ovarian dysfunction, and recently the **vinca alkaloids** have been implicated. Testicular failure has been documented with cyclophosphamide, busulfan, nitrogen mustard, **nitrosoureas, procarbazine,** and **chlorambucil.** The toxicity of other cytotoxic agents, such as doxorubicin, bleomycin, cisplatin, nitrosoureas, and cytosine arabinoside, is unclear.

    d. Dose. Gonadal dysfunction is related to the **cumulative dose** of cytotoxic agents. Although gonadal failure is common following high-dose therapy, low-dose therapy over a prolonged period also may cause failure of sex hormone production.

  2. Radiation-induced dysfunction. Both the testes and ovaries are highly radiosensitive, requiring **doses of only 50–150 cGy** to produce some dysfunction. **Doses of 200–500 cGy** generally cause reversible dysfunction; function is regained after a period equal (in years) to the number of grays of radiation given (eg, 3 years following 300 cGy, 5 years following 500 cGy). **Sterility and complete cessation of sex hormone production** develop following **cumulative doses greater than 600 cGy.** As with chemotherapy-induced dysfunction, the impact of irradiation on gonadal function increases not only with dose but also with the addition of cytotoxic therapy and with age: only 30% of females below the age of 20 years are rendered infertile by radiation therapy, compared with 80% at age 30 and 100% at age 40.

II. Presentation. Signs and symptoms of sex hormone deficiency vary, depending on the hormone involved and the duration of the deficiency.

  A. Estrogen. Signs and symptoms of acute estrogen deficiency include **hot flashes; vaginal dryness,** itching, burning, discomfort, and bleeding; dyspareunia; **emotional lability** with anxiety, depression, and feelings of fatigue; urinary urgency, frequency, and incontinence; change in libido and orgasmic function; **amenorrhea;** symptoms of pelvic relaxation; and loss of skin turgor and resultant increased wrinkling. Chronic estrogen deficiency often results in **osteoporosis,** increased serum low-density lipoproteins, and decreased serum high-density lipoproteins leading to an increased risk of cardiovascular disease.

  B. Testosterone. The signs and symptoms of acute androgen deficiency are **hot flushes, decreased testicular volume, impotence,** oligo- or azoospermia, decreased libido, irritability, inattentiveness, and depression. Chronic androgen deficiency produces a demasculinization syndrome.

III. Diagnosis. In patients at risk for gonadal failure, the diagnosis is confirmed simply by determining **serum levels of estrogen or testosterone.** In addition, pituitary causes can be excluded merely by ascertaining the levels of **serum follicle-stimulating hormone and luteinizing hormone.**

IV. Therapy. Although many symptoms of sex hormone deficiency can be treated successfully without restoration of normal serum hormone levels, both the majority of symptoms and the deficiency itself can be reversed easily and quickly with exogenous replacement of the specific hormone.

  A. Estrogen

    1. Replacement therapy

      a. Patients who have had a hysterectomy. Either **oral** or **transcutaneous estrogen (dermal patches)** (1.25–7.5 mg/d **continuously**) may be used to treat these patients.

      b. Patients who have not had a hysterectomy. These patients should be given **concomitant continuous or cyclic (days 1–12) progesterone** to limit estrogen-induced endometrial hyperplasia and neoplasia.

    2. Other therapy. Patients with an absolute (breast cancer) or relative (endometrial carcinoma) contraindication to estrogen administration must rely on other, sometimes multiple, nonestrogenic agents to palliate the symptoms of gonadal failure. For example, **vaginal dryness** may be corrected with special lubricating preparations (eg, Replens), **vasomotor instability** may be remedied with progestins as well as dopaminergic and vasodilatory drugs. In addition, new calcitonin analogs may prove to be effective in preventing the **osteoporosis** that follows chronic hypoestrogenism.

  B. Androgens

    1. Replacement therapy. Testosterone cypionate (50–400 mg every 2–4 weeks IM) can be given to patients without prostate cancer, which is an absolute contraindication to testosterone administration. This therapy is highly effective and well tolerated. **Side effects** of testosterone replacement that may occur include prostatic hypertrophy, liver function abnormalities, and erythrocytosis.

    2. Other therapy. There are few alternatives for patients who are unable to receive testosterone. Vasomotor instability and accelerated osteoporosis can be treated as described for estrogen deficiency (see **A.2,** above).

PROBLEMS WITH FERTILITY

I. **Etiology.** Fertility problems associated with cancer or cancer therapy can be classified as gonadal failure (loss of sperm or oocyte production) or anatomic alterations of the genitalia.

   A. **Gonadal failure.** Sex hormone deficiency almost universally precipitates **germ cell failure** (inability to produce viable sperm or oocytes); however, germ cell failure is not always accompanied by sex hormone deficiency. Frequently, **chemotherapy** and **radiation therapy** cause infertility. In addition, the **psychosexual and neuroendocrinologic impact of many cancers** often leads to reproductive problems; for instance, 50% of males with testicular carcinoma or lymphoma have impaired semen production (< 20 million/mL or < 50% motility).

   B. **Anatomic alterations of the genitalia.** A major goal of cancer therapy is to maintain a functionally intact genital tract whenever possible. Normal pregnancy requires at least one functioning gonad that maintains a physiologic connection with the body surface (in both male and female) and an appropriate receptacle (womb) for the fertilized ovum. Although unilateral oophorectomy (even with resection of the uterine cornua) and orchiectomy (even when accompanied by prostatectomy) do not preclude successful reproduction, many surgical procedures decrease or eliminate the possibility of pregnancy. For example, radical **prostatectomy** and **cystoprostatectomy** for prostate and bladder cancer, **hypogastric artery ligation,** and **modified bilateral retroperitoneal lymphadenectomy** for testicular carcinoma produce vasogenic impotence or ejaculatory dysfunction in 20–50% of patients. In females, **pelvic adhesions and infection** following intra-abdominal and pelvic surgery also lower fertility significantly. Although some mutilating procedures (eg, radical vulvectomy, forequarter amputation, colostomy) do not physically prevent pregnancy, the **psychological repercussions** interfere with normal reproductive activities. Finally, some radical procedures (**bilateral orchiectomy, oophorectomy, hysterectomy, and penectomy**) do completely eliminate the possibility of successful reproduction.

II. **Presentation.** Many patients do not express their concerns regarding the consequences of cancer and cancer therapy on their reproductive ability. The initial complaint of women is usually the **inability to achieve or maintain a normal pregnancy.** Clinical complaints among men include loss of libido, impotence, and regression of secondary sexual characteristics.

III. **Diagnosis.** The diagnosis of infertility is established only **after 1 year of unprotected coitus (ie, without conception).** Semen analysis may exclude impaired semen production (< 20 million sperm/mL or < 50% motility). Further workup, including serum hormone levels, radiographic studies, and psychological evaluation, may be indicated.

IV. **Therapy.** Treatment of infertility in cancer patients consists of primary prevention of unnecessary gonadal damage, correction of sex hormone deficiencies, psychological counseling, and in vitro fertilization techniques.

   A. **Gonadal preservation**

   1. **Protection from radiation-induced injury**

   a. **Testes.** Although relocation of the testes to areas outside the proposed radiation field (**orchiopexy**) is theoretically possible, it is not practical, and, until recently, testicular shielding was unsatisfactory because of radiation scatter. Currently, however, **improved radiation equipment combined with gonadal shielding** may reduce the testicular dose to less than 10% of the total radiation dose.

   b. **Ovaries.** Since effective shielding of the ovary is frequently impossible, efforts have focused on **relocating the ovaries to areas outside the radiation field (oophoropexy).** Following surgical mobilization of the ovaries, suspensory ligaments, and blood vessels, the ovaries can be rotated out of the pelvis or placed in the midline (behind the uterus), or microsurgical techniques can be used to "transplant" the ovaries to a remote anatomic location. These maneuvers decrease ovarian irradiation in up to 50% of females receiving pelvic irradiation; however, in vitro fertilization techniques may be required to achieve a successful pregnancy following ovarian oophoropexy.

   2. **Protection from chemotherapy-induced injury.** Theoretically, chemotherapy-induced gonadal toxicity may be minimized by pretreatment germ cell suppression because nondividing cells are relatively resistant to cytotoxic therapy. Oral contraceptives in females, parenteral testosterone in males, and gonadotropin-releasing hormone (Gn-RH) analogs in both sexes have been tried, but results have been limited by the frequent need for immediate chemotherapy

administration before full germ cell suppression is achieved. Despite promising early results, no definite benefit has been documented with this approach.

3. **Cryopreservation of sperm or oocytes.** Sperm and oocyte banking is now widely available for individuals undergoing cytotoxic therapy. This approach is hampered, however, by its expense, the time required to donate adequate sperm (rarely limiting) or oocytes (commonly limiting), the low viability (30–50% of sperm, oocytes, and embryos are viable after freezing) and the resulting low conception rate (50–60%), and by the fact that 80–90% of male cancer patients cannot produce adequate semen. In addition, the cryopreservation of embryos raises ethical and legal questions about custodial rights in case of parental death or divorce.

B. **Preservation of sexual function.** Several standard radical surgical procedures have been modified to improve postoperative sexual function in men. Specifically, **anterior displacement of the lateral pelvic fascial incision** during radical prostatectomy or cystoprostatectomy preserves ejaculation in 70–80% of patients, and **avoidance of the sympathetic fibers in the area of the aortic bifurcation and sacral promontory** during retroperitoneal lymphadenectomy maintains antegrade ejaculation in 50–70% of patients. Similarly, individual modifications of radical hysterectomy, radical vulvectomy, and the formation of a neovagina in women who have undergone vaginectomy help to maintain or re-establish coital and orgasmic function.

C. **Alternative reproductive methods.** Several options exist for both male and female patients with fertility problems.
1. **Females.** After bilateral oophorectomy, females may still become pregnant following in vitro **fertilization and implantation of a donated ovum.** After hysterectomy, females with functional ovaries may reproduce using a **surrogate uterus.**
2. **Males.** In males with ejaculatory dysfunction, **electroejaculation** may provide enough semen for subsequent insemination; however, the only option for males with poor semen is **artificial insemination** with donor sperm.

PROBLEMS OF SEXUAL (COITAL AND ORGASMIC) FUNCTION

Aside from the physical impact that cancer and its treatment has on the reproductive system, the psychological trauma of a diagnosis of cancer may be profound and, in and of itself, may lead to sexual dysfunction. Data indicate that **30–90% of women treated for gynecologic malignancies experience sexual dysfunction** and desire information and help to regain a satisfying sex life.

I. **Etiology.** Dysfunction can occur at any or all phases of the sexual response cycle (sexual desire, excitement, orgasm, and resolution). The cause of the problem usually is multifactorial and may involve (1) alteration of normal genital anatomy, (2) sex hormone deficiency, (3) disruption of body image both independently of and contingent upon disfiguring surgery, and (4) depression.

II. **Presentation.** Although patients with sexual dysfunction present with a wide range of complaints, careful questioning frequently reveals the exact nature of the problem.

III. **Diagnosis.** The diagnosis is confirmed by obtaining an **accurate sexual history**. In addition, a pretreatment history is invaluable in determining what is "normal" and desirable for the patient.

IV. **Therapy**
A. **General considerations.** The single most important element necessary for the successful treatment of sexual dysfunction is a caring health professional. The issue of sexual function and gratification is highly personal, often striking at the core of an individual's identity. Although certain social, economic, and racial groups discourage conversation regarding sexual function, **professional openness and empathy** facilitate discussion and treatment of these problems.

B. **Specific treatment**
1. **Altered anatomy.** Safe reductions in the extent of radical surgical procedures have led to better preservation of sexual function. For example, the **combined modality therapy for vulvar carcinoma, using irradiation and wide local excision** instead of traditional radical vulvectomy, dramatically improves postoperative sexual function. In addition, improved methods of **vaginal reconstruction following vaginectomy** greatly enhance the acceptance and function of the neovagina. Occasionally, however, coital function cannot be maintained. In these unfortunate cases, the patient and his or her partner should be encouraged to explore and develop alternative methods of sexual gratification.

2. **Sex hormone replacement.** (See p 114, **IV.**)
3. **Altered body image.** Disorders involving body image are treated primarily with **behavior modification techniques.** A professional experienced in the sexual and family therapy of cancer patients is essential.

4. **Depression.** Although numerous physiologic causes (eg, anemia, pain, cata-
bolic state with weight loss) may account for the general malaise, dysphoria,
decreased libido, and depression often observed in cancer patients, psychological causes must not be overlooked, and referral to individuals skilled in the
counseling of cancer patients and their partners should not be delayed.

CANCER AND PREGNANCY

Cancer During Pregnancy
The incidence of cancer during pregnancy is **1 per 2205, or 0.45 per 1000 pregnancies.**
Knowledge of all the implications and available options is crucial to the successful manage-
ment of this relatively common problem.
  I. **Leukemia.** Fetuses exposed to antileukemia chemotherapy during the **first trimester**
     are compromised, and therapeutic abortion in these cases is recommended; however,
     data indicate that treatment during the **second and third trimesters** does not ad-
     versely affect fetal viability or subsequent pediatric growth and development. Moreover,
     no increased incidence of cancer has been observed in offspring of mothers treated
     with chemotherapy during pregnancy.
 II. **Cervical carcinoma**
     A. **Microinvasive carcinoma (stage IA).** Microinvasive disease diagnosed by cone
        biopsy should be followed closely with **serial colposcopy** every 4–6 weeks during
        pregnancy. The pregnancy may be allowed to proceed to term, and definitive ther-
        apy withheld until after cesarean or vaginal delivery.
     B. **Invasive carcinoma.** The treatment of invasive cervical cancer is determined by
        the gestational age of the fetus. **Before 20–24 weeks' gestation,** therapy should
        be instituted immediately and the fetus sacrificed. **After 28 weeks' gestation,** the
        fetus can be evaluated by amniocentesis for pulmonary maturity, treated with corti-
        costeroids to accelerate surfactant production, and delivered when viable. Between
        20 and 28 weeks' gestation, the situation must be discussed with the patient. Delay
        in instituting therapy until 28 weeks (when delivery is possible) is an alternative with
        some risk to the patient. Once counseled, the patient can make an informed deci-
        sion regarding her therapy.

Pregnancy Following Cancer
The incidence of birth defects in the offspring of cancer survivors is 4%; only 0.3% are purely
genetic disorders. Although the statistical power to detect small increases in the incidence of
genetic defects in this population is limited by the available data, the incidence is essentially
identical to that of the general population.

PARANEOPLASTIC SYNDROMES

Inappropriate secretion of gonadotropins—ie, follicle-stimulating hormone (FSH), luteinizing hormone (LH), and human chorionic gonadotropin (hCG)—may cause distinct clinical
syndromes in both males and females as well as children. All 3 hormones have a common
alpha subunit but are distinguished by their beta subunits. Because FSH and LH are present
at varying levels in normal adults (and, in particular, at elevated levels in cancer patients with
gonadal failure) and because hCG is produced only by placental tissue, clinical studies have
focused on hCG levels in cancer patients. Elevated serum levels are documented in patients
with **lung (large-cell and adenocarcinoma), breast, and gastrointestinal (hepatoma,
carcinoids, pancreatic endocrine tumors) carcinoma** as well as the better-known tumors:
pituitary, gestational trophoblastic, and germ cell. Moreover, these studies found elevated
hCG levels in 5–10% of chronic benign diseases (eg, uremia, pregnancy). Inappropriate gonadotropin production may produce the following clinical "paraneoplastic" syndromes.
  I. **Males. Precocious puberty** in children as well as **painful gynecomastia** and **hyper-
     thyroidism** in adult males occur as a result of inappropriate serum gonadotropin levels.
     If elevated serum hCG is documented in an adult male without known malignancy, a
     search for testicular, lung, and extragonadal germ cell neoplasms is warranted.
 II. **Females. Precocious puberty** in children as well as **oligomenorrhea, hirsutism,** and
     hyperthyroidism in premenopausal females occur as a result of excess serum gonad-
     otropin. In postmenopausal females, symptoms are rare.

REFERENCES

Catanzarite VA, Ferguson JE: Acute leukemia and pregnancy: A review of management and outcome, 1972–1982. *Obstet Gynecol Surg* 1984;**39:**663.

20 Malignant Melanoma

Robert B. Cameron, MD, and Jan Wong, MD

I. **Epidemiology.** Melanoma is the **eighth** most common malignancy in the United States, accounting for **3% of all cancers**. In 1985, **11.2** cases per 100,000 males and **8.4** cases per 100,000 females were diagnosed, leading to 2.8 and 1.5 deaths, respectively. Estimates indicate that **32,000 new cases** and **6800 deaths** would be diagnosed in 1993. During the past decade, the incidence of melanoma has increased faster than that of any other malignant neoplasm, averaging **5–7% per year** (doubling every 10–15 years). By the year 2000, **1 of every 75 individuals** (compared with 1 in 1500 in 1935) will develop cutaneous melanoma. Worldwide, the incidence varies from a high of **28.4** per 100,000 population in **Australia** to 0.2 per 100,000 in Japan.

II. **Risk factors**
   A. **Age.** The incidence of melanoma gradually increases from less than 1 per 100,000 before 20 years of age to **26.8** per 100,000 by **age 80**.
   B. **Sex.** The risk for males is **1.3 times** greater than that for females.
   C. **Race.** The risk for caucasians is **17 times** greater than that for blacks and amounts to a **1% lifetime risk**. Asian, Hispanic, and American Indian populations are at intermediate risk.
   D. **Genetic factors**
      1. **Family history.** The risk of melanoma in first-degree relatives of patients with melanoma is **4 times** greater than that of the general population.
      2. **Familial syndromes.** True mendelian-inherited, familial melanoma syndromes constitute **8–12%** of all cases of cutaneous melanoma. These lesions typically occur **earlier** than noninherited lesions and are often **multiple** (11–27%).
      3. **Genetic abnormalities.** In general, melanoma cells are **highly aneuploid** and often contain chromosomal alterations (deletions) involving **chromosome 1p**, as well as **chromosomes 6 and 7**. In addition, activated ras oncogenes have been reported in melanoma.
   E. **Skin complexion.** Individuals with fair complexions, particularly those with **blond or red hair** (1.6–3 times), **fair skin** (2 times), and **poor tanning ability**, are at substantially higher risk of developing melanoma than the general population.
   F. **Previous dermal pathology**
      1. **Freckles and nevi.** The risk of malignant melanoma for individuals with **freckles or more than 20 nevi** is **3 times** greater than for those without these traits.
      2. **Actinic keratosis.** The presence of actinic keratoses is associated with an increased risk of malignant melanoma.
      3. **Pigmented precursor lesions**
         a. **Dysplastic nevus syndrome.** This disorder is characterized by an **increased risk of melanoma, multiple nevi (< 100)**, at least **1 nevus more than 8 mm**, and at least 1 junctional or compound nevus with **atypical** features, both grossly (ie, variegation, irregularity, asymmetry, and diameter < 6 mm) and microscopically (eg, melanocytic hyperplasia and rete ridge elongation; enlarged, hyperchromatic melanocytic nuclei; rete ridge bridging of aggregated melanocytes; lamellar and concentric dermal fibroplasia; and a lymphocytic infiltrate). A common familial variant is the **familial atypical multiple mole-melanoma (FAMMM) syndrome** (or B-K mole syndrome, from the first letter of the last names of the first 2 families studied). Originally believed to be an autosomal dominant disease with incomplete penetration, this syndrome is transmitted by an **unknown mechanism** but probably involves a locus on **chromosome 1p**.
         b. **Congenital nevi.** Congenital melanocytic nevi occur in **1%** of neonates and are classified as **small (< 1.5 cm)**, medium (1.5–20 cm), or large (> 20

cm). Clinical features of these hamartomas include: (1) grossly **irregular** surface, (2) **hyperpigmentation**, and (3) **hypertrichosis**. Melanomas can arise within any congenital nevi, regardless of size (lifetime risk is **6–20%**), although it is likely that the risk is proportional to diameter. Therefore, all congenital nevi must be either removed or monitored closely and require a biopsy if any change is noted.

c. **Melanoma.** The risk of melanoma in patients previously diagnosed with melanoma is **900 times** that of the population at large, or a **3–5% lifetime risk.**

d. **Xeroderma pigmentosum.** This rare **autosomal recessive** disease features a genetic defect in the **repair of DNA damage caused by ultraviolet (UV) radiation**. These patients are at extremely high risk for cutaneous melanoma, basal and squamous cell carcinomas, and sarcomas. Most patients die before the age of 25.

G. **Radiation exposure.** The high incidence of melanoma in people living near the **equator**, in people who **migrate** to sunny climates, in individuals with **3 or more blistering sunburns or outdoor summer jobs** before age 20, and in sun-exposed anatomic sites all suggest that cumulative exposure to **UV light** is an important risk factor for cutaneous melanoma. The recent **depletion of ozone** may be partially responsible for the increasing incidence of cutaneous melanoma. However, the exact relationship between UV light and melanoma remains unclear, because melanoma can occur in relatively **unexposed** areas of the skin (eg, palms, soles, and areas of the trunk covered by a bathing suit) and in **young** patients without a long history of sun exposure. Most likely, melanoma is related to periods of **acute, intense, and intermittent sun exposure** manifested by blistering sunburns.

H. **Hormones.** Some data suggest that females who use **oral contraceptives for more than 5 years** and who have a **first child after age 30** are at increased risk of developing melanoma. Furthermore, anecdotal reports describe rapid proliferation and dissemination of melanoma during **pregnancy**.

I. **Diet.** No dietary factors have been identified.

J. **Smoking.** Tobacco has not been implicated in the pathogenesis of cutaneous melanoma.

K. **Urbanization.** Melanoma is more frequent among urban **white collar** workers who work indoors and enjoy outdoor recreational activities than people in agricultural and **blue-collar** occupations who work primarily outdoors.

III. **Presentation**

A. **Signs and symptoms**

1. **Local manifestations.** Clinical signs and symptoms of cutaneous melanoma include **change** in a particular pigmented lesion. Changes that should be noted are (1) **color** (particularly variegated shades of red, white, blue, brown, and black), (2) **size**, (3) **shape** (especially irregular borders), (4) **surface** (particularly scaling, crusting, ulceration, nodularity, and oozing), (5) **surrounding skin** (eg, especially pigmented satellite lesion, erythema), (6) **sensation** (particularly itching and pain), (7) **elevation** (ie, sudden elevation of a macular nevus), and (8) **consistency** (especially softening). Therefore, changing pigmented lesions always require a biopsy to exclude malignant melanoma.

2. **Systemic manifestations.** Distant **"in transit"** skin lesions (ie, dermal lymphatic metastases) may be noted along with enlarged regional lymph nodes (lymph node metastases), jaundice and hepatomegaly (liver metastases), pulmonary nodules and dyspnea (lung metastases), focal and generalized neurologic symptoms (brain metastases), and bone pain (bone metastases).

B. **Paraneoplastic syndromes.** No true paraneoplastic syndromes have been associated with cutaneous melanoma; however, **melanosis** may occur (see p 108, **IX**).

IV. **Differential diagnosis.** The vast majority of patients who have melanoma present with a **pigmented dermal lesion**; however, a multitude of benign pigmented lesions exist, including inflammatory lesions (eg, eczema, lichen planus, systemic lupus erythematosus), pigmented lesions of **Peutz-Jeghers**, **Albright's**, and **Leopard syndromes**, congenital nevi (eg, nevi of Ota and Ito), seborrheic keratosis, poikiloderma, incontinentia pigmenti, urticaria pigmentosa, and, in rare cases, common freckles (ephelis).

V. **Screening programs.** Cutaneous melanoma is uniquely suited for mass screening because all lesions are **easily visible** by physical inspection. A 2-tiered approach with frequent self-examinations and annual physician examinations has been proposed, particularly for patients with known risk factors.

A. **Self-examination.** All patients should be instructed on the systematic inspection of the entire dermal surface. The only requirements are full-length and hand-held mirrors, 2 chairs, and a blow dryer. Protocols for complete self-examination, published by the American Cancer Society as well as other organizations, require little time and stress the mnemonic **ABCD**: **A** symmetry, **B** order irregularity, **C**olor variegation, **D**iameter of more than 6 mm. Periodic self-examinations (**every 1-2 months**) are recommended, with patients reporting any **new or changing lesion** to a physician.

B. **Physician examination.** In addition to patient self-examination, inexpensive screening can be accomplished by simple **annual total cutaneous examinations by a physician**. This is highly recommended, especially for high-risk patients because, with training, meticulous total cutaneous examination has a **97% sensitivity** (although only a **40% specificity**) in detecting cutaneous melanoma.

VI. **Diagnostic workup**

A. **Medical history and physical examination.** A thorough medical history (documenting risk factors) and a complete physical examination should be performed in all patients with suspected cutaneous melanoma. Particular attention should be directed at the following areas:

1. **General appearance.** An evaluation of the patient's general functional (see Appendix A) and nutritional status should be included (see also p 1, **I** and **III**).

2. **Eyes.** Both of the patient's eyes should be examined with an ophthalmoscope for evidence of ocular melanoma.

3. **Lymph nodes.** The number, consistency, tenderness, and distribution of all cervical, supraclavicular, axillary, and inguinal lymph nodes must be carefully documented.

4. **Chest.** Evidence for pleural effusions and pulmonary metastases (eg, decreased or absent breath sounds, pleural friction rub) should be excluded on pulmonary examination.

5. **Abdomen.** Hepatosplenomegaly, ascites, and all masses (intraperitoneal metastases) must be fully described.

6. **Rectum.** The anus should be carefully inspected for **perianal melanoma**, and metastatic rectal masses (**Blumer's shelf lesions**) must be excluded. In addition, stool should be tested for **occult blood**.

7. **Nervous system.** A thorough neurologic examination must be carefully documented.

B. **Primary tests and procedures.** The following diagnostic tests and procedures should be performed initially in all patients with suspected ovarian carcinoma.

1. **Blood tests** (see p 1, **IV.A**)
   a. Complete blood count.
   b. Hepatic enzymes.
   c. Alkaline phosphatase.
   d. BUN and creatinine.
   e. Albumin.

2. **Urine tests. Routine urinalysis** (see p 3, **IV.B**) may demonstrate urine that turns black on exposure to air as a result of systemic **melanosis** (see p 108, **IX**).

3. **Imaging studies. A chest x-ray** should be obtained (see p 3, **IV.C.1**).

4. **Invasive procedures**
   a. **Dermoscopy.** Examination of the integument with the aid of an **epiluminescence microscope** (eg, dermatoscope) may increase the diagnostic accuracy of physical inspection. Each lesion is viewed under oil with a 10x magnifying lens.
   b. **Biopsy.** Any suspicious or changing lesion, particularly in high-risk patients, requires a biopsy (see, also, p 123, **IX.A.1.c**).

C. **Optional tests and procedures.** The following examinations may be indicated by previous diagnostic findings or clinical suspicion.

1. **Blood tests** (see p 1, **IV.A**)
   a. **5-nucleotidase**.
   b. **GGTP**.

2. **Imaging studies**
   a. **Computed tomography** (see p 3, **IV.C.2**). CT scan of the abdomen and pelvis provide useful information regarding the liver, genitourinary tract, retroperitoneal lymph nodes, and peritoneal disease.
   b. **Magnetic resonance imaging** (see p 3, **IV.C.3**).
   c. **Upper gastrointestinal series.** Occasionally, this study is necessary because patients may present with symptoms of gastrointestinal obstruction (uncommon).
   d. **Technetium-99m bone scan** (see p 3, **IV.C.5**).
   e. **Lymphoscintigraphy.** Cutaneous lymphoscintigraphy with gold 198- or

technetium-99m–labeled **albumin or dextran** (injected into the area of the original lesion) may identify which regional **lymph node basins** are **at risk** for harboring occult metastatic disease. In addition, lymphoscintigraphy with **monoclonal antibody** (conjugated to ^{131}I, ^{111}In, or ^{99m}Tc) raised to melanoma antigens may specifically detect regional as well as distant metastases.

3. **Fine needle aspiration** can be used to assess suspicious supraclavicular or inguinal lymph nodes and lung, liver, and pelvic masses.

VII. **Pathology**

A. **Location.** Malignant melanomas may arise anywhere, but **90%** occur in the **skin** (most commonly on the **lower extremities in females** and increasingly on the **trunk in males**) and **10%** originate in the eye, meninges, respiratory tract, gastrointestinal tract, urethra, and vagina. Currently, **52%** of melanomas are located on the **head, neck, and trunk**, whereas **46%** are on the **upper and lower extremities**. Melanomas that arise from **dysplastic nevi**, however, may appear anywhere on the body, especially the trunk and those areas of the body that are normally **covered** (eg, **buttocks, scalp, and breasts**). No primary lesion is identified in **4–10%** of cases.

B. **Multiplicity.** Multiple synchronous and metachronous primary melanomas occur in **4–5%** of patients and usually present **within 1 year**.

C. **Gross appearance.** The American Joint Committee on Cancer recognizes the following 5 distinct forms of extraocular melanoma, each with discrete clinical and biologic characteristics.

1. **Radial (superficial) spreading melanoma (SSM; 70%).** Generally, SSM arises **slowly** (over 1–5 years) in **pre-existing** lesions (in particular, **dysplastic nevi**). SSM initially appears **macular, variegated**, and **irregular**, with characteristic **notching** of the borders (radial growth phase). Subsequently, these lesions become nodular (vertical growth phase). In addition, **amelanotic** regions represent areas of **regression**. SSM occurs on the head, neck, and trunk of adult males and on the lower extremities of adult females, with a peak incidence in the fifth decade.

2. **Lentigo maligna melanoma (LMM; 4–10%).** Typically, LMM originates in **elderly** patients (median age of 70 years) from **long-standing** (eg, 5–20 years old) lentigo maligna lesions (ie, **melanotic freckle of Hutchinson** or **melanosis of Dubreuilh**). These **large** (> 3 cm in diameter), **flat, irregular** lesions occur on the sun-exposed areas of the head and neck with no sex predilection. As with SSM, **amelanotic** regions represent areas of **regression**.

3. **Nodular melanoma (NM; 8–20%).** Commonly, NM develops **rapidly** (over 1–24 months) on the trunk of middle-aged males (median age of 49) and is biologically **aggressive**. Lesions appear **dark, symmetric, 1–2 cm** in diameter, and **uniform in color**, with no melanocytic abnormalities visible in the adjacent epidermis. Nearly **5%** of NM are **amelanotic**.

4. **Acral lentiginous melanoma (ALM; 3–5%).** Although uncommon, ALM arises **quickly** (over 3–36 months) on the **palms, soles, subungual regions**, and, in rare cases, in the oral cavity, anus, vagina, and conjunctiva (ie, **mucosal** lentiginous melanoma) of **older** patients (mean age of 59), particularly blacks, Asians, and Hispanics. Characteristically, ALM is **aggressive, large** (> 3 cm), tan to dark brown in color, **irregular**, and rarely ulcerating or fungating. **Subungual** melanoma typically occurs on the **great toe** or **thumb**.

5. **Unclassified melanoma (UM; 0–5%).** A melanoma that does not fall into one of the above 4 categories is an **unclassified** melanoma.

D. **Histology.** Melanomas arise from melanocytes that reside at the **epidermal-dermal junction** of the skin and contain a variable number of melanosomes with the pigment, **melanin**. Nearly **1%** of melanomas, however, are **amelanotic**. Both **radial** (ie, prolonged and **not** associated with metastases) and **vertical** (ie, brief and frequently associated with metastatic spread) growth phases often exist.

E. **Metastatic spread**

1. **Modes of spread.** Melanoma generally spreads via 3 basic mechanisms:

   a. **Direct extension.** Melanoma characteristically spreads **horizontally** into the surrounding skin during the **radial growth phase** and **deep** into the deep dermis and subcutaneous fat (rarely muscle) in the **vertical growth phase**.

   b. **Lymphatic metastasis.** Melanoma may embolize through **intradermal lymphatics** to both adjacent and distant skin sites (**"satellitosis"** and **"in transit"** metastases) as well as regional lymph nodes in 41%, 74%, and 89% of Clark's level III, IV, and V lesions, respectively.

   c. **Hematogenous metastasis.** Cutaneous melanoma frequently gains access to blood vessels and subsequently disseminates to distant sites.

2. **Sites of spread.** Autopsy series demonstrate that once it enters the vertical growth phase, melanoma quickly metastasizes to the following wide array of distant organs: **dermis,** 50–75%; **lung,** 70–87%; **liver,** 54–77%; **central nervous system (CNS),** 36–54%; **bone,** 23–49%; **gastrointestinal tract,** 26–58%; **adrenals,** 36–54%; **pancreas,** 38–53%; **kidneys,** 35–48%; and **heart,** 40–45%.

VIII. **Staging.** In 1987, the Union Internationale Contre le Cancer and the American Joint Committee on Cancer adopted a joint TNM staging system that combined the previous 3-tiered clinical staging system with important prognostic information available from primary **tumor thickness (Clark's level** and **Breslow's depth** of invasion). Clark's and Breslow's microstaging systems, the former clinical staging system, and the new pathologic TNM staging system are outlined below.

A. **Microstaging systems**
   1. **Clark's system.** Clark's method of microstaging is based on a qualitative description of the increasing levels of penetration through the dermis to the subcutaneous fat. Its accuracy is directly related to the experience of the pathologist.
      a. **Level I.** Tumor remains above an intact basal lamina (melanoma in situ).
      b. **Level II.** Tumor invades into the papillary dermis.
      c. **Level III.** Tumor reaches the papillary-reticular dermis interface.
      d. **Level IV.** Tumor invades into the reticular dermis.
      e. **Level V.** Tumor invades into the subcutaneous fat.
   2. **Breslow's system.** Breslow's microstaging method uses an ocular micrometer to quantitate the vertical **depth of invasion** (in mm) from the granular layer of the epidermis (or the base of an ulcer) to the deepest identifiable contiguous melanoma cell. This method is clearly **more accurate and reproducible** than Clark's level of invasion.
      a. **0 mm** (Clark's level I).
      b. **No larger than 0.75 mm** (Clark's level II).
      c. **0.76–1.5 mm** (Clark's level III).
      d. **1.6–3.9 mm** (Clark's level IV).
      e. **4 mm or more** (Clark's level V).

B. **Clinical staging system.** The most commonly utilized staging system for melanoma involves 3 stages:
   1. **Stage I.** Localized melanoma, including satellite lesions less than 5 cm from the primary.
   2. **Stage II.** Regional lymph node metastases with or without "in-transit" metastases.
   3. **Stage III.** Disseminated melanoma.

C. **TNM staging system**
   1. **Tumor stage**
      a. **TX.** The primary tumor cannot be assessed.
      b. **T0.** No evidence of a primary tumor exists.
      c. **Tis.** Melanoma in situ (eg, atypical melanocyte hyperplasia, severe melanocytic dysplasia) but no invasion (Clark's level I).
      d. **T1.** Tumor no more than 0.75 mm in thickness and invading the papillary dermis (Clark's level II).
      e. **T2.** Tumor more than 0.75 mm but less than 1.5 mm in thickness, invading the papillary-reticular dermal interface, or both (Clark's level III).
      f. **T3.** Tumor more than 1.5 mm but less than 4 mm in thickness, invading the reticular dermis, or both (Clark's level IV).
         (1) **T3a.** Tumor more than 1.5 mm but less than 3 mm in thickness.
         (2) **T3b.** Tumor more than 3 mm but less than 4 mm in thickness.
      g. **T4.** Tumor more than 4 mm in thickness, invading the subcutaneous tissue (Clark's level V), satellites less than 2 cm of the primary tumor, or all of these.
         (1) **T4a.** Tumor more than 4 mm in thickness, invading the subcutaneous tissue, or both.
         (2) **T4b.** Satellite or satellites less than 2 cm of the primary tumor.
   2. **Lymph node stage**
      a. **NX.** The regional lymph nodes cannot be assessed.
      b. **N0.** No regional lymph node metastases exist.
      c. **N1.** Metastases no larger than 3 cm in greatest dimension are present in any regional lymph node area.
      d. **N2.** Metastases larger than 3 cm in greatest dimension are present in any regional lymph node area, in-transit metastases are present, or both.
         (1) **N2a.** Metastasis larger than 3 mm in greatest dimension is present in any regional lymph node area.
         (2) **N2b.** In-transit metastases are present.

       (3) N2c. Both N2a and N2b metastases are present.
3. **Metastatic stage**
    a. **MX.** The presence of distant metastases cannot be assessed.
    b. **M0.** No distant metastases exist.
    c. **M1.** Distant metastases are present.
       (1) M1a. Metastases are present in the skin or subcutaneous tissue or the lymph node or nodes beyond the regional lymph node areas.
       (2) M1b. Visceral metastases are present.
         Note: In-transit metastases involve the skin or subcutaneous tissue more than 2 cm from the primary tumor but not beyond the regional lymph nodes.
4. **Histopathologic grade**
    a. **GX** The grade cannot be assessed.
    b. **G1** Well differentiated.
    c. **G2** Moderately well differentiated.
    d. **G3** Poorly differentiated.
    e. **G4** Undifferentiated.
5. **Stage groupings**
    a. **Stage I (47%).** T1–2, N0, M0.
    b. **Stage II (38%).** T3, N0, M0.
    c. **Stage III (13%).** T4, N0, M0; any T, N1–2, M0.
    d. **Stage IV (2%).** Any T, any N, M1.

IX. Treatment
A. Surgery
1. **Primary malignant melanoma**
    a. **Indications.** Presently, the only effective therapy for melanoma is surgical resection.
    b. **Approaches.** The surgical approach to each lesion varies considerably and depends on the location and depth of the primary lesion. Therefore, treatment must be individualized.
    c. **Procedures.** Surgical procedures vary widely depending on the specific circumstances. Generally, once the diagnosis of melanoma is established by biopsy, a wide excision of the primary lesion is performed, and lymphadenectomy is considered based on clinical findings and risk factors.
       (1) Biopsy. A biopsy of **all suspicious dermal lesions** should be performed to exclude the possibility of melanoma. A **full-thickness** sample of dermis and subcutaneous fat must be obtained for accurate **microstaging** (Breslow's thickness and Clark's level). Although excisional and incisional biopsies are both acceptable, **shave or curette biopsies are absolutely contraindicated**.
         (a) Excisional biopsy. Complete excision of lesions **less than 1.5–2 cm** in diameter is recommended unless the lesion is situated in a critical location (eg, the face, hand, foot) and sufficient skin is not available for primary closure. **Margins of 2 mm** are satisfactory, and the orientation of the incision should not compromise subsequent wide excision.
         (b) Incisional biopsy. A biopsy of lesions in **critical areas** (the face, hands, and feet) as well as **large lesions** is performed best with a **6-mm dermal punch**. A full-thickness core from a **central area** is preferred. No data suggests that incisional biopsies increase the risk of local recurrence or distant metastases.
       (2) Wide excision. Re-excision is required following simple biopsy because a **40% local recurrence rate** may be expected in the absence of wide excision. Skin and subcutaneous tissue around the primary site are excised down to the underlying fascia, and the wound is closed primarily or with a skin graft. Originally, **5-cm** margins were used empirically, and initial data supported this; yet several subsequent studies suggest that the width of excision did not influence the pattern of recurrence or patient survival. If, however, patients are stratified based on Breslow's depth of invasion, recent data indicate that the **risk of local recurrence is directly related to the thickness of the primary lesion**. A randomized trial conducted by the **World Health Organization (WHO)** found that **1 cm margins** were adequate in all patients with thin melanomas (**< 1 mm thick**) but not in those with invasions of more than 1 mm. Therefore, **the width of surgical margins should be guided by the depth of the primary melanoma** (see Table 20–1), particularly

TABLE 20–1. THE REQUIRED EXTENT OF WIDE EXCISION FOR MALIGNANT MELANOMA

Depth of Invasion	Width of Excision
0 mm (in situ)	1 cm
0–1.0 mm	1–2 cm
1.0–3.0 mm	3 cm
> 3.0 mm	3–5 cm

because minimal cosmetic differences with "narrow" and "wide" excisions if **rotation and advancement flap techniques** are used for primary closure. Certain anatomic sites, however, merit special consideration. **Subungual melanomas**, for instance, should be treated with distal interphalangeal (small lesions) or ray (extensive lesions) **amputation**. For lesions of the **ear helix, wedge excision** with plastic closure or **partial amputation** is recommended. Due to cosmetic considerations and the fact that most lesions are thin, **facial melanomas** generally are excised with a **1–2.5 cm margin**. They have a **4% recurrence rate**, depending on location and the microstage. No evidence suggests that a long time interval between biopsy and wide excision adversely affects outcome.

(3) Regional lymphadenectomy

(a) **Therapeutic (delayed) lymphadenectomy.** Melanoma frequently metastasizes to regional lymph nodes, and removal of the involved nodes (lymphadenectomy) currently remains the **only effective and potentially curative treatment** for these patients. In the absence of metastatic disease, a biopsy (fine needle aspiration or open biopsy) and lymphadectomy of **clinically suspicious lymph nodes** should be performed. Standard lymphadenectomy procedures include the following:

(i) **superficial inguinal lymphadenectomy** (triangle bounded by the sartorius muscle, inguinal ligament, and adductor muscle group), may require extension to the **deep inguinal (pelvic) nodes** if the highest inguinal node (**Cloquet's node**) is involved.

(ii) **axillary lymphadenectomy** (pyramid defined by the pectoralis and latissimus dorsi muscles, chest wall, skin, humerus, and axillary vein), often sacrifices the intercostobrachial cutaneous nerve but spares the **long thoracic nerve (of Bell)** and the **thoracodorsal nerve**.

(iii) **anterior cervical lymphadenectomy** (triangle delineated by the midline, sternocleidomastoid muscle, and mandible).

(iv) **posterior cervical lymphadenectomy** (triangle confined by the sternocleidomastoid and trapezius muscles and the clavicle).

(v) **radical cervical lymphadenectomy** (bordered by the midline, mandible, trapezius muscle, and clavicle), can be modified to preserve the **internal jugular vein, sternocleidomastoid muscle, and accessory spinal nerve**.

(vi) **superficial parotidectomy** (for scalp and face lesions that arise anterior to the pinna of the ear and superior to the commissure of the lip), is often combined with radical cervical lymphadenectomy.

(b) **Elective (immediate or prophylactic) lymphadenectomy.** Considerable controversy surrounds the management of clinically uninvolved regional lymph nodes. Theoretically, early lymphadenectomy **may prevent distant dissemination** and increase survival in patients with microscopic nodal disease but without distant metastases: ie, Clark's levels III and IV (0.76–3.99 mm) lesions. In addition to microstaging, other prognostic factors such as anatomic site, ulceration, and gender may identify patients who harbor regional microscopic metastases. Prospective nonrandomized data from the Sydney Melanoma Unit and the University of Alabama as well as retrospective information from Duke Medical Center and Memorial Sloan-Kettering Cancer Center suggest that **10-year survival** in patients with **intermediate thickness (0.76–3.99 mm)** melanomas is **improved by 16–31%** with elective lymphadenectomy. However, two large, **prospective, randomized trials** sponsored by the WHO (extremity melanomas only) and the Mayo Clinic failed to substantiate these findings, although the WHO study did demonstrate a small (10% at 5 years and 20% at 10 years) but statistically insignificant advantage to elective lymphadenectomy in patients with 3–3.9 mm lesions. Currently, 2 international cooperative surgical trials are evaluating the efficacy of elective lymph node dissection in patients with melanoma.

- (c) **Selective lymphadenectomy.** Although elective lymphadenectomy may not increase survival (see above), lymphadenectomy is required for **optimal staging, prognosis, and treatment planning** (particularly in clinical trials). Yet many patients do not have lymph node metastases and, therefore, are subjected needlessly to the substantial morbidity of elective lymphadenectomy (particularly **inguinal** lymphadenectomy; see below). To overcome this limitation, patients at UCLA were studied by **intraoperative isosulfan blue lymphoscintigraphy** to identify **"sentinel"** lymph nodes that were at risk for occult metastatic disease. If prompt pathologic inspection (including **S-100 stain**) demonstrated melanoma, **immediate lymphadenectomy was performed**; however, if no tumor was detected, the procedure was terminated. Preliminary results suggest that this technique accurately identifies patients who may benefit from elective lymphadenectomy. However, the results from a multicenter clinical trial designed to confirm this observation are not yet available. Therefore, it should still be considered **experimental**.

2. **Locally advanced and metastatic melanoma**
    a. **In-transit metastases.** Dermal and subcutaneous metastases between the area of the primary tumor and the regional lymphatics, in-transit metastases, occur in **1–2% of patients**. These lesions are much more common on the **lower extremity** and are associated with lymph node metastases in **67%** of patients and systemic disease in most patients. Treatment depends on the **number** and **location** of the metastases and may include simple excision (for limited numbers or residual disease), radiation therapy, chemotherapy, intra-lesional immunotherapy, and isolated limb perfusion, but almost always includes **regional lymphadenectomy**. Isolated limb perfusion may be the **treatment of choice** for most patients who have no distant metastases (see p 127, **IX.C.3.b**).
    b. **Distant metastases.** Despite widespread dissemination, excision of metastatic melanoma may provide excellent palliation in **selected patients**.
        (1) **Subcutaneous metastases.** Subcutaneous and lymph node metastases occur in **50–75% of patients** and may be the only manifestation of disease. Simple excision of these disease sites is associated with a **median survival of 17–31 months and 5-year survival of 5–10%**.
        (2) **Pulmonary metastases.** Although the lungs are involved in **70–87%** of patients with melanoma, **5–22%** will present with a **solitary** pulmonary nodule as the sole manifestation of disease. Although controversial, in patients with tumor **doubling times of more than 40 days, thoracotomy is indicated** following 1–3 months of observation (to allow other metastases time to present) because **33–50%** of patients will have a **benign** nodule or a **second primary lesion** (eg, lung carcinoma) and because **median survival of 16–24 months and 5-year survival of 12–35%** have been reported in this setting.
        (3) **Central nervous system metastases.** Although intracranial metastases occur in **36–54%** of patients with disseminated melanoma, solitary cerebral metastases are **uncommon (25% of patients)** but are associated with a high rate of hemorrhage and seizure activity. However, retrospective and prospective data suggest that if a solitary brain metastasis is discovered, resection (followed by postoperative radiation therapy) **improves symptoms in 87%** of patients and occasionally **may prolong survival** to as long as 3 years.

(4) Gastrointestinal metastases. Most commonly, patients with gastrointestinal metastases present with **occult blood loss**. However, **obstruction** (often caused by **intussusception**), also occurs frequently and, along with **acute** hemorrhage, is a common indication for surgery. Because widespread disease is present in most patients and prolonged survival is unusual, surgery should be considered strictly **palliative**.

3. **Morbidity and mortality.** Most complications of lymphadenectomy are wound-related; their nature and severity vary with the surgical site.

  a. **Superficial parotidectomy.** Overall, problems following this procedure are uncommon.
    (1) Facial nerve paralysis (10–20% temporary; 1–3% permanent).
    (2) Gustatory sweating (**Frey's syndrome**; 5%).
    (3) Seroma (uncommon).
    (4) Salivary fistulae (uncommon).
    (5) Infection (rare).

  b. **Cervical lymphadenectomy. Acute** complications occur in **10–19%** of patients, whereas **chronic** complaints arise in only **6–7%**.
    (1) Pain (acute; common).
    (2) Seroma (acute; uncommon).
    (3) Skin necrosis (acute; uncommon).
    (4) Chyle leak (acute; uncommon; stops within 10 days if < 50 mL/d).
    (5) Infection (acute; rare).
    (6) Spinal accessory nerve damage (chronic; 30%).
    (7) Unsatisfactory cosmetic result (chronic; common).
    (8) Neck pain (chronic; uncommon).

  c. **Axillary lymphadenectomy.** Complications following this operation are uncommon but increase with age.
    (1) Seroma (27%).
    (2) Nerve pain or dysfunction (temporary or permanent; 22%).
    (3) Hemorrhage (1%).
    (4) Functional deficit (chronic; 9%).
    (5) Chronic pain (6%).
    (6) Arm edema (1%).

  d. **Inguinal lymphadenectomy.** The most debilitating problem following this procedure is **leg edema**, particularly if the iliac and obturator nodes are removed along with the superficial inguinal nodes. However, with **prophylactic measures** (eg, perioperative antibiotics, leg elevation, elastic stockings, diuretics) the incidence of **acute edema** may be reduced from **46% to 7%** and **chronic edema, to 2–5%**. Other complications increase with age and include the following difficulties:
    (1) Seroma (23%).
    (2) Chronic pain (5%).
    (3) Functional deficit (3%).
    (4) Skin necrosis (uncommon).

B. **Radiation therapy**

1. **Primary malignant melanoma.** Currently, conventional radiation therapy is not indicated in the treatment of primary melanoma; however, several European reports suggest that **superficial contact x-ray therapy** at extremely high doses (**> 10,000 cGy**) with rapid fall-off (> 50% at 1 mm) may be indicated for large, superficial lesions in critical areas (eg, lentigo maligna melanoma of the head and neck).

2. **Adjuvant radiation therapy**

  a. **Preoperative radiation therapy.** Radiation therapy in this setting has not been fully evaluated.

  b. **Postoperative radiation therapy.** Limited data suggests that radiation therapy (**4500 cGy over 10 days**) following local excision of **nodular head and neck melanomas** may improve local tumor control. Moreover, one study of postoperative radiation therapy (**2400–3000 cGy over 4–5 days**) in **high-risk** head and neck melanomas reported better regional tumor control with the addition of radiation therapy, although no impact on disease-free or overall survival was documented.

3. **Locally advanced and metastatic melanoma.** Although malignant melanoma was considered "radioresistant" for many years, recent evidence suggests that radiation therapy may be effective in many clinical situations. **Large-dose and fractional-dose strategies** yield **50% complete response rates** with **subcu-**

taneous and lymph node metastases, **50%** with **bone** metastases, and **67%** with **brain** metastases. Furthermore, the addition of **hyperthermia** increases the complete response rate to **70–80%. Fast neutron therapy** also produces high complete response rates (**71%**) but with a **22% morbidity rate**. New data also indicate that radiation may control **in-transit** melanoma that has failed other therapy. Finally, initial response rates may be **underestimated** because the gross disappearance of melanoma may take several months and residual masses may be composed of nondividing cells and fibrous stroma.

C. **Chemotherapy**
1. **Primary malignant melanoma.** No role has been documented for chemotherapy in the initial treatment of primary melanoma.
2. **Adjuvant chemotherapy**
   a. **Isolated limb perfusion.** The use of isolated limb perfusion in the adjuvant setting is **controversial.** Results from several **nonrandomized institutional** studies suggest that the combination of surgery and hyperthermic isolated limb perfusion with phenylalanine mustard substantially **improves the recurrence and survival rates** of patients with localized or regionally metastatic melanoma when compared to surgery alone. The only **prospective randomized trial** comparing surgery (wide excision with regional lymphadenectomy) alone to surgery with hyperthermic (42° C) isolated limb perfusion using phenylalanine mustard was closed prematurely as a result of a highly statistically significant **improvement in recurrence rate** in the isolated limb perfusion group; however, because of poor results in the control arm, the entire trial has been questioned. Currently, randomized multi-institutional studies sponsored by the WHO and the North American Perfusion Group are attempting to define the role, if any, that isolated limb perfusion plays in the adjuvant treatment of melanoma.
   b. **Systemic chemotherapy.** Numerous clinical trials with **dacarbazine (DTIC)**, either alone or in combination with other chemotherapeutic (nitrosourea) and immunomodulatory agents, have demonstrated **no survival benefit** over therapy with surgery alone. However, because 90% of patients present with localized disease and many are at high risk for local, regional, and systemic recurrence, adjuvant therapy should remain an active area of research.
3. **Locally advanced and metastatic melanoma.** Despite limited success, chemotherapy remains the **only systemic treatment** option available to most patients with metastatic melanoma. Chemotherapy, however, rarely is effective or indicated in the management of in-transit melanoma unless systemic disease is present.
   a. **Regional chemotherapy.** The intra-arterial infusion of chemotherapeutic agents (**DTIC or cisplatin**) for locally recurrent and regional **in-transit** melanoma has produced **brief responses in 40–50%** of patients, but this approach has never been directly compared with intravenous therapy.
   b. **Hyperthermic (42° C) isolated limb perfusion** with phenylalanine mustard (1 mg/kg) is highly successful in controlling **in-transit** metastases, with **76%** of patients achieving **long-term eradication of local or regional disease**. No improvement, however, is observed in survival because patients die of distant metastases. Unfortunately, phenylalanine mustard is no longer available for this use; other drugs have been substituted but do not have the same degree of success. Finally, surgical excision of residual lesions, particularly if they are large and symptomatic, is often indicated.
   c. **Single agents.** Of 30 drugs tested in the treatment of metastatic melanoma, only **2 (DTIC and nitrosoureas)** yielded response rates greater than 10%, with **DTIC** (850 mg/m^2 IV every 3 weeks, 250 mg/m^2 IV for 5 days every 3 weeks, or 4.5 mg/kg/day IV for 10 days every 4 weeks) considered to be the single most active agent (**15–25% overall and 4.5% complete response rate**). **Nitrosoureas** such as carmustine (BCNU), lomustine (CCNU), and semustine (methyl-CCNU) produced **10–18% overall response rates. Skin, subcutaneous, lymph node, and lung metastases** responded significantly better than liver and brain disease. Other agents with response rates of 10% included cisplatin, vinca alkaloids, mitolactol (Dibromodulcitol), vindesine, doxorubicin, and taxol. Phase II studies are required to more clearly define the activity of new agents, but it appears that none exceed the activity of DTIC.
   d. **Combination chemotherapy.** Historically, combination chemotherapy regimens have not enhanced response rates over DTIC alone in multi-institutional cooperative group trials; however, a recent pilot study combining **high-**

dose cisplatin with the thiol derivative **WR-2721** ([S-2-3-amino-propylamino] ethyl phosphorothionic acid), to deliver a more effective dose with less normal tissue toxicity, reported a **53% objective response rate** with improved activity at doses of **more than 150 mg/m²**. Other trials of high-dose cisplatin (200 mg/m²) have yielded more modest response rates (28% and 29%). In addition, the **combination of DTIC, carmustine, cisplatin**, and **tamoxifen** produced a **response rate of more than 50%** in an initial series as well as a subsequent confirmatory study. However, as a result of thrombotic complications, **tamoxifen was omitted** in an intervening series of 20 patients and the **response rate fell to 10%**. Combinations of DTIC, cisplatin, and tamoxifen as well as cisplatin, carmustine, and vinblastine are currently under study; however, randomized trials comparing these new promising combinations to DTIC alone will be necessary before they can be recommended.

D. **Hormonal therapy.** Although unproven, melanoma has long been suspected of being an **estrogen-dependent tumor** based on the following observations: (1) it is **rare** before puberty, (2) the **peak incidence** in females occurs during the **childbearing years**, (3) widespread **dissemination** may occur during **pregnancy**, (4) spontaneous **regressions** have been reported following **parturition**, and (5) survival rates favor **postmenopausal females**. Furthermore, **estrogen receptors** were found recently on **both** tumor cells and benign nevi of melanoma patients but **not** on nevi of normal individuals. The antiestrogen **tamoxifen** by itself, at standard or high doses, has little objective antitumor activity. However, when combined with DTIC alone (Italian Cooperative Multicenter Oncology Group) or DTIC, cisplatin, and carmustine, **synergistic response rates** have been documented in **preliminary** trials. The mechanism of this synergy may involve calcium channel activity or an interaction with DTIC, cisplatin, or carmustine. Further study is required to confirm these findings.

E. **Immunotherapy.** A well-recognized, albeit uncommon occurrence in melanoma is **spontaneous regression**. This phenomenon implies the presence of an immunologic influence on tumor growth and is the impetus to the development of immunomodulatory therapy. The types of immunotherapy currently being investigated for specific immunity are (1) monoclonal antibodies (MoAb), tumor cell vaccine, and interleukin-2 (IL-2) (active immunity), (2) tumor-infiltrating lymphocytes (TIL) (adoptive immunity), and (3) conjugated MoAb (ricin,[131]I) (passive immunity). Nonspecific investigational immunotherapy includes (1) IL-2, interferon (IFN), IL-6, and bacillus Calmette-Guerin (BCG) (active immunity), (2) lymphokine-activated killer (LAK) cells (adoptive immunity), and (3) chemotherapy (passive immunity) (see Table 20–2).

1. **Primary malignant melanoma.** As a result of the tremendous effectiveness of surgery in the treatment of primary melanoma, the use of immunotherapy as the initial treatment of malignant melanoma cannot be justified.

2. **Adjuvant immunotherapy.** Adjuvant immunotherapy continues to generate interest, because in some cases it is associated with **minimal toxicity**. However, the value of adjuvant immunotherapy in the treatment of high-risk melanoma patients remains to be determined.

   a. **Tumor cell vaccine.** Although early trials of **allogeneic whole melanoma cell vaccine** demonstrated antibody responses in some patients and an apparent improvement in survival, subsequent studies by the WHO and others have failed to substantiate this finding. An oncolysate vaccinia has also been used in a prospective randomized trial without success.

   b. **Interferon-alpha (IFN-alpha).** The Eastern Cooperative Oncology Group

TABLE 20–2. CURRENT EXPERIMENTAL IMMUNOTHERAPY FOR MALIGNANT MELANOMA

Specificity	Passive	Active	Adoptive
Specific	Conjugated MoAb (ricin, ^{131}I, etc.)	MoAb Tumor cell vaccine ?IL-2	TIL
Nonspecific	Chemotherapy	IL-2 IFN IL-6 BCG	LAK

(ECOG) and the North Central Cancer Treatment Group (NCCTG) sponsored adjuvant trials of **IFN-alpha-2 at maximum tolerated doses in patients with either regional lymph node metastases or T4 primary lesions**. In the ECOG study, 20×10^6 units/m² per day for 5 of 7 days each of the first 4 weeks (**induction**) followed by 10×10^6 units/m² every other day for 11 months (**maintenance**) were given, whereas 12×10^6 units/m² every other day for 3 months was administered in the NCCTG study. Both trials included concomitant controls but currently are not mature enough to analyze. In addition, to exploit the **maximum antiproliferative activity** generated by prolonged IFN-alpha exposure and the **maximum natural killer (NK) cell activation** produced by 3×10^6 units of IFN-alpha per dose, ECOG recently instituted a second trial comparing the previous regimen as well as observation alone to low-dose therapy (3×10^6 units/m² 3 times weekly) for an indefinite period. A similar trial in patients with lymph node metastases was recently opened by the WHO, comparing observation alone to low-dose therapy (3×10^6 units/m² every other day) for 2 years. Results from these 4 studies will provide important information, not only on the therapeutic efficacy of IFN-alpha in the adjuvant treatment of malignant melanoma, but also on the optimum effective in vivo dose.

   c. **Interferon-gamma (IFN-gamma).** The Southwest Oncology Group (SWOG) **terminated** its trial of adjuvant IFN-gamma in patients with T2–T4 (> 0.76 mm) primary lesions or regional lymph node metastases because of a trend toward increased relapse and earlier death among subjects receiving IFN-gamma (**58.6% vs 37.8% in controls**), although the difference was **not** statistically significant. A larger, ongoing study by the European Organization for Research and Treatment of Cancer comparing IFN-gamma (at the same dose as the SWOG study) to IFN-alpha and controls, however, has demonstrated no adverse trends. Although the SWOG IFN-gamma **dose and subcutaneous (SC) route of administration** have been questioned, it is difficult to interpret the failure of this trial in the absence of any immunologic monitoring, especially because the patients most likely to benefit from immunotherapy are those with the **lowest tumor burden**, who experience late relapse and require long-term follow-up to observe antitumor effects. Further follow-up from both trials should help define the role of adjuvant IFN-gamma therapy.

3. **Locally advanced and metastatic melanoma**
   a. **Tumor cell vaccine.** Based on the observation that antibodies in sera of melanoma patients recognized cell surface antigens on melanoma cells, numerous attempts have been made to develop a vaccine to induce active immunity against melanoma in an effort either to cause the regression of established tumors or, more frequently, to influence the natural history of high-risk individuals by preventing recurrence. The majority of these vaccines have utilized either whole melanoma cells or extracts obtained from melanoma cells.
   b. **Interferon-alpha.** As a result of **low doses** and **brief treatment intervals**, clinical trials with **purified natural** IFN-alpha were **inadequate** to fully evaluate the antitumor activity of this agent. With recombinant cytokine, however, phase I and II trials using up to the maximum tolerated dose of IFN-alpha ($10–50 \times 10^6$ units/dose SC, IM, or IV daily) in a variety of doses, routes, and schedules have yielded response rates between 14.4% (IFN-alpha-2a) and 22.6% (IFN-alpha-2b). The optimum dose, however, has not been determined. Although **intermittent** therapy is associated with **worse** response rates, results with the different types of recombinant IFN-alpha are **identical (overall response rate of 17.5%). Small** tumor masses respond more frequently than large ones, and some responses are observed only after a protracted period of therapy.
   c. **Interferon-gamma.** Although numerous studies of IFN-gamma have been reported, **none have demonstrated significant antitumor activity in malignant melanoma**. The optimum dose, route, and schedule of administration for antitumor activity, however, have not been defined. A recent ECOG phase I and II(B) study began to examine **doses over a long range, administered 3 times weekly for 3 months in 80–160 patients at each dose** to identify the optimal immunomodulatory dosage for antitumor activity. Once this is known, meaningful clinical trials will be possible.
   d. **Interleukin-2.** Based on a variety of animal tumor models demonstrating **dose-dependent IL-2 antitumor activity**, clinical trials were instituted by

the Surgery Branch of the National Cancer Institute (NCI) as well as 6 extramural clinical research centers (IL-2 Extramural Working Group [EMWG] to evaluate **high-dose IL-2 therapy** (100,000 Cetus units/kg or $1-6 \times 10^6$ Hoffmann-LaRoche units/m^2 every 8 hrs for 5 days and repeated after 7–10 days) in the treatment of metastatic melanoma. A **24% overall response rate** was observed with **no** complete responses. However, the toxicity of high-dose bolus IL-2 administration (due to a **capillary leak syndrome**; see, also, p 23, **I.A.3.c**), including a 1.5% treatment-related mortality, has been a major obstacle to more widespread application of this therapy. West et al have reported the use of continuous infusions of 3×10^6 Cetus units/m^2 per day (18×10^6 IU/m^2 per day), with diminished toxicity by continuous infusion and comparable antitumor activity.

e. **Lymphokine-activated killer (LAK) cells.** The incubation of CD3$^-$, CD16$^+$ peripheral blood mononuclear cells (including large granular lymphocytes) in IL-2 for 3–5 days activates the cells to lyse a variety of **fresh and cultured tumor cells** but not fresh normal cells. The adoptive transfer of these **LAK cells** with IL-2 in animal models mediates greater antitumor activity than either IL-2 or LAK cells alone. Clinical trials were instituted by the Surgery Branch of the NCI as well as the EMWG to evaluate IL-2 and LAK cell therapy in the treatment of metastatic melanoma. An **overall response rate (21%)** identical to that of IL-2 alone was found; however, the addition of LAK cells did increase the **complete response rate (8.3%)**. Some of the complete responses have been durable (up to 52 months). Again, the EMWG has reproduced these findings. Efforts are ongoing to increase the efficacy of LAK cells by **purifying LAK cell populations** (eg, through plastic adherence yielding "A-LAK") and by **increasing LAK cell localization** at the site of tumor (eg, by MoAb), but until more progress is made, LAK cell therapy must be considered highly experimental.

f. **Tumor-infiltrating lymphocytes (TIL).** TIL are lymphocytes isolated from tumor deposits and expanded to large numbers in vitro in the presence of **autologous tumor cells and IL-2**. Murine experiments suggest that these CD3$^+$ cells are 50–100 times more potent than LAK cells, require less IL-2, persist for longer periods of time, and specifically migrate to sites of tumor. Early clinical trials indicate that patients treated with TIL and IL-2 have as high as a **55% response rate**; however, further work must be done to confirm these results.

g. **Combination therapy.** Combinations of various immunomodulatory and chemotherapeutic agents in animal models demonstrate improved and occasionally synergistic therapeutic efficacy. Combinations of IL-2 and other agents, such as IFN-alpha and more recently IFN-gamma, tumor necrosis factor (TNF), low-dose cyclophosphamide, DTIC, cisplatin, and WR2721 are specific examples. IL-2 and either cyclophosphamide or TNF have produced disappointing response rates of 10% or less in early trials, whereas the addition of **IFN-alpha to IL-2 improves the response rate from 24% to 36%**. In addition, the combination of IL-2 and IFN-gamma enhances LAK generation, although this has not yet been shown to improve therapy.

h. **Monoclonal antibodies (MoAb).** MoAb studies have centered on 4 melanoma antigens: the **gangliosides GD$_2$ and GD$_3$, p97 antigen, and melanoma chondroitin-sulfated proteoglycan**. If given alone, murine IgG3 MoAbs that activate complement and mediate antibody-dependent cellular cytotoxicity (ADCC) produce **19% (anti-GD$_3$) and 22% (anti-GD$_2$) response rates**. However, murine MoAb conjugated to the **ricin A chain** (inhibitor of protein synthesis) demonstrated only a **9% response rate** in phase II trials, and murine MoAb **Fab fragments** (anti-p97) conjugated to ^{131}I have not yet been tested. Problems stemming from the development of **human anti-mouse antibodies (HAMA)** have led to the exploration of human as well as chimeric MoAb (murine Fab fragments bound to human Fc segments). **Intralesional injection of human** MoAb (anti-GD$_2$) resulted in complete clinical and histologic regression of **90%** of **in-transit** melanoma lesions. Despite promising early results, therapy with MoAb remains strictly experimental.

i. **Bacillus Calumette-Guerin (BCG).** One of the earliest examples of successful immunotherapy was the regression of **60–90%** of recurrent cutaneous melanoma lesions with **intralesional** BCG. Moreover, 20% of nearby untreated nodules regressed simultaneously. Unfortunately, no concomitant **systemic** activity resulted. Other agents that have been used as nonspecific immunostimulants include **dinitrochlorobenzene**, purified protein derivatives, and methanol-extracted residue.

X. Prognosis

A. **Risk of recurrence.** The risk of recurrence may be separated into the risk of local and the risk of distant recurrence.

1. **Local manifestations.** The risk of local recurrence (within 5 cm of the primary lesion) is **3.2% overall** but is increased by the following factors: **thickness of more than 4 mm,** 13%; **ulceration,** 11.5%; and **face, scalp, hand, or foot location,** 5–12%.

2. **Systemic manifestations.** The risk of systemic (lymph node and distant) recurrence depends on the depth of penetration by Breslow's staging.
   a. **Less than 0.75 mm,** 2–3% lymph node and distant metastases.
   b. **0.76–1.50 mm,** 25% lymph node and 8% distant metastases.
   c. **1.51–4 mm,** 57% lymph node and 15% distant metastases.
   d. **More than 4 mm,** 62% lymph node and 72% distant metastases.

B. **Five-year survival.** The 5-year survival by TNM stage is outlined below:
1. **Stage I,** 97%.
2. **Stage II,** 74%.
3. **Stage III,** 41%.
4. **Stage IV,** less than 10%.

C. **Adverse prognostic factors.** A multitude of prognostic factors influence the ultimate prognosis. The **most important** characteristics, however, are the presence of **lymph node metastases**, the **depth of invasion** of the primary lesion, and **ulceration**. In addition, the following factors may adversely affect the prognosis:

1. **Age. Advanced age** is associated with a poor outcome.

2. **Sex. Males** have a worse prognosis than females, primarily as a result of a higher incidence of truncal and ulcerating lesions.

3. **Site of primary lesion.** For equivalent lesions, **trunk** melanomas do poorly compared to those on the **head and neck**, which also do poorly compared to **extremity** lesions. In addition, primary lesions located on the skin of the upper back, posterior arm, neck, and scalp ("**BANS" area**), particularly if associated with regional lymph node metastases, have a uniquely poor prognosis for unclear reasons.

4. **Ulceration.** Ulceration decreases **5-year survival from 77% to 52%** for lesions larger than 3 mm in diameter.

5. **Histology.** A **high rate of mitosis per square millimeter** and the presence of **lymphatic or vascular invasion** signify a poor prognosis.

6. **Growth pattern.** Nodular melanomas do worse than **superficial spreading melanomas** which, in turn, do worse than lentigo maligna melanoma.

7. **Clark's level.** Increasing Clark's levels are associated with a **greater** likelihood of lymph node and distant metastases and a poor overall prognosis.

8. **Breslow's depth.** Tumor thickness of more than 0.75 mm, which correlates with the incidence of **lymph node and distant metastases** and the **overall prognosis**, is more accurate than Clark's level. In the presence of **regression**, however, the prognostic value of tumor thickness (and Clark's level) is diminished.

9. **Pregnancy.** Although controversial, melanomas arising during pregnancy are associated with a particularly aggressive clinical course and a grave prognosis.

10. **Lymph node metastases.** The **number** of involved lymph nodes, as determined by immunohistologic (S-100) staining, is the **single most important prognostic factor**. Irrespective of the level or depth of the primary lesion, the 5-year survival rate is **73%** for patients with pathologically **negative** nodes, **55%** for those with **1–3 positive** nodes, and only **26%** for those with **4 or more nodes** involved. In addition, some evidence suggests that **macroscopic** (clinically positive) nodal involvement (**21% 5-year and 12% 10-year survival**) signifies a worse outcome than **microscopic** (clinically negative) disease (**44% 5-year and 28% 10-year survival**). Finally, patients with lymph node metastases from a **known primary site** exhibit worse survival than those from an **unknown** source, particularly **after 5 years**.

11. **Number of metastatic sites. Multiple** metastatic sites signify a worse prognosis than a **single** metastatic site (**7–12 month** median survival). The median survival is 2–8 months for the former and 7–12 months for the latter.

12. **Brief disease-free interval.** Patients with a disease-free interval of **less than 12 months** have an expected **median survival of 3 months** compared to **7.1 months** for a disease-free survival of **more than 12 months**.

13. **First site of metastatic disease.** The prognosis for patients with **CNS or he-**

patic metastases is worse than for those with **subcutaneous, lymph node, or pulmonary** metastases. The median survival is 2–4 months for the former and 10–11 months for the latter.

XI. Patient follow-up

A. **General guidelines.** Patients with melanoma should be followed every 3 months for 2 years, every 6 months for an additional 3 years, and then annually for evidence of tumor recurrence. Patients with metastatic disease should be followed every 1–2 months for symptoms requiring further palliative measures and for nutritional monitoring, but diagnostic tests should be limited to symptomatic areas that are amenable to further palliation. Each clinic visit should include the following examinations:

1. **Medical history and physical examination.** An interval medical history and thorough physical examination should be performed during each office visit.
2. **Blood tests** (see p 1, **IV.A**)
   a. **Complete blood count.**
   b. **Hepatic transaminases.**
   c. **Alkaline phosphatase.**
3. **Chest x-ray** (see p 3, **IV.C.1**)

B. **Optional evaluation.** The following examinations may be indicated depending on previous findings or clinical suspicion.

1. **Blood tests** (see p 1, **IV.A**)
   a. **5-Nucleotidase.**
   b. **GGTP.**
2. **Imaging studies** (see p 3, **IV.C**)
   a. **Chest CT.** Chest CT scan remains a good method of detecting mediastinal adenopathy and pulmonary metastases. In patients with no residual tumor, a chest CT scan should be obtained if suspicious findings are identified on medical history, physical examination, or chest x-ray.
   b. **Abdominal CT.** CT scan of the abdomen is the most sensitive test to exclude liver metastases and should be ordered if symptoms or blood tests suggest the possibility of liver disease.
   c. **Magnetic resonance imaging.**
   d. **Technetium-99m bone scan.**
3. **Invasive diagnostic procedures.** In a patient without known residual cancer, a biopsy of any suspicious or abnormal mass detected on physical examination, chest x-ray, or routine blood testing is indicated.

REFERENCES

Comis RL: DTIC (NSC 45388) in malignant melanoma: a perspective. *Cancer Treat Rep* 1976; **60**:165–176.

Del Prete SA et al: Combination chemotherapy with cisplatin, carmustine, dacarbazine, and tamoxifen in metastatic melanoma. *Cancer Treat Rep* 1984;**68**:1403–1405.

Fossati G et al: Immune response to autologous human melanoma: implication of class I and II MHC products. *Biochem Biophys Acta* 1986;**865**:235–251.

Ghussen F et al: The role of regional hyperthermic cytostatic perfusion in the treatment of extremity melanoma. *Cancer* 1988;**61**:654–659.

Glover D et al: WR-2721 and high-dose cisplatin: an active combination in the treatment of metastatic melanoma. *J Clin Oncol* 1987;**5**: 574–578.

Harwood AR: Conventional fractionated radiotherapy for 51 patients with lentigo maligna and lentigo maligna melanoma. *Int J Radiat Oncol Biol Phys* 1983;**9**:1019–1021.

Overgaard J, von der Masse H, Overgaard MA: A randomized study comparing two high-dose per fraction radiation schedules in recurrent or metastatic melanoma. *Int J Radiat Oncol Biol Phys* 1985;**11**:1837–1839.

Rosenberg SA et al: Experience with the use of high-dose interleukin-2 in the treatment of 652 cancer patients. *Ann Surg* 1989;**210**:474–485.

Sim FH et al: Lymphadenectomy in the management of stage I malignant melanoma: a prospective randomized study. *Mayo Clin Proc* 1986;**61**:697–705.

Storm FK, Morton DL: Value of therapeutic hyperthermic limb perfusion in advanced recurrent melanoma of the lower extremity. *Am J Surg* 1985;**150**:32–35.

Veronesi U et al: Primary cutaneous melanoma 2 mm less in thickness: results of a randomized study comparing wide with narrow surgical excision. A preliminary report. *N Engl J Med* 1988;**318**:1159–1162.

Veronesi U et al: Delayed regional lymph node dissection in stage I melanoma of the skin of the lower extremities. *Cancer* 1982;**49**:2420–2430.

21 Malignancies of the Skin

Andres Taleisnik, MD

I. **Epidemiology.** Basal cell carcinoma (**BCC**) and **squamous cell carcinoma (SCC)** are the most common forms of nonmelanoma skin cancer in the United States. In 1985, more than 208 cases per 100,000 males and females were diagnosed, leading to 12 deaths per 100,000 population. It is estimated that more than 600,000 new cases and 2000 deaths will occur in 1993. Although BCC outnumbers SCC by 3 to 1, SCC accounts for 75% of skin cancer deaths (1% of SCC cases). Geographically, the incidence of skin cancer increases as latitude decreases; however, the relative incidence of BCC compared to SCC is higher in northern (90% vs 10%) than in southern climates (75% vs 25%). The highest incidence of skin cancer occurs in whites at latitudes near the equator, while its occurrence in noncaucasian populations is often associated with unusual etiologic factors and anatomic sites.

II. **Risk factors**
   A. **Age.** The incidence of BCC and SCC steadily increases (33% per decade) after the age of 50 with more than 95% of lesions occurring in patients over 40 years of age.
   B. **Sex.** The risk of BCC and SCC is 1.5–2 and 2–3 times greater, respectively, in males than in females.
   C. **Race.** The risk in whites (232.6 per 100,000) is markedly higher than in blacks (3.4 per 100,000). Asian populations are at intermediate, albeit low risk.
   D. **Genetic factors**
      1. **Family history.** First-degree relatives of patients with skin cancer do not appear to be at increased risk.
      2. **Familial syndromes**
         a. **Xeroderma pigmentosum.** This autosomal recessive disease, affecting 0.4 people per 100,000, is associated with **defective repair of ultraviolet light-induced DNA damage** and strongly predisposes individuals to skin cancer, both BCC and SCC. Despite complete avoidance of sun exposure, patients often die from cutaneous malignancies before age 20.
         b. **Nevoid basal cell carcinoma syndrome.** This autosomal dominant symptom complex includes epidermoid cysts, 1–3 mm palmar and plantar "pits" (65%), and multiple BCCs that appear between puberty and age 35 in association with mild hypertelorism, rib anomalies, calcified falx cerebri, medulloblastoma, and fibrosarcoma of the jaw.
         c. **Gardner's syndrome** is inherited as an autosomal dominant disorder marked by epidermal and sebaceous cysts.
         d. **Nevus sebaceus syndrome of Jadassohn.** This distinctive syndrome is detected initially in affected children as a solitary, oval, yellow plaque on the scalp associated with alopecia. This area becomes verrucous during puberty, and multiple skin cancers of all types subsequently develop.
         e. **Torres's syndrome.** This hereditary disease is characterized by numerous BCC and nonmetastasizing sebaceous carcinomas arising in patients with multiple keratoacanthomas. **Carcinoma of the colon and ampulla of Vater** are frequent associated findings.
         f. **Epidermodysplasia verruciformis.** This rare autosomal recessive disorder manifests in childhood as multiple, disseminated, scaly, red-brown macules mimicking tinea versicolor. Human papillomavirus is commonly identified in these lesions, and 30% of patients develop SCC in sun-exposed areas by age 40.
         g. **Albinism.** Oculocutaneous albinism is an autosomal recessive disease distinguished by hypomelanosis or amelanosis of the skin, iris, fundus, and hair with photophobia, nystagmus, decreased visual acuity, and multiple cutaneous malignancies, including BCC, SCC, and melanoma.

E. **Skin complexion.** Fair skin that freckles, green or blue eyes, red or light blond hair, and poor tanning ability are all correlated with an increased risk of skin cancer.
F. **Previous dermatologic pathology**
   1. **Freckles.** The risk of skin cancer is elevated in patients with freckles.
   2. **Actinic keratoses.** Also known as **senile** or **solar keratoses**, these well-circumscribed macules are distinguished by a rough, thickened, scaly surface that may be brown, red, gray, or black and several millimeters to several centimeters in diameter. They arise on the head, neck, and extremities and are considered to be precancerous, although the exact rate of malignant transformation is unknown.
   3. **Disease of pigmentation** (see **2a** and **2g,** above).
   4. **Infection.** Viral infection with human papillomavirus (particularly type 5) is associated with both benign (eg, epidermodysplasia verruciformis) and malignant skin diseases.
   5. **Chronic inflammation and trauma.** SCC (and rarely BCC) that does not occur in sun-exposed skin often arises in areas chronically inflamed for years, ie, burn wounds (Marjolin's ulcers), draining wounds, chronic granulomas, fistulas, decubitus ulcers, and osteomyelitic sinuses. Infrared burns from hot pots worn next to the body for warmth (Kangri ulcers of India and Kairo ulcers of Japan), hot beds (Kang ulcers of China), and open fires (leading to chronic dermatitis known as erythema ab igne in China) predispose to skin cancer. Furthermore, old scars (eg, vaccination scars, tattoos, and scars on the scalp, trunk, and extremities that are more than 20 years old) are additional sites where tumor can arise. **Lymph node metastases are more** common in these patients, reflecting frequent delay in diagnosis and perhaps a more aggressive tumor.
G. **Radiation exposure**
   1. **Ultraviolet (UV) radiation.** UV radiation is the chief risk factor for skin cancer (both BCC and SCC) and is divided into 3 wavelength bands: UV-A (320–400 nm), UV-B (290–320 nm) and UV-C (200–290 nm). UV-C is effectively filtered by atmospheric ozone, while UV-B is only partially screened, resulting in sunburn, chronic skin damage, and skin cancer. Moreover, UV-B exposure is increasing as ozone is progressively eroded by pollutants, such as fluorocarbons used in refrigerants and aerosol propellants. UV-A, the wavelength used in tanning salons, induces additional damage beyond that of UV-B. Most likely, carcinogenesis involves photochemical alterations of DNA (formation of cross-linked pyrimidine dimers that block normal DNA synthesis) and alterations in immunity (modified Langerhans cell function as well as decreased helper and increased suppressor lymphocytes).
   2. **Ionizing radiation.** In the past, superficial irradiation (> 1000 cGy) administered (often inappropriately) for benign conditions such as acne, psoriatic keratosis, hemangioma, and hirsutism produced radiodermatitis, characterized by skin atrophy, depigmentation, telangiectasia, alopecia, and keratosis. Following a long latency period, 20–40% of these patients develop SCC (or BCC if the lesion is on the face). In addition, poor shielding commonly led to SCC of the hands of radiologists, dentists, and technicians. With improved equipment, technique, and radiation precautions, the risk of radiation-induced skin cancer has decreased dramatically. Interestingly, skin cancer is uncommon (5%) in areas of radiodermatitis from high-dose therapy for malignant disease. More dead cells, fewer genetically injured but viable cells, and shorter patient survival have been implicated as possible explanations for this difference.
H. **Chemical carcinogens.** Although rare today, chemically-induced skin cancers are known to occur in workers exposed to **soot** (scrotal cancer in chimney sweeps), **paraffin, pitch, coal tars, anthracene, creosote, asphalt, and lubricating oils.** Ingestion of **quinacrine hydrochloride or arsenic** (in drinking water, pesticides, Fowler's or Donovan's medicinal solutions for psoriasis, and Asiatic pills for asthma) and the use of **psoralens** (photosensitizers, similar to those found in tanning accelerators, used to treat psoriatic lesions) have been shown to increase the risk of skin carcinoma. Chemical carcinogens probably initiate cancers that subsequently are promoted nonspecifically.
I. **Immunosuppression.** The risk of skin malignancies in organ (particularly kidney) transplant recipients (patients with acquired immunodeficiency syndrome [AIDS]) and cancer patients who are taking cytotoxic agents and corticosteroids is up to 16 times greater than in the normal population. These tumors are more aggressive and are often multiple, with SCC 1.9 times more likely than BCC. In addition, limited data suggest that UV exposure multiplies the carcinogenic potential of immunosup-

pressive drugs. Recently, however, with the use of **cyclosporin,** the incidence of skin cancer in these patients appears to be decreasing.

   J. **Urbanization.** Workers in rural uranium mines and some urban manufacturing industries involved in metal ore smelting are known to be at risk for skin cancer from exposure to **ionizing radiation** and **arsenic,** respectively.

III. **Presentation**
   A. **Signs and symptoms**
      1. **Local manifestations**
         a. **Basal cell carcinoma.** Classically, basal cell carcinoma presents as raised, palpable, slow-growing lesions most commonly found on sun-exposed skin (face, neck, and extremities) with pearly, translucent edges, bluish pigmentation, and telangiectasias.
         b. **Squamous cell carcinoma.** Squamous cell carcinoma may manifest de novo as erythematous, slow-growing papules (surrounded by normal skin) that become nodular and frequently ulcerate. In areas of skin injury or damage (see p 134, **II.F.5**), induration that extends beyond the original lesion is frequently the first sign of malignancy; however, unlike BCC, SCC does not have a typical appearance. Chronic lower extremity ulcers with heaped-up borders found in locations atypical for venous stasis or arterial disease must be biopsied. On mucosal surfaces (conjunctiva, nose, mouth, vagina, and rectum), SCC initially may appear as an erythematous or whitish macule.
      2. **Systemic manifestations.** Since only 10–35% of SCC and 0.0028% of BCC metastasize, systemic manifestations of these neoplasms are uncommon. Weight loss, anorexia, lethargy, pleural effusions (lung metastases), ascites (liver metastases), neurologic symptoms (brain metastases), and bone pain (bone metastases) are rare.
   B. **Paraneoplastic syndromes.** No specific paraneoplastic syndromes have been associated with skin cancer, although SCC, particularly if metastatic, may present with symptoms similar to those observed with squamous neoplasms originating at other sites, such as the esophagus (see p 221, **III.B**).

IV. **Differential diagnosis.** Skin cancer (both BCC and SCC) most commonly presents as a superficial ulcer, and a biopsy is indicated for any persistent lesion. Benign cutaneous ulcers are common, particularly on the lower extremity, and may be an indication of infection (eg, fungus, tularemia, syphilis, anthrax), inflammation (pyoderma gangrenosum, gout), venous stasis and arterial ulcerations, neuropathic ulcers (malum perforans), as well as psoriatic, seborrheic, and premalignant keratoses. Other malignancies (amelanotic melanoma and adnexal skin tumors) also may mimic BCC and SCC.

V. **Screening programs.** No specific screening programs exist, but an **annual complete cutaneous examination** is recommended. More frequent skin self-examination and inspection by a physician (every 3–6 months) are appropriate for high-risk patients, such as those with xeroderma pigmentosum.

VI. **Diagnostic workup**
   A. **Medical history and physical examination.** In addition to a detailed medical history documenting risk factors, a thorough physical examination must be performed on all patients with suspected skin malignancies. Specific attention should be focused on the following areas.
      1. **General appearance.** An assessment of the overall functional and nutritional status should be made (see also p 1, **I** and **III**).
      2. **Skin.** The entire integument (including scalp, oral cavity, intertriginous and perianal areas, and genitalia) should be carefully inspected. All benign and malignant lesions as well as evidence of solar damage, such as the presence of telangiectasias, freckles, or solar lentigines, should be fully described. If multiple lesions are present, their exact appearance, location, and nature can be documented best by pictures of those areas. In addition, the presence of palmar pitting in patients with nevoid basal cell carcinoma syndrome should be noted.
      3. **Neck.** Palpation of the neck for evidence of local extension and lymph node metastases is important.
      4. **Lymph nodes.** Regional and distant lymph nodes must be palpated and assessed for evidence of metastatic disease.
      5. **Chest.** Auscultation and percussion of the chest may reveal evidence of chronic pulmonary disease (barrel chest, distant breath sounds, wheezing), pleural effusions, or lung metastases.
      6. **Abdomen.** Masses and hepatomegaly are important findings.

    7. **Extremities.** All areas of scarring (including vaccination scars, tattoos) should be recorded for serial examination.

B. Primary tests and procedures. All patients with suspected skin cancers should have the following diagnostic tests performed.

    1. **Blood tests** (see p 1, **IV.A**)
       a. Complete blood count.
       b. Hepatic transaminases.
       c. Alkaline phosphatase.

    2. **Imaging studies.** A baseline chest x-ray film should be obtained (see p 3, **c.1**).

    3. **Invasive procedures.** Biopsy of all suspicious lesions should be performed by one of the following 4 principal biopsy techniques. All may be performed as simple office procedures under local anesthesia.

       a. Shave biopsy. The shave biopsy technique involves removing a superficial portion of the lesion with a scalpel; however, in general, shave biopsies should be avoided unless an obvious nodulo-ulcerative, superficial, or cystic BCC is present for which a shave biopsy is adequate.

       b. Punch biopsy. During this procedure, a circular scalpel blade is used to excise a small sample of the lesion down to the subcutaneous tissue. For small lesions, this may be equivalent to an excisional biopsy (see c, below). The wound may be closed or left open to heal by secondary intention. Punch biopsies are appropriate for *all* lesions, including those suspicious for SCC, BCC (particularly morphea-form), malignant melanoma, and adnexal carcinomas.

       c. Excisional biopsy. A simple scalpel excision is indicated for small lesions (especially those < 3 mm) that are suspicious for BCC, SCC, keratoacanthoma, malignant melanoma, and adnexal carcinoma.

       d. Incisional biopsy. Removal of only part of the lesion is recommended as the initial biopsy procedure for large lesions (> 0.5–1.0 cm) and for lesions suspicious for benign keratoacanthomas that require a paramedian wedge biopsy extending from the edge to the center of the lesion.

C. Optional tests and procedures. The following examinations may be indicated by previous diagnostic findings or clinical suspicion.

    1. **Blood tests** (see p 1, **IV.A**)
       a. Nucleotidase.
       b. GGTP.

    2. **Imaging studies** (see p 3, **IV.C**)
       a. Computed tomography (CT). CT scans may be useful to assess (1) the **extent of the primary lesion,** (2) the **amount of underlying bone involvement** (particularly with the orbit), and (3) the **regional lymph nodes** as well as the **liver** and **lung** for the presence of metastatic disease. With prior radiotherapy, however, radiographic bone changes may occur even in the absence of neoplastic invasion.
       b. Magnetic resonance imaging (MRI).
       c. Bone scan.

    3. **Invasive procedures.** Regional or distant lymphadenopathy as well as intra-abdominal, hepatic, and pulmonary nodules can be evaluated with fine needle aspiration cytology to exclude a metastatic neoplasm.

VII. Pathology. SCCs are more aggressive than BCCs and tend to ulcerate earlier, grow more rapidly, and invade underlying structures earlier.

A. Location. Most cutaneous neoplasms occur on **sun-exposed areas: the head, neck,** and **extremities.** Nearly 80% of BCCs arise on the upper face, nose, ears, and lower face, whereas most SCCs are found (in order of frequency) on the ears, hands, and upper face. Although both BCC and SCC are more common on the lower extremities of females than males, BCC rarely occurs on the extremities. In the United States, BCC is slightly more common on the left face in males and the right face in females; in Great Britain, the opposite is true, probably because of driving habits (males are more likely to drive cars, whereas females are more likely to be passengers). SCC of the trunk and extremities has a different etiology and prognosis than most head and neck SCC, and, with the exception of SCC of the hand, these lesions frequently occur at sites of chronic inflammation.

B. Multiplicity. Multiple synchronous or metachronous primary BCCs and SCCs develop in 30% of females, 50% of males, and nearly 80% of patients with skin cancers induced by ionizing radiation. In addition, a high incidence of multiple cutaneous neoplasms occurs in nevoid basal-cell carcinoma syndrome and xeroderma pigmentosum. True multicentric disease does not exist because continuous nests of tumor cells extend along the rete ridges.

C. **Histology**

1. **Basal-cell carcinoma.** BCC arises from pluripotent cells located in the basal layer of the epidermis. The following types of BCC exist:

   a. **Nodulo-ulcerative ("rodent ulcer") BCC.** This is the most common type of BCC and appears as a waxy pink papule with prominent telangiectasias, central ulceration, and a pearly border. Hyperchromatic nuclei, peripheral palisading, fibroblastic stroma, amyloid deposits, and an absence of abnormal mitoses and intercellular bridges are characteristic.

   b. **Pigmented BCC.** These lesions resemble nodulo-ulcerative BCC, with the exception of color, which is tan, blue, brown, or black and often indistinguishable grossly from malignant melanoma.

   c. **Superficial BCC.** Superficial BCC occurs on the trunk and manifests as red scaly macules that occasionally ulcerate. Microscopically, peripheral palisading and buds of neoplastic cells invading from the deep epidermis are typical.

   d. **Morphea-form (sclerosing) BCC.** Flat or slightly elevated, indurated, whitish single macules mark this form of BCC, which is more common in patients who form keloids or contractures (eg, Dupuytren's). Histology reveals basal-like cells imbedded in a dense fibrous connective tissue stroma.

   e. **Infiltrative BCC.** This variant arises as an opaque, yellow, poorly defined lesion that is contained within the reticular dermis and subcutaneous tissue.

   f. **Fibroepithelial tumor of Pinkus.** This type of BCC presents as a truncal pink papule. Biopsy demonstrates long cords of cells stretching from the bottom of the epidermis to a dense fibrous connective tissue stroma.

2. **Squamous cell carcinoma.** Although SCC is a malignancy of the **epidermis, dermal invasion is characteristic.** Superficial SCC is confined to the upper reticular dermis, whereas infiltrating SCC involves the lower reticular dermis and subcutaneous tissue. SCC consists of both mature and anaplastic squamous cells (horn cells), with keratin pearl formation. Both the degree of differentiation and the depth of penetration determine the malignant potential. Low-grade well-differentiated SCC exhibits horn pearls, an inflammatory dermal infiltrate, limited invasion (not beyond level of adnexa), and at least partial preservation of the basement membranes. In anaplastic tumors, most cells are atypical and lack intercellular bridges. Several variants of SCC have special features, which are discussed below:

   a. **Basosquamous cell carcinoma (BSCC).** BSCC is identical in behavior (metastatic and local recurrence rates) to SCC and should be treated aggressively like a squamous, not a basal cell malignancy.

   b. **Verrucous carcinoma.** This slow-growing, exophytic, fungating lesion occurs in the oral cavity (florid papillomatosis) and the perianal region (giant condyloma acuminatum of Buschke and Lowenstein) and on the plantar surface of the foot (epithelioma cuniculatum) and the penis.

   c. **Erythroplakia.** This red, well-demarcated patch of SCC or SCC in situ occurs in the oral cavity, often accompanied by leukoplakia, and is delineated by the application of a 1% toluidine blue solution.

3. **Other cutaneous malignancies**

   a. **Apocrine carcinoma.** This rare adenocarcinoma appears as a reddish-purple firm or cystic nodular mass up to 8 cm in diameter that may metastasize to lymph nodes and distant organs. It occurs most commonly after age 50.

   b. **Eccrine carcinoma.** Primary eccrine adenocarcinomas are rare. The mean age at presentation is 60 years and 5 histologic variants have been described (porocarcinoma, syringoid, mucinous, clear cell, and microcystic adnexal carcinoma). These malignancies are locally aggressive and may metastasize to regional lymph nodes.

   c. **Merkel cell carcinoma.** Merkel cells are characteristic of this neuroendocrine carcinoma, which may recur locally or metastasize to lymph nodes as well as distant sites.

   d. **Paget's disease (extramammary).** Lesions ranging from erythematous scaly patches of the vulva, scrotum, and perianal area to erythematous, crusted, pruritic plaques represent adenocarcinoma of the epidermis. A visceral malignancy is associated with 12% of these patients.

      e. Sebaceous carcinoma. Representing < 5% of all cutaneous neoplasms, sebaceous carcinoma typically arises as a slow-growing, firm, yellow nodule of the Meibomian glands or glands of Zeis of the eyelid.

D. Metastatic spread. Overall, 0.0028% of BCCs and 2–5% of SCCs metastasize. Certain sites (ears, nostrils, and mucosal surfaces) and settings (Marjolin's ulcers), however, metastasize more frequently (up to 35%, depending on differentiation, size, penetration (> 4 mm), and previous treatment).

  1. Modes of spread. BCC and SCC can spread by 3 mechanisms.

    a. Direct extension. Both BCC and SCC invade underlying structures by direct extension. Growth can be either **superficial and spreading** or **localized and invasive.**

    b. Lymphatic metastasis. Tumor emboli lodge in regional lymphatics in most (68–90%) of patients with metastatic spread.

    c. Hematogenous metastasis. Although spread through blood vessels to distant organs is uncommon, it does occur in 20% of patients who develop metastatic disease.

  2. Sites of spread. Although uncommon, metastases do occur and involve the following organs: regional lymph nodes, lung, bone, liver, brain, and kidneys.

VIII. Staging. Because no widely accepted staging system has been developed, numerous staging systems based on depth of invasion (similar to Clark's levels for melanoma) and grading systems based on the extent of differentiation (Broder's system) have been proposed. In an effort to standardize staging and reporting of therapeutic results, the American Joint Committee on Cancer has outlined the following TNM staging system:

A. Tumor stage

  1. TX. The minimum requirements to assess the primary tumor are not met.

  2. Tis. Carcinoma in situ.

  3. T0. No primary tumor is present.

  4. T1. Tumor of no more than 2 cm in its largest dimension, strictly superficial or exophytic.

  5. T2. Tumor of more than 2 cm but no larger than 5 cm in largest dimension or with minimal infiltration of the dermis, irrespective of size.

  6. T3. Tumor of more than 5 cm in its largest dimension or with deep infiltration of the dermis, irrespective of size.

  7. T4. Tumor involving other structures such as cartilage, muscle, or bone.

B. Lymph node stage

  1. NX. The minimum requirements to assess the regional nodes are not met.

  2. N0. No evidence of regional lymph node involvement exists.

  3. N1. Movable ipsilateral regional lymph nodes are present.

  4. N2. Movable contralateral or bilateral regional lymph nodes are present.

  5. N3. Fixed regional lymph nodes are present.

     Note: Nodal involvement for cervical nodes is identical to that for head and neck cancers.

C. Metastatic stage

  1. MX. The presence of distant metastases cannot be assessed.

  2. M0. No distant metastases are present.

  3. M1. Distant metastases are present.

D. Histopathologic grade

  1. GX. Grade cannot be assessed.

  2. G1. Well differentiated.

  3. G2. Moderately well differentiated.

  4. G3–4. Poorly to very poorly differentiated.

E. Stage groupings

  1. Stage I. T1, N0, M0.

  2. Stage II. Any T, N1–3, M0.

  3. Stage III. Any T; any N, M1.

IX. Treatment

A. Surgery

  1. Primary cutaneous carcinoma. In general, **SCC should be treated more aggressively than BCC,** with wider margins (both superficial and deep) and serious consideration given to possible **lymph node metastases.** Because of the extreme rarity of metastases with BCC, control of local disease constitutes cure.

    a. Indications. Surgical resection is indicated for any BCC larger than 2 cm and any SCC larger than 1 cm. Smaller lesions, however, can be treated successfully by curettage and electrodesiccation.

b. **Approaches.** The surgical approach depends on the anatomic location but includes an assessment of the **three-dimensional extent** of the tumor, including invasion into contiguous structures such as the parotid gland, the facial musculature, and the nasal cartilage. The approach then can be tailored to the individual situation to assure a successful en bloc resection with uninvolved margins.

c. **Procedures**

(1) **Curettage and electrodesiccation (E and D).** Under local anesthesia, small tumors are readily separated from normal dermis and removed with a cutaneous curette. Electrodesiccation or carbon dioxide laser vaporization of the area follows. The procedure is then repeated carefully 2 or more times. Typically, cure rates of 95–100% (lesions < 1 cm) are obtained. Although this approach is preferred for superficial lesions of less than 0.5 cm in diameter and is the primary therapeutic modality used by dermatologists in the United States, it is **contraindicated for morphea-form and recurrent tumors.** In addition, the adequacy of resection cannot be determined because no specimen is provided for histopathologic examination.

(2) **Surgical excision**

(a) **Basal cell carcinoma.** Previously untreated small lesions (< 2.0 cm) may be excised adequately with 0.2–0.5 cm margins (> 95% cure rate). For tumors > 2 cm or those with a long clinical history and indistinct borders, margins of 0.5–1.0 cm are advisable. Recurrent and morphea-form BCC demand 1–2 cm margins. Although not generally necessary, frozen section examination of the specimen may be required to confirm complete tumor removal, particularly if the tumor is large or a flap reconstruction is planned (flaps make the detection of deep recurrence difficult). Other indications for frozen section examination include recurrent tumor, aggressive or complex pathology, and difficult anatomic locations.

Because only a 25–35% 5-year recurrence rate is expected with positive margins (with no additional therapy), both **observation and immediate re-excision** are acceptable options. Moreover, delayed closure or temporary split-thickness skin graft can be used until final pathology is available if bone margins are in question (frozen sections are not possible).

(b) **Squamous cell carcinoma.** For small lesions (< 1 cm), a clinical margin of 1 cm is sufficient (90–100% cure rate), but more extensive SCCs require larger (2–3 cm) margins (70–90% cure rate). The depth of resection is dictated partly by underlying structures. For example, tumors overlying the maxilla and orbit necessitate resection of bone if osseous involvement exists. Similarly, parotidectomy and dissection of the seventh cranial nerve may be crucial for tumors of the cheek. Adequate resection, however, should almost never be compromised by preservation of expendable structures. Several anatomic sites require special consideration:

Frontal scalp. Advanced tumors in this region frequently necessitate resection of the outer table of the skull to achieve cure. If radiographic evidence of bone involvement exists, however, full-thickness bone resection should be considered.

External ear. Because of a 14% local recurrence rate and a high incidence of lymph node metastases (12% overall, 6% at presentation), superficial parotidectomy is often necessary. Cervical lymphadenectomy, however, is indicated only for palpable nodal involvement.

Trunk and extremities. SCCs of the trunk and extremities frequently arise in areas of chronic inflammation (see p 134, **F.5**). Because of their aggressive nature, tumors in these locations should be removed with generous (2–3 cm) margins and, in the presence of palpable lymph nodes, regional lymphadenectomy. Lymphadenectomy in the absence of palpable nodes, however, is controversial. Accurate orientation of the specimen is critical, and frozen section examination of the surgical margins is advisable, although this is limited if the margin involves bone. If final pathologic assessment reveals tumor at the margin, an immediate **second surgical**

excision, if technically feasible, should be performed; otherwise, **radiation therapy** must be considered.

(3) **Mohs' micrographic (chemo)surgery.** With this technique, a staged excision (previously after fixation in situ with zinc chloride) of the lesion is performed guided by immediate examination of the entire margin in serial horizontal sections that have been carefully mapped with regard to orientation and location. Mohs's surgery is particularly well-suited for removing selected SCCs as well as recurrent and morphea-form BCCs, which tend to be more extensive than their perceptible borders. For example, the incidence of metastatic disease following Mohs's resection of SCC of the lip is only 50% of that after conventional surgery. Moreover, the overall cure rate is 99.9% for small previously untreated BCCs and 90.5% for tumors > 3 cm.

d. **Reconstruction.** As a result of a high cure rate, most patients with BCCs and selected patients with SCCs are candidates for immediate reconstruction. With moderate-sized tumors, split- or full thickness skin grafts and local flaps can be used, whereas large tumors may require transposition flaps (random or myocutaneous), microvascular free flaps, or both. Tissue expansion is an option that ultimately allows for excision of skin grafts.

2. **Locally advanced and metastatic cutaneous cancer**

   a. **Locally advanced and recurrent disease.** Recurrent disease may develop a few weeks to 10 years or more after primary therapy, and the recurrence rate following retreatment is 5–8 times higher (24%) than for the initial resection. Mohs's micrographic surgery produces the best results, with a cure rate of 85–96.8%. Surgical margins in the setting of recurrent disease should be 1.5–3 cm, and involved skin grafts and flaps must be removed. In addition, full-thickness resection of the cheek, nose, or calvarium may be necessary.

   b. **Metastatic disease.** Although metastases from SCC are uncommon and those from BCC are rare, patients occasionally develop distant disease. **Lymph node metastases** are most common and may be managed by **regional lymphadenectomy,** which produces some cures. Distant visceral metastases, however, are *not* amenable to surgical intervention.

3. **Morbidity and mortality.** The major morbidity rate after surgical therapy is 10% and is primarily related to scar formation. Common problems include the following complications:

   a. **Hemorrhage.** Although rare, hemorrhage may occur 5–7 days postoperatively with curettage.

   b. **Infection.**

   c. **Scar contraction.** This is particularly troublesome with large lesions involving the nasal tip and ala, the canthi and eyelids, and the lip vermilion treated with curettage and electrodesiccation. Such lesions are better treated with radiation therapy, which maintains superior cosmesis and function.

   d. **Hypertrophic scarring.** This can be treated with intralesional triamcinolone acetonide suspension. (Keloid is rare, even in susceptible patients.)

   e. **Changes in pigmentation.** Persistent hypopigmentation may occur, especially after curettage and electrodesiccation on actinic skin.

B. **Radiation therapy**

   1. **Primary cutaneous carcinoma.** Radiotherapy (3400 cGy in 680 cGy fractions 3 times a week for BCC and 5400 cGy in 600 cGy fractions 3 times a week for SCC) controls more than 92% of most small (< 2 cm) SCCs of the face and ears and 95% of BCCs of the same size, a success rate comparable with conventional surgery. A 5–10 mm margin of normal tissue is included in the treatment field, and radiation with a half-value depth (D1/2 = tissue depth in mm at which 50% of the surface dose is absorbed) equal to the tumor thickness should be used. **Radiation is preferred for areas where tissue preservation and cosmesis are important,** such as the eyelids, ears, nose, and lip, whereas **surgery yields superior results for lesions invading bone or cartilage and for morphea-form BCC.** Unfortunately, recurrences following radiation therapy do not respond to retreatment and should be surgically excised. In patients older than 60 years of age who require extensive surgical resection, primary radiotherapy can be substituted with good results.

   2. **Adjuvant radiation therapy.** If the pathologist finds that the surgical margins are inadequate and additional surgery is impractical because of the presence

of vital structures, postoperative radiation should be added to the treatment regimen.

3. **Locally advanced and metastatic cutaneous cancer.** Older patients with large lesions requiring a major resection and patients with inoperable disease or symptomatic metastases can be controlled remarkably well with proper palliative radiation therapy.

4. **Morbidity and mortality.** Initially, the cosmetic result is acceptable, but, with time, the following delayed complications may develop and effectively limit therapy to patients over 40 years of age: depigmentation, alopecia, skin atrophy, ulceration (late), and injury to adjacent structures (eg, eye, lacrimal glands).

C. **Cryotherapy.** This technique involves the application of liquid nitrogen ($-196.5°$ C) to cutaneous neoplasms, either as a spray or a direct probe to achieve tumor destruction. The entire tumor is frozen to a depth of 5 mm with 4–5 mm of normal surrounding skin to between $-25°$ C and $-50°$ C, as monitored by clinical appearance, a thermocouple (requires local anesthesia), or electrical impedance (eutectic point). Two freeze-thaw cycles (each requiring 1–2 minutes for freezing as well as thawing) are recommended and result in a cure rate of more than 96% for small noninvasive lesions. In addition, cryotherapy can be used to remove fungating, foul-smelling, portions of large inoperable tumors; however, **treatment of tumors larger than 2 cm, recurrent tumors, and morphea-form BCC is contraindicated.** Complications include edema, blistering and skin necrosis, subsequent hypopigmentation, skin atrophy, and scarring.

D. **Chemotherapy**
  1. **Primary cutaneous carcinoma**
     a. **Chemoprophylaxis. Sunscreens** are recommended for all individuals, particularly those with a previous cutaneous malignancy who are at high risk for additional primary tumors. These compounds either reflect (zinc oxide) or absorb (para-aminobenzoic acid or PABA) ultraviolet radiation. A minimum sun protection factor (SPF) of 15—the additional UVB energy required with sunscreen to produce a minimal erythematous reaction—is adequate for most outdoor activities, although SPFs as high as 50 can be used. In addition, existing actinic skin damage may be improved with daily use of tretinoin cream for weeks or months.
     b. **Topical chemotherapy.** Topical chemotherapy with 5-fluorouracil cream (1–5% cream twice a day for 4–6 weeks) has been effective in therapy of precancerous as well as small superficial BCCs. The cure rate (93%), however, is inferior to that rendered by standard surgical therapy; therefore, this approach should be used with caution.
     c. **Systemic chemotherapy.** Therapy with systemic cytotoxic agents has no role in the treatment of primary localized skin cancer. However, an **experimental approach** utilizing systemic administration of **hematoporphyrin derivatives** followed by phototherapy with red laser light (**photodynamic therapy**) does hold promise because the photosensitizing substances used are selectively retained in the cancer cells and mediate a photodynamic reaction that destroys only those cells.
  2. **Adjuvant chemotherapy.** No data exists to support the use of chemotherapy in the adjuvant setting, either topically for patients at high risk for local recurrence (eg, positive surgical margins) or systemically for patients at risk for distant metastases (scar SCC).
  3. **Locally advanced and metastatic cutaneous cancer.** The administration of 5-fluorouracil, cisplatin, doxorubicin, and isotretinoin (a vitamin A derivative) for metastatic BCC and SCC has been reported. Currently, however, no evidence supports the use of systemic cytotoxic agents in patients with cutaneous malignancies.

E. **Immunotherapy.** Encouraging results with intralesional alpha-2-interferon and topical 2, 4-dinitrochlorobenzene (DNCB) have been reported in the treatment of superficial BCC. More data is required, however, before the efficacy of these treatments is known.

X. **Prognosis**
  A. **Risk of recurrence.** Recurrence rates vary, depending on location and depth of penetration. The highest recurrence rates occur with lesions of the face (especially the nose) and neck. In addition, neoplasms of the trunk and extremities with a depth of invasion greater than 4 mm have a high local recurrence rate; SCC with a depth of invasion greater than 8 mm has a high incidence of lymph node metastases.

Most recurrences or metastases occur within 3 years of treatment. Furthermore, new primary lesions develop in 20–40% of patients.

B. **Five-year survival.** Long-term (5–10 year) survival depends on histology and stage.

1. **Basal cell carcinoma.** Death from BCC is rare, and usually occurs only from long-standing untreated disease that invades the periorbital bone and eventually the brain. Overall long-term survival for primary disease is 98.6%, whereas that for recurrent disease is 96%.

2. **Squamous cell carcinoma.** Although only 2–6.6% of patients develop distant metastases, 55–94% of them die of their disease (94–99% overall long-term survival). Because of a higher metastatic potential, survival for SCC that arise in areas of scarring is only 70–85%.

C. **Adverse prognostic factors.** The following characteristics have been associated with a poor prognosis, independent of tumor stage:

1. **Size greater than 3 cm.** A tumor of this size decreases cure rate from 99.5% (< 1 cm) to 59%.
2. **Invasion deeper than 4 mm.**
3. **Duration longer than 1 year.**
4. **Previous treatment.**
5. **Poorly differentiated histology.** Undifferentiated tumors, regardless of size, have a 5–20% greater mortality rate than do well-differentiated tumors.
6. **Acantholytic cells.** These nonadherent cells are more likely to metastasize, decreasing prognosis.
7. **Perineural invasion.** Paresthesias, pain, numbness, and paralysis may indicate growth along nerve sheaths that occurs in 2.5–5% of SCCs and is associated with a particularly poor prognosis.
8. **Mucous membrane location.** Mucous membrane SCC, particularly of the lip, is more likely to metastasize or spread along nerves to the middle cranial fossa.
9. **Ear lesion.** SCC of the external ear may metastasize, even if small, and it has a high recurrence rate (8%–14%).
10. **SCC arising in scar or an irradiated field.** This is primarily the result of delayed diagnosis, which results in advanced lesions in these locations.

XI. **Patient follow-up**

A. **General guidelines.** Patients with SCC or BCC carcinoma should be followed closely every 3 months for the first year, every 6 months for an additional 4 years, and then annually for recurrent disease and new primary lesions. Recurrent disease following curative resection may be "salvaged" with further therapy, if detected at an early stage. Specific guidelines for patient follow-up are outlined below.

B. **Medical history and physical examination.** An interval medical history and a complete physical examination, including a detailed cutaneous inspection should be performed during every clinic visit. Attention is focused on those areas discussed under **VI.A, above.**

C. **Routine evaluation.** Patient with BCC and SCC who have undergone potentially curative therapy do not require routine blood tests or imaging studies.

D. **Additional evaluation.** A chest x-ray should be obtained every 6–12 months for 3–5 years in patients with high risk SCC to exclude pulmonary metastases.

E. **Optional evaluation.** The following tests and procedures may be indicated on the basis of previous diagnostic findings or clinical suspicion.

1. **Blood tests** (see p 1, **IV.A**)
   a. **Complete blood count.**
   b. **Hepatic transaminases.**
   c. **Alkaline phosphatase.**
   d. **Nucleotidase.**
   e. **GGTP.**
2. **Imaging studies** (see p 3, **IV.C**)
   a. **Computed tomography (CT).**
   b. **Magnetic resonance imaging.**
   c. **Technetium-99m Bone scan.**

REFERENCES

Abide JM, Nahai F, Bennett RG: The meaning of surgical margins. *Plast Reconst Surg* 1984;**73:**492–497.

Bennett RG: *Fundamentals of Cutaneous Surgery.* St. Louis, MO: CV Mosby; 1988.

Binns JH, Sherriff HM: Low incidence of recurrence in excised but non-irradiated basal cell carcinomas. *Br J Plast Surg* 1975;**28**:133–134.

Casson PR, Robins P: Malignant tumors of the skin. In McCarthy J (editor): *Plastic Surgery. Volume 5: Tumors of the Head & Neck and Skin.* Philadelphia: WB Saunders; 1990:3614–3662.

Conway H, Hugo NE: Metastatic basal cell carcinoma. *Am J Surg* 1965;**110**:620–624.

Cottel WI: Skin tumors I: basal and squamous cell carcinoma (Overview). *Selected Readings in Plastic Surgery* 1988;**5**(6):1–25.

Dellon AL et al: Prediction of recurrence in incompletely excised basal cell carcinoma. *Plast Reconstr Surg* 1985;**75**:860–871.

Dubin N, Kopf AW: Multivariate risk score for recurrence of cutaneous basal cell carcinomas. *Arch Dermatol* 1983;**119**:373–377.

Fitzpatrick PJ et al: Basal and squamous cell carcinoma of the eyelids and their treatment by radiotherapy. *Int J Radiat Oncol Biol Phys* 1984;**10**:449–454.

Greenway HT et al: Treatment of basal cell carcinoma with intralesional interferon. *J Am Acad Dermatol* 1986;**15**:437–443.

Hayes H: Basal cell carcinoma: the East Grinstead experience. *Plast Reconstr Surg* 1962;**30**:273–280.

Immerman SC et al: Recurrent squamous cell carcinoma of the skin. *Cancer* 1983;**51**:1537–1540.

Kopf AW et al: Curettage-electrodesiccation treatment of basal cell carcinomas. *Arch Dermatol* 1977;**113**:439–443.

Lever WF: *Histopathology of the Skin.* 5th ed. Philadelphia: JB Lippincott; 1975.

Litwin MS et al: Use of 5-fluorouracil in the topical therapy of skin cancer: a review of 157 patients. *Proc Natl Cancer Conf* 1973;**7**:549–561.

Mohs FE: *Chemosurgery: Microscopically Controlled Surgery for Skin Cancer.* Springfield, IL: Charles C Thomas; 1978.

Mohs FE, Jones DL, Bloom RF: Tendency of fluorouracil to conceal deep foci of invasive basal cell carcinoma. *Arch Dermatol* 1978;**114**:1021–1022.

National Cancer Institute. *1987 Annual Cancer Statistics Review.* Bethesda, MD: National Institutes of Health; 1987.

Penn I. Cancers following cyclosporin therapy. *Transplantation* 1987;**43**(4):32–35.

Popkin GL. Tumors of the skin: a dermatologist's viewpoint. In McCarthy J (editor) *Plastic Surgery, V. tumors of the Head & Neck and Skin.* Philadelphia: WB Saunders; 1990;3599–3607.

Rank BK, Wakefield AF: Surgery of basal cell carcinoma. *Br J Surg* 1959;**45**:531.

Sakura CY, Calamel PM: Comparison of treatment modalities for recurrent basal cell carcinoma. *Plast Reconstr Surg* 1979;**63**:492–496.

Shanoff LB, Spira M, Hardy SB: Basal cell carcinoma: a statistical approach to rational management. *Plast Reconstr Surg* 1967;**39**:619–624.

Stromberg BV et al: Scar carcinoma: prognosis and treatment. *South Med J* 1977;**70**:821–822.

Von Essen CF. Roentgen therapy of skin and lip carcinoma: factors influencing success and failure. *Am J Roentgenol* 1960;**83**:556–570.

Zacarian SA: Cryosurgery of cutaneous carcinomas: an 18-year study of 3,022 patients with 4,228 carcinomas. *J Am Acad Dermatol* 1983;**9**:947–956.

22 Malignancies of the Eye

J. Michael Lahey, MD

I. **Epidemiology.** Ocular malignancies are **rare,** accounting for less than 0.2% of all cancers if nonmelanoma skin cancer is excluded. The most common intraocular tumor is **uveal melanoma,** which comprises 70% of all neoplasms of the eye. In the United States, 0.6 cases per 100,000 population, resulting in 0.1 deaths, were reported in 1985. It was estimated that 1225 new cases and 175 deaths would occur in 1993. Previously, the incidence of uveal melanoma was one-eighth that of cutaneous melanoma; however, with the recent surge in cutaneous disease (and stable incidence of ocular melanoma), the incidence of uveal melanoma is now 1/27th that of melanoma of the skin. Worldwide, the incidence of uveal melanoma is not known to vary significantly.

II. **Risk factors**
   A. **Age.** The incidence of ocular melanoma increases slowly from less than 1.0 per 100,000 before age 55 to no more than 2.0 per 100,000 by age 80. The median age at the time of diagnosis is 55 years. Uveal melanoma is rare in children and uncommon after the age of 70.
   B. **Sex.** The risk is slightly greater in males than in females.
   C. **Race.** The risk in whites is 8 and 3 times greater than that in blacks and Asians, respectively.
   D. **Genetic factors**
      1. **Family history.** The risk in first-degree relatives is not significantly increased, and multiple family members are rarely affected.
      2. **Chromosomal anomalies.** Deletions of chromosome 2 have been reported in a few patients; however, the relationship of these genetic aberrations to the pathogenesis of uveal melanoma is unclear.
   E. **Diet.** No dietary factors have been identified.
   F. **Smoking.** Smoking is not believed to be a risk factor.
   G. **Iris pigmentation.** The risk is 1.7 times greater in patients with lightly pigmented irides (eg, blue eyes) than in more heavily pigmented (brown-eyed) individuals.
   H. **History of previous ocular pathology**
      1. **Ocular nevi.** Many ocular melanomas arise in pre-existing **choroidal nevi.** In addition, the **nevus of Ota (oculodermal melanosis)** is associated with occasional uveal melanomas; however, the risk of developing melanoma in a known choroidal nevus is low.
      2. **Ocular scarring.** Melanomas originating in chorioretinal scars from previous cryotherapy have been reported.
   I. **Radiation.** The role of ultraviolet (UV) radiation in the pathogenesis of ocular melanoma is controversial.
   J. **Urbanization.** No predilection for urban or rural populations has been documented.

III. **Clinical presentation**
   A. **Signs and symptoms**
      1. **Local manifestations.** Loss of vision from exudative retinal detachment or posterior pole involvement is a frequent presenting symptom. Patients also commonly complain of "floaters," flashes of light, or visual field defects. In rare instances, asymptomatic patients may be discovered incidentally.
      2. **Systemic manifestations.** Although patients rarely present initially with systemic metastases, **hepatomegaly** and **jaundice** (liver metastases) are common complaints in the presence of advanced disease. Other frequent findings include pulmonary nodules (lung metastases), bone pain or pathologic fractures (bone metastases), and skin nodules (cutaneous metastases).
   B. **Paraneoplastic syndromes.** Although ocular melanoma is not associated with known paraneoplastic syndromes, certain malignancies (lung, pancreatic, colon, and ovarian cancer) may induce multiple small areas of choroidal melanocytic pro-

liferation, known as the "super nevus" syndrome, which may result in vision loss from exudative retinal detachment.

IV. **Differential diagnosis.** Although uveal melanoma must be excluded in any patient with a pigmented intraocular lesion, the following also must be considered: (1) congenital abnormalities (retinal pigment epithelial hypertrophy), (2) vascular abnormalities (hemangiomas), (3) extramacular disciform scar, (4) choroidal detachment, (5) benign neoplasms (nevi, melanocytomas, and choroidal osteomas), and (6) other malignancies (breast or lung metastases).

V. **Screening programs.** Although general screening programs are impractical because of the rarity of ocular melanoma, a **dilated fundus examination** and **scleral depression** may identify small melanomas or pre-existing suspicious nevi.

VI. **Diagnostic workup**
   A. **Medical history and physical examination.** A thorough medical history and complete physical examination, with emphasis on the following areas, is required for all patients with suspected ocular malignancies:
      1. **General appearance.** A simple assessment of the patient's functional and nutritional status should be performed (see, also, p 1, **I** and **III**).
      2. **Skin.** A complete cutaneous examination must be performed to exclude the possibility of a primary cutaneous melanoma.
      3. **Head.** A thorough search for primary scalp neoplasms, including melanomas, is mandatory.
      4. **Eyes.** A meticulous ocular examination, including a dilated fundus examination and scleral depression, is mandatory. In addition, gonioscopy and contact lens examination are useful in most cases.
      5. **Lymph nodes.** Cervical, supraclavicular, axillary, epitrochlear, inguinal, and abdominal lymph node areas should be carefully examined to exclude metastatic disease from a cutaneous primary melanoma.
      6. **Breasts.** Careful breast examination is required to detect primary lesions that may metastasize to the eye.
      7. **Chest.** Auscultation and percussion may reveal evidence of pulmonary metastases or primary lung cancer.
      8. **Abdomen.** Hepatomegaly (liver metastases) and abdominal masses should be fully described.
      9. **Rectum.** Occult fecal blood and pelvic masses (Blumer shelf lesions), suggesting metastatic disease should be excluded in all patients.
      10. **Extremities.** All dermal lesions must be described and biopsied if malignancy is suspected.
      11. **Nervous system.** Cranial and peripheral nerve deficits suggesting central nervous system metastases should be documented.
   B. **Primary tests and procedures.** The following tests and procedures are indicated in all patients with suspected ocular malignancies.
      1. **Blood tests** (see p 1, **IV.A**)
         a. **Complete blood count.**
         b. **Hepatic transaminases.**
         c. **Alkaline phosphatase.**
         d. **Blood urea nitrogen and creatinine.**
      2. **Imaging studies**
         a. **Chest x-ray studies.** (see p 3, **IV.C**)
         b. **Mammography.** Bilateral screening mammography should be ordered on all females to eliminate the possibility of breast cancer with metastatic involvement of the eye.
         c. **Fluorescein angiography.** The significant findings of double circulation and multiple punctate hot spots on fluorescein angiography are characteristic, but not diagnostic, of uveal melanoma.
      3. **Invasive procedures.** Trans-scleral (rarely transvitreal) fine-needle aspiration (FNA) (25-gauge needle) can be used in selected patients who have atypical lesions without increased risk of dissemination. An experienced cytopathologist, however, is crucial for accurate diagnosis.
   C. **Optional tests and procedures.** The following examinations may be indicated by previous diagnostic findings or clinical suspicion.
      1. **Blood tests** (see p 1, **IV.A**)
         a. **Nucleotidase**
         b. **GGTP**
      2. **Imaging studies** (see p. 3, **IV.C**).
         a. **Computed tomography (CT).** Abdominal CT scan may be necessary to

exclude the presence of hepatic metastases, particularly if elevated serum alkaline phosphatase or liver enzymes are detected. Routine CT scans, however, are controversial.

    b. Magnetic resonance imaging. Occasionally, MRI may distinguish melanomas from other malignancies and may demonstrate optic nerve involvement.

    c. Ultrasonography. Transillumination and ultrasound examination may differentiate hemorrhage, choroidal effusions, and neoplasia.

VII. Pathology

  A. Location. Uveal melanomas may arise from **melanocytes of the choroid, ciliary body,** and **rarely the iris.** Neoplasms of the anterior choroid and ciliary body regularly become large and metastasize before presentation. Consequently, both carry a poor prognosis, as do cases in which sheets of malignant cells extend diffusely throughout the uveal tract, making diagnosis difficult. In contrast, posterior tumors often cause early visual symptoms and are associated with a more favorable outcome.

  B. Multiplicity. Although multicentric and bilateral uveal melanomas do occur in rare instances, metastatic disease from an extraocular primary neoplasm or "super nevus" syndrome should be suspected in the presence of multiple ocular lesions.

  C. Gross appearance. Melanomas are classified on the basis of their size. Small tumors are 10 mm or less in diameter (base) and up to 3 mm in height. Medium tumors are between 10 and 15 mm in diameter and larger than 3 mm but no deeper than 5 mm. Large tumors are more than 15 mm in diameter and above 5 mm in height.

  D. Histology. Uveal melanomas often arise from pre-existing **choroidal nevi,** although it may be difficult to distinguish small melanomas from nevi even histologically. Generally, uveal melanomas can be classified into 4 types.

    1. Spindle A cell melanomas (5% of uveal melanomas). These tumors consist of cells with small indistinct nucleoli, a prominent chromatin stripe, and few mitotic figures. Some spindle A cell melanomas may be nevi.

    2. Spindle B cell melanomas (39% of uveal melanomas). Spindle B cell melanomas are distinguished by slightly larger cells and a single round, prominent nucleolus. Again, mitotic figures are uncommon.

    3. Epithelioid cells (3% of uveal melanomas). Epithelioid melanomas are highly anaplastic neoplasms marked by cellular pleomorphism, round nuclei, and one or more prominent nucleoli. The cells resemble epithelial cells because of their conspicuous eosinophilic cytoplasm; however, they are not cohesive. In contrast to spindle cell melanomas, these tumors contain frequent mitotic figures and have a poor prognosis.

    4. Mixed melanomas (45% of uveal melanomas). Melanomas with both spindle and epithelioid cells are common. In addition, 7% of melanomas cannot be categorized because of extensive necrosis.

  E. Metastatic spread

    1. Modes of spread. Because the eye has no lymphatic drainage, uveal melanoma, unlike cutaneous melanoma, can spread by only 2 routes.

      a. Direct extension. Nearly 6% of uveal melanomas involve the sclera either directly or through emissary or vortex veins. The extent of scleral extension is an important prognostic factor. Vitreous infiltration, however, is rare.

      b. Lymphatic metastasis. As noted above, the eye has no lymphatics.

      c. Hematogenous metastasis. In more than 50% of patients, uveal melanoma regularly spreads through the vortex veins or other involved blood vessels to distant sites.

    2. Sites of metastases. Metastases from melanoma may occur anywhere in the body.

      a. Liver is the most common site (30% of all patients with uveal melanoma).

      b. Lung.

      c. Bone.

      d. Subcutaneous tissue.

VIII. Staging. There is no standardized staging system for uveal melanoma. Prognosis and treatment are based on tumor size, location, cell type, and the presence of scleral infiltration or extrascleral extension. The presence of metastases found on screening imaging studies markedly changes the treatment of the primary ocular tumor.

IX. Treatment

  A. Surgery

    1. Primary uveal melanoma

    a. Indications. Surgical resection of localized uveal melanoma is indicated in a few selected patients. Initially, distant metastases should be excluded before any procedure is considered.

    b. Procedures

        (i) Local resection. Local eye wall resection can be used in highly selected patients, particularly those with small anterior tumors.

        (ii) Enucleation. Enucleation represents the mainstay of surgical treatment for uveal melanoma. Although a "gentle touch technique" has been advocated to avoid dislodging tumor cells during surgery, this technique is controversial. A 20 mm silicone prosthesis may be implanted into the orbit simultaneously, although recently developed integrated hydroxyapatite implants may provide better ocular movements and cosmesis.

        (iii) Orbital exenteration. Orbital exenteration may be indicated for extrascleral tumor infiltration and often can be performed without removing the eyelid, which is less disfiguring; however, the effect of this radical procedure on survival is unclear.

2. Locally advanced and metastatic uveal melanoma. Because more than 80% of patients with metastatic disease die within 1 year, primary uveal melanomas in the presence of distant metastases generally are not resected, primarily because of the obligate vision deficit. If **neovascular glaucoma** or extensive **extrascleral tumor infiltration** results in a painful blind eye, palliative enucleation or orbital exenteration, respectively, may be warranted.

3. Morbidity and mortality. Most problems in these patients develop secondary to the accompanying general anesthesia, but the complications listed below occasionally arise.

    a. Implant migration or extrusion.

    b. Superior sulcus syndrome.

    c. Vitreous hemorrhage (eye wall resection).

    d. Retinal detachment (eye wall resection).

B. Radiation therapy. Although radiation therapy makes surgery unnecessary for many malignancies, radiotherapy for uveal melanoma **requires surgery first** to expose or delineate the target area.

1. Primary uveal melanoma

    a. Brachytherapy. Tumors less than 15 mm in diameter may be treated successfully with brachytherapy (enucleation or particle irradiation is preferred for larger neoplasms). This involves suturing a radioactive plaque to the eye wall for 4 days. Although a number of isotopes have been used, the most common is I^{125}. At least one study demonstrated no difference in survival between brachytherapy and enucleation.

    b. Charged-particle irradiation. If enucleation is not necessary or desirable in selected patients with large (> 15 mm) neoplasms, charged-particle therapy can be used. The highly localized dose distribution characteristic of such particles as protons and helium ions permits the delivery of a uniform dose of irradiation. Before irradiation, tantalum rings are placed on the sclera at the edges of the tumor. Subsequently, 7000 cGy in 5 fractions over 7–10 days is delivered using a computer-assisted 3-dimensional treatment program that minimizes radiation to the lens, optic nerve, and fovea.

    c. Enucleation. Local recurrence following charged particle and brachytherapy generally requires **enucleation,** although selected patients may be treated with additional radiation or with **photocoagulation,** which destroys the tumor's blood supply.

2. Adjuvant radiation therapy

    a. Preoperative radiotherapy. Although preoperative irradiation potentially may lower the rate of distant metastasis, decrease the extent of surgical resection required, and improve survival, studies of irradiation before enucleation have failed to show any benefit. Further studies are ongoing.

    b. Intraoperative radiotherapy. Outside of the placement of radioactive plaques for brachytherapy, intraoperative radiotherapy has not been studied extensively.

    c. Postoperative radiotherapy. Though used in rare circumstances, postoperative irradiation generally is not recommended.

3. Locally advanced and metastatic uveal melanoma. Palliative radiation therapy is considered only in exceptional cases with localized symptomatic metastases.

   4. **Morbidity and mortality.** Local irradiation (both charged particle and brachytherapy) causes radiation retinopathy, a vasculopathy that usually begins 1 year after treatment. Retinal or iris neovascularization secondary to radiation retinopathy may require pan retinal photocoagulation. Anterior segment problems such as **cataract,** neovascular glaucoma, lash loss, dry eye, epiphoria, and keratopathy occur more commonly with charged particle therapy.
C. **Chemotherapy** (see also p 127, **IX.C**)
   1. **Primary uveal melanoma.** Chemotherapy has not proved to be useful in the treatment of primary uveal melanoma.
   2. **Adjuvant chemotherapy.** Chemotherapy in the adjuvant setting is not effective.
   3. **Locally advanced and metastatic uveal melanoma.** Although numerous chemotherapeutic agents have been studied in the treatment of systemic melanoma, the results have been disappointing.
D. **Immunotherapy.** Experimental data on the treatment of metastatic melanoma is encouraging (see also p 128, **IX.D**).
E. **Combined modality therapy.** Early data combining hyperthermia with irradiation is promising, but further study is necessary.
X. **Prognosis**
A. **Risk of recurrence**
   1. **Local recurrence.** In the absence of extrascleral extension, local recurrence after enucleation is rare. After radiation therapy, however, the recurrence rate is 1%. Depending on the adequacy of surgical margins, local recurrence also may occur following eye wall resection.
   2. **Distant recurrence.** Distant metastases develop in 50% of patients, usually within 3–5 years.
B. **Five-year survival.** The 5- and 10-year overall survival is 55% and 38–50%, respectively, and is determined by the incidence of distant metastases.
C. **Adverse prognostic factors.** The following features are associated with a poor outcome:
   1. **Cell type.** The prognosis depends on the predominant cell type present in the melanoma (see **VII.D**). An 85%, 71%, 33%, and 14% 10-year survival rate is associated with spindle cell A, spindle cell B, mixed, and epithelioid melanomas, respectively.
   2. **Extrascleral extension.** The presence of extrascleral extension reduces survival from 78% to 26%.
   3. **Tumor size.** The 6-year survival for small tumors (< 10 mm) is 87%, whereas that for medium and large tumors (> 12 mm) drops to 30%.
   4. **Anterior location.** Anterior tumors that involve the ciliary body have a poor prognosis.
XI. **Patient follow-up**
A. **General guidelines.** Patients must be followed closely (every 4–6 months) if an in situ lesion is being observed for growth. After treatment of an established lesion, patients should be followed every 3 months for 2 years, every 6 months for an additional 3 years, and then annually for evidence of tumor recurrence. Specific guidelines are outlined below.
B. **Routine evaluation.** Each clinic visit should include the following examinations:
   1. **Medical history and physical examination.** A pertinent medical history, thorough physical examination, and a meticulous bilateral ocular examination, should be performed during each office visit. Large **fundus drawings** are helpful, and **photographs** can be invaluable in documenting growth or regression of posterior tumors. Areas for particular attention are discussed in (**VI.A**, above).
   2. **Blood tests** (see p 1, **IV.A**)
      a. **Complete blood count.**
      b. **Hepatic transaminases.**
      c. **Alkaline phosphatase.**
   3. **Imaging studies** (see p 3, **IV.C**)
      a. **Chest x-ray.**
      b. **Ultrasonography.** Often an ocular ultrasound examination is used to follow the response to therapy.
C. **Optional evaluation.** The following examinations may be indicated, depending on previous diagnostic findings or clinical suspicion.
   1. **Blood tests** (see p 1, **IV.A**)
      a. **5′-Nucleotidase.**
      b. **GGTP.**

2. **Imaging studies** (see p 3, **IV.C**)
   a. **Computerized tomography.**
      (i) **Chest CT.** Chest CT scan remains a good method of detecting medi-astinal adenopathy and pulmonary metastases. In patients with no re-sidual tumor, a chest CT scan should be obtained if suspicious findings are identified on medical history, physical examination, or chest x-ray films.
      (ii) **Abdominal CT.** A CT scan of the abdomen is the most sensitive test for excluding liver metastases and should be ordered if symptoms or blood tests suggest the possibility of liver disease.
   b. **Magnetic resonance imaging.**
   c. **Technetium-99m bone scan.**
3. **Invasive diagnostic procedures.** In a patient without known residual cancer, a biopsy of any suspicious or abnormal mass is mandatory.

REFERENCES

Brown GC et al: Radiation retinopathy. *Ophthalmology* 1982;**89:**1494.

Char DH: *Clinical Ocular Oncology.* New York: Churchill Livingstone, 1988.

Char DH et al: Helium ion therapy for choroidal melanoma. *Ophthalmology* 1983;**90:**1219.

Foulds WS: The local excision of choroidal melanomata. *Trans Ophthalmol Soc UK* 1973;**93:**343.

Gass JDM: *Stereoscopic Atlas of Macular Disease.* St. Louis: CV Mosby, 1987.

Legha SS: Interferons in the treatment of malignant melanoma: A review of recent trials. *Cancer* 1986;**57:**1675.

Ryan SJ: *Retina,* vol 1. St. Louis: CV Mosby, 1989;625–736.

Sellami M et al: Chemotherapy in ocular malignant melanoma: Study of 20 cases. *Oncology* 1986;**43:**221.

Shields JA: *Diagnosis and Management of Intraocular Tumors.* St. Louis: CV Mosby, 1983.

Shields JA et al: Cobalt plaque therapy of uveal melanomas. *Ophthalmology* 1982;**89:**1201.

Zimmerman LE et al: Does enucleation of the eye containing a malignant melanoma prevent or accelerate the dissemination of tumor cells? *Br J Ophthalmol* 1978;**62:**420.

23 Malignancies of the Lip, Oral Cavity, & Pharynx

Matthew J. Lando, MD, and James K. Bredenkamp, MD

I. **Epidemiology.** Malignancies of the lip, oral cavity, and pharynx (oropharynx) constitute 4% of all cancers. In the United States, **16.5** cases per 100,000 males and **6.8** cases per 100,000 females were reported in 1985, resulting in 5 and 1.8 deaths, respectively. It is estimated that **29,800 new cases and 7,700 deaths** will occur in 1993. Worldwide, the incidence varies from areas of high frequency—eg, Canada, France, India, Romania, Hong Kong, Singapore, and Hawaii—to regions of low incidence—eg, Japan, Norway, Czechoslovakia, and Yugoslavia.

II. **Risk factors**

   A. **Age.** Carcinoma of the oral cavity and pharynx rapidly increases from less than 1 per 100,000 before age 30 to a peak of **51 cases per 100,000 by age 70**.

   B. **Sex.** In males, the risk is **2 times** (lip), **1.8 times** (tongue), **1.5 times** (mouth), and **2.3 times** (pharynx) greater than in females.

   C. **Race.** Although the risk of carcinoma of the oral cavity and pharynx in **blacks ages 35–65** is **2.8 times** greater than in whites, the risk in **whites older than 65 years** is nearly **2.1 times** greater than in blacks of the same age.

   D. **Genetic factors.** First-degree relatives are **not** at increased risk of developing oropharyngeal carcinoma.

   E. **Diet**

   1. **Alcohol.** Ingestion of ethanol significantly increases the risk of oropharyngeal cancer and, if combined, with **smoking**, the risk increases **synergistically**.

   2. **Iron deficiency.** A link between **sideropenic (iron deficiency) dysphagia** and the development of oropharyngeal cancer is well established.

   3. **Vitamin deficiency.** Some studies suggest that deficiencies of **vitamin A** and **vitamin C** may contribute to the pathogenesis of oral and pharyngeal cancer.

   F. **History of previous oropharyngeal pathology**

   1. **Dental hygiene.** Reports of an association between oral cancer and either **poor oral hygiene** or chronic irritation from **ill-fitting dentures** are numerous, although anecdotal. Proof of such a relationship, however, has not been documented.

   2. **Infection**

      a. **Fungi.** Although **candidiasis** often occurs in patients with oral cancer, whether chronic inflammation from this infection contributes to or results from the development of an oral malignancy is uncertain.

      b. **Spirochetes.** *Treponema pallidum* infection (**syphilis**) increases the risk of cancer of the **tongue** (particularly the anterior two-thirds of the dorsum) **4-fold**.

      c. **Viruses**

         (1) **Epstein-Barr virus (EBV).** Epidemiologic data strongly implicates EBV in the pathogenesis of **nasopharyngeal carcinoma**. Anti-EBV titers in some populations reach 100%.

         (2) **Herpes simplex virus (HSV).** Although serum antibodies to **HSV Type I** are elevated in patients with head and neck cancers, an etiologic role is unproved.

         (3) **Human immunodeficiency virus.** Oral cancer is more prevalent among patients with **AIDS** than in immunocompetent patients.

   G. **Radiation.** Exposure to sunlight (**ultraviolet radiation**) is believed to explain the relatively high incidence of lip cancer found on the **lower** (compared to the upper) lip, in **fair skinned** populations, and **outdoor workers**.

   H. **Tobacco. Smoking or chewing** tobacco greatly increases the risk of oropharyngeal carcinoma. **Cigarette smoking** correlate most strongly with cancer of the **floor of the mouth; cigar smoking**, with carcinoma of the **tongue and pharynx**; and **chewing tobacco**, with cancer of the **alveolus, pharynx, and salivary glands**. The habit of **reverse smoking**, especially prevalent in India, substantially increases the incidence of **palate cancer**, but accompanying **thermal injury** also may contribute.

  I. **Urbanization.** For unknown reasons, certain urban occupations such as **food service, mechanics, and carpentry** are associated with a high incidence of oral, hypopharyngeal, and nasopharyngeal cancers.

III. Presentation
A. Signs and symptoms
  1. Local manifestations
- **a. Lip.** Initially, carcinoma develops as a **thickening** most frequently on the **lower lip midway between the midline and the commissure**, which develops into an **ulcerative or exophytic lesion**.
- **b. Oral cavity.** Although early lesions often are **asymptomatic**, progression may lead to **pain, dysphagia, dysarthria**, and, ultimately, to **otalgia**, halitosis, necrosis, ulceration, and hemorrhage.
- **c. Pharynx.** Patients often complain initially of a persistent **sore throat** and subsequently of **otalgia**, odynophagia, and hemorrhage. A **neck mass (50%)** is common and often is the first sign of an otherwise silent nasopharyngeal carcinoma. Eustachian tube obstruction and resulting serous otitis media may cause **unilateral hearing loss**, and erosion into the cavernous sinus and base of the skull may lead to **cranial nerve deficits** (most commonly the sixth cranial nerve).

  2. Systemic manifestations. General signs and symptoms other than **weight loss** are infrequent.

B. Paraneoplastic syndromes. No paraneoplastic syndromes are associated with oropharyngeal carcinomas.

IV. Differential diagnosis. Vascular abnormalities (hemangiomas), anatomic variations such as osteomas (torus palitinus and torus mandibularis), ranulae (sublingual gland retention cyst), ectopic thyroid, infections (eg, tuberculosis, syphilis, histoplasmosis, blastomycosis), inflammation (lichen planus), and benign neoplasms (fibromas, papillomas, and pyogenic granulomas) can be confused with malignancy and require a biopsy to exclude cancer.

V. Screening programs. No formal screening programs exist for the early detection of oropharyngeal carcinomas; however, patients with significant risk factors (heavy use of tobacco and ethanol) are encouraged to undergo a **periodic head and neck examination**.

VI. Diagnostic workup
A. Medical history and physical examination. A detailed medical history and thorough physical examination are essential in the evaluation of all patients with suspected oral and pharyngeal malignancy.
  1. General appearance. An assessment of the general functional and nutritional status should be made (see p 1, **I**, and **III**).

  2. Oropharynx. The **size** and **location** of the primary lesion must be documented, and careful examination of the entire head and neck should be performed to **assess dentition** and to **exclude synchronous primary lesions**.

  3. Neck. Palpation of the neck for evidence of local extension and lymph node metastases is important.

  4. Chest. Auscultation and percussion may reveal signs of chronic pulmonary disease or occult lung neoplasms, either primary or metastatic.

  5. Heart. Cardiac examination frequently uncovers indications of ischemic heart disease, which often coexists in these patients because of common risk factors (eg, smoking).

  6. Abdomen. A small liver, splenomegaly, and ascites suggest the presence of **cirrhosis** which, because of common risk factors such as heavy alcohol consumption, also often occur in patients with oropharyngeal cancer. Hepatomegaly and other abdominal masses, however, may indicate metastatic disease.

  7. Nervous system. Extensive cervical disease may involve the cranial nerves and cervical sympathetic plexus.

B. Primary tests and procedures. The following diagnostic tests and procedures should be obtained in all patients with suspected oropharyngeal carcinoma.
  1. Blood tests (see p 1, **IV.A**)

       a. Complete blood count.
       b. Hepatic transaminases.
       c. Alkaline phosphatase.
   2. Imaging studies (see p 3, **IV.C**)
       a. Chest x-ray.
       b. Magnetic resonance imaging. Currently, MRI surpasses CT and is the imaging modality of choice in head and neck cancer because of its ability to define the extent of the primary tumor and demonstrate disruption of soft tissue planes.
   3. Invasive procedures
       a. Laryngoscopy. Direct laryngoscopy with biopsy is essential (except in lip cancers) to ascertain the extent of the lesion, confirm the diagnosis, and look for synchronous primary tumors.
       b. Biopsy. Diagnostic biopsy of any abnormal area is imperative. Usually, this is accomplished at the time of head and neck examination or during direct laryngoscopy. **Fine needle aspiration** should be used to evaluate neck masses or swellings because open biopsy may convert **intracapsular** to **extracapsular** disease and significantly decrease prognosis.
  C. Optional tests and procedures. The following tests and procedures may be indicated by previous diagnostic findings or clinical suspicion.
   1. Blood tests (see p 1, **IV.A**)
       a. 5-Nucleotidase.
       b. GGTP.
   2. Imaging studies
       a. Computed tomography (see p 3, **IV.C.2**). CT scan of the head and neck may give valuable information regarding the extent of the primary lesion, especially if bone involvement is suspected.
       b. Esophagogram. Barium esophagography may be useful to assess the extent of disease and exclude the existence of synchronous esophageal neoplasms.
       c. Technetium-99m bone scan (see p 3, **IV.C.5**).
   3. Invasive procedures
       a. Esophagoscopy. In patients with hypopharyngeal tumors, esophagoscopy is required to delineate the extent of disease. Routine esophagoscopy to exclude synchronous esophageal malignancies is controversial.
       b. Bronchoscopy. In high-risk patients, examination of the respiratory tree may identify synchronous bronchogenic carcinoma. Routine bronchoscopy is not recommended, however.
VII. Pathology
  A. Location. Tumor location has important prognostic and therapeutic implications.
   1. Lip (25–30%). The vermilion lip is the **most common site** of oral cavity cancer; more than **90%** arise on the **lower** lip.
   2. Floor of mouth (10–15%).
   3. Tongue (25%). The most common location for carcinoma of the tongue is along the **posterolateral aspect of the middle third of the tongue**. Because of their different embryologic origins, **anterior tongue (ectoderm)** lesions generally are more exophytic and differentiated than those arising in the **posterior tongue (endoderm)**.
   4. Tonsils and pharynx. The **tonsil and tonsillar fossa** is the most common site for **oropharyngeal** neoplasms which, in time, involve the palate and nasopharynx superiorly and the base of tongue and hypopharynx inferiorly. The **piriform sinus (70%)** and **posterior pharyngeal wall (25%)** are the most frequent sites of **hypopharyngeal** tumors.
   5. Nasopharynx. Although rare in most ethnic groups, nasopharyngeal carcinoma is common in Chinese (particularly **Cantonese**) populations regardless of geographic location. The most common primary **sites** of nasopharyngeal carcinoma are the **roof of the nasopharynx (35%)** and the **fossa of Rosenmuller (30%)**.
  B. Multiplicity. Because of common risk factors, synchronous primary carcinomas occur in **15–20%** of all patients and in as many as **37%** of those with **palate** and **floor of mouth** lesions.
  C. Histology. The vast majority of oropharyngeal cancers are **squamous cell carcinomas**, but adenocarcinoma, chordoma, plasmacytoma, and lymphoma of the nasopharynx and tonsils also occur.
  D. Metastatic spread

1. **Modes of spread**
   a. **Direct extension.** Squamous cell carcinoma of the oropharynx most commonly spreads directly to adjacent compartments and contiguous structures.
   b. **Lymphatic metastasis.** The **nasopharynx, base of the tongue, hypopharynx, and tonsillar fossa** frequently involve lymph nodes at the time of presentation (**75–87%**). In addition, the **oropharynx, retromolar trigone, and soft palate** also commonly present with metastases (**45–60%**), whereas only 33% of patients with lesions on the **tongue and floor of the mouth** present with lymph node metastases. Certain patterns of lymphatic metastasis are common, depending on the primary site (see Table 23–1).

VIII. **Staging.** The American Joint Committee on Cancer and the Union Internationale Contre le Cancer have adopted a joint TNM staging system for most head and neck cancers. Minor changes in the staging of these tumors were approved in 1987; and these modifications and the full staging systems for malignancies of the lip, oral cavity, and oropharynx are outlined below.

A. **Tumor stage**
   1. **Lip.** The lip extends from the skin-vermilion junction and only includes the surface that contacts the opposing lip. The mucosal surfaces of the lip are included with the oral cavity for staging purposes.
      a. **TX.** The primary tumor cannot be assessed.
      b. **T0.** No evidence of a primary tumor exists.
      c. **Tis.** Carcinoma in situ.
      d. **T1.** Tumor is limited to the lip and is no larger than 2 cm in its greatest dimension.
      e. **T2.** Tumor is limited to the lip and is larger than 2 cm but no larger than 4 cm in its greatest dimension.
      f. **T3.** Tumor is limited to the lip and is larger than 4 cm in its greatest dimension.
      g. **T4.** Tumor invades beyond the lip to contiguous structures (bone, tongue, skin of neck).
   2. **Oral cavity.** The oral cavity extends from mucosal surfaces of lip to the junction of the hard and soft palate superiorly and the line of circumvallate papillae inferiorly. The oral cavity is subdivided into buccal mucosa, lower and upper alveo-

TABLE 23–1. INCIDENCE AND LOCATION OF NODAL METASTASES FOR PRIMARY TUMORS

Site	Ipsilateral Metastases (%)	Contralateral Metastases (%)	Initial Nodal Groups
Lower lip	5–15	< 5	Submandibular (lateral), submental (medial)
Upper lip	40–50	< 5	Submandibular, buccal, parotid
Buccal mucosa	25–47	< 5	Submandibular, submental, subdigastric
Lower gingiva	35–71	< 5	Submandibular, submental, subdigastric
Upper gingiva and hard palate	35–46	< 5	Submandibular, retropharyngeal, buccal, parotid
Retromolar trigone	12–68	< 5	Submandibular, subdigastric
Floor of mouth	11–54	10–47	Submandibular, subdigastric
Oral tongue	14–76	5–27	Submandibular, subdigastric, jugular, omohyoid
Base of tongue	70–84	30	Subdigastric, jugular
Soft palate	8–67	16	Subdigastric, jugular
Tonsil	70–90	5	Submandibular, jugular, junctional, spinal accessory
Nasopharynx	83–97	50	Prevertebral, jugular
Oropharynx	25–76	30	Subdigastric, jugular
Hypopharynx	63–79	10–19	Subdigastric, jugular, retropharyngeal

lar ridges, retromolar gingiva (mucosa overlying the ascending ramus of the mandible), floor of mouth, hard palate, and anterior two thirds of tongue.

    a. **TX.** The primary tumor cannot be assessed.
    b. **T0.** No evidence of a primary tumor exists.
    c. **Tis.** Carcinoma in situ.
    d. **T1.** Tumor is no larger than 2 cm in its greatest dimension.
    e. **T2.** Tumor is larger than 2 cm but no larger than 4 cm in its greatest dimension.
    f. **T3.** Tumor is larger than 4 cm in its greatest dimension.
    g. **T4.** Tumor invades contiguous structures (cortical bone, deep muscle of the tongue, maxillary sinus, skin).

3. **Oropharynx.** The oropharynx extends from the plane of the hard palate superiorly to the plane of the hyoid inferiorly.

    a. **TX.** The primary tumor cannot be assessed.
    b. **T0.** No evidence of a primary tumor exists.
    c. **Tis.** Carcinoma in situ.
    d. **T1.** Tumor is no larger than 2 cm in its greatest dimension.
    e. **T2.** Tumor is larger than 2 cm but no larger than 4 cm in its greatest dimension.
    f. **T3.** Tumor is larger than 4 cm in its greatest dimension.
    g. **T4.** Tumor invades contiguous structures (cortical bone, deep muscle of the tongue, soft tissues of the neck).

4. **Nasopharynx.** The inferior limit of the nasopharynx is the level of the hard palate and the superior boundary lies at the base of the skull.

    a. **TX.** The primary tumor cannot be assessed.
    b. **T0.** No evidence of a primary tumor exists.
    c. **Tis.** Carcinoma in situ.
    d. **T1.** Tumor is limited to 1 subsite of the nasopharynx.
    e. **T2.** Tumor involves more than 1 subsite of the nasopharynx.
    f. **T3.** Tumor invades the nasal cavity, the oropharynx, or both.
    g. **T4.** Tumor invades the skull, cranial nerves, or both.

        Note: The subsites of the nasopharynx include the **posterosuperior wall** (extending from the level of the junction of the hard and soft palates to the base of the skull), the **lateral wall** (including the fossa of Rosenmuller), and the **inferior (anterior) wall** (consisting of the superior surface of the soft palate).

5. **Hypopharynx.** The hypopharynx extends from the plane of the hyoid bone superiorly to the plane of the lower border of the cricoid cartilage and is composed of three areas: the piriform sinus, postcricoid area, and posterior pharyngeal wall.

    a. **TX.** The primary tumor cannot be assessed.
    b. **T0.** No evidence of a primary tumor exists.
    c. **Tis.** Carcinoma in situ.
    d. **T1.** Tumor is limited to 1 subsite of the hypopharynx.
    e. **T2.** Tumor invades more than 1 subsite of the hypopharynx or an adjacent site **without fixation of the hemilarynx**.
    f. **T3.** Tumor invades more than 1 subsite of the hypopharynx **with fixation of the hemilarynx**.
    g. **T4.** Tumor invades contiguous structures (eg, cartilage or soft tissues of the neck).

        Note: The subsites of the hypopharynx include the **pharyngoesophageal junction or postcricoid area** (extending from the level of the arytenoid cartilages and connecting folds to the inferior border of the cricoid cartilage), the **pyriform sinus** (stretching from the pharyngoepiglottic fold to the upper end of the esophagus and bounded laterally by the thyroid cartilage and medially by the surface of the aryepiglottic fold and the arytenoid and cricoid cartilages), and the **posterior pharyngeal wall** (ranging from the level of the floor of the vallecula to the level of the cricoarytenoid junction).

B. **Lymph node stage**

1. **NX.** Regional lymph nodes cannot be assessed.
2. **N0.** No regional lymph nodes are involved.
3. **N1.** Metastasis involves a single ipsilateral lymph node no larger than 3 cm in its greatest dimension.
4. **N2.** Metastasis involves a single ipsilateral lymph node larger than 3 cm but no larger than 6 cm in its greatest dimension or multiple ipsilateral lymph nodes no larger than 6 cm in their greatest dimension.

    a. **N2a.** Metastasis involves a single ipsilateral lymph node larger than 3 cm but no larger than 6 cm in its greatest dimension.

        b. N2b. Metastases involve multiple ipsilateral lymph nodes no larger than 6 cm in their greatest dimension.
    5. N3. Metastases involve ipsilateral nodes larger than 6 cm in their greatest dimension, bilateral lymph nodes, or contralateral lymph nodes.
        a. N3a. Metastases involve ipsilateral lymph nodes and are larger than 6 cm in their greatest dimension.
        b. N3b. Metastases involve bilateral lymph nodes.
        c. N3c. Metastases involve only contralateral lymph nodes.
C. Histopathologic grade
    1. GX. The grade cannot be assessed.
    2. G1. Well differentiated.
    3. G2. Moderately well differentiated.
    4. G3. Poorly differentiated.
    5. G4. Undifferentiated.
D. Metastatic stage
    1. M0. No distant metastases are present.
    2. M1. Distant metastases are present.
E. Stage groupings
    1. Stage 0. Tis, N0, M0.
    2. Stage I. T1, N0, M0.
    3. Stage II. T2, N0, M0.
    4. Stage III. T3, N0, M0; T1–3, N1, M0.
    5. Stage IV. T4, N0-1, M0; any T, N2–3, M0; any T, any N, M1.
IX. Treatment. Squamous cell carcinoma of the oral cavity and pharynx is treated primarily with **surgery, radiation therapy**, or a **combination** of the two modalities.
  A. Surgery. In general, surgery produces results **equivalent** to those of radiation therapy for **T1 and T2** lesions. **T3 and T4** lesions are best managed by **surgery** with or without radiation therapy.
    1. Primary oropharyngeal carcinoma
      a. Lip
        (1) Indications. Although radiation therapy that combines interstitial implants and external-beam irradiation yields cure rates comparable to those for surgical therapy, **surgery produces better cosmetic results** and lower morbidity and local recurrence rates, particularly in the presence of extensive disease.
        (2) Approaches. Lip resurfacing (**vermilionectomy**) is ideal for **diffuse** precancerous lesions and for carcinoma in situ. Simple **"V" or "W" excision** with primary closure provides excellent cosmetic and functional results and is indicated for **small lesions (< 1.5 cm)** involving no more than **33% of the lower** lip or **25% of the upper** lip. Larger lesions (occupying 33–70% of lip) require flaps such as the **Abbe-Estlander cross-lip flap** for reconstruction, whereas **cheek advancement flaps** are required when **more than 70%** of the lip is excised.
        (3) Procedures. For the best cosmetic results, **vermilionectomy** excises the entire mucosa of the involved (usually lower) lip, widely undermining, advancing, and suturing the oral mucosa to the vermilion-dermal border. Simple "V" or "W" excision and primary closure can be facilitated by removal of bilateral **Burrow's triangles** at the apexes or by rotation of V-shaped **cross-lip flaps** (50% of the size of the defect) based on the **labial artery**, which is ligated 14 days later. Complex excisions and reconstructions for large lesions may involve **cheek advancement flaps**, bilateral **commissurotomies, buccal flap** advancement, resection of the superior **Burrow's triangle**, and reconstruction of the vermilion lip with a **staged tongue flap**.
      b. Buccal mucosa
        (1) Indications. Surgery is indicated for **both early and advanced lesions** because radiation therapy, despite providing high cure rates with early lesions, often is complicated by **mucositis** and **osteoradionecrosis** of underlying bone.
        (2) Approaches. Small lesions can be excised **transorally**, whereas large lesions may require an **external approach** via a **Weber-Fergusson** or **lip-splitting incision**, particularly if the maxilla or mandible also must be resected.
        (3) Procedures. Simple excision and primary closure is appropriate for early lesions, whereas advanced lesions may require partial **maxillectomy,**

mandibulectomy, and flap closure. The method of reconstruction depends on the size of the defect. Small defects can be closed with **split-thickness skin grafts**, but intermediate defects often necessitate **palatal or tongue flaps**. Frequently, large lesions need full-thickness cheek removal and reconstruction with a **pectoralis myocutaneous flap**.

c. **Gingival ridge**
   (1) **Indications.** Unless discovered at an early stage, alveolar ridge carcinoma usually invades bone. Because of possible **osteonecrosis** from radiation therapy, surgery is indicated for nearly all lesions.
   (2) **Approaches.** As with buccal mucosal lesions, a **transoral** or **transbuccal** approach can be used.
   (3) **Procedures.** The surgical options are similar to those with buccal mucosa lesions. However, **resection of bone is common** and requires reconstruction with bone graft or a prosthesis.

d. **Floor of mouth**
   (1) **Indications.** The same general principle of surgery or radiation applies for Stage I or II lesions. Combination therapy is required for advanced lesions.
   (2) **Approaches.** Small lesions can be approached transorally, whereas more advanced lesions generally are removed using a **combined transoral and transcervical** approach.
   (3) **Procedures.** Early lesions that do not extend to the mandible can be **widely excised** and closed with a split-thickness skin graft. Advanced lesions, however, necessitate resection of the underlying mandible. This can be performed **in continuity** with a cervical lymphadenectomy (**pull-through operation**). Often, a **pectoralis myocutaneous flap** is required for reconstruction.

e. **Hard palate**
   (1) **Indications.** Except for diffuse superficial lesions, **surgery is preferred** as the initial therapy for carcinoma of the hard palate.
   (2) **Approaches.** Most lesions are amenable to a **transoral** approach.
   (3) **Procedures.** Wide excision usually is performed; if maxillectomy is included, reconstruction often is accomplished with a **prosthetic obturator**.

f. **Oral tongue**
   (1) **Indications.** Although surgery and radiation are **equally** successful for most lesions, **radiation therapy** generally produces **superior function**, particularly in early lesions. Surgery is indicated if **irradiation fails** or **lymph node metastases** are detected.
   (2) **Approaches.** Early (T1) neoplasms can be excised transorally; however, more extensive lesions are best managed with a simultaneous **transoral** and **transcervical (pull-through operation)** approach.
   (3) **Procedures.** Like floor-of-mouth tumors, these cancers (if early) can simply be excised transorally or (if extensive) removed with an **in-continuity** cervical lymphadenectomy (**pull-through operation**).

g. **Oropharynx**
   (1) **Indications.** Because most malignancies in this region are advanced with submucosal spread at the time of diagnosis, **surgery often is combined with radiation** for maximum benefit. Early lesions, however, can be treated with either surgery or primary radiation.
   (2) **Approaches.** Small accessible lesions can be excised transorally, whereas excision of larger or inaccessible neoplasms can be accomplished with a **transcervical midline translingual, lateral, or transhyoid pharyngotomy**, depending on the location of the tumor. The pharyngotomy usually can be performed through the upper limb of the **radical neck incision**. A composite mandibular resection or a mandibular osteotomy (if no bony involvement exists) can be used for lesions in close proximity to the ramus of the mandible.
   (3) **Procedures.** Transcervical transpharyngeal tumor resection is the primary goal. During the procedure, the superior laryngeal nerves must be identified and preserved. A **transhyoid pharyngotomy** is made for **small posterior** lesions and **laterally or translingually** for large and anterior lesions. The pharyngotomy must be performed well away from the tumor. Reconstruction is achieved with a deltopectoral, sternocleidomastoid, or pectoralis myocutaneous flap.

h. **Hypopharynx**
   (1) **Indications.** Because malignancies in this region are often asympto-

matic until locally advanced and metastatic to regional lymph nodes, **surgery is combined most often with adjuvant radiation therapy**.

    (2) Approaches. Most malignancies in this location are approached through a variety of **cervical incisions**.

    (3) Procedures. Most lesions require a **laryngopharyngectomy** and **cervical lymphadenectomy**, although advanced tumors may necessitate **laryngopharyngoesophagectomy** and reconstruction with a **gastric pull-up procedure**.

   i. Nasopharynx

    (1) Indications. Because primary treatment for these neoplasms is radiation therapy, surgery is **reserved for radiation failure** and is only moderately successful.

    (2) Approaches. Although access to the nasopharynx is limited, a **transpalatal** or **infratemporal** approach can be used.

    (3) Procedures. Resection of nasopharyngeal cancers are not widely performed and the **results are mixed**.

2. Locally advanced and metastatic oropharyngeal cancer

   a. Lymph node metastases. Generally, cervical lymph node metastases are treated best by surgical excision. Metastases smaller than 2 cm in their greatest dimension, however, may respond well to **radiation therapy. Radical or modified radical cervical lymphadenectomy** (see Table 26–5) should be performed if **clinically obvious nodal metastases** are present (> 50% of patients with nasopharynx, hypopharynx, base of tongue and tonsillar cancers) and if the **risk of occult metastases is judged to be greater than 25–30%**, as with piriform sinus (35–40%), oral tongue (35%), and floor-of-mouth (30%) lesions.

   b. Distant metastases. Few indications for surgery exist in the presence of metastases to distant organs; however, isolated pulmonary metastases, symptomatic soft tissue masses, and rare solitary brain metastases can be removed after careful and thorough patient evaluation.

3. Morbidity and mortality. The surgical morbidity depends heavily on the **extent and location** of the primary neoplasm. Large lesions in highly functional areas are subject to significant postoperative deficits. In addition to the problems arising from the primary tumor, the following complications may arise from cervical lymphadenectomy as well as any cervical operation:

   a. Nerve injury of uninvolved nerves—particularly the facial, vagus, spinal accessory, hypoglossal, and phrenic—may be damaged inadvertently.

   b. Thoracic duct injury occurs in 1–2% of cases and may produce a chylous fistula.

   c. Aspiration is especially common with lingual and pharyngeal tumors.

   d. Hemorrhage is infrequent.

   e. Skin flap necrosis occurs in 4% of cases and is more common in irradiated patients.

   f. Pneumothorax is infrequent.

   g. Chronic pain and decreased range of shoulder motion can be the result of sacrificing the spinal accessory nerve.

B. Radiation therapy

  1. Primary oropharyngeal carcinoma. Radiation therapy (**6500-7000 cGy over 7 weeks** via an external beam with or without brachytherapy) is highly effective in the treatment of squamous cell carcinoma **limited to the mucosa (Stage I and II disease)** and is equivalent to surgery. **Verrucous carcinoma** (most commonly of the buccal mucosa), however, does **not** respond well to radiation, even if detected early. Furthermore, **advanced disease** generally requires **surgery or combined modality** therapy, with the exception of advanced **nasopharyngeal** carcinoma, which is routinely treated with **radiation therapy**. In addition, **occult** primary head and neck malignancies may be adequately controlled with radiation (**5000 cGy over 5 weeks**). Brachytherapy in combination with chemotherapy in the therapy of advanced lesions currently is under study.

  2. Adjuvant radiation therapy. Adjuvant radiation therapy is widely used for advanced lesions and provides superior local and regional tumor control. Radiation complements surgery because **radiation fails in the center** of large lesions and **recurrences after surgery** typically occur at the **margins**. The superiority of preoperative versus postoperative radiation therapy is controversial. In practice, however, both methods yield similar results (locoregional control in as many as **80%** of patients).

   a. Preoperative radiation therapy. Preoperative radiation therapy (**6000–**

6500 cGy over 6–7 weeks) is followed by an interval of **4–6 weeks** to allow for maximal tumor regression before surgery. Preoperative therapy is particularly useful for patients with **borderline resectable neck masses**, planned **gastric reconstruction** (stomach radiation tolerance ≤ 4000 cGy), and previous **open biopsy** of a neck mass.

  b. **Postoperative radiation therapy.** Postoperative radiation therapy (**5500 cGy over 6 weeks**) typically begins **3–4 weeks after surgery** (to allow for wound healing) and is indicated if the **risk of recurrence** is believed to **exceed 20–30%** (ie, in patients with close or involved margins, cartilage or bony invasion, high grade, and perineural extension).

3. **Locally advanced and metastatic oropharyngeal cancer**

  a. **Lymph node metastases.** Radiation successfully controls cervical lymph node metastases in **98%** of patients with **occult disease** and in **85%** with **clinically apparent** but small (< 2–3 cm) lymph node metastases; however, large (> **2 cm**) lymph nodes do not respond well and are an indication for surgery.

  b. **Distant metastases.** Palliative radiation therapy, both alone and in combination with chemotherapy, may be useful for symptomatic metastases.

4. **Morbidity and mortality.** Significant complications following radiation therapy often are related to advanced disease and a patient's poor health rather than to the radiation therapy itself. Dental care **before therapy** is essential to avoid **dental caries** and **osteoradionecrosis**, particularly because dental extraction **after** radiation therapy greatly increases the risk of osteoradionecrosis. Other major complications include **skin desquamation** and **orocutaneous fistulae**. Frequent minor side effects include xerostomia, transient mucositis, dysphagia, and odynophagia.

C. **Chemotherapy**

1. **Primary oropharyngeal carcinoma.** Currently, chemotherapy plays no role in the treatment of primary squamous cell carcinoma of the upper aerodigestive tract.

2. **Adjuvant chemotherapy**

  a. **Preoperative chemotherapy.** A multi-institutional, prospective, randomized trial conducted by the Head and Neck Contracts Program compared **surgery and postoperative radiation (standard therapy)** to standard therapy following **induction** chemotherapy with **cisplatin and bleomycin**. One group also received 6 months of **maintenance** chemotherapy with **cisplatin**. Although maintenance chemotherapy may have slightly reduced the rate of distant relapses, **no change occurred in disease-free and overall survival**. Further studies are in progress.

  b. **Postoperative chemotherapy.** Recent data suggests that postoperative chemotherapy with **cisplatin and fluorouracil** administered before radiation may reduce distant relapse rates in squamous cell carcinoma; however, clinical trials designed to verify this finding are not yet available.

3. **Locally advanced and metastatic oropharyngeal cancer**

  a. **Single agents. Methotrexate** has been the most extensively studied single agent. **Overall response rates** (> 50% reduction) with methotrexate vary from **12–65%**, depending on the study. High-dose methotrexate with leucovorin rescue, despite increased toxicity, does not significantly increase the response rate over low dose therapy. **Bleomycin** and **cisplatin** have also been studied and used extensively as single agents. Some studies report response rates as high as **40%**, but neither agent alone is considered as effective as methotrexate.

  b. **Combination chemotherapy.** Many chemotherapeutic combinations, particularly cisplatin-based regimens, have been used for palliation. **Response rates** as high as **70%** with **cisplatin and fluorouracil** have been reported, but conclusive results comparing long-term survival of single-agent versus multiagent palliative chemotherapy are unavailable.

D. **Immunotherapy.** No significant trial of immunotherapy with head and neck squamous carcinoma have been conducted.

X. **Prognosis**

A. **Risk of recurrence.** The risk of recurrence is most closely related to the nodal stage with a **10%** risk for patients with **N0-1 disease** and up to **60%** for patients with **N2–3 disease**.

B. **Five-year survival.** The 5-year survival varies with the **stage** and **location** of the primary tumor (see Table 23–2).

C. **Adverse prognostic factors.** The following pathologic features are associated with a particularly poor outcome:

TABLE 23–2. FIVE-YEAR SURVIVAL BY STAGE OF VARIOUS HEAD AND NECK PRIMARY TUMORS

Primary Site	Stage I (%)	Stage II (%)	Stage III (%)	Stage IV (%)
Lip	90	> 90	70	30
Floor of mouth, anterior tongue	80–90	60–70	40	20
Soft palate, uvula, anterior pillar	85	70	40	20
Tonsil	80	60	50	20
Hypopharynx	65	60	40	25
Base of tongue	60	60	40	10–20
Nasopharynx	80	> 50	> 50	20

      1. **Vascular invasion.**
      2. **Local recurrence,** supraclavicular recurrence **doubles** the risk of distant metastases (17% vs 8%).
      3. **Distant metastases.**
XI. Patient follow-up
    A. General guidelines. Patients with oropharyngeal carcinoma should be examined monthly for 1 year, every 2–3 months for the following 2 years, every 4–6 months for an additional 2 years, and then annually because early detection of recurrent disease may permit salvage. The following specific guidelines are recommended.
    B. Routine evaluation. Although routine blood tests, imaging studies, and invasive procedures are not indicated for patients with oropharyngeal cancer, an interval history and complete physical examination are mandatory during every office visit. Special attention should be paid to those areas listed on p 151, **VI.A**.
    C. Optional evaluation. The following tests and procedures may be indicated by previous diagnostic findings or clinical suspicion.
      1. **Blood tests** (see p 1, **IV.A**)
        a. Complete blood count.
        b. Hepatic transaminases.
        c. Alkaline phosphatase.
        d. Epstein-Barr virus antibody titer. The levels of this antibody can be followed to detect early relapse of **nasopharyngeal** cancer.
        e. 5-Nucleotidase.
        f. GGTP.
      2. **Imaging studies** (see p 3, **IV.C**)
        a. Chest x-ray.
        b. Magnetic resonance imaging.
        c. Computed tomography.
        d. Technetium-99m bone scan.
      3. **Endoscopy.** Direct laryngoscopy, esophagoscopy, and bronchoscopy may be indicated if **suspicious masses, swellings, or ulcerations** occur in areas that cannot be assessed adequately by direct physical examination.
      4. **Biopsy.**

REFERENCES

Adelstein DJ et al: Simultaneous radiotherapy and chemotherapy with 5-fluorouracil and cisplatin for locally confined squamous cell head and neck cancer. *NCI Mono* 1988;**6**:347–351.

Calcaterra TC, Juillard GJF: Oral cavity and oropharynx. In: Haskell CM (editor), *Cancer Treatment*, 3rd ed. Philadelphia, PA: WB Saunders; 1990:373–401.

Cummings CW (editor): *Otolaryngology: Head and Neck Surgery*, vol 2. Philadelphia, PA: CV Mosby; 1986.

English GM (editor): *Otolaryngology*, vol 5. Philadelphia, PA: JB Lippincott; 1990.

Guerry TL, Silverman S, Dedo HH: Carbon dioxide laser resection of superficial oral carcinoma: indications, technique, and results. *Ann Otol Rhinol Laryngol* 1986;**95**:547–555.

Levine PH et al: Epstein-Barr virus serology in the control of nasopharyngeal carcinoma. *Cancer Detect Prevent* 1988;**12**:357–362.

Peters LJ, Ang KK, Thames HD: Accelerated fractionation in the radiation treatment of head and neck cancer: a critical comparison of different strategies. *Acta Oncologica* 1988;**27**:185–194.

Spiro RH, Spiro JD, Strong EW: Surgical approach to squamous cell carcinoma confined to the tongue and the floor of mouth. *Head Neck Surg* 1986;**9**:27–31.

Stockwell HG, Lyman GH: Impact of smoking and smokeless tobacco on the risk of cancer of the head and neck. *Head Neck Surg* 1986;**9**:104–110.

Thawley SE, Panje WR (editors): *Comprehensive Management of Head and Neck Tumors*, vol 2. Philadelphia, PA: WB Saunders; 1987.

Vaughn TL: Occupation and squamous cell cancers of the pharynx and sinonasal cavity. *Am J Indust Med* 1989;**16**:493–510.

24 Malignancies of the Larynx

Matthew J. Lando, MD, and James K. Bredenkamp, MD

I. **Epidemiology.** Although laryngeal carcinoma constitutes **less than 2% of all cancers**, it comprises **25% of all head and neck malignancies**. In 1985, **8.6 cases per 100,000 males and 1.7 cases per 100,000 females** were reported, resulting in 2.5 and 0.4 deaths per 100,000 males and females, respectively. It is estimated that **12,600 new cases and 3,800 deaths** will be reported in 1993. Worldwide, the incidence of laryngeal carcinoma parallels the prevalence of smoking, with a high incidence among males in Sao Paulo, Brazil; Bombay, India; and the northeastern and Gulf coasts in the United States.

II. **Risk factors**
   A. **Age.** The incidence of laryngeal carcinoma increases from less than 1 case per 100,000 population before age 40 to a peak of **24 per 100,000 by age 65**. Most laryngeal cancers occur in people between 50 and 70 years of age.
   B. **Sex.** The risk for males is **5.1 times** greater than for females, although the incidence is currently increasing more rapidly among females.
   C. **Race.** In the United States, the risk for blacks is **1.4 times** greater than for whites, regardless of sex.
   D. **Genetic factors.** In Syrian hamsters, genetic determinants result in an incidence of laryngeal cancer in carcinogen-susceptible and resistant strains of 50% and 4%, respectively. In humans, however, first-degree relatives are not known to be at increased risk.
   E. **Diet**
      1. **Alcohol.** Alcohol ingestion increases the risk of laryngeal carcinoma by **5 times**.
      2. **Vitamin A.** A vitamin A deficient diet has been implicated as an etiologic factor.
   F. **Smoking.** Epidemiologic, clinical, and laboratory evidence all demonstrate that **tobacco smoke** causes squamous cell carcinoma of the upper aerodigestive tract. Because tobacco is weakly carcinogenic, exposure over many years may be required.
   G. **Previous laryngeal pathology**
      1. **Inflammation.** Chronic reflux laryngitis may produce inflammatory changes that are associated with atypia and dysplasia as well as frankly invasive carcinoma.
      2. **Infection**
         a. **Viral infection.** Laryngeal infection with **human papilloma virus** predisposes to squamous cell carcinoma. In contrast, Herpes and Epstein-Barr virus infections do not correlate with the development of cancer.
         b. **Other infections.** Laryngeal involvement with **tuberculosis** and **syphilis** has been correlated with an increased incidence of laryngeal malignancies.
      3. **Neoplasms.** As a result of generalized epithelial damage from heavy smoking and alcohol abuse, patients with other respiratory tract neoplasms develop laryngeal carcinoma more frequently than does the general population.

III. **Presentation**
   A. **Signs and symptoms**
      1. **Local manifestations.** The most common presenting symptom is **hoarseness** (> 90%). Sore throat (10%), dysphagia (10%), and dyspnea (10%) from respiratory obstruction also may occur with vocal cord fixation or large tumors. **Otalgia** indicates involvement of the **glossopharyngeal or vagus nerve** and, in adults, should always prompt a thorough head and neck examination. Neck mass, persistent cough, halitosis, and hemoptysis are late presenting symptoms.
      2. **Systemic manifestations.** Although a **weight loss of 8%** is a relatively common presenting complaint, other systemic signs and symptoms such as pleural

161

effusion (lung metastases), ascites (liver metastases), and bone pain (bony metastases) are infrequent.

B. Paraneoplastic syndromes. No paraneoplastic syndromes are associated with laryngeal cancer.

IV. **Differential diagnosis.** Patients presenting with laryngeal carcinoma almost always complain of **hoarseness**. Hoarseness can be caused by a wide variety of both benign and malignant lesions, including:

A. Infection

1. **Tuberculosis.** *Mycobacterium tuberculosis* can cause laryngeal edema, erythema, and exophytic masses that commonly involved the posterior commissure, whereas carcinoma usually presents along the anterior larynx.

2. **Syphilis.** This venereal disease commonly involves the epiglottis, ventricles, and arytenoids and produces edema (early stage) or ulcers and gummas (late).

3. **Blastomycosis.** *Blastomyces dermatitidis* infection can mimic laryngeal carcinoma.

B. Inflammation. Lupus erythematosus of the larynx may present with ulcers and irregular raised nodules.

C. Benign neoplasms. Polyps, singer's nodules, and contact ulcers, which may be confused with carcinomas, generally present as **pedunculated masses**.

D. Other diseases. Leukoplakia, pachydermia laryngitis sicca, and other chronic laryngeal lesions can be difficult to differentiate from carcinoma except on biopsy.

V. **Screening programs.** No screening programs exist for the early detection of laryngeal carcinoma.

VI. **Diagnostic workup**

A. Medical history and physical examination. A complete medical history and thorough physical examination are essential when evaluating patients with suspected laryngeal carcinoma.

1. **General appearance.** An assessment of the patient's general functional and nutritional status should be made (see p 1, **I** and **II**).

2. **Oral cavity and pharynx.** Careful palpation and visual examination of the base of tongue and pharynx is important to exclude local extension and other synchronous primary lesions.

3. **Larynx. Indirect laryngoscopy** is mandatory and gives valuable information regarding the extent of the lesion and vocal cord mobility, both of which have important therapeutic and prognostic implications.

4. **Neck.** Careful palpation of the neck for **masses** (local extension and lymph node metastases), including a midline pretracheal lymph node (**Delphian node**), is important.

5. **Chest.** Auscultation and percussion of the chest may reveal evidence of tobacco-induced chronic pulmonary disease (eg, barrel chest, distant breath sounds, wheezing) or lung metastases.

6. **Heart.** Cardiac examination may uncover signs of ischemic heart disease, which is frequently found in patients with laryngeal cancer because of common risk factors such as smoking.

7. **Abdomen.** A small liver, splenomegaly, and ascites suggest coexisting cirrhosis, which often is present from alcohol ingestion.

B. Primary tests and procedures. The following tests and procedures should be performed on all patients with suspected laryngeal carcinoma:

1. **Blood tests** (see p 1, **IV.A**)
   a. Complete blood count.
   b. Hepatic transaminases.
   c. Alkaline phosphatase.
   d. Albumin.

2. **Pulmonary function tests.** PFTs and, in particular, flow-volume loops are used to assess candidates for conservative laryngeal surgery. Partial laryngectomy should not be considered in patients with FEV_1 less than 50% of predicted volume. The ability to climb 2 flights of stairs without difficulty is a simple clinical test for adequate pulmonary reserve.

3. **Imaging studies** (see p 3, **IV.C**)
   a. **Chest x-ray.**
   b. **Computed tomography. CT scan of the neck** often gives valuable information regarding the extent of both local (ie, cartilaginous, paralaryngeal, and pre-epiglottic invasion) and metastatic disease that may not be apparent on physical examination.
   c. **Magnetic resonance imaging.** MRI surpasses CT in the ability to differen-

tiate the extent of tumor and disruption of soft tissue planes. New high resolution MRI scanners using solenoid surface coils can now accurately delineate the extent of disease in the larynx and neck.
   4. **Invasive procedures. Direct laryngoscopy** with biopsy is essential to ascer-
      tain the extent of the lesion and to confirm the diagnosis.
C. **Optional tests and procedures.** The following tests may be indicated by previous
   diagnostic findings or clinical suspicion:
   1. **Blood tests** (p 1, **IV.A**)
      a. 5'Nucleotidase.
      b. GGTP.
   2. **Imaging studies**
      a. **Barium swallow esophagography.** Barium esophagography can be use-
         ful to assess the extent of disease and to exclude the existence of esopha-
         geal synchronous tumors.
      b. **Laryngography.** Laryngography occasionally can be useful in assessing
         the extent of disease.
      c. **Technetium-99m bone scan** (see p 3, **IV.C.5**).
   3. **Invasive procedures**
      a. **Esophagogastroscopy.** In certain patients, esophagogastroscopy may be
         required to delineate esophageal involvement and exclude synchronous
         esophageal malignancies. The merits of routine esophagogastroscopy are
         debated, however.
      b. **Bronchoscopy.** Examination of the respiratory tree may identify synchro-
         nous tracheobronchial carcinomas in high-risk patients, but routine bron-
         choscopy is not recommended.
      c. **Biopsy. Fine needle aspiration** should be used to evaluate neck masses
         or swellings because open biopsy may convert **intracapsular** to **extra-
         capsular** disease and significantly reduce the chance of a positive prog-
         nosis.
VII. **Pathology**
   A. **Location.** The location of the tumor has important prognostic and therapeutic impli-
      cations. Although **transglottic tumors** (those involving the ventricle, false cord,
      and true cord) **account for almost 20%** of tumors, carcinoma of the larynx gener-
      ally is divided into the following 3 regions:
      1. **Supraglottis (25–40%).** This region extends from the tip of the epiglottis
         through the false cords and includes the epiglottis (both lingual and laryngeal
         surfaces), the arytenoids, aryepiglottic folds, and the ventricular bands (false
         cords).
      2. **Glottis (50–75%).** This region extends from the floor of the ventricle to 1 cm
         below the edge of the true vocal cords, including anterior and posterior commis-
         sures. Nearly **75% of cancer involve the anterior half of the true vocal
         cords.**
      3. **Subglottis (1–5%).** This region extends from 1 cm below the edge of the true
         vocal cords to the inferior border of the cricoid cartilage.
   B. **Multiplicity.** Synchronous primary carcinomas (other upper aerodigestive tract ma-
      lignancies that are identified within 6 months of the initial diagnosis) occur in **10–
      15% of patients** and are probably related to common risk factors.
   C. **Histology. Squamous cell carcinoma represents 95–98% of all laryngeal ma-
      lignancies.** The remaining 2–5% are predominantly adenocarcinomas and sarco-
      mas.
   D. **Metastatic spread**
      1. **Modes of spread**
         a. **Direct extension.** Laryngeal carcinoma spreads via direct extension to in-
            volve other portions of the larynx and the paraglottic space, frequently caus-
            ing vocal cord fixation.
         b. **Lymphatic metastasis.** Compartmentalization of the lymphatic system di-
            rects the spread of carcinoma to four compartments: glottic, supraglottic,
            ventricular, and infraglottic. The degree and pattern of lymphatic spread
            varies greatly, depending primarily on tumor location, but also on tumor size
            and cellular differentiation.
            (1) **Tumor location**
               (a) **Supraglottic tumors**. Lymphatics are abundant in the supraglottic
                  region, and ipsilateral as well as contralateral lymph node metas-
                  tases commonly occur (**21–60%, with 7–20% representing oc-
                  cult disease**). This location is most often associated with bilateral

neck disease (late **contralateral metastases** appear in **33%** of patients with ipsilateral nodal involvement initially).

- **(b) Glottic tumors.** Because vocal cords have few lymphatics, lymph node metastases are **unusual (0.4–2%)**; however, this rate increases to 16% if there is anterior commissure, arytenoid, or more than 5 mm of subglottic extension.
- **(c) Subglottic tumors.** Primary or secondary involvement of the subglottis produces lymph node metastases in **10–25%** of cases.
- **(d) Extralaryngeal extension.** Involvement of the vallecula and the base of the tongue leads to **bilateral cervical lymph node metastases in 10%** of cases.

- **(2) Tumor size.** The incidence of lymph node metastases varies with tumor size. For example, the incidence of lymph node metastases from tumors confined to the glottis range from 1–5% of T1 tumors to 60% for T3 and T4 lesions.
  - **c. Hematogenous metastasis.** Spread through systemic blood vessels generally does not occur until late in the disease. At autopsy, metastases below the clavicle are found in 46.7% of patients who die of epidermoid carcinoma of the head and neck.
- **2. Sites of spread.** Autopsy studies demonstrate that carcinoma of the larynx commonly metastasizes to the following distant sites: **lung,** 50%; **liver,** 27%; **kidney,** 20%; **adrenal glands,** 14%; and **bone,** 3%.

VIII. Staging. In 1987, the American Joint Committee on Cancer and the Union Internationale Contre le Cancer jointly developed a TNM staging system for laryngeal carcinoma.

- **A. Tumor stage**
  - **1. Supraglottic tumor**
    - **a. TX.** Primary tumor cannot be assessed.
    - **b. T0.** No evidence of primary tumor exists.
    - **c. Tis.** Carcinoma in situ.
    - **d. T1.** Tumor is confined to 1 supraglottic site of origin; vocal cord mobility is normal.
    - **e. T2.** Tumor invades the glottis or more than 1 supraglottic site; vocal cord mobility is normal.
    - **f. T3.** Tumor is limited to the larynx with vocal cord fixation or extends to the postcricoid area, the medial wall of the piriform sinus, or the pre-epiglottic space.
    - **g. T4.** Tumor invades thyroid cartilage or beyond the larynx to involve the oropharynx or soft tissues of the neck.
  - **2. Glottic tumor**
    - **a. TX.** Primary tumor cannot be assessed.
    - **b. T0.** No evidence of primary tumor.
    - **c. Tis.** Carcinoma in situ.
    - **d. T1.** Tumor confined to vocal cord(s) with normal vocal cord mobility (includes involvement of anterior or posterior commissures).
      - **(1) T1a.** Tumor is limited to 1 vocal cord.
      - **(2) T1b.** Tumor involves both vocal cords.
    - **e. T2.** Tumor extends to the supraglottis or subglottis or impairs vocal cord mobility.
    - **f. T3.** Tumor is confined to the larynx with cord fixation.
    - **g. T4.** Tumor invades through the thyroid cartilage or extends beyond the larynx to the oropharynx or soft tissues of the neck.
  - **3. Subglottic tumor**
    - **a. TX.** Primary tumor cannot be assessed.
    - **b. T0.** No evidence of primary tumor.
    - **c. Tis.** Carcinoma in situ.
    - **d. T1.** Tumor is confined to the subglottis.
    - **e. T2.** Tumor extends to the vocal cords with normal or impaired vocal cord mobility.
    - **f. T3.** Tumor is limited to the larynx with vocal cord fixation.
    - **g. T4.** Tumor invades beyond the cricoid or thyroid cartilage or extends to the oropharynx or soft tissues of the neck.
- **B. Lymph node stage**
  - **1. NX.** Regional lymph nodes cannot be assessed.
  - **2. N0.** No regional nodes are involved.

3. **N1.** A single ipsilateral node no larger than 3 cm in its greatest diameter contains metastatic tumor.

4. **N2.** Metastasis involves a single ipsilateral lymph node larger than 3 cm but no larger than 6 cm in its greatest dimension or multiple ipsilateral lymph nodes no larger than 6 cm in their greatest dimension.

   a. **N2a.** Metastasis involves a single ipsilateral lymph node larger than 3 cm but no larger than 6 cm in its greatest dimension.

   b. **N2b.** Metastases involve multiple ipsilateral lymph nodes no larger than 6 cm in their greatest dimension.

5. **N3.** Metastases involve ipsilateral nodes larger than 6 cm in their greatest dimension, bilateral lymph nodes, or contralateral lymph nodes.

   a. **N3a.** Metastases involve ipsilateral lymph nodes and are larger than 6 cm in their greatest dimension.

   b. **N3b.** Metastases involve bilateral lymph nodes.

   c. **N3c.** Metastases involve only contralateral lymph nodes.

C. **Metastatic stage**
   1. **M0.** No distant metastases are present.
   2. **M1.** Distant metastases are present.

D. **Histopathologic grade**
   1. **GX.** Grade cannot be assessed.
   2. **G1.** Well differentiated.
   3. **G2.** Moderately well differentiated.
   4. **G3.** Poorly differentiated.
   5. **G4.** Undifferentiated.

E. **Stage groupings**
   1. **0.** Tis, N0, M0.
   2. **I.** T1, N0, M0.
   3. **II.** T2, N0, M0.
   4. **III.** T3, N0, M0; T1–3, N1, M0;
   5. **IV.** T4, N0–1, M0; any T, N2–3, M0; any T, any N, M1.

IX. **Treatment.** Laryngeal carcinoma is treated primarily with surgery, radiation therapy, or a combination of the 2 modalities.

A. **Surgery**
   1. **Primary laryngeal carcinoma**
      a. **Indications.** Surgery, either alone or in combination with radiation therapy, is indicated for **T4, T3, and extensive T2 glottic tumors as well as most supra- and subglottic lesions.** For Tis, T1, and limited T2 tumors, both surgery and radiotherapy produce excellent 5-year survival rates. Radiation therapy is preferred because the resulting vocal quality is superior to that after partial laryngectomy. For these early lesions, surgery is an acceptable alternative when (1) radiation therapy is not available, (2) the tumor histology is relatively resistant to radiation therapy (ie, adenocarcinoma, verrucous carcinoma, and sarcoma), (3) regional lymph node metastases exist, or (4) the patient refuses radiation therapy.

      b. **Approaches** (see also p 185, **IX.A.1.b**). Two approaches are available: **laryngectomy and radical cervical lymphadenectomy.** Although laryngectomy can be accomplished through several different approaches, an incision that combines both procedures is generally used.

      c. **Procedures. Conservative surgical procedures** that avoid the severe communication handicap accompanying laryngectomy can be used for **60%** of all laryngeal lesions without compromising survival. Surgical therapy normally involves one of the following operations:

         (1) **Local excision. Preinvasive carcinoma** can be excised using suspension laryngoscopy and an operating microscope. The supravital stain, **toluidine blue (2%),** is readily absorbed by superficial cancers as well as carcinoma in situ and can be used to guide complete resection of these tumors. **Cordectomy and laser excision** also can be used for treatment of Tis and T1 lesions. (*Caution:* great care should be exercised in resection of anterior commissure lesions, which may be more extensive than appreciated). **Cure rates from both surgical and laser excision approach 90%** and are comparable to those obtained with radiation therapy.

         (2) **Partial vertical hemilaryngectomy.** This procedure is used primarily for **T1, T2, and limited T3 glottic carcinomas.** A perichondrial strap muscle flap is elevated bilaterally, and a vertical laryngofissure is cre-

ated away from the tumor. Then, under direct vision, the tumor is resected. Glottic reconstruction is performed with a sternohyoid or omohyoid muscle flap. Tracheostomy is mandatory. Variations have been described for anterior and advanced lesions. **Contraindications to this procedure include: (1) subglottic extension greater than 1 cm, (2) cartilage invasion, (3) bilateral arytenoid or interarytenoid involvement, and (4) supraglottic extension greater than 2 mm at the petiole.**

- (3) **Supraglottic laryngectomy.** This approach is indicated in early supraglottic lesions and involves construction of an inferior perichondrial muscle flap. A horizontal laryngofissure is developed, and the larynx is entered at the vallecula on the side opposite the tumor. To avoid injuring the vocal cords, the aryepiglottic fold is incised first, followed by the tumor at the ventricular level. Modifications have been reported for more extensive lesions that include ipsilateral true vocal cord resection. **Contraindications to this procedure include (1) invasion of laryngeal ventricle, piriform apex, postcricoid, and interarytenoid regions, (2) tumor that extends to within 5 mm of the anterior commissure, (3) cartilage invasion, and (4) regional lymph node metastases requiring bilateral neck dissections.** Supraglottic laryngectomy predisposes to aspiration and dysphagia to a much greater degree than does vertical partial laryngectomy and should not be performed if the patient has **severe pulmonary disease**.
- (4) **Total laryngectomy.** For extensive disease, the entire larynx is removed, including the strap muscles. Controlled vallecular or piriform entry is used so that tumor resection can be performed under direct vision. Piriform and esophageal mucosa should be preserved to prevent stricture and permanent deglutition problems. **Contraindications to this procedure include (1) the existence of conservative surgical options, (2) tumor extension into the vertebral fascia or carotid sheath, and (3) distant metastases.**
- (5) **Radical neck dissection.** Although many modifications for radical neck surgery exist, a large **"apron" flap** is used most commonly in association with laryngeal surgery. Extent of the dissection is defined by the **superior belly of the omohyoid** anteromedially, the **trapezius** posteriorly, the **supraclavicular fossa** inferiorly, the **submandibular space** superiorly, and the **scalenus fascia** deeply. **Modified** neck dissections can be performed when the disease is less extensive and involves **preservation of the spinal accessory nerve, the sternocleidomastoid muscle, and the jugular vein** in certain cases. Neck metastases are generally best treated by surgery, although involved lymph nodes less than 2 cm in diameter respond well to radiation. In the absence of clinically evident lymph node metastases, prophylactic lymph node dissection is indicated if radiation therapy is not planned and the incidence of occult metastases is estimated to be greater than 25%. **Contraindications to radical neck dissection are an untreatable primary lesion, distant metastases, and invasion of prevertebral fascia, base of the skull, or the carotid artery.**

d. **Speech rehabilitation.** Speech rehabilitation is essential in patients undergoing total laryngectomy and may restore effective speech in the majority of patients. Customarily, one of the following basic methods of speech is chosen:

- (1) **Esophageal speech.** Esophageal speech involves exhalation of air from the stomach through the pharyngoesophagus. This creates sound by **mucosal vibration** that is then articulated by the palate, tongue, and lips.
- (2) **Artificial larynx.** These electronic devices transmit sound to the airspaces of the neck, where it is articulated.
- (3) **Speech with tracheo-esophageal puncture.** A small valved prosthesis is placed in a **fistula** between the trachea and cervical esophagus, allowing air to flow into the esophagus and resulting in improved speech that more closely resembles laryngeal speech.

2. **Locally advanced and metastatic laryngeal cancer.** Usually, surgery provides no benefit in locally advanced and metastatic disease, although local measures (eg, cryotherapy) are occasionally useful for controlling exophytic neck lesions.

3. **Mortality and morbidity.** The risk of complications and death varies with the procedure performed:
   a. **Total laryngectomy. Mortality for total laryngectomy is 2%**, and complications include the following problems:
      (1) Pharyngocutaneous fistula, 15% (most common).
      (2) Wound infection, 1%.
      (3) Hemorrhage, 1%.
      (4) Pharyngoesophageal stenosis (late).
      (5) Tracheostomal recurrence, 3.8-20%—particularly if delayed more than 24 hrs after tracheostomy for malignant obstruction.
   b. **Partial laryngeal surgery.** Serious morbidity following partial laryngeal procedures stems from **chronic aspiration pneumonitis** or the **inability to decannulate.**
   c. **Radical neck dissections.** Cervical lymphadenectomy significantly increases the morbidity and mortality of laryngeal surgery because of the following problems:
      (1) **Nerve injury,** (< 1%) injury to uninvolved nerves, especially facial, vagus, spinal accessory, hypoglossal, or phrenic.
      (2) **Thoracic duct injury** (1-2%), with resulting chylous fistula.
      (3) **Hemorrhage,** 1%.
      (4) **Skin necrosis** (4%), which is particularly common in irradiated patients.
      (5) **Pneumothorax,** < 1%.
      (6) **Chronic pain and numbness of the neck.**
B. **Radiation therapy**
   1. **Primary laryngeal carcinoma. T2 lesions limited to the mucosa, T1, and Tis tumors should be treated with radiation therapy.** Although surgery and radiation produce equal results, radiotherapy in these early lesions is preferred because of better preservation of vocal quality. **T3 and T4 neoplasms are treated best with combined surgery and radiation therapy.** Cobalt or megavoltage radiation is used with a dose of **6000–7000 cGy over approximately 6–7 weeks**. Occult nodal disease is cured in 85-90% of cases with this regimen; however, lymph nodes larger than 2 cm and **verrucous carcinoma** do not respond well to radiation therapy; thus, surgical therapy rather than radical radiotherapy is recommended for these lesions.
   2. **Adjuvant radiation therapy**
      a. **Preoperative radiotherapy.** Preoperative radiotherapy has been advocated for advanced laryngopharyngeal cancer to increase the cure rate from radical surgery. Radiation ports include the primary tumor and all cervical nodes bilaterally. Usually, **5500 cGy** is delivered, followed by a **rest interval of 3–6 weeks** to allow for maximal tumor regression. Because reduction in the extent of resection diminishes the benefit of combined therapy, radical surgery is planned on the basis of the **original tumor size**.
      b. **Intraoperative radiotherapy.** No intraoperative teletherapy or brachytherapy is currently in use.
      c. **Postoperative radiotherapy.** Postoperative radiation therapy is advocated for malignancies with close surgical margins or confirmed lymph node metastases. Typically, **5000–7000 cGy is administered over a period of 6 weeks**.
   3. **Locally advanced and metastatic laryngeal cancer.** Radiation therapy is indicated for symptoms associated with unresectable or metastatic tumor. Combinations of radiotherapy and chemotherapy currently are under study.
   4. **Mortality and morbidity.** Most of the severe complications of radiation therapy are related to advanced disease and poor patient health rather than to the radiotherapy itself and include the following problems:
      a. **Odynophagia or dysphagia,** secondary to mucositis or ulceration (100%).
      b. **Xerostomia with dental caries,** unless pretherapy dental care is instituted.
      c. **Laryngeal edema,** with transient worsening of voice (100%).
      d. **Desquamation of skin.**
      e. **Osteochondronecrosis.**
      f. **Radiation myelitis** (rare).
C. **Chemotherapy**
   1. **Primary laryngeal carcinoma.** There is currently no role for chemotherapy in the treatment of primary laryngeal carcinoma.
   2. **Adjuvant chemotherapy**
      a. **Preoperative chemotherapy.** The Head and Neck Contracts Program, a

multi-institutional, prospective randomized trial, compared three treatment options: (1) induction chemotherapy with cisplatin (100 mg/m^2) on day 1 and bleomycin (15 mg/m^2 continuous infusion) on days 3-7, followed by standard therapy (surgery and post-op radiation), (2) induction chemotherapy and standard therapy followed by maintenance chemotherapy for 6 months with cisplatin, and (3) standard therapy alone. Distant relapse rates were slightly reduced with maintenance chemotherapy, but no change occurred in disease-free or overall survival. Further studies are in progress.

- **b. Postoperative chemotherapy.** Currently, no role exists for the administration of chemotherapy after potentially curative surgery.

3. **Locally advanced and metastatic laryngeal cancer**
   - **a. Single agents.** Many drugs have been used to treat patients who have failed primary surgery and radiation therapy. Single agents are as effective but less toxic than are combination regimens (see below). However, response rates remain poor, with methotrexate (40–60 mg/m^2 weekly), cisplatin (80–120 mg/m^2), and bleomycin (0.25–0.5 units/kg twice weekly) producing responses in 35%, 25–30%, and 30–40% of patients, respectively.
   - **b. Combination chemotherapy.** Although early results with the combination of **cisplatin** (80–120 mg/m^2 followed by **fluorouracil** (800–1000 mg/m^2) are encouraging (**50–70% overall** and **10–20% complete response rates**), no large prospective randomized trials to date have demonstrated a survival advantage for patients treated with any chemotherapeutic combination.

D. **Immunotherapy.** No significant trials of immunotherapy have been conducted with laryngeal carcinoma.

X. Prognosis

A. **Risk of recurrence.** Recurrent disease after radiation and partial laryngectomy can be **salvaged** by further therapy in **50–75%** of patients. The risk of recurrence by T stage is listed below:
   1. **T1.** 10%.
   2. **T2.** 29%.
   3. **T3.** 39–49%.
   4. **T4.** 51–70%.

B. **Five-year survival.** The prognosis by TNM stage is summarized below:
   1. **Stage I.** 93–100%.
   2. **Stage II.** 85–95%.
   3. **Stage III.** 53–67%.
   4. **Stage IV.** 30–40%.

C. **Adverse prognostic factors.** The presence of the following factors decreases the likelihood of long-term survival of patients:
   1. **Lymph node metastases.** Survival declines to 40% when lymph nodes are involved.
   2. **Black race.** The overall 5-year survival rate for **blacks is 53%** compared with **68% for whites**.

XI. Patient follow-up

A. **General guidelines.** Patients with laryngeal carcinoma should be followed closely every month for the first year, every 3 months for the following 2 years, every 6 months for an additional 2 years, and then annually. Recurrent disease after curative resection may be "salvaged" with further therapy if detected at an early stage. Specific guidelines for patient follow-up are outlined below:

B. **Medical history and physical examination.** An interval medical history and a complete physical examination, including a detailed head and neck inspection should be performed during every clinic visit. Attention is focused on those areas discussed on p 162, **VI.A**, and, in particular, on indirect laryngoscopy with videotaped records that allow serial comparisons.

C. **Routine evaluation.** Patients with laryngeal carcinoma who have undergone potentially curative therapy do not require routine blood tests or imaging studies.

D. **Optional evaluation.** The following tests and procedures may be indicated by previous diagnostic findings or clinical suspicion:
   1. **Blood tests** (see p 1, **IV.A**).
      - a. Complete blood count.
      - b. Hepatic transaminases.
      - c. Alkaline phosphatase.

    d. 5'-Nucleotidase.
    e. GGTP.
  2. Thyroid function tests. Free T_4 index, T_3RIA, T_4RIA, and TSH may be indicated if signs and symptoms of hypothyroidism develop.
  3. Imaging studies (see p 3, **IV.C**)
    a. Chest x-ray.
    b. Technetium-99m bone scan.
  4. Direct laryngoscopy. Direct laryngoscopy and biopsy is indicated when suspicious masses, swelling, or ulcerations occur. Fine needle aspiration can be used to evaluate neck masses or swelling. Open biopsy of suspicious neck masses should not be performed because it may significantly decrease prognosis as intracapsular disease is converted to extracapsular disease.

REFERENCES

Adjuvant chemotherapy for advanced head and neck squamous carcinoma. Final report of the head and neck contracts program. *Cancer* 1987;**60**:301–311.

Brandenburg JH, Condon KG, Frank TW: Coronal sections of larynges from radiation-therapy failures: a clinical-pathologic study. *Otolaryngol Head Neck Surg* 1986; **95**:213–218.

Chang TM: Induction chemotherapy for head and neck cancers: a literature review. *Head Neck Surg* 1988;**10**:150–159.

Cummings CW et al: *Atlas of Laryngeal Surgery.* Philadelphia, PA: CV Mosby; 1984.

English GM (editor): *Otolaryngology,* vol.5. Philadelphia, PA: JB Lippincott; 1990.

Hoover LA et al: Magnetic resonance imaging of the larynx and tongue base: clinical applications. *Otolaryngol Head Neck Surg* 1987;**97**:245–256.

Mendenhall W et al: The role of radiation therapy in laryngeal cancer. *CA-A Cancer J Clin* 1990;**40**:150-165.

Silver C, Moisa I: The role of surgery in the treatment of laryngeal cancer. *CA-A Cancer J Clin* 1990;**40**:134-149.

Singer M, Blom E: Medical techniques for voice restoration after total laryngectomy. *CA-A Cancer J Clin* 1990;**40**:166-182.

Wetmore SJ, Key JM, Suen JY: Laser therapy for T1 glottic carcinoma of the larynx. *Arch Otolaryngol Head Neck Surg* 1986;**112**:853–855.

25 Malignancies of the Salivary Glands

James J. Bredenkamp, MD, and Matthew J. Lando, MD

I. **Epidemiology.** Salivary carcinoma represents 3–6% of all head and neck tumors. In the United States, 1–2 cases per 100,000 population were reported in 1985. In 1993, 2000 new cases and 790 deaths are predicted; however, the true incidence is difficult to determine because of the rare nature of these tumors. Worldwide, the incidence of malignant tumors of the salivary glands varies only slightly.

II. **Risk factors**
   A. **Age.** Although the average age at presentation is 55 years, nearly 2% of tumors occur in children between the ages of 1 month and 10 years, and 16% develop in patients older than 30 years. Almost 33% of all pediatric salivary gland neoplasms are malignant (most frequent is mucoepidermoid carcinoma). Undifferentiated tumors occur most commonly in patients in their sixth or seventh decade of life.
   B. **Sex.** Although generally there is no gender predilection, the risk in noncaucasian females in the United States and Africa is slightly greater than that in males. The risk of mucoepidermoid carcinoma and acinic cell carcinoma is 2–4 times more common in females than in males.
   C. **Race.** No known racial predisposition exists for these tumors.
   D. **Genetic factors.** First-degree relatives of patients with salivary carcinomas are not at increased risk. In addition, there are no known associated familial syndromes.
   E. **Diet.** No association exists between diet or alcohol intake and salivary cancers.
   F. **Smoking.** Generally, tobacco is not a risk factor.
   G. **Previous salivary pathology.** No relationship exists between prior trauma, chronic infection, or sialolithiasis and the subsequent development of salivary neoplasms; however, pleomorphic adenomas (a benign tumor) may undergo malignant transformation to a carcinoma ex-pleomorphic adenoma (malignant mixed tumor).
   H. **Radiation.** Studies of atomic bomb survivors and patients irradiated for acne demonstrate that low-dose radiation (< 300 cGy) increases the incidence of both benign and malignant salivary malignancies by 9 times. Tumors develop after a latent period of 15–20 years and occur more often in the parotid gland than in other sites.

III. **Presentation**
   A. **Signs and symptoms.** Because the salivary glands occupy the entire upper aerodigestive tract, salivary gland tumors may present with a variety of signs and symptoms.
      1. **Local manifestations.** A slowly-enlarging, rubbery, painless mass (pre- or infra-auricular, submandibular, or submucosa) is the only symptom of a salivary gland tumor in 60–85% of patients. The mass may be noted incidentally while washing or shaving and may have been present for more than 5 years (20%). Facial nerve paresis or paralysis (see Table 25–1), skin or deep fixation (28%), pain (sensory nerve involvement), and ulceration are presumptive evidence of a parotid malignancy and a poor prognosis.
      2. **Systemic manifestations.** Neck masses (cervical node metastases) are identified in 18%, 28%, and 15% of patients with carcinoma of the parotid, submandibular, and minor salivary glands, respectively. Other rare signs and symptoms include pulmonary masses and shortness of breath (lung metastases); bony pain, masses, and pathologic fractures (bony metastases); renal masses (metastases); and weakness, malaise, and weight loss. Ultimately, 33% of patients with malignant salivary tumors develop distant disease.
   B. **Paraneoplastic syndromes.** No known paraneoplastic syndromes are associated with salivary neoplasms.

IV. **Differential diagnosis.** It is frequently impossible to distinguish clinically between benign and malignant salivary masses. Nearly 27% of excised parotid masses are caused by non-neoplastic conditions, whereas 73% are neoplastic in origin (11% malignant and 62% benign). For submandibular masses, 85% are non-neoplastic and 15% represent neoplasm (8% benign and 7% malignant). As a rule, rapidly growing tumors are

TABLE 25-1. INCIDENCE OF FACIAL NERVE PARALYSIS IN PAROTID TUMORS

Histology	Incidence of paralysis (%)
Mucoepidermoid carcinoma	9
Acinic cell carcinoma	1
Adenoid cystic carcinoma	17
Adenocarcinoma	11
Carcinoma ex-pleomorphic adenoma	7
Squamous cell carcinoma	19
Undifferentiated carcinoma	24
Total	12

more likely than slowly-growing masses to be malignant. Other processes that may produce salivary gland masses include (1) inflammatory diseases (acute and chronic sialoadenitis such as epidemic parotitis or mumps), (2) retrograde infections (staphylococcus or streptococcus), (3) necrotizing sialometaplasia, granulomatous diseases (chronic progressive granulomatosis, tuberculosis, cat scratch disease, actinomycosis, histoplasmosis, toxoplasmosis, syphilis, and sarcoid), (4) AIDS, (5) salivary cysts, (6) autoimmune disorders (localized B-cell lymphoepithelial lesions in Sjögren's syndrome), (7) occlusive disease (sialithiasis, Kussmaul's disease, and strictures), (8) congenital anomalies (branchial cleft or mucus retention cysts), and (9) normal anatomic variants (masseter muscle hypertrophy and a prominent transverse process of the atlas). Benign neoplasms (pleomorphic adenomas, Warthin's tumors, oncocytomas, basal cell adenomas, hemangiomas, and lymphangiomas) as well as metastatic lesions (head and neck squamous cell carcinoma and melanoma, lymphoma, leukemia, and, rarely, lung, breast, and renal cancer) also may simulate primary salivary tumors.

V. Screening programs. Programs to actively screen patients are not practical because of the rare nature of these neoplasms. Currently, patient education and increased physician awareness remain the only methods of increasing early detection.

VI. Diagnostic workup

  A. Medical history and physical examination. A thorough medical history that emphasizes common presenting complaints and a complete head and neck examination is essential to exclude the presence of primary salivary malignancies.

  1. **General appearance.** The functional status of the patient may be quickly assessed by his or her general appearance.

  2. **Head.** Mass size and mobility should be assessed, although this does not help to distinguish benign from malignant processes. However, skin fixation or infiltration, facial nerve dysfunction, pain, or trismus are often indicative of malignancy. Tumors presenting in the deep lobe of the parotid may bulge into the oropharynx and cause obstruction of the airway or dysphagia. Salivary flow is not affected by either benign or malignant disease. The skin and scalp regions should be examined carefully for skin tumors such as melanoma because of the high incidence of parotid metastases.

  3. **Neck.** All masses should be described and may represent primary or lymphatic metastatic disease.

  4. **Chest.** On occasion, wheezing, decreased breath sounds, and rales may indicate the presence of pulmonary metastases.

  5. **Abdomen.** Hepatomegaly and masses are important findings.

  B. Primary tests and procedures. The following tests and procedures should be performed on all patients with suspected salivary gland malignancies.

  1. **Blood tests** (see p 1, **IV.A**)

     a. **Complete blood count.**

     b. **Hepatic transaminases.**

     c. **Alkaline phosphatase.**

  2. **Imaging studies** (see p 3, **IV.C**)

     a. **Chest x-ray.**

     b. **Magnetic resonance imaging.** MRI scans provide superior results to CT scans since MRI can (1) better distinguish intra- from extraglandular masses, deep parotid tumors from primary parapharyngeal lesions, and tumor from normal muscle, (2) directly image the facial nerve, (3) be obtained without motion artifact and interference from dental fillings, (4) generate multiplanar images, (5) enhance tumor images with gadolinium, and (6) be obtained without ionizing radiation and i.v. contrast.

3. **Invasive procedures.** Fine needle aspiration of salivary gland masses poses minimal risk and discomfort to the patient and should be obtained in all patients. With the aid of an experienced cytopathologist, an overall accuracy rate of 80–90% (false negative rate of 5% and false positive rate of 4%) has been reported. Specimens can be collected either extraorally or perorally. Preoperative knowledge of the diagnosis permits an informed operative plan and patient consent.

C **Optional tests and procedures.** The following examinations may be indicated by prior diagnostic tests or by clinical suspicion.

1. **Blood tests** (see p 1, **IV.A**)
   a. **Nucleotidase.**
   b. **GGTP.**

2. **Imaging studies.** Although useful information rarely is gained from preoperative radiographic studies, imaging studies may be indicated in certain situations.
   a. **Plain radiographs.** If calculi are suspected, plain radiographs can be useful in evaluating salivary gland masses, particularly of the submandibular gland (> 80% of submandibular calculi are radiopaque).
   b. **Sialography.** Sialography rarely distinguishes benign from malignant processes. It is most useful in the evaluation of chronic inflammatory conditions.
   c. **Computed tomography (CT).** CT scans may be helpful in evaluating involvement of the deep parotid gland, parapharyngeal space, and bone. CT sialography may provide better delineation of glandular tissue from neoplastic growth, but its role has not been clearly defined.
   d. **Ultrasonography** (see p 3, **IV.C.3**).
   e. **Salivary scan.** Although these studies are "hot" in Warthin's tumors and oncocytomas, the specificity is low, and at present, these technetium-99m studies are not indicated in the diagnosis of parotid tumors.
   f. **Technetium-99m bone scan** (see p 3, **IV.C.4**).

3. **Invasive procedures.** Incisional and true cut needle biopsy of major salivary tumors should be avoided since they increase the local recurrence rate and make later en bloc resection more difficult. **Parotidectomy** remains the procedure of choice for biopsy of most parotid tumors if FNA fails to establish a diagnosis.

VII. **Pathology**
   A. **Location.** The salivary glands are divided into major and minor glands. Tumor distribution parallels that of normal glandular tissue (see Table 25–2).

   1. **The major salivary glands.** The parotid, submandibular, and sublingual glands comprise the major salivary glands. The parotid gland consists of a superficial lobe (90% of parotid tissue and tumors) and a deep lobe (10%). The most frequent site of parotid neoplasms is in the **tail of the superficial lobe.**

   2. **The minor salivary glands.** Between 700 and 1,000 small salivary glands are located throughout the pharynx, larynx, trachea, nose, paranasal sinuses, and the oral mucosa. Nearly 33% of minor salivary gland tumors are located in the **palate,** and 20% are located in the tongue, floor of the mouth, and gingiva. The remainder occur in the paranasal sinuses, cheeks, lips, and nose.

TABLE 25–2. INCIDENCE OF SALIVARY NEOPLASMS BY SALIVARY GLAND LOCATION

Gland	Proportion of all Salivary Tumors (%)	Benign (%)	Malignant (%)
Parotid	80	80	20
Submandibular	10	50	50
Sublingual and minor	10	20	80

B. **Multiplicity.** Multiple tumors within the same gland are rare except for benign Warthin's tumors and acinic cell carcinoma, which are bilateral in 10–15% and 3% of patients, respectively. Metastasis within the gland or seeding from a recurrent pleomorphic adenoma also occurs. Approximately 11% of patients have a synchronous second primary malignancy, and the incidence of breast cancer is increased 8 times in women.

C. **Histology.** A variety of histopathologic neoplasms arise in salivary tissue (see Table 25–3). Malignancies are divided into either low or high grades.

   1. **Low-grade neoplasms**
      a. **Acinic cell carcinoma.** Acinic cell carcinomas are slow-growing neoplasms, occurring almost exclusively in the parotid gland.
      b. **Low-grade mucoepidermoid carcinoma.** These tumors make up 67% of all mucoepidermoid cancers, have a high mucous cell content and cystic architecture, and are locally aggressive but rarely metastatic.

   2. **High-grade neoplasms**
      a. **High-grade mucoepidermoid carcinoma.** This malignancy resembles squamous cell carcinoma and constitutes 33% of all mucoepidermoid tumors. It is more likely to metastasize than low grade mucoepidermoid tumors and carries a worse prognosis.
      b. **Adenoid cystic carcinoma (cylindroma).** These tumors fall into 3 histologic patterns: tubular (most favorable), cribriform (intermediate), and solid (least favorable).
      c. **Malignant mixed tumor.** These neoplasms occur de novo or arise in a previously benign mixed tumor (approximately 2–5% of all mixed tumors undergo malignant transformation) and are highly aggressive. The appearance of this tumor is similar to those that occur in other tissues. The lack of mucin differentiates it from a high-grade mucoepidermoid carcinoma.
      d. **Adenocarcinoma.** The adenocarcinoma is a heterogeneous group of neoplasms, including mucinous adenocarcinoma, salivary duct carcinoma, and intercalated duct carcinoma.
      e. **Undifferentiated carcinomas.** These neoplasms are divided into large- and small-cell types.

   3. **Lymphoma.** Primary lymphoma of the salivary glands occurs most commonly in the parotid gland and its frequency is increasing in AIDS patients.

D. **Metastatic spread.** Metastases are identified in 33% of patients and are more common in patients with high grade malignancies and facial nerve paralysis (60% incidence of metastases).

   1. **Modes of spread.** Salivary carcinomas spread via one or more of the following mechanisms.
      a. **Direct extension.** Salivary neoplasms frequently grow into adjacent normal tissues, including the facial nerve, mandible, oral cavity, and palate. Adenoid cystic carcinomas may spread for long distances along nerves.
      b. **Lymphatic metastasis.** The rate of regional lymph node metastasis varies with the location of the cancer (see Table 25–4). Intraparotid, infra-auricular, preauricular, and deep cervical lymph nodes are most commonly involved with parotid tumors. The rate of lymph node metastasis among patients with

TABLE 25–3. INCIDENCE OF SALIVARY MALIGNANCIES BY GLAND AND HISTOLOGIC TYPE

Histologic Type	Parotid Gland (%)	Submandibular Gland (%)	Sublingual and Minor Glands (%)	All Glands (%)
Mucoepidermoid carcinoma	50	30	25	34
Adenoid cystic carcinoma	7	36	35	22
Carcinoma expleomorphic adenoma	18	19	6	12
Adenocarcinoma	10	16	29	17
Acinic cell carcinoma	12	2	1	5
Squamous cell carcinoma	3	6	< 1	4
Undifferentiated carinoma	1	< 1	4	3

TABLE 25–4. INCIDENCE OF LYMPH NODE METASTASES BY SALIVARY GLAND LOCATION

Gland	At Presentation (%)	At Autopsy (%)
Parotid	20	25
Submandibular	33	37
Sublingual and minor	13	22

parotid carcinoma varies with histologic appearance (see Table 25–5). Submandibular malignancies often spread to the submandibular, upper cervical, submental, and deep cervical lymph nodes. Overall, 20–25% of patients present with lymph node metastases.

    c. Hamatogenous metastasis. Metastatic spread through blood vessels is uncommon.

  2. Sites of spread. The most common distant metastatic sites include the following organs: lymph nodes (20–25%), lung (most frequent), bone, and liver.

VIII. Staging. The American Joint Committee on Cancer and the Union Internationale Contre le Cancer recently proposed a joint TNM staging system.

  A. Tumor stage

    1. TX. Primary tumor cannot be assessed.

    2. T0. No clinical evidence of primary tumor.

    3. T1. Tumor no larger than 2 cm in size.

    4. T2. Tumor larger than 2 cm but no larger than 4 cm in size.

    5. T3. Tumor larger than 4 cm but no larger than 6 cm in size.

    6. T4. Tumor larger than 6 cm in size.

      Note: All tumor categories are further subdivided in either "a" (no local extension) or "b" (local extension present). Local extension is defined as clinical or macroscopic involvement of skin, soft tissues, bone, or nerves.

  B. Lymph node stage

    1. NX. Regional lymph nodes cannot be assessed.

    2. N0. No regional lymph node metastasis are present.

    3. N1. Metastasis in a single ipsilateral lymph node no larger than 3 cm in size.

    4. N2. Metastases in a single ipsilateral lymph node larger than 3 cm but no larger than 6 cm in size, or in multiple ipsilateral lymph nodes no larger than 6 cm in size, or in bilateral or contralateral lymph nodes no larger than 6 cm in size.

      a. N2a. Metastasis in a single ipsilateral lymph node larger than 3 cm but no larger than 6 cm in size.

      b. N2b. Metastases in multiple ipsilateral lymph nodes no larger than 6 cm in size.

      c. N2c. Metastases in bilateral or contralateral lymph nodes no larger than 6 cm in size.

    5. N3. Metastases in lymph nodes larger than 6 cm in size.

  C. Metastatic stage

TABLE 25–5. INCIDENCE OF REGIONAL LYMPH NODE AND DISTANT METASTASES

Histologic Type	Lymph Node Metastases (Occult) (%)	Distant Metastases (%)
Mucoepidermoid carcinoma (high grade)	44 (16)	8
Acinic cell carcinoma	13 (0)	14
Adenoid cystic carcinoma	5 (0)	42
Adenocarcinoma	26 (9)	27
Carcinoma ex-pleomorphic adenoma	21 (0)	21
Squamous cell carcinoma	37 (40)	15
Undifferentiated carcinoma	23 (—)	36

      1. **MX.** Metastases cannot be assessed.
      2. **M0.** No evidence of distant metastases is present.
      3. **M1.** Distant metastases are present.
  D. Histopathologic grade
      1. **GX.** Grade cannot be assessed.
      2. **G1.** Well differentiated.
      3. **G2.** Moderately well differentiated.
      4. **G3.** Poorly differentiated.
      5. **G4.** Undifferentiated.
  E. Stage groupings
      1. **Stage I.** T1–2a, N0, M0.
      2. **Stage II.** T1–2b or T3a, N0, M0.
      3. **Stage III.** T3b or T4a, N0, M0; any T except T4b, N1, M0.
      4. **Stage IV.** T4b, any N, M0; any T, N2–3, M0; any T, any N, M1.
IX. Treatment
  A. Surgery
    1. Primary salivary carcinoma
      a. Indications. Surgery remains the preferred treatment for essentially all neoplasms of the salivary glands.
      b. Approaches. Most parotid neoplasms are approached through a vertical incision in the preauricular skin crease that extends inferiorly into the upper neck, although tumors in the deep lobe (parapharyngeal space) also can be attacked through either a submandibular approach or a mandibular osteotomy (midline or ramus). Submandibular neoplasms are removed through an incision parallel with and 3 cm below the mandible.
      c. Procedures. The type of procedure required depends on the site of the tumor.
        (1) Parotid malignancies
          (a) Parotidectomy. After the initial skin incision is made and skin flaps (anterior and posterior) are raised, the greater auricular nerve is identified and divided. The parotid is separated from the sternocleidomastoid and digastric muscles as well as the external auditory canal. After identifying the facial nerve in the tympanomastoid sulcus, the superficial gland is meticulously dissected along each branch of the nerve. For low-grade T1 and T2 neoplasms (mucoepidermoid and acinic cell carcinoma), removal of the superficial gland (superficial parotidectomy) is all that is required. For high-grade T1 and T2 malignancies and tumors extending into the deep gland, resection of the superficial and deep lobes (total parotidectomy), with or without the facial nerve [see **IX.A.1.c.(i),(b), below**], is necessary. In addition, extension beyond the parotid capsule and invasion of contiguous structures (mandible, zygoma, temporal bone, and masseter muscle) may mandate removal of these involved tissues.
          (b) Facial nerve resection. Usually, the facial nerve is identified at the stylomastoid foramen in the tympanomastoid sulcus. Occasionally, however, the nerve cannot be identified in this location and must be approached alternatively from within the temporal bone or traced back retrograde from a distal branch. Traditionally, facial nerve resection (with immediate reconstruction) was mandatory for all high-grade salivary malignancies. Recent data, however, indicates that in the absence of clinical or histologic involvement, the nerve can be preserved without adversely affecting survival. If the nerve is invaded, the involved segment is resected until clear margins are obtained, as determined by immediate frozen section pathologic examination. Then, immediate reconstruction is achieved [see p 176, **IX.A.1.d.(i)**].
          (c) Temporal bone resection. If invasion of the facial nerve extends to the stylomastoid foramen, the mastoid bone itself should be removed until pathologic clear margins are obtained. This may entail lateral or complete temporal bone resection.
        (2) Submandibular malignancies. This procedure excises the entire submandibular gland and possibly involved adjacent structures such as the digastric and mylohyoid muscles, hypoglossal and lingual nerves, mandible, and the floor of the mouth. Initially, an incision is

made in a skin crease 3 cm below the mandible. Skin flaps deep to the platysma muscles are then raised, and the mandibular branch of the facial nerve is identified and preserved, dividing the posterior facial vein. After preliminary mobilization of the gland, the facial artery and vein are divided. Next, the submandibular ganglion and Wharton's duct are sequentially ligated, and the submandibular gland is removed, carefully preserving the lingual and hypoglossal nerves.

(3) Sublingual and minor salivary gland malignancies. The extent of resection for these neoplasms depends on the size, histologic type, and location. Every effort must be made to confirm the diagnosis before instituting definitive surgical therapy. The basic surgical oncology tenet of wide excision should be faithfully observed during all procedures.

(4) Radical neck dissection. A standard radical neck dissection excises all cervical lymph nodes, sternocleidomastoid muscle, jugular vein, submandibular gland, and spinal accessory nerve. However, a modified radical neck dissection preserves one or more of these structures. Therapeutic neck dissection is indicated for all patients with clinically palpable cervical lymph nodes, whereas prophylactic lymph node dissection may be beneficial for those with advanced stage, high-grade squamous cell carcinoma, mucoepidermoid carcinoma, adenocarcinoma, anaplastic carcinoma, and malignant mixed tumors, even in the absence of clinically palpable nodes. Although the exact indications for neck dissection remain controversial, regional control is highly desirable even in the presence of documented distant metastases because uncontrolled regional disease is responsible for a major portion of the morbidity and mortality of this disease.

d. Reconstruction

(1) Facial nerve. Immediate reconstruction with a primary anastomosis or a sensory nerve conduit (greater auricular or sural nerve) is preferred. In unusual circumstances, a hypoglossal- or facial-facial nerve crossover may be necessary. Partial or complete recovery generally occurs in 6–12 months and is unaffected by postoperative radiation. Muscle tone is normally good, although some motor synkinesis is expected. Corneal protection must be provided with lubricants, tape on the eyelids at night, gold weights or springs on the upper eyelid for adequate closure, and tarsorrhapy as necessary. Furthermore, static or dynamic muscle slings, unilateral rhytidectomy, and forehead lifts may be required.

(2) Soft tissues. Tumor resections that include removal of large, functionally important blocks of soft tissue and bone often require complex individualized reconstructions using bone grafts, dental or prosthetic appliances, myocutaneous flaps, and skin grafts.

2. Locally advanced and metastatic salivary carcinoma. Pulmonary metastases from adenoid cystic carcinoma typically present after long disease-free intervals (up to 10 years) and progress extremely slowly. Thoracotomy and resection of these metastatic lesions is recommended.

3. Mortality and morbidity. The complications of salivary gland procedures include the following problems:

a. Hemorrhage (4%, including wound hematomas).

b. Infection.

c. Scar.

d. Poor cosmetic result.

e. Weakness or pain of the shoulder (loss of cranial nerve XI function).

f. Skin flap necrosis.

g. Chylous fistula.

h. Cranial nerve dysfunction (15%, particularly temporary VII nerve palsy).

i. Salivary fistulae (2%, usually closes spontaneously).

j. Gustatory sweating (Frey's syndrome) (1–59%, characterized by sweating in the area of distribution of the auriculotemporal nerve in response to sialogogues) usually minor and self-limiting.

B. Radiation therapy. The major role of radiation therapy in the treatment of salivary gland tumors is adjunctive to surgery in the form of postoperative irradiation.

1. Primary salivary carcinoma. Patients with inoperable lesions, those with resectable lesions but medical contraindications to surgery, and those who refuse surgery should be considered for curative primary radiation. With conventional radiation therapy (5000 cGy over 7 weeks) local or regional control is achieved in 25–33% of patients. With fast neutrons, up to 67% of patients are cured locally; however, few long-term cures have been reported because of distant metastases.

2. **Adjuvant radiotherapy**
   a. **Preoperative radiation.** Patients with large, unresectable neoplasms may undergo preoperative radiation therapy to reduce tumor mass and increase resectability.
   b. **Intraoperative radiation.** Currently, no data are available to support intraoperative radiation therapy of salivary carcinomas.
   c. **Postoperative radiation.** Several nonrandomized studies support the use of postoperative radiotherapy (5000 cGy over 6 weeks) to decrease the risk of recurrence (9%, compared with 30% without radiotherapy), to increase facial nerve preservation, and, possibly, to increase overall survival. Although conventional therapy is most widely used, interstitial implantation also can be used. Indications for postoperative irradiation include the following:
      (1) **Advanced stage** (Stage III and IV).
      (2) **High grade lesions.**
      (3) **Responsive histology** (mucoepidermoid carcinoma, acinic cell carcinoma, and adenoid cystic carcinoma).
      (4) **Recurrent, bulky, or fixed tumors.**
      (5) **Minimal or positive surgical margins.**
      (6) **Perineural invasion.**
      (7) **Regional cervical lymph node metastases.**
      (8) **Lesions of the deep parotid gland.**
      (9) **Proximity to facial nerve.**
      (10) **Paranasal sinus minor salivary gland tumors.**
3. **Locally advanced and metastatic salivary cancer.** Radiation therapy (5000 cGy over 7 weeks) for inoperable salivary gland tumors provides local control in 25–33% of patients. Metastatic disease, in general is not amenable to radiation therapy.
4. **Mortality and morbidity.** Although facial nerve grafts are not compromised with postoperative radiation, complications do occur. Careful exclusion of the eyes and opposite salivary glands from the field of therapy minimizes the risks, which include the following: xerostomia, trismus, otitis media, alopecia, osteoradionecrosis of the mandible (5%), dental complications, skin changes, loss of taste, mucositis, and hypothyroidism, (1% overt and 10% chemical disease).

C. **Chemotherapy**
   1. **Primary salivary carcinoma.** Chemotherapy has not proved to be effective in this setting and is not indicated.
   2. **Adjuvant chemotherapy.** The high incidence of distant salivary gland metastases (higher than that seen in squamous cell carcinoma of the head and neck) suggests the need for adjuvant chemotherapy to decrease the chance of failure at distant sites. At present, little experience is available in this area.
   3. **Locally advanced and metastatic salivary cancer.** Overall, palliative chemotherapy produces response rates of 10% (complete) and 32% (partial). Fifty-eight percent of patients will have no response. Adenocarcinoma, adenoid cystic carcinoma, carcinoma ex-pleomorphic adenoma, and acinic cell respond best to doxorubicin, cisplatin, and fluorouracil. Squamous cell carcinoma and mucoepidermoid carcinoma respond best to methotrexate and cisplatin. Other regimens with 50% response rates include cyclophosphamide combined with doxorubicin as well as cyclophosphamide combined with doxorubicin and cisplatin (squamous cell carcinoma).

X. **Immunotherapy.** This area awaits experimental findings.
XI. **Prognosis**
   A. **Risk of recurrence.** The risk of tumor recurrence depends on the histologic type of malignancy, the extent of surgical resection, as well as the adjuvant therapy administered. Malignant mixed tumors have a recurrence rate of 40–70% after surgery alone.
   B. **Five-year survival.** The paucity of these neoplasms has produced variability in published incidence and survival figures; however a general summary of survival data is included in Tables 25–6 and 25–7. Because of the addition of adjuvant radiotherapy, survival rates recently have nearly doubled. The overall 10-year survival by disease stage is as follows: Stage I (90%), Stage II (65%), Stage III–IV (22%).

TABLE 25–6. TEN-YEAR SURVIVAL RATES BY HISTOLOGIC TYPE AND RISK FACTOR

Factors	Mucoepidermoid (%)	Adenoid Cystic (%)	Acinic Cell (%)	Malignant Mixed (%)
Tumor size				
T1	97	47	68	36
T2	83	11	68	—
T3	28	21	—	13
Nodal status				
Negative	80	32	99	30
Positive	20	22	44	10
Histologic grade				
Low	66	70	71	—
Intermediate	—	51	—	—
High	36	12	33	—
Surgical margins				
Negative	43	8	37	—
Positive	97	34	86	—
Site				
Parotid	64	77	61	26
Submandibular	45	29	—	20

C. **Adverse prognostic factors.** The following characteristics are associated with a poor outcome: advanced stage, large tumor size, high-grade histology, tumor ulceration or fixation, facial nerve involvement, lymph node and distant metastasis, and advanced age.

XII. **Patient follow-up**

   A. **General guidelines.** Salivary gland tumors frequently exhibit a prolonged disease course. Patients with these tumors should be followed every 3 months for 2 years, every 6 months for an additional 3 years, and then annually for evidence of tumor recurrence. Specific guidelines for patients with salivary gland malignancies are listed below.

   B. **Routine evaluation.** The following examinations should be included with each clinic visit:

   1. **Medical history and physical examination.** An interval medical history and a thorough physical examination is essential to every office visit. Particular attention should be directed to those areas outlined above (see p 171, **VI.A**).

   2. **Blood tests** (see p 1, **IV.A**)
      a. **Complete blood count.**
      b. **Hepatic transaminases.**
      c. **Alkaline phosphatase.**

   3. **Chest x-ray** (see p 3, **IV.C.1**).

   C. **Optional evaluation.** The following tests and procedures may be indicated by previous diagnostic findings or clinical suspicion.

   1. **Blood tests** (see p 1, **IV.A**)
      a. **Nucleotidase.**
      b. **GGTP.**

   2. **Imaging Studies** (see p 3, **IV.C**)

TABLE 25–7. FIVE-, 10-, AND 20-YEAR SURVIVAL FOR ADENOID CYSTIC CARCINOMA

Histologic Grade	5-Year Survival (%)	10-Year Survival (%)	20-Year Survival (%)
Low grade (tubular pattern)	92	78	40
Intermediate grade (cribiform pattern)	78	51	18
High grade (solid pattern)	25	12	5

a. **Computed tomography.** A CT scan can be useful in evaluating recurrent cervical masses.
b. **Magnetic resonance imaging.** Like CT scans, MRI scans can be instrumental for assessing patients who have recurrent neck masses.
c. **Technetium-99m bone scan.**
3. **Invasive procedures.** Fine needle aspiration may provide essential information about the nature of recurrent neck masses. This procedure is particularly helpful in the hands of experienced cytopathologists armed with pathologic material obtained from previous surgical procedures.

REFERENCES

Bardwill JM et al: Report of one hundred tumors of the minor salivary glands. *Am J Surg* 1966;**112**:493–497.

Batsakis J: Salivary tumors. In: Batsakis J (editor), *Tumors of the head and neck: clinical and pathological considerations.* 2nd ed. Baltimore, MD: Williams and Wilkins; 1979:1–99.

Beahrs OH, Woods JE, Weland CH. Surgical management of parotid tumors. *Adv Surg* 1978;**12**:301–311.

Conley J, Hamaker RC: Prognosis of malignant tumors of the parotid gland with facial nerve paralysis. *Arch Otolaryngol* 1975;**101**:39–45.

Conley J, Tinsley PP: Treatment and prognosis of mucoepidermoid carcinoma in the pediatric age group. *Arch Otolaryngol* 1985;**111**:322–324.

Elkon D et al: Radiation therapy in the treatment of malignant salivary gland tumors. *Cancer* 1978;**41**:502–509.

Eneroth CM: Facial nerve paralysis: a criterion of malignancy in parotid tumors. *Arch Otolaryngol* 1972;**95**:300–311.

Friedman M et al: Malignant tumors of the major salivary glands. *Otolaryngol Clin North Am* 1986;**19**:625–636.

Jenkins JR et al: Minor salivary gland tumors: the role of radiotherapy. *Am J Otolaryngol* 1989;**10**:250–256.

Matsuba HM et al: High-grade malignancies of the parotid gland: effective use of planned combination surgery and irradiation. *Laryngoscope* 1985;**95**:1059–1063.

McKenna RJ: Tumors of the major and minor salivary glands. *CA-A Cancer J Clin* 1984;**34**:24–39.

Million RR, Cassisi NJ (editors): *Management of Head and Neck Cancer: A Multidisciplinary Approach.* Philadelphia, PA: JB Lippincott; 1984:1139–1150.

Posner MR et al: Chemotherapy of advanced salivary gland neoplasms. *Cancer* 1982;**50**:2261–2264.

Rentschler R, Burgess MA, Byers R: Chemotherapy of malignant salivary gland neoplasms. *Cancer* 1977;**40**:619–624.

Rice DH, Hemenway WG, Canalis RF: Malignant neoplasms of the salivary glands. In: English GM (editor), *Otolaryngology.* Philadelphia, PA: JB Lippincott; 1989.

Sener SF, Scanlon EF: Irradiation-induced salivary gland neoplasms. *Ann Surg* 1980;**138**:46–53.

Shah JP, Ihde JK: Salivary gland tumors. *Curr Prob Surg* 1990;**27**:775–883.

Shidnia et al: Carcinoma of major salivary glands. *Cancer* 1980;**45**:693–699.

Simpson JR, Thawley SE, Matsuba HM: Adenoid cystic salivary gland carcinoma: treatment with irradiation and surgery. *Radiology* 1984;**151**:509–512.

Sismanis A et al: Diagnosis of salivary gland tumors by fine needle aspiration biopsy. *Head Neck Surg* 1981;**3**:482–489.

Suen JY, Johns ME: Chemotherapy for salivary gland cancer. *Laryngoscope* 1982;**92**:235–239.

Tapley H, Guillamordequi OM, Byers RM: The place of irradiation in the treatment of malignant tumors of the salivary glands. *Curr Probl Cancer* 1976;**1**:13–30.

Tu B et al: The superiority of combined therapy (surgery and postoperative irradiation) in parotid cancer. *Arch Otolaryngol* 1982;**108**:710–713.

26 Malignancies of Undetermined Head & Neck Primary Site

James J. Bredenkamp, MD, and Matthew J. Lando, MD

I. **Epidemiology.** Head and neck malignancies of undetermined primary site (occult cancers) account for **5% of all metastatic squamous cell carcinomas** of the head and neck. Often, the primary neoplasm either regressed spontaneously or is too small to be identified, despite a thorough search.

II. **Risk factors.** The risk of occult head and neck primary malignancies, in general, reflects the overall risk of head and neck neoplasms with known primary site (see Chpts 23, 24, and 25).

III. **Presentation**
   A. **Signs and symptoms**
      1. **Local manifestations.** Patients most often complain of a solitary, unilateral, mobile (or predominantly mobile) neck mass (70-84%). This finding occurs in 25%, 23%, and 47% of patients with known oropharyngeal, thyroid, and nasopharyngeal carcinoma, respectively. In addition, multiple ipsilateral and bilateral lymph nodes are each present in 10% of patients. Although any lymph node group may be affected, the upper jugular nodes are most commonly involved, followed by the midjugular and supraclavicular chains. Furthermore, supraclavicular, lower jugular, and lower posterior triangle neck masses most commonly represent metastatic disease originating below the clavicle.
      2. **Systemic manifestations.** Weight loss, fever, night sweats, malaise, anorexia, and manifestations of impaired cellular immunity are common.
   B. **Paraneoplastic syndromes.** No known paraneoplastic syndromes are associated with occult head and neck neoplasms.

IV. **Differential diagnosis.** A multitude of benign (including congenital and inflammatory) as well as malignant processes may present as a solitary neck mass (see Table 26–1).

V. **Screening.** Due to the rare nature of these neoplasms, screening of the general population is not practical. Patients with known head and neck cancers, however, must be screened carefully for synchronous second primaries which occur in up to 10% of patients.

VI. **Diagnostic workup**
   A. **Medical history and physical examination.** A thorough medical history (emphasizing risk factors) and a complete (often repeated) head and neck examination, including inspection, palpation, and fiberoptic endoscopy, identifies the location of the primary head and neck malignancy in 85-90% of patients (see Figure 26–1).
      1. **General appearance.** The functional status of the patient as well as the ability to tolerate diagnostic procedures and therapy may be quickly assessed by his/her general appearance. This is particularly important since alcohol and tobacco abuse is prevalent in these patients.
      2. **Head.** The size, position, and mobility of all masses must be documented. Careful inspection and palpation of the lip, oral cavity (buccal and gingival mucosa, tongue, posterior trigone, and floor of mouth), pharynx, and larynx should be included.
      3. **Neck.** All masses should be fully described.
      4. **Chest.** On occasion, wheezing, decreased breath sounds, etc. may indicate the presence of a primary lung cancer or pulmonary metastases.
      5. **Abdomen.** Hepatomegaly and masses are important findings.
   B. **Primary tests and procedures.** The following tests and procedures should be performed on all patients with suspected salivary gland malignancies.
      1. **Blood tests**
         a. **Complete blood count.** (see p 1, **IV.A.1**).
         b. **Hepatic transaminases.** (see p 1, **IV.A.2**).
         c. **Alkaline phosphatase.** (see p 1, **IV.A.3**).

TABLE 26-1. DIFFERENTIAL DIAGNOSIS OF CERVICAL MASSES

Inflammatory
    Odontogenic abscesses
    Cervical lymphadenitis
        Bacterial
        Granulomatous: tuberculosis, actinomycosis, sarcoidosis
        Viral: Infectious mononucleosis
Congenital
    Thyroglossal duct cyst
    Branchial cleft cysts
Neoplasms
    Benign
        Vascular; hemangioma, lymphangioma, arteriovenous malformation, aneurysms
        Chemodectomas: glomus tumors, carotid body tumors
        Neural tumors: neurofibroma, schwannoma
        Miscellaneous: lipoma, fibroma, teratoma
    Malignant
        Primary: lymphoma, sarcoma, thyroid, salivary gland, branchial cleft and thyroglossal duct cyst carcinomas
    Metastatic
        Supraclivicular: mucosal, skin, salivary gland, thyroid
        Infraclavicular: lung, kidney, prostate, germ cell, gastrointestinal, breast
Miscellaneous
    Zenker's diverticulum
    External laryngocele
    Amyloidosis
Normal structures
    Hyoid bone
    Carotid bulb
    Transverse vertebral process

---

      d. Calcium. The serum level of this cation may be elevated due to tumor production of parathormone-like substances.
  2. Imaging studies.
    a. Chest X-ray. (see p 3, **IV.C.1**).
    b. Magnetic Resonance Imaging (MRI). (see p 3, **IV.C.1**).
  3. Invasive procedures
    A. Endoscopy. Diagnostic evaluation should include an exhaustive examination under general anesthesia, including nasopharyngoscopy and "triple" endoscopy (direct laryngoscopy, esophagoscopy, and bronchoscopy). Directed or random biopsies should be obtained, and tonsillectomy should be considered. In addition to locating primary lesions, panendoscopy identifies 50% of **second primary neoplasms.**
    B. Diagnostic biopsy. If noninvasive evaluation fails to locate a primary malignancy, diagnostic material should be obtained from the presumed metastatic focus by either fine needle aspiration or excisional biopsy.
      (1) Fine-needle aspiration (FNA). FNA is a safe technique with an accuracy of 80-96% and a false positive and negative rate of 0-0.7% and 2.1-12%, respectively. In certain circumstances, CT or MRI guidance may enhanced its utility; however, if the diagnosis is inconclusive or seemingly inappropriate, it should be repeated or disregarded.
      (2) Excisional biopsy. An excisional biopsy is required in 5% of patients (incisional and core needle biopsies of neck masses are avoided) and should be performed only after all alternative diagnostic methods have been exhausted since this type of biopsy increases the incidence of local recurrence and distant metastases and reduces patient survival. The skin incision must be planned with the definitive surgical procedure in mind, and immediate surgical intervention may be indicated.

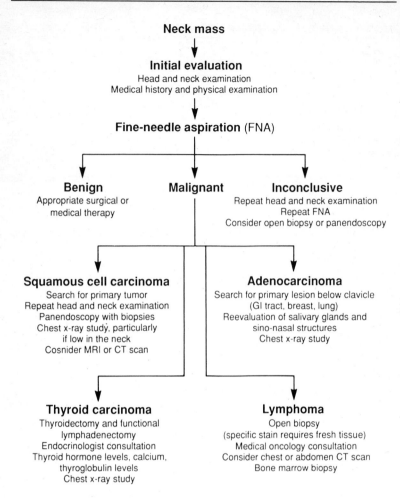

Figure 26–1. Algorithm for the evaluation of neck masses.

C. **Optional tests and procedures.** The following examinations may be indicated by prior diagnostic tests or clinical suspicion.
   1. **Blood tests**
      a. **5′nucleotidase.** (see p 2, **IV.A.4**).
      b. **GGTP.** (see p 2, **IV.A.5**).
      c. **Albumin.** (see p 3, **IV.A.7**).
      d. **Epstein-Barr virus (EBV) antibody titers.** The levels of anti-EBV antibodies are frequently increased in patients with undifferentiated and non-keratinizing nasopharyngeal carcinoma.
   2. **Imaging studies**
      a. **Plain radiographs.** Plain radiographs of the neck are of limited value.
      b. **Computed tomography (CT).** CT may be useful in evaluating areas of possible metastatic disease. (see also p 3, **IV.C.2**)
      c. **Barium swallow esophagram.** This radiographic test is indicated in patients with swallowing symptoms.

      d. Ultrasonography. B-mode ultrasonography may be helpful in identifying occult metastasis and carotid involvement (see also p 3, **IV.C.4**).

      e. Thyroid scan. This nuclear scan may be helpful in the evaluation of masses with a position or biopsy suggesting thyroid cancer.

      f. Bone scan. (see also p 3, **IV.C.5**).

VII. Pathology

  A. Location. The site-specific incidence of cervical metastasis from various head and neck primary (squamous cell) cancers is summarized in Table 26–2. The nasopharynx, base of tongue, tonsillar area, and pyriform sinus are the most common sites of occult primary lesions. In addition, the location of the adenopathy frequently correlates with the location of the occult primary lesion (see Table 26–3). Of tumors identified following definitive therapy, **67% originate above the clavicle** and 33% of these arise from the naso- and oropharynx, 33% emanate from the tonsil and base of tongue, and 20% start in the hypopharynx. Nearly **50% of infraclavicular neoplasms begin in the lung** with the remainder divided equally between the gastrointestinal tract, breast, prostate, ovary, bladder, and kidney.

  B. Multiplicity. Synchronous (those identified within 6 months) second primary neoplasms (lung, esophagus, hypopharynx, etc.) occur in 10% of patients, while **metachronous** tumors (those found after 6 months) arise in 20%.

  C. Histology. Table 26–4 outlines the site-specific incidence of the different histologies.

    1. Squamous cell carcinoma (most common). Metastatic cervical squamous cell carcinoma arises from head and neck primary sites in 90% of patients.

    2. Adenocarcinoma (non-thyroid). Most commonly found in the supraclavicular fossa, adenocarcinoma often represents an **infraclavicular neoplasm** (lung, breast, gastric, prostate, pancreas, ovary, etc.) but occasionally originates from the ethmoid sinuses or salivary glands.

    3. Thyroid carcinoma. Cervical metastases are the initial manifestation in up to 60% of patients with papillary thyroid carcinoma.

    4. Lymphoma. Hodgkin's disease will present with a **cervical mass** in 70-80% of cases, while non-Hodgkin's lymphoma will present as a cervical mass in 30-70% of cases.

    5. Undifferentiated carcinoma. This histology usually arises from the nasopharynx.

  D. Metastatic spread

    1. Modes of spread. Since the primary lesion cannot be determined in cases of occult head and neck malignancies and the initial manifestation is that of metastatic disease, the specific avenues of spread cannot be discussed but most commonly include lymphatic and hematogenous metastasis.

    2. Sites of spread. Distant metastasis from a head and neck primary are most likely to be found in the **lung and liver**. Nasopharyngeal carcinoma most commonly metastasizes to bone.

VIII. Staging. For head and neck malignancies of undetermined primary site, the American

TABLE 26–2. SITE-SPECIFIC INCIDENCE OF HEAD AND NECK MALIGNANCIES BY SITE OF PRESENTING ADENOPATHY [1]

Involved Lymph Nodes	OC	OP	HP	NP	LX	THY	Lung	OS	OI
Submandibular	71%	22%	0%	2%	3%	0%	0%	2%	0%
High jugular	22%	23%	15%	12%	9%	9%	<1%	11%	0%
Mid jugular	13%	38%	21%	7%	13%	11%	<1%	<1%	0%
Low jugular	8%	14%	25%	12%	13%	27%	1%	<1%	0%
Supraclavicular	1%	4%	4%	0%	4%	23%	40%	4%	30%
High posterior	0%	30%	12%	55%	2%	3%	0%	0%	0%
Low posterior	3%	19%	25%	24%	8%	17%	3%	0%	2%

[1]OC, oral cavity; OP, oropharynx; HP, hypopharynx; NP, nasopharynx; LX, larynx; THY, thyroid; OS, other supraclavicular sites; OI, other infraclavicular sites. (Data from Lindberg R. Distribution of cervical lymph node metastases from squamous cell carcinoma of the upper respiratory and digestive tracts. Cancer 229:1446, 1972.)

TABLE 26–3. SITE OF ORIGIN BASED ON LOCATION OF METASTATIC DISEASE

Involved Nodes	Probable Site of Origin
Submandibular	Skin of the upper face, scalp, and temple
Submental	Skin of the lateral face, anterior tongue, floor of mouth
Preauricular	Anterior floor of mouth, lip
Jugular-digastric	Posterior third and lateral tongue, palate, middle and posterior thirds of the floor of mouth, tonsils
Midjugular	Posterior and lateral pharyngeal wall, pyriform sinus, thyroid, supra-glottic larynx
Low jugular	Thyroid, cervical esophagus, lung, breast, stomach, kidney, prostate, pancreas
Posterior	Nasopharynx, thyroid
Scalene/supraclavicular	Lung, breast, stomach, kidney, prostate, pancreas

Joint Committee on Cancer (AJCC) and Union Internationale Contre le Cancer (UICC) joint TNM staging system assigns stage based on nodal and metastatic status.

A. Tumor stage. Tumor stage, by definition, is TX (primary tumor cannot be assessed.)

B. Lymph node stage
1. **NX** Regional lymph nodes cannot be assessed.
2. **N0** No regional lymph node metastasis are present.
3. **N1** Metastasis in a single ipsilateral lymph node <3 cm in size is present.
4. **N2** Metastases in a single ipsilateral lymph node >3 cm but <6 cm in size, or in multiple ipsilateral lymph nodes <6 cm in size, or in bilateral or contralateral lymph nodes <6 cm in size are present.
   a. **N2a** Metastasis in a single ipsilateral lymph node >3 cm but <6 cm in size is present.
   b. **N2b** Metastases in multiple ipsilateral lymph nodes <6 cm in size are present.
   c. **N2c** Metastases in bilateral or contralateral lymph nodes <6 cm in size are present.
5. **N3** Metastases in lymph node(s) >6 cm in size are present.

C. Metastatic stage
1. **MX** Metastases cannot be assessed.
2. **M0** No evidence of distant metastases is present.
3. **M1** Distant metastases are present.

D. Histopathologic grade
1. **GX** Grade cannot be assessed.
2. **G1** Well differentiated.
3. **G2** Moderately well differentiated.
4. **G3** Poorly differentiated.
5. **G4** Undifferentiated.

E. Stage groupings
1. **Stage I:** T1-2a, N0, M0.

TABLE 26–4. RELATIVE INCIDENCE OF VARIOUS HISTOLOGIES (EXCLUDING LYMPHOMA)

Histology	Supraclavicular	Infraclavicular
Squamous cell carcinoma	47%	9%
Adenocarcinoma	2%	17%
Undifferentiated carcinoma	14%	8%
Thyroid carcinoma	2%	2%
Total	67%	33%

  2. Stage II: T1-2b or T3a, N0, M0.
  3. Stage III: T3b or T4a, N0, M0; Any T except T4b, N1, M0.
  4. Stage IV: T4b, any N, M0; Any T, N2-3, M0; Any T, Any N, M1.
IX. **Treatment**
  A. **Surgery**
    1. **Primary head and neck carcinoma.** If a primary tumor is identified, surgical therapy is determined by the histologic type, location, and stage of the primary lesion (see Chpts 23, 24, and 25).
    2. **Locally advanced and metastatic head and neck cancer**
      a. **Indications.** Although surgery is indicated for any undiagnosed, suspicious neck mass, the surgical treatment of cervical lymph node metastases from occult head and neck malignancies is controversial. Most neck masses <3 cm (N1 disease) may be treated by either **surgery or radiation** with similar results. If surgery is employed, postoperative cervical radiation (including the neck and potential primary sites) generally is employed. Neck masses 3 cm or greater (N2 and N3 disease) may be treated with **surgery, radiation, or chemotherapy** alone or with combined modality approaches. Persistent resectable disease following radiation and chemotherapy, however, is an indication for salvage lymphadenectomy.
      b. **Approaches.** Cervical lymphadenectomy may be accomplished through a variety of incisions, and although each has advantages and disadvantages, the choice often depends on the personal preference of the surgeon and the presumed primary tumor site.
      c. **Procedures**
        (1) **Excisional biopsy.** Simple excision of a single cervical metastasis albeit occasionally diagnostically useful, is rarely therapeutically helpful.
        (2) **Radical cervical lymphadenectomy.** A standard radical lymphadenectomy removes all cervical lymph nodes and soft tissue from the clavicle to the mandible and skull base, including the sternocleidomastoid muscle, jugular vein, submandibular gland, and the spinal accessory nerve (specific steps involved in a standard radical lymphadenectomy are outlined in Table 26–5). A modified cervical lymphadenectomy preserves at least one of the above normal structures, and a functional lymphadenectomy spares all of them. The advantages and disadvantages of various lymphadenectomies remain controversial.
    3. **Mortality and morbidity.** The complications of cervical lymphadenectomy include the following problems:
      a. **Hemorrhage.**
      b. **Infection.**
      c. **Poor cosmetic result.**
      d. **Skin flap necrosis.**
      e. **Chyle fistula.**
      f. **Cranial nerve dysfunction,** particularly XI with weakness or pain of the shoulder.
  B. **Radiation therapy**
    1. **Primary head and neck carcinomas.** Neck masses <3 cm (N1 disease) may be successfully treated with radiation therapy alone. Although the role of prophylactic irradiation of potential primary sites is controversial, most patients receive radiotherapy to all potential head and neck primary sites.
    2. **Adjuvant radiation therapy**
      a. **Preoperative radiotherapy.** Rarely, large unresectable and fixed neck disease may benefit from preoperative radiation therapy in an attempt to reduce the tumor mass. Treated masses may become smaller, more discrete and ultimately more easily resected.
      b. **Intraoperative radiotherapy.** No data supports the use of intraoperative radiation therapy in the treatment of head and neck malignancies of undetermined primary site.
      c. **Postoperative radiotherapy.** Most patients are treated with postoperative irradiation to both sides of the neck and to the potential primary sites.
    3. **Morbidity and mortality.** In addition to mucositis and loss of taste that may occur during therapy, the following complications may occur and should prompt shielding of the contralateral eye and salivary glands:
      a. **Xerostomia.**
      b. **Trismus.**

TABLE 26–5. SURGICAL TECHNIQUES FOR RADICAL CERVICAL LYMPHADENECTOMY

Incisions

The skin incision (ie Schrobinger, MePhee, utility flap, etc) is based on location of the primary tumor, cosmesis, need for specific surgical exposures, carotid protection, and specific needs of the reconstruction.

Skin flaps

Skin flaps are developed in the subplatysmal plane to the anterior boarder of the trapezius muscle, clavicle, midline neck, and inferior edge of mandible (exposes the tail of the parotid). The facial artery and vein are ligated and the submandibular gland fascia is reflected superiorly to protect the marginal mandibular nerve.

Inferomedial dissection

The sternocleidomastoid (SCM) muscle is transected at its clavicular and sternal heads thus exposing the jugular vein and carotid sheath (with its contents). The omohyoid muscle is resected and the jugular vein doubly ligated at the thoracic inlet. Care is taken not to damage the thoracic trunk, carotid artery, and vagus nerve.

Inferolateral dissection

A plane is developed over the scalene muscle above the deep layer of the deep cervical fascia. The phrenic nerve is identified as it runs obliquely across the anterior scalene muscle deep to this fascia layer. Laterally, the supraclavicular fat pad and its lymphatics are dissected to the anterior border of the trapezius muscle. Multiple transverse cervical vessels are ligated. The brachial plexus is deep to these structures and should not be injured.

Posterior dissection

The dissection is continued along the anterior border of the trapezius muscle up to the level of the SCM muscle. The spinal accessory nerve is cut as it enters the trapezius muscle at the junction of the lower and middle thirds. Superiorly, the SCM muscle is divided near its attachments to the mastoid.

Superomedial dissection

Dissection of the specimen is continued superiorly along the carotid artery. The sensory nerve roots are sacrificed laterally, while the vagus nerve is protected. The submandibular gland and contents of the submandibular and submental spaces are removed, while the hypoglossal nerve is identified at the level of the carotid bifurcation and preserved. The diagastric muscle is preserved in most instances. Often the carotid sinus must be blocked with lidocaine to prevent reflex bradycardia and hypotension.

Superior dissection

The tail of the parotid is resected taking care to stay lateral to the posterior belly of the digastric muscle in order to prevent inadvertent injury to the great vessels and the facial and hypoglossal nerves. The jugular vein is doubly ligated and the spinal accessory nerve transected at the skull base, while the carotid artery and hypoglossal and vagus nerves are preserved.

Optional identification of CN IX

The spinal accessory nerve is most commonly identified along the posterior border of the SCM muscle at the junction of the superior and middle thirds. Alternatively, the nerve can be identified along the anterior boarder of the trapezius muscle or at the jugular foramen. Once the nerve is identified, a nerve hook is utilized to carefully dissect it from the surrounding tissue. Perforating nerve branches to the SCM muscle may be sacrificed.

Closure

After hemostatis is achieved, a chyle leak is excluded by applying positive pressure ventilation. Closure is performed in 2 layers, and pressure dressings and/or suction drains are utilized.

---

       c. **Otitis media.**

       d. **Alopecia.**

       e. **Osteoradionecrosis of the mandible,** 5%.

       f. **Hypothyroidism,** subclinical in 10% and clinical in 1%.

       g. **Dental complications.**

       h. **Skin changes.**

   C. **Chemotherapy**

     1. **Primary head and neck carcinoma.** Chemotherapy as the initial therapy for head and neck cancers of undetermined primary site has not been widely employed and should be used only within approved clinical trials.

     2. **Adjuvant chemotherapy**

       a. **Preoperative chemotherapy.** Chemotherapy given prior to surgery or radiation therapy (neoadjuvant) may be successful in reducing the size of tumors and may extend disease-free intervals. Its effect on long-term survival has yet to be proven.

       b. **Postoperative chemotherapy.** Although early data with "maintenance" chemotherapy appears promising, the utility of chemotherapy following successful surgical resection is unproven and should be reserved for patients with residual disease.

3. **Locally advanced and metastatic head and neck cancer.** Chemotherapy should be considered in patients with residual disease following surgery and radiotherapy; however, the optimal role of chemotherapy in the management of head and neck cancer remains to be defined.

   a. **Single agents.** The most effective agents include **cyclophosphamide, methotrexate, hydroxyurea, and bleomycin** with response rates of 34-40%. Cisplatin, vinblastine, doxorubicin, and carboplatin also are useful, producing objective responses in 24-30% of patients. 5-Fluorouracil (15% response rate), however, is only marginally effective.

   b. **Combination chemotherapy.** Initial combination regimens (most containing bleomycin, methotrexate, and various other drugs) as well as recent combinations of cisplatin and bleomycin, methotrexate, or 5-fluorouracil produce higher response rates (20-67% and 30-60%, respectively) than single agents. Randomized trials comparing these combinations to single agent therapy with cisplatin or methotrexate, however, have failed to demonstrate superior response duration or survival.

4. **Immunotherapy.** Systemic and regional IL-2 administration has been investigated but remains experimental.

X. **Prognosis**

A. **Risk of recurrence.** Within 3 years, 16-30% of patients ultimately manifest a primary lesion; however following radiotherapy, the rate of detection of primary lesions is lower. In those patients whose primary neoplasm is **never identified,** the prognosis is **more favorable.** In addition, patients who continue to abuse tobacco following therapy are more likely to die from a second primary carcinoma than from their original cancer.

B. **5-year survival.** Although 5-year survival statistics vary depending on the definition of "occult" tumors, the intensity of the search for the primary lesion, and the therapy employed, the overall 3-year survival is 33% for patients with squamous cell carcinoma metastatic to cervical lymph nodes.

C. **Adverse prognostic factors.** The 4 most important adverse prognostic factors include the following features:

   1. **Advanced nodal stage.** Large, multiple, bilateral, or fixed nodes are associated with a poor prognosis.

   2. **Supraclavicular site.** Supraclavicular lymph node involvement heralds a 3-12% 3-year survival.

   3. **Adenocarcinoma histology.** Although well differentiated thyroid carcinoma is associated with a good long-term outlook, the prognosis for patients with metastatic adenocarcinoma, in general, is poor.

   4. **Well differentiated tumor.** Excluding thyroid cancer, outcome with well differentiated carcinomas is worse than with poorly differentiated tumors.

XI. **Patient follow-up**

A. **General guidelines.** Patients with head and neck malignancies of undetermined primary site should be followed every month for 1 year, every 2, 3, 4, 6 months for an additional year each, and then annually for evidence of the primary neoplasm or tumor recurrence. Specific guidelines are listed below.

B. **Routine evaluation.** The following examinations should be included with each clinic visit.

   1. **Medical history and physical examination.** An interval medical history, emphasizing weight change, swallowing function, diet, and physical activity, and a thorough physical examination is essential to every office visit. Particular attention should be directed to those areas outlined above (VI,A.).

   2. **Complete blood count.** (see p 1, **IV.A.1**).

   3. **Hepatic transaminases.** (see p 1, **IV.A.2**).

   4. **Alkaline phosphatase.** (see p. 1, **IV.A.3**).

   5. **Calcium.** (see **VI,B,1,d.** above).

   6. **Chest X-ray.** (see p 3, **IV.C.1**).

C. **Optional evaluation.** The following tests and procedures may be indicated by previous diagnostic findings or clinical suspicion.

   1. **5'nucleotidase.** (see p 2, **IV.A.4**).

   2. **GGTP.** (see p 2, **IV.A.5**).

   3. **EBV antibody titers.** (see **VI,C,1,d.** above).

   4. **Magnetic Resonance Imaging (MRI).** (see also **VI,B,2,b.** above).

   5. **Computed tomography (CT).** (see **VI,C,2,b**. above).

6. **Barium swallow esophagram.** (see **VI,C,2,c.** above).
7. **Ultrasound.** B-mode ultrasound examination may be used routinely to detect early tumor recurrence. It also may differentiate tumor from postoperative scar (see also **VI,C,2,d.** above).
8. **Bone scan.** (see p 3, **IV.C.5**).
9. **Biopsy.** Fine needle aspiration (FNA) may provide essential information as to the nature of recurrent neck masses. This procedure, however, requires an experienced cytopathologist.
10. **Endoscopy.** Certain suspicious signs or symptoms (dysphagia, odynophagia, hemoptysis, etc.) may require specific endoscopic examination.

REFERENCES

Abemayor E, Ljung B, Ward PH, et. al: CT-directed fine needle aspiration biopsies of masses in the head and neck. *Laryngoscope* 1985;**95**:1382–1386.

Batsakis J: The pathology of head and neck tumors: The occult primary and metastases to the head and neck. *Head Neck Surg* 1983;**3**(10):409–423.

Batsakis J: *Tumors of the Head and Neck: Clinical and Pathological Considerations*, 2nd ed. Baltimore: Williams & Wilkins, 1979:1–99.

Carlson LS, Fletcher GH, Oswald MJ: Guidelines for radiotherapeutic techniques for cervical metastasis from an unknown primary. *Int J Radiat Oncol Biol Phys* 1986;**12**:2101–2110.

Chang TM: Induction chemotherapy for advanced head and neck cancers: A literature review. *Head Neck Surg* 1988;**10**:150–159.

DeSanto LW, Neel NB: Squamous cell carcinoma metastasis to the neck from an unknown or undiscovered primary. *Otolaryngol Clin N Amer* 1985;**18**:505–513.

Final Report of the Head and Neck Contracts Program: Adjuvant chemotherapy for advanced head and neck squamous carcinoma. *Cancer* 1987;**60**:301–311.

Harper CS, Mendenhall WM, Parsons JT, et. al: Cancer in neck nodes with unknown primary site: Role of mucosal radiotherapy. *Head Neck* 1990;**12**:463–469.

Lindberg R: Distribution of cervical lymph node metastases from squamous cell carcinoma of the upper respiratory and digestive tracts. *Cancer* 1972;**229**:1446–1449.

Lingeman RE, Shellhamer RH: Surgical management of tumors of the neck. In Thawley SE, Panje WR (editors): *Comprehensive Management of Head and Neck Tumors.* Philadelphia: WB Saunders, 1987:1325–1350.

Luna MA: The occult primary and metastatic tumors to and from the head and neck. In Barnes L (editor): *Surgical Pathology of the Head and Neck.* New York: Dekker; 1985:

Million RR, Cassisi NJ: The unknown primary. In *Management of Head and Neck Cancer: A Multidisciplinary Approach.* Philadelphia: JB Lippincott; 1984:231–238.

Nesthofen M: Ultrasound B-scans in the follow-up of head and neck tumors. *Head Neck Surg* 1991;**9**:272–278.

27 Malignancies of the Lung

Robert B. Cameron, MD

I. **Epidemiology.** In the United States, lung cancer is the second most common malignancy in males and third in females, but it is the most frequent cause of cancer-related deaths in both sexes. In 1985, **82.6 cases per 100,000 males and 34.7 cases per 100,000 females** were diagnosed, resulting in 74.0 and 26.4 deaths, respectively. In 1993 estimates indicate that **170,000 new cases** will be diagnosed and **149,000 patients will die,** representing **15% of all new cancer cases** and **28% of all cancer deaths.** In addition, the incidence of lung cancer is increasing slowly in males and rapidly in females: Between 1973 and 1984, it rose 14.3% among males and 81% among females. Between 1984 to 1985, however, the incidence in males actually decreased from 86.4 to 82.6 per 100,000, reflecting the recent decrease in smoking behavior. Worldwide, more than 590,000 people develop lung cancer each year. The incidence in males varies from a high of 108.5 in Scotland to 25.3 per 100,000 in Chile, and the incidence in females ranges from 30.4 in Hong Kong to 5.9 per 100,000 in Switzerland. Other areas of high incidence include Northern Europe (Netherlands, England, Ireland, Austria, West Germany, Denmark, and Poland), the United States, Canada, New Zealand, and Australia. Areas of low incidence include Japan, Norway, Israel, and Sweden.

II. **Risk factors.** Although genetic factors may predispose patients to develop lung carcinoma, environmental exposure to carcinogens (predominantly through cigarette smoke) is responsible for the vast majority of cases.

   A. **Age.** The incidence of lung carcinoma rises rapidly from less than 1 per 100,000 before the age of 30 to a peak of **329.9 per 100,000** between the ages of 70 and 74. The average age at diagnosis is 60 years.

   B. **Sex.** Males are **2.4 times** more likely to develop lung cancer than females, primarily the result of different patterns of cigarette consumption.

   C. **Race.** Blacks are **1.4 times** more likely than whites to develop a lung malignancy.

   D. **Genetic factors**
   1. **Family history.** Although circumstantial, some evidence indicates that first-degree relatives of patients with lung cancer are at **2.4 times** greater risk of developing either lung or some other nonsmoking-related cancer.
   2. **Genetic traits.** Several genetic characteristics found in lung cancer cells may favor the development of lung carcinoma:
      a. **Debrisoquine metabolic phenotype.** High activity of 4-debrisoquine hydroxylase has been implicated in a **10 times greater risk** of lung cancer than are normal "metabolizers." The mechanism for this is unknown.
      b. **Autocrine growth factor production.** In many cases, lung cancer cells (especially small cell) produce growth factors that stimulate growth of the tumor by calcium fluxes and activation of tyrosine kinases. These factors include **insulin-like (IGF)** and **transferrin-like (TGF)** growth factors, but the most important factor is a fetal lung growth protein, **gastrin-releasing peptide (GRP or bombesin).**
      c. **Tumor suppressor genes.** In both lung and renal cell carcinoma, strong data exists that chromosomal deletions in **11p, 13q, 17p,** but especially **3p,** contribute to oncogenesis by eliminating certain gene products such as aminoacylase, thyroid hormone receptor ErbAb, and retinoic acid-receptor-like gene Hap-1.
      d. **Oncogenes.** Nuclear changes that cause constitutive, high-level expression of c-, N-, and L-myc, c-myb, p53, H-ras, N-ras, and K-ras-2 proto-oncogenes may be responsible for gene amplification, rearrangement, and loss of intragenic attenuator signals. In addition, c-raf-1, which exists on the frequently deleted chromosome 3p, has been identified in all types of lung carcinoma.

   E. **Diet.** Diets deficient in **vitamin A** and beta-carotene have been shown to increase

189

the risk of lung cancer in animal models and in humans. The mechanism for the protective effect of vitamin A is unknown. Other potential protective agents include vitamin E and selenium.

F. **Smoking.** Tobacco smoking accounts for **85%** of all lung cancer cases, and the risk of developing lung carcinoma is directly proportional to the amount of tobacco smoked. The effect is greatest for cigarettes, less for cigars, and least for pipe smoking. After the cessation of smoking, the risk declines exponentially beginning 5–6 years after cessation and asymptotically approaching that of nonsmokers after 15 years. In addition, **"passive"** exposure to cigarette smoke increases the risk of lung cancer in nonsmokers **2–3 times** and accounts for **25%** of lung cancer cases in nonsmokers. Recent reductions of tar in cigarettes has not affected lung cancer rates.

G. **Previous pulmonary pathology.** An excessively high risk of lung cancer has been associated with the following benign pulmonary diseases.

1. **Chronic obstructive pulmonary disease (COPD).** Patients with bronchitis and emphysema (COPD) appear to be at a substantial risk of developing lung carcinoma; as many as **8.8%** developing cancer within **10 years.** Many of these are **"scar carcinomas"** with adenocarcinoma histology.

2. **Progressive systemic sclerosis (scleroderma).** Patients with progressive systemic sclerosis are at a significantly increased risk of developing lung cancer, especially **bronchoalveolar carcinoma.**

H. **Radiation**

1. **Radon.** Exposure to radon and its alpha-emitting daughter isotopes has been correlated with a high incidence of lung cancer in uranium miners. Many cases of lung cancer in the general population may be caused by recently discovered high levels of radon in many homes. This is the result of a high radon content in the soil in some areas and decreased ventilation from better insulation and weatherproofing. Although variable, the exposure can exceed that of uranium miners.

2. **Ionizing radiation.** An increased risk of lung carcinoma has been claimed in patients who have received radiation therapy to the thorax.

I. **Urbanization**

1. **Occupational exposure.** Occupations that have been linked to an increased risk of lung cancer are bakers, cooks, construction workers, cosmetologists, leather workers, pitchblende miners, plumbers, printers, pottery workers, rubber workers, shipyard workers, and truck drivers.

a. **Asbestos.** Occupational exposure to asbestos among shipyard workers, insulation, cement makers, truck drivers, and plumbers may account for as many as **23%** of lung cancer cases. All forms of asbestos (amosite, chrysotile, and crocidolite) have been implicated and cause all types of lung cancer, although small cell and squamous cell are the most common. The risk is especially pronounced in smokers and can occur with nonoccupational exposure as well.

b. **Other carcinogens.** A myriad of substances have been associated with an excess risk of lung cancer, including arsenic (smelter workers, artesian well water), cadmium (batteries), chromium (masons), chloromethyl ether (wood workers), and formaldehyde.

2. **Air pollution.** Although environmental pollution has been incriminated in the development of lung cancer, this may reflect the presence of other urban carcinogens.

III. **Presentation**

A. **Signs and symptoms.** Although lung cancer can be **asymptomatic in 6%** of patients, the following signs and symptoms are common:

1. **Local manifestations.** Patients may complain of symptoms associated with growth of the primary tumor (27%), and these symptoms will differ, depending on the location of the tumor.

a. **Central.** Central tumors can produce **cough, hemoptysis,** respiratory difficulty (wheezing, dyspnea, stridor), pain, and symptoms of pneumonia.

b. **Peripheral.** Peripheral lesions cause cough; pain in the chest wall, shoulder, and arm (Pancoast tumor); respiratory difficulty (dyspnea); pleural effusions; symptoms of pulmonary abscess (cavitary squamous tumor); and **Horner's syndrome** (ipsilateral miosis, ptosis, and anhydrosis; Pancoast tumor).

2. **Regional.** Direct extension from the primary tumor and extracapsular spread from lymphatic metastases can result in **hoarseness** from recurrent paralysis

of the laryngeal nerve (left more commonly than right because of a longer intrathoracic course), dyspnea secondary to phrenic paralysis, dysphagia resulting from compression or invasion of the esophagus, superior vena cava (SVC) syndrome from compression or invasion of the SVC (see p 50, Superior Vena Cava Syndrome) and signs of pericardial tamponade (pulsus paradoxicus, distended neck veins, tachycardia, pericardial rub, distant heart tones, and Kussmaul's sign).

   3. **Systemic manifestations.** Systemic manifestations of lung cancer stem from distant metastases as well as the systemic effects of cancer. These signs and symptoms include jaundice, abdominal pain, or mass; bony pain or fracture; neurologic deficits, mental status changes, or seizures; soft tissue masses; weight loss; anorexia; weakness; and malaise.

B. **Paraneoplastic syndromes.** Lung cancer has been associated with numerous common paraneoplastic syndromes that may be the sole manifestation of disease.

   1. **Cardiovascular**
      a. **Thrombophlebitis** (see p 81, Coagulation abnormalities, II).
      b. **Nonbacterial thrombotic endocarditis** (see p 52, Paraneoplastic syndromes).
   2. **Neuromuscular** (see p 57, Paraneoplastic syndromes)
      a. **Subacute cerebellar degeneration.**
      b. **Dementia.**
      c. **Limbic encephalitis.**
      d. **Optic neuritis/retinopathy.**
      e. **Subacute necrotic myelopathy.**
      f. **Peripheral sensorimotor neuropathy.**
      g. **Autonomic neuropathy.** This entity is particularly associated with small cell lung cancer.
      h. **Myasthenic (Eaton-Lambert) syndrome.** This syndrome occurs with small cell carcinoma.
      i. **Polymyositis.**
   3. **Nephrotic syndrome** (see p 64, Paraneoplastic syndromes).
   4. **Gastrointestinal** (see p 72, Paraneoplastic syndromes, II and IV.A).
      a. **Carcinoid syndrome.** Carcinoid symptoms are associated with small cell malignancies.
      b. **Anorexia/cachexia.**
   5. **Hematologic**
      a. **Erythrocytosis** (see p 77, Erythrocyte abnormalities).
      b. **Leukocytosis** (see p 78, Leukocyte abnormalities, I).
   6. **Metabolic**
      a. **Inappropriate ACTH.** This syndrome occurs primarily in small-cell lung carcinoma (see p 90, Paraneoplastic syndromes, V).
      b. **Inappropriate ADH.** This syndrome usually develops in small-cell cancers (see p 89, Paraneoplastic syndromes, IV).
      c. **Hypercalcemia.** This syndrome occurs with squamous-cell carcinoma (see p 87, Paraneoplastic syndromes, I).
      d. **Inappropriate gonadotropins** (see p 117, Paraneoplastic syndromes).
   7. **Fever** (see p 99, Paraneoplastic syndromes).
   8. **Hypertrophic pulmonary osteoarthropathy.** This entity is reported in squamous, adenocarcinoma, and large-cell lung cancers.
   9. **Dermatologic** (see p 108, Paraneoplastic syndromes).
      a. **Acanthosis nigricans.** This finding is associated with adenocarcinoma.
      b. **Dermatomyositis.**
      c. **Erythema gyratum.**
      d. **Ichthyosis.**

IV. **Differential diagnosis.** Patients with lung cancer often present with radiographic evidence of a solitary pulmonary nodule and minimal or no symptoms. Solid proof that the nodule does not represent malignancy must be obtained. In general, malignant nodules grow rapidly, often with **surface umbilication or notching** and eccentric excavation; lack calcium (CT Hounsfield units < 175); occur in smokers older than 40 years; and are associated with negative skin tests (although positive tests do not exclude cancer). In contrast, benign masses are stable (> 2 years), often calcified (CT Hounsfield units > 175), and associated with positive skin tests in patients older than 35 years of age. Frequently, a combination of factors exists and the following diagnostic possibilities should be carefully considered: (1) infection with mycobacteria (tuberculosis), fungus (histoplasmosis, coccidioides), and parasites (echinococcus granulosus), (2) inflammation (rheumatoid arthritis, focal pneumonitis, and Wegener's granulomatosis), (3) congenital anomalies (bronchogenic cysts and arteriovenous malformations), (4) neoplasms, both benign (hamartomas, hemangiomas, papillary tumors, and benign mesotheliomas) and malignant (metastatic cancer, bronchial adenomas, and malignant mesotheliomas), and (5) miscellaneous causes (hematoma, pulmonary infarct, nipple shadows, pleural plaque, chest wall masses, and loculated interlobar pleural effusions).

V. Screening programs. Multiple randomized, prospective clinical trials screening asymptomatic male smokers older than 45 years have been conducted at Johns Hopkins, the Mayo Clinic, Memorial Sloan-Kettering, and the University of Cincinnati. All trials have used chest x-rays to detect peripheral lesions and sputum cytologies to discover more central lesions. The results can be summarized as follows.

A. Chest x-ray. Chest x-rays every 4–12 months have been used to screen high-risk groups in an attempt to detect early lung carcinoma. These x-rays can detect 67–82% of asymptomatic lung cancers, and as many as 24% of these have simultaneously abnormal sputum cytologies. When combined with sputum cytologies, chest x-rays aid in detecting earlier resectable lung cancer; however, the mortality rate does not change significantly. Therefore, screening with chest x-rays even in high-risk groups cannot be advocated.

B. Sputum cytology. Cytologic examination of expectorated sputum every 4 months as a screening test for lung cancer has been carefully evaluated. Between 26% and 40% of patients with asymptomatic lung carcinoma will have positive cytologies, and as many as 45% of these will also have abnormal chest x-rays. When combined with chest x-rays, sputum cytologies aid in detecting earlier resectable lung cancer; however, the mortality rate does not change substantially. Thus, screening with sputum cytologies, even in high-risk groups, cannot be recommended.

C. Biochemical serum markers. Many biochemical substances, including ACTH, calcitonin, beta-human chorionic gonadotropin (beta-hCG), parathormone, carcinoembryonic antigen (CEA), ferritin, sialic acid, lipotropin, and beta-2-microglobulin, have been evaluated as serum markers for lung cancer. None have proved to be useful because levels required for high sensitivity have low specificity and vice versa.

VI. Diagnostic workup

A. Medical history and physical examination. A complete medical history emphasizing presenting symptoms (eg, cough, hemoptysis, smoking history) and a thorough physical examination are essential for a complete evaluation.

1. **General appearance.** Evidence for cancer cachexia/anorexia, weight loss, overall energy level, and mental status are important findings.

2. **Skin.** Pallor (anemia); jaundice; hyperpigmentation of the neck, axillae, or anorectal areas (acanthosis nigricans); and inflammatory lesions (dermatomyositis, erythema gyratum, and ichthyosis) should be recorded.

3. **Eyes.** Unilateral miosis and ptosis may accompany facial anhydrosis as a manifestation of an ipsilateral lung carcinoma invading the stellate ganglion **(Horner's syndrome).** In addition, scleral icterus suggests hepatic metastases.

4. **Mouth and throat.** Associated oral, pharyngeal, and laryngeal carcinomas may be found, and vocal cord paralysis indicating recurrent laryngeal nerve involvement should be excluded in hoarse patients.

5. **Neck.** The presence of a signal node (also called Virchow's or Troisier's node) as well as other masses must be noted.

6. **Chest.** The quality of the breath sounds, presence of wheezing, and evidence of consolidation, pleural effusions, or both are all important findings indicating ongoing pulmonary disease.

7. **Heart.** The presence of a pericardial rub should raise the suspicion of a pericardial effusion.

8. **Abdomen.** Mass lesions can be detected in the presence of liver metastases.

9. **Rectum.** Guiaic-negative stool can help eliminate gastrointestinal blood loss as a source of anemia and the colon as a source of metastatic disease to the lung.

10. **Extremities.** Muscle strength, nerve function, distribution of fat, striae, and clubbing are important findings to note.

B. Primary tests and procedures. All patients with suspected lung cancer should have the following tests performed.

1. Blood tests
   a. Complete blood count (see p 1, **IV.A.1**).
   b. Hepatic transaminases (see p 1, **IV.A.2**).

    c. Alkaline phosphatase (see p 1, **IV.A.3**).

    d. BUN and creatinine (see p 3, **IV.A.6**).

    e. Calcium and phosphorus. Elevated levels of calcium and decreased levels of phosphorus suggest inappropriate parathormone secretion that may require preoperative therapy.

    f. Arterial blood gas. Measurement of the arterial oxygen and carbon dioxide partial pressures can be helpful in predicting postresection function. $P_aO_2 <$ 55 torr and $P_aCO_2 > 45$ torr suggest a high risk of postresection pulmonary failure.

2. Sputum cytology. Sputum collected for cytologic examination can confirm the diagnosis of malignancy in 45–90% of patients. The yield with central lesions is superior to that with small peripheral lesions. The sputum can either be induced or be obtained at the time of bronchoscopy.

3. Pulmonary function tests (PFTs). These parameters are obtained to predict the maximum tolerated resection and the postresection ventilatory capacity. The forced vital capacity (FVC) and the forced expiratory volume in 1 second (FEV_1) are the most commonly measured. If the $FEV_1 > 2.5$ L, then all resections, including pneumonectomy, are possible. If the $FEV_1 < 0.8$ L, all resections are contraindicated. If the FEV_1 falls between 0.9 and 2.4 L, the maximum tolerated resection possible and the risk are subject to surgical judgment. Age, extent of tumor-induced respiratory impairment, coexisting pulmonary disease, patient cooperation, contribution of associated infection, and cardiac status must be considered in the surgical decision. In addition, further testing with **scintigraphic ventilation-perfusion scan** may be helpful.

4. Electrocardiography (ECG). An ECG should be obtained to exclude coexistent cardiac disease, including ischemia, arrhythmias, and conduction defects.

5. Imaging studies

    a. Chest x-ray. This simple test is important in localizing and characterizing **pulmonary masses** as well as in detecting evidence of **hilar and mediastinal lymph node metastases.** Additional critical findings include **atelectasis,** collapse (bronchial obstruction), **rib notching** (SVC syndrome), and a high diaphragm (phrenic nerve paralysis). Special oblique or lordotic views may be necessary to view the paramediastinal and superior sulcus areas, respectively, and fluoroscopy may be required to evaluate diaphragmatic excursion.

    b. Computed tomography. Chest CT scans are useful to exclude benign causes of pulmonary nodules **(Hounsfield units > 175 = benign),** to evaluate the mediastinum for the presence of metastatic lymph nodes (nodes < 1 cm = negative; 1–2 cm = indeterminant; > 2 cm = positive), and to document vertebral body involvement in superior sulcus tumors. In addition, chest CT scans should extend to include the **liver and adrenal glands** to evaluate these two common sites of metastases. Overall, CT scans are **73% sensitive and 80% specific** in staging lung cancer.

6. Invasive procedures

    a. Bronchoscopy. Fiberoptic bronchoscopy is indicated in all patients to evaluate the extent of disease—with the possible exception of small peripheral lesions with widely metastatic disease since they rarely produce significant findings. Bronchoscopy will provide evidence of malignancy in more than 90% of visible tumors and should include bronchial washings and brushings for cytologic examination as well as forceps or needle biopsy, if indicated. With peripheral tumors, the diagnostic yield is less than 60%; it is less than 30% if the lesion is smaller than 2 cm.

    b. Fluoroscopy-guided transbronchial needle aspiration. This procedure can yield positive findings in as many as 80% of peripheral lesions smaller than 2 cm. Complications, including **bronchospasm, hemorrhage, and pneumothorax,** occur in 0.15%, and the mortality rate is lower than 0.05%.

    c. Transthoracic percutaneous needle biopsy. TTPNB is indicated in peripheral tumors that have had nondiagnostic sputum cytologies. Although this procedure has an accuracy rate of more than 95%, it also has a 20% risk of pneumothorax and a 6% risk of pneumothorax requiring chest tube placement.

C. Optional tests and procedures. The following tests and procedures may be indicated based on previous diagnostic findings or clinical suspicion.

    1. Blood tests

        a. Nucleotidase (see p 2, **IV.A.4**).

    b. GGTP (see p 2, **IV.A.5**).

    c. **Carcinoembryonic antigen (CEA).** Serum levels of this tumor marker are elevated in many lung cancer patients, but the false negative rate exceeds 50%. Extremely high titers (> 15 ng/mL), however, do correlate with unresectable disease, and the marker may be useful in following the response to therapy.

2. Imaging studies

    a. **Full-lung tomograms (FLTs).** This series of tomograms has almost been displaced by CT scans; however, in some circumstances (eg, superior sulcus tumors), they still may be useful.

    b. **Barium esophagram.** Radiologic evaluation of the esophagus is indicated if symptoms of dysphagia or odynophagia are present.

    c. **Magnetic resonance imaging.** For areas, such as the hilum, MRI may be superior to CT (see, also, p 3, **IV.C.2**).

    d. **Pulmonary angiography.** Involvement of the pulmonary arteries, pericardium, and other great vessels may require angiography. However, the angiogram, should never be used as exclusive evidence of unresectability.

    e. **Ventilation-perfusion scan.** This nuclear medicine study aids in the evaluation of patients with marginal lung function. Using fractional measurements of right-and-left lung ventilation (and perfusion), an estimated postresection FEV_1 can be obtained by multiplying the ventilation fraction of the uninvolved side by the measured FEV_1. If the product is > 0.8 resection can be considered.

    f. **Technetium-99m bone scan.** (see p 3, **IV.C.5**).

    g. **Gallium[67] scan.** Although controversial, gallium scans, which localize inflammatory as well as neoplastic lung lesions and hilar and mediastinal nodes, are obtained to evaluate patients with small-cell carcinoma.

    h. **Indium[111] monoclonal antibody imaging.** Localization of tumor with anti-CEA and anti-c-myc antibodies as well as the 791T/36 antibody has been of limited success. This type of imaging should be considered strictly **experimental.**

3. Invasive procedures. Many of the following procedures are indicated in staging patients with indeterminant findings on previous diagnostic studies.

    a. **Bone marrow biopsy.** Previously, bone marrow biopsy was performed on all patients with **small-cell carcinoma.** However, in the absence of clinical evidence of bone marrow involvement, **only 10–15% of these tests will yield positive results.** Thus, their routine use it is not recommended at present.

    b. **Scalene lymph node biopsy.** This procedure is indicated solely with palpable supraclavicular adenopathy or with superior sulcus tumors because only **4–10%** of other situations generate **positive findings.** Complications occur in 2% and include infection, hemorrhage, pneumothorax, phrenic and recurrent laryngeal nerve damage, and thoracic duct injury.

    c. **Mediastinoscopy.** Although preoperative evaluation with mediastinoscopy is performed routinely in some centers, other centers perform the procedure only **if lymph nodes larger than 1 cm are present** on CT scan. The technique involves a 3–4 cm incision just superior to the suprasternal notch. After careful dissection, the mediastinoscope is passed along the pretracheal fascia to the area below the azygous vein. **Biopsy of the aortopulmonary and anterior hilar nodes cannot be accomplished** with this approach, and aspiration must precede any biopsy not clearly visualized to prevent biopsy of the pulmonary artery, azygous vein, or aorta. Large series have demonstrated that 42% of central lesions and 30% of peripheral tumors have nodal metastases on mediastinoscopy. In addition, negative findings are associated with a curative resection rate of 88%.

       Findings that contraindicate surgery include extensive extracapsular ipsilateral lymph node involvement; lymph node metastases above the midtrachea, in the anterior mediastinum, or in the contralateral mediastinum; fixed metastases; or metastases invading the proximal pulmonary artery. The complication rate is 1.6%, with a death rate of 0.08%. Potential complications include hemorrhage, mediastinitis, recurrent laryngeal nerve damage, esophageal perforation, bradycardia, myocardial infarction, stroke, and air embolism.

    d. **Anterior parasternal mediastinotomy (Chamberlain procedure).** This procedure is performed through a 6-cm parasternal incision and is indicated in patients requiring evaluation of the **left mediastinum, hilum, and aortopulmonary window** for lymph node metastases and direct tumor extension. As with mediastinoscopy, the complication rate is extremely low.

VII. Pathology

A. **Location.** Lung cancer is more common in the **right lung** than the left, and the **upper lobes** are involved more often than the lower (or right middle) lobes. The location of tumors is generally divided into central and peripheral, and the location of lesions depends on the histologic type (see Table 27–1).

B. **Multiplicity.** Patients with lung cancer have a 1.5 times greater risk of developing a second lung primary than do identical patients without lung cancer. **Synchronous lung carcinoma** occurs in 1–7% of patients, whereas **metachronous second primary tumors** arise in approximately 10%. In addition, an increased incidence of cancer in the upper respiratory tract, oral cavity, bladder, and kidney has been noted in patients with the diagnosis of lung carcinoma.

C. **Histology.** Four main histologic types of lung cancer exist, **squamous cell carcinoma, adenocarcinoma, large-cell (anaplastic) carcinoma, and small-cell (oat-cell) carcinoma.** Recently the incidence of squamous cell carcinoma has declined, whereas that of adenocarcinoma has increased.

   1. **Squamous cell carcinoma.** These malignancies constitute 33–64% of all lung cancers. Most occur **centrally,** invading the bronchial cartilage and causing obstruction. Peripheral lesions can cavitate and mimic a pulmonary abscess. Microscopically, they are highly differentiated tumors with abundant keratin, and they metastasize relatively late.

   2. **Adenocarcinoma.** Between 15% and 35% of all lung tumors are adenocarcinomas. Most arise peripherally and present as firm, gray-white pipestemmed structures that tend to invade the overlying pleura. The **bronchoalveolar variant** represents 1.5–6% of adenocarcinomas and grossly occurs as the solitary-nodule, **multinodular, or diffuse (pneumonic) type.** It is associated with previous lung damage from chronic pneumonia, granulomatous disease, progressive pulmonary fibrosis, asbestosis, fibrosing alveolitis, systemic sclerosis, and Hodgkin's disease. Osmiophilic lamellar bodies containing surfactant have linked these tumors to **Type II alveolar cells.** In addition, papillary tumors develop in areas of scar and can contain psammoma bodies in 5–15% of cases. Hematogenous metastases occur early, whereas lymphatic metastases develop later.

   3. **Large-cell carcinoma.** These tumors make up about 5–20% of all lung malignancies. They consist of poorly differentiated squamous and adenocarcinoma components and occur both centrally and peripherally. A **giant-cell variant** is rapidly fatal, and a **clear-cell variant** containing areas of glycogen can be confused with metastatic renal cell carcinoma.

   4. **Small-cell carcinoma.** Approximately 19–35% of all lung cancers are composed of small submucosal anaplastic cells. Three subtypes—**oat cell** (lymphocyte-like), **intermediate,** and **combined** (oat cell and squamous or adenocarcinoma)—have been described. Oat cells are smaller than intermediate or combined cells and have a higher nucleus-to-cytoplasm ratio. The chromatin exhibits a typical **salt-and-pepper** distribution. These anaplastic tumors generally arise centrally and metastasize early and widely to a variety of organs, including bone marrow (10–15%), pituitary (15%), thyroid (8%), testes (7%), and parathyroid (1%). Metastases to bone may be **osteoblastic** in appearance.

D. **Metastatic spread**

TABLE 27–1. LOCATION OF LUNG CANCER BY HISTOLOGIC TYPE

Histology	Central (%)	Peripheral (%)
Squamous cell carcinoma	64–81	19–36
Adenocarcinoma	5–29	71–95
Large-cell carcinoma	42–49	51–58
Small-cell carcinoma	74–83	17–26
Overall	63	37

1. **Modes of spread.** Lung cancer spreads by three distinct mechanisms.
   a. **Direct extension.** Direct growth frequently leads to involvement of visceral and parietal pleura, great vessels, pericardium, diaphragm, the chest wall, and vertebral column.
   b. **Lymphatic metastasis.** Initial lymphatic spread occurs to **bronchial** and then to **hilar lymph nodes,** especially near the bronchus intermedius on the right and the area between the upper lobe bronchus and the superior segmental bronchus of the lower lobe on the left. Subsequently, right-sided tumors spread to the **subcarinal, tracheobronchial, and paratracheal nodes.** Left-sided tumors metastasize to the **tracheobronchial, aortic window, and anterior mediastinal nodes,** and in 10% of upper lobe lesions and 25% of lower lobe tumors, spread across the mediastinum to subcarinal and right paratracheal nodes.
   c. **Hematogenous metastasis.** Vascular spread of tumor cells to distant organs occurs early and widely, sparing no organs.
2. **Sites of spread.** Although every organ has been reported as a site of metastatic lung cancer, the following sites of metastasis are more common: lung, liver, bone (ribs, spine, pelvis, humerus, and femur), brain, pancreas, kidney, skin and subcutaneous tissue, myocardium, spleen, intestines, ovary, testes, soft tissues, endocrine glands (thyroid, parathyroid, and pituitary), and adrenal glands.

VIII. **Staging.** By 1987 the American Joint Committee on Cancer and the Union Internationale Contre le Cancer had developed a joint staging system for lung carcinoma to help unify reporting of end results and to facilitate comparisons between different centers. The recommended TNM staging system is listed below.
   A. **Tumor stage**
      1. **TX.** Primary tumor cannot be assessed, including proved disease by cytologies but negative imaging studies.
      2. **T0.** No evidence of primary tumor.
      3. **Tis.** Carcinoma in situ.
      4. **T1.** Tumor **no larger than 3 cm** in its greatest dimension, surrounded by lung or visceral pleura, and without bronchoscopic evidence of invasion more proximal than lobar bronchi (ie, the tumor does not invade the main bronchus; with the exception of superficially invasive tumor limited to the bronchial wall).
      5. **T2.** The tumor (1) is **larger than 3 cm** in its greatest dimension, (2) invades the mainstem bronchus but is **no closer than 2 cm to the carina,** (3) invades the **visceral pleura,** or (4) is associated with **atelectasis** or obstructive pneumonitis that extends to the hilum but does not involve the entire lung.
      6. **T3.** A tumor of any size that invades the chest wall (including superior sulcus tumors), the diaphragm, the mediastinal or parietal pleura, or the **mainstem bronchus within 2 cm of the carina** (but does not involve the carina) or one of any size that is associated with atelectasis or **obstructive pneumonitis** of the entire lung.
      7. **T4.** A tumor of any size that invades the mediastinum, heart, great vessels, trachea, esophagus, vertebral bodies, or carina or one that is associated with a malignant pleural effusion.
   B. **Lymph node stage**
      1. **NX.** Regional nodes cannot be assessed.
      2. **N0.** No regional lymph node metastases are present.
      3. **N1.** Ipsilateral peribronchial, hilar lymph nodes, or both, including direct extension, are present.
      4. **N2.** Ipsilateral mediastinal subcarinal lymph nodes or both are present.
      5. **N3.** Contralateral mediastinal or hilar nodes or both, ipsilateral or contralateral scalene nodes, or supraclavicular lymph nodes are present.
         Note: supraclavicular, scalene, paratracheal, pretracheal, paraesophageal, carinal, subcarinal, aortic, anterior and posterior mediastinal, hilar, intrapulmonic, and peribronchial lymph nodes are considered regional nodes.
   C. **Metastatic stage**
      1. **MX.** The presence of distant metastases cannot be assessed.
      2. **M0.** No distant metastases are present.
      3. **M1.** Distant metastases are present.
   D. **Histopathologic grade**
      1. **GX.** Grade cannot be assessed.
      2. **G1.** Well differentiated.
      3. **G2.** Moderately well differentiated.

      4. G3. Poorly differentiated.
      5. G4. Undifferentiated.
  E. Stage groupings
      1. Occult carcinoma. TX, N0, M0.
      2. Stage 0. Tis, N0, M0.
      3. Stage I. T1–2, N0, M0.
      4. Stage II. T1–2, N1, M0.
      5. Stage IIIA. T1–2, N2, M0; or T3, N0–2, M0.
      6. Stage IIIB. Any T, N3, M0 or T4; any N, M0.
      7. Stage IV. Any T; any N, M1.
IX. Treatment
  A. Surgery
    1. Primary lung carcinoma
      a. Indications. The indications for surgery can be divided into three distinct situations: those with an undiagnosed pulmonary nodule, those with occult disease, and those with documented lung carcinoma.
        (1) Solitary nodules. Surgery is indicated for all patients **over age 30,** particularly smokers, who present with an indeterminant pulmonary nodule. In these patients, 35–55% of nodules represent malignancies, and 85% of these are primary bronchogenic carcinomas.
        (2) Occult lung cancer. Cytologic findings suggest carcinoma, but no gross lesions can be detected in the nose, throat, or tracheobronchial tree. These patients should be followed with repeated bronchoscopies, with selective bronchial washings, until localized tumor is identified. Advances with tantalum powder, hematoporphyrin derivatives, and photodynamic therapy may improve the localization and treatment of these small occult tumors.
        (3) Documented lung cancer. Excluding small-cell lung cancer, surgery provides the best chance of cure in lung cancer patients. Generally, resection is indicated in patients whose gross disease can be resected technically (ie, **Stage I, II, or IIIA** without mediastinal or subcarinal lymph node metastases) and whose existing pulmonary reserve can compensate adequately for the loss of pulmonary parenchyma required by the resection. Approximately 20–25% of patients with non-small-cell carcinoma fall into this category. Contraindications to surgery indicating unresectable disease or high surgical risk are listed in Table 27–2. Although small-cell lung cancer is a contraindication to surgery, recent data analysis indicates that resection of primary tumors in Stage I and II disease may increase local control.

TABLE 27–2. MEDICAL AND SURGICAL CONTRAINDICATIONS TO SURGERY

Surgical contraindications
  Symptoms
    Head and upper extremity edema (superior vena cava syndrome)
    Hoarseness (recurrent laryngeal nerve paralysis)
    Ptosis, anhydrosis, and miosis (Horner's syndrome)
  Findings
    Small cell histology
    Tumor < 2 cm from carina
    Bilateral endobronchial tumor
    Metastasis to midtracheal lymph nodes and above
    Contralateral lymph node metastases
    Contralateral pulmonary metastases
    Pulmonary artery involvement
    Pericardial involvement
    Malignant pleural effusion
    Distant metastases
Medical contraindications
  $FEV_1 < 0.8$
  $FEV_1 = 0.9–2.4$ and insufficient pulmonary reserve to compensate for required resection
  Myocardial infarction within last 3 months

b. **Preoperative patient evaluation.** Patients with lung cancer often have co-existing chronic pulmonary and cardiac disease. Therefore, before surgery all patients should have complete physiologic staging, including assessment of their general and cardiopulmonary status.

   (1) **Performance status.** The patient's general performance status or functional classification is probably the most useful factor in predicting which patients can tolerate surgery. Fully ambulatory patients (Karnofsky status > 80; see Appendix A) tolerate aggressive resection much better than do patients who are partially or totally bedridden. In addition, advanced age, by itself, does not adversely affect performance status or mortality and is not a contraindication to surgery. Instead, **physiologic age** rather than chronologic age is important.

   (2) **Pulmonary status.** Each patient's ability to tolerate resection of pulmonary parenchyma is evaluated with **pulmonary function tests, arterial blood gas measurements,** and, occasionally, **ventilation-perfusion scanning** or pulmonary arterial pressure measurements. Patients are not surgical candidates if they have an **FEV_1 less than 0.8 L** (or an estimated postresection FEV_1 less than 0.8 L based on ventilationperfusion scanning), a **maximum voluntary ventilation less than 50% of the predicted amount, P_aCO_2 greater than 45 mm Hg,** or a mean pulmonary arterial pressure higher than 30 mm Hg after unilateral pulmonary artery occlusion. Patients who have an FEV_1 greater than 2.5 L usually can tolerate all resections, including pneumonectomy, and patients with an FEV_1 between 0.9 and 2.4 L are at high risk but can be considered surgical candidates, depending on the extent of surgery planned and their pulmonary reserve. Resection in the latter group requires sound clinical judgment regarding the patient's ability to tolerate the planned resection.

   (3) **Cardiac status.** Lung cancer patients frequently have cardiac disease because of the presence of common risk factors. **Myocardial infarction** within the previous 3 months is associated with a 20% perioperative mortality and is an absolute contraindication to surgery. Other high-risk findings include myocardial infarction within the previous 6 months, arrhythmias, and heart block, especially left posterior fascicular block.

c. **Approaches.** Four different approaches are used; however, the vast majority of surgeons prefer the standard posterolateral thoracotomy because of the superior hilar exposure it affords.

   (1) **Posterolateral thoracotomy.** This approach involves an incision from below the nipple extending to the vertebral column passing below the tip of the scapula. The **latissimus dorsi** and **serratus anterior muscles** generally are divided, although muscle-sparing incisions have been used. Excellent exposure of the mainstem bronchus and pulmonary vessels is facilitated by using a **double-lumen endotracheal tube** that allows unilateral ventilation. The major problem with this approach is postoperative **pain,** which can compromise respiratory function.

   (2) **Anterolateral thoracotomy.** This approach uses an incision from the sternum to the lateral thorax in the second or third intercostal space. It is **less painful** than a posterolateral incision, but it also provides **less exposure** of the hilar structures.

   (3) **Median sternotomy.** This technique involves a midline incision over and through the sternum. Although the posterior mediastinum cannot be visualized well and lesions involving the posterior and superior chest walls cannot be excised with this approach, some surgeons favor it because it results in **minimal postoperative pain,** which may allow a slightly more extensive resection in borderline surgical candidates.

   (4) **Prone.** This approach is rarely used because of the inability to perform cardiac resuscitation while the patient is in this position.

d. **Procedures.** The choice of procedure often is made intraoperatively on the basis of the extent of the primary tumor, the presence or absence of lymph node metastases, and involvement of contiguous organs such as the pericardium, trachea, diaphragm, and chest wall. Three basic procedures are possible.

   (1) **Segmental resection.** Limited segmental resections for Stages I and

II "early" disease (in a manner similar to segmental mastectomy in early breast carcinoma) has been attempted, with reported local recurrence rates of 12–19% and mortality rates lower than 6%. No decrease in long-term survival has been shown when compared to lobectomy. A recent randomized trial sponsored by the Lung Cancer Study Group demonstrated a 2.7 times increased local recurrence rate–but identical survival–in patients undergoing limited resections compared to patients undergoing lobectomy.

  (2) Lobectomy. Resection of an intact lobe is indicated when the entire tumor is confined to one lobe with a 1-cm margin of normal proximal bronchus and no distant nodal metastases are identified. Samples of the bronchopulmonary, hilar, subcarinal, aortopulmonary window (left-sided lesions), and paratracheal lymph nodes are submitted for immediate pathologic examination. The pulmonary vessels and bronchus are ligated with nonabsorbable suture or an automatic stapling device. A modification of the lobectomy that includes a **"sleeve" resection** of the mainstem bronchus (or trachea in some circumstances) when the lobar bronchus is involved with tumor (most common with right upper-lobe lesions) has been described. This parenchyma-sparing operation replaces pneumonectomy, but it is associated with a 7% mortality rate and a 7–16% local recurrence rate. The final step in any lobectomy includes testing the bronchial closure underwater with 30 cm H_2O pressure and the placement of pleural drainage catheters (chest tubes). These chest tubes are removed when no air leak is detected and the drainage is less than 200 mL/day.

  (3) Pneumonectomy. Removal of the entire lung may be required if lobectomy does not achieve adequate margins on the primary tumor or bronchopulmonary and hilar lymph node metastases. Occasionally, the surgery can include mediastinal lymph node dissection, intrapericardial ligation of the pulmonary vessels, or tracheal sleeve resection. After pneumonectomy, 0 or 1 pleural drainage catheters are placed, and air is aspirated from the pleural space until negative intrapleural pressure balances the contralateral intrathoracic pressure (mediastinum is midline or minimally shifted toward the side of resection on postresection chest x-ray).

2. **Metastatic lung carcinoma.** Generally, surgery is not indicated in metastatic lung cancer because radiation therapy can be used to palliate symptomatic metastatic lesions. However, several new procedures with potential therapeutic applications are being evaluated.

   a. **Laser therapy.** Neodymium yttrium-aluminum-garnet (Nd-YAG) and CO_2 lasers have been used experimentally to reopen bronchi obstructed by tumor. Although the technique needs to be refined, it is a promising procedure that may help significantly in the palliation of obstructing malignancies.

   b. **Photodynamic therapy.** A particularly promising procedure involves exposure of a surface containing malignancy to light at a wavelength that causes damage to areas such as tumor which have selectively concentrated a hematoporphorin derivative that absorbs light in the emitting range. Surfaces most amenable to this type of therapy are the pleural cavity and the endobronchial lining.

3. **Morbidity and mortality.** With improvements in preoperative evaluation of patients and perioperative anesthetic management, the mortality of patients undergoing **segmental resection, lobectomy, and pneumonectomy** have decreased recently to 1.4%, 2.9%, and 6.2%, respectively. Common causes of postoperative morbidity and mortality include the following complications.

   a. **Respiratory insufficiency.**
   b. **Hemorrhage.** (More than 100 mL/hr for 4 hrs from chest tubes necessitates more surgery).
   c. **Infection** (pneumonia, empyema).
   d. **Cardiac arrhythmias and myocardial infarction.**
   e. **Bronchopleural fistula.**
   f. **Pulmonary embolism.**

B. **Radiation therapy**
  1. **Non-small-cell lung carcinoma**
     a. **Primary radiation therapy.** Radiation therapy with curative intent is indicated in patients with **Stage I or II disease** who refuse or medically cannot

tolerate surgery and in patients with **Stage IIIa (N2) or IIIb (unresectable) disease.** Total doses of 5500–6000 cGy through small ports but encompassing the entire tumor with 2 cm margins and the entire superior mediastinum to 6 cm below the carina are recommended. Continuous 200 cGy daily fractions, "split-dose" 250–300 cGy daily fractions for 4 weeks with a 2-week rest in the middle, and weekly 500 cGy fractions have been tried without clear superiority of any regimen. The recurrence rates in the irradiated and nonirradiated fields at this dose are both less than 30%. Even with aggressive radiotherapy, however, 75% of the patients develop distant metastases, and 10% survive less than 5 years.

   b. Adjuvant radiation therapy
   (1) Preoperative radiation. Although preoperative radiation (4000–5000 cGy) has been shown to sterilize 46% of early lung tumors and rarely converts an unresectable lesion into a resectable one, no study to date, including two randomized trials (a Veterans Administration cooperative and an NIH collaborative) as well as multiple retrospective studies, has established a survival benefit for preoperative radiotherapy. In fact, some studies demonstrate a mortality rate as high as 22% and a 5-year survival as low as 13% in Stage I and II patients.
   (2) Intraoperative radiation. Intraoperative external beam radiation therapy with 2500 cGy to lymph node beds at high risk for metastases has been attempted; however, the **rate of severe complications has been prohibitively high.** In addition, **interstitial radiation therapy (brachytherapy)** with ^{192}Ir, ^{198}Au, and ^{125}I has been tried with good local control (78% in Stages I and II, 71% in node-negative Stage III, and 63% node-positive Stage III) but no improvement in long-term survival. Currently, these approaches cannot be recommended outside of approved clinical trials.
   (3) Postoperative radiation. Retrospective trials using historic controls, although inconclusive, suggested that postoperative radiotherapy may improve survival of patients with adenocarcinoma. One study suggested that postoperative radiation may improve the survival of patients with squamous cell carcinoma as well. However, two randomized trials, including one by the Lung Cancer Study Group in 1986 confirmed a **decreased local and overall recurrence rate** with N2 disease, but **no survival advantage** was noted.

2. **Small-cell lung carcinoma.** Because 70% of patients with small-cell carcinoma present with metastases and more than 90% die with distant disease, radiotherapy as a single agent is theoretically useless, and studies have confirmed this. However, seven randomized clinical trials have been performed comparing chemotherapy alone to chemotherapy with concurrent, alternating, or sequential radiotherapy (4000–5000 cGy, in patients with limited-stage small-cell lung carcinoma. None of the methods of radiation administration was shown to be superior. The chemotherapy varied but all regimens included cyclophosphamide and 6 of 7 included doxorubicin, vincristine, or both. Four of the 7 studies demonstrated modest (3–4 month) increases in median survival for patients treated with combined radiation and chemotherapy. In addition, significantly increased local control rates in 3 of 4 studies reporting this data were recorded. Yet, all reported increased toxicity (radiation pneumonitis, esophagitis, pericardial constriction, death) in the combined modality group. Therefore, although radiation therapy can **potentially increase local control and modestly prolong survival,** routine use cannot be overwhelmingly recommended, especially in patients with margin pulmonary function or functional status. In extensive-stage small-cell carcinoma, randomized studies have shown minimal effect of radiation on disease progression in the thorax and no effect on median, 2-year, or 5-year survival. In this setting, radiation should be limited to (1) **prophylactic brain irradiation** (PBI) in patients with **complete responses** to chemotherapy alone (although controversial, PBI decreases cerebral symptoms from 25% to 6% but does not prolong survival), (2) to therapeutic brain irradiation in **symptomatic patients,** 60–85% of whom are substantially palliated, and (3) **therapeutic spinal irradiation** (combined with intrathecal methotrexate through an Ommaya reservoir) for symptomatic spinal cord compression.

3. **Metastatic lung carcinoma.** Approximately 90% of patients with metastatic lung cancer require **symptomatic palliation** with radiotherapy, particularly in the case intrathoracic, intracranial, or bony metastases. In addition, radiotherapy is very successful in the palliation of hemoptysis (80% improved), cough

and dyspnea (60–70% improved), **and bony pain** (> 50% improved). In addition, **neurologic symptoms from brain metastases and edema from superior vena cava syndrome** are improved in 75% of patients. Although some physicians favor palliation of potentially symptomatic lesions, in general, patients can be followed closely without instituting radiation therapy until symptoms develop.

4. **Morbidity and mortality.** Morbidity and mortality are determined by the dose-limiting thoracic structures: ie, the lung, spinal cord, and heart. In addition, other non-dose-limiting structures can contribute significantly to the morbidity of radiation therapy. The following complications can occur during or after completion of therapy:

   a. **Dysphagia.**
   b. **Chronic pericardial fibrosis** (constriction, tamponade).
   c. **Radiation pneumonitis.**
   d. **Pulmonary fibrosis.**
   e. **Transverse myelitis.**
   f. **Dermatitis.**

C. **Chemotherapy**

1. **Non-small-cell lung carcinoma**

   a. **Primary lung carcinoma.** Although chemotherapy is not used as primary therapy for non-small cell lung cancer, **combinations of radiation therapy and chemotherapy** have been evaluated. Single agents (**cyclophosphamide, fluorouracil, nitrogen mustards, and vinblastine**) and combination regimens (**cisplatin and etoposide**) have not improved long-term survival over that observed with radiotherapy alone, and in some instances, survival was actually decreased. Thus, no rationale exists supporting the use of chemotherapy as the primary form of treatment in resectable non-small cell lung cancer.

   b. **Adjuvant chemotherapy**

      (1) **Preoperative chemotherapy.** Renewed interest in preoperative chemotherapy has been generated by recent reports of **47–56% response rates** in patients (with disease limited to the thorax) receiving **cisplatin and etoposide** or **cisplatin with either mitomycin-C and vinblastine or cyclophosphamide and doxorubicin.** Early results from trials using preoperative chemotherapy demonstrate **a high number of responses (56–75%), an increased resectability rate (0–35% before chemotherapy and 18–92% after), and possible survival advantages in Stage I, II, and III disease.** However, caution should be exercised since these studies were **not** randomized, the chemotherapy-related **mortality was as high as 5%,** and the long-term survival is unknown.

      (2) **Postoperative chemotherapy.** A large number of randomized and nonrandomized as well as prospective and retrospective trials of postoperative chemotherapy in the treatment of non-small cell lung carcinoma have been reported without any success. Recently spurred by initial high response rates with cisplatin of 23–56%, the LCSG conducted a randomized, prospective trial comparing **surgery combined with BCG and levamisole to surgery with cyclophosphamide, doxorubicin, and cisplatin (CAP) in Stage II and III patients.** The group receiving **surgery and chemotherapy had a significantly longer median survival** compared to the surgery and immunotherapy arm (**20 vs 12.7 months**). Although this study remains to be confirmed, it provides hope that with new active chemotherapeutic agents, increased long-term survival can be attained in the treatment of non-small cell lung cancer.

2. **Small-cell lung carcinoma**

   a. **Single-agent chemotherapy.** Cyclophosphamide, carboplatin (CBDCA), doxorubicin, etoposide (VP-16), hexamethylmelamine, Mechlorethamine, Methotrexate, Teniposide (VM-26), and vincristine have been shown to produce **partial responses in 30–90% and complete responses in** less than 5% of patients as single agents. Cisplatin, ifosfamide, nitrogen mustards (except mechlorethamine), procarbazine, and vindesine produce marginal response rates. **Response rates to all agents in relapsing patients are generally less than 15%.** New drugs with higher, more consistent response rates are clearly needed.

   b. **Combination chemotherapy.** Combinations of active single agents produce **85–95% and 75–85% overall responses in limited-stage and extensive-stage disease,** respectively. In addition, **50–60% and 15–30% complete responses, median survivals of 12–16 months and 7–11 months, and 2-year disease-free survivals of 15–20% and less than 5% are attainable in limited- and extensive-stage tumors,** respectively. The efficacy appears to be related to the total antiproliferative effect as measured by bone marrow suppression. **Three or four drugs have been shown to be optimal,** however, higher doses of one or two drugs may be equivalent. Early and late intensive therapy and alternating drug regimens have been tried without definitive improvement in the above response rates. The combination of **etoposide and cisplatin** may prove superior to all other regimens for salvage therapy, producing **50% responses after failure** of initial chemotherapy. Currently, the most effective and widely used regimen combines **cyclophosphamide (1000 mg/M^2), doxorubicin (45 mg/M^2), and vincristine (2 mg).** The duration of therapy has not been completely defined, although the majority of effect seems to take place **within the first 4 cycles.**

3. **Metastatic lung carcinoma.** No benefit to the use of chemotherapy in the setting of advanced metastatic disease has been demonstrated. Chemotherapeutic agents normally active in limited disease (ie, cisplatin and etoposide) lack therapeutic efficacy once distant metastases develop (23–28% response compared to 47–56% without distant metastases). In addition, **several randomized studies have examined the benefit of chemotherapy when compared to supportive care. These demonstrated slight but significant improvements (+14 weeks) in survival but with significant toxicity.** Therefore, palliative therapy for metastatic disease primarily should utilize radiation therapy, and until more solid evidence of benefit exists, chemotherapy should be tried only in the setting of an approved clinical trial.

4. **Morbidity and mortality.** Intensive chemotherapy for non-small cell and small cell carcinoma of the lung produces substantial toxicity, with **hospitalization required in as many as 30–50%.** Following are many of the specific problems: myelosuppression; febrile neutropenia; thrombocytopenia and hemorrhage; infections (opportunistic and otherwise); nausea, vomiting, mucositis; alopecia; cardiomyopathy (doxorubicin); neuropathy (vincristine, cisplatin); hemorrhagic cystitis (cyclophosphamide); acute tumor lysis syndrome; acute myeloblastic leukemia; pulmonary toxicity (methotrexate); and death (0–8%).

D. **Immunotherapy.** Immunotherapy with BCG and levamisole has not proven useful despite some evidence that lung cancers can be immunogenic. Newer forms of adoptive immunotherapy (lymphokines, tumor-infiltrating lymphocytes) are currently being developed for the experimental treatment of small cell as well as non-small-cell lung cancer, however initial reports are not particularly encouraging.

E. **Combined modality therapy.** Patients with Stage II and III disease (N2 disease: mediastinal metastases) have been the target of two studies of multimodality therapy. Although the data is conflicting, there is some evidence for efficacy of combined therapy, especially in the early postoperative period. However, **routine use of combined modality treatment cannot be encouraged** outside of approved clinical trials.

X. **Prognosis**

A. **Risk of recurrence.** The risk of recurrence after attempted curative therapy with either surgery or radiation in non-small-cell carcinoma is outlined in Table 27–3 and in both cases depends on the likelihood of distant metastases since metastatic non-small-cell is refractory to therapy by any modality.

B. **Five-year survival.** The survival of patients with non-small-cell carcinoma depends on the status of mediastinal nodes and distant metastases. In general, overall survival reflects the surgical curability of the lesions because radiotherapy and chemotherapy, in most instances, do not substantially change the final outcome. In patients with small-cell lung cancer, the major determinant of long-term survival is the extent of disease, either limited- or extensive-stage. The survival rates for **non-small-cell carcinoma** at 5 years are 43–53% for Stage I disease, 27–31% for Stage II, 15–25% for Stage IIIA, 5–7% for Stage IIIB, and less than 2% for Stage IV. With small-cell carcinoma, survival depends on the extent of disease: patients with **limited-stage cancer** have a median survival of 12–16 months and 5–25% 2-year survival; those with extensive disease achieve a median survival of 7–11 months and 2-year survival of 1–3%.

C. **Adverse prognostic factors.** The following factors have independent adverse prognostic significance: poor performance status, short duration of symptoms, male

TABLE 27–3. RISK OF RECURRENCE BY TUMOR STAGE

Stage	Recurrence Rate (%)
I	36
T1, N0	30
T2, N0	42
II	70–80
T1, N1	68
T2, N1	—
IIIA	80–90
T3, N0–1	57–85
T1–3, N2	75–95
IIIB	> 95
Any T, N3	> 95
T4, any N	> 95
IV	—
Overall	8.6%/yr

      sex, small-cell histology, metastatic disease at the time of diagnosis, and rising or persistently elevated CEA (> 15 ng/mL).

XI. Patient follow-up
  A. General guidelines. Because of the high risk of recurrence with lung cancer, patients should be followed very closely every 3 months for the first 3 years, every 6 months for an additional 2 years, then annually to exclude evidence of recurrence and a second respiratory tract primary lesion.
  B. Routine evaluation. Each clinic visit should include the following examinations:
    1. Medical history and physical examination. An interim medical history and complete physical examination with particular attention focused on the areas outlined on p 192 (**VI.A**) should be performed at each clinic visit.
    2. Blood tests
      a. Complete blood count (see p 1, **IV.A.1**).
      b. Hepatic transaminases (see p 1, **IV.A.2**).
      c. Alkaline phosphatase (see p 1, **IV.A.3**).
      d. BUN and creatinine (see p 3, **IV.A.6**).
      e. Calcium and phosphorus (see **IV.B.1,** above).
    3. Chest x-ray. A simple posterior-anterior and lateral chest x-ray can detect suture line recurrences, second primary tumors, pleural effusions, atelectasis and pneumonias secondary to bronchial obstruction, and bony metastases in the ribs and vertebral bodies.
  C. Additional evaluation. Other tests and procedures that are indicated at regular intervals include **a computed tomography (CT) scan of the chest.** These scans are useful to exclude local recurrences or intrathoracic metastatic disease. In addition, chest CT scans should extend to **include the liver and adrenal glands** to evaluate these two common sites of metastases. These scans should be obtained **every 6–12 months** in patients undergoing curative resection to detect early recurrence that may benefit from palliative radiation therapy.
  D. Optional evaluation. The following examinations may be indicated by previous diagnostic findings or clinical suspicion.
    1. Blood tests
      a. Nucleotidase (see p 2, **IV.A.4**).
      b. GGTP (see p 2, **IV.A.5**).
      c. Carcino embrionic antigen (CEA) (see above, **VI.C.1.c**).
    2. Imaging studies
      a. Barium esophagram (see above, **VI.C.2.b**).
      b. Magnetic Resonance Imaging (MRI) (see p 3, **VI.C.2.c**).
      c. Technetium-99m bone scan (see p 3, **IV.C.5**).
      d. Bone marrow biopsy (see above, **VI.C.3.a**).

REFERENCES

Aisner J et al: role of chemotherapy in small cell lung cancer: A consensus report of the International Association for the Study of Lung Cancer workshop. *Cancer Treat Rep* 1983;**67**:37–43.

Choi NC: Curative radiation therapy of unresectable non-small cell carcinoma of the lung: indications, techniques, results, and role of postoperative radiation therapy in lung cancer with either metastases to regional lymph nodes (N1 or unforseen N2) or direct invasion beyond visceral pleura (T3). In: Grillo H, Choi NC (editors), *Thoracic Oncology.* New York: Raven Press; 1983:163–199.

Cox JD, Byhardt RW, Komaki R: The role of radiotherapy in squamous, large cell, and adenocarcinoma of the lung. *Semin Oncol* 1983;**10**:81–94.

Cox JD et al: Cisplatin and etoposide before definitive radiation therapy for inoperable carcinoma of the lung: a phase II study of the RTOG. *Cancer Treat Rep* 1986;**70**:1219–1220.

Friess GG et al: Effect of initial resection of small cell carcinoma of the lung: a review of Southwest Oncology Group Study 7628. *J Clin Oncol* 1985; **3**:964–968.

Holmes EC: Surgical adjuvant therapy of non-small cell lung cancer. *Chest* 1986;**89**(suppl):295s–298s.

Holmes EC, Gail M: Lung Cancer Study Group: surgical adjuvant therapy for stage II and stage III adenocarcinoma and large-cell undifferentiated carcinoma. *J Clin Oncol* 1986;**4**:702–709.

Jensik RJ: The extent of resections for localized lung cancer: Segmental resection. In: Kulle CF (editor), *Current Controversies in Thoracic Surgery.* Philadelphia, PA: WB Saunders; 1986:175–182.

Johnson DH, Greco FA: Small cell carcinoma of the lung. *CRC Crit Rev Oncol/Hematol* 1986;**4**:303–336.

Kjaer M: Radiotherapy of squamous, adeno- and large cell carcinoma of the lung. *Cancer Treat Rev* 1982;**9**:1–20.

Kradin RL et al: Tumor-derived interleukin-2 dependent lymphocytes in adoptive immunotherapy of lung cancer. *Cancer Immunol Immunother* 1987;**24**:76–85.

Lowe JE et al: The role of bronchoplastic procedures in the surgical management of benign and malignant pulmonary lesions. *J Thorac Carciovasc Surg* 1982;**83**:227–234.

Lung Cancer Study Group. Effects of postoperative mediastinal radiation on completely resected stage II and stage III epidermoid cancer of the lung. *N Engl J Med* 1986;**315**:1377–1381.

Morstyn G et al: Small cell lung cancer 1973–1983: early prognosis and recent obstacles. *Int J Radiat Oncol Biol Phys* 1984;**10**:515–539.

Nagasaki F, Flehinger BJ, Martini N: Complications of surgery in the treatment of carcinoma of the lung. *Chest* 1982;**82**:25–29.

Pearson FG: Radical surgery for N2 disease. *Chest* 1986;**89**(suppl):339s–340s.

Seifter EJ, Ihde DC: Therapy of small cell lung cancer: a perspective on two decades of clinical research. *Semin Oncol* 1988;**15**:278–299.

Shields TW: Carcinoma and other lung tumors. In: Hardy JD, Kukora JS, Pass HI (editors), *Hardy's Textbook of Surgery.* 2nd ed. Philadelphia, PA: JB Lippincott; 1988:856–875.

28 Malignancies of the Pleura

Robert B. Cameron, MD

I. **Epidemiology.** Malignancies of the pleura (**mesotheliomas**) are rare tumors. In 1985, **1.2 cases per 100,000 males and 0.2 cases per 100,000 females** were reported, leading to 0.6 and 0.1 deaths, respectively. Estimates indicate that **more than 3600 new cases and more than 2400 deaths** would occur in 1993 and that the incidence will peak between 3600 and 4200 cases per year by 1995. Worldwide, the incidence parallels the use of asbestos (see below).

II. **Risk factors**
   A. **Age.** The incidence of pleural neoplasms increases from less than 1 per 100,000 population before age 55 to **5.1 per 100,000 by age 75.** The majority of mesotheliomas occur between the ages of 50 and 70 years.
   B. **Sex.** The risk in males is **2.5–3 times** that in females presumably because of occupational exposure to asbestos.
   C. **Race.** No racial predilection has been reported.
   D. **Genetic factors.** No true hereditary predisposition has been identified, although the lifetime risk in **first-degree relatives** of asbestos workers is **1%** because of incidental exposure to asbestos.
   E. **Diet.** No dietary factors are associated with the pathogenesis of pleural malignancies.
   F. **Previous pulmonary pathology. Tuberculosis, beryllium exposure, and chemical and lipoid aspiration pneumonia** have been implicated anecdotally in the development of pleural neoplasms.
   G. **Smoking.** Unlike the case for lung carcinoma, **no** data exists linking cigarette smoking to the development of mesothelioma.
   H. **Asbestos.** Asbestos, a silicate fiber used in insulation, was first implicated in the pathogenesis of mesothelioma by Wagner in 1960. The carcinogenic potency of asbestos fibers varies with cross-sectional diameter. Thick **serpentine** fibers (**chrysotile**) are deposited **proximally** in the respiratory tract and are easily cleared, thus posing less of a risk than the thin needle-like **amphibole** fibers (**crocidolite and amosite**) that lodge in the terminal airways. In addition, **zeolite,** a soil silicate related to asbestos, is associated with a high incidence of mesothelioma in the **Antoli region of Turkey (220 per 100,000).** The risk of mesothelioma in workers exposed to asbestos and their family members is **8–13%** and **1%,** respectively, and the incidence increases with time to 5.5 cases per 1000 person-years 40 to 45 years after exposure—a **300 times** increased risk. Generally, the **latency period** ranges from **15–50 years.** Estimates indicate that nearly 8 million people in the United States have been exposed to significant amounts of asbestos. The Occupational Safety and Health Act established exposure standards as **less than 0.2 fibers that are more than 5 mμ-in length/mL of air** while ignoring fibers less than 5 mcm in length.
   I. **Radiation.** A small number of mesotheliomas arise 7–36 years (**median 16 years**) following exposure to ionizing radiation.
   J. **Urbanization.** Mesothelioma is more common in urban areas as a result of occupational exposure to asbestos in the shipbuilding, construction, automobile, and textile industries. Asbestos is found in cement water conduits, roofing shingles, flooring products, insulation in public and private buildings, plastics, brake linings, and some textiles.

III. **Presentation**
   A. **Signs and symptoms**
      1. **Local manifestations.** The initial symptoms is **dyspnea** that is related primarily to the presence of a **pleural effusion** and **chest wall discomfort** (restrictive pulmonary disease in "dry" mesothelioma). **Pleural thickening** and other characteristic radiographic findings (see p 207, **VI.B.3.a**) are evident in only **20–50%** of patients. A nonproductive cough, malaise, anorexia, weight loss, dys-

phagia (esophageal involvement), Horner's syndrome, superior vena cava syndrome, pericardial tamponade (pericardial effusion), severe chest wall pain (direct invasion), and abdominal distention and discomfort (peritoneal involvement) also may occur.

   2. **Systemic manifestations.** Pulmonary nodules, liver masses, and painful bone lesions (all indicating metastatic disease) have been documented on autopsy, but they rarely become clinically apparent.

   B. **Paraneoplastic syndromes.** Although **hypertrophic pulmonary osteoarthropathy and hypoglycemia** are present in **35% and 4%** of **benign** mesotheliomas, respectively, **fever** is the only paraneoplastic syndrome that has been associated with **malignant** mesothelioma.

IV. **Differential diagnosis.** Although malignant mesothelioma should be suspected clinically in any patient with a **unilateral pleural effusion, thickening** or both associated with progressive symptoms and a history of **prior asbestos exposure** (> 15 years previously), mesotheliomas account for only 1 of every 3000 newly diagnosed pleural effusions, whereas other malignancies are identified in 400. Other inflammatory (benign) and malignant diseases that are associated with mesothelial hyperplasia include infections (chronic empyema), inflammation (asbestos, rheumatoid and idiopathic pleuritis), benign neoplasms (benign mesotheliomas and solitary fibrous tumor), and other malignant neoplasms (bronchogenic carcinoma, metastatic adenocarcinoma, and primary sarcomas of the chest wall).

V. **Screening programs.** Despite a well-defined high-risk population, screening programs have not been developed because early detection does not alter the almost uniformly fatal outcome of this disease.

VI. **Diagnostic workup**
   A. **Medical history and physical examination.** A complete medical history, including a history of asbestos exposure and common symptoms of mesothelioma (eg, dyspnea, chest discomfort) as well as a thorough physical examination are essential to a complete evaluation.

      1. **General appearance.** Evidence of anorexia, weight loss, and malaise are important findings.
      2. **Skin.** Pallor (anemia) and jaundice, albeit rare, should be noted.
      3. **Eyes.** Unilateral miosis, ptosis, and facial anhydrosis (**Horner's syndrome**), which indicate invasion of the **stellate ganglion,** and scleral icterus, which suggests hepatic metastases, must be described.
      4. **Mouth and throat.** Vocal cord paralysis, signifying **recurrent laryngeal nerve** involvement, must be excluded in hoarse patients.
      5. **Neck.** The presence of a signal node (also called **Virchow's or Troisier's node**) as well as other masses must be noted.
      6. **Chest.** The quality of the breath sounds, presence of wheezing, and evidence of consolidation, pleural effusions, or both are important findings of pulmonary disease.
      7. **Breasts.** Masses suggesting breast cancer with metastatic pleural disease should be fully described.
      8. **Heart.** The presence of a pericardial rub should raise the suspicion of pericardial effusion and tamponade.
      9. **Abdomen.** In rare cases, masses may be detected in the presence of liver metastases.
      10. **Rectum.** Prostatic nodules, rectal masses, and occult fecal blood raises the possibility of a prostatic or colorectal source of metastatic disease to the pleura.
      11. **Extremities. Hypertrophic pulmonary osteoarthropathy** associated with pulmonary disease and benign mesothelioma should be noted.

   B. **Primary tests and procedures.** All patients with suspected mesothelioma should have the following diagnostic tests performed.

      1. **Blood tests**
         a. Complete blood count (see p 1, **IV.A.1**).
         b. Hepatic transaminases (see p 1, **IV.A.2**).
         c. Alkaline phosphatase (see p 1, **IV.A.3**).
         d. BUN and creatinine (see p 3, **IV.A.6**).
         e. Arterial blood gas. Measurement of the arterial oxygen and carbon dioxide partial pressures may be useful in assessing existing intrapulmonary shunts and in predicting postresection function. $P_aO_2 < 55$ torr and $P_aCO_2 > 45$ torr suggest a high risk of postresection pulmonary failure.
      2. **Pulmonary function tests (PFTs).** This test measures the restrictive defect

often associated with mesothelioma and assists in estimating the extent of pulmonary resection possible (see, also, p 193, **VI.B.3**).

3. **Imaging studies**
   a. **Chest x-ray.** In addition to the frequent finding of **pleural effusion,** a chest x-ray often reveals **contraction** of the ipsilateral hemithorax, irregular **pleural thickening, thickening** of the interlobar **fissures,** a **fixed central mediastinum** despite a large effusion, **contralateral pleural plaques** suggesting asbestos exposure (20% of patients), and, in advanced disease, **rib destruction.** Further critical findings include **atelectasis, rib notching** (superior vena cava syndrome), and a **high diaphragm** (phrenic nerve paralysis). Special oblique or lordotic views may be necessary to view the paramediastinal and superior sulcus areas, respectively, and fluoroscopy may be required to evaluate diaphragmatic excursion.
   b. **Computed tomography.** Chest CT scans are useful to detect **early contraction** of the hemithorax, irregular **pleural thickening,** and **contralateral pleural plaques** suggesting asbestos exposure (50% of patients). In addition, unsuspected **lobar collapse** caused by an underlying endobronchial lesion may be demonstrated. Because **chest wall invasion** and **peritoneal penetration** also may be detected, the CT scan should visualize the upper abdomen to exclude metastases to the liver, adrenal glands, and kidneys.
4. **Invasive procedures.** In general, **pleural biopsy** remains the most reliable method of establishing the diagnosis of mesothelioma and can be accomplished either **open or closed** as outlined below.
   a. **Pleural fluid cytology.** This approach is highly dependent on the cytopathologist's experience and yields evidence **suggestive** of mesothelioma in 0–77% of patients. **In rare cases, a definitive diagnosis is made.**
   b. **Fine needle aspiration cytology.** As with pleural fluid cytology, cytologic findings **suggest** mesothelioma, at best, and are **rarely diagnostic.**
   c. **Closed transthoracic needle biopsy of the pleura.** Closed needle biopsy, including trephine pleural biopsy, produces a definitive diagnosis in **21–54%** of patients.
   d. **Thoracoscopy-guided pleural biopsy.** In patients with pleural effusions, thoracoscopy-guided pleural biopsy confirms the diagnosis of mesothelioma in **57%** of patients.
   e. **Open surgical biopsy of the pleura.** Open surgical biopsy with **immediate frozen pathologic tissue examination** and **definitive resection** (see p 209, **IX.A.1.d** is the **most reliable** method of establishing a pathologic diagnosis. Moreover, unlike other biopsy techniques that potentially seed the chest wall with malignant cells, this procedure **avoids chest wall contamination** and is recommended for all patients who have no evidence of spread beyond the parietal pleura (Stage I disease).
C. **Optional tests and procedures.** The following tests and procedures may be indicated on the basis of previous diagnostic findings or clinical suspicion.
   1. **Blood tests**
      a. 5-Nucleotidase (see p 2, **IV.A.4**).
      b. GGTP (see p 2, **IV.A.5**).
      c. Carcinoembryonic antigen (CEA). This tumor marker may be elevated with metastatic adenocarcinoma but not with mesothelioma.
   2. **Imaging studies**
      a. Barium esophagram. Radiologic evaluation of the esophagus is indicated if symptoms of **dysphagia** or **odynophagia** are present.
      b. Magnetic resonance imaging (see p 3, **IV.C.2**).
      c. Ventilation-perfusion scan (see p 194, **VI.C.2.e**).
      d. Technetium-99m bone scan (see p 3, **IV.C.4**).
   3. **Invasive procedures**
      a. **Laparoscopy.** Direct visualization of the peritoneum and liver often is useful to exclude involvement of these organs during the staging process.
      b. **Bronchoscopy.** Although rarely indicated for the workup of mesothelioma, rigid or fiberoptic bronchoscopy may be necessary to exclude a synchronous bronchogenic carcinoma.

VII. **Pathology**
   A. **Location.** Mesotheliomas arise in the **right hemithorax in 60%** of patients and most commonly involve the lower lung fields. Nearly **35%** originate in the **left hemithorax,** and 5% are bilateral. Although 81% of all mesotheliomas occur in the thorax, 19% are primary neoplasms of the peritoneum.

B. **Multiplicity.** Localized, solitary disease is rare, and most malignant mesotheliomas are **diffuse** in nature. In addition, **5% are bilateral.**

C. **Histology.** On microscopic examination, 4 types of mesothelioma may be identified.

1. **Epithelial (tubopapillary).** This type is associated with **pleural effusions** and constitutes **35–40%** of all mesotheliomas. A **variant** marked by abundant mucoid stroma and small numbers of loosely arranged cells with poorly formed tubules, clefts, and cystic spaces is associated with a slightly **better prognosis.**

2. **Mesenchymal (fibrosarcomatous).** These types of mesotheliomas are characterized by **pleural thickening** without effusion (**"dry" mesothelioma**) and represent **20%** of all mesotheliomas.

3. **Mixed.** Tumors with both epithelial and mesenchymal elements represent **35–40%** of all mesotheliomas. Mixed neoplasms with predominantly epithelial components produce pleural effusions, whereas those with primarily mesenchymal constituents present as "dry" mesotheliomas.

4. **Undifferentiated.** These primitive neoplasms represent **5–10%** of all mesotheliomas.

D. **Metastatic spread**

1. **Modes of spread.** Although mesotheliomas spread primarily by direct invasion, lymphatic and hematogenous metastases do occur in advanced disease.

   a. **Direct extension.** Direct invasion of the **chest wall and ribs (most common), mediastinum (including esophagus, trachea, and great vessels), diaphragm, and pericardium** often occurs as the disease progresses.

   b. **Lymphatic metastasis.** Lymphatic emboli to the regional lymph nodes have been documented in **70%** of patients at autopsy; however, these metastases rarely become clinically evident.

   c. **Hematogenous metastasis.** Although spread through blood vessels to distant organs is common in advanced disease, these metastases usually remain clinically silent.

2. **Sites of spread.** Spread to distant sites often involve the following organs: **liver, lung, bone, kidney,** and **adrenal gland.**

VIII. **Staging.** The staging of malignant mesotheliomas is based on the extension beyond the confines of the parietal pleura. An initial staging system was proposed by Butchart in 1976. Recently, however, the Union Internationale Contre le Cancer proposed a TNM staging system. The American Joint Committee on Cancer has yet to adopt a formal staging system of mesotheliomas.

A. **Butchart staging system**

1. **Stage I.** Tumor is confined within the **"capsule"** of the parietal pleura: ie, involving the ipsilateral pleura, lung, diaphragm, and **external** surface of the pericardium within the pleural reflection only.

2. **Stage II.** Tumor invades the chest wall or mediastinum (esophagus, trachea, or great vessels). Alternately, lymph nodes **within the chest** are involved with metastatic disease.

3. **Stage III.** Tumor penetrates the diaphragmatic muscle to involve the peritoneum or retroperitoneum, the pericardium to involve the internal surface or heart, and the mediastinum to involve the contralateral pleura. Alternately, lymph nodes **outside the chest** are involved with metastatic disease.

4. **Stage IV.** Distant hematogenous metastases are present.

B. **TNM staging system**

1. **Tumor stage**

   a. **TX.** The primary tumor cannot be assessed.

   b. **T0.** No evidence of a primary tumor exists.

   c. **T1.** The primary tumor is limited to the ipsilateral parietal and/or visceral pleura.

   d. **T2.** Tumor invades any of the following: ipsilateral lung, endothoracic fascia, diaphragm, and pericardium.

   e. **T3.** Tumor invades any of the following: ipsilateral chest wall muscle, ribs, and mediastinal organs or tissues.

   f. **T4.** Tumor extends to any of the following: contralateral pleura or lung by direct extension, peritoneum or intra-abdominal organs by direct extension, and cervical tissues.

2. **Lymph node stage**

   a. **NX.** Regional lymph nodes cannot be assessed.

   b. **N0.** No regional lymph node metastases are present.

    c. **N1.** Metastases are present in ipsilateral bronchopulmonary or hilar lymph nodes.

    d. **N2.** Metastases are present in ipsilateral mediastinal lymph nodes.

    e. **N3.** Metastases are present in contralateral mediastinal, internal mammary, supraclavicular, or scalene lymph nodes.

3. **Metastatic stage**
    a. **MX.** The presence of distant metastases cannot be assessed.
    b. **M0.** No distant metastases exist.
    c. **M1.** Distant metastases are present.

4. **Stage groupings**
    a. **Stage I.** T1–2, N0, M0.
    b. **Stage II.** T1–2, N1, M0.
    c. **Stage III.** T3, N0–1, M0; T1–3, N2, M0.
    d. **Stage IV.** T4, any N, M0; any T, N3, M0; any T, any N, M1.

IX. **Treatment**
  A. **Surgery**
    1. **Primary malignant mesothelioma**
      a. **Indications.** Although controversial, initial radical surgery is recommended in **physically fit patients with Stage I disease** who potentially may be **cured** by surgery (with or without postoperative adjuvant radiation and/or chemotherapy).

      b. **Preoperative patient evaluation.** Because patients are often of advanced age (> 60 years) and frequently have coexisting chronic pulmonary and cardiac disease, all patients should have complete physiologic staging, including an assessment of their general and cardiopulmonary status in a manner similar to that outlined for bronchogenic carcinoma (see p 197, **IX.A.1.b**).

      c. **Approaches.** A standard **posterolateral thoracotomy** (see p 198, **IX.A.1.c**) is preferred, using **2 levels of access** to the thorax (**6th and 10th intercostal spaces** through a single skin incision) to facilitate removal of the diaphragm and placement of a diaphragmatic prosthesis.

      d. **Procedures.** The only potentially curative surgical procedure for mesothelioma consists of an initial diagnostic biopsy, followed by immediate radical pleuropneumonectomy.

        (1) **Open pleural biopsy.** Because of the risk of seeding the chest wall during transthoracic needle biopsies of the pleura, patients with highly **suspicious symptoms and physical findings** and no evidence of spread beyond the parietal pleura (**Stage I**) should undergo **initial open pleural biopsy** through a limited posterolateral thoracotomy with immediate pathologic evaluation. If the diagnosis of mesothelioma is confirmed, **immediate radical pleuropneumonectomy** is performed.

        (2) **Radical pleuropneumonectomy.** This procedure should be contemplated only in patients with Stage I disease. All pleural surfaces are removed including the parietal and visceral pleura. (The parietal pleura requires removal of the **diaphragm and pericardium,** and the visceral pleura necessitates **pneumonectomy.**) Initially, the parietal pleura is mobilized from the chest wall and mediastinum, the pericardium and diaphragm are excised (sparing the peritoneum), then a standard intrapericardial pneumonectomy is performed. If **extrapleural (eg, chest wall, mediastinal) invasion** or **intrapericardial or intraperitoneal extension** is encountered during this dissection, the operation is terminated. If part of the peritoneum is removed and the remaining peritoneum is inadequate to isolate the thorax from the abdominal cavity, a **prosthetic diaphragm** is constructed. No chest drainage catheters are required postoperatively. With this radical procedure, **10–37% 2-year and 3.5–10% 5-year survival** have been reported in retrospective series. However, the extent of survival benefit (if any) directly attributable to surgery is unknown.

    2. **Locally advanced and metastatic mesothelioma**
      a. **Locally advanced disease.** The goals of palliative surgery are to (1) **drain and prevent** recurrent pleural **effusions,** which frequently are not treated adequately with chest drainage catheters, (2) **relieve respiratory embarrassment,** and (3) **alleviate pain.** Removal of the parietal pleura (**pleurectomy**) with **decortication,** sparing the diaphragmatic pleura and lung, has been strongly advocated, especially at Memorial Sloan-Kettering Cancer Center. With this procedure, **88%** of effusions are controlled and acceptable

relief of pain and dyspnea is achieved for a period of weeks to months. Its use in **Stage I** patients also has been proposed because similar survival rates (**32–40% 2-year survival**) and lower morbidity and mortality rates have been reported in retrospective series as compared with radical pleuropneumonectomy.

   b. **Metastatic disease.** Because most metastases occur in advanced disease and remain asymptomatic, surgery is rarely indicated in these patients.

3. **Morbidity and mortality.** Although published **mortality rates** for pleuropneumonectomy vary from **0–32%**, improvements in preoperative patient evaluation and selection and perioperative anesthetic management have reduced recent mortality rates to **5–9%**, whereas mortality following **pleurectomy** is only **1%**. Common causes of postoperative morbidity include the following complications: **respiratory insufficiency; hemorrhage; infection (pneumonia, empyema); cardiac arrhythmias and myocardial infarction; bronchopleural fistula; pulmonary embolism; chylothorax, cardiac herniation,** which occurs through a pericardial defect; **tension pneumoperitoneum; and intrathoracic herniation** (abdominal contents).

B. **Radiation therapy**

1. **Primary malignant mesothelioma.** The use of radiotherapy as initial therapy in the treatment of malignant mesothelioma has been reported in several retrospective series using either external beam or intracavitary irradiation. Although the putative goal is cure, **long-term survival remains anecdotal** and palliation of pain and dyspnea is a more practical goal. Results have been independent of histologic type (eg, epithelial, mesenchymal, mixed).

   a. **External beam radiotherapy.** External beam radiotherapy (> **4000–6500 cGy over 35–45 days**) yields symptomatic relief in **67%** of patients compared with **22%** in patients receiving **less than 4000 cGy.** Furthermore, localized **electron** beam radiation (**2100 cGy over 3 days**) administered to **biopsy sites** reduces the risk of wound and needle track seeding from **44%** to approximately **1%**.

   b. **Intracavitary radiotherapy.** Anecdotal experience with intrapleural instillation of ^{198}Au and ^{32}P indicates that **67% of malignant pleural effusions** can be controlled with this approach; however, the available data suggests that survival is unaffected.

2. **Adjuvant radiation therapy**

   a. **Preoperative radiation.** No significant experience has been reported with this approach.

   b. **Postoperative radiation.** External beam irradiation, ^{125}I and ^{192}I implantation, and ^{32}P instillation have been administered **after palliative debulking surgery (pleurectomy and decortication)** in an effort to improve survival. The resulting median survival (**17.5–25 months**), however, does **not** differ substantially from the reported median survival of patients receiving either no therapy (16.5 months) or surgery alone (21 months).

3. **Locally advanced and metastatic mesothelioma.** No data exist to support the use of radiotherapy in the treatment of localized bulky or metastatic disease. Although distant metastases rarely become symptomatic, radiation therapy may be useful in the palliation of **painful bone metastases.**

4. **Morbidity and mortality.** Morbidity and mortality are determined primarily by the dose-limiting thoracic structures, ie, the lung, spinal cord, and heart. The following complications can occur during or after completion of therapy: **dysphagia, chronic pericardial fibrosis** (constriction, tamponade), **radiation pneumonitis, pulmonary fibrosis, transverse myelitis,** and **dermatitis.**

C. **Chemotherapy**

1. **Primary mesothelioma.** Although not used extensively for Stage I disease, chemotherapy has been administered to patients with more advanced primary lesions. The results are similar to those observed in locally advanced and metastatic lesions (see **C.3**).

2. **Adjuvant chemotherapy**

   a. **Preoperative chemotherapy.** No significant experience with this modality has been reported. Recently, however, a trial of preoperative doxorubicin, cyclophosphamide, and dacarbazine was initiated at M. D. Anderson Hospital and Tumor Institute.

   b. **Postoperative chemotherapy.** A limited number of studies have failed to improve disease-free or overall survival compared with retrospective historical controls. Recently, the Lung Cancer Study Group instituted a trial of intrapleural chemotherapy (cisplatin), followed by systemic cisplatin and mitomycin C for mesothelioma grossly resected by radical "decortication." However, results are not yet available.

3. **Locally advanced and metastatic mesothelioma**
   a. **Single agents.** Multiple trials of systemic single cytotoxic agents involving up to 164 patients reveal low overall response rates and only a few active drugs, such as **detorubicine response rates for only a few drugs, such as detorubicine (43%), cyclophosphamide (28%), doxorubicin (18%), mitomycin C (17%), fluorouracil (14%),** and cisplatin (10%).
   b. **Combination chemotherapy.** Initial response rates of 30–40% for various combinations based on either **doxorubicin or cisplatin** were not confirmed by subsequent large cooperative randomized studies that demonstrated response rates no different from those for single agents **(0–18%).**
4. **Morbidity and mortality.** Limited data is available on the toxicity of chemotherapy in patients with mesothelioma. Agents with **pulmonary toxicity** (eg, mitomycin-C), in particular, must be administered cautiously in these patients because of the risk of respiratory compromise.

D. **Immunotherapy.** Immunomodulatory agents have not been tried in the treatment of mesothelioma.

E. **Combined modality therapy.** Combinations of surgery, radiotherapy, and chemotherapy hold the most promise in the treatment of mesothelioma; however, early data from studies at several centers do not demonstrate improved survival.

X. **Prognosis**

A. **Risk of recurrence.** Re-exploration following pleurectomy and decortication often demonstrates residual disease on the visceral pleura (51%), diaphragm (49%), mediastinum (49%), chest wall (27%), and lung (5%). In **87% of patients,** the disease recurs **within 2 years,** regardless of therapy.

B. **5-year survival.** The 1-, 2-, and 5-year survival rates for patients treated with surgery, chemotherapy, radiation, and no therapy are summarized in Table 28–1. Although the overall rate of survival is poor, it is relatively unpredictable: some patients live as long as **16 years** with their disease.

C. **Adverse prognostic factors.** The following factors have independent adverse prognostic significance: **male sex; poor performance status; short duration of symptoms** (< 6 months); **history of chest pain; and mesenchymal, mixed,** and **undifferentiated histologies.**

XI. **Patient follow-up**

A. **General guidelines.** Because of the high risk of recurrence with mesothelioma, patients should be followed closely every 3 months for the first 2 years, every 6 months for an additional 3 years, then annually to exclude evidence of recurrence.

B. **Routine evaluation.** Each clinic visit should include the following examinations.
   1. **Medical history and physical examination.** An interim medical history and complete physical examination, with particular attention focused on the areas outlined under **VI.A** above should be performed at each clinic visit.
   2. **Blood tests** (p 1, **IV.A**).
      a. Complete blood count.
      b. Hepatic transaminases.
      c. Alkaline phosphatase.
      d. BUN and creatinine.
   3. **Chest x-ray.** This simple test can detect pleural effusions, atelectasis, bony metastases (ribs), and recurrent pleural thickening. Its sensitivity, however, is inferior to that of CT.

C. **Additional evaluation.** Other tests and procedures that are indicated at regular

Table 28–1. 1-, 2-, and 5-year survival rates by treatment strategy

Therapy	1-year	2-year	5-year
None	77%	31%	<10%
Surgery	82%	31%	<10%
Radiation	100%	33%	<7%
Chemotherapy	75%	33%	0%

(Data from Law MR, Gregor A, Hodson ME, et al: Malignant mesothelioma of the pleura: A study of 52 treated and 64 untreated patients. Thorax 39:255–259, 1984.)

intervals include a **CT scan of the chest.** These scans are useful to exclude local recurrences or intrathoracic metastatic disease. In addition, CT scans of the chest should **include the liver, kidneys, and adrenal glands** to evaluate these common sites of metastases. These scans should be obtained **every 6–12 months** to detect early recurrence that may benefit from palliative therapy.

  D. Optional evaluation.
    1. Blood tests (see p 2, **IV.A**)
      a. 5-Nucleotidase.
      b. GGTP.
    2. Barium esophagram (see p 207, **VI.C.2.a**).
    3. Imaging studies (see p 3, **IV.C**)
      a. Magnetic resonance imaging (MRI).
      b. Technetium-99m bone scan.
    4. Biopsy. In patients without known active disease, new suspicious masses should be biopsied by fine needle aspiration, core needle biopsy, or open surgical biopsy to confirm recurrent disease.

REFERENCES

Antman KH, Aisner J: Chemotherapy of malignant mesothelioma. In: Roth JA, Ruckdeschel JC, Weisenburger TH (editors), *Thoracic Oncology*. Philadelphia, PA: WB Saunders; 1989:588–593.

Butchart EG: Surgery of mesothelioma of the pleura. In: *Thoracic Oncology*. Philadelphia, PA: WB Saunders; 566–583.

Law MR et al: Malignant mesothelioma of the pleura: a study of 52 treated and 64 untreated patients. *Thorax* 1984;**39**:255–259.

Probst G et al: The role of pleuropneumonectomy in the treatment of diffuse malignant mesothelioma of the pleura. In: Deslauriers J, Lacquet LK (editors), *Thoracic Surgery: Surgical Management of Pleural Diseases,* vol 6. Philadelphia, PA: CV Mosby; 1990:344–350.

Rusch VW, Ginsberg RJ: New concepts in the staging of mesotheliomas. In: Deslauriers J, Lacquet LK (editors), *Thoracic Surgery: Surgical Management of Pleural Diseases,* vol 6. Philadelphia, PA: CV Mosby; 1990:336–343.

Wilkins MF, Adams M: Radiotherapy of malignant pleural mesothelioma. In: Roth JA, Ruckdeschel JC, Weisenburger TH (editors), *Thoracic Oncology*. Philadelphia, PA: WB Saunders; 1989:584–587.

29 Malignancies of the Mediastinum

Robert B. Cameron, MD

I. **Epidemiology.** Although a variety of neoplasms occur in the mediastinum (eg, lymphoma, germ-cell neoplasms, neurogenic tumors, carcinoids), malignancies of the thymus (thymomas) are unique in this location and constitute **20% of all adult mediastinal masses.** Worldwide, the incidence of thymoma is not known to vary significantly.

II. **Risk factors**
   A. **Age.** Thymomas are rare before age 20, and the peak incidence occurs between 40 and 60 years of age. Nearly **70% arise after age 40.**
   B. **Sex.** There is no known sex predilection.
   C. **Race.** The risk of thymoma is identical in blacks and whites.
   D. **Genetic factors.** The risk in first-degree relatives is not increased, and no genetic abnormalities or hereditary syndromes have been associated with the development of thymomas.
   E. **Diet.** No dietary factors have been identified.
   F. **Smoking.** Smoking is not a known risk factor.
   G. **Radiation.** Thymomas have not been associated with radiation exposure.
   H. **Previous immunologic pathology.** A large number of immune-mediated diseases have been associated with thymoma, including dermatomyositis, polymyositis, Raynaud's disease, regional enteritis, rheumatoid arthritis, sarcoid, scleroderma, Sjögren's syndrome, systemic lupus erythematosus, Takaysu's syndrome, thyroiditis, and ulcerative colitis. The 3 most common disorders, however, are **myasthenia gravis, red-cell aplasia, and hypogammaglobulinemia.**
      1. **Myasthenia gravis.** This disease is characterized by ocular (ptosis), oropharyngeal (dysphagia), respiratory (dyspnea), and, occasionally, generalized (proximal to distal) muscle weakness. Circulating antibodies to the acetylcholine neuromuscular receptor are present, and 70% of patients develop thymic lymphoid hyperplasia. Reports indicate that **8.5–15% of patients with myasthenia develop a thymoma;** however, **15–59% of patients with thymomas have myasthenia.** The peak incidence of myasthenia in the absence of thymoma occurs at age 30 and that of myasthenia with thymoma is the same as thymoma itself: ages 40–60 years. Whereas **68–75% of patients with myasthenia improve with thymectomy** (a 20–37% rate of complete remission), **only 25% of patients with myasthenia and thymoma experience improvement.**
      2. **Red-cell aplasia.** This syndrome, marked by the nearly complete absence of erythropoiesis, is associated with leukopenia and thrombocytopenia (30%), the presence of a thymoma (50%), and improvement following thymectomy (25–33%). Nearly **5% of all patients with thymoma** are found to have red-cell aplasia.
      3. **Hypogammaglobulinemia.** This disorder of both cellular and humeral immunity occurs in 5% of patients with thymoma. Improvement with thymectomy is rare, however.
   I. **Urbanization.** No difference in the incidence of thymoma between urban and rural populations has been reported.

III. **Clinical presentation**
   A. **Signs and symptoms**
      1. **Local manifestations.** Although **50–70% of patients experience symptoms** from the presence of a mediastinal mass, the **symptoms are vague** and include dyspnea, chest discomfort, cough, dysphagia, anorexia, weight loss, and fever. An **asymptomatic** mediastinal mass, however, is discovered on routine chest x-ray in **33–50% of patients.** In advanced disease, recurrent laryngeal and phrenic nerve paralysis as well as superior vena cava syndrome may be present.
      2. **Systemic manifestations.** More than **70% of patients** present with an asso-

ciated autoimmune disease (see p 213, **II.H**); however, hepatomegaly, abdominal masses, bone pain, and neurologic symptoms resulting from metastatic disease are extremely rare.

B. Paraneoplastic syndromes. Although thymomas are associated with numerous autoimmune disorders (see **II.H**), the only true paraneoplastic syndrome that has been reported is myasthenia gravis (see p 213, **II.H.1,** and p 59, **II**).

IV. Differential diagnosis. Many thymomas are discovered as asymptomatic mediastinal masses. The differential diagnosis of these masses depends on their location in the mediastinum. Diagnostic possibilities include the following:

A. Anterosuperior mediastinum (54% adult, 26% pediatric). This portion of the mediastinum extends from the thoracic inlet (superiorly) to the diaphragm (inferiorly) and from the sternum (anteriorly) to the anterior pericardium and great vessels (posteriorly). Lesions in the anterosuperior mediastinum include **congenital abnormalities** (substernal or ectopic **thyroid** in 5%; pericardial fat pads, and cysts in 7%), inflammation and infection (benign lymphadenopathy), **vascular abnormalities** (innominate or subclavian aneurysm or ectasia), **benign neoplasms (parathyroid adenomas,** lipomas, hemangiomas, chondromas, carotid body paragangliomas, lymphangiomas, and myxomas), and **malignancies** (thymic tumors in 30%, teratomas in 18%, and thyroid carcinoma and ["terrible"] lymphomas in 20% as well as lung cancer, rhabdomyosarcoma, thymic carcinoid, and metastatic carcinoma). In addition, **substernal hernia of Morgagni** may be identified as a lower anterior mediastinal mass.

B. Middle mediastinum (20% adult; 11% pediatric). This compartment is bounded by the thoracic inlet (superiorly), the diaphragm (inferiorly), the anterior pericardium and great vessels (anteriorly), and the anterior aspect of the vertebral bodies (posteriorly). Masses in this area may represent **congenital abnormalities** (thoracic duct; bronchogenic, pericardial, and foregut duplication **cysts** in 60%; and epicardial fat pad), **inflammation and infection** (eg, lymphadenopathy from sarcoid, AIDS), **benign neoplasms** (angiomas and lipomas), **malignant neoplasms** (lymphoma in 21%, bronchogenic carcinoma, esophageal carcinoma, tracheal neoplasms, myeloma, or vagal and phrenic nerve tumors), **metastatic carcinoma,** and, in rare cases, **thymoma,** esophageal diverticula, and hiatal hernias.

C. Posterior mediastinum (26% adult, 63% pediatric). This part of the mediastinum stretches from the thoracic inlet (superiorly) to the diaphragm (inferiorly) and from the anterior border of the vertebral bodies (anteriorly) to the costovertebral sulci (posteriorly). Abnormalities in this area may be the result of **congenital abnormalities** (meningoceles or ectopic thyroid as well as thoracic duct, bronchogenic, and foregut duplication cysts in 34%), **inflammation and infection** (paravertebral abscesses), **vascular abnormalities** (aneurysmal dilation of the azygous and hemiazygous veins as well as the descending aorta), **benign neoplasms** (paragangliomas, **neurogenic tumors,** myxomas, chondromas, and lipomas), **malignancies** (neurogenic tumors in 53%; lymphomas, fibrosarcomas, pheochromocytomas, lung cancer, and esophageal carcinoma, and other diseases (esophageal diverticula and hiatal hernias).

V. Screening programs. All patients with a history of myasthenia gravis, red-cell aplasia, and agammaglobulinemia should be screened periodically with CT of the chest; however, because of the low incidence of mediastinal tumors, screening tests, including chest x-ray, are not warranted in the general population.

VI. Diagnostic workup

A. Medical history and physical examination. A complete medical history emphasizing presenting symptoms (eg, dyspnea, chest discomfort, cough) and a thorough physical examination are essential to a complete evaluation.

1. **General appearance.** Evidence for cancer cachexia/anorexia, weight loss, overall energy level, and mental status are important findings.

2. **Eyes.** Ptosis suggests the presence of myasthenia gravis.

3. **Larynx.** Vocal cord paralysis indicating recurrent laryngeal nerve involvement should be excluded in hoarse patients.

4. **Neck.** The presence of a signal node (also called Virchow's or Troisier's node) as well as other masses must be noted.

5. **Lymph nodes.** Diffuse lymphadenopathy must be described in detail and may indicate an infectious etiology or lymphoma.

6. **Chest.** The quality of the breath sounds, the presence of wheezing, and evidence of consolidation, pleural effusions, or both are important indications of ongoing pulmonary disease.

7. **Abdomen.** Mass lesions can be detected in the presence of liver metastases.

In addition, a palpable pulsatile mass may indicate the presence of a thoracoabdominal aneurysm.

8. **Extremities.** Muscle strength and nerve function are important findings to note.

B. **Primary tests and procedures.** All patients with suspected thymomas should have the following diagnostic tests performed.

1. **Blood tests**
   a. Complete blood count (see p 1, **IV.A.1**).
   b. Hepatic transaminases (see p 1, **IV.A.2**).
   c. Alkaline phosphatase (see p 1, **IV.A.3**).
   d. Calcium and phosphorus: Elevated calcium levels and decreased phosphorus levels suggest the presence of a parathyroid adenoma that may be located in the mediastinum.

2. **Imaging studies**
   a. **Chest x-ray.** This simple test is important to localize and characterize mediastinal masses. Additional findings include **linear calcifications,** which are found in 20% of **thymoma capsules;** atelectasis; collapse (bronchial obstruction); rib notching (SVC syndrome); and a high diaphragm (phrenic nerve paralysis). Special oblique or lordotic views may be necessary to view the paramediastinal area.
   b. **Computed tomography.** A CT scan of the chest provides valuable information regarding the size, location, and nature (cystic vs solid) of mediastinal masses, the presence of calcifications, and involvement of contiguous structures. CT is particularly helpful for imaging lesions in the area of the heart and great vessels. Chest CT is indicated in the workup of all patients with mediastinal masses on chest x-ray as well as myasthenia gravis and red-cell aplasia. In addition, chest CT should include the upper abdomen (liver, spleen, and kidneys) to exclude metastatic disease.

C. **Optional tests and procedures.** The following tests and procedures may be indicated on the basis of previous diagnostic findings or clinical suspicion:

1. **Blood tests**
   a. **Nucleotidase** (see p 2, **IV.A.4**).
   b. **GGTP** (see p 2, **IV.A.5**).
   c. **Tumor markers.** Serum levels of alpha-fetoprotein (alpha-FP), beta-human chorionic gonadotropin (beta-hCG), and neuron-specific enolase (NSE) should be measured if a **mediastinal teratoma** or another germ-cell neoplasm is suspected (see also, p 334, **VI.B.1.d**).
   d. **Arterial blood gas (ABG) analysis.** Patients with pulmonary disease may require preoperative ABG to determine whether the patient is a surgical candidate.

2. **Urine tests.** A 24-hour collection of urine measuring epinephrine, norepinephrine, vanillylmandelic acid, and metanephrines must be ordered for patients with significant hypertension or suspicion of **mediastinal pheochromocytoma** (see also, p 462, **VI.B.2.b**).

3. **Pulmonary function tests (PFTs).** The forced vital capacity (FVC) and the forced expiratory volume in 1 second (FEV_1) are commonly measured in patients with myasthenia gravis. These parameters are followed closely postoperatively as a measure of pulmonary function and response to thymectomy.

4. **Imaging studies**
   a. **Barium esophagram.** Radiologic evaluation of the esophagus is indicated if symptoms of dysphagia or odynophagia are present.
   b. **Magnetic resonance imaging.** MRI is superior to chest CT in evaluating **posterior mediastinal neurogenic tumors** to exclude extension into the spinal canal. Furthermore, excellent imaging of vascular structures is achieved without use of IV contrast. Moreover, the mass/liver signal ratio on T_2-weighted spin echo scans can definitely diagnose pheochromocytomas (ratio > 3.0). (See also, p 3, **IV.C.3**, and p 462, **VI.B.3.c**.)
   c. **Pulmonary angiography.** Involvement of the pulmonary arteries, pericardium, and other great vessels may require angiography.
   d. **[125]I thyroid scan.** If a **substernal or ectopic thyroid** is suspected, a ^{125}I thyroid scan (rather than technetium-99m scan because of high mediastinal background counts) is indicated.
   e. **Technetium-99m bone scan** (see p 3, **IV.C.4**).
   f. **[123]Metaiodobenzylguanidine (MIBG) scan.** If pheochromocytoma is suspected and urinary catecholamines and the MRI scan are equivocal, a

MIBG scan may be necessary to exclude this possibility (see also, p 463, **VI.C.2.d**).

5. Invasive procedures

    a. Esophagoscopy. This endoscopic procedure is indicated if esophageal symptoms are present or if esophageal invasion or a primary esophageal carcinoma is suspected.

    b. Bronchoscopy. Symptoms or radiographic indications that suggest bronchogenic carcinoma or bronchial invasion require fiberoptic bronchoscopy.

    c. Bone marrow aspiration. Patients with either suspected **lymphoma or myasthenia gravis with red-cell aplasia** require bone marrow aspiration to exclude malignant involvement and aplastic anemia, respectively.

    d. Mediastinoscopy. In cases of suspected **lymphoma, sarcoidosis,** and unresectable lesions, a limited procedure such as cervical mediastinoscopy may establish the diagnosis. Biopsy of the aortopulmonary and anterior hilar nodes cannot be accomplished with this approach, however, and needle aspiration must precede any biopsy to prevent inadvertent injury to the pulmonary artery, azygous vein, or aorta (see, also, p 194, **VI.C.3.c**).

    e. Anterior parasternal mediastinotomy (Chamberlain procedure). This procedure is indicated in patients with suspected **lymphoma, sarcoidosis,** and unresectable lesions located in the **aortopulmonary window or left anterior pulmonary hilum.** All other patients require thoracotomy for diagnosis and definitive resection (see, also, p 194, **VI.C.3.d**).

    f. Transthoracic percutaneous needle biopsy. TTPNB is indicated in rare patients who are not surgical candidates because of medical contraindications or the presence of extensive, clearly unresectable lesions. TTPNB also is appropriate for patients with suspected metastatic carcinoma before radiation or chemotherapy is initiated.

VII. Pathology

    A. Location. Although thymomas rarely are found in the neck and posterior mediastinum, 95% of them occur in the **anterosuperior mediastinum** between the level of the suprasternal notch and the xiphoid.

    B. Multiplicity. Multiple primary thymomas are extremely rare.

    C. Histology. More than 95% of **thymomas** consist of a **mixture of epithelial cells and lymphocytes,** with pure epithelial tumors constituting less than 5%. Cystic areas (40–60%) and necrosis (25%) may be present in some tumors. Most thymomas (50–70%) are encapsulated neoplasms 5–10 cm in diameter; however, 30–50% are **invasive,** and this distinction is determined best at the time of surgery, not on histologic appearance. Calcium is often present in the capsule, and the presence of tonofibrils, desmosomes, elongated cytoplasmic processes, and Hassall's bodies help distinguish thymoma from lymphoma, seminoma, and small-cell carcinoma. Based on the predominant cell type (> 80% of cells), the following histologic types have been described:

        1. Epithelial predominant (40%). This type consists mainly of epithelial cells and includes the variants: spindle-cell thymoma (22%) and pseudorosette thymoma.

        2. Lymphocytic predominant (23–35%). Most thymomas associated with myasthenia gravis are lymphocytic thymomas, which are associated with a slightly better prognosis.

        3. Mixed lymphoepithelial (25–35%).

    D. Metastatic spread

        1. Modes of spread. Thymoma potentially may spread by 3 different mechanisms:

            a. Direct extension. Direct invasion of contiguous structures is the **most common** mode of spread. Local extension is determined best by the gross findings at the time of surgery.

            b. Lymphatic metastasis. Lymphatic spread is uncommon with all types of thymoma, including lymphocytic predominant.

            c. Hematogenous metastasis. Thymomas rarely spread through blood vessels to distant organs.

        2. Sites of spread. Metastases to the following organs have been reported: liver, bone, kidney, brain, spleen, and colon.

VIII. Staging. Although no formal TNM staging system has been developed by the American Joint Committee on Cancer or the Union Internationale Contre le Cancer, 2 similar staging systems have been proposed.

A. **Bergh staging system**
   1. **Stage I** (40%). Tumor growth within the intact capsule.
   2. **Stage II** (19%). Tumor penetrates the capsule and invades the mediastinal fat tissues.
   3. **Stage III** (41%). Tumor invades contiguous organs, intrathoracic metastases are present, or both.
B. **Japanese staging system**
   1. **Stage I** (40%). Tumor is macroscopically encapsulated and microscopically does not invade the capsule.
   2. **Stage II** (14%). Tumor penetrates the capsule, invades the mediastinal fat or pleura, or both.
      a. **Stage IIa.** Tumor invades the mediastinal fat, the pleura, or both.
      b. **Stage IIb.** Tumor penetrates the capsule.
   3. **Stage III** (34%). Tumor macroscopically invades contiguous organs (pericardium, great vessels, and lung).
   4. **Stage IV.** Pleural, pericardial, or distant metastatic disease is present.
      a. **Stage IVa** (9%). Pleural or pericardial dissemination is present.
      b. **Stage IVb** (3%). Lymphatic or hematogenous metastases are present.
IX. **Treatment**
A. **Surgery**
   1. **Primary thymoma**
      a. **Indications.** Surgery is indicated in all patients with mediastinal masses unless the lesion is clearly unresectable. The **goals are both definitive diagnosis and complete resection.**
      b. **Perioperative management.** Patients with myasthenia gravis pose a special problem in perioperative management. Preoperatively, they should be well controlled on **pyridostigmine** (Mestinon) or **plasmapheresis** should be considered. Intraoperatively, aminoglycoside antibiotics and paralyzing anesthetic agents must be avoided, and "stress doses" of **corticosteroids** (hydrocortisone 100 mg IV) must be administered if the patient has been maintained on prednisone. Postoperatively, the patient can be extubated immediately or within 24–48 hours, depending on pulmonary status, but low levels of intermittent mandatory ventilation for prolonged periods should be avoided because this increases the required respiratory effort and leads to exhaustion. **Pyridostigmine** can be resumed after 12–24 hrs, but at a reduced dose (⅓ to ½ the preoperative dose) because of **increased neuromuscular sensitivity.**
      c. **Approaches.** In general, 2 approaches are used for mediastinal masses.
         (1) **Median sternotomy.** A midline sternum-splitting incision is preferred for most patients with thymomas and other anterosuperior mediastinal masses. Lateral extension may be necessary in selected cases. Patients with myasthenia, in particular, benefit from the reduced pain associated with this approach.
         (2) **Posterolateral thoracotomy.** Lesions of the middle and posterior mediastinum as well as tumors of the anterosuperior mediastinum that invade posteriorly are approached best through a standard posterolateral thoracotomy on the side of the lesion. A cervical approach, however, has also been described.
      d. **Procedures.** Complete thymectomy, including resection of the anterior mediastinal fat pad is the procedure of choice for all patients with thymoma. **Biopsy should be avoided.** Invasive thymomas should be aggressively treated with resection of involved structures if possible, such as the innominate vein, superior vena cava, pericardium, vagus nerve, and lung. In patients with myasthenia, however, the phrenic nerve should be preserved since the resulting pulmonary compromise is often catastrophic.
   2. **Locally advanced and metastatic thymoma.** Subtotal resection of bulky unresectable lesions and removal of pleural and pericardial metastases may be considered, although this is somewhat controversial. Distant metastases almost never require surgery since they occur only in advanced disease and rarely manifest clinically.
   3. **Morbidity and mortality. Pulmonary complications** are the primary source of morbidity and mortality—particularly in patients with myasthenia gravis—and include the following problems: hemorrhage, atelectasis, pulmonary insufficiency, pneumonia, cardiac arrhythmias, and sternal infection.
B. **Radiation therapy**

1. **Primary thymoma.** With the exception of lymphoma, radiation is not indicated for the initial management of patients with mediastinal tumors, including those with thymoma.
2. **Adjuvant radiation therapy**
   a. **Preoperative radiotherapy.** Although no randomized trials or definitive data on preoperative radiotherapy are available, small series suggest that, in general, this approach is not useful, although it may be tried in lesions with borderline resectability.
   b. **Intraoperative radiotherapy.** This unique modality may avoid radiation pneumonitis; however, its usefulness has not been proved, and clinical trials are currently in progress.
   c. **Postoperative radiotherapy.** Postoperative radiation therapy (4500–6000 cGy over 4–6 weeks) is indicated in patients with **invasive thymomas,** regardless of the extent of resection (ie, complete vs incomplete). This **reduces the risk of local recurrence** from 28% to 5%. In addition, patients with persistent symptoms of myasthenia gravis after thymectomy may respond to mediastinal radiation.
3. **Locally advanced and metastatic thymoma.** Palliative radiation therapy (5000–6000 cGy over 5–6 weeks) may provide some benefit. A **median survival rate of 4.1 years** has been reported, and **23% of patients survive for 10 years.**

C. **Chemotherapy**
1. **Primary thymoma.** Currently, chemotherapy plays no role in the initial management of resectable thymoma.
2. **Adjuvant chemotherapy.** The use of chemotherapy in the adjuvant setting has not been studied extensively because of the high success rate of surgery and postoperative radiotherapy.
3. **Locally advanced and metastatic thymoma**
   a. **Single agents.** Although a paucity of information is available on the effectiveness of single cytotoxic agents, the general impression is that cisplatin, doxorubicin, cyclophosphamide, and nitrogen mustard are active as single agents. Furthermore, anecdotal reports indicate that continuous glucocorticoid (prednisone) administration achieves 57% partial and 25% complete (82% overall) responses in patients, many of whom failed to respond to radiation.
   b. **Combination chemotherapy.** Numerous combination chemotherapy regimens, including some known to be effective in lymphomas, have been tried in advanced thymoma. Overall, **cisplatin-based combinations** such as bleomycin, doxorubicin, cisplatin, and prednisone (BAPP) produce a 77–79% response rate, whereas **cyclophosphamide-based regimens** such as cyclophosphamide, vincristine, procarbazine, and prednisone (COPP) yield a 67–75% response rate. The true value of chemotherapy in thymoma, however, remains to be defined by prospective randomized trials.

D. **Immunotherapy.** Although lymphocytes constitute a significant portion of most thymomas (95%), immunotherapy has not been explored in these patients.

X. **Prognosis**
A. **Risk of recurrence.** The risk of recurrence for encapsulated thymomas is low (2–6%), whereas the risk for **invasive thymomas** is 28–36% without and 5% with postoperative radiotherapy.
B. **Five-year survival.** The 5- and 10-year survival rates for encapsulated and invasive thymoma are 84% and 80% and 52% and 35%, respectively. In addition, the 10-year survival for invasive thymoma associated with myasthenia is only 8.7%.
C. **Adverse prognostic factors.** The following tumor and patient characteristics are associated with a poor prognosis:
   1. **Symptoms of myasthenia gravis.** This has been questioned by recent data.
   2. **Mixed or epithelial histology.**
   3. **Capsular invasion.**

XI. **Patient follow-up**
A. **General guidelines.** To exclude evidence of recurrence, patients should be followed closely every 3 months for the first 2 years, every 6 months for an additional 3 years, and then annually.
B. **Routine evaluation.** Each clinic visit should include the following examinations:
   1. **Medical history and physical examination.** An interim medical history and complete physical examination with particular attention focused on the areas should be performed at each clinic visit (see p 214, **VI.A**).

      2. **Blood tests** (see p 1, **IV.A**)
         a. Complete blood count.
         b. Hepatic transaminases.
         c. Alkaline phosphatase.
      3. **Chest x-ray.** A chest x-ray may detect local recurrences, second primary tumors, pleural effusions, atelectasis, and bony metastases in the ribs and vertebral bodies.
   C. Additional evaluation. Other tests and procedures that are indicated at regular intervals include a **computed tomography (CT) scan of the chest.** These scans are useful to exclude local recurrences or intrathoracic metastatic disease. In addition, chest CT scans should include the liver, spleen, and kidneys to evaluate these two common sites of metastases. These scans should be obtained every 6–12 months to detect early recurrence that may benefit from palliative radiation, chemotherapy, or both.
   D. Optional evaluation. The following tests and procedures may be indicated based on previous diagnostic findings or clinical suspicion.
      1. **Blood tests** (see p 2, **IV.A**)
         a. Nucleotidase.
         b. GGTP.
      2. **Imaging studies** (see p 3, **IV.C**)
         a. Magnetic resonance imaging.
         b. Technetium-99m bone scan.
      3. **Biopsy.** Fine needle aspiration of new mediastinal masses to exclude recurrent disease requiring radiation, chemotherapy, or both, should be considered.

REFERENCES

Almog C, Horowitz M, Burke M: Steroid therapy in inappropriate secretion of anti-diuretic hormone due to malignant thymoma. *Respiration* 1983;**44**:382–386.

Ariaratnam LS et al: The management of malignant thymoma with radiation therapy. *Int J Radiat Oncol Biol Phys* 1979;**5**:77–80.

Batata MA et al: Thymomas: clinicopathologic features, therapy and prognosis. *Cancer* 1974;**34**:389–396.

Bergh NP et al: Tumors of the thymus and thymic region: I. clinicopathological studies on thymomas. *Ann Thorac Surg* 1978;**25**:91–98.

Bernatz et al: Thymoma: factors influencing prognosis. *Surg Clin North Am* 1973;**53**:885–892.

Chahinian AP et al: Treatment of invasive or metastatic thymoma: report of eleven cases. *Cancer* 1981;**47**:1752–1761.

Evans WK et al: Combination chemotherapy in invasive thymoma: role of COPP. *Cancer* 1980;**46**:1523–1527.

Hu E, Levine J: Chemotherapy of malignant thymoma: a case report and review of the literature. *Cancer* 1986;**57**:1101–1104.

McKenna WG et al: Malignancies of the thymus. In: Roth JA, Ruckdeschel JC, Weisenburger TH (editors), *Thoracic Oncology*. Philadelphia, PA: WB Saunders; 1989:466–477.

Mulder DG, Haskell CM: Mediastinal tumors. In: Haskell CM (editor). *Cancer Treatment*. Philadelphia, PA: WB Saunders; 1990:192–205.

Phillips TL, Bushke F: The role of radiation therapy in myasthenia gravis. *Calif Med* 1967;**106**:282–289.

Rosenberg JC: Neoplasms of the mediastinum. In: DeVita VT, Hellman S, Rosenberg SA (editors), *Cancer: Principles and Practice of Oncology*. 3rd ed. Philadelphia, PA: JB Lippincott; 1989:706–724.

30 Malignancies of the Esophagus

Robert B. Cameron, MD

I. **Epidemiology.** Esophageal carcinoma is an uncommon malignancy in the United States; it constitutes only 1.0% of all cancers and 1.9% of all cancer deaths, excluding skin cancer. In 1985, 6.3 cases per 100,000 males and 1.9 cases per 100,000 females were diagnosed, resulting in 5.7 and 1.4 deaths, respectively. Estimates indicate that **11,300 new cases and 10,200 deaths will occur** in 1993 in the **United States.** The worldwide incidence of esophageal cancer varies tremendously. In China, for example, mortality rates as high as 436 per 100,000 males and 22.5 per 100,000 females have been reported in Honan Province, whereas mortality rates in Yunan Province were only 1.4 and 0.7 per 100,000 males and females. Furthermore, in South Africa the incidence among black males age 35–64 is 246 per 100,000, compared with a rate of only 3 per 100,000 in West Africa. A distinct **esophageal "cancer belt"** extends from northern Iran and the Caspian Sea through central Asia to Mongolia and northern China. Other areas of high incidence include France, Switzerland, Finland, Iceland, and Puerto Rico. Low incidence rates are found in Great Britain, Scandinavia, and Australia.

II. **Risk Factors**

A. **Age.** Esophageal carcinoma is rare before age 40 and increases from fewer than 3 cases per 100,000 at age 50 to a **peak of 20.4 per 100,000** between the ages of 75 and 79.

B. **Sex.** Males are at greater risk than females for esophageal cancer. The increased risk varies from 9 times greater in South Africa to only 1.7 times greater in Iran. In the United States, the risk is **3.3 times greater for males** than for females.

C. **Race.** In the United States, the risk is **3.4 times greater for blacks** than for whites regardless of sex.

D. **Genetic factors**
   1. **Family history.** First-degree relatives are not at increased risk.
   2. **Familial syndromes. Tylosis palmaris et plantaris** is a syndrome consisting of hyperkeratosis of the palms and soles and papillomata of the esophagus. This autosomal dominant syndrome carries a 40–70% lifetime risk of esophageal cancer.

E. **Diet**
   1. **Alcohol consumption.** Alcohol increases the risk of esophageal cancer, especially when it is in home-brewed beverages made from maize, as noted in Bantu, Africa, or when it is used in conjunction with **tobacco smoking.**
   2. **Nitrosamine compounds.** An association between esophageal cancer and nitrosamine compounds was identified in Linhsien County, Honan Province, China. In this area, both people and chickens have a high incidence of esophageal carcinoma related to high levels of these compounds in the food.
   3. **Croton flaveus.** When eaten or used to brew tea, leaves from this shrub increase the risk of esophageal cancer. This was noted in the population of Curacao, where such practices are common.
   4. **Betel nuts.** In India consumption of these nuts is known to be associated with a greater incidence of esophageal carcinoma.
   5. **Thermal injury.** Drinking hot tea may increase the risk of esophageal cancer, but the evidence has not been convincing.

F. **Smoking**
   1. **Tobacco.** Cigarette smoking, especially when **combined with alcohol,** greatly increases the risk of esophageal carcinoma.
   2. **Bidi smoking.** This Indian cigarette also is associated with an increased risk of esophageal malignancies.
   3. **Opium consumption.** In Afghanistan the practice of eating residue from opium pipes has been linked to a high incidence of esophageal cancer.

G. **History of previous esophageal pathology**

1. **Inflammatory conditions**
   a. **Lye esophagitis.** Patients with this condition have been reported to carry a 5–30% lifetime risk of esophageal cancer.
   b. **Peptic esophagitis.** Chronic irritation caused by reflux of gastric acid is associated with a 1% lifetime risk of esophageal carcinoma. If peptic esophagitis is associated with a **short esophagus,** the risk can be as high as 5%.
   c. **Barrett's esophagus.** The existence of columnar epithelium in the lower esophagus, known as Barrett's esophagus, is associated with chronic inflammation, metaplasia, and an increased risk of adenocarcinoma. Some, however, consider this to be a neoplasm of ectopic gastric mucosa rather than a malignancy of the esophagus.
   d. **Plummer-Vinson syndrome.** This syndrome of **sideropenic anemia, atrophic glossitis, esophagitis, and dysphagia** is more common among females than males and is associated with a **10–16%** lifetime risk of esophageal malignancies.
2. **Anatomic abnormalities**
   a. **Achalasia.** As many as 2–7% of patients with a 25-year history of achalasia develop esophageal carcinoma. This may be the result of chronic inflammation in the dilated proximal esophagus.
   b. **Esophageal webs.** These uncommon abnormalities are associated with a risk of esophageal carcinoma as high as **20%.**
   c. **Epiphrenic diverticula.** An increased risk of cancer in patients with esophageal diverticula has been reported.
   H. **Urbanization.** The risk of esophageal malignancies is greater for urban dwellers than for the rural population. **Bartenders, waiters, and construction** workers are specifically at high risk, probably because of exposure to common risk factors such as tobacco smoke and alcohol.
III. **Clinical presentation**
   A. **Signs and symptoms.** Signs and symptoms of malignant esophageal disease are often subtle and insidious. Frequently, an obvious problem develops before a patient realizes the chronic nature of his or her symptoms.
      1. **Local manifestations.** The most common presenting local symptom of esophageal carcinoma is **dysphagia** (90%). Patients with esophageal cancer typically present with progressive dysphagia, initially for solids but eventually for liquids as well. Other common local signs and symptoms are **odynophagia** (50%), regurgitation, hematemesis, hemoptysis or cough (tracheoesophageal fistula), melena (10%), dysphonia (recurrent laryngeal nerve involvement), edema of the upper torso and extremities (superior vena cava obstruction), aspiration pneumonia, and shortness of breath (phrenic nerve and diaphragmatic paralysis).
      2. **Systemic manifestations.** General signs and symptoms commonly identified at presentation are **weight loss** (90%), pleural effusions, cervical adenopathy, Horner's syndrome (miosis, ptosis, and anhydrosis), bony pain (bony metastases), hepatomegaly (liver metastases), and ascites (alcoholic cirrhosis).
   B. **Paraneoplastic syndromes.** Esophageal cancer may present with one of the following paraneoplastic syndromes as the only manifestation of disease:
      1. **Hypercalcemia** (see p 87).
      2. **Inappropriate ACTH** (see p 90).
      3. **Inappropriate gonadotropins** (see p 117).
IV. **Differential diagnosis.** Although progressive dysphagia in an elderly patient is highly suggestive of esophageal carcinoma the following also should be considered: **vascular abnormalities** (thoracic aneurysms and an aberrant right subclavian artery or **dysphagia lusoria**), **inflammatory strictures** (lye and peptic), and **anatomic abnormalities** (achalasia and esophageal webs), infections (tuberculosis, pemphigus, syphilis, and acute viral laryngitis), **neurologic diseases** (bulbar paralysis, syphilitic medullary degeneration, hysteria, and anterior poliomyelitis), **neuromuscular disorders** (botulism and myasthenia), and **poisonings** (lead, alcohol, and fluoride).
V. **Screening programs.** Screening programs for esophageal cancer have not been actively developed in the United States because of its low incidence of esophageal cancer. However, in areas of high prevalence, such as Linhsien County, China, attempts have been made to screen the general population. **Annual esophageal brushings** are obtained with a brush that is swallowed and then retrieved with an attached string. This approach has had good success, with an accuracy of 80–90% and a **cure rate approaching 90%** because of the large number of limited early tumors found.
VI. **Diagnostic work-up**

A. Physical examination. In addition to a thorough medical history documenting risk factors as well as signs and symptoms of esophageal disease, a complete physical examination should be performed, with particular attention paid to the following areas:

1. **General appearance.** An assessment of the general functional and nutritional status should be made (see p 1, **I, III**).
2. **Skin.** The palms and soles should be examined for evidence of hyperkeratosis suggesting **tylosis palmaris et plantaris.**
3. **Lymph nodes.** The presence of a signal node (also referred to as Virchow's or Troisier's node) may be associated with esophageal carcinoma in rare cases.
4. **Abdomen.** The liver should be examined for hepatomegaly because of distant metastases. Ascites and splenomegaly indicating cirrhosis are often found in patients with esophageal cancer resulting from a common risk factor (alcohol).
5. **Rectum.** A stool specimen should be examined for occult blood.

B. Primary tests and procedures. The following diagnostic tests and procedures should be performed initially in all patients with suspected esophageal carcinoma.

1. **Blood tests** (see p 1, **IV.A**).
   a. Complete blood count.
   b. Hepatic transaminases.
   c. Alkaline phosphatase.
   d. Albumin.
2. **Imaging studies**
   a. Chest x-ray (see p 3, **IV.C.**).
   b. Barium swallow esophagography. In patients with malignant disease, barium swallow esophagography demonstrates an intraluminal mass or abrupt irregular strictures larger than 20 mm that are usually diagnostic of cancer, whereas benign strictures are usually smaller than 20 mm with gradually tapering ends. Small lesions (< 3.5 cm) may escape detection as often as 40% of the time.
3. **Esophagogastroscopy with biopsy.** This procedure is the primary method of establishing a definitive (tissue) diagnosis. Flexible endoscopes are generally used, but documenting malignant disease on biopsy may be difficult because of submucosal spread of tumor. In such circumstances, an examination with a rigid esophagoscope for further multiple deep biopsies may be needed.

C. Optional tests and procedures. The following tests and procedures may be indicated by either previous diagnostic findings or clinical suspicion to (1) assess the extent and resectability of the primary tumor, (2) evaluate metastatic spread, (3) exclude other associated malignancies, or (4) evaluate associated complications of esophageal cancer.

1. **Blood tests**
   a. Nucleotidase (see p 2, **IV.A.4**)
   b. GGTP (see p 2, **IV.A.5**).
   c. Calcium (see p. 87).
   d. Cortisol (see p 90).
   e. Gonadotropins (see p 117).
2. **Imaging studies**
   a. **Computed tomography**
      (1) **Chest CT.** A CT scan of the chest is the best imaging technique for evaluating the extent of the primary tumor, mediastinal nodal metastases, and pulmonary metastases and can reliably predict resectability. Yet, 10–20% of **lesions deemed unresectable** by CT scan because of contiguous organ invasion **are actually resectable.** Therefore, these findings should not preclude operation.
      (2) **Abdominal CT.** A CT scan of the abdomen can be used to assess metastatic involvement of the celiac nodes and liver.
   b. **Magnetic resonance imaging** (see p 3, **IV.C.**).
   c. **Hepatic ultrasound** (see p 3, **IV.C.**).
   d. **Technetium-99m bone scan** (see p 3, **IV.C.**).
3. **Invasive procedures.** The following invasive procedures may be required in the workup of patients with esophageal cancer:
   a. **Laryngoscopy.** This procedure is reserved for documenting suspected vocal cord paralysis and ruling out other associated malignancies such as laryngeal carcinoma.

b. **Bronchoscopy.** The possibility of tracheal extension and coexisting lung cancer should be evaluated with this procedure.

VII. Pathology

A. **Location.** The frequency of carcinomas occurring in various segments of the esophagus can be summarized as follows: **upper third,** 10–20%; **middle third,** 50%; and **lower third,** 30–40%.

B. **Multiplicity.** Synchronous esophageal "skip" lesions can be found **up to 8 cm** from a primary tumor because of submucosal lymphatic spread. In addition, there is a relatively high incidence of **synchronous** (1–3%) or **metachronous** (4–9%) associated primary malignancies (pharynx, oral cavity, larynx, and lung), which are probably related to common risk factors.

C. **Histology.** A wide variety of epithelial, nonepithelial, and metastatic lesions can involve the esophagus. Some of these histologic types are summarized in Table 30–1.

D. **Metastatic spread**

1. **Modes of spread.** Esophageal carcinoma can spread via three distinct mechanisms:

   a. **Direct extension.** Because of the absence of a serosa and the proximity of other vital structures, direct growth into contiguous structures, including trachea, aorta, diaphragm, pericardium, pleura, lung, and mediastinal nerves, occurs in many lesions.

   b. **Lymphatic metastasis.** Interconnected longitudinal submucosal and muscular lymphatics provide a fertile route for spread to internal jugular, cervical, supraclavicular, paratracheal, hilar, subcarinal, paraesophageal, paraortic, gastric, and celiac nodes.

   c. **Hematogenous metastasis.** Spread through systemic and portal vessels results in metastases to a wide variety of organs.

2. **Sites of metastatic spread.** Esophageal cancer often metastasizes to at least one of the following sites:

   a. **Regional lymph nodes.** The most commonly involved draining lymph nodes are the celiac nodes. The incidence of celiac lymph node metastases varies with the involved segment of esophagus: **upper third lesions,** celiac involvement in 10%; **middle third lesions,** celiac involvement in 44%; and **lower third lesions,** celiac involvement in more than 50%.

   b. **Liver,** 32%.

   c. **Lung,** 21%.

   d. **Bone,** 1%.

   e. **Pleura,** 1%.

   f. **Kidney,** 1%.

   g. **Central nervous system,** 1%.

TABLE 30–1. HISTOLOGIC CLASSIFICATION OF ESOPHAGEAL MALIGNANCIES[a]

Epithelial Malignancies (%)		Nonepithelial Malignancies (%)		Metastatic Malignancies (%)	
Squamous cell carcinoma	96	Leiomyosarcoma	< 1	Lesions from other primaries	< 1
Squamous cell variants		Rhabdomyosarcoma	< 1		
Spindlecell carcinoma	< 1	Fibrosarcoma	< 1		
Carcinosarcoma	< 1	Coriocarcinoma	< 1		
Verrucouscarcinoma	< 1	Malignant melenoma	< 1		
Carcinoma in situ	< 1				
Adenocarcinoma	< 2				
Adenoid cystic carcinoma	< 1				
Mucospidermoid carcinoma	< 1				
Carcinoid	< 1				
Undifferentiated carcinoma	< 1				

[a] Adapted from DeVita V, Hellman S, Rosenberg S: *Cancer: Principles and Practice of Oncology.* Philadelphia, PA: JB Lippincott; 1989:726, with permission.

VIII. Staging. In 1987 the American Joint Committee on Cancer and the Union Internationale Contre le Cancer published a unified staging system for esophageal carcinoma. Although not an integral part of the staging system, the committees divided the esophagus into 4 regions. These regions and the TNM staging system are listed below:

A. Esophageal regions
1. **Cervical esophagus.** This portion begins at the **cricoid cartilage** and ends **18 cm from the incisors** at the thoracic inlet (suprasternal notch).
2. **Thoracic esophagus.** The thoracic esophagus is further subdivided into 3 regions:
   a. **Upper thoracic esophagus.** This portion extends from the **thoracic inlet** to the **tracheal bifurcation** 24 cm from the incisors.
   b. **Midthoracic esophagus.** Extending from the **tracheal bifurcation** half the distance to the gastroesophageal junction, this portion ends at a distance of **32 cm from the incisors.**
   c. **Lower thoracic esophagus.** This segment spans from midway between the tracheal bifurcation and the gastroesophageal junction to the gastroesophageal junction itself, ending **40 cm from the incisors.**

B. Tumor stage
1. **TX.** Primary tumor cannot be assessed.
2. **T0.** No primary tumor is present.
3. **T1s.** Carcinoma in situ.
4. **T1.** Tumor invades the lamina propria or submucosa.
5. **T2.** Tumor invades the muscularis propria.
6. **T3.** Tumor invades the adventitia.
7. **T4.** Tumor invades adjacent structures.

C. Lymph node stage
1. **NX.** Regional lymph nodes are not assessed.
2. **N0.** No regional nodal involvement is present.
3. **N1.** Regional lymph node involvement is present.
   Note: For cervical lesions, cervical, internal jugular, superior mediastinal, periesophageal, and supraclavicular nodes are considered regional nodes. In upper and midthoracic lesions, regional nodes include internal jugular, tracheobronchial, peritracheal, carinal, hilar, posterior mediastinal, periesophageal, and perigastric. For lower thoracic lesions, posterior mediastinal, lesser curvature, perigastric, cardiac, and left gastric nodes are considered regional. All other nodes are considered distant metastases.

D. Metastatic stage
1. **MX.** Presence of distant metastases not assessed.
2. **M0.** No distant metastases are present.
3. **M1.** Distant metastases are present.

E. Histopathologic grade
1. **GX.** Grade cannot be assessed.
2. **G1.** Well differentiated.
3. **G2.** Moderately-well differentiated.
4. **G3.** Poorly differentiated.
5. **G4.** Undifferentiated.

F. Stage groups
1. **Stage 0.** Tis, N0, M0.
2. **Stage I.** T1, N0, M0.
3. **Stage IIA.** T2 or 3, N0, M0.
4. **Stage IIB.** T1 or 2, N1, M0.
5. **Stage III.** T3, N1, M0 or T4; any N, M0.
6. **Stage IV.** Any T; any N, M1.

IX. Treatment

A. Surgery
1. **Resectable primary esophageal carcinoma.** As with most gastrointestinal cancers, the only true curative therapy for esophageal carcinoma is surgery. In the United States, however, most lesions present at an advanced stage so that **palliation of esophageal obstruction** is the major concern. Because of coexisting chronic pulmonary, vascular, and liver diseases from previous heavy use of alcohol and tobacco and malnutrition from esophageal obstruction, **only 50% of patients are candidates for surgery.** However, as many as 87% of all explored patients are resectable for either cure or, more commonly, palliation. Because surgical palliation of obstructive symptoms is successful in as many as 93% of resected patients and is **superior to other forms of palliation,**

every attempt should be made to resect the primary lesion even when the likelihood of cure is low.

a. **Indications.** Generally, resection for either cure or palliation is indicated in anyone with esophageal carcinoma even in the presence of metastatic disease.

b. **Contraindications.** Contraindications to operation include:

   (1) **Direct invasion of contiguous vital structures:** ie, the trachea, spine, or great vessels.

   (2) **Fixed cervical lymph node metastases** (with cervical lesions).

   (3) **Widespread metastases,** with an expected survival of less than 6 weeks.

   (4) **Expected high operative mortality from pulmonary disease,** with minimal reserve (FEV1 < 1.0); cardiac disease, with little or no reserve (ejection fraction < 40% or one that decreases with exercise), and general nutritional debility.

   Note: Advanced age alone is not an absolute contraindication for surgical resection.

c. **Surgical approaches.** Surgical approaches generally fall into one of four distinct categories, each with specific advantages.

   (1) **Left thoracoabdominal incision (Sweet approach).** This is an excellent approach for **lower thoracic and GE junctional lesions.** However, when dissection needs to be carried into the upper thorax, the aortic arch obscures vision and hampers dissection. The division or ribs and cartilage is also painful.

   (2) **Right thoracotomy/laparotomy (Lewis approach).** This is a common approach involving an **initial laparotomy** for assessment of celiac and other intraabdominal lymph nodes as well as abdominal viscera. If widespread distant metastases are not present, the lower esophagus and stomach are isolated and mobilized. Following division, the stomach is passed into the right chest and the laparotomy incision is closed. A **separate posterolateral thoracotomy** is then required for resection of the thoracic esophagus and anastomosis of the cervical or upper thoracic esophagus to the stomach (or colon, if an interposition segment is used). A modification introduced by Fisher utilizes an anterolateral thoracotomy for **simultaneous thoracic and abdominal dissection.** However, dissection of the lower esophagus is more difficult with this approach.

   (3) **Right thoracotomy alone (Belsey approach).** Esophagectomy with esophagogastrostomy is performed by sequential ligation of gastric vessels through the esophageal hiatus. Although this technique affords good exposure for thoracic anastomoses, no abdominal lymph node dissection can be performed. Thus, its use is limited to the setting of palliative resections.

   (4) **Laparotomy and cervical incision (Turner approach).** This **transhiatal method** is used extensively for benign disease, but because of the frequent palliative nature of resections, this approach has been proposed for use in malignant disease as well. A laparotomy is combined with a neck incision. Dissection of the thoracic esophagus is performed blindly. This blunt dissection does not achieve wide margins on the tumor, but it does avoid the necessity of a thoracotomy and its accompanying pain. Such an approach, however, cannot be performed in the presence of **tracheobronchial, great vessel, or pericardial involvement.** Some surgeons claim that the results are similar to transthoracic approaches, but this is controversial.

d. **Procedures.** The type of procedure necessary is dictated, in part, by the location of the primary tumor. Lesions of the cervical esophagus require a slightly different approach than do thoracic lesions. Almost all procedures require a **gastric drainage procedure,** either **pyloroplasty or pyloromyotomy.** Yet some surgeons believe that drainage procedures are not absolutely necessary.

   (1) **Cervical esophagus.** Lesions located in the cervical esophagus act more like head and neck tumors than gastrointestinal malignancies. They directly invade vital structures early in their course, often precluding resection, and they metastasize to cervical rather than thoracic and abdominal, lymph nodes. In many instances, resection is possible ei-

ther initially or after radiation therapy and is associated with a slightly **longer survival** (15 vs 9 months) and an improved quality of life. Morbidity from the procedure, however, can be great because resection almost always includes total esophagectomy, pharyngectomy, laryngectomy, tracheal resection, bilateral modified radical neck dissections, and, occasionally, mediastinal tracheostomy (after resection of the manubrium and both clavicular heads). Head and neck, thoracic, plastic, and general surgeons are frequently required for successful resection and reconstruction.

   (2) Thoracic esophagus. Because of the potential for distant spread of tumor in the esophageal lymphatics, **subtotal or total esophagectomy rather than segmental resection** should be performed. Although some surgeons favor more radical procedures involving mediastinal and abdominal lymph node dissections for thoracic lesions, they generally only increase the morbidity and mortality of the procedure and do not improve survival. The overall 5-year survival rate in the United States remains 6.2% despite attempts at curative resection. However, in Asia, where screening programs have increased the number of early carcinomas detected, a higher success rate has been attained. Overall 5-year survival as high as 34.6% has been reported with radical esophagectomy in Japan.

e. Reconstruction. There are several methods of reestablishing gastrointestinal continuity after esophageal resection.

   (1) Esophagogastrostomy. The stomach can be used as a conduit for as many as 93% of cases of thoracic esophageal resection. Occasionally, it also is appropriate for cervical lesions, although colon interposition, gastric tubes, musculocutaneous flaps, jejunal grafts, and other less successful techniques are often used in these situations.

      (a) Cervical anastomosis. Cervical anastomosis of the stomach and esophageal remnant is a **safer** procedure than thoracic anastomosis because leaks are limited to subcutaneous tissues, are detected earlier, and are easily drained. However, not all gastric remnants can be mobilized enough to reach the cervical esophagus.

      (b) Thoracic anastomosis. Intrathoracic anastomoses are more difficult to manage if such complications occur as anastomotic leakage, which then necessitates drainage of the entire involved hemithorax. Some surgeons believe that tacking the gastric serosa to the prevertebral fascia reduces anastomotic tension and the complication rate; however, this has not been subjected to critical study.

   (2) Colon interposition. Although the gastric remnant is used in the majority of cases, segments of colon offer an alternate method of reestablishing gastrointestinal continuity. Both iso- and antiperistaltic segments have been used without any clear benefit. The preoperative evaluation in patients considered for these types of reconstruction must include a barium enema, mesenteric angiography, and an adequate antibiotic-based bowel preparation (see p 277, **I.A.2.**).

      (a) Left colon. Left colonic segments are usually longer, better vascularized, and closer in diameter to the esophagus, which makes them more popular. An antiperistaltic position is most commonly used.

      (b) Right colon. Right colonic segments also are frequently used. These segments can be placed in an isoperistaltic position, and an intact ileocecal valve can theoretically decrease the incidence of reflux. These segments can be limited by the length of the blood supply, however.

      (c) Transverse colon. This segment of bowel is a rare source of interposition grafts but is used on occasion for this purpose if the left and right colon segments are not acceptable.

   (3) Reversed gastric tube. This is created by constructing a tube the length and size of the normal esophagus from the **greater curvature of the stomach.** The tube remains attached to the stomach at the fundus, and the **antral end** is anastomosed to the cervical esophagus.

   (4) Jejunal interposition. A loop of jejunum is interposed, with or without constructing a pouch, in the same manner as a colon interposition.

f. **Mortality and morbidity.** The mortality rate from esophageal surgery ranges from 1.4% to 37.5%. The mortality and morbidity rates depend on the location and size of the primary lesion and the type of resection and reconstruction used. Many complications are associated with esophageal resection, including the following: **anastomotic problems** (leaks and strictures); **respiratory insufficiency** from preexisting pulmonary disease or esophageal reflux and chronic aspiration; **dysphagia; wound infection; hemorrhage; subphrenic abscess; obstruction** at the esophageal hiatus; and **torsion, gangrene, or rupture of the neoesophagus.**

2. **Locally advanced esophageal carcinoma.** Esophageal lesions that are not resected due to various factors (see above, **IX.A.1.b**) lead to esophageal obstruction. Although a number of approaches for palliation of symptomatic obstruction are available, none of them consistently produce satisfactory results.

a. **Gastrostomy and cervical esophagostomy.** Palliation with these two procedures is rarely indicated because cervical esophagostomy produces an unsightly and cumbersome fistula and gastrostomy merely serves to prolong the patient's suffering.

b. **Bypass.** Intra- or extrathoracic gastric or colonic bypass of an unresectable esophageal lesion can be considered in certain situations. If this option is used, some form of **drainage of the excluded esophagus** must be established because peristalsis and mucous secretion continue, ultimately resulting in staple-line disruption and abscess formation. A **tracheoesophageal fistula** can serve as the site of drainage in patients with this problem. Bypass procedures carry a 7–42% mortality rate.

c. **Intraluminal intubation.** Tubes designed to maintain esophageal patency may be the only option in patients who are unable to tolerate extensive surgical procedures. These esophageal tubes provide limited palliation with significant risk.

(1) **Types of tubes.** Esophageal tubes fall into one of two categories. The first type, the **"pull-through" tube,** requires endoscopic or surgical placement of a guide wire and includes Celestin, Mousseau-Barbin, Fell, and Haering tubes. A second type, **"push-through" tubes,** relies on blind passage and includes Mackler and Stoutter tubes.

(2) **Mortality and morbidity.** Intraluminal intubation is associated with a significant mortality of 10–40%. Many complications can occur, including **obstruction** by food, **migration, perforation** with mediastinitis, and **aspiration pneumonia** caused by regurgitation of stomach contents through the tube. In addition, palliation is only slight with 60–90% of patients tolerating a semisolid diet after intubation.

d. **Esophageal dilation.** Dilation of a malignant stricture can be accomplished, often without undue morbidity if dilation is done **slowly** over a period of days to weeks. Most people do not experience dysphagia until the esophageal diameter is **less than 12 mm.** To prevent this, the esophagus is dilated to **17 mm** (50 French) in increments of no more than 3 sizes during one session. Like intraluminal tubes, 2 types of dilators exist: those that require guide wires (eg, Eder-Preston and Savary dilators) and those that do not (eg, Maloney Bougies).

e. **Laser therapy.** The neodymium yttrium-aluminum-garnet (Nd-YAG) laser has been used recently to palliate malignant esophageal obstruction. Successful increases in lumen diameter (to as large as 16 mm) after 3 **laser treatments** have been reported in 80% of patients. Exophytic lesions respond better, and palliation lasts 8–10 weeks without further treatment.

3. **Metastatic esophageal carcinoma.** Except for palliative resection of primary esophageal carcinoma, surgery in patients with metastatic esophageal cancer should be avoided. Gastric and jejunal feeding tubes should not be placed merely to prolong life.

B. **Radiation**

1. **Primary esophageal carcinoma.** Radiation therapy for possible cure is indicated for the rare patient who has unresectable lesions **less than 5 cm in length** and **no distant metastases** or **tracheoesophageal fistulae.** Patients with resectable lesions who are poor surgical candidates or who refuse surgery also should be considered for curative radiation. Typically, 5000–7000 cGy are delivered over a period of 4–7 weeks. Despite radiation's curative potential, however, good **local control** of tumor growth is achieved in only 20–50% of patients, and patients rarely survive 5 years.

2. **Adjuvant radiation therapy**
    a. **Preoperative radiation therapy.** Preoperative radiation therapy commonly consists of 4000 cGy delivered over 4 weeks with a 4–6 week waiting period before surgery. Initially, an increase from 58% to 79% in the resectability rate was claimed; however, 3 recent randomized prospective trials have failed to substantiate this. Most studies also indicate that **no difference in operative mortality or morbidity** exists despite caution expressed about performing an anastomosis in an irradiated field. Although one prospective randomized study noted a statistically significant increase in 5-year survival from 25% to 45.5% for patients with midthoracic lesions (Huang et al, 1986), 2 other prospective randomized studies indicate that overall survival is unaffected.
    b. **Intraoperative radiation therapy (IORT).** Intraoperative radiation with dosages of 1500–3500 cGy delivered by electron beam to nodal beds has been proposed, but its benefit has not been proved. No randomized studies have been performed, and animal data is scarce.
    c. **Postoperative radiation therapy.** Radiation therapy is indicated if **gross or microscopic tumor remains, lymph nodes are involved, or the chance of recurrence is deemed to be high.** Radiation doses of 4500–4800 cGy are limited by the presence of stomach, colon, lung, heart, and spinal cord in the radiation field. Mediastinal and neck recurrences can be decreased with postoperative radiation and, if no lymph node metastases are present, **survival** can be improved from 16% to 35% (Kasai, Mori, & Watanabe, 1978). Yet, in the presence of lymph node or distant metastases, no survival benefit has been demonstrated.
3. **Locally advanced and metastatic esophageal cancer.** Radiation therapy for palliation of symptoms is indicated for patients with unresectable lesions larger than 5 cm or those who have distant metastases. Generally, 4500–4800 cGy are given over 4–6 weeks, and as many as 75% of patients attain **good short-term symptomatic relief;** however, 11% achieve no palliation. Patients with tumor invading the tracheobronchial tree are not good candidates for radiation because radiation may hasten the development of a fistula. Even in patients without tracheobronchial encroachment, **fistulae** develop in 5–18% of them during therapy. Radiation sensitizing drugs such as misonidazole and a nitroimadazole derivative, SR–2508, have not improved the response rate attained with radiation alone.
4. **Complications of radiation therapy.** Complications from radiation therapy occur to some extent in nearly every patient. The following are some of the more frequent problems: **odynophagia or dysphagia;** esophagitis, esophageal hemorrhage, or stricture; pericarditis and pericardial tamponade; radiation pneumonitis and fibrosis; transverse myelitis with doses higher than 5000 cGy; and **fistulae.**

C. **Chemotherapy**
1. **Primary esophageal carcinoma.** Because surgery and radiation therapy are usually used to treat primary esophageal carcinoma, limited data exists on the use of chemotherapy in this setting. Although information extrapolated from other studies suggests that 50% of patients may respond to chemotherapy, this form of therapy cannot currently be recommended.
2. **Adjuvant chemotherapy**
    a. **Preoperative chemotherapy.** Studies of preoperative therapy with various combinations of bleomycin, cisplatin, fluorouracil, vindesine, and mitoguazone have documented **response rates** of 14–76%, with 0–9% complete responses and median survivals of 8.5–17.6 months. A single randomized trial with bleomycin, cisplatin, and vindesine, however, failed to demonstrate a difference in resectability or survival.
    b. **Postoperative chemotherapy.** Little information is available on the use of postoperative chemotherapy in patients resected for cure. Until sound data are available, this form of treatment cannot be recommended.
3. **Locally advanced and metastatic esophageal cancer**
    a. **Single agents.** Ten chemotherapeutic agents, including bleomycin, cisplatin, fluorouracil, mitomycin-C, etoposide, mitoquazone, and vindesine, have demonstrated 6–48% **response rates as single agents. Symptomatic relief of dysphagia** was attained in 35–73%. No single agent has proved to be consistently superior to other agents.
    b. **Combination chemotherapy.** When combinations of 2 or more of the

above agents are used, **response rates** of 26–63% with a duration of 3.5–7.5 months can be expected. The highest response rates (40–63%) are obtained with combinations of cisplatin and mitoquazone. At present, however, no evidence exists for a survival benefit from chemotherapy alone. This is true in both adjuvant and metastatic settings.

D. **Immunotherapy.** No significant trials of immunotherapy of any type have been conducted with esophageal carcinoma. The responsiveness to this kind of therapy is unknown and remains experimental.

E. **Combined modality treatment.** Combination therapy with surgery, chemotherapy, and radiation therapy offers the best hope of prolonged survival. The exact dosage schedule and sequence, however, remains to be defined.

1. **Primary esophageal carcinoma.** Aggressive **radiochemotherapy without surgery** has been attempted as a primary treatment for esophageal carcinoma. Different combinations of **fluorouracil, cisplatin, mitomycin-C, and bleomycin** with radiation therapy (2000–6000 cGy) have produced clinical response rates of 71–100% (up to 84% complete responses) and rates of 25–47% for 2-year survival. One study reported a 32% actuarial 5-year survival rate. Median survivals range from 12 to more than 30 months. Although these studies suggest that surgery may not be required for treatment of esophageal cancer, confirmation of improved survival rates awaits randomized clinical trials.

2. **Adjuvant radiochemotherapy.** Adjuvant radiochemotherapy has been used almost exclusively in the **preoperative setting.** Most protocols have combined radiation therapy (3000 cGy over 3 weeks) with fluorouracil and either mitomycin-C (Wayne State University protocol, WP) or cisplatin (modified WP). After radiochemotherapy, 38–100% of patients were able to undergo surgery, and **pathologic complete responses** were documented in 17–55% of these patients. Median survival was 12–26 months. Although 2-year survival was improved when compared with historical controls (50% vs 18%), long-term survival (5 years) in patients completing therapy was lower than 13% because of distant recurrence in 88% of patients. In addition, a **high surgical mortality rate** (11–30%) and serious morbidity was reported with these protocols. A single randomized trial comparing preoperative bleomycin and radiotherapy to radiation therapy alone failed to show significant differences in survival.

X. **Prognosis**

A. **Risk of recurrence.** The risk of local and distant recurrence after maximal treatment with combined surgery, radiotherapy, and chemotherapy is summarized in Table 30–2.

B. **Five-year survival.** The outlook for patients with esophageal cancer is uniformly dismal regardless of stage. Most patients die within 6–12 months, and the overall 5-year survival is only 6.2%, with 78% of all 5-year survivors eventually dying of recurrent disease.

C. **Adverse prognostic factors.** Patients who do survive long term generally have **mid or lower thoracic lesions** and do *not* have any of the following adverse prognostic factors: a **tumor longer than 5 cm, an obstruction, or distant metastases** at the time of diagnosis.

XI. **Patient follow-up**

A. **General guidelines.** Patients with esophageal carcinoma, whether resected for cure or palliation, should be followed every 3 months for 2 years, every 6 months for an additional 3 years, and then annually for evidence of tumor recurrence. Patients with metastatic disease should be followed every 1–2 months for symptoms requir-

TABLE 30–2. RISK OF LOCAL AND DISTANT RECURRENCE AFTER THERAPY

Site	Frequency of Recurrence	
	Local (%)	Distant (%)
Alone	12	68
With distant recurrence	20	—
With local recurrence	—	20
Total	**32**	**88**

ing further palliative measures and for nutritional monitoring, but diagnostic tests should be limited to symptomatic areas that are amenable to further palliation. Specific guidelines for following patients with esophageal cancer are listed below.

B. Routine evaluation. Each clinic visit should include the following examinations:
1. **Medical history and physical examination.** An interval medical history and thorough physical examination should be performed during each office visit. (Areas for particular attention are discussed on p 222, **VI.A.**)
2. **Blood tests** (see p 1, **IV.A.**)
    a. Complete blood count.
    b. Hepatic transaminases.
    c. Alkaline phosphatase.
    d. Albumin.
3. **Chest x-ray** (see p. 3, **IV.C.**).

C. Additional evaluation. Other tests that should be obtained at regular intervals include the following:
1. **Barium swallow esophagography.** After resection, this test should be ordered every 6–12 months to monitor for stricture and anastomotic recurrence.
2. **Esophagogastroscopy.** Performed every 6 months, this procedure is a direct way to monitor for esophagitis, stricture, and tumor recurrence.

D. Optional evaluation. The following examinations may be indicated, depending on previous findings or clinical suspicion.
1. **Blood tests** (see p 2, **IV.A.**)
    a. Nucleotidase.
    b. GGTP.
2. **Imaging studies** (see p 3, **IV.C**)
    a. **Chest CT.** Chest CT scan remains a good method to detect recurrent esophageal masses, mediastinal adenopathy, and pulmonary metastases. In patients with no residual tumor, a chest CT scan should be obtained if suspicious findings are identified on medical history, physical examination, chest x-ray, or barium swallow esophagography.
    b. **Abdominal CT.** A CT scan of the abdomen is the most sensitive test to exclude liver metastases and should be ordered if symptoms or blood tests suggest the possibility of liver disease.
    c. **Magnetic resonance imaging**
    d. **Technetium-99m bone scan.**
3. **Invasive diagnostic procedures.** In a patient without known residual cancer, a biopsy of any suspicious or abnormal mass detected on physical examination, chest x-ray, barium swallow esophagography, esophagogastroscopy, or routine blood testing is indicated.

REFERENCES

Akiyama H et al: Principles of surgical treatment for carcinoma of the esophagus. *Ann Surg* 1981; **194**:438–446.

Akiyama H et al: Use of the stomach as an esophageal substitute. *Ann Surg* 1978;**188**:606–610.

Boyce HW: Palliation of advanced esophageal cancer. *Semin Oncol* 1984;**11**:186–195.

Collin CF, Spiro RH: Carcinoma of the cervical esophagus: changing therapeutic trends. *Am J Surg* 1984;**148**:460–466.

DeMeester TR, Barlow AP: Surgery and current management for cancer of the esophagus and cardia: part I and II. *Curr Probl Surg* 1988;**25**:480–605.

Fein R et al: Adenocarcinoma of the esophagus and gastroesophageal junction: prognostic factors and results of therapy. *Cancer* 1985;**56**:2512–2518.

Gignoux M et al: The value of preoperative radiotherapy in esophageal cancer: results of a study of the E.O.R.T.C. *World J Surg* 1987;**11**:426–432.

Hancock SL, Glatstein E: Radiation therapy of esophageal cancer. *Semin Oncol* 1984;**11**:144–158.

Huang G et al: Experience with combined preoperative irradiation and surgery for carcinoma of the esophagus. *Gann Monograph on Cancer Res* 1986;**31**:159–164.

Kasai M, Mori S, Watanabe T: Follow-up results after resection of thoracic esophageal carcinoma. *World J Surg* 1978;**2**:543–551.

Martini N et al: Tracheoesophageal fistula due to cancer. *J Thorac Cardiol Surg* 1970;**59**:318–324.

Orringer MB: Transhiatal esophagectomy without thoracotomy for carcinoma of the thoracic esophagus. *Ann Surg* 1984;**200**:282–288.

Pietrafitta JJ, Dwyer RM: Endoscopic laser therapy of malignant esophageal obstruction. *Arch Surg* 1986;**121**:395–400.

Postlethwait RW et al: Colon interposition for esophageal substitution. *Ann Thorac Surg* 1971; **12**(1):89–109.

31 Malignancies of the Stomach

Robert B. Cameron, MD

I. **Epidemiology.** Excluding skin cancer, stomach cancer is the **ninth most common malignancy** in the United States **among males** and 15th among females. However, it is the sixth most common cause of cancer-related mortality in men and the eighth most common in women. In 1985, 11.9 cases per 100,000 males and 5.3 per 100,000 females were reported, leading to 7.4 and 3.4 deaths, respectively. In 1993, **24,000 people** in the United States will develop stomach cancer, and **13,600 patients will die** from the disease. For unexplained reasons, however, the incidence of stomach cancer in the western world has decreased 73% since 1930, when it was the most common malignancy in the United States, and the **mortality rate has fallen 75%.** The decline in incidence and mortality has been attributed to environmental factors. The worldwide incidence varies tremendously with geographic locale. In Japan, where stomach cancer is the number one cause of cancer deaths, the incidence is as high as 84 per 100,000 males. Costa Rica, Colombia, Singapore, and Iceland also have high incidence rates. In Hong Kong, however, only 5.8 cases occur per 100,000 males. Epidemiologic studies reveal that first-generation migrants from areas of high incidence to areas of low incidence generally have an intermediate risk, whereas second-generation migrants carry the same risk as the general population.

II. **Risk factors**
   A. **Age.** The incidence of stomach cancer increases progressively after age 35 from fewer than 1 per 100,000 to **96.1 per 100,000 after age 85.**
   B. **Sex.** In the United States, the risk for **males is 2.2 times greater** than that of females. Worldwide, the increased risk for males over females varies from 9 times greater in South Africa to 1.7 times greater in Iran.
   C. **Race.** American **blacks** of either sex have a **3-fold greater risk** than whites.
   D. **Genetic factors.** Although genetic traits have been associated with increased risk, they cannot be clearly separated from environmental influences.
      1. **Family history.** In one study, a family history of gastric carcinoma was associated with a 2- to 3-fold increase in the risk of stomach cancer in first-degree relatives.
      2. **Blood types.** Equivocal data suggests that patients with **blood group A** or **Lewis group-specific substance** carry a 15–20% increased risk of gastric malignancies.
      3. **Familial syndromes.** The autosomal dominant **Peutz-Jeghers syndrome** (multiple gastrointestinal (GI) hamartomatous polyps associated with melanic pigmentation of the buccal mucosa, lips, and digits) has been variably linked to an increased risk of stomach cancer but only if **gastric hamartomas** are present.
   E. **Diet.** Dietary factors are strongly associated with stomach cancer.
      1. **Dietary nitrates.** Nitrates found in preserved foods (pickled, salted, or smoked) when ingested are converted to nitrites and then to **nitrosamines,** which are potent carcinogens. Better refrigeration has reduced the need for nitrates and, as a consequence, the incidence of stomach cancer.
      2. **Fresh fruits and vegetables.** Foods containing vitamins A and C inhibit the conversion of dietary nitrates to nitrosamines and are associated with a decreased risk of gastric carcinoma.
   F. **History of previous gastric pathology**
      1. **Pernicious anemia.** This disease of the elderly is associated with **achlorhydria** and a 5–10% risk of stomach cancer.
      2. **Gastric polyps.** Gastric polyps vary in size and histology (Table 31–1). All polyps should be biopsied, and growths **larger than 2 cm** should be removed, whereas benign polyps smaller than 2 cm can be followed.
      3. **Ulcer diathesis**
         a. **Chronic gastric ulcers.** Malignancies develop in less than 3% of chronic

TABLE 31-1. FREQUENCY AND MALIGNANT POTENTIAL OF GASTRIC POLYPS

Type of Polyp	Polyps (%)	Malignant Potential (%)
Hyperplastic	88	0.6
Hamartomatous adenomatous	10	0
Villous adenomas	2	69

gastric ulcers; therefore, chronic ulcer disease does not necessarily imply cancer.

    b. Previous ulcer surgery. Partial gastric resections for ulcer diatheses have been associated with cancer in the gastric remnant 15–40 years later. Chronic inflammation from bile reflux has been cited as a possible etiologic factor.

   4. Gastritis. In the past, an association between stomach cancer and both **atrophic gastritis and Menetrier's disease** (giant hypertrophic gastritis) was described. These associations are now believed to be dubious.

  G. Ionizing radiation. Atomic bomb survivors and patients treated with x-ray therapy for spinal cord disorders have been found to have a higher incidence of stomach cancer than does the general population.

  H. Urbanization. Several factors common among city dwellers have been associated with an increased risk of stomach cancer.

   1. Industrial occupations. Workers with high levels of exposure to **nickel, rubber, and asbestos** are at increased risk.

   2. Socioeconomic status. People of **low socioeconomic status,** for uncertain reasons, are twice as likely to develop stomach cancer as those of higher status.

III. Presentation

  A. Signs and symptoms. Stomach cancer produces few signs and symptoms until late in the disease, and, when symptoms do occur, they are generally nonspecific. The most common signs and symptoms associated with local-regional and systemic disease are listed below:

   1. Local manifestations. Weight loss (80%), abdominal pain (69%), emesis (43%), change of bowel habits (40%), anorexia (30%), dysphagia (17%), massive hemorrhage (10%), and early satiety (5%) are common findings.

   2. Systemic manifestations. Evidence of systemic disease includes weakness (19%), hepatic mass (10%); abdominal or bony pain; jaundice; ascites; rectal urgency or obstruction (from Blumer's rectal shelf metastases); supraclavicular, axillary, or periumbilical adenopathy; and pulmonary, ovarian, or central nervous system (CNS) masses.

  B. Paraneoplastic syndromes. A number of syndromes have been described in association with stomach cancer. Although uncommon, the following symptom complexes may be the sole manifestation of disease:

   1. Dermatomyositis (see p 59, 110, **III**).

   2. Acanthosis nigricans (see p 109).

   3. Thrombophlebitis (see p 81).

   4. Erythema gyratum repens (see p 108).

   5. Eaton-Lambert syndrome (see p 59, **II**).

   6. Dementia and cerebellar ataxia. (see p 57, **I**).

   7. Inappropriate ACTH (see p 90).

   8. Carcinoid syndrome (see p 73).

IV. Differential diagnosis. Adenocarcinomas of the stomach frequently develop ulcerations that can be confused with benign gastric ulcers on barium upper GI x-ray studies. Although patients with gastric ulcers usually undergo endoscopy with biopsy for diagnosis, certain radiologic characteristics aid in the diagnosis of **benign versus malignant disease** (Table 31-2).

V. Screening programs. Although screening for stomach cancer is not feasible in the United States because of its low incidence, mass screening with upper GI x-rays and endoscopy in Japan has increased the detection of early mucosal lesions from 3.8% in 1955 to 34.5%. Patients with this early-stage disease have a rate of 5-year survival better than 90%.

TABLE 31–2. RADIOLOGIC CRITERIA FOR BENIGN VS MALIGNANT GASTRIC ULCERS

Characteristic	Benign Ulcers	Malignant Ulcers
Penetration	Beyond the stomach wall	Into a filling defect but not beyond the stomach wall
Appearance of rugal folds	Converge toward ulcer	Do not converge
Location	Can occur anywhere	Can occur anywhere (most occur in antrum or along lesser curvature)
Borders	Elevated	Flat

VI. Diagnostic workup

  A. Physical examination. A complete history and physical examination are essential in the evaluation of any patient but, when stomach cancer is suspected, extra care should be exercised in examining the following areas:

    1. General appearance. An assessment of the nutritional status and recent changes in weight should be made.

    2. Skin. Evidence of jaundice from liver metastases should be noted, and specific evidence of hyperpigmentation and hyperkeratosis indicating **acanthosis nigricans** should be sought.

    3. Lymph nodes. All lymph node areas require close examination for metastatic disease, including cervical, supraclavicular (**Virchow's or Troisier's node** in left supraclavicular area), axillary (**Irish's node** in left anterior axilla), and inguinal adenopathy.

    4. Abdomen. A search should be made for intra-abdominal masses caused by the primary tumor or hepatic metastases. Abdominal distention from malignant ascites and periumbilical masses **(Sister Mary Joseph nodule)** also should be recorded.

    5. Pelvis. Bimanual examination of the ovaries may reveal metastatic deposits of tumor referred to as Krukenberg's tumor.

    6. Rectum. Digital examination of the rectal shelf should be performed to ascertain the presence of "drop" metastases called **Blumer's shelf lesions.** Occult blood in the stool also should be evaluated.

    7. Nervous system. A full examination of sensorium, cranial nerves, and peripheral motor and sensory function is mandatory. If localizing signs are present, carcinomatous meningitis should be suspected.

  B. Primary tests and procedures. All patients with suspected gastric carcinoma should have the following diagnostic tests performed:

    1. Blood tests (see p 1, **IV.A**)

      a. Complete blood count.

      b. Hepatic transaminases.

      c. Alkaline phosphatase.

      d. Albumin.

    2. Imaging studies

      a. Chest x-ray (see p 3, **IV.C.1**).

      b. Barium upper GI series (UGI). This test provides anatomic details of the extent of the primary tumor and can accurately detect malignant lesions in more than 90% of the cases.

      c. Computed tomography. CT scans of the chest and abdomen are excellent methods of resolving questions of pulmonary or intra-abdominal metastases. They also can provide useful information as to involvement of contiguous organs and existence of lymph node metastases.

    3. Invasive procedures. Esophagogastroduodenoscopy is essential to obtain tissue for pathologic confirmation of malignancy. Either brush or needle biopsy may establish the diagnosis in more than 92% of **exophytic carcinomas** and 50% of **infiltrating lesions.**

  C. Optional tests and procedures. The following tests may be indicated by previous diagnostic findings or clinical suspicion:

    1. Blood tests

      a. Nucleotidase (see p 2, **IV.A.4**).

      b. GGTP (see p 2, **IV.A.5**).

  c. **Carcinoembryonic antigen** (CEA). This fetal antigen is elevated in as many as 60% of advanced cases, but it is nonspecific because elevations occur in a wide variety of malignant as well as benign diseases.

  d. **Alpha-fetoprotein.** Elevations in this fetal antigen are found in 15–20% of stomach cancer patients but are not helpful for routine patient management.

 2. **Imaging studies** (see p 3, **IV.C**)

  a. **Ultrasound.**

  b. **Magnetic resonance imaging.**

  c. **Technetium-99m bone scan.**

 3. **Invasive procedures.** Any suspiciously enlarged lymph node or nodule should be biopsied to rule out metastatic disease. If liver nodules are found, percutaneous needle biopsy may be indicated.

VII. Pathology

 A. Location. The distribution of malignancies in the stomach has been well characterized and is listed below: cardia and gastroesophageal junction, 7%; body of the stomach, 18%; lesser curvature, 22%; greater curvature, 3%; and antrum, 50%.

 B. Multiplicity. Synchronous primary lesions are reported in approximately 2% of all cases; however, as many as 22% of patients with **pernicious anemi**a may have multicentric disease.

 C. Gross appearance. Bormann first divided gastric malignancies into four classes, depending on gross pathologic appearance. Verse later modified this classification (see below). A rough correlation with outcome has been attempted but is better correlated with stage.

  1. **Ulcerative.** This type of appearance occurs in 75% of tumors and is characterized by a mass with a central necrotic crater.

  2. **Polypoid.** Only 10% of malignancies fall into this category, yet this type of appearance is associated with well-differentiated noninvasive tumors and a relatively good prognosis.

  3. **Scirrhous.** This gross appearance is better known as linitis plastica or **"leather bottle" appearance.** It occurs 10% of the time and unfortunately is uniformly fatal.

  4. **Superficial.** This appearance is associated with sheetlike cells replacing the normal gastric mucosa and occurs in 5% of cases.

 D. Histology. Adenocarcinomas, frequently of the **signet-ring** variety, make up 95% of all gastric malignancies. Other common histologies include lymphomas (3%), leiomyosarcomas (1%), adenoacanthomas (< 1%), squamous cell carcinoma (< 1%), and carcinoid tumors (< 1%).

 E. Metastatic spread.

  1. **Modes of spread.** Stomach cancer at the time of diagnosis has spread beyond the stomach wall in 88% of the cases and generally spreads by four distinct mechanisms.

   a. **Direct extension.** Because of the lack of symptoms, primary tumors frequently grow to involve adjacent structures such as the omentum, colon, pancreas, and spleen. In 27% this is the only mode of spread at the time of diagnosis, but it is a **component of spread** in 56%.

   b. **Nodal metastasis.** Present in 50–60% of patients at the time of diagnosis, this is the sole site of extragastric spread 11% of the time. Nodal groups can be divided into regional and distant.

    (1) Regional nodes. These node groups include gastric, gastroduodenal, pancreatic, pancreaticoduodenal, hepatic, and celiac nodes.

    (2) Distant nodes. Node groups that are considered sites of distant spread include supraclavicular **(Virchow's or Troisier's node),** axilla **(Irish's node),** and periumbilical **(Sister Mary Joseph nodule)** nodes.

   c. **Hematogenous metastasis.** Vascular spread through portal, portovertebral, or portosystemic (esophageal) vessels occurs in 35% of patients before the time of diagnosis.

   d. **Direct implantation.** Direct physical implantation on structures remote from the primary tumor occurs in the peritoneum. The **ovary** is involved in 10% of all cases **(Krukenberg's tumor),** but the **rectal shelf** (Blumer's shelf) and the entire peritoneum can be involved, occasionally resulting in malignant ascites.

  2. **Sites of spread.** The organ most frequently involved in distant spread is the **liver.** Table 31–3 lists the other most frequent sites of metastatic spread. **Carcinomatous meningitis** is the most common form of metastatic spread to the CNS.

TABLE 31-3. FREQUENCY OF METASTATIC SITES FROM GASTRIC CARCINOMA

Site	Incidence of Metastases (%)	Site	Incidence of Metastases (%)
Liver	45	Bone	5
Peritoneum	25	GI tract	5
Lungs	20	Spleen	2
Adrenals	12	CNS	2
Pancreas	10	GU tract	< 1

VIII. **Staging**
   A. **Hoerr classification.** A surgical classification system based on extent of local disease and the presence of distant spread has been used at some centers.
      1. **Stage of primary lesion**
         a. **Stage I.** This stage is limited to disease involving only the mucosa, submucosa, and muscularis and occurs in 10.9% of cases.
         b. **Stage II.** This stage involves the serosa and is found in 33.3% of patients.
         c. **Stage III.** This advanced stage includes contiguous spread, which occurs in 55.8%.
      2. **Metastatic stage**
         a. **Stage A.** No metastases are evident (12.7% of cases).
         b. **Stage B.** Regional nodal metastases are present (39.2% of cases).
         c. **Stage C.** Distant metastases beyond regional nodal groups has occurred (35.6% of cases).
   B. **TNM classification.** In 1987 the American Joint Committee on Cancer and the Union Internationale Contre le Cancer in cooperation developed a joint TNM staging system that provides the basis for future studies. Uniform use will assure accurate direct comparisons between studies performed in different centers. The proposed staging system is a amalgamation of previous staging systems and is reproduced below:
      1. **Tumor stage**
         a. **TX.** Primary tumor cannot be assessed.
         b. **T0.** No evidence of tumor.
         c. **Tis.** Intraepithelial tumor without invasion of lamina propria or carcinoma in situ.
         d. **T1.** Tumor invades the lamina propria or submucosa.
         e. **T2.** Tumor invades the muscularis propria or subserosa.
         f. **T3.** Tumor penetrates the serosa but does not invade adjacent structures.
         g. **T4.** Tumor invades adjacent structures.
      2. **Lymph node stage**
         a. **NX.** Cannot be assessed.
         b. **N0.** No regional nodal metastases are present.
         c. **N1.** Metastases are present in the perigastric lymph nodes **within 3 cm** of the edge of the primary tumor.
         d. **N2.** Metastases are present in the perigastric lymph nodes **more than 3 cm** from the edge of the primary tumor or in lymph nodes along the left gastric, common hepatic, splenic, or celiac arteries.
             Note: Nodes formerly classified as N3 nodes (eg, para-aortic, retropancreatic) are now considered distant metastases.
      3. **Metastatic stage**
         a. **MX.** The presence of distant metastases cannot be assessed.
         b. **M0.** No distant metastases are present.
         c. **N1.** Distant metastases are present.
      4. **Histopathologic grade**
         a. **GX.** Grade cannot be assessed.
         b. **G1.** Tumor is well differentiated.
         c. **G2.** Tumor is moderately well differentiated.
         d. **G3.** Tumor is poorly differentiated.
         e. **G4.** Tumor is undifferentiated.

5. **Stage groupings**
   a. **Stage 0.** Tis, N0, M0.
   b. **Stage IA.** T1, N0, M0.
   c. **Stage IB.** T1, N1, M0 or T2, N0, M0.
   d. **Stage II.** T1, N2, M0; T2, N1, M0; or T3, N0, M0.
   e. **Stage IIIA.** T2, N2, M0; T3, N1, M0; or T4, N0, M0.
   f. **Stage IIIB.** T3, N2, M0 or T4, N1, M0.
   g. **Stage IV.** T4, N2, M0 or any T, any N, M1.

IX. **Treatment**
   A. **Surgery**
      1. **Primary gastric carcinoma.** Surgery remains the only therapy with curative potential for gastric malignancies. Even in the face of metastatic disease, resection of the primary lesion improves the patient's quality and duration of survival and therefore should be contemplated in selected patients.
         a. **Indications.** Resection of primary gastric carcinoma for cure or palliation is generally indicated in any operative candidate with a resectable lesion. Involvement of the distal esophagus, proximal duodenum, distal pancreas, spleen, lymph nodes, omentum, or colon does **not** constitute contraindications to resection because these organs can be removed en bloc with the primary lesion. Resection is not indicated, however, in patients with **widely metastatic disease, malignant ascites, or a brief life expectancy.**
         b. **Approaches.** The majority of resections can be accomplished through a standard midline abdominal laparotomy incision. However, proximal lesions may pose problems similar to those associated with lower esophageal malignancies and may require one of the approaches used for this malignancy (see p 225, **IX.A.1.C**).
         c. **Procedures.** Two major procedures have been used in the surgical treatment of gastric carcinoma. The choice of which type to use is determined by the size, location, histology, and extent of the primary tumor as well as the surgeon's preference.
            (1) **Subtotal gastrectomy.** This procedure involves removal of the **distal 50–85% of the stomach,** including a 5–6 cm margin of normal stomach around the lesion, the first part of the duodenum, and omentum. In addition, except in the rare case of leiomyosarcoma, which rarely metastasizes to lymph nodes, **extensive lymph node dissections** are performed in the areas of the porta hepatis and celiac lymph node groups. The **spleen is generally not removed** unless obvious involvement occurs or the primary lesion encroaches on the proximal portion of the stomach. In nonrandomized studies radical **subtotal gastrectomy** was associated with a 5-year survival of 30–46%, whereas radical **total gastrectomy** was associated with a survival of only 10–16%. This difference, however, may be related to a greater number of advanced lesions in patients undergoing radical total gastrectomy because more recent Japanese reports indicate that subtotal and radical total gastrectomies result in 11.1–17.1% and 26.3–33.3% 5-year survival, respectively. Proximal subtotal gastrectomy is sometimes used with GE junctional lesions. In this case, 80–85% of the proximal stomach is removed and an esophagogastrostomy is performed.
            (2) **Radical total gastrectomy.** Resection of the entire stomach, distal esophagus or proximal duodenum (depending on the location of the primary tumor), omentum, and, frequently, the spleen is an integral part of radical total gastrectomy. Lymph node dissection of the porta hepatis and celiac axis also is included, except with leiomyosarcoma, as noted above. Occasionally, the **distal pancreas, peripancreatic nodes, and colon also are removed (extended total gastrectomy).** Total gastrectomy is most often used for lesions involving the proximal stomach, a large portion of the gastric corpus, or both.
         d. **Reconstruction.** Recreating gastrointestinal continuity can be achieved several ways, depending on the situation, the operation performed, and expertise of the surgeon. Some include the construction of a substitute gastric reservoir.
            (1) **Gastroduodenostomy.** Direct anastomosis of the proximal portion of the stomach to the duodenum **(Billroth I)** is a common method of reconstruction after a **radical subtotal gastrectomy.** This method has

the advantage of creating near-normal anatomy, but **bile reflux** is a frequent complication.

(2) **Gastrojejunostomy.** Anastomosis of the proximal stomach remnant to a simple or Roux-en-Y loop of jejunum **(Billroth II)** is another popular method of reconstruction after radical subtotal gastrectomy. The resulting anatomy deviates farther from normal than gastroduodenostomy, but the incidence of bile reflux is decreased.

(3) **Esophagoduodenostomy.** After radical total gastrectomy, continuity can be reestablished by direct end-to-end anastomosis of the esophagus and duodenum in a small number of patients. The usefulness of **this approach is limited,** however, because the duodenum often cannot be mobilized enough to guarantee a tension-free anastomosis.

(4) **Esophagojejunostomy.** The most frequently used method of gastrointestinal reconstruction after radical total gastrectomy involves the anastomosis of a simple or Roux-en-Y loop of jejunum to the esophagus. A jejunal pouch or reservoir can be created in an attempt to palliate the obligatory dumping that occurs postoperatively, but it can also be fashioned as a separate procedure at a later time.

2. **Unresectable primary gastric carcinoma.** Gastric lesions that are too large to resect are difficult to palliate; therefore, every effort should be made to remove the primary tumor. Unresected gastric malignancies can cause **bleeding, perforation, obstruction, and pain.** If attempts at removal fail and impending obstruction exists, one of the following procedures may be indicated:

   a. **Gastroenterostomy.** Because a high percentage fail to function, simple loop or Roux-en-Y gastrojejunostomy **only rarely** provides adequate palliation for malignant obstruction of the stomach. As a result of this high failure rate and a high complication rate, this procedure is generally **not recommended.**

   b. **Tube gastrostomy.** Relief of gastric obstruction can sometimes be achieved by tube gastrostomy either surgically or endoscopically. However, when gastric malignancies are advanced and involve a large portion of the stomach, an adequate portion of normal stomach is often not available as a site for gastrostomy placement.

3. **Metastatic gastric carcinoma.** In the presence of metastatic disease, palliative resection of gastric malignancies has been shown to double mean survival from 4.5 to 9 months, probably from improved nutrition, and is recommended in patients who are reasonable candidates for surgery. However, there is no indication for surgery in patients with life expectancies that are shorter than the recovery time from major procedures unless life-threatening complications such as perforation or bleeding develop.

4. **Mortality and morbidity.** Most acute complications resulting from gastrectomy are related to infection and anastomotic disruption. Chronic complications usually relate to altered gastrointestinal function and malnutrition. The following are some more commonly encountered causes of morbidity and mortality after gastric resection:

   a. **Anastomotic leaks and strictures,** 3%.

   b. **Wound infection, subphrenic abscess, or both,** 5%.

   c. **Postprandial dumping syndrome.** This syndrome is a result of rapid fluid shifts created by the hyperosmolar effects of carbohydrates. Measures that should be taken to prevent these unpleasant symptoms include reclining after meals, small frequent feedings, and a high protein, high fat, low carbohydrate diet.

   d. **Megaloblastic anemia.** Inadequate or absent production of gastric intrinsic factor results in a deficiency of vitamin B_{12} absorption and is easily preventable with **monthly B_{12} injections** (100 mcg IM).

B. **Radiation**

1. **Primary gastric carcinoma.** Generally, radiation therapy has no role as a curative modality in gastric carcinoma. Theoretically, small lesions are curable with external-beam radiation therapy; however, these lesions also are amenable to surgical extirpation, the treatment of choice. Gastric lymphoma, when isolated, also is usually treated by resection with postoperative radiation therapy but, when part of disseminated disease, can be treated with primary radiation with curative intent.

2. **Adjuvant radiation therapy**

   a. **Preoperative radiation therapy.** Preoperative external beam therapy has not been used in this country. In Japan, however, it has been attempted with some degree of success. Preoperative therapy could potentially increase the resectability rate among the 30–50% of patients who are found to have **unresectable lesions** at laparotomy.

b. **Intraoperative radiation therapy (IORT).** Electron-beam radiation therapy performed intraoperatively theoretically could reduce the incidence of complications since the small bowel, liver, and colon can be displaced from the fields. In Japan, encouraging results from nonrandomized trials indicate a possible survival benefit for patients receiving intraoperative radiation therapy when compared with surgery alone. However, this can be accomplished only in large centers and may not be superior to standard postoperative external-beam radiation therapy because the retracted organs also can be frequent sites of local recurrences. In this type of therapy, 1500–3500 cGy is commonly delivered to each field by electron beam.

c. **Postoperative radiation therapy.** As many as 50–80% of patients undergoing gastric resection for adenocarcinoma of the stomach subsequently **develop local recurrences.** Postoperative radiation therapy with or without chemotherapy is often recommended to reduce the number of recurrences, especially in patients with positive lymph nodes. Doses in the range of 4500–5500 cGy are typically delivered in 180 cGy fractions over 4–5 weeks. Although a sound rationale exists for the use of postoperative radiation therapy in gastric cancer, clinical trials to date have **not** definitively demonstrated any benefit for such treatment.

3. **Locally advanced and metastatic gastric carcinoma.** In the setting of metastatic stomach cancer, radiation therapy with or without chemotherapy may be useful for palliation of **painful bony metastases,** occasionally for palliation of large unresectable **symptomatic primary lesions,** and for palliation of **carcinomatous meningitis** in conjunction with intrathecal methotrexate.

4. **Morbidity and mortality.** Most complications that develop are related to the gastrointestinal tract, although the following organ systems also may be involved: anastomotic leak and disruption, diarrhea, transverse myelitis with doses of 5000 cGy to the spinal cord, radiation nephritis, and radiation hepatitis.

C. **Chemotherapy**

1. **Primary gastric carcinoma.** No data are available to justify the use of chemotherapy as the initial therapy in surgically resectable gastric malignancies.

2. **Adjuvant chemotherapy**

a. **Single agent therapy.** No studies, including several randomized prospective trials, have demonstrated any survival benefit of single-agent adjuvant chemotherapy. Agents that have been evaluated include fluorouracil, floxuridine, thiotepa, and mitomycin-C.

b. **Combination chemotherapy.** Combination chemotherapy holds more promise than single agent therapy because of the higher response rates seen in advanced disease. One randomized prospective study by the Gastrointestinal Tumor Study Group (1982c) evaluating **fluorouracil and semustine** demonstrated an improved 4-year survival of 59% compared with a control group with 44% (p < 0.03). In a similar trial, however, the Eastern Cooperative Oncology Group was unable to verify these results. Multiple randomized prospective trials in Japan have failed to show any benefit to other combination chemotherapy regimens such as mitomycin-C and fluorouracil. Further work needs to be done before any one regimen can be recommended.

Note: **Semustine** is associated with secondary hematogenous malignancies and is currently available only in an approved clinical trial.

3. **Locally advanced and metastatic gastric carcinoma**

a. **Single agent therapy.** Many agents have been evaluated over the past 20 years. The most active agents include fluorouracil, mitomycin-c, carmustine, semustine, and doxorubicin, all of which have response rates of 17% to 24%. Newer agents such as **cisplatin and triazinate** have been reported recently to have **response rates** of 26% and 15%, respectively. All have short durations of response (< 6 months), and complete responses are rare.

b. **Combination chemotherapy.** Combinations of the single agents discussed above have produced slightly higher response rates. The most widely studied regimens involve **fluorouracil, doxorubicin, mitomycin-C, and semustine.** Fluorouracil combined with semustine (FMe) produced responses in 21–40% of patients. Fluorouracil, doxorubicin, and mitomycin-C

(FAM) was shown to produce responses in 25–55%, whereas fluorouracil, doxorubicin, and semustine (FAMe) resulted in a 30–47% response rate. According to the Gastrointestinal Tumor Study Group (1982a), small significant survival advantages (4–17 weeks) have been observed with these last two regimens; however, these occur only when the data are heavily weighted toward earlier time points. In addition, the findings have not been shown consistently in other prospective randomized trials. Phase II studies involving new regimens, though, suggest that fluorouracil, doxorubicin, and cisplatin (FAP) may improve survival because of a **higher complete response rate.**

D. **Immunotherapy.** To date, no trials of immunotherapy of any type have been conducted on patients with gastric carcinoma. The responsiveness of this tumor to immunomodulatory agents is completely unknown and cannot be recommended outside of an approved clinical trial.

E. **Combined modality treatment.** Combination of chemotherapy to combat systemic disease and radiation therapy to eradicate the high incidence of local recurrences are being examined at several cancer centers. So far, the results have been disappointing. The combinations of fluorouracil plus carmustine or fluorouracil, doxorubicin, and mitomycin-C before or after radiation therapy have been tried without success. In one study, the Gastrointestinal Tumor Study Group (1982b) found an early advantage to fluorouracil and semustine over chemotherapy combined with radiation, however, after 4 years the survival of the combined modality group was superior to that of the chemotherapy alone arm. Although most results with combined modality therapy have been discouraging, the combination of therapeutic modalities, nonetheless, represents the best chance of successful treatment of gastric carcinoma in the future.

X. **Prognosis**

A. **Risk of recurrence.** For patients undergoing potentially curative resection, the risk of recurrence and prognosis corresponds to the extent of disease found at surgery. Typical 5-year survival rates based on extent of disease at surgery are listed below. The current TNM system has not been in use long enough to have accurate data by TNM stage.
   1. **Negative nodes with involvement of mucosa only,** 85%.
   2. **Negative nodes with involvement of gastric wall,** 52%.
   3. **Negative nodes with involvement of gastric serosa,** 47%.
   4. **Positive regional lymph nodes,** 17%.
   5. **Positive distant lymph nodes,** 5%.

B. **Patterns of failure.** The sites of failure after attempted curative resection of gastric carcinoma can be local or regional, peritoneal, or distant.
   1. **Recurrence at a single site.** The incidence of isolated recurrences at different sites is summarized below:
      a. **Local/regional.** Twenty-nine percent of patients fail with **only local or regional disease.**
      b. **Peritoneal.** Nearly 4% of all patients with failure have only peritoneal metastases.
      c. **Distant.** Six percent of patients fail with only distant disease.
   2. **Recurrence in multiple areas.** The incidence of recurrence at various sites as a component of multisite failure are listed below:
      a. **Local/regional.** Eighty-eight percent of patients fail with local or regional disease as one component.
      b. **Peritoneal.** Fifty-four percent of all patients with multiple areas of failure have peritoneal metastases.
      c. **Distant.** Twenty-nine percent of patients develop distant metastases as one of several areas of recurrence.

C. **Five-year survival.** The 5-year survival rate by stage is summarized as follows: Stage I, 70.6%, Stage II, 38.6%, Stage III, 15.4%, and Stage IV, 7.7%.

D. **Prognostic factors.** The prognosis for all patients with stomach cancer is poor: only 15% of all patients survive 5 years. The most important adverse prognostic factor is the presence of metastases, either nodal or distant. The following factors also adversely affect the prognosis:
   1. **A short history of symptoms.**
   2. **Advanced age and poor performance status.**
   3. **A poorly differentiated histology or linitis plastica.**
   4. **A locally advanced unresectable primary lesion.**
   5. **Proximal lesions requiring total gastrectomy.**

XI. Patient follow-up
  A. General guidelines. Patients with gastric carcinoma should be followed every 3 months for the first 2 years and every 6 months thereafter, although patients with symptomatic metastases may require more frequent visits for coordination of palliative efforts. General guidelines for patient follow-up are listed below.
  B. Routine evaluation. Each clinic visit should include the following tests and procedures:
    1. Physical examination. A general physical examination should be performed with each clinic visit and should include evaluation of those areas initially assessed at the time of presentation (see p 233, **VI.A**).
    2. Blood tests (see p 1, **IV.A**)
      a. Complete blood count.
      b. Hepatic transaminases.
      c. Alkaline phosphatase.
    3. Chest x-ray (see p 3, **IV.C.1**).
    4. Administration of vitamin B$_{12}$. With large gastric resections, inadequate intrinsic factor is produced to maintain normal absorption of vitamin B$_{12}$. Thus, parenteral administration of 100 mcg of this vitamin every month is required to prevent megaloblastic anemia.
  C. Additional evaluation. Other tests that should be obtained at regular intervals include the following examinations:
    1. Barium upper gastrointestinal series. The UGI exam is required 6 months after surgical resection and every year thereafter to rule out local recurrences and obstruction.
    2. Endoscopy. Direct visualization and evaluation of the esophagus, gastric remnant, and proximal small bowel for local recurrence should be performed every 6–12 months. This test is often alternated with barium studies.
  D. Optional evaluation. The following tests and procedures may be indicated by previous findings or clinical suspicion:
    1. Blood tests (see p 2, **IV.A**)
      a. Nucleotidase.
      b. GGTP.
      c. Carcinoembryonic antigen (CEA).
    2. Imaging studies (see p 3, **IV.C**)
      a. Computed tomography.
      b. Magnetic responance imaging.
      c. Technectium-99m bone scan.
    3. Invasive procedures. Biopsy of any suspicious mass or lymph node is indicated in anyone with a history of gastric carcinoma.

REFERENCES

Douglass HO, Nava HR: Gastric adenocarcinoma—management of the primary disease. *Semin Oncol* 1985;**12**(1):32–45.

Gastrointestinal Tumor Study Group: A comparative clinical assessment of combination chemotherapy in the management of advanced gastric carcinoma. *Cancer* 1982a;**49**:1362–1366.

Gastrointestinal Tumor Study Group: A comparison of combination chemotherapy with combined modality therapy for locally advanced gastric carcinoma. *Cancer* 1982b;**49**:1771–1777.

Gastrointestinal Tumor Study Group: Controlled trial of adjuvant chemotherapy following curative resection for gastric cancer. *Cancer* 1982;**49**:1116–1122.

Glimelius B: Radiation therapy in upper GI tract tumours. *Acta Chir Scand* 1988;**541**(suppl):32–38.

Gunderson LL, Sosin H: Adenocarcinoma of the stomach—areas of failure in a reoperation series [second or symptomatic looks]: clinicopathologic correlation and implications for adjuvant therapy. *Int J Radiat Oncol Biol Phys* 1982;**8**:1–11.

Hallissey MT et al: Palliative surgery for gastric cancer. *Cancer* 1988;**62**:440–444.

Howson CP, Hiyama T, Wynder EL: The decline in gastric cancer: epidemiology of an unplanned triumph. *Epidemiol Rev* 1986;**8**:1–27.

Macdonald JS, Gohmann JJ: Chemotherapy of advanced gastric cancer: present status, future prospects. *Semin Oncol* 1988;**15**(3):42–49,

Schein PS et al: Current management of advanced and locally unresectable gastric carcinoma. *Cancer* 1982;**50**:2590–2596.

Weissberg JB: Role of radiation therapy in gastrointestinal cancer. *Arch Surg* 1983;**118**:96–104.

Wils JA: Current status of chemotherapy for advanced gastric cancer. *Anticancer Res* 1987;**7**:755–760.

32 Malignancies of the Small Intestine

Robert B. Cameron, MD

I. **Epidemiology.** Cancer of the small intestine is relatively uncommon: It accounts for less than 5% of all gastrointestinal malignancies. In 1985 approximately 1.4 males and 0.8 females per 100,000 of the population were diagnosed with small bowel cancer, and it was estimated in 1993 that **3,600 new cases and 925 deaths** would occur because of small intestinal malignancies. The incidence worldwide is uniform, with little geographic variation.

II. **Risk factors**

A. **Age.** The incidence gradually increases from less than 1 per 100,000 to 6.1 per 100,000 between the ages of 80 and 84. The mean age at the time of diagnosis is 59 years. A slightly increased incidence of primary small bowel lymphoma also occurs in patients younger than 10 years.

B. **Sex.** American **males are at 1.75 times higher risk** than females for **adenocarcinomas** and **1.5 times higher risk for** primary small-bowel **lymphomas.** There is no sex preponderance for sarcomas or carcinoids.

C. **Race.** No significant differences exist between ethnic groups. However, primary small intestinal lymphomas are more common among ethnic groups in the Middle East.

D. **Genetic factors**

1. **Family history.** No increased risk has been demonstrated in first-degree relatives.

2. **Familial syndromes**

   a. **Familial polyposis.** Multiple adenomatous polyps of the small and large bowel mark this autosomal dominant disease, which increases the risk of small intestinal malignancies.

   b. **Peutz-Jeghers syndrome.** This autosomal dominant disease is characterized by **small intestinal hamartomas** and excessive melanin pigmentation of the skin and mucous membranes. Although benign hamartomas are common in this disorder, there is **no increased risk for malignant neoplasms.**

   c. **Gardner's syndrome.** Colonic and small intestinal polyposis with supernumerary teeth, cranial fibrous dysplasia, osteomas, fibromas, and sebaceous cysts distinguish this autosomal dominant disease, which predisposes to **small intestinal adenocarcinomas.**

   d. **Neurofibromatosis.** This autosomal dominant disease is distinguished by spots of increased skin pigmentation **(cafe au lait spots)** and multiple neurofibromas. These neurofibromas can occur in the gastrointestinal tract and rarely undergo malignant degeneration.

E. **Diet.** No dietary factors have been linked with the development of small intestinal tumors. The rapid transit of ingested food through the small bowel has been proposed as an explanation for this finding.

F. **Previous intestinal pathology**

1. **Inflammatory bowel disease. Crohn's disease** has been associated with a slightly higher risk of malignancies of the small intestine than in the general population.

2. **Celiac disease.** Celiac disease (also known as nontropical sprue or gluten-induced enteropathy) has been shown to increase the risk of small intestinal tumors, especially **lymphomas.**

3. **Immunodeficiency syndromes.** For unknown reasons, syndromes associated with chronic immunodeficiency states are associated with a higher incidence of small bowel malignancies.

III. **Presentation**

A. **Signs and symptoms.** As many as 75% of patients present with one or more of the following signs or symptoms:

1. **Local manifestations.** Common signs and symptoms of localized tumor in-

clude **pain** (65%), nausea and vomiting (40%), **gastrointestinal hemorrhage** (75%), obstruction (20–35%), perforation, palpable mass (30–50%), and jaundice (duodenal tumors).

    2. Systemic manifestations. Frequent systemic signs and symptoms are weight loss (30%), weakness, **fever (lymphomas),** and anemia.

B. Paraneoplastic syndromes. The carcinoid syndrome is associated with metastatic small bowel carcinoid tumor.

IV. Differential diagnosis. Small bowel tumors often produce **intestinal obstruction** associated with an intramural mass, but other causes of small bowel obstruction are much more common and include internal or external **herniation, inflammatory diseases** (Crohn's disease and graft-versus-host disease), **infections** (*Ascaris*), **benign tumors** (adenomas, leiomyomas, lipomas, hemangiomas, neurofibromas, fibromas, pseudolymphomas, and hamartomas), and **vascular strictures** (atherosclerosis and radiation).

V. Screening programs. Screening programs for small bowel malignancies are not cost-efficient because of their low prevalence.

VI. Diagnostic workup

  A. Medical history and physical examination. A complete medical history emphasizing the common presenting signs and symptoms outlined above and a thorough physical examination are essential.

    1. Skin. Pallor indicating anemia and jaundice indicating biliary obstruction as well as **carcinoid flushing** should be noted.

    2. Lymph nodes. The presence of a signal node (also called **Virchow's or Troisier's node)** must be recorded.

    3. Abdomen. Masses and hepatomegaly are important findings.

    4. Rectum. A digital examination for masses and occult blood should be performed.

  B. Primary tests and procedures. All patients with suspected small bowel malignancies should undergo the following diagnostic tests and procedures:

    1. Blood tests

      a. Complete blood count (see p 1, **IV.A.1**).

      b. Hepatic transaminases (see p 1, **IV.A.**).

      c. Alkaline phosphatase (see p 1, **IV.A.**).

      d. Bilirubin. Elevation of the serum direct bilirubin may indicate obstruction from duodenal tumors.

      e. Amylase. Hyperamylasemia may be associated with obstruction of the pancreatic duct caused by duodenal malignancies.

      f. 5-hydroxyindoleacetic acid (5-HIAA). This breakdown product of **serotonin** is elevated in the urine in 17%, 72%, and 88% of patients with duodenal, ileal, and jejunal **carcinoid tumors,** respectively, regardless of the presence of the carcinoid syndrome.

    2. Imaging studies

      a. Chest x-ray (see p 3, **IV.C.1**).

      b. Abdominal series. This set of plain x-rays of the abdomen, although nonspecific, can suggest the presence of small bowel tumors by **demonstrating obstruction** with intestinal dilation, air-fluid levels, or possibly abdominal masses.

      c. Barium upper GI series with small bowel follow through. This common examination may demonstrate as many as 50% of **small intestinal malignancies.** Adenocarcinomas frequently appear as ulcerated intraluminal masses, whereas lymphomas and sarcomas are often visualized as intramural masses.

  C. Optional tests and procedures. The following tests and procedures may be indicated on the basis of previous diagnostic findings or clinical suspicion.

    1. Blood tests

      a. Nucleotidase (see p 2, **IV.A.4**).

      b. GGTP (see p 2, **IV.A.5**).

      c. Carcinoembryonic antigen (CEA). This tumor antigen is rarely elevated in malignancies of the small intestine and generally is not useful.

    2. Imaging studies

      a. Enteroclysis. This test, which involves direct instillation of barium into the small intestine through a long intestinal tube, is the most useful one for visualizing the small bowel mucosa. However, the considerable effort required to pass a long intestinal tube precludes its routine use.

   b. **Barium enema.** Reflux of barium into the terminal ileum during a barium enema may aid in diagnosing **terminal ileal tumors.**
   c. **Computed tomography.** Abdominal CT is not worthwhile in small intestinal malignancies unless distant metastases are suspected or large abdominal masses are present.
   d. **Magnetic resonance imaging.** Abdominal MRI scans may demonstrate small bowel tumors that can appear as masses with **brighter signal intensities** than normal small bowel or liver.
   e. **Visceral angiogram.** In rare cases, angiography may be helpful in the diagnosis of small intestinal malignancies if a tumor blush or area of hypovascularity can be demonstrated.
   f. **Technetium-99m bone scan** (see p 3, **IV.C.4**).
  3. **Invasive procedures.** In patients with biliary, pancreatic or duodenal obstruction, esophagogastroduodenoscopy is indicated to visualize the duodenum directly and biopsy any suspicious lesions.
VII. **Pathology**
  A. **Location.** The location of tumors vary depending on the histologic type of malignancy (see Table 32–1).
  B. **Multiplicity. Synchronous lesions** are found in as many as **30% of patients with carcinoids.** In addition, as many as **47% of carcinoid patients** may have **non-carcinoid intra-abdominal malignancies.**
  C. **Histology.** There are four frequent histologic types of small bowel cancer:
   1. **Adenocarcinomas.** These malignancies of the glandular epithelium make up **50% of small intestinal cancers.** They tend to extend through the bowel wall, ulcerate, and metastasize in a manner similar to large bowel carcinomas.
   2. **Carcinoid tumors.** These tumors arise from the argentaffin cells in the submucosa and account for **30% of small intestinal malignancies.** They are usually solitary, slow growing, and **asymptomatic** 70% of the time. Circulating and urinary levels of 5-hydroxyindoleacetic acid are often increased, and, in 10% of patients who develop liver metastases, this leads to the carcinoid syndrome of cutaneous flushing, episodic watery diarrhea, and paroxysmal dyspnea associated with bronchospasm.
   3. **Sarcomas.** These mesenchymal tumors make up **20% of all small bowel malignancies** and usually present as large intramural masses, 75% of which are **more than 5 cm in diameter.** The most frequent subtypes are **leiomyosarcoma** (75%), fibrosarcomas (10%), angiosarcomas, and, in rare cases, liposarcomas, neurofibrosarcomas, and malignant schwannomas.
   4. **Primary lymphomas.** Lymphomas originating in the small intestine account for **less than 1% of all small bowel malignancies** and should be considered only if mesenteric lymph node involvement is localized to the involved bowel, the white-blood-cell count is normal, and no peripheral or mediastinal lymphadenopathy exists. In 70% of the cases, these tumors occur as a **discrete intramural mass more than 5 cm in diameter.** Extension to the mucosa and serosa may occur, and mesenteric lymph nodes may be involved. Although symptoms of partial small bowel obstruction are frequent complaints, **complete intestinal obstruction is uncommon.**
  D. **Metastatic spread**
   1. **Modes of spread.** Small bowel malignancies spread by three distinct mechanisms.
    a. **Direct extension.** Growth of tumor into contiguous organs is particularly

TABLE 32–1. LOCATION OF SMALL INTESTINAL MALIGNANCIES

Site	Adenocarcinoma (%)	Carcinoids (%)	Sarcomas (%)	Lymphomas (%)
Duodenum	40[a]	8	10	10
Jejunum	35	8	35	10
Ileum	25	84	55	80

[a]Sixty-five percent occur in the periampullary region, 20% occur proximal to the ampulla, and 15% occur distal to the ampulla.

important in duodenal carcinomas, which commonly involve the pancreas and biliary tree. Carcinomas and sarcomas of the jejunum and ileum often invade the mesentery, retroperitoneum, abdominal wall, adjacent bowel, and other viscera.

- b. **Lymphatic metastasis.** Metastatic spread to regional lymph nodes commonly occurs in **carcinomas** and **lymphomas** but is an uncommon route of spread for sarcomas.
- c. **Hematogenous metastasis.** All histologic types of small intestinal malignancies may spread through portal and systemic veins to distant organs.

2. **Sites of spread.** Distant spread of small bowel tumors may involve one or more of the following organs: liver, lung, distant lymph nodes (lymphomas), bone, and peritoneum.

VIII. **Staging.** Except for primary lymphoma of the small intestine, no formal staging system has been developed for malignancies of the small intestine. The staging for **primary lymphomas** is outlined below.

- A. **Stage I.** Tumor is confined to a single area in the gastrointestinal tract; no nodal involvement.
- B. **Stage II.** Tumor is confined to a single area in the gastrointestinal tract; nodal involvement; no perforation or peritonitis.
- C. **Stage III.** Tumor in the gastrointestinal tract has invaded adjacent structures, with or without free perforation or peritonitis.
- D. **Stage IV.** Tumor arises in the gastrointestinal tract and distant metastases are present.

IX. **Treatment**

- A. **Surgery**
  1. **Primary small intestinal malignancies**
     - a. **General considerations.** Surgical resection of primary small bowel malignancies remains the only therapy with curative potential regardless of histology. The objective of surgery is to remove the tumor along with margins of at least 6 inches of normal proximal and distal small bowel as well as a wide segment of mesentery containing draining lymph nodes (not required with sarcomas, which do not usually metastasize to lymph nodes). Surgery for primary small bowel **lymphoma** should include **liver and lymph node biopsy,** but **splenectomy is not indicated.** Only about **50%** of all small bowel tumors are **resectable for cure.**
     - b. **Bowel preparation.** Adequate bowel preparation with isotonic lavage solutions and oral antibiotics are preferred (see also p 277, **I.A.2**); however, many patients present with acute intestinal obstruction, which obviates any attempt to cleanse the intestines.
     - c. **Approaches.** The vast majority of surgeons prefer a **midline approach** for the resection of small bowel tumors because it affords the greatest exposure and latitude if additional, unplanned surgery must be performed.
     - d. **Procedures.** The precise nature of the surgical procedure required depends on the location of the primary tumor.
       - (1) **Duodenal tumors.** Most tumors in the duodenum are adenocarcinomas, and most occur **in or near the papilla of Vater.** As a result of early invasion of surrounding structures such as the pancreas, the distal common bile duct, and the stomach, most malignancies of the duodenum should be resected by **pancreaticoduodenectomy,** followed by choledochojejunostomy, pancreaticojejunostomy, and gastrojejunostomy **(Whipple procedure).** A small number of lesions in the proximal or distal duodenum may be amenable to segmental small bowel resection with adequate margins.
       - (2) **Jejunal tumors. Segmental resection** with margins of at least **6 inches** of normal bowel on either side of the lesion is the treatment of choice for jejunal malignancies.
       - (3) **Ileal tumors.** Segmental resection of ileal tumors in a manner similar to that described for jejunal cancer is preferred for ileal malignancies unless the tumor invades and compromises the lymphovascular mesenteric pedicle to the right colon. In this situation, a distal ileal resection with right hemicolectomy should be performed.
  2. **Locally advanced and metastatic small bowel tumors**
     - a. **Curative surgery.** In general, surgery is not a viable treatment modality for locally advanced or metastatic small intestinal malignancies. However, if a

single distant metastasis is detected in a patient with a previously resected primary lesion, surgical resection of the metastatic focus may be of some benefit. In addition, symptomatic small bowel obstruction from metastases from malignancies outside the gastrointestinal tract, such as melanoma and ovarian carcinoma, may require small bowel resection, bypass, or both.

    b. **Palliative surgery.** Surgery is often indicated in patients with locally advanced (unresectable) and metastatic small bowel tumors, predominantly to **relieve obstruction.** Gastroenterostomy, enteroenterostomy, enterocolostomy, and choledochoenterostomy are occasionally required.

  3. **Mortality and morbidity.** Operative mortality for elective small bowel resection is less than 1%, and morbidity ranges from 5% to 20% With emergent small bowel resection, mortality and morbidity increase significantly. Complications include the following: wound infection and sepsis, anastomotic dehiscence and fistulae, prolonged ileus, anastomotic stricture, pneumonia, thrombophlebitis and pulmonary embolism, and myocardial infarction.

B. Radiation therapy

  1. **Primary tumor therapy.** Because of the relatively radiation-resistant nature of small bowel malignancies (especially carcinoma) and the relative radiosensitive small bowel mucosa, radiation therapy has not found a role in the primary treatment of small intestinal malignancies except in patients with small bowel lymphoma, which is secondary to systemic disease.

  2. **Adjuvant therapy**

    a. **Preoperative radiation therapy.** Preoperative irradiation has no role in small bowel cancer.

    b. **Intraoperative radiation therapy.** High doses of radiation can be delivered intraoperatively to areas suspected of harboring residual tumor while shielding normal tissues that are radiosensitive. This modality, however, has not yet proved to be of practical benefit.

    c. **Postoperative radiation therapy.** Postoperative radiation therapy has limited usefulness, except in patients with **primary small bowel lymphoma** who demonstrate involvement of regional nodes (stages II and III) who may benefit from adjuvant radiation therapy.

  3. **Palliative radiation therapy.** External beam radiation therapy can be used to palliate symptomatic lesions that cause intestinal bleeding, obstruction, and pain. **Liver irradiation** can also improve symptoms associated with the **carcinoid syndrome.** In addition, there is limited evidence that occasional remissions can be obtained with radiation therapy alone.

  4. **Doses.** Typically, 4000–5000 cGy are delivered in small fractions over 4–6 weeks using multiple fields, although toxicity from small and large bowel irradiation may impose a much lower limit.

  5. **Morbidity and mortality.** Side effects are almost universal with high-dose abdominal radiation and usually occur as a result of one of the following complications: fatigue and generalized weakness, anemia, enteritis and diarrhea with malabsorption, intestinal obstruction, or perforation.

C. Chemotherapy. Various cytotoxic agents have been used with some success, depending on the histologic type of small bowel cancer.

  1. **Adenocarcinoma.** The nitrosoureas and fluorouracil have been used alone and in combination with limited rates of response carcinoma of the small intestine. Adjuvant chemotherapy after surgical resection is currently under investigation.

  2. **Carcinoid. Streptozotocin and fluorouracil** have demonstrated some responses in the treatment of metastatic carcinoid tumor. In addition, **intrahepatic arterial therapy** has occasionally improved the symptoms of the carcinoid syndrome.

  3. **Sarcoma.** In metastatic disease, **doxorubicin, cyclophosphamide, vincristine, and imidazole carboxamide** have a response rate as high as 65%. Adjuvant therapy with these agents is currently being evaluated.

  4. **Lymphoma.** Agents commonly used for systemic lymphomas, such as **methotrexate, cyclophosphamide, vincristine, and 6-mercaptopurine,** should be tried in patients with unresectable primary small bowel lymphoma or systemic disease. Adjuvent therapy after resection of a single focus of primary intestinal lymphoma is the topic of considerable debate.

D. Immunotherapy. No forms of immunotherapy, specific or nonspecific, have been evaluated in patients with small bowel malignancies. This new form of therapy holds promise as an additional therapeutic modality in the treatment of small bowel cancer.

X. Prognosis

A. Five-year survival. The outcome of small intestinal tumors depends on both the histologic type and the extent of the malignancy (see Table 32–2).

B. Adverse prognostic factors. As a result of the variation in histologic types and locations of small bowel malignancies as well as their infrequent occurrence, correlating specific independent adverse prognostic factors has been difficult. Some factors that may signify a poor prognosis include the following: intestinal obstruction, jaundice, invasion of contiguous structures, grade of the tumor (sarcomas, carcinomas), and perforation with peritonitis.

XI. Patient follow-up

A. General guidelines. Patients should be followed closely every 3–4 months for 2 years, every 6 months for an additional 3 years, then annually for evidence of local or systemic recurrence. The following guidelines are recommended.

B. Routine evaluation. Each clinic visit should include the following tests and procedures:

    1. History and physical examination. A full-interval history and physical examination is required during each clinic appointment. Areas that should receive specific attention are listed on p 242, **VI.A.**

    2. Blood tests (see p 1, **IV.A**)
       a. Complete blood count.
       b. Hepatic transaminases.
       c. Alkaline phosphatase.

    3. Chest x-ray (see p 3, **IV.C**).

C. Additional evaluation. Other tests that should be done at regular intervals include an upper-gastrointestinal series with small bowel follow through. This radiologic test should be obtained 6 months after surgical resection and annually thereafter to monitor for anastomotic and local recurrence.

D. Optional evaluation. The following tests may be indicated on the basis of previous diagnostic findings or clinical suspicion.

    1. Blood tests (see p 2, **IV.A**)
       a. Nucleotidase.
       b. GGTP.

    2. Imaging studies (see p 3, **IV.C**)
       a. Computed tomography. If signs or symptoms of liver or lung metastases develop, CT is useful in evaluating these organs; however, this test is not universally obtained in routine follow-up of patients.
       b. Magnetic resonance imaging
       c. Technetium-99m bone scan

TABLE 32–2. FIVE-YEAR SURVIVAL OF PATIENTS WITH TUMORS IN THE SMALL INTESTINE

Histologic Type	Resected Disease (%)	Unresected, Metastatic Disease, or Both (%)
Carcinoma	20	< 5
Lymph node negative	70	
Lymph node positive	15	
Carcinoid	45–65	20
Noninvasive	100	
Invasive	45–65	
Sarcoma	50	< 5[a]
Lymphoma	40	25
Stage I	75	
Stage II	35–50	
Stage III	25	
Stage IV	10	

[a]As many as 25% of patients with resectable pulmonary metastases may survive 5 years.

3. **Biopsy.** In patients resected for cure, biopsy of any abnormal tissue should be obtained with biopsy forceps, by needle aspiration, or by surgical exploration, if necessary.

REFERENCES

Feldman JM: Carcinoid tumors and the carcinoid syndrome. *Curr Probl Surg* 1989;**26:**835–885.

Lillemoe KD: Small bowel tumors. In: Cameron JL (editor), *Current Surgical Therapy-3,* 3rd ed. Philadelphia, PA: BC Decker; 1989;88–91.

Shaffer HA: Small bowel diseases: diagnosis using radiographic pattern analysis. *Curr Probl Diag Radiol* 1984;**13**(3):1–71.

Wright JC: Update in cancer chemotherapy: gastrointestinal cancer, cancer of the small intestines, gallbladder, liver, and esophagus. *J Nat Med Assoc* 1986;**78:**753–766.

33 Malignancies of the Exocrine Pancreas

Robert B. Cameron, MD

I. **Epidemiology.** Although cancer of the pancreas in the United States is the eighth most common malignancy in males and the seventh most common cancer in females, it is the **fourth leading cause of cancer deaths.** In 1985, 11.1 cases per 100,000 males and 8.2 cases per 100,000 females were diagnosed, resulting in 10.3 and 7.1 deaths, respectively. In 1993 it is estimated that 27,700 new cases are now reported each year, leading to 25,000 deaths. During the last 30 years, the **mortality rate has increased** 12% for males and 26% for females because of unidentified factors. The worldwide incidence of pancreatic cancer varies from as high as 18.3 per 100,000 population in the San Francisco Bay area among black males to 14.8 per 100,000 in Maori, New Zealand, to fewer than 1 per 100,000 in Bombay, India. Studies of immigrants show that the incidence rate rapidly increases toward the rate of the host country in first-generation immigrants but that a persistent difference may remain.

II. **Risk factors.** Environmental factors have been predominantly implicated in the pathogenesis of pancreatic cancer. The following have either been causally linked to or associated with the development of pancreatic malignancies.
   A. **Age.** The incidence of pancreatic cancer increases from fewer than 1 per 100,000 after the age of 35 to **96.1 per 100,000 after age 85.** The median age of presentation is 69 years.
   B. **Sex. Males** in the United States are at **1.35–1.5 times greater risk** than females.
   C. **Race. Blacks** in the United States are at **1.5 times greater risk** than whites. Hawaiians, American Indians, Polynesians, and Jews also are at higher risk.
   D. **Genetic factors.** No distinct genetic predisposition for pancreatic cancer is known.
   E. **Smoking.** Cigarette smoking (at least two packs per day) **doubles the risk** of pancreatic carcinoma.
   F. **Diet.** Although a number of dietary factors have been implicated in the pathogenesis of pancreatic cancer, all have been questioned and none have been definitively proved.
      1. **Coffee consumption.** A single study demonstrated a positive correlation between coffee consumption and pancreatic carcinoma. To date, the results of this study remain unconfirmed.
      2. **Alcohol.** Although one Finnish study suggested an association between alcohol consumption and pancreatic cancer, most studies fail to show a correlation.
      3. **Dietary fat.** Some studies have implicated dietary fat as a risk factor for pancreatic carcinoma, but these results have not been widely accepted.
   G. **Previous pancreatic pathology**
      1. **Pancreatitis.** An increased incidence of pancreatic cancer among patients with **chronic pancreatitis** suggests that prolonged inflammation may predispose to the development of pancreatic malignancies.
      2. **Diabetes mellitus.** Diabetes has been associated with pancreatic carcinoma; however, because pancreatic cancer can directly cause diabetes, the magnitude of the increased risk, if any, is unknown.
   H. **Urbanization**
      1. **Socioeconomic status.** Pancreatic carcinoma is more prevalent among people in **lower socioeconomic groups** than among those in higher income brackets.
      2. **Industrial toxin exposure. Chemists, coke and metal workers, and gas plant workers** have as much as a **5 times greater risk** because of exposure to solvents and petroleum compounds such as benzidine, beta-naphthylamine, nitrosamines, and azaserine.

III. **Presentation**
   A. **Signs and symptoms.** Presenting signs and symptoms are usually **insidious and nonspecific** and often result in a delayed diagnosis.
      1. **Local manifestations**

       a. Lesions of the pancreatic head. Common signs and symptoms include
        weight loss (92%), **jaundice** (87%), **enlarged liver** (83%), **pain** (72%),
        anorexia (64%), **dark urine** (63%), **light stools** (62%), nausea (45%), em-
        esis (37%), weakness (35%), palpable gallbladder (**Courvoisier's sign;**
        29%), pruritus (24%), ascites (14%), abdominal mass (13%), steatorrhea
        (10%), and diabetes (10%).
       b. Lesions of the pancreatic body and tail. Common presenting signs and
        symptoms include weight loss (100%), pain (87%), weakness (43%), nau-
        sea (43%), emesis (37%), anorexia (33%), enlarged liver (33%), constipa-
        tion (27%), abdominal mass (23%), ascites (23%), jaundice (13%), and fatty
        foods intolerance (7%).
     2. Systemic manifestations. Many of the systemic symptoms above reflect local
      disease. In addition, hepatomegaly (liver metastases), pulmonary nodules
      (lung metastases), neurologic symptoms (metastases to the central nervous
      system), and weight loss can be manifestations of metastatic pancreatic can-
      cer.
  B. Paraneoplastic syndromes. The following paraneoplastic syndromes have been
    associated with pancreatic carcinoma and, although uncommon, may be the sole
    manifestation of an underlying malignancy:
    1. Migratory thrombophlebitis (Trousseaus' sign) (see p 81).
    2. Panniculitis-arthritis-eosinophilia syndrome. This syndrome (also called
      systemic nodular panniculitis and Weber-Christian disease) is manifested
      by **recurrent fever, eosinophilia, polyarthritis, and groups of erythema-
      tous subcutaneous nodules** that may be accompanied by abdominal pain
      and fat necrosis in bone, lungs, and other organs. The subcutaneous nodules
      are variably erythematous and sometimes necrotic. Although benign pancreatic
      disease also is associated with this phenomenon because of elevated levels of
      circulating pancreatic lipase, malignancy must be excluded.
IV. Differential diagnosis. Pancreatic masses are associated with a number of acute and
   chronic pancreatic diseases. In the presence of a pancreatic mass, the diagnosis of
   carcinoma must be pursued. Occasionally, however, carcinoma can be extremely difficult to prove; even with substantial biopsy samples, the difference between inflammation and carcinoma can be obscure. Benign pathologic processes that may be associated with a pancreatic mass include pancreatitis, pseudocysts, benign pancreatic
   exocrine tumors (adenoma, cystadenoma, fibroadenoma, oncocytoma, lipoma,
   leiomyoma, hemangioma, and lymphangioma), and islet cell neoplasms.
V. Screening programs. To date, no effective screening programs have been developed; however, detection of serum antigens associated with visceral malignancies
   have been identified and provide hope that future research will lead to simple screening
   assays that are both sensitive and specific.
VI. Diagnostic workup
  A. Medical history and physical examination. A complete medical history empha-
    sizing common presenting symptoms (eg, weight loss, abdominal pain, and jaun-
    dice) and a thorough physical examination are essential to a complete evaluation.
    1. General appearance. The level of nutrition and overall health can be quickly
      assessed.
    2. Skin. The presence of pallor (anemia), jaundice (biliary obstruction), evidence
      of thrombophlebitis **(Trousseau's sign),** and erythematous subcutaneous nod-
      ules **(systemic nodular panniculitis)** should be noted.
    3. Lymph nodes. The presence of a signal node (also called **Virchow's or
      Troisier's node**) must be recorded.
    4. Abdomen. A thorough search for hepatomegaly, a palpable gallbladder
      (Courvoisier's sign), ascites, and palpable abdominal masses should be made.
    5. Rectum. Stool should be examined for occult blood, and pelvic masses
      (Blumer's shelf lesions) must be excluded.
  B. Primary tests and procedures. All patients with suspected pancreatic malignan-
    cies should have the following diagnostic tests performed:
    1. Blood tests (see p 1, **IV.A**).
      a. Complete blood count.
      b. Hepatic transaminases.
      c. Alkaline phosphatase.
    2. Imaging studies (see p 3, **IV.C**).
      a. Chest x-ray.
      b. Computerized tomography (CT). CT is the standard test for assessing the
        extent of disease because the pancreas, regional lymph nodes, and other

abdominal organs such as the liver can be evaluated for tumor involvement. CT scans have demonstrated a greater than **77% sensitivity and an 82% specificity** in identifying pancreatic masses.

   3. **Invasive procedures. Percutaneous transabdominal needle aspiration** is a simple procedure that provides the diagnosis in 87–100% of patients with minimal morbidity (< 5%).

C. **Optional tests and procedures.** The following tests and procedures may be indicated on the basis of previous diagnostic results or clinical suspicion:

   1. **Blood tests**
      a. **Nucleotidase** (see p 2, **IV.A.**).
      b. **GGTP** (see p 2, **IV.A.**).
      c. **Carcinoembryonic antigen** (CEA). Elevated serum levels of this tumor marker occur in more than 80% of patients with pancreatic malignancies, but because 40% of patients with benign pancreatic disease also have increased levels, this is a **nonspecific** finding. **Levels that are greater than 10 ng/mL,** however, are almost always associated with advanced malignant disease. Conversely, 70% of patients with advanced disease are found to have levels greater than 10 ng/mL.
      d. **Alpha-fetoprotein.** Elevated serum levels of AFP have been noted in as many as **25%** of pancreatic cancer patients, but this fetal antigen also is increased in germ cell malignancies.
      e. **Pancreatic oncofetal antigen.** POA is a glycoprotein with a molecular weight of 800,000 daltons, which is increased in **77–90% of patients** with **malignant** pancreatic disease, but **only 0–17% of patients with benign pancreatic or extrapancreatic disease.**
      f. **Ca 19–9 antigen.** This tumor-associated antigen has been detected by a murine monoclonal antibody raised against a human colon carcinoma. This antigen can be detected in **80% of patients** with pancreatic **malignancy** versus only **8%** of patients with **benign** pancreatic disease and 1% of normal subjects.

   2. **Imaging studies**
      a. **Abdominal ultrasonography** (ULTZ). ULTZ is an excellent screening examination for the presence of pancreatic masses. It boasts a **82% sensitivity and 84% specificity.**
      b. **Barium upper gastrointestinal examination.** This dye study may demonstrate anterior displacement of the stomach, **widening of the "C" duodenal loop, or a "reverse three"** duodenal abnormality caused by lesions of the pancreatic head. This examination is less useful for lesions of the body and tail.
      c. **Magnetic resonance imaging** (see p 3, **IV.C.3**).
      d. **Angiography.** This special examination is used to identify encasement of the superior mesenteric, hepatic, or celiac arteries, as well as any abnormal vascular anatomy, but it is only required when a question regarding resectability arises.
      e. **Technetium-99m bone scan** (see p 3, **IV.C.5**).

   3. **Invasive procedures**
      a. **Endoscopic retrograde cholangiopancreatography (ECRP).** ERCP is capable of visualizing periampullary carcinoma as well as tumor encasement or obstruction of the pancreatic duct. The **diagnostic accuracy** can be as high as 85% and, when combined with biliary cytologies, can be as high as 90%.
      b. **Percutaneous transhepatic cholangiography.** This invasive procedure is particularly useful in the presence of biliary obstruction if a question arises about the proximal extent of the tumor into the common bile duct.

VII. **Pathology**
A. **Location.** The location of the primary pancreatic tumor often determines the resectability as well as the presenting signs and symptoms.
   1. **Lesions of the pancreatic head,** 73%.
   2. **Lesions of the pancreatic body,** 20%.
   3. **Lesions of the pancreatic tail,** 7%.
B. **Multiplicity. Synchronous primary lesions** (usually carcinoma in situ) are found in as many as 25% of resected specimens.
C. **Histology.** The common histology types of pancreatic carcinoma are listed in Table 33–1, along with their frequencies.

TABLE 33–1. HISTOLOGIC TYPES OF CARCINOMA OF THE PANCREAS

Histologic Type	Frequency (%)
Adenocarcinoma	80
Adenosquamous carcinoma	4
Giant cell carcinoma	4
Cystadenocarcinoma	2
Acinar cell carcinoma	2
Pancreaticoblastoma	1
Papillary cystic carcinoma	1
Anaplastic carcinoma	1
Microadenoma	1
Lymphoma	1
Sarcoma	1

D. **Metastatic spread.** Metastases to distant sites are present in as many as 50% of patients at the time of diagnosis.
 1. **Modes of spread.** Pancreatic cancer can spread by four distinct mechanisms:
  a. **Direct extension.** At the time of diagnosis, pancreatic neoplasms frequently have spread by direct extension to the following organs:
   (1) Lesions of the pancreatic head. These tumors spread into the **duodenum** (19%) and the **stomach** (11%).
   (2) Lesions of the pancreatic body. These malignancies extend to the **spleen** (14%), **transverse colon** (12%), **stomach** (5%) and **duodenum** (5%).
   (3) Lesions of the pancreatic tail. These neoplasms grow into the left adrenal gland (24%), spleen (14%), transverse colon (14%), stomach (5%), left kidney (5%), and jejunum (5%).
  b. **Lymphatic metastasis.** Malignant cells can spread readily through lymphatic channels to superior and inferior pancreatic, gastric, pyloric, mesenteric, and anterior pancreaticoduodenal lymph nodes.
  c. **Hematogenous metastasis.** Tumor cells that are dislodged and attain access to the vascular system can travel through portal, portovertebral, and portosystemic vessels to distant organs.
  d. **Direct implantation.** Tumor cells shed into the peritoneal cavity can implant on the peritoneal surfaces of any intra-abdominal viscera.
 2. **Sites of spread.** At autopsy, frequent sites of metastatic spread include the following organs:
  a. **Regional lymph nodes,** 50–75%.
  b. **Liver,** 70%.
  c. **Lungs,** 15–30%.
  d. **Peritoneal surfaces,** 25%.
  e. **Adrenal glands,** 29% (body and tail lesions); 13% (lesions of the head).
  f. **Duodenum,** 67% (lesions of the head); 24% (body and tail lesions).
  g. **Stomach,** 25–40% (lesions of the body and head); 7% (tail lesions).
  h. **Spleen,** 12–36% (body and tail lesions); 6% (lesions of the head).
  i. **Gallbladder,** 10% (lesions of the head); less than 1% (body and tail lesions).
  j. **Kidney,** 7%.
  k. **Small intestine,** 7%.
VIII. **Staging.** The American Joint Committee on Cancer and the Union Internationale Contre le Cancer recently revised their TNM staging systems. The result is a single international standard for future studies that allows direct comparison of different treatment regimens. The staging of ampullary carcinoma differs slightly from that of the rest of the pancreas. Each system is presented below:
 A. **Ampulla of Vater**
  1. **Tumor stage**
   a. **TX.** Primary tumor cannot be assessed.

      b. T0. No evidence of a primary tumor exists.
      c. Tis. Carcinoma in situ.
      d. T1. Tumor is limited to the ampulla of Vater.
      e. T2. Tumor invades the duodenal wall.
      f. T3. Tumor invades less than 2 cm into the pancreas.
      g. T4. Tumor invades more than 2 cm into the pancreas, other adjacent organs, or both.

  2. Lymph node stage
      a. NX. Regional lymph nodes cannot be assessed.
      b. N0. No regional lymph node metastases are present.
      c. N1. Regional lymph node metastases are present.
          Note: Regional lymph nodes include superior and inferior pancreatic, anterior and posterior pancreaticoduodenal, pyloric, proximal mesenteric, and common bile duct but do not include splenic lymph nodes or nodes near the pancreatic tail, which are considered distant metastases.

  3. Metastatic stage
      a. MX. Distant metastases cannot be assessed.
      b. M0. No distant metastases are present.
      c. M1. Distant metastases are present.

  4. Histopathologic grade
      a. GX. Grade cannot be assessed.
      b. G1. Well differentiated.
      c. G2. Moderately well differentiated.
      d. G3. Poorly differentiated.
      e. G4. Undifferentiated.

  5. Stage groupings
      a. Stage 0. Tis, N0, M0.
      b. Stage I. T1, N0, M0.
      c. Stage II. T2–3, N0, M0.
      d. Stage III. Any T, N1, M0.
      e. Stage IV. T4; any N, M0 or any T; any N, M1.

B. Exocrine pancreas

  1. Tumor stage
      a. TX. The primary tumor cannot be assessed.
      b. T0. No evidence of a primary tumor.
      c. T1. The tumor limited to the pancreas:
          (1) T1a. Tumor is smaller than 2 cm in diameter.
          (2) T1b. Tumor is larger than 2 cm in diameter.
      d. T2. Tumor extends directly into the duodenum, bile duct, or peripancreatic tissues.
      e. T3. Tumor extends directly into the stomach, spleen, colon, or adjacent large blood vessels.

  2. Lymph node stage
      a. NX. Regional lymph nodes cannot be assessed.
      b. N0. No regional lymph node metastases are present.
      c. N1. Regional lymph node metastases are present.
          Note: Regional lymph nodes include peripancreatic, hepatic, retroperitoneal, superior mesenteric, and lateral aortic. Infrapyloric, subpyloric, and celiac nodes are included for tumors only in the head. Pancreaticolienal and splenic nodes are included only for tumors of the body and tail.

  3. Metastatic stage
      a. MX. Distant metastases cannot be assessed.
      b. M0. No distant metastases are present.
      c. M1. Distant metastases are present.

  4. Histopathologic grade
      a. GX. Grade cannot be assessed.
      b. G1. Well differentiated.
      c. G2. Moderately well differentiated.
      d. G3. Poorly differentiated.
      e. G4. Undifferentiated.

  5. Stage groupings
      a. Stage I. T1–2, N0, M0.
      b. Stage II. T3, N0, M0.
      c. Stage III. Any T, N1, M0.
      d. Stage IV. Any T, any N, M1.

IX. Treatment
A. Surgery
1. Primary pancreatic carcinoma

a. **Indications.** Surgical resection remains the only chance of cure for patients with pancreatic carcinoma. Surgery should be contemplated in any medically fit patient whose disease is believed to be resectable. **Contraindications** that may or may not be identified preoperatively include **distant metastases** (eg, liver, lung), **peritoneal implants** (Blumer's shelf lesions), **nodal metastases** (particularly with islet cell or ampullary cancers), **encasement of the superior mesenteric or celiac vessels, and invasion of the portal vein or inferior vena cava.** Advanced age alone is not a contraindication to surgery. Using these criteria, approximately 75% of patients are operative candidates; however, only 20% are ultimately resectable. The resectability rates are the highest for ampullary (70%) and islet cell tumors (33%) and lower for adenocarcinoma of the pancreas (13%).

b. **Preoperative biliary decompression.** Preoperative surgical or percutaneous biliary decompression in patients with obstructive jaundice was formerly thought to decrease the morbidity and mortality of definitive surgery. This belief was based on retrospective studies using historical controls, which demonstrated a decrease in perioperative mortality from 20–50% to 4–18%. However, three subsequent randomized prospective trials have failed to show any clear benefit to preoperative biliary decompression. In addition, decompression (either percutaneously or endoscopically) is associated with a mortality rate of 2–13%.

c. **Approaches.** Most surgeons prefer to approach the pancreas for possible resection through a **bilateral subcostal "chevron" incision.** An additional upper midline "Mercedes-Benz" extension also can be made. A standard midline incision also can be used, but it is usually considered to be suboptimal.

d. **Procedures**

(1) **Pancreaticoduodenectomy (Whipple procedure).** This procedure removes the distal stomach, duodenum, gallbladder, distal common bile duct, head of the pancreas (to the level of the superior mesenteric vein), and proximal jejunum. A significant portion of the procedure is devoted to assessing resectability and to establishing a diagnosis (if not known preoperatively) by **transduodenal core needle biopsy.** After confirming the diagnosis of pancreatic carcinoma and ruling out liver or nodal metastases, surgical dissection is carried out to mobilize the head of the pancreas and to assess involvement of inferior vena cava and the celiac, hepatic, mesenteric, and portal vessels. If one of these situations is encountered, the procedure is terminated and palliative bypass is undertaken. More recent modifications of the Whipple procedure include **pylorus-preserving procedures** that also do not require truncal vagotomy.

(2) **Regional (total) pancreatectomy.** Some surgeons argue that the multicentric nature of pancreatic carcinoma demands that a total pancreatectomy be performed as part of a pancreaticoduodenectomy. They also point out that this avoids the morbidity associated with **pancreatic fistulae** resulting from pancreaticoenteric anastomoses. On the other hand, opponents argue that the **brittle diabetes** which develops in 25% of patients after this procedure and a lack of improved survival outweigh all the proposed benefits and that, in general, this procedure is warranted only if the **pancreatic remnant is friable, the margin is positive for tumor, or if preexisting severe diabetes is present.**

(3) **Distal pancreatectomy and splenectomy.** Twenty-five percent of pancreatic malignancies occur in the **body or tail of the pancreas** and do not require a Whipple procedure. However, because of their location, few symptoms are produced until late in the course: therefore, only a small fraction of these malignancies are resectable. In these few resectable tumors, distal pancreatectomy and splenectomy are generally indicated.

e. **Reconstruction**

(1) **Biliary reconstruction.** A **choledochojejunostomy** is usually the first anastomosis performed during the reconstruction phase of the opera-

tion. The end of the common bile duct is carefully sutured to the mucosa of the jejunum with fine **absorbable suture** (e.g. 4–0 maxon). Preoperative placement of biliary drainage catheters can be extremely useful because it facilitates the intraoperative identification of the common bile duct and acts as a stent for the anastomosis, thereby obviating any need for T-tube placement. The choledochojejunostomy is generally performed **proximal to the gastric anastomosis** to help prevent **marginal ulceration** of the gastrojejunostomy.

- **(2) Pancreatic reconstruction.** Most commonly, the distal pancreas is sewn to the most proximal portion of the jejunum with fine **nonabsorbable suture** and the proximal pancreatic duct is anastomosed with extremely fine nonabsorbable suture (e.g., 5–0 prolene) to the mucosa of the jejunum. Extreme care must be taken with this anastomosis to avoid the development of postoperative pancreatic fistulae. This pancreaticojejunostomy, like the choledochojejunostomy, is performed **proximal to the gastrojejunostomy** to prevent **marginal ulceration** caused by non-neutralized gastric acid.
- **(3) Enteric reconstruction.** The last step in reconstruction is to fashion a standard two-layer (inner absorbable and outer nonabsorbable) **gastrojejunostomy.** The remaining stomach is carefully sewn to the jejunum distal to the other two anastomoses. If a pylorus-preserving procedure is not used, a truncal vagotomy is performed as well.

2. **Locally advanced and metastatic carcinoma**
   a. **Curative surgery.** Currently, surgery is not an option for locally advanced or metastatic tumor, although some centers are now investigating the combination of surgical resection and intraoperative radiation therapy for locally advanced pancreatic carcinoma.
   b. **Palliative (bypass) surgery.** Palliative bypass procedures should be performed in all unresectable patients who are medically able to undergo surgery. The procedure should include both a biliary-enteric and gastro-enteric bypass. Much debate has centered on what type of biliary bypass should be used in pancreatic carcinoma patients. Some surgeons favor a **cholecysto-jejunostomy** because of its technical ease. Others, however, favor a **choledochojejunostomy** and cite the frequency of diseased gallbladders and a 10–15% rate of **delayed cystic duct obstruction.** When analyzed in light of the short expected survival of patients with pancreatic carcinoma, either method of biliary bypass is acceptable. In addition, chronic back and abdominal pain can be substantially, and occasionally permanently, relieved in 90% of patients by intraoperative celiac nerve block. This can be done without increased morbidity or mortality simply by injecting 50 mL of **50% alcohol or 6% phenol** in the area of the celiac plexus. This procedure can play a crucial role in palliating the usually difficult problem of pancreatic cancer pain.
   c. **Nonoperative palliation.** Percutaneous transhepatic or endoscopic placement of **biliary catheters and stents** offers an alternative to surgical bypass in pancreatic carcinoma patients. Because 80% of patients fail to develop duodenal obstruction, significant palliation can be afforded by these techniques alone. In experienced hands, these techniques can be performed in 70–90% of cases with acceptable morbidity and 2–5% mortality. Internal stents can often be placed without the need for external catheters. The **stents and catheters must be changed every three months;** however, most patients do not require more than one catheter change.

3. **Morbidity and mortality.** The worldwide mortality rate for pancreaticoduodenectomy ranges from 15–20%. At specialized centers in the United States, recent mortality figures range from 2–5%. Morbidity rates vary from 20–50%. Several common causes of postoperative morbidity and mortality are **sepsis and wound infection, pancreatitis and pancreatic fistulae,** biliary or gastric anastomotic leak, hemorrhage, anastomotic stricture, marginal ulceration, dumping syndrome, diabetes mellitus, and pancreatic exocrine insufficiency.

B. **Radiation therapy**
   1. **Primary radiation therapy.** Radiation therapy as a primary treatment modality for potentially resectable pancreatic carcinoma should be reserved only for patients who refuse surgery.
   2. **Adjuvant radiation therapy**

a. **Preoperative radiation therapy.** Two small studies suggest that preoperative radiation therapy may permit **delayed resection** in as many as 33% of selected patients with localized but unresectable disease. The possible long-term survival advantage of this approach, however, has not been investigated.

b. **Intraoperative radiation therapy.** Administration of 2000 cGy immediately after pancreatic resection can spare radiosensitive normal tissues and, according to a single prospective randomized trial at the National Cancer Institute, may result in **prolonged survival**—20 months vs 12 months without radiation (p = 0.1) (Sindelar & Kinsela, 1986). This method of therapy, however, requires specialized equipment that is currently available in only a few centers worldwide.

c. **Postoperative radiation therapy.** Administration of standard external beam radiation therapy postoperatively after resection of pancreatic carcinoma (4000 cGy over 6 weeks) has been evaluated in a single prospective randomized trial by the Gastrointestinal Tumor Study Group (1985) in conjunction with postoperative administration of fluorouracil. Significant improvement in 2-year survival was observed (43% versus 18% in controls; p = 0.5) and in median survival (21 months versus 11 in controls; p = 0.5). This study, however, has yet to be confirmed.

3. **Radiation therapy of locally advanced unresectable disease**

a. **External beam radiation therapy.** External beam radiation therapy, typically using a 3 field approach and fractions of 180–200 cGy, is a viable method of **palliating pain** associated with locally advanced pancreatic carcinoma. Patients considered for this therapy should be free of distant disease and demonstrate an adequate nutritional status (weight loss < 10% of body weight). Results depend on the total dose delivered: 25% of patients receive palliation after 4000 cGy; 33%, after 5000 cGy; and 67%, after more than 6000 cGy. **Tumor growth, however, is controlled in fewer than 50%** of patients even with doses as high as 7000 cGy.

b. **Interstitial radiation therapy.** Three different series have described the use of implanted ^{125}I in the therapy of locally advanced pancreatic carcinoma. Although no clear survival advantages were noted in any of the studies, significant morbidity was reported, including pancreatitis, pancreatic fistulae, abscesses, and duodenal ulcerations and perforation. Without further studies, this form of treatment **cannot be recommended.**

c. **Intraoperative radiation therapy.** Results of intraoperative radiation therapy are available from 3 American centers and from Japan. Doses of 2000–3000 cGy have been used, and postoperative external-beam therapy, radiation sensitizers (misonidazole), and chemotherapy (fluorouracil) have often been added to the treatment package. Although few side effects other than duodenal ulceration and hemorrhage have been noted, **no therapeutic benefit** has been established.

d. **Other methods of radiation therapy.** High-energy-transfer radiation (neutrons), helium ions, and negative pi mesons have been used experimentally in the treatment of pancreatic carcinoma. To date, no improvement over standard external-beam radiation therapy has been shown.

4. **Metastatic disease.** Because survival is extremely limited, radiation therapy is rarely indicated for patients with metastatic pancreatic carcinoma.

C. **Chemotherapy.** Because of the large number of patients presenting with unresectable and metastatic disease, chemotherapy has been investigated as a primary treatment modality in pancreatic carcinoma. Unfortunately, **host debility, advanced disease, and tumor cell resistance** have limited the success of chemical agents and generated widespread pessimism about their usefulness in pancreatic cancer.

1. **Single-agent therapy.** More than 33 different agents have been evaluated as single agents in the treatment of pancreatic carcinoma. Although no single agent produces dramatic effects, several result in moderate response rates: for example, **fluorouracil** (26%), **ifosfamide** (26%), **epirubicin** (22%), **mitomycin-C** (21%), lomustine (16%), and streptozotocin (11%).

2. **Combination chemotherapy.** Fluorouracil has been combined with a variety of agents in 2-drug regimens that have not proved to be superior to fluorouracil alone. Two 3-drug regimens—SMF (streptozotocin, mitomycin-C, and fluorouracil) and FAM (fluorouracil, doxorubicin, and mitomycin-C)—have been examined extensively without consistent therapeutic efficacy. Thus, no 2- or 3-

drug combination regimens can be recommended outside of formal clinical trials.

   3. Adjuvant chemotherapy. Fluorouracil has been used in combination with radiation therapy after surgical resection of pancreatic carcinoma without clear benefit and cannot be recommended at this time.

  D. Immunotherapy. A murine IgG2a monoclonal antibody, 17–1A, raised against a human colorectal carcinoma cell line has been used alone and in combination with FAM chemotherapy in the treatment of patients with pancreatic malignancies. Although initial, albeit brief, responses were reported, **no therapeutic benefit** has been demonstrated. Additional antibodies, including DU-PAN-1 through DU-PAN-5 and ACI, as well as other forms of immunotherapy (lymphokine-activated killer cells and tumor infiltrating lymphocytes) may be of value, but the efficacy of this form of biologic therapy in pancreatic carcinoma has not been proved.

X. Prognosis

  A. Five-year survival. The prognosis for nearly all patients with pancreatic carcinoma is dismal. Overall 2 year-survival is approximately 10%, and a 5-year survival of 1–5% is typical. Patients with resectable ampullary tumors, however, have an improved outlook: as many as 40–60% survive 5 years. In addition, patients with cystadenocarcinomas, which usually occur in the pancreatic tail, have a 5-year survival rate as high as 30–60% if totally resected, whereas those with giant cell carcinoma of the "epulis" type have only a slightly improved prognosis.

  B. Adverse prognostic factors. Several factors adversely affect the prognosis in patients with pancreatic carcinoma: tumor located in the body or tail, high-grade tumors, short duration of symptoms, and distant metastases present at the time of diagnosis.

XI. Patient follow-up

  A. General guidelines. Patients with resected and unresected disease should be followed every 2–3 months or more often for symptoms that may require further palliation. Patients who survive more than 2 years can be followed less frequently, depending on their clinical status. The following guidelines are offered for patient follow-up.

  B. Routine evaluation. Each clinic visit should include the following tests and procedures.

    1. Complete history and physical examination. An interval history should be taken and a complete physical examination should be performed during all clinic appointments. Particular attention should be focused on the areas discussed earlier above (see p 249, **VI.A**).

    2. Blood tests (see p 1, **IV.A**).

      a. Complete blood count.

      b. Hepatic transaminases.

      c. Alkaline phosphatase.

    3. Chest x-ray (see p 3, **IV.C.1**).

  C. Additional evaluation. Computerized tomography (CT) scans of the abdomen should be obtained every 4–6 months in patients resected for cure to detect any evidence of local recurrence that may be amenable to radiation therapy.

  D. Optional evaluation. The following tests and procedures may be indicated by previous diagnostic findings or clinical suspicion.

    1. Blood tests (see p 2, **IV.A**)

      a. Nucleotidase.

      b. GGTP.

    2. Imaging studies (see p 3, **IV.C**)

      a. Magnetic resonance imaging (MRI).

      b. Techneticum-99m bone scan.

    3. Biopsy. In patients resected for cure, biopsy of any abnormal tissue should be obtained with biopsy forceps or by needle aspiration. Surgical exploration as an attempt to make a diagnosis, however, is almost never indicated.

REFERENCES

Cullinan SA et al: A comparison of chemotherapeutic regimens in the treatment of advanced pancreatic and gastric carcinoma. *JAMA* 1985;**253**:2061.

Gastrointestinal Tumor Study Group: Further evidence of effective adjuvant combined radiation and chemotherapy following curative resection of pancreatic cancer. *Cancer* 1987;**59**:2006.

Gastrointestinal Tumor Study Group: Pancreatic cancer: adjuvant combined radiation and chemotherapy following curative resection. *Arch Surg* 1985;**120**:899.

Gastrointestinal Tumor Study Group: Phase II studies of drug combinations in advanced pancreatic carcinoma: fluorouracil plus doxorubicin plus mitomycin-C. *J Clin Oncol* 1986;**4**:1794.

Howard JM, Jordan GL, Reber HA (editors): *Surgical Diseases of the Pancreas.* Philadelphia, PA: Lea & Febiger; 1987.

Moossa AR: Pancreatic cancer—approach to diagnosis, selection for surgery, and choice of operation. *Cancer* 1982;**50**:2689–2698.

Moossa AR: Periampullary cancer. In: Cameron JL (editor), *Current Surgical Therapy–3,* 3rd ed. Philadelphia, PA: BC Decker; 1989:331–339.

Oster MW et al: Chemotherapy for advanced pancreatic cancer: a comparison of 5-fluorouracil, Adriamycin, and mitomycin-C (FAM) with 5-fluorouracil, streptozotocin, and mitomycin-C (FSM). *Cancer* 1986;**57**:29.

Schein PS: The role of chemotherapy in the management of gastric and pancreatic carcinoma. *Semin Oncol* 1985;**12**:49.

Sindelar WF, Kinsella TJ: Randomized trial of intraoperative radiotherapy in resected carcinoma of the pancreas. *Int J Radiat Oncol Biol Phys* 1986;**12**(suppl):148.

34 Malignancies of the Liver & Intrahepatic Biliary Tract

Terence P. Wade, MD, and Robert B. Cameron, M.D.

I. **Epidemiology.** Primary hepatic neoplasms are uncommon in the United States, constituting **less than 1% of both new cancer cases and deaths,** excluding skin cancer. In 1985, **3.9 males and 1.3 females per 100,000** population were diagnosed with hepatocellular carcinoma. Combined with extrahepatic biliary malignancies, estimates indicated that 7,800 new cases and 6,500 deaths will occur in 1993, nearly double the number of cases that occurred 20 years ago. The worldwide incidence of liver cancer varies dramatically. Areas of Asia and of Africa, such as Mozambique, where hepatitis B is endemic, have a peak incidence as high as 164 cases per 100,000, whereas areas such as Australia and Wales have fewer than 0.6 cases per 100,000 population.

II. **Risk factors**

  A. **Age.** The incidence of hepatocellular carcinoma increases from less than 1.0 per 100,000 before age 45 to **16.2 per 100,000 by age 80.** In areas where the incidence of hepatocellular carcinoma is high, eg, in sub-Saharan Africa, the peak incidence occurs earlier between the ages of 20 and 50 years. The **fibrolamellar variant** of hepatocellular carcinoma also occurs in a younger population with a mean age of less than 30 years.

  B. **Sex.** Independent of preexisting liver disease, there is no sex predilection. The **male:female ratio of 3:1** in the United States reflects the increased incidence of liver disease in males.

  C. **Race.** The risk in **American Blacks is 1.5 times** that of the white population, and Asian Americans have an 8 times higher risk than Caucasians.

  D. **Genetic factors.** No independent genetic factors have been identified, but inherited diseases such as **alpha-1-antitrypsin deficiency** produce **cirrhosis** and therefore predispose to liver cancer. Familial clustering of hepatic adenomas and even carcinomas have been reported in the literature.

  E. **Diet**

   1. **Aflatoxins.** These substances are by-products of the fungus, *Aspergillus flavus,* which contaminates grains, dairy products, and **peanuts** and is a potent hepatic carcinogen.

   2. **Alcohol.** Heavy ethanol use, especially when resulting in cirrhosis, has been implicated as a major predisposing factor for hepatocellular carcinoma in the United States.

  F. **Smoking.** Tobacco has not been identified as an independent risk factor in hepatocellular carcinoma.

  G. **Steroids. Anabolic steroids and birth control pills** have been associated with a higher than normal incidence of hepatic tumors, many of which are **adenomas.**

  H. **History of previous hepatic pathology**

   1. **Cirrhosis.** In the United States, cirrhosis is often associated with the development of hepatocellular carcinoma. In patients with a history of heavy ethanol use, 10–55% who die of **cirrhosis** are found to have **hepatocellular carcinoma** at autopsy. In patients with **cirrhosis secondary to hemochromatosis,** 10–20% develop an hepatic neoplasm. The mechanism is unclear, but chronic inflammation accompanying cirrhosis is believed to play a critical role.

   2. **Infection**

    a. **Hepatitis B.** Approximately 70–80% of patients with hepatocellular carcinoma in Asia and Africa and 21% of patients in the United States harbor the hepatitis B virus. Although the association between hepatitis B and liver cancer has been well documented, whether direct nuclear changes or indirect chronic inflammation and cirrhosis are the inciting factor is unknown.

b. **Liver flukes. Cholangiocarcinoma** (bile duct cancer) occurs in the liver in association with parasitic infestations of the bile ducts by the Asian liver fluke *Clonorchis sinensis.*

c. **Bacterial infections.** The chronic **typhoid carrier state** has been identified with an increased risk of liver cancer.

3. **Congenital abnormalities.** An association between Caroli's disease (cystic dilation of the intrahepatic biliary system) and intrahepatic bile duct carcinoma has been reported in the literature.

l. **Urbanization.** Poor sanitation and overcrowding associated with urban areas increases the risk of hepatitis, cirrhosis, and hepatocellular cancer. In addition, exposure to hepatotoxins such as **mycotoxins, plant alkaloids, and vinyl chloride** has been implicated in the etiology of hepatocellular carcinoma.

III. **Presentation**

A. **Signs and symptoms**

1. **Local manifestations.** Dull **pain in the right upper quadrant (57%), pain in the right shoulder (diaphragmatic involvement), hepatomegaly (52%),** abdominal mass (41%), rapidly progressive ascites from hepatic venous occlusion (**Budd-Chiari Syndrome,** 3%), and acute abdominal pain (tumor rupture, hemorrhage, or both, 4%) are typical signs and symptoms from hepatic tumors. In patients with preexisting cirrhosis, hepatocellular cancer can present as acute hepatic failure.

2. **Systemic manifestations.** Fatigue (46%), anorexia and weight loss (33%), fevers, and night sweats (15%) are common systemic symptoms of hepatoma. About 5% of patients present with metastatic lesions, which usually present as mass lesions and usually occur in the lungs.

B. **Paraneoplastic syndromes.** Hepatic carcinoma can be associated with paraneoplastic disorders, especially hematologic and endocrine abnormalities.

1. **Porphyria cutanea tarda.** This unusual syndrome of **painful, pruritic, skin lesions** that vary from slight fragility to photosensitive severe chronic scarring is associated with excessive skin deposition of porphyrins, urinary excretion of uroporphyrin and coproporphyrin, and, in rare cases, with hepatocellular carcinoma.

2. **Hypercalcemia** (see p 87).

3. **Inappropriate ACTH** (see p 90).

4. **Inappropriate gonadotropins** (see p 117).

IV. **Differential diagnosis.** The major difficulty in the diagnosis of hepatic masses is to differentiate between primary hepatocellular tumors and the **more common metastatic lesions.** In addition, abscesses (bacterial or amoebic), regenerating nodules, vascular abnormalities (hemangiomas), and other benign tumors (adenomas) can mimic hepatocellular carcinoma.

V. **Screening programs.** Screening of large populations at risk for hepatic cancer with alpha-fetoprotein has been attempted in China and may result in an increase in the discovery of resectable tumors.

VI. **Diagnostic workup**

A. **Medical history and physical examination.** A complete medical history covering known risk factors such as heavy ethanol use, hepatitis exposure, transfusions, sexual preference, and known congenital disorders must be obtained. Furthermore, a detailed physical examination should be performed, with particular attention to the following areas:

1. **General appearance.** The level of nutrition is important to note.

2. **Skin.** Spider angiomata, palmar erythema, jaundice, and caput medusae are all important findings indicating chronic ethanol abuse.

3. **Head.** The sclera and palate are the most sensitive areas to note clinical jaundice. **Fetor hepaticus,** a particular odor of the breath, is characteristic of liver disease.

4. **Lymph nodes.** The presence of a signal node (also called **Virchow's or Troisier's node**) as well as other lymphadenopathy should be recorded.

5. **Lungs.** Rales associated with fibrosis from ethanol-induced chronic aspiration pneumonias can be detected in some patients.

6. **Abdomen.** Right upper-quadrant masses, bruits, or both should be adequately documented. In addition, the presence of ascites and hepatosplenomegaly should be noted.

7. **Nervous system.** The functional status and the presence or absence of hepatic encephalopathy must be known before any therapeutic intervention is initiated.

B. **Primary tests and procedures.** All patients with known or suspected hepatocellular carcinoma require the following diagnostic tests:
 1. **Blood tests**
    a. **Complete blood count.** This is a good indicator of splenic sequestration of platelets caused by portal hypertension (see also p 1, **IV.A.1**).
    b. **Hepatic transaminases.** These enzymes may be unreliable in the presence of cirrhosis because of limited hepatic reserve (see also p 1, **IV.A.2**).
    c. **Alkaline phosphatase.** (see p 1, **IV.A.3**).
    d. **Albumin.** Albumin is one variable in the nutritional assessment (see p 1, **III**) and Child's classification of liver disease (see Table 34–1).
    e. **Alpha-fetoprotein (AFP).** Elevated levels of this fetal serum marker (> 10 ng/ml) are found in 75–90% of **patients with hepatoma** as well as in patients with hepatitis, cirrhosis, and germ-cell cancers. AFP may return to normal after successful resection and, in this case, may be a useful postoperative test to monitor patients for recurrences.
    f. **Coagulation studies.** The **prothrombin time** is obtained to assess the synthetic function of the liver as well as to anticipate perioperative bleeding problems.
 2. **Imaging studies**
    a. **Chest x-ray.** (see p 3, **IV.C.1**).
    b. **Computed tomography scan (CT).** When obtained with the administration of IV contrast, CT study can detect lesions **as small as 1 cm.** It also can allow directed diagnostic needle biopsy.
    c. **Angiography.** Preoperative hepatic angiography can be helpful to exclude the possibility of hemangioma, detect multiple hepatic lesions, and to delineate vascular anatomy before operation.
 3. **Invasive procedures.** Various types of needle liver biopsy can be utilized to make a pre-operative diagnosis of hepatic malignancy. Although it is accompanied by the risk of hemorrhage and tumor seeding, it can be particularly effective when done under CT or ultrasonic guidance. However, biopsy and assessment of resectability are best performed at laparoscopy/laparotomy.
C. **Optional tests and procedures.** The following examinations may be indicated by diagnostic findings or clinical suspicion.
 1. **Blood tests**
    a. **Nucleotidase** (see p 2, **IV.A.4**).
    b. **GGTP** (see p 2, **IV.A.5**).
    c. **Carcinoembryonic antigen levels** (CEA). Elevated levels of this serum marker are found in some patients with intrahepatic carcinoma of the bile ducts but are uncommon in sera from patients with hepatocellular carcinoma and extrahepatic biliary cancer. Therefore, it occasionally may help to distinguish the histology.
 2. **Imaging studies**
    a. **Ultrasound** (see p 3, **IV.C.3**).
    b. **Magnetic resonance imaging (MRI).** MRI can frequently distinguish between hepatocellular carcinoma, hemangioma, and cirrhosis (see also, p 3, **IV.C.2**).
    c. **Dimethyl-iminodiacetic acid (HIDA) scan.** This study can help evaluate liver function by assessing bile excretion; however, it plays only a peripheral role in the preoperative assessment of hepatocellular carcinoma.
    d. **Technetium-99m bone scan** (see p 3, **IV.C.4**).
 3. **Invasive procedures.** Laparoscopy can be used effectively to directly visualize and biopsy lesions, controlling the risk of bleeding. It also allows visualization of

TABLE 34–1. CHILD'S CLINICAL AND LABORATORY CLASSIFICATION OF HEPATIC FUNCTION

Child's Class	Albumin	Bilirubin	Nutrition	Ascites	Encephalopathy
A	>3.5 mg/dL	< 2.0 mg/dL	Excellent	None	None
B	3.0–3.5 mg/dL	2.0–3.0 mg/dL	Good	Easily controlled	Mild
C	< 3.0 mg/dL	>3.0 mg/dL	Poor	Poorly controlled	Severe (coma)

the liver, the peritoneal cavity, and lymph nodes. However, it requires general anesthesia for most patients and a skilled operator.

VII. Pathology

A. Location. There is no predilection for a specific hepatic lobe in the occurrence of hepatocellular carcinoma.

B. Multiplicity. In cirrhotic patients, hepatomas are frequently accompanied by **multifocal satellite lesions** that can be difficult to distinguish from regenerative nodules. In noncirrhotic patients, however, multiplicity is less characteristic.

C. Histology. Hepatocellular carcinoma and cholangiocarcinoma make up the vast majority of primary hepatic malignancies. Therapeutically, there is no need to differentiate between the two tumors because they are treated identically.

1. **Hepatocellular carcinoma.** This histologic cell type accounts for approximately **90% of primary hepatic malignancies.** Most hepatomas have a trabecular histologic appearance, but the less common **fibrolamellar variant** has a more favorable prognosis, even without resection or even if lymph nodes are involved (if resected).

2. **Cholangiocarcinoma.** Cancer of the intrahepatic bile ducts (cholangiocarcinoma) accounts for about **7% of hepatic malignancies.** This carcinoma is associated with liver fluke infestation in the Orient and has a **female:male predominance of 2:1.** These lesions are more common in patients with **ulcerative colitis** and are hard to distinguish histologically from sclerosing cholangitis.

3. **Other primary tumors.** Bile duct cystadenocarcinoma, squamous cell carcinoma, and sarcoma are other rare histologic types of primary liver cancer. **Angiosarcoma** has been associated with **vinyl chloride and Thorotrast** (a thorium-containing contrast agent that is no longer used) exposure. Hepatoblastoma is a tumor of early childhood discussed in Chapter 68.

D. Metastatic spread

1. **Modes of spread.** Primary hepatic malignancies spread by three distinct mechanisms:

   a. **Direct extension.** In 14% of patients, tumor grows directly into adjacent organs, including adjacent liver, gallbladder, diaphragm, stomach, duodenum, colon, portal and hepatic veins, and the inferior vena cava (IVC). **Satellite lesions** frequently develop from direct extension of small nests of cells.

   b. **Lymphatic metastasis.** Metastatic spread through lymphatics to hepatic, celiac, and other regional nodes occurs in as many as 40% of patients.

   c. **Hematogenous metastasis.** Metastatic spread through portal and systemic vessels occurs much less frequently than does lymphatic metastasis; only 10% of patients have distant organ involvement at autopsy.

2. **Sites of spread.** At autopsy, a variety of distant organs can be involved with tumor, including those listed below. However, most patients develop intraabdominal problems (eg, gastrointestinal and intra-abdominal bleeding, biliary obstruction) secondary to local tumor growth and spread: lung; bone, including sternum (with inferior vena cava obstruction); adrenal gland; and central nervous system.

VIII. Staging.

In 1988 the American Joint Committee on Cancer and the Union Internationale Contre le Cancer adopted a joint TNM staging system that may aid in the comparison of future treatment protocols.

A. Tumor stage

1. **TX.** Primary tumor cannot be assessed.
2. **T0.** No evidence of a primary tumor exists.
3. **T1.** A solitary tumor smaller than 2 cm without vascular invasion.
4. **T2.** A solitary tumor smaller than 2 cm with vascular invasion, a solitary tumor larger than 2 cm without vascular invasion, or multiple unilobar tumors smaller than 2 cm without vascular invasion.
5. **T3.** A solitary tumor larger than 2 cm with vascular invasion, multiple unilobar tumors smaller than 2 cm with vascular invasion, or multiple unilobar tumors larger than 2 cm with or without vascular invasion.
6. **T4.** Multiple tumors involving more than one lobe or a major branch of the portal or hepatic vein.

B. Lymph node stage

1. **NX.** Regional lymph nodes cannot be assessed.
2. **N0.** No regional lymph node metastases.
3. **N1.** Regional lymph node metastases are present.

C. **Metastatic stage**
   1. **MX.** Distant metastases cannot be assessed.
   2. **M0.** No distant metastases are present.
   3. **M1.** Distant metastases are present.
D. **Histopathologic grade**
   1. **GX.** Grade cannot be assessed.
   2. **G1.** Well differentiated.
   3. **G2.** Moderately well differentiated.
   4. **G3.** Poorly differentiated.
   5. **G4.** Undifferentiated.
E. **Stage groupings**
   1. **Stage I.** T1, N0, M0.
   2. **Stage II.** T2, N0, M0.
   3. **Stage III.** T1 or T2, N1, M0, or T3; any N, M0.
   4. **Stage IVA.** T4, any N, M0.
   5. **Stage IVB.** Any T, any N, M1.
IX. **Treatment**
   A. **Surgery**
      1. **Primary hepatocellular carcinoma**
         a. **General considerations.** Even with the advanced techniques of modern surgery, only about **33% of patients with hepatoma are candidates for resection;** of these, **only 33% (10–12%) will be resectable** at operation and, of those resected, **only 33% (3–4%) will survive long-term.**
         b. **Preoperative assessment.** Successful resection of hepatic malignancies depends on accurate preoperative assessment of the size, location, and vascular anatomy of the lesion as well as on the functional capacity of the remaining hepatic parenchymal. CT scans and angiographic studies answer most of the questions, but accurate assessment of remaining hepatic synthetic function in cirrhotic livers is, at present, imprecise. In patients without ascites and with normal bilirubin, albumin, and transaminases (Child's class A; see Table 34–1 for Child's classification), lobar resection, in most instances, can be performed. However, a patient who has **known cirrhosis and ascites** with even mildly abnormal liver function often will not tolerate lobar or even segmental hepatic resection.
         c. **Approaches.** Hepatic masses are usually explored through a **long midline or bilateral subcostal (chevron) incision.** Most resections can be accomplished transabdominally, though some surgeons prefer a **thoracoabdominal incision** for large right-sided lesions. On the basis of the preoperative arteriogram, hilar dissection is performed first to assess regional nodes and involvement of portal structures supplying the contralateral hepatic lobe and to allow ligation of the hepatic arterial and porta venous supply and bile duct to the involved lobe. The parenchyma is then resected, often with the aid of an **ultrasonic scalpel (CUSA).** The hepatic veins are either ligated when encountered during resection of the parenchyma or ligated at the level of the vena cava before resection. Drains are frequently placed to prevent the formation of large collections of serum and bile that can subsequently form abscesses.
      2. **Locally advanced hepatocellular carcinoma.** Because of a short life expectancy, surgery should be avoided in most patients with unresectable hepatocellular carcinoma. In unusual cases, biliary or gastric bypass procedures can be performed, and, in some patients with metastatic disease, resection of the primary tumor (when possible) may afford significant palliation.
      3. **Metastatic hepatocellular carcinoma.** Resection of metastatic hepatoma is rarely indicated because curative resections are rarely possible. Thus, resection of hepatoma metastases should be considered only in the rare instance in which there is a single lesion and a particularly long disease-free interval. Resection of metastatic cholangiocarcinoma also is indicated only rarely.
      4. **Transplantation.** Hepatic transplantation has been attempted for treatment of unresectable hepatocellular carcinoma, but no significant long-term survival has been reported. Patients with the fibrolamellar variant, however, do slightly better, with as long as a 20-month disease-free survival. In contrast, patients with hepatocellular carcinoma **discovered incidentally** at transplantation have a **uniformly excellent prognosis.**
      5. **Morbidity and mortality.** Currently, the mortality rate in noncirrhotic patients after lobar resection is **less than 5%,** with a morbidity rate of about 10%. Com-

mon complications are listed below. Both morbidity and mortality rates increase significantly in patients with cirrhosis and with more extensive resections. The mortality by Child's class is 4% for class A, 11% for Class B, and 50% for Class C.
   a. **Wound infection,** 4%.
   b. **Abscess,** 4%.
   c. **Sepsis,** 4%.
   d. **Biliary leakage,** 2%.
   e. **Hemorrhage,** 4%.
   f. **Hepatic insufficiency,** especially hypoglycemia (3%).
B. **Radiation therapy**
   1. **Primary hepatocellular carcinoma.** External-beam radiation therapy for primary treatment of hepatocellular carcinoma is limited by the development of radiation hepatitis with **doses in excess of 3000 cGy** over 3 weeks. Even when combined with chemotherapy, no more than a 15% partial response rate has been demonstrated. ^{131}I-antiferritin, which is preferentially taken up by hepatic malignancies because of increased blood flow to the tumor and large tumor ferritin stores has not proved to be more beneficial than other forms of therapy.
   2. **Adjuvant radiation therapy.** This modality has not been studied extensively because of the limited hepatic reserve of most patients undergoing resection and to the poor response rate to radiation therapy in general.
   3. **Locally advanced and metastatic hepatocellular carcinoma.** In some circumstances, radiation therapy can relieve symptoms of pressure and pain but otherwise offers little in the palliation of hepatocellular carcinoma.
C. **Chemotherapy**
   1. **Primary hepatocellular carcinoma.** Patients with resectable hepatocellular carcinoma should not be treated initially with chemotherapy because chemotherapy is only minimally effective.
   2. **Adjuvant chemotherapy.** Adjuvant chemotherapy involves the same drugs that have little effect on established disease; thus, no significant responses have been observed. **Doxorubicin** is again the most promising agent, and several trials are currently in progress.
   3. **Locally advanced and metastatic hepatocellular carcinoma**
      a. **Systemic chemotherapy.** Patients with unresectable hepatic malignancies have been treated with a variety of single chemotherapeutic agents such as fluorouracil, VP-16, mitoxantrone, lomustine, cytarabine, and doxorubicin as well as combination regimens. **Doxorubicin,** alone, produces response rates between 2% and 22%. No other single agent or combination of agents produces responses in more than 10% of patients. No prolongation of survival has been claimed with any regimen.
      b. **Local hepatic infusion chemotherapy.** After initial encouraging results with methotrexate and other agents, no studies have demonstrated superior results with intra-arterial infusion over those attained with systemic administration.
D. **Combined modality treatment.** Combinations of chemotherapy and radiation therapy have been tried without significant success.
E. **Immunotherapy.** The response of hepatocellular carcinoma to various forms of immunotherapy remains completely unknown.
X. **Prognosis**
A. **5-year survival.** The prognosis for hepatoma of any type is poor, although the **fibrolamellar or encapsulated type** is more encouraging: 5-year survival has been reported in about 25% of patients in some series. In the face of cirrhosis and hepatoma, 5-year survival is essentially zero. In resectable patients, operative mortality and 5-year survival are about 10–15% each in most series. Even after successul resection, **mean survivals are measured in months,** with death resulting from local and systemic recurrence.
B. **Adverse prognostic factors.** Although cirrhosis is associated with a poor outcome, it is not an independent prognostic indicator when sex and age are taken into account. The following factors, however, are associated with a poorer than normal prognosis: **male sex, advanced age, poor performance status, jaundice, and anorexia.**
XI. **Patient follow-up**
A. **General guidelines.** Patients with hepatocellular carcinoma should be followed every 3 months for the first 2 years and every 6 months thereafter. Guidelines for interval evaluation of patients are outlined below:

B. **Routine evaluation.** Each clinic visit should include the following examinations:
   1. **Medical history and physical examination.** A complete history should be taken and a physical examination should be performed at each visit and should include the areas discussed in **VI.A.** above.
   2. **Blood tests**
      a. **Complete blood count** (see p 1, **IV.A.1**).
      b. **Hepatic transaminases** (see p 1, **IV.A.2**).
      c. **Alkaline phosphatase** (see p 1, **IV.A.3**).
      d. **Alpha-fetoprotein** (AFP). Levels of this marker should return to normal after complete resection or after a complete response to chemotherapy. Serum levels are routinely followed after treatment because increasing levels are associated with recurrence (however, low levels do not exclude the existence of disease). Elevation of AFP to abnormal levels, or 2–3 times the lowest postoperative level, is usually an indication for a more extensive metastatic evaluation.
   3. **Chest x-ray** (see p 3, **IV.C.1**).
C. **Additional evaluation.** Other tests that should be performed at regularly scheduled intervals include a CT scan of the abdomen, which should be obtained every 6 months in patients resected for cure to evaluate the liver for recurrences amenable to further resection.
D. **Optional evaluation.** The following examinations may be indicated by previous findings or clinical suspicion:
   1. **Blood tests** (see p 2, **IV.A**)
      a. **Nucleotidase.**
      b. **GGTP.**
   2. **Imaging studies** (see p 3, **IV.C**).
      a. **Magnetic resonance imaging (MRI).**
      b. **Technetium-99m bone scan.**
   3. **Biopsy.** In patients resected for cure, any suspicious or abnormal mass is an indication for diagnostic biopsy. The type of biopsy depends on the location and size of the mass, but needle biopsies are generally preferred to open biopsies.

REFERENCES

Cady B: Natural history of primary and secondary tumors of the liver. *Semin Oncol* 1983;**10:**127–134.

Cady B: Liver tumors. In: Cameron JL (editor), *Current Surgical Therapy-3,* 3rd ed. Philadelphia, PA: JB Lippincott; 1989;212–216.

Choi TK, Lee NW, Wong J: Chemotherapy for advanced hepatocellular carcinoma: Adriamycin versus quadruple chemotherapy. *Cancer* February 1984;**53:**104–105.

Farhi DC et al: Hepatocellular carcinoma in young people. *Cancer* 1983;**52:**1516–1525.

Forbes A, Williams R: Chemotherapy and radiotherapy of malignant hepatic tumors. *Baillieres Clin Gastroenterol* 1987;**1**(1):151–169.

Friedman MA: Hepatic intraarterial chemotherapy-current status and future prospects. *Gan To Kagaku Ryoho* 1983;**10:**1209–1224.

LaBerge JM et al: Hepatocellular carcinoma: assessment of resectability by computed tomography and ultrasound. *Radiology* 1984;**152:**485–490.

Malt RA: Surgery for hepatic neoplasms. *N Engl J Med* 1985;**313:**1591–1596.

Meyers WC: The liver. In: Sabiston DC (editor), *Textbook of Surgery,* 13th ed. Philadelphia, PA: WB Saunders; 1986.

Nagorney DM et al: Primary hepatic malignancy: surgical management and determinants of survival. *Surgery* 1989;**106:**740–749.

35 Malignancies of the Gallbladder & Extrahepatic Biliary Tract

Terence P. Wade, MD, and Robert B. Cameron, MD

I. **Epidemiology.** Although cancer of the extrahepatic biliary tree is uncommon in the United States, carcinoma of the gallbladder is the **fifth most common gastrointestinal malignancy,** accounting for 1–2% of all cancers. In 1985, **1.8 females and 1.0 males per 100,000** of the population were diagnosed with gallbladder carcinoma. Estimates indicated that almost 6000 new cases of gallbladder cancer and nearly 2000 new cases of bile duct carcinoma will be diagnosed in 1993. The worldwide incidence of gallbladder carcinoma varies from as low as 0.9 per 100,000 in Bombay, India, to as high as 22.2 per 100,000 females in areas of Latin America, Israel, Europe, Japan, and New Mexico.

II. **Risk factors**
- A. **Age.** Both gallbladder and bile duct carcinoma increase from less than 1 per 100,000 before age 50 to **19.1 and 16.7 per 100,000 respectively, after age 85.** The average age of onset for these tumors is 60 years of age.
- B. **Sex. Bile duct tumors** are diagnosed **1.5 times more frequently in males** than in females, whereas **gallbladder cancer is 2–3 times more common in females** than in males.
- C. **Race.** In the United States, gallbladder carcinoma is more prevalent among American Indians, Mexican Americans, and native Alaskans. With rates as high as 22.2 cases per 100,000 among American Indians, the increased risk correlates with an increased incidence of cholelithiasis.
- D. **Genetic factors.** No clear genetic predisposition has been demonstrated for either malignancy.
- E. **Diet. Aflatoxins** have been demonstrated to cause bile duct cancers in animals.
- F. **Tobacco.** Smoking has not been shown to be an independent risk factor in the etiology of either malignancy.
- G. **History of previous biliary disease**
  1. **Inflammation**
     - a. **Cholelithiasis.** Cholelithiasis is present in between 65% and 90% of patients with gallbladder carcinoma but in only 30% of patients with **primary bile duct cancer.** This is reflected in the increased risk of gallbladder cancer in the elderly, female, and native American populations. **Porcelain (calcified) gallbladders** also have a high incidence of associated malignancies, as do cholecystoenteric fistulae. Approximately 1% of all gallbladders removed for symptomatic cholelithiasis are found to contain malignancy.
     - b. **Ulcerative colitis.** Patients with ulcerative colitis are at **10 times greater risk** for developing malignant biliary tract disease, including bile duct and gallbladder cancer. **Total colectomy does not eliminate this increased risk.**
     - c. **Sclerosing cholangitis.** Sclerosing cholangitis is associated with both bile duct and gallbladder malignancies.
  2. **Infection**
     - a. **Parasitic disease.** Patients infected with the **common Asian liver fluke,** *Clonorchis sinensis,* face an increased risk of biliary cancer.
     - b. **Bacterial infections. Thyphoid carriers** have been noted to be at high risk for developing carcinoma of the biliary tree.

III. **Presentation**
- A. **Signs and symptoms**
  1. **Local manifestations**
     - a. **Bile duct cancer.** Findings consistent with cancer of the bile ducts include **elevated alkaline phosphatase (94%), painless jaundice (84%), liver**

265

enzyme abnormalities (SGOT, SGPT; 50%), pruritus, fatigue, fever, abdominal pain (distention of the liver capsule), and hepatomegaly.

  b. **Gallbladder cancer.** Gallbladder carcinoma produces **pain (80%), nausea and vomiting (53%), right upper-quadrant abdominal mass (50%),** anorexia/weight loss (42%), jaundice (33%), pruritus, fatigue, and fever, although many cases are discovered incidentally after routine cholecystectomy for cholelithiasis.

 2. **Systemic manifestations.** In both bile duct and gallbladder malignancies, splenomegaly and ascites may signal portal vein obstruction, lymph node metastases, and unresectable disease.

IV. **Differential diagnosis.** Bile duct cancer must be separated from other causes of extrahepatic biliary obstruction, which include **choledocholithiasis, gallbladder carcinoma, inflammatory strictures** (sclerosing cholangitis, pancreatitis), **congenital abnormalities** (choledochal cysts), and **other malignancies** (periampullary pancreatic cancer, lymphoma, and metastatic celiac lymph nodes).

V. **Screening programs.** Because of the low incidence of gallbladder and biliary malignancies, methods of screening for these cancers have not been developed.

VI. **Diagnostic workup**

 A. **Medical history and physical examination.** A complete medical history emphasizing common presenting complaints such as jaundice, pruritus, pain, and anorexia/weight loss as well as a thorough physical examination are mandatory for all patients presenting with possible biliary malignancies.

  1. **General appearance.** The examination should include an assessment concerning the patient's general nutritional and functional status.

  2. **Skin.** The integument should be examined for evidence of jaundice as well as physical trauma that reflects scratching caused by pruritus.

  3. **Lymph nodes.** The presence of a signal node (also called **Virchow's or Troisier's node**) must be recorded.

  4. **Abdomen.** Masses (especially in the right upper quadrant), tenderness, hepatosplenomegaly, and ascites should be noted.

  5. **Rectum.** Occult blood indicating possible hemobilia should be excluded.

 B. **Primary tests and procedures.** All patients with known or suspected biliary and gallbladder cancer should have the following diagnostic tests performed:

  1. **Blood tests**

   a. **Complete blood count.** Elevated WBC may indicate **cholangitis or cholecystitis,** and anemia may occur from hemobilia (see also, p 1, **IV.A.1**).

   b. **Hepatic transaminases.** SGOT and SGPT levels are abnormal in as many as 50% of patients with biliary tract cancer; however, these enzymes are usually normal with gallbladder carcinoma, except in advanced cases (see, also, p 1, **IV.A.2**).

   c. **Alkaline phosphatase.** Serum levels of the heat-stable fraction of this enzyme are significantly elevated in 94% patients with **bile duct cancer** but in fewer than 50% of patients with **gallbladder carcinoma** (see also, p 1, **IV.A.3**).

   d. **Bilirubin.** Bilirubin levels are almost uniformly increased in biliary tract malignancies and in advanced cases of gallbladder cancer.

  2. **Imaging studies**

   a. **Chest x-ray** (see p 3, **IV.C.1**).

   b. **Ultrasonography.** This rapid and safe examination can reliably detect biliary obstruction as well as the level of the obstructing lesion.

   c. **Computed tomography (CT).** CT scan of the abdomen provides information about mass lesions of the liver, gallbladder, porta hepatis, and head of the pancreas. Lesions in any one of these areas may cause similar symptoms.

  3. **Invasive procedures**

   a. **Percutaneous transhepatic cholangiography (PTC).** This special radiologic procedure requires dilated intrahepatic bile ducts. It involves cannulating an intrahepatic biliary radical, sampling bile for cytologic analysis, and injecting contrast dye to visualize the anatomy of the biliary tree proximal to the obstructing lesion. In addition, **stents can be passed through malignant obstructions** or allowed to drain to external bags to **decompress** the biliary ductal system.

   b. **Endoscopic retrograde cholangiopancreatography (ERCP).** This special gastrointestinal procedure can be used in place of PTC to evaluate the biliary system and does not require dilated biliary ducts. However, it does involve **upper gastrointestinal endoscopy** to collect bile for cytologic analysis and to inject contrast dye directly into the biliary and pancreatic ducts to evaluate the level of obstruction and distal duct structure. As with PTC, stents can be passed beyond some obstructing lesions in the distal common bile duct to decompress the biliary tree; however, ERCP **does not usually visualize the biliary anatomy proximal to the obstruction.**

  C. **Optional tests and procedures.** The following tests and procedures may be indicated by previous diagnostic findings or clinical suspicion.

   1. **Blood tests**
    a. **5′-Nucleotidase** (see p 12, **IV.A.4**).
    b. **GGTP** (see p 2, **IV.A.5**).
   2. **Imaging studies**
    a. **Magnetic resonance imaging (MRI)** (see p 3, **IV.C.2**).
    b. **Angiography.** Celiac angiograms are used to evaluate tumors and the anatomy of their blood supply only in unusual cases for which resection is contemplated.
    c. **Dimethyl-iminodiacetic acid (HIDA) scan.** This nuclear medicine scan can demonstrate extrahepatic biliary obstruction and provide a gross estimate about the functional status of different areas of the liver by the degree of uptake of the HIDA dye.
   3. **Invasive procedures.** Percutaneous ultrasound- or CT-guided needle biopsy is **rarely indicated** in patients with either type of biliary malignancy because a combination of the above tests and procedures will yield the diagnosis in 90–95% of cases.

VII. Pathology
  A. **Location.** Most gallbladder carcinomas occur in the **fundus of the gallbladder.** Bile duct carcinomas occur anywhere in the ductal system; nearly 50% are found in the upper third; 25%, in the middle third; and 15–19%, in the lower third of the extrahepatic bile ducts. **Six percent to 10% of tumors are diffuse** in nature. Tumors at the confluence of the right and left hepatic ducts are termed **"Klatskin" tumors.**
  B. **Multiplicity.** Distinct synchronous and metachronous lesions in the biliary tract generally do not occur.
  C. **Histology.** Adenocarcinoma represents 85% of gallbladder and bile duct malignancies and includes papillary, intestinal, pleomorphic giant cell, signet ring, clear cell, and colloid subtypes. Other cell types include squamous and adenosquamous (10%), oat cell, and various sarcomas.
  D. **Metastatic spread**
   1. **Modes of spread.** Malignancies of the gallbladder and bile ducts spread primarily by two mechanisms, although three modes are possible:
    a. **Direct extension.** Both carcinoma of the bile ducts and gallbladder spread by direct extension to the surrounding structures, primarily **the liver (63%) and the duodenum, stomach, and pancreas (55%)** in virtually all patients.
    b. **Lymphatic metastasis.** Local lymph node metastases, including cholecystic, periduodenal, para-aortic, and celiac nodes, occur in as many as 70% of patients with these malignancies, whereas distant lymph node metastases (eg, supraclavicular and mediastinal lymph nodes) occur less often.
    c. **Hematogenous metastasis.** Spread of malignant cells through the circulatory system to distant organs is **relatively uncommon:** Fewer than 33% of all patients harbor distant metastases at the time of autopsy.
   2. **Sites of spread.** At autopsy, organs likely to be involved in distant metastatic spread include the following sites: lymph nodes, 35–70%; liver, 63%; lung, 30%; and peritoneum, 24%.

VIII. Staging. The American Joint Committee on Cancer and the Union Internationale Contre le Cancer proposed a joint staging system for bile duct cancers in 1988. At the same time, a separate system was developed for gallbladder carcinoma.
  A. **Gallbladder carcinoma**
   1. **Tumor stage**
    a. **TX.** Primary tumor cannot be assessed.
    b. **T0.** No evidence of a primary tumor.
    c. **Tis.** Carcinoma in situ.
    d. **T1.** Tumor invades into mucosa or muscularis.
     (1) T1a. Tumor invades into the mucosa.

       (2) T1b. Tumor invades into the muscularis.
- **e. T2.** Tumor invades the perimuscular tissue but does not extend beyond the serosa or into the liver.
- **f. T3.** Tumor invades beyond the serosa, into one adjacent organ (liver extension must be < 2 cm).
- **g. T4.** Tumor invades into two or more adjacent organs (stomach, duodenum, colon, pancreas, omentum, extrahepatic bile ducts, and liver) or extends more than 2 cm into the liver.

2. **Lymph node stage**
   - **a. NX.** Regional lymph nodes cannot be assessed.
   - **b. N0.** No evidence of regional lymph node metastases.
   - **c. N1.** Regional lymph node metastases are present.
     - **(1) N1a.** Nodal metastases are present in the cystic duct, pericholedochal, or hilar lymph nodes.
     - **(2) N1b.** Nodal metastases are present in the peripancreatic, periduodenal, periportal, celiac, or superior mesenteric lymph nodes.

3. **Metastatic stage**
   - **a. MX.** Distant metastases cannot be assessed.
   - **b. M0.** No distant metastases are present.
   - **c. M1.** Distant metastases are present.

4. **Histopathologic grade**
   - **a. GX.** Grade cannot be assessed.
   - **b. G1.** Well differentiated.
   - **c. G2.** Moderately well differentiated.
   - **d. G3.** Poorly differentiated.
   - **e. G4.** Undifferentiated.

5. **Stage groupings**
   - **a. Stage 0.** Tis, N0, M0
   - **b. Stage I.** T1, N0, M0.
   - **c. Stage II.** T2, N0, M0.
   - **d. Stage III.** T1 or T2, N1, M0, or T3, any N, M0.
   - **e. Stage IV.** T4, any N, M0, or any T, any N, M1.

B. Bile duct carcinoma
1. **Tumor stage**
   - **a. TX.** Primary tumor cannot be assessed.
   - **b. T0.** No evidence of a primary tumor exists.
   - **c. Tis.** Carcinoma in situ.
   - **d. T1.** Tumor invades the mucosa or muscularis.
     - **(1) T1a.** Tumor invades the mucosa.
     - **(2) T1b.** Tumor invades the muscularis.
   - **e. T2.** Tumor invades outside the muscularis.
   - **f. T3.** Tumor invades adjacent organs including liver, pancreas, duodenum, gallbladder, colon, and stomach.

2. **Lymph node stage**
   - **a. NX.** Regional lymph nodes cannot be assessed.
   - **b. N0.** No regional lymph node metastases are present.
   - **c. N1.** Regional lymph node metastases are present.
     - **(1) N1a.** Lymph node metastases in the cystic duct pericholedochal, hilar lymph nodes, or both.
     - **(2) N1b.** Lymph node metastases in the peripancreatic, periduodenal, periportal, celiac, or superior mesenteric lymph nodes.

3. **Metastatic stage**
   - **a. MX.** Distant metastases cannot be assessed.
   - **b. M0.** No distant metastases are present.
   - **c. M1.** Distant metastases are present.

4. **Histopathologic grade**
   - **a. GX.** Grade cannot be assessed.
   - **b. G1.** Well differentiated.
   - **c. G2.** Moderately well differentiated.
   - **d. G3.** Poorly differentiated.
   - **e. G4.** Undifferentiated.

5. **Stage groupings**
   - **a. Stage 0.** Tis, N0, M0
   - **b. Stage I.** T1, N0, M0.
   - **c. Stage II.** T2, N0, M0.

   d. Stage III. T1 or T2, N1, M0.
   e. Stage IVA. T3, any N, M0.
   f. Stage IVB. Any T, any N, M1.
IX. Treatment
 A. Surgery
  1. Primary tumor
   a. General considerations. Although in theory, radiation therapy has curative potential in localized biliary malignancies, surgery provides the best chance, albeit small, of achieving long-term survival. In addition, surgery also may provide good palliation of biliary obstruction through bypass procedures.

    (1) Indications. Any patient with a localized lesion should be explored for possible curative resection. If the lesion is obviously **not resectable** because of contiguous or distant organ involvement, however, **attempts at percutaneous or endoscopic stent placement are preferable** to palliative surgery. In addition, **surgical exploration may be required for definitive tissue diagnosis** when bile cytologies and other studies do not clearly demonstrate malignancy.

    (2) Preoperative biliary decompression. Although intuitively preoperative biliary decompression should improve liver function and surgical morbidity and mortality, 2 recent randomized, prospective trials have failed to demonstrate any benefit to biliary drainage prior to definitive surgery.

    (3) Approaches. Most surgeons prefer either a **bilateral subcostal (chevron) incision or a midline incision** that can be extended into a thoracoabdominal incision if necessary.

   b. Gallbladder carcinoma. Because of the low incidence of this malignancy and the frequently incidental nature of its discovery at the time of cholecystectomy, the optimal surgical procedure has not been defined. A reasonable surgical approach is to biopsy any area that is not completely compatible with cholecystitis and to aspirate bile for cytologic examination, particularly in high-risk patients such as the elderly or those with gallstones and a thickened or calcified gallbladder wall. If carcinoma is found, **a 3–4 cm wedge of normal liver** surrounding the gallbladder fossa should be resected along with the gallbladder. No evidence to date indicates that a right hepatic lobectomy provides better control than does a more limited resection. In addition, an extensive lymph node dissection should be performed, including common duct, porta hepatis, periportal, perihepatic artery, and superior and inferior peripancreatic nodes. **If the margins or lymph nodes are positive or if the disease extends into the liver, postoperative radiation, chemotherapy, or both should be considered.** For clinically occult lesions noted only postoperatively after cholecystectomy, **reexploration with resection of the gallbladder bed and lymph-node dissection should be considered** for all patients except in medically high-risk patients with disease limited to the mucosa or submucosa.

   c. Bile duct carcinoma. The initial step in the surgical management of bile duct tumors is to establish the diagnosis in patients without previous tissue diagnosis. Direct biopsy of palpable masses is often adequate, although endoscopic biopsy using a choledochoscope is occasionally required. The remaining surgical treatment varies, depending on the location of the tumor, but can be divided into three main categories:

    (1) Proximal bile ducts. Malignancies of the proximal bile ducts, including lesions at the confluence of the right and left hepatic ducts **(Klatskin's tumor)** are amenable to resection in only 20% of patients and are rarely curable. If only **one hepatic duct is involved,** resection of that **duct and** a corresponding **hepatic lobectomy is the treatment of choice.** If both sides are involved, as in Klatskin's tumor, resection of the involved ductal system and draining lymph nodes with a 60 cm Roux-en-Y hepaticojejunostomy or hepaticocholedochostomy is preferred. **Preoperative percutaneous biliary stents** can be placed to decompress the biliary system preoperatively, to aid in the intraoperative identification of the bile ducts, to act as stents for biliary-enteric anastomoses, and to provide permanent drainage access to the biliary tree.

    (2) Middle bile ducts. Carcinoma of the middle third of the extrahepatic biliary tree defies curative resection because of the proximity of vital structures such as the portal vein and hepatic artery. These tumors are **uniformly fatal** and amenable only to palliative measures.

(3) **Distal bile ducts and papilla of Vater.** Small tumors of the distal common bile duct are **most amenable to curative surgery** because the length of the proximal ducts allows wide margins and adequate biliary-enteric bypass procedures. **Radical pancreaticoduodenectomy** (Whipple procedure) is the preferred surgical procedure and may be pylorus-preserving. Reconstruction is usually accomplished with a 60 cm Roux-en-Y choledocho-, pancreatico-, and gastrojejunostomy.

2. **Locally advanced and metastatic biliary tract cancer.** Metastatic disease to the liver and lung generally is not amenable to surgical therapy unless all disease is limited to one hepatic lobe, which can be resected in continuity with the involved bile duct.

a. **Stenting.** In patients with unresectable disease, **percutaneous or intraoperative placement of biliary stents** prevent many of complications of biliary obstruction, including sepsis, hepatic dysfunction, and even the pruritus associated with dermal deposition of bile salts. If initial attempts to pass a catheter beyond a malignant obstruction are unsuccessful, a **second attempt should be made 3–5 days later** when the associated edema has improved. Palliation with this approach can be substantial because many biliary malignancies grow relatively slowly.

b. **Bypass.** Many types of biliary enteric bypass procedures depend on the level of obstruction. However, there is little benefit of these procedures over percutaneous stent placement in patients with clearly unresectable disease. All bypass procedures include the use of a 60 cm Roux-en-Y loop of jejunum.

(1) **Hepaticojejunostomy.** This procedure involves the anastomosis between a Roux-en-Y loop of jejunum and either the **right or left hepatic duct** or a dilated biliary radical that is isolated in the superficial hepatic parenchyma. This bypass procedure is commonly used for **proximal and middle-third biliary lesions.**

(2) **Choledochojejunostomy.** This operation consists of an anastomosis between a Roux-en-Y loop of jejunum and the **common bile duct.** This is the procedure of choice for **distal bile duct cancers.**

(3) **Cholecystojejunostomy.** This procedure entails the anastomosis between the **gallbladder** and a Roux-en-Y jejunal loop. Except in rare instances, it is **not an acceptable bypass procedure because the cystic duct may become obstructed,** thereby leaving the bypass nonfunctional.

3. **Morbidity and mortality.** The complication rate depends on the location of the tumor, the operation performed, and the patient's condition. Overall morbidity has been reported to be as high as 67%, with **mortality** ranging from 10% after palliative procedures to 13% after resection. Pancreaticoduodenectomy was associated with a mortality as high as 24% but is now often accomplished with less than 5% mortality. Most postoperative complications are related to wound and intra-abdominal infections.

B. **Radiation therapy**

1. **Primary bile duct or gallbladder carcinoma.** Recent preliminary evidence suggests that radiotherapy may provide curative potential in patients with local-regional disease. External-beam radiation with doses of 6000–7000 cGy over 6–7 weeks can control gross tumor with **proximal bile duct lesions;** with more distal lesions, however, stomach, duodenum, kidney, and spine limit the ability to deliver such high doses. Lower doses of external-beam therapy (5000 cGy) combined with brachytherapy (iridium or radium wire) delivered through the biliary drainage tube may offer promise for more distal lesions. Because of the incidental discovery of most gallbladder carcinomas, primary radiation therapy is seldom a consideration.

2. **Adjuvant therapy**

a. **Preoperative therapy.** The theoretical advantages of preoperative radiation therapy, including tumor shrinkage and an increased resectability rate, remain unproved.

b. **Intraoperative therapy.** Japanese studies in patients with bile duct carcinoma indicate that single intraoperative doses of 2500–4000 cGy offer significant palliation, with **90% of patients radiographically demonstrating**

recanalization of the bile ducts. In addition, potentially curative responses were observed in patients receiving more than 3500 cGy, but median survival was only 13 months.

    c. Postoperative therapy. Despite scant data, postoperative radiation therapy appears to **prolong the survival** of patients with **gallbladder cancer** from a **median of 29 months to 63 months.** In patients with **bile duct carcinoma,** increased survival also has been reported; **nonirradiated patients** survive a mean of **6 months,** and **irradiated patients** survive a mean of **11–20 months.** Radiation doses range from 3800–7225 cGy using external-beam irradiation, brachytherapy, or a combination of the two.

  3. Palliative therapy. In many studies, good palliation from malignant biliary obstruction was attained with external-beam irradiation, brachytherapy, or a combination, with as many as **90% of patients** receiving **some relief** from symptoms.

  4. Morbidity and mortality. The complications observed with high-dose radiation therapy involve organs present in the area and include radiation hepatitis, gastritis, duodenitis, colitis, and transverse myelitis. The use of multiple fields and brachytherapy tend to reduce the severity of the observed complications.

C. Chemotherapy. The paucity of data on chemotherapy in the treatment of biliary tract malignancies underscores the need for further clinical trials before solid recommendations can be made.

  1. Systemic administration. Chemotherapy has been used in both the adjuvant and metastatic setting with little success. Response rates vary, but none last longer than a few weeks.

    a. Single agents. Limited data suggest that a small number of objective responses to several agents, including **fluorouracil** (13–24%) and **mitomycin-C** (0–42%), as well as anecdotal reports of responses with doxorubicin and carmustine do occur. In all cases, however, responses were extremely short-lived.

    b. Combination chemotherapy. Combinations of various single agents, such as FAM (fluorouracil, doxorubicin, and mitomycin-C), **FAB** (ftorafur, doxorubicin, and carmustine), and **doxorubicin with bleomycin** have been tried, with responses no greater than single-agent therapy (ie, 20–43% response rate).

  2. Local hepatic artery infusion. A single trial of intrahepatic infusion of **fluorouracil and mitomycin-C** demonstrated a **response rate of 69%,** which suggested a higher response rate than other systemically administered single agents or combination therapies.

D. Immunotherapy. There is no data to support the use of immunotherapy in the treatment of biliary tract malignancies.

E. Combined modality therapy. Combinations of radiation therapy and chemotherapy in the adjuvant setting offer the best chance at the successful treatment of biliary malignancies, however, the data are extremely limited.

X. Prognosis

A. Five-year survival. Long-term survival with bile ducts and gallbladder malignancies depends on the location and extent of the tumor.

  1. Gallbladder carcinoma. The 5-year survival by TNM stage is best if the carcinoma is found incidentally and if invasion does not extend outside the gallbladder itself: Stage I, 55–64%; Stage II, 20–33%; Stage III, 10–13%; and Stage IV, 4–7%.

  2. Bile duct carcinoma. The 5-year survival of patients with bile duct cancer depends on the histologic type and location of the primary tumor and is listed below.

    a. Histologic type. Papillary, 31%; sclerosing cholangiocarcinoma, 20%; well differentiated, 8%; and undifferentiated, 0%.

    b. Location. Upper-third lesions, 10%; middle-third lesions, 0%; and lower-third lesions, 28%.

B. Adverse prognostic factors. The following factors are associated with a poor prognosis.

  1. Gallbladder carcinoma

    a. Jaundice.

    b. Hepatic enzyme abnormalities.

    c. Ascites.

  2. Bile duct carcinoma

    a. Adverse histologic type (see **X.A.2.a** above).

      b. **Upper- and middle-third lesions.**
      c. **Ascites.**

XI. **Patient follow-up**
    A. **General guidelines.** Patients should be followed closely every 3 months for 2 years, every 6 months for an additional 3 years, and then annually thereafter. Specific guidelines for patient evaluation are outlined below.
    B. **Routine evaluation.** Each clinic visit should include the following tests and procedures.
        1. **Medical History and physical examination.** A full history and physical examination must be performed during each clinic appointment. Special emphasis should be focused on those areas listed earlier on p. 266, **VI.A** above.
        2. **Blood tests**
            a. **Complete blood count** (see p 266, **VI.B.1.a** above).
            b. **Hepatic transaminases** (see p 266, **VI.B.1.b** above).
            c. **Alkaline phosphatase** Elevated serum levels of this enzyme are the most sensitive test for recurrent biliary tract carcinoma (see p 266, **VI.B.1.c** above).
            d. Bilirubin (see p 266, **VI.B.1.d** above).
        3. Chest x-ray (see p 3, **IV.C.1**).
    C. **Additional evaluation.** Other tests which should be obtained at regular intervals include the following examinations.
        1. **Computed tomography.** CT scan should be performed every 3–6 months initially (see, also, p 266, **VI.B.2.c** above).
        2. **Biliary drainage tube replacement.** Patients with percutaneous biliary drainage tubes in place should have them **changed** over a wire under fluoroscopic guidance **every 3 months.** Internal stents should be changed every 3 months as well, using endoscopic techniques. Both procedures can be accomplished on an **outpatient basis,** but **antibiotics** should be administered immediately before any manipulation.
    D. **Optional tests and procedures.** The following tests and procedures may be indicated by previous diagnostic findings or clinical suspicion:
        1. **Blood tests** (see p 2, IV.A).
            a. **5′nucleotidase.**
            b. **GGTP.**
        2. **Imaging studies**
            a. **Ultrasonography** (see p 266, **VI.B.2.b** above).
            b. **Magnetic resonance imaging** (see p 3, **IV.C.2**).
        3. **Percutaneous transhepatic cholangiography (PTC).** This special radiologic procedure may be required to evaluate new episodes of jaundice to exclude recurrent tumor, benign strictures, and other biliary pathology (see also p 266, **VI.B.3.a** above).
        4. **Endoscopic retrograde cholangiopancreatography** (see p 266, **VI.B.3.b**).
        5. **Percutaneous ultrasound-guided or CT-guided needle biopsy.** This procedure is indicated in patients with either type of biliary malignancy whenever a recurrent mass is identified and histologic confirmation of recurrence is desired.

REFERENCES

Buskirk SJ et al: Analysis of failure following curative irradiation of gallbladder and extrahepatic bile duct carcinoma. *Int J Radiat Oncol Biol Phys* 1984;**10**:2013–2023.

Donohue JD et al: Carcinoma of the gallbladder. *Arch Surg* 1990;**125**:237–244.

Fields JN, Emami B: Carcinoma of the extrahepatic biliary system—results of primary and adjuvant radiotherapy. *Int J Radiat Oncol Biol Phys* 1987;**13**:331–338.

Lai ECS et al: Proximal bile duct cancer. *Ann Surg* 1987;**205**:111–118.

Morrow CE et al: Primary gallbladder carcinoma. *Surgery* 1983;**94**:709–714.

Oberfield RA, Rossi RL: The role of chemotherapy in the treatment of bile duct cancer. *World J Surg* 1988;**12**(1):105–108.

Ottow RT, August DA, Sugarbaker PH: Treatment of proximal biliary tract carcinoma. *Surgery* 1985;**97**:251–261.

Wanebo HJ, Schwalke MA: Gallbladder cancer. In: Cameron JL (editor), *Current Surgical Therapy-3,* 3rd ed. Philadelphia, PA: BC Decker; 1989;291–297.

Zinner MJ: Bile duct tumors. In: Cameron JL (editor), *Current Surgical Therapy-3,* 3rd ed. Philadelphia, PA: BC Decker, 1989;289–291.

36 Malignancies of the Colon

Robert B. Cameron, MD

I. **Epidemiology.** Excluding skin cancer, cancer of the colon (not including the rectum) is the **third most common malignancy of both males and females** in the United States. It is also the third leading cause of cancer deaths. In 1985, **42.5 cases per 100,000 males and 33.2 cases per 100,000 females** were diagnosed, resulting in **21.4 and 15.3 deaths,** respectively. Estimates indicated that 109,000 new cases will be reported in 1993, leading to 50,000 deaths and accounting for 15% of all cancer diagnoses and 12% of all cancer deaths. Because of unknown factors, the incidence in the United States has increased 19% since 1950. Mortality, however, has decreased by 20% during the same period, primarily as a result of better anesthesia and surgical care. The worldwide incidence of colon cancer varies substantially—as many as 33 cases per 100,000 are diagnosed each year in the Northeastern United States, Northern Europe, Australia, and New Zealand and as few as 1.3 per 100,000 are diagnosed in Ibadan, Nigeria. Because migrants generally adopt the risk of the population in their new locale, dietary, environmental factors, or both, may play a role in this phenomenon.

II. **Risk factors.** Both environmental and genetic factors have been implicated in the pathogenesis of colon cancer. All of the following have either been associated with or been causally linked to the development of colon malignancies.

A. **Age.** The incidence of colon cancer steadily increases after age 35 from less than 2 per 100,000 to more than **400 per 100,000 after age 85.** Approximately 2 out of 3 cases occur in people older than 50.

B. **Sex.** The **risk for males is 1.3 times that of females** in the United States.

C. **Race.** Since 1950 there has been no overall difference between the incidence of colon cancer in blacks and whites, regardless of gender.

D. **Genetic factors.** Certain familial polyposis syndromes and a family history of colon carcinoma predispose patients for the disease. This may be related to an inherited genetic abnormality such as a mutated ras oncogene, which recently has been found in as many as 50% of patients with colon cancer.

1. **Family history.** A family history of colon cancer increases the risk in first-degree relatives by about 3-fold.

2. **Family cancer syndrome.** An **autosomal dominant** predisposition for adenocarcinomas of all types, most commonly of the colon, breast, and endometrium, has been described in the literature.

3. **Familial polyposis syndromes**

a. **Familial polyposis coli.** Multiple adenomatous polyps of the colon beginning at puberty mark this autosomal dominant disorder. These polyps have a high malignant potential: **nearly 100%** of these patients **develop carcinoma by age 55.** Similar familial syndromes of hereditary colon carcinoma without the development of polyposis also have been described.

b. **Gardner's syndrome.** Colonic polyposis with **supernumerary teeth, cranial fibrous dysplasia, osteomas, fibromas, and sebaceous cysts** distinguish this autosomal dominant disease.

c. **Turcot's syndrome.** This autosomal dominant syndrome is characterized by colonic polyposis accompanied by **gliomas.**

d. **Oldfield's syndrome.** Colonic polyposis with **multiple sebaceous cysts** marks this autosomal recessive disease.

E. **Diet**

1. **Dietary fiber.** Epidemiologic data, primarily from Africa, suggests that certain types of dietary fiber may reduce the risk of colon cancer. **Dilution or binding of carcinogens and reduced transit time** of the stool (thereby decreasing the exposure to carcinogens) have been proposed as possible explanations.

2. **Dietary fat.** Experimental and epidemiologic data have implicated dietary fat,

273

particularly **unsaturated fat, cholesterol, and colonic bile salts,** as possible factors in the etiology of colon carcinoma.

F. **Previous colonic pathology**

1. **Unresected adenomatous polyps.** Many large studies indicate that the presence of an adenomatous polyp increases the risk of colon cancer. The increased risk depends on **polyp type and size** (Table 36–1). In addition, multiple polyps pose a 2–2.5 times greater risk than does a single polyp. Thus, whenever possible, all nonhyperplastic polyps should be removed.

2. **Inflammatory bowel disease**

   a. **Ulcerative colitis.** Risk of colon carcinoma in patients with ulcerative colitis increases with the duration and severity of the disease. The **risk after 10 years is between 10% and 20%.**

   b. **Crohn's colitis.** Overall, Crohn's colitis minimally increases the risk of colon cancer, but the risk can reach **20 times normal** in patients with early onset of disease (age < 21).

G. **Urbanization.** Industrialized areas are associated with a higher risk of colon cancer, but this may be related to other factors, including diet.

III. **Presentation**

A. **Signs and symptoms.** Presenting signs and symptoms vary with location of the primary lesion and presence or absence of metastases.

1. **Local manifestations**

   a. **Left colonic lesions.** Common signs and symptoms include **pain** (75%), **bleeding** (50%), constipation or decreased stool diameter (40%), and obstruction (25%).

   b. **Right colonic lesions.** Common signs and symptoms include **pain** (75%), bleeding (30%), weakness or anemia (30%), obstruction (25%), and abdominal mass (25%).

2. **Systemic manifestations.** Signs and symptoms include pain; hepatic, pulmonary, or ovarian masses; weight loss; and weakness.

B. **Paraneoplastic syndromes.** Paraneoplastic syndromes have been associated with colon carcinoma. Although uncommon, these symptom complexes may be the sole manifestation of disease.

1. **Dermatomyositis/myositis** (see p 59, **III**).
2. **Acanthosis nigricans** (see p 109, **II.A**).
3. **Subacute cerebellar degeneration** (see p 58, **II.A**).
4. **Thrombophlebitis** (see p 81).
5. **Nonbacterial thrombotic endocarditis** (see p 52).
6. **Erythema gyratum repens** (see p 108).
7. **Hypertrichosis languinosa** (see p 110).
8. **Leser-Trelat syndrome** (see p 109).

IV. **Differential diagnosis.** On barium enema, colon carcinoma usually appears as a **constricting ("apple-core") or mass (filling defect) lesion.** Malignant constriction, as a rule, abruptly changes the bowel lumen, whereas the lumen caliber gradually tapers in benign lesions. Although such a lesion in any patient older than 40 is likely to represent cancer, benign conditions, such as **diverticulitis,** Crohn's and ulcerative **colitis,** periappendiceal **abscesses,** unusual **infections** (actinomycosis, tuberculosis, and amoebiasis), **extrinsic masses** (pancreatitis, endometriosis, lymphoma, and ovarian carci-

TABLE 36–1. FREQUENCY AND MALIGNANT POTENTIAL OF COLONIC POLYPS

Type of Polyp/Size of Polyp	Polyps (%)	Malignant Potential
Hyperplastic	90	0
Adenomas	8	3
Villous	0.4	20
Villotubular	1.6	10
Tubular	6	3
< 1 cm	80	1
1–2 cm	15	3
> 2 cm	5	7.5

noma), **vascular compromise,** and, in rare cases, physiologic **muscular sphincters, foreign bodies, and colitis cystica profunda** also should be considered.

V. **Screening programs.** Everyone older than 20 years should undergo a general physical examination, including a digital rectal examination, every three years. After age 40, this should be done annually.

A. **Stool guiaic test.** A formal test for occult fecal blood should be done annually after age 40. This involves **restriction of dietary meat** beginning 24 hours before the test, which reduces false positives resulting from blood, and consumption of large quantities of fruits, vegetables, and cereals, which reduces false negatives by inducing bleeding from any existing lesion via mechanical irritation). In addition, to increase accuracy, 2 samples from different areas of a fecal mass are sampled on three consecutive days (total of 6 samples). When administered properly, hemoccult tests have a **0.5% false positive rate and a 50% predictive value** in patients older than 40 (50% of positives will turn out to have either adenomas or carcinomas). However, a **20% false negative rate** limits the usefulness of the test.

B. **Sigmoidoscopy.** Rigid sigmoidoscopy has been proposed as a screening procedure for colon carcinoma; however, the yield in asymptomatic patients under 50 is extremely low (< 0.2%). In addition, nearly two-thirds of cancers are out of reach of this instrument. Therefore, rigid sigmoidoscopy should be performed on all patients, but only **every 3–5 years after the age of 50 and after 2 initial negative examinations** are done 1 year apart. Flexible sigmoidoscopy can visualize approximately three times the length of bowel as the rigid exam and is better tolerated by patients. Although the flexible examination requires more training, and although its usefulness has not been fully evaluated, the greater patient acceptance and increased detection potential makes it the preferred approach whenever possible.

VI. **Diagnostic workup**

A. **Medical history and physical examination.** A complete medical history emphasizing common presenting symptoms (eg, weight loss, change in bowel habits) and a thorough physical examination are essential to a complete evaluation.

1. **Skin.** Pallor (anemia), hyperpigmentation of the neck, axillae, or anorectal area **(acanthosis nigricans),** or inflammatory lesions **(dermatomyositis and erythema gyratum repens)** should be noted.

2. **Lymph nodes.** The presence of a signal node (also called **Virchow's or Troisier's node)** must be recorded.

3. **Abdomen.** Masses and hepatomegaly are important findings.

4. **Rectum.** A digital examination to exclude masses and **occult fecal blood** is mandatory in all patients.

B. **Primary tests and procedures.** All patients with suspected colon cancer should have the following diagnostic tests performed.

1. **Blood tests**
   a. **Complete blood count** (see p 1, **IV.A.1**).
   b. **Hepatic transaminases** (see p 1, **IV.A.2**).
   c. **Alkaline phosphatase** (see p 1, **IV.A.3**).
   d. **Carcinoembryonic antigen (CEA).** Elevated serum levels of this antigen after resection of the primary tumor or after an initial postoperative normalization of levels correlates with the presence of tumor.

2. **Imaging studies**
   a. **Chest x-ray** (see p 3, **IV.C.1**).
   b. **Barium enema (BE).** A **double-contrast enema (air/barium)** is useful for small mucosal lesions and a single contrast enema (barium alone) is most useful for constricting and large-mass lesions. Although sensitive, barium enemas **miss 5–10% of lesions;** however, they provide a "road map" that is often extremely useful for the surgeon.

3. **Invasive procedures**
   a. **Sigmoidoscopy.** Sigmoid examination should be performed for left-sided lesions. As discussed above, **flexible examinations are preferred** because they visualize more lesions and are better tolerated by patients. Barium enemas also are required to evaluate the remaining colon for synchronous primary lesions.
   b. **Colonoscopy.** Examination of the entire colon is indicated to biopsy suspicious lesions or polyps, to diagnose right-sided lesions, or to exclude synchronous primary lesions or polyps.

C. **Optional tests and procedures.** The following tests and procedures may be indicated on the basis of previous diagnostic findings or clinical suspicion.

1. **Blood tests** (see p 2, **IV.A**)

   a. **Nucleotidase.**
   b. **GGTP.**
2. **Imaging studies** (see p 3, **IV.C**)
   a. **Computed tomography.**
   b. **Magnetic resonance imaging.**
   c. **Ultrasound.**
   d. **Technetium-99m bone scan.**
3. **Invasive procedures.** If symptoms of pneumaturia or recurrent urinary tract infections are elicited, **cystoscopy** is indicated to evaluate the possibility of a **colovesical fistula.**

VII. Pathology

A. **Location.** The location of primary colonic lesions has changed recently, with an increasing propensity for proximal lesions: **sigmoid and descending colon, 52%; transverse colon, 16%; and cecum and ascending colon, 32%.**

B. **Multiplicity. Synchronous** primary lesions are found in 3% of colon cancer patients; another 2% develop a **metachronous lesion.** This high frequency of second primaries necessitates an evaluation of the entire colon before and periodically after therapy.

C. **Histology.** Adenocarcinoma constitutes more than 98% of all colonic malignancies. Other malignancies include signet-ring carcinoma, adenosquamous carcinoma, squamous cell carcinoma, sarcoma, lymphoma, carcinoid, and undifferentiated carcinomas (all < 1%).

D. **Metastatic spread**
   1. **Modes of spread.** Colon cancer spreads by 4 mechanisms.
      a. **Direct extension.** Tumor may grow directly into adjacent organs and structures and may extend along nerves and vessels.
      b. **Lymphatic metastasis.** Malignant cells readily spread through **circular lymphatics** of the colon and create the common "apple-core" lesion. **Longitudinal spread** is much **less extensive** and is **unusual more than 5 cm from the primary tumor.** Regional and distant lymph node metastases are common when the primary tumor extends beyond the muscularis propria. Tumors that do not extend outside this layer rarely metastasize (3–5%) and, usually, only when the lesions are poorly differentiated.
      c. **Hematogenous metastasis.** Tumor cells dislodge and are carried through portal, portovertebral, and portosystemic (hemorrhoidal) vessels to distant organs. Approximately **25% of patients** present with synchronous hematogenous metastases.
      d. **Implantation.** Direct implantation can occur in distant colonic sites, the **ovaries, peritoneum,** and possibly to anastomoses.
   2. **Sites of spread.** At autopsy, many organs are likely to be involved in metastatic spread of colon carcinoma: **liver** (60–71%), **lung** (25–40%), vertebral body and other bony sites (5–10%), ovary (3–5%), adrenal gland (1%), and central nervous system (1%).

VIII. Staging.
In 1932 Cuthbert Dukes, a pathologist at St. Mark's Hospital in London, first realized that colorectal cancer spreads in an orderly fashion from a primary lesion to regional lymphatics and finally to distant organs. With this in mind, he proposed a staging system made up of 3 stages. Multiple revisions of Dukes' original system have been proposed, including one by Astler and Coller in 1954 which is still commonly used. The American Joint Committee on Cancer recently revised its TNM staging system in cooperation with the Union Internationale Contre le Cancer. Thus, a single international standard based on Dukes' original staging system now exists. This standard allows direct comparison of most past and any future studies. All three of these staging systems are compared below.

A. **Dukes system**
   1. **Stage A.** Disease does not extend beyond the muscularis propria.
   2. **Stage B.** Disease extends through the entire bowel wall.
   3. **Stage C.** Any primary tumor with positive lymph nodes.

B. **Astler-Coller modification of the Dukes classification**
   1. **Stage A** (2%). Disease is limited to the mucosa.
   2. **Stage B1** (11%). Disease extends through muscularis mucosa but not through muscularis propria.
   3. **Stage B2** (30%). Disease extends beyond muscularis propria.
   4. **Stage C1** (2%). Stage B1 with positive regional lymph nodes.
   5. **Stage C2** (22%). Stage B2 with positive regional lymph nodes.
   6. **Stage D** (33%). Distant metastases.

C. **TNM classification**
  1. **Tumor stage**
     a. **TX.** Primary tumor cannot be assessed.
     b. **T0.** No evidence of tumor.
     c. **Tis.** Carcinoma in situ.
     d. **T1.** Tumor invades into but not through submucosa.
     e. **T2.** Tumor invades into but not through muscularis propria.
     f. **T3.** Tumor invades through muscularis propria into subserosa.
     g. **T4.** Tumor perforates visceral peritoneum or invades other organs or structures (including other loops of bowel).
  2. **Lymph node stage**
     a. **NX.** Regional lymph nodes cannot be assessed.
     b. **N0.** No regional lymph nodes are involved.
     c. **N1.** One to 3 pericolic lymph nodes are involved.
     d. **N2.** Four or more pericolic lymph nodes are involved.
     e. **N3.** Regional nodes along named vascular trunks are involved.
  3. **Metastatic stage**
     a. **MX.** The presence of distant metastases cannot be assessed.
     b. **M0.** No distant metastases are present.
     c. **M1.** Distant metastases are present.
  4. **Histopathologic grade**
     a. **GX.** Grade cannot be assessed.
     b. **G1.** Well differentiated.
     c. **G2.** Moderately well differentiated.
     d. **G3.** Poorly differentiated.
     e. **G4.** Undifferentiated.
  5. **Stage groupings**
     a. **Stage 0.** Tis, N0, M0.
     b. **Stage I** (Duke's A). T1 or T2, N0, M0.
     c. **Stage II** (Duke's B). T3 or T4, N0, M0.
     d. **Stage III** (Duke's C). Any T, N1, N2, or N3, M0.
     e. **Stage IV.** Any T; any N, M1.

IX. **Treatment**
  A. **Surgery**
    1. **Primary colon carcinoma**
       a. **General considerations.** Surgery remains the mainstay of therapy for primary colon carcinoma. The goal is to remove en bloc the involved segment of bowel and the regional lymph nodes. **Right hemicolectomy** is indicated for lesions of the cecum, right colon, and hepatic flexure. **Transverse colectomy** should be performed for lesions of the transverse colon, although many surgeons prefer to treat these lesions with a formal extended right hemicolectomy that includes the transverse colon.

       Lesions of the splenic flexure, left colon, and sigmoid are routinely removed by **left hemicolectomy**. If the morbidity of a formal hemicolectomy is deemed excessive, a smaller segmental resection may then become the procedure of choice. Patients with **familial polyposis or inflammatory bowel diseases,** however, should be considered for **total proctocolectomy** because the risk of multiple primary lesions is exceedingly high. **Bowel margins** both proximally and distally should be generous, but under no circumstances should the bowel be transected within **5 cm** of the tumor mass because tumor cells readily spread this distance within the bowel wall lymphatics. The paracolic and intermediate lymph nodes should be removed along with the mesentery down to the base of the vascular pedicle. Local invasion into adjacent organs should be treated by wedge resection of the involved portion when feasible. In 1967 Turnbull proposed a **"no-touch technique"** with an associated improvement in survival; however, this could not be confirmed by others. An integral part of Turnbull's technique was **wide resection of bowel mesentery and lymphatics,** which is currently credited with the improved survival.
       b. **Bowel preparation.** Proper bowel preparation is essential for acceptable morbidity and mortality in surgery of the large bowel. Regimens generally involve both mechanical and antibiotic preparation. Oral antibiotics have been shown to reduce rates of septic complications and wound infections from 43% and 35% to 9% and 9%, respectively. Supplemental intravenous antibiotics are widely used, although no additional benefit has been shown over oral antibiotics alone. Two typical regimens are shown in Table 36–2.

TABLE 36–2. COMMON BOWEL PREPARATION REGIMENS

Day	Diet	Cathartic
Condon bowel preparation		
1	Low residue	6 pm: 1 tablet bisacodyl sodium
2	Low residue	10 am, 2 and 6 pm: 30 cc magnesium sulfate (50% solution)
3	Clear liquids	10 am and 2 pm: 30 cc magnesium sulfate (50% solution)
Lavage bowel preparation		
1	Clear liquids	6 pm: 4 liters isotonic polyethylene glycol solution over 4 hrs.
2	Clear liquids	7 am: 2–4 liters isotonic polyethylene glycol solution over 2–4 hrs.

Robert Condon described a cathartic-based mechanical and antibiotic preparation that produced excellent results. Lavage-based preparations were not widely used because of dehydration that was often produced by the normal saline or Ringer's solution used in the preparation. However, this problem has been averted by the invention of **polyethylene glycol solutions** (GoLYTELY, COLYTE) that are isotonic and therefore do not cause dehydration.

   c. **Staged procedures.** Many patients may require staged procedures for removal of a primary colonic lesion. Three approaches have been advocated in various circumstances.

      (1) One-stage procedure. A single operation is performed during which the primary lesion is resected and the colon is reanastomosed primarily. This procedure is used almost exclusively in elective resections, although right-sided obstructing lesions can be treated with a 1-stage right hemicolectomy. In addition, reports of a one-stage procedure combined with **intraoperative colonic irrigation** in cases of left-sided acute obstruction have surfaced in the literature.

      (2) Two-stage procedure. Commonly used in cases of acute obstruction, the 2-stage procedure initially involves **primary resection** of the tumor and **colostomy formation.** The colostomy is created either at the site of transection or proximally as a diverting colostomy with reanastomosis of the bowel at the primary transection site. Later, a **second procedure** is performed to **take down the colostomy.** Alternatively, only a proximal colostomy is performed at the initial operation. Following bowel preparation, a **second procedure** is performed to **resect the tumor and reanastomose the bowel.**

      (3) Three-stage procedure. Formerly used for patients with acute obstruction, this approach includes **initial decompression** of the bowel by colostomy formation followed by a **second operation to resect the primary tumor.** A **third procedure** was required to **take down the colostomy.** This approach is uncommon today.

  2. **Metastatic colon carcinoma**

   a. **Curative surgery.** Surgery is usually not an option for patients with metastatic colon cancer. Recently, however, several groups have demonstrated a 25–30% 5-year survival for patients with **1–4 resectable liver metastases** if all lesions are resected. Furthermore, some benefit has been demonstrated from resection of pulmonary metastases. **Second-look laparotomies** for elevated CEA levels have been evaluated with mixed results. Some studies indicate that as many as 59% of recurrences can be resected with a 5-year survival rate as high as 37%. However, similar percentages have been reported for laparotomies of clinically manifested recurrences.

   b. **Palliative surgery.** Surgery is often indicated for palliation of symptoms from metastatic colon carcinoma. "Second-look" laparotomy for elevated CEA levels without localizable tumor is controversial because no definitive evidence exists for improvement in survival over treatment instituted when symptomatic localized recurrences occur. Frequent indications for surgery include the conditions listed below:

(1) **Malignant gastric outlet or small bowel obstruction. Gastrostomy** is often performed in this situation because it is simple and affords good palliation. **Small-bowel resection, bypass, or both** are also frequently used options if feasible.

(2) **Malignant colonic obstruction. Proximal diverting colostomy** is usually the procedure of choice for unresectable lesions because it allows the patient to resume eating and quickly leave the hospital.

3. **Mortality and morbidity.** Operative mortality for **elective colon resection is 1–3%.** Morbidity ranges from 15–20% and often includes one of the following complications: sepsis and wound infection, 5–10%; anastomotic leak, 2–5%; stomal complications; urinary retention, with extensive pelvic dissection; or impotence, with extensive pelvic dissection.

B. **Radiation therapy**

1. **Primary colon carcinoma.** Radiation has no role in the initial treatment of colon cancer.

2. **Adjuvant therapy**

a. **Preoperative therapy.** Radiation therapy has been used preoperatively in attempts to convert marginally unresectable lesions to resectable status and to decrease dissemination at the time of surgery. The data, however, are not convincing.

b. **Postoperative therapy.** Radiation therapy has been used postoperatively in an attempt to decrease the incidence of local recurrence. The advantages of postoperative therapy include an **operating field free of radiation** effects at the time of surgery, **no delay in tumor resection, improved staging, and delineation of the extent of the tumor** by intraoperatively placed clips. Furthermore, patients who have no lymph node metastases (approximately 50%) can be **spared unnecessary radiation.** Although no definitive study exists on this mode of therapy, possible indications for postoperative radiation therapy include the following findings: **lymph node involvement, known residual disease, and adherence to adjacent structures** (ie, pelvic side walls or retroperitoneum).

c. **Combined preoperative and postoperative therapy.** A combination of low-dose preoperative therapy (500 cGy in one fraction or 200 cGy in 5 daily fractions) and postoperative therapy in a **"sandwich" technique** has recently generated much enthusiasm as a means of using the advantages of both pre- and postoperative therapy.

d. **Doses and responses.** Generally, 4500–5000 cGy are delivered over 5–6 weeks using multiple fields, although more accelerated schedules are also used. Several nonrandomized studies have shown a **decrease in local recurrence rates** from 30–40% to less than 10% with postoperative radiation therapy for **sigmoid carcinomas.** Actuarial **5-year survivals improved** from 60–64% to 70–100% in **patients with Dukes B2 lesions,** and a slight survival benefit was seen in **patients with C2 lesions** in one study as well (Kopelson, 1983).

3. **Palliative therapy.** Radiation therapy has been used in attempts to palliate symptomatic metastases. **Bony metastases** may respond especially well to radiotherapy on a short-term basis.

4. **Morbidity and mortality.** The incidence of complications from postoperative external beam radiation therapy is dose dependent and is related mostly to the gastrointestinal tract. Complications occur 5–10% of the time and include small bowel **obstruction,** intestinal **fistulization,** and intestinal **perforation.**

C. **Chemotherapy.** Chemotherapy has had limited success in the treatment of colon carcinoma and cannot be recommended as routine therapy outside of approved clinical trials. Two major approaches to the delivery of chemotherapeutic agents have been used:

1. **Systemic chemotherapy**

a. **Primary colon carcinoma.** Chemotherapy has not proved to be useful in the initial treatment of resectable colon cancer.

b. **Adjuvant chemotherapy.** Despite a number of randomized prospective trials by cooperative groups such as the Veterans Administration Surgical Oncology Group, the Central Oncology Group, the Gastrointestinal Tumor Study Group, the Southwestern Oncology Group, and the National Surgical Adjuvant Breast and Bowel Project (NSABP), no definitive answer on adjuvant chemotherapy has been forthcoming. **Methyl-CCNU and fluorouracil** have been tested most extensively, and vincristine and levamisole also have been tried (see **X.D.1**). An **improved disease-free (p = 0.02) and overall survival (p = 0.05)** in patients receiving **fluorouracil, methyl-CCNU, and vincristine** was demonstrated in the NSABP study; however, the magnitude of the improvement was small (58% vs 51% disease-free survival and 67% vs. 59% overall survival), and the period of administration was up to 80 weeks (Wolmark et al, 1988). One study demonstrated a 41% reduction in recurrence rate and a 33% reduction in the overall death rate by administration of fluoracil and levamistole in patients with Dukes C cancer; however, appropriate control groups were not included. In another study, the Central Oncology Group noted an improvement in disease-free survival (but not overall survival) in patients who received fluorouracil. Although only one study has shown an overall survival benefit, reports consistently have demonstrated a small benefit for patients receiving fluorouracil. Therefore, if a patient is willing to accept the morbidity of chemotherapy with fluorouracil, it may be reasonable to administer this drug even though there is only a slight chance of survival benefit.

   Note: Methyl-CCNU is associated with secondary hematogenous malignancies and is currently available only in an approved clinical trial.

   c. **Locally advanced and metastatic colon cancer.** No single agent, including fluorouracil, has proved to be beneficial in the setting of metastatic disease. However, recent reports indicate a small but statistically significant benefit to combination therapy with **fluorouracil and leucovorin** (O'Connell, 1989).

2. **Local hepatic infusion chemotherapy.** Initial studies indicated that hepatic artery chemotherapy infusion was associated with a **40–80% response rate.** Subsequent prospective randomized trials failed to demonstrate any advantage over systemically administered therapy. More recent reports from England suggest a survival benefit with **portal vein infusion of fluorouracil** in patients with **Dukes B carcinoma** resected for cure. In this randomized study, 5-year survival of 95% with perfusion and 65% without were noted (Taylor et al, 1985). The results of this study has not yet been confirmed by others. Although no consistent benefit has been seen, significant toxicities such as chemical hepatitis, cholangitis, and cholecystitis (when a cholecystectomy is not performed) are common.

D. **Immunotherapy**

1. **Nonspecific therapy.** Both Bacillus Calmette-Guerin (BCG) and a methanol extract of BCG have been tested in clinical trials without any evidence of efficacy. Most recently, the NSABP demonstrated **no benefit to BCG scarification** in tumor-related mortality (Wolmark et al, 1988). **Adjuvant levamisole, when combined with fluorouracil, reduced the recurrence rate of Dukes C lesions by 41% and the overall death rate by 33%.** However, the chance that the observed effect was the result of fluorouracil alone cannot be excluded because appropriate control groups were not included. Trials with interferon-alpha and interleukin-2 (alone, with lymphokine-activated killer cells, or with tumor-infiltrating lymphocytes) also have begun, with some early reports of responses.

2. **Specific therapy.** The use of monoclonal antibodies, such as **17–1A, B72.3, and 44 × 14,** either alone or combined with other immunomodulatory agents have undergone preliminary trials and some objective responses have been reported.

X. **Prognosis**

A. **Risk of recurrence.** Prognosis closely correlates with recurrence because few patients are cured of recurrent disease. Table 36–3 lists the likelihood of failure after potentially curative surgical resection.

B. **Five-year survival** (by Astler-Coller modified Dukes stage)

   1. **Dukes stage A,** 75–100%.
   2. **Dukes stage B1,** 65%.
   3. **Dukes stage B2,** 50%.
   4. **Dukes stage C1,** 40%.
   5. **Dukes stage C2,** 15%.
   6. **Dukes stage D,** < 5%, unless the patient has only 1–4 resectable liver metastases, which carry a 25–30% survival probability.

TABLE 36–3. PATTERNS OF COLON CARCINOMA RECURRENCE: LIKELIHOOD OF FAILURE BY DUKES STAGE

Dukes Stage	Local Only (%)	Distant Only (%)	Local and Distant Failure (%)
A	0	0	3
B1	1	7	1
B2	15	20	26
C1	0	25	0
C2	22	27	59
Total	6	11	13

*Adapted from Willet CG et al: Failure patterns following curative resection of colonic carcinoma. Ann Surg 1984;**200**:685.*

    C. Adverse prognostic factors. Multiple factors that carry an adverse prognostic significance for patients with colon cancer are listed below:
        1. Ulceration or perforation of the primary lesion.
        2. Circumferential obstructing primary lesion.
        3. Invasion of contiguous structures, including nerves and blood vessels.
        4. CEA levels higher than 5 ng/mL.
        5. Age younger than 30 years at the time of diagnosis.
        6. High-grade (undifferentiated) lesions.
XI. Patient follow-up
    A. General guidelines. Patients should be followed every 3 months for 2 years, every 6 months an additional 3 years, and then annually for recurrence because local disease and limited (1–4 metastases) hepatic disease can be treated successfully with surgery. The following specific guidelines are recommended.
    B. Routine evaluation. Each clinic visit should include the following tests and procedures:
        1. Medical history and physical examination. A complete examination should be performed during routine clinic appointments. Particular attention should be paid to the areas listed on p 275, **VI.**
        2. Complete blood count (see p 1, **IV.A.1**).
        3. Hepatic transaminases (see p 1, **IV.A.2**).
        4. Alkaline phosphatase (see p 1, **IV.A.3**).
        5. Carcinoembryonic antigen (CEA). Serum CEA levels are used to monitor for recurrence. This test should be ordered during every clinic visit, but it is useful only if the preoperative CEA was elevated and subsequently returned to normal within 4–6 weeks postoperatively (half-life = 24 hrs and, therefore, **5–7 days are required for elevated levels to return to normal**). Nonmalignant causes of elevated CEA levels include liver disease, smoking, chronic pulmonary diseases, and inflammatory bowel disease.
        6. Chest x-ray (see p 3, **IV.C.1**).
    C. Additional evaluation. Other examinations that should be performed at regular intervals include the following:
        1. Barium enema. A barium enema is required every year to evaluate the remaining colon for **metachronous primary carcinomas and for suture line recurrences.**
        2. Endoscopy. Sigmoidoscopy or colonoscopy should be performed every year to assess the colon for anastomotic recurrence and metachronous primary lesions. Colonoscopy and barium enema alone miss 5–10% of colonic neoplasms; therefore, a regimen of alternating colonoscopy and barium enema every 6 months is useful to increase the number of lesions detected.
    D. Optional evaluation. The following tests may be indicated by previous diagnostic findings or clinical suspicion.
        1. Blood tests (see p 2, **IV.A**)
           a. Nucleotidase.
           b. GGTP.

2. **Imaging studies** (see p 3, **IV.C**)
   a. **Computerized tomography.**
   b. **Magnetic resonance imaging.**
   c. **Technetium-99m bone scan.**
3. **Biopsy.** A sample of any abnormal tissue should be obtained with biopsy forceps using either a colonoscope or a sigmoidoscope if any colonic or anastomotic abnormalities are noted or with needle aspiration if any pelvic, hepatic, pulmonary, or other visceral masses are noted.

REFERENCES

Dent TL, Kukora JS, Nejman JH: The colon, rectum, and anus. In: Hardy JD, Kukora JS, Pass HI (editors), *Hardy's Textbook of Surgery,* 2nd ed. Philadelphia, PA: JB Lippincott; 1988:582–636.

Dukes CE: The classification of cancer of the rectum. *J Pathol Bacteriol* 1932;**35:**323–332.

Ferguson E: Operations of choice for cancer of the colon and rectum: an overview. *Am Surg* 1984;**50:**121–127.

Gastrointestinal Tumor Study Group: Adjuvant therapy of colon cancer—results of a prospectively randomized trial. *N Engl J Med* 1984;**310:**737–743.

Gunderson LL, Beart RW, O'Connell MJ: Current issues in the treatment of colorectal cancer. *Crit Rev Oncol/Hematol* 1986;**6:**223–260.

Kopelson G: Adjuvant postoperative radiation therapy for colorectal carcinoma above the peritoneal reflection, I. sigmoid colon. *Cancer* 1983;**51:**1593–1598.

Lise M et al: Adjuvant therapy for colorectal cancer: the EORTC experience and a review of the literature. *Dis Colon Rect* 1988;**30:**847–854.

Moertel CG et al: Levamisole and fluorouracil for adjuvant therapy of resected colon carcinoma. *N Engl J Med* 1990;**322:**352–358.

O'Connell MJ: A phase III trial of 5-fluorouracil and leucovorin in the treatment of advanced colorectal cancer: a Mayo Clinic/North Central Cancer Treatment Group study. *Cancer* 1989;**63**(suppl 6):1026–1030.

Sugarbaker PH et al: A simplified plan for followup of patients with colon and rectal cancer supported by prospective studies of laboratory and radiologic test results. *Surgery* 1987;**102**(1):79–87.

Taylor I et al: A randomized controlled trial of adjuvant portal vein cytotoxic perfusion in colorectal cancer. *Br J Surg* 1985;**72:**352–358.

Tepper JE: Adjuvant irradiation of gastrointestinal malignancies: impact on local control and tumor cure. *Int J Radiat Oncol Biol Phys* 1986;**12:**667–671.

Turnbull RB, Kyle K, Watson FR: Cancer of the colon: the influence of the no-touch technic on survival rates. *Ann Surg* 1967;**166:**420–427.

Willett CG et al: Failure patterns following curative resection of colonic carcinoma. *Ann Surg* 1984;**200:**685–690.

Wolmark N, Fisher B, other NSABP investigators: Postoperative adjuvant chemotherapy or BCG for colon cancer: results from NSABP protocol C–01. *JNCI* 1988;**80:**30–37.

37 Malignancies of the Rectum

Robert B. Cameron, MD

I. **Epidemiology.** Cancer of the rectum (excluding the colon) is the **fifth most common malignancy** in both males and females in the United States. When combined with colon carcinoma, colorectal cancer is the second most common malignancy after lung cancer in males and breast cancer in females and the third most frequent cause of death in both sexes. In 1985, **19.5 cases per 100,000 males and 11.6 cases per 100,000 females** were diagnosed, resulting in **3.7 and 2.2 deaths,** respectively. In 1993, 43,000 new cases will be diagnosed leading to 7,000 deaths. Worldwide, the variation in the incidence of rectal cancer follows a pattern similar to that of colon carcinoma. Areas of high incidence include the Northeastern United States, Austria, Australia, Belgium, Czechoslovakia, Denmark, Hungary, New Zealand, and Switzerland. In contrast, Barbados, Chile, Ecuador, Greece, Kuwait, Panama, Peru, and Suriname report fewer than 10 cases per 100,000 population annually.

II. **Risk factors.** Most risk factors are identical to those of colon carcinoma; however, some differences do exist.
   A. **Age.** The number of cases of rectal carcinoma gradually increase after the age of 35 from less than 1 per 100,000 to **120.3 per 100,000 by the age of 80.**
   B. **Sex.** Males are at **1.7 times greater risk** than females in the United States.
   C. **Race.** In the United States, the risk among **whites is 1.4 times** that of blacks.
   D. **Genetic factors.** As with colon cancer, a family history of colorectal carcinoma and specific familial syndromes predispose patients to rectal cancer through an unidentified genetic mechanism.
      1. **Family history.** A history of rectal carcinoma increases the risk in first-degree relatives by a **factor of 3.**
      2. **Familial polyposis syndromes**
         a. **Familial polyposis coli.** This autosomal dominant disease is marked by the progressive development of multiple adenomatous polyps throughout the colon and rectum. By age 40, 80% of those affected will have at least one carcinoma; **by age 55, 100% will have developed cancer.**
         b. **Gardner's syndrome.** A variant of familial polyposis with autosomal dominant inheritance, this syndrome is characterized by pancolorectal polyposis, **supernumerary teeth, cranial fibrous dysplasia, osteomas, fibromas, and sebaceous cysts.**
         c. **Turcot's syndrome. Gliomas** associated with pancolorectal polyposis distinguish this autosomal dominant syndrome.
         d. **Oldfield's syndrome.** Inherited through an autosomal recessive mechanism, this syndrome is characterized by polyposis of the colon and rectum and **multiple sebaceous cysts.**
   E. **Diet**
      1. **Dietary fiber.** African epidemiologic evidence implicates a low-fiber diet as a major factor in the development of colorectal carcinoma. It has been proposed that fiber may **dilute or bind fecal carcinogens** (fecapentaenes and benzopyrene), **decrease bowel transit time, and lower fecal Ph,** all of which have been associated with a decreased incidence of colorectal carcinoma.
      2. **Dietary fat.** Increased dietary fat may promote secretion of bile acid and the formation of **ketosteroids,** both of which are incriminated in the genesis of colorectal cancer.
   F. **Previous rectal pathology**
      1. **Rectal polyps.** Rectal polyps can be either hyperplastic or adenomatous. Adenomas are divided into three types: tubular, villous, or mixed tubular and villous.
         a. **Hyperplastic polyps.** These are the most common type of polyps; however, they are of little consequence because they harbor **no malignant potential.**
         b. **Tubular polyps.** These polyps are usually small, carry a variable risk of

283

rectal carcinoma depending on size, and do not differ from those found in the colon (see Table 36–1).

    c. **Villous polyps.** These polyps occur more frequently in the rectum than in the colon, and between **25% and 40% will contain carcinoma** in situ or invasive carcinoma.

    d. **Mixed tubular/villous polyps.** These polyps have characteristics of both villous and tubular adenomas.

  2. **Inflammatory bowel disease**

    a. **Ulcerative colitis.** The rectum is involved in ulcerative colitis in **more than 90% of cases,** and the risk of malignancy increases with the duration and severity of disease. **After 10 years, the risk of adenocarcinoma is at least 10%.**

    b. **Crohn's colitis.** Involvement of the rectum and anus with Crohn's disease may increase the risk of carcinoma. Like ulcerative colitis, the risk increases with the severity and duration of symptoms.

III. **Presentation**

  A. **Signs and symptoms.** Presenting signs and symptoms of patients with rectal cancer include the following.

    1. **Local manifestations.** Common complaints and findings include **bleeding** (50%), constipation, decreased stool caliber, diarrhea, rectal urgency, tenesmus, urinary frequency or burning, pneumaturia, and perineal or buttock pain.

    2. **Systemic manifestations.** Signs and symptoms indicating advanced metastatic disease are pain in the right upper quadrant and right shoulder, hepatomegaly, and hepatic and pulmonary masses.

  B. **Paraneoplastic syndromes.** Like colon carcinoma, rectal cancer has been rarely associated with paraneoplastic symptom complexes, which may represent the patient's sole presenting complaint.

    1. **Dermatomyositis/myositis** (see p 59, **III**).

    2. **Acanthosis nigricans** (see p 109).

    3. **Thrombophlebitis** (see p 81).

    4. **Erythema gyratum repens** (see p 108).

    5. **Hypertrichosis languinosa** (see p 110).

    6. **Leser-Trelat syndrome** (see p 109).

IV. **Differential diagnosis.** Many rectal tumors present as a **rectal mass** on digital rectal examination. However, **the cervix, pelvic abscesses, and other pelvic neoplasms** (uterine leiomyomas, pelvic sarcomas, chordomas, and cervical, uterine, bladder, and prostate tumors) as well as **benign rectal tumors** (villous adenomas) can be confused with rectal carcinoma.

V. **Screening programs**

  A. **Physical examination.** A digital rectal examination can detect most rectal carcinomas and is a simple, but reliable, screening test. The American Cancer Society recommends that **everyone 40 years of age or older** should be examined annually with a digital rectal examination.

  B. **Stool guiaic test.** Annual stool testing for occult blood can detect many rectal carcinomas because they often cause gastrointestinal bleeding. However, previous studies have shown that fecal testing is cost-effective only in high-risk populations (eg, patients older than 50 or patients with a family history of colon cancer). When performed properly, this test has a good predictative value for adenomas and carcinomas (see p 275, **V**) and is a suggested part of a yearly physical examination for patients older than 50.

  C. **Proctosigmoidoscopy.** Several studies have shown that annual screening with proctosigmoidoscopy can detect early tumors of the distal sigmoid and rectum. However, most malignancies occur in patients over 50 years of age; therefore, the American Cancer Society recommends proctosigmoidoscopy (preferably with a 60-cm flexible endoscope) **every 3–5 years** in people **after age 50 after 2 initial examinations have normal results.**

VI. **Diagnostic workup**

  A. **Medical history and physical examination.** A complete medical history with reference to common presenting signs and symptoms should be obtained along with a thorough physical examination.

    1. **General appearance.** Some indication as to a patient's nutritional status can be obtained by simply observing the patient's appearance.

    2. **Skin.** Pallor (anemia), hyperpigmentation of the neck axillae, or anorectal area **(acanthosis nigricans),** or inflammatory lesions **(dermatomyositis and erythema gyratum repens)** should be noted.

3. **Lymph nodes.** The presence of a signal node (also called **Virchow's or Troisier's node**) must be recorded.
4. **Abdomen.** Low abdominal or right upper-quadrant masses or hepatomegaly may indicate advanced disease.
5. **Rectum.** This is the most important aspect of the physical examination because **1/3–1/2 of rectal tumors are within reach of the examining finger.**
6. **Pelvic examination.** Pelvic examination in females is crucial for determining the anterior extent of rectal tumors. Adherence of the tumor to the uterus or vagina alters the magnitude of the required surgical procedure.

B. **Primary tests and procedures.** The following diagnostic tests and procedures should be performed on all patients with suspected rectal carcinoma.
   1. **Blood tests**
      a. **Complete blood count** (see p 1, **IV.A.1**).
      b. **Hepatic transaminases** (see p 1, **IV.A.2**).
      c. **Alkaline phosphatase** (see p 1, **IV.A.3**).
      d. **Carcinoembryonic antigen** (CEA). Levels of this oncofetal antigen should always be obtained preoperative and again **2–6 weeks postoperatively**. Persistently elevated levels after primary tumor resection may indicate persistent tumor, whereas increased levels after an initial postoperative normalization of levels often correlates with recurrence or with the presence of a nonmalignant cause of elevated CEA levels such as liver or pulmonary disease, smoking, and inflammatory bowel disease.
   2. **Imaging studies**
      a. **Chest x-ray** (see p 3, **IV.C.1**).
      b. **Barium enema.** An air-contrast barium enema is useful to **exclude synchronous lesions** in other parts of the colon. However, because it may miss 5–10% of small mucosal lesions, it should be combined with flexible proctosigmoidoscopy or be replaced by **colonoscopy**.
      c. **Computerized tomography (CT).** A CT scan of the abdomen and pelvis should be obtained in all cases except those of small mucosal lesions. This examination can be used to evaluate the **extent of local tumor** as well as the existence of **nodal and hepatic metastases.** In addition, evidence of ureteral involvement (eg, hydroureter, hydronephrosis) can be obtained with an intravenous contrast-enhanced CT. This also eliminates the need for preoperative intravenous pyelograms.
   3. **Invasive procedures**
      a. **Flexible proctosigmoidoscopy.** This endoscopic examination should be performed to obtain a **biopsy** of the primary tumor for histologic confirmation and to exclude synchronous lesions in the sigmoid. This procedure should be **combined with an air-contrast barium enema** to examine the entire colon.
      b. **Colonoscopy.** This procedure can be substituted for the combination of air-contrast barium enema and flexible proctosigmoidoscopy with similar results. Approximately **5–10% of lesions may be missed because of blind corners** and an inability to visualize the right colon and cecum.
      c. **Biopsy.** Diagnostic biopsy of any lesion seen on proctosigmoidoscopy or colonoscopy should be performed before a final treatment plan is recommended to the patient.

C. **Optional tests and procedures.** The following tests and procedures may be indicated by previous diagnostic findings or clinical suspicion.
   1. **Blood tests** (see p 2, **IV.A**)
      a. **Nucleotidase.**
      b. **GGTP.**
   2. **Imaging studies**
      a. **Ultrasound examination.** Transrectal ultrasound may assess accurately the depth of tumor penetration and the presence of lymph node metastases (see, also, p 3, **IV.C.4**).
      b. **Magnetic resonance imaging** (see p 3, **IV.C.4**).
      c. **Technetium-99m bone scan** (see p 3, **IV.C.5**).
      d. **Monoclonal antibody imaging.** Early studies with radiolabeled **monoclonal antibodies 17–1A and B72.3** have shown expression in up to 85% of colorectal cancers; however, variable expression on individual tumor cells has limited the usefulness of such scans to the research setting.
   3. **Invasive procedures. Cystoscopy** is indicated to evaluate the possibility of bladder invasion and **colovesical fistula** if symptoms of pneumaturia or recurrent urinary tract infections are elicited.

VII. Pathology
  A. Location. There is no site predilection for rectal carcinoma.
  B. Multiplicity. Except in ulcerative colitis and the familial polyposis syndromes, when the incidence of multiple carcinomas is unusually high, **synchronous** primary lesions are found in 3% of patients and an additional 2% will subsequently develop a **metachronous** lesion.
  C. Histology. Adenocarcinoma (mucinous, signet-ring, adenosquamous, and undifferentiated) accounts for 95% of all rectal malignancies. **Carcinoids** are the second most frequent tumor type; these tumors are noted as a **small yellowish nodule** found 4–13 cm from the dentate line along the **anterior or lateral walls.** Other histologic types that occasionally can be found are sarcomas and lymphomas.
  D. Metastatic spread
    1. Modes of spread. Four distinct mechanisms can be involved in the spread of rectal carcinoma.
      a. Direct extension. Tumor growth may extend **circumferentially** around the rectum as well as cephalad and caudad. However, **longitudinal spread occurs less often than previously believed.** At least one study has shown an absence of distal submucosal extension in more than 88% of patients.
      b. Lymphatic metastasis. Tumor cells spread readily through circumferential lymphatics in the submucosa. Subsequently, pararectal, superior hemorrhoidal, inferior mesenteric, middle hemorrhoidal, obturator, hypogastric, and iliac chains may become involved.
      c. Hematogenous metastasis. Malignant cells can drain through the superior hemorrhoidal vessels and the portal system to the liver or through middle and inferior hemorrhoidal vessels and the inferior vena cava to the lungs. On occasion, drainage through **vertebral veins** leads to the development of spinal metastases.
      d. Implantation. Direct implantation of tumor cells into **hemorrhoids** as well as areas of surgical dissection (eg, bowel anastomoses and abdominal wounds) have been explained by the intraluminal and intraoperative spread of tumor cells.
    2. Sites of spread. Autopsy studies have produced evidence of metastatic spread to the following organs: **liver, 60–70% (40% as the sole site of metastasis);** lung, 25%; regional lymph nodes, 23%; vertebral and bony metastases, 10%; and central nervous system, 1%.
VIII. Staging. The staging for rectal carcinoma is identical to colon carcinoma (see p 276, **VIII**).
  IX. Treatment
    A. Surgery
      1. Primary rectal carcinoma
        a. General considerations. The backbone of therapy for rectal carcinoma is surgical resection. En bloc removal of the tumor, the involved segment of rectum, and the local lymph nodes is indicated in all patients with resectable lesions and without medical contraindications. Even in the presence of metastatic disease, surgery offers the **best palliation** from bleeding and pain for all but extremely small rectal lesions. A **proximal margin** of at least **5 cm** and a **distal margin** of at least **2–5 cm** is required.
        b. Bowel preparation. A combination of mechanical and antibiotic bowel preparation is recommended (see p 277, **IX.A.1.b**).
        c. Radical procedures. Several different procedures and approaches have been used for rectal carcinoma. The choice of the most appropriate procedure depends on the location and size of the tumor, patient body habitus, concomitant colorectal diseases, and the surgeon's preference and experience.
          (1) Low anterior resection. This sphincter-sparing technique is performed through a **midline, anterior, transabdominal approach.** If a question about the possible need for abdominoperineal resection exists, or if a stapled anastomosis is planned, the patient should be draped in the **modified lithotomy position.** After mobilizing the rectum to the levators, a segmental resection is performed that includes the **superior hemorrhoidal vessels** and lymph node chain to the **origin of the left colic artery.** Ligating the inferior mesenteric artery at the level of the aorta is unnecessary. End-to-end or side-to-end reconstruction is accomplished through a two-layered, hand-sewn technique or with the use of the circular stapler.

(2) **Abdominosacral resection.** This sphincter-sparing technique is performed through a simultaneous **anterior midline** as well as a **transsacral approach** with the patient in the lateral position. The rectum is first mobilized to the levator muscles. The sacrum is then removed through a second perineal incision just posterior to the anus. An end-to-end anastomosis is fashioned through the perineal incision to reconstruct gastrointestinal continuity.

(3) **Posterior transsacral resection (Kraske procedure).** This sphincter-preserving procedure is performed with the patient in the **prone position.** A midline incision is made over the sacrum, and the nonarticular sacrum is isolated and removed. **Waldeyer's fascia** is opened, exposing the rectum. After mobilizing the rectum, the appropriate resection is performed and the rectum and wound are closed.

(4) **Posterior trans-sphincteric resection (Bevan or York Mason procedure).** This sphincter-preserving procedure is performed with the patient in the prone position. A midline or slightly oblique incision is made over the sacrum and the **coccyx is removed,** as is done in the Kraske procedure. The external sphincter complex and levator muscles **(somatic tube)** are divided and tagged with identifying suture for accurate reapproximation. The anorectum **(visceral tube)** is then mobilized and the appropriate resection is performed. The **external sphincter complex and levator muscles are carefully repaired** and the wound is closed.

(5) **Coloanal resection (endorectal pull-through).** This combined abdominal and perineal procedure involves complete rectal mobilization and resection as well as a **mucosal proctectomy.** Bowel continuity is reestablished by pulling the colon through the demucosalized anal canal and constructing a **coloanal anastomosis** in a sphincter-sparing manner.

(6) **Abdominoperineal resection (Miles operation).** This procedure removes the entire rectum and anus and creates a permanent colostomy. With the patient in the modified lithotomy position, the abdomen is explored and the rectum is mobilized. The superior hemorrhoidal vessels are ligated just distal to the left colic artery. In females, the rectum is mobilized from the vagina; if any vaginal involvement is suspected, however, a **posterior vaginectomy and hysterectomy** is included. The anus and pelvic floor muscles are excised and a colostomy is formed.

d. **Treatment of specific lesions**

(1) **Upper-third lesions.** These malignancies lie more than **10–11 cm from the anal verge** and are routinely treated with a **low anterior resection** as long as 2–5 cm of normal rectum can be excised distal to the tumor. A hand-sewn or stapled anastomosis is then fashioned and the rectal sphincter is preserved.

(2) **Middle-third lesions.** These lesions, which extend **5–11 cm from the anal verge,** are the most controversial because the results from abdominoperineal resection are not superior to those of sphincter-preserving operations. **Abdominosacral, posterior transsacral, posterior transsphincteric, coloanal, and even low anterior resections** can be used successfully, depending on the type and size of the tumor, the patients body habitus, the presence of concomitant colonic disease, the surgeon's expertise, and the patient's wishes.

(3) **Lower third lesions.** These tumors are within approximately **5–6 cm of the anal verge** and are almost universally treated with an **abdominoperineal resection.** Extremely small lesions or carcinoid tumors can be excised with an abdominosacral or posterior sphincter-sparing approach, but adequate margins can be difficult to obtain.

e. **Local procedures.** In medically poor-risk patients with lesions **smaller than 3 cm that are limited to the mucosa,** several local procedures with only a **10% 5-year tumor-related mortality** can be used.

(1) **Local excision.** Submucosal or full-thickness local excision can be performed with a **transanal or posterior** (transsacral or transsphincteric) **approach,** depending on the location of the primary tumor.

(2) **Fulguration.** Single- or multiple-staged **cauterization procedures** can be used successfully in 50–90% of lower-third rectal lesions. **De-**

layed hemorrhage can develop in as many as 20% of cases, however.

    (3) Laser ablation. A newer modality of neodymium yttrium-aluminum-garnet (Nd-YAG) laser ablation of low-lying rectal lesions may represent a viable alternative in the future treatment of rectal carcinoma.

2. **Locally advanced and recurrent carcinoma.** The presence of locally advanced or recurrent cancer does not preclude resection. Even with minimal distant metastatic disease, resection should be contemplated because it affords **excellent palliation from rectal pain and hemorrhage**. Advanced tumors require more radical procedures. If posterior extension of the tumor exists, resection of the nonarticular sacrum is an option. Anterior involvement of the vagina necessitates hysterectomy and posterior vaginectomy. With anterior extension into the bladder in females or the prostate and bladder in males, pelvic exenteration is required. Even with these radical procedures for extensive tumor, as many as **30% of patients without distant metastases are cured**. In addition, adjuvant radiation therapy may improve the results.

3. Metastatic carcinoma

    a. **Curative surgical therapy.** Previously, surgery has had little application in the cure of metastatic disease. However, several recent studies indicate that as many as **32% of patients with 1–4 resectable liver metastases** from colorectal carcinoma **can be cured** if all lesions are resected. In addition, resection of **single pulmonary metastases**—if isolated and, particularly, if detected after a long disease-free interval—may result in a **5-year survival** rate of **as high as 20%**.

    b. **Palliative surgical therapy.** Symptoms of primary rectal carcinoma are palliated best by excising the primary tumor. Metastatic foci may cause malignant obstruction of the stomach, small bowel, or colon that requires gastrostomy, small-bowel resection or bypass, or colostomy, respectively. However, **colostomy as a palliative procedure for primary rectal lesions is not recommended** because rectal pain and hemorrhage are not adequately treated.

4. **Mortality and morbidity.** The mortality for all radical procedures is identical and varies between **2% and 6%**. The morbidity, especially from abdominoperineal resection, is considerable: as many as **65% of patients develop one of the following** postoperative complications: **hemorrhage** (2–6%); **perineal wound problems,** including infection (17–35%); abdominal wound and intra-abdominal infection (2–5%); stomal complications (11%); **neurogenic bladder** (30%); **sexual dysfunction** (retrograde ejaculation, impotency; 20–61%); or general surgical complications (eg, myocardial infarction, pulmonary embolism, hepatitis; 2–5%).

B. Radiation therapy

1. **Primary rectal carcinoma.** Radiation therapy has been used as a primary treatment for early rectal carcinoma in high-risk patients. Excluding poorly differentiated lesions, superficial tumors **smaller than 4.5 cm** can be treated successfully with **intracavitary** (contact) **radiation** (Papillon technique). This type of radiation is administered by the transanal insertion of a low energy x-ray unit until it almost abuts (contacts) the tumor. It results in **local control** in 95% of patients and **5-year survival rates of 76%**. One advantage of this procedure is that the resulting scar is soft and easily assessed for recurrence during follow-up examinations.

2. Adjuvant radiation therapy

    a. **Preoperative radiotherapy.** At least 4 nonrandomized trials and 3 randomized trials have shown that **preoperative radiation therapy decreases local recurrence from 15–35% in groups receiving surgery alone to 4–15%** in groups receiving surgery plus radiation. In addition, no tumor was identified in surgical specimens in as many as 17% of cases, and a decrease in the number of patients with positive lymph nodes from 30–40% to 20–25% was noted. In one randomized study, **improvement in 5-year survival from 64% to 80%** was noted (Kutzner, Bruckner, & Kampf, 1984). In all studies, however, preoperative doses in excess of 2500 cGy were required for therapeutic efficacy. In patients with locally advanced disease, the advantage of preoperative radiation is less clear because of a higher incidence of distant metastatic spread. Other potential benefits of preoperative radiotherapy include the following:

        (1) Improved toxicity. Because the small bowel remains out of the pelvis, fewer gastrointestinal symptoms result. In addition, the surgical complication rate has been **no greater** than that following surgery without preoperative radiation.

    (2) Increased resectability rate. With decreased tumor size and lymph node involvement, patients with borderline tumors may be resectable after radiation therapy.

    (3) Increased radiosensitivity. With fewer ischemic cells present than in the postoperative period, the effectiveness of radiotherapy should increase.

    (4) Decreased intraoperative seeding. Fewer viable cells exist for intraoperative implantation into local tissues, anastomoses, and incisions.

  b. Intraoperative radiotherapy. Intraoperative radiation therapy using photon beams, electron beams, or interstitial implants has been used in combination with preoperative radiation therapy in patients with locally advanced disease. Doses between 1000 and 1500 cGy have been used. Results, although inconclusive, suggest improved local control and possibly survival in selected patients, and morbidity has been low except with interstitial implants.

  c. Postoperative radiotherapy. At least 3 nonrandomized and 3 randomized studies, including studies from the Gastrointestinal Tumor Study Group and the National Surgical Adjuvant Bowel and Breast Cancer Project (NSABP), has demonstrated a **decrease in the local recurrence rate in patients with Dukes stage B2 and C lesions from 13–67% to 0–53%.** Survival benefits, however, have not been convincingly demonstrated. Few studies of locally advanced disease with positive margins have been reported, but some evidence is available on the efficacy of postoperative radiation therapy in these patients. Potential benefits of postoperative radiation therapy over preoperative therapy include the following.

    (1) More appropriate patient selection. Surgical staging can exclude those patients (ie, those with Dukes A lesions) who would probably not benefit from radiation. In addition, intraoperative placement of clips can help define the extent of tumor involvement more clearly.

    (2) Smaller tumor volume. A much smaller amount of tumor (often microscopic tumor only) can be treated postoperatively with better results.

    (3) Prompt surgery. Definitive surgical resection is not delayed.

  d. "Sandwich" radiotherapy. Three nonrandomized studies have demonstrated that combined pre- and postoperative "sandwich" radiation therapy (500–1500 cGy pre- and 4140–6500 cGy post-operatively) **increases local control in a manner similar to that of high-dose postoperative therapy.** In addition, one study suggests that the preoperative component may reduce the number of distant metastases that presumably occur because of surgical manipulation and thus may increase patient survival (Mohiuddin et al, 1985). However, this requires confirmation.

3. Palliative therapy. Radiation therapy may provide acceptable palliation from pain and hemorrhage in unresectable primary or locally recurrent rectal carcinoma. However, no proof exists of any survival benefit.

4. Morbidity and mortality. The side effects of radiotherapy can be considerable and life threatening. Significant complications from pelvic radiation include the following: intestinal obstruction, intestinal perforation, intestinal fistulae, decreased wound healing, increased postoperative infection rate, cystitis, and radiation fibrosis and ureteral obstruction.

C. Chemotherapy

1. Primary rectal carcinoma. To date, there is no indication for chemotherapy in the initial treatment of primary rectal carcinoma.

2. Adjuvant chemotherapy. The data regarding the use of adjuvant chemotherapy is limited. Almost all trials have failed to show a survival advantage to postoperative chemotherapy. One trial sponsored by the NSABP demonstrated a statistically significant disease-free and overall survival benefit in selected subsets of patients receiving **methyl-CCNU, vincristine, and 5-fluorouracil** (MOF; Fisher, 1988). These findings have not been confirmed by additional studies, however, and methyl-CCNU remains available only for approved clinical trials.

3. Locally advanced and metastatic disease. The experience with chemotherapy of rectal carcinoma has been no different from that with colon carcinoma (see p 280, **IX.c**).

D. Immunotherapy. No distinction has been made between the treatment of colon cancer and the therapy of rectal carcinoma in immunotherapy trials. The results of nonspecific and specific immunotherapy in the treatment of colorectal carcinoma are summarized on p 280, **IX.D**).

E. Combined modality therapy. Combinations of chemotherapy and radiation therapy, especially in the postoperative adjuvant setting, have produced promising results. Studies by the Gastrointestinal Tumor Study Group and the North Central Cancer Treatment Group have suggested an **increase in overall survival** from 43–49% in controls to 55–59% in patients treated with adjuvant radiotherapy, methyl-CCNU, and fluorouracil. Although the benefit is slight, variations in the delivery of the chemotherapy in current ongoing trials may improve the advantage.

X. Prognosis

A. Risk of recurrence. The risk of recurrence, both locoregional and distant, depends on the extent of the primary tumor and the presence or absence of nodal metastases. The approximate risk of local recurrence is 0% for Dukes stage A, 15–30% for stage B, and 21–49% for stage C. The risk for distant recurrence is 15% for Dukes stage A, 24% for stage B, and 58% for stage C.

B. Five-year survival. The 5-year survival rates after definitive surgery by Dukes stage are as follows: Dukes A, 78–93%; Dukes B, 40–65%; Dukes C, 15–33%; and Dukes D, 0–5%.

C. Adverse prognostic factors. The following factors can adversely affect the prognosis for patients with rectal cancer: age younger than 40 years at the time of diagnosis, male gender, CEA level greater than 5 ng/mL, short duration of symptoms (< 6 months), circumferential obstructing primary lesion, ulceration or perforation of the primary lesion, involvement of adjacent organs, colloid or mucinous histology, high-grade (poorly differentiated) lesions, lymphatic and perineural invasion, aneuploidy and more than 19.7% tumor cells in S-phase, and lack of immune response (lymphocytic tumor infiltrate, reactive lymph nodes).

XI. Patient follow-up

A. General guidelines. Patients should be followed closely every 3 months for 3 years, every 6 months for an additional 2 years, then annually thereafter. Local recurrences and limited distant metastases can be treated successfully if detected early.

B. Routine evaluation. Each clinic visit should include the tests and procedures listed below:

1. **Medical history and physical examination.** An interval history and complete physical examination should be performed during each office visit. Specific areas listed on p 284 **VI.A**) should be carefully checked.

2. **Blood tests**
   a. **Complete blood count** (see p 1, **IV.A.1**).
   b. **Hepatic transaminases** (see p 1, **IV.A.2**).
   c. **Alkaline phosphatase** (see p 1, **IV.A.3**).
   d. **CEA** (see p 285, **VI.B.1.d**).

3. **Chest x-ray** (see p 3, **IV.C.1**).

C. Additional evaluation. Other examinations that should be obtained at regular intervals include the following:

1. **Barium enema.** An annual air-contrast barium enema should be obtained to exclude the presence of **metachronous colon lesions** as well as suture-line recurrences or strictures.

2. **Computerized tomography (CT).** A CT scan of the pelvis should be obtained within 6 months of surgery and every 6–12 months thereafter to identify local recurrence that may be amenable to surgical extirpation.

3. **Sigmoidoscopy.** Flexible sigmoidoscopy should be performed annually after surgical resection to exclude suture-line recurrences as well as metachronous lesions.

D. Optional evaluation. The following tests may be indicated by previous diagnostic findings or clinical suspicion:

1. **Blood tests** (see p 2, **IV.A**)
   a. **Nucleotidase.**
   b. **GGTP.**

2. **Imaging studies** (p 3, **IV.C**)
   a. **Magnetic resonance imaging**
   b. **Technetium-99m bone scan.**

3. **Biopsy.** In patients treated for cure, any abnormal tissue should be biopsied by the most appropriate method to determine whether recurrence has occurred. However, postoperative abnormalities in the sacral hollow, should be followed by CT scan and biopsied only if increasing in size.

REFERENCES

Douglass HO et al: Survival after postoperative combination treatment of rectal cancer. *N Engl J Med* 1986;**315:**1294–1295.

Fisher B et al: Postoperative adjuvant chemotherapy or radiation therapy for rectal cancer: results from NSABP protocol R-01. *JNCI* 1988;**80**(1):21–29.

Hoover HC: Colorectal tumors. In: Cameron JL (editor), *Current Surgical Therapy-3,* 3rd ed. Philadelphia, PA: BC Decker; 1989:150–155.

Krook J et al: Radiation vs. sequential chemotherapy-radiation-chemotherapy: a study of the North Central Cancer Treatment Group. *Proc Am Soc Clin Oncol* 1986;**5:**82.

Kutzner J, Bruckner R, Kempf P: Preoperative strahlentherapie beim rektum karzinomen. *Strahlentherapie* 1984;**160:**236–238.

Localio SA, Eng K, Coppa GF: Abdominosacral resection for midrectal cancer. *Ann Surg* 1983;**198:**320–324.

Mohiuddin M et al: Results of adjuvant radiation therapy in cancer of the rectum: Thomas Jefferson University Hospital experience. *Cancer* 1985;**55:**350–353.

Papillon J: New prospects in the conservative treatment of rectal cancer. *Dis Colon Rect* 1984;**27:**695–700.

Westbrook KC et al: Posterior surgical approaches to the rectum. *Ann Surg* 1982;**195:**677–685.

38 Malignancies of the Anus

Robert B. Cameron, MD

I. **Epidemiology.** In the United States, cancer of the anus is relatively uncommon, accounting for **less than 2% of all colorectal carcinomas.** The world-wide incidence of anal cancer varies only slightly, although males in New Delhi, India have an unusually high incidence.

II. **Risk factors.** Environmental rather than genetic factors are predominantly implicated in the development of anal carcinoma.
   A. **Age.** The incidence of anal cancer increases with age, with **80% of anal canal tumors and 50% of anal margin carcinomas** occurring in **patients over 60 years of age.** The incidence increases from < 1 per 100,000 under the age of 50 to **6.1 per 100,000 by the age of 80**.
   B. **Sex.** Overall, U.S. females are twice as likely to develop anal carcinoma. With anal canal lesions, females are at 2.3 times greater risk, however with anal margin lesions males are at 2 times greater risk.
   C. **Race.** There is no known racial biases in the incidence of anal cancer.
   D. **Genetic factors.** There is no known genetic predisposition to anal cancer, and first degree relatives of patients with anal tumors are not at increased risk.
   E. **Diet.** There are no dietary factors involved in the pathogenesis of anal carcinoma.
   F. **Smoking.** Cigarette smoking may increase the risk of anal cancer by as much as 2 times, however, there remains some doubt as to this association.
   G. **Previous anal pathology**
      1. **Infections.** Various infectious agents have been associated with an increased risk of anal carcinoma.
         a. **Viral infections. Papillomaviruses** (condylomata acuminata) and **herpes simplex virus, type 2,** have both been implicated in the genesis of anal malignancies. In addition, the **human immunodeficiency virus** (HIV) has recently been implicated with an increased risk of anal tumors. This association has been postulated to be due to viral infection, immunosuppression, or anal-receptive intercourse. Further studies are required to delineate this relationship.
         b. **Bacterial infections.** Gonorrhea and chlamydia infections have been reported to mildly increase the risk of anal cancer.
      2. **Inflammation.** Various pathologic processes that cause chronic inflammation in and around the anal area are associated with a higher than expected incidence of anal cancer. These include fistulae, fissures, abscesses, and hemorrhoids.
   H. **Immunosuppression.** A 100 times increased incidence of anal malignancies has been noted in renal transplant and AIDS patients. This increased risk, however, may be due to coexisting viral and opportunistic infections present in these populations.
   I. **Radiation exposure.** Some reports have linked the development of anal cancer with previous radiation exposure.

III. **Presentation**
   A. **Signs and symptoms.** The initial symptoms of anal malignancies are identical to those of more common benign anal conditions, and this frequently leads to delayed diagnosis.
      1. **Local manifestations.** Common presenting complaints and findings include **bleeding, pain, sensation of an anal mass, and pruritus**.
      2. **Systemic manifestations.** Systemic signs and symptoms are uncommon since only a minority of patients develop distant metastases from these tumors. If present, these findings are usually related to pulmonary or liver metastases.
   B. **Paraneoplastic syndromes.** No defined paraneoplastic syndromes have been associated with anal cancer.

IV. **Differential diagnosis.** Anal malignancies present with bleeding, pain, and the sensation of an anal mass. Many common benign conditions also produce similar complaints and may be confused with cancer. Generally, **benign diseases improve within 2 weeks** with conservative therapy and include **thrombosed hemorrhoids, perirectal or crypt abscesses, fissures, and fistula in ano**. Condyloma acuminata, anal papilloma, and rectal carcinoma also may mimic anal cancer.

V. **Screening programs.** Unlike most malignancies, anal carcinoma is readily accessible to the examining physician. While no widespread screening programs have been developed, simple physical examination of high-risk populations (i.e., homosexual, immunosuppressed, etc.) will identify most tumors.

VI. **Diagnostic workup**

A. **Medical history and physical examination.** A complete medical history eliciting symptoms of high risk behavior, anal bleeding, pain, and mass sensation, and a thorough physical examination are essential to an adequate evaluation.

1. **General appearance.** Evidence of chronic disease and immunosuppression can occasionally be noted on general inspection of the patient.

2. **Skin.** Kaposi's lesions suggesting HIV infection should be recorded.

3. **Lymph nodes.** The rare presence of a signal node (also called **Virchow's or Troisier's node**) must be excluded, since this may represent another coexisting visceral malignancy.

4. **Abdomen.** Evidence of hepatic masses should be sought.

5. **Groin.** Examination of the groin to exclude palpable lymphadenopathy is an integral part of the examination.

6. **Anus.** Visualization and digital examination of the anus is the most important diagnostic step in anal cancer.

B. **Primary tests and procedures.** The following diagnostic tests should be obtained in all patients with suspected anal malignancies.

1. **Blood tests** (see p 1, **IV.A**)
   a. **Complete blood count.**
   b. **Hepatic transaminases.**
   c. **Alkaline phosphatase.**

2. **Imaging studies**
   a. **Chest x-ray** (see p. 3, **IV.C**).
   b. **Barium enema.** A double **contrast barium enema** (air/barium) should be obtained to exclude **synchronous** colon carcinoma, especially with **perianal Bowen's and Paget's diseases** which are associated with visceral malignancies.

3. **Invasive procedures**
   a. **Anoscopy.** Examination of the entire anus, including the anal canal under direct vision is mandatory in all patients.
   b. **Sigmoidoscopy.** Rigid or flexible sigmoidoscopy should be performed to exclude coexisting disease in the rectum and distal sigmoid colon.
   c. **Biopsy.** An **incisional biopsy** of any abnormal area in or around the anus is mandatory. This can be accomplished relatively easily in most circumstances with **local anesthesia**. Complete excisional biopsies should be avoided unless the lesion is very small and superficial.

C. **Optional tests and procedures.** Based on previous diagnostic findings or clinical suspicion, the following tests and procedures may be indicated.

1. **Blood tests** (see p 2, **IV.A**)
   a. **Nucleotidase.**
   b. **GGTP.**

2. **Imaging studies**
   a. **Computerized tomography.** CT is useful in the evaluation of the lungs and liver, as well as pelvic and inguinal lymph nodes, if metastases to these organs are suspected; however, this test is not universally obtained in the routine workup of patients.
   b. **Magnetic resonance imaging (MRI)** (see p 3).
   c. **Ultrasound** (see p 3).
   d. **Intravenous pyelogram.** Although IVP is useful if obstruction of the urinary tract is suspected, a CT scan performed with the injection of i.v. contrast more thoroughly evaluates the urinary tract.

3. **Invasive procedures**
   a. **Examination under anesthesia (EUA).** Some patients may require examination and biopsy under anesthesia due to **extreme anal pain**. This proce-

dure should be utilized liberally in such circumstances, since an accurate diagnosis depends on an adequate examination and representative biopsy.
  b. **Biopsy.** Palpable inguinal lymphadenopathy should be evaluated with either a fine needle aspiration or excisional biopsy to exclude the presence of cancer. Liver and lung lesions should be evaluated with fine needle aspiration cytology, if feasible.

VII. **Pathology**
  A. **Location.** The anus extends from the **dentate line** out onto the perianal skin to a distance of **5 cm from the anal verge**. Anal carcinomas can occur anywhere along this distance, and the histology varies depending on the epithelium present in the following zones.
    1. **The dentate line.** The **dentate or pectinate line** marks the transition zone from a stratified squamous epithelium to the columnar epithelium of the rectum. Some areas of cuboidal epithelium also exist.
    2. **Anal canal.** The anal canal ranges from the dentate line to the anal verge and consists of a **hairless stratified squamous epithelium**.
    3. **Anal margin.** This portion of the anus runs from the anal verge onto the perianal skin to a distance of **5 cm from the anal verge**. The epithelium is a stratified squamous epithelium containing hair follicles.
  B. **Multiplicity.** Certain histologies (i.e., **perianal Bowen's and Paget's diseases**) are associated with as much as 75% incidence of coexisting visceral malignancies.
  C. **Histology.** Although many different types of cancer can occur in the anus, the most frequent histologies include **squamous cell carcinoma (65%),** transitional (cloacogenic) **carcinoma (25%), adenocarcinoma (<10%),** Paget's disease (<1%), melanoma (<1%), lymphoma (<1%), basal cell carcinoma (<1%), and small cell carcinoma (<1%). Despite a wide variety of cell types, the clinical outcome does not depend on the histologic appearance of the tumor.
  D. **Metastatic spread**
    1. **Modes of spread.** Anal carcinoma may spread via any one of three mechanisms.
      a. **Direct extension.** Local invasion can lead to involvement of the rectum, urethra, bladder, bony sacrum or pelvis, prostate, and vagina.
      b. **Lymphatic metastasis.** The **dual lymphatic drainage** of the anal area allows for spread to both the inguinal as well as the obturator, hypogastric, and mesenteric lymph nodes, depending on the site of the primary lesion.
        (1) **Anal canal tumors.** With tumors in the anal canal as many as 30–50% of patients develop pelvic nodal metastases, however, these tumors do not commonly metastasize to inguinal lymph nodes.
        (2) **Anal margin tumors.** Anal margin tumors, especially if > 4 cm^2, metastasize to **inguinal nodes** in approximately 30% of cases but rarely spread to pelvic nodes.
        (3) **Malignant melanoma.** Melanoma of the anorectum frequently metastasizes to both **inguinal** (20%) and **pelvic** (50%) **lymph nodes.**
      c. **Hematogenous metastasis.** Due to the dual drainage system of this region, tumor cells may dislodge and can be carried to distant organs by both the portal and systemic circulations. This occurs infrequently with most histologies, however, with malignant melanoma, early metastases occur to a wide variety of distant organs.
    2. **Sites of spread.** Although metastatic disease is uncommon, distant sites that can become involved include the following organs: lung, liver, peritoneum, and bone.

VIII. **Staging.** Several attempts have been made to devise a meaningful staging system for anal carcinoma. Previous systems were proposed by groups at the Mayo clinic, Roswell Park Memorial Institute, and the Union Internationale Contre le Cancer (UICC). However, none was widely accepted. Recently the UICC and the American Joint Committee on Cancer (AJCC) jointly proposed a practical staging system for cancer of the anal canal. Carcinoma of the anal margin is staged identically to squamous cell skin cancer. The staging system for both tumors is outlined below.
  A. **Tumors of the anal canal**
    1. **Tumor stage**
      a. **TX.** Primary tumor cannot be assessed.
      b. **T0.** No evidence of a primary tumor can be found.
      c. **Tis.** Carcinoma *in situ.*
      d. **T1.** Tumor ≤2 cm in greatest dimension.
      e. **T2.** Tumor >2 cm but ≤5 cm in greatest dimension.

      f. T3. Tumor >5 cm in greatest dimension.

      g. T4. Tumor of any size that invades adjacent organs (not including rectal sphincter muscle).

  2. Lymph node stage

    a. NX. Regional lymph nodes cannot be assessed.

    b. N0. No regional lymph node metastases are present.

    c. N1. Metastases in perirectal lymph nodes are present.

    d. N2. Metastases in unilateral internal iliac and/or inguinal lymph nodes are present.

    e. N3. Metastases in perirectal and inguinal lymph nodes and/or bilateral internal iliac and/or inguinal lymph nodes are present.

  3. Metastatic stage

    a. MX. The presence of distant metastases cannot be assessed.

    b. M0. No distant metastases are present.

    c. M1. Distant metastases are present.

  4. Histopathologic grade. The following grading scheme applies to all histologies, except melanoma.

    a. GX. Grade cannot be assessed.

    b. G1. Well differentiated.

    c. G2. Moderately well differentiated.

    d. G3. Poorly differentiated.

    e. G4. Undifferentiated.

  5. Stage groupings

    a. Stage 0. Tis, N0, M0.

    b. Stage I. T1, N0, M0.

    c. Stage II. T2 or 3, N0, M0.

    d. Stage IIIA. T4, N0, M0; or T1, 2, or 3, N1, M0.

    e. Stage IIIB. T4, N1, M0; or any T, N2 or 3, M0.

    f. Stage IV. Any T; any N, M1.

B. Tumors of the anal margin

  1. Tumor stage

    a. TX. Primary tumor cannot be assessed.

    b. T0. No evidence of a primary tumor can be found.

    c. Tis. Carcinoma *in situ.*

    d. T1. Tumor ≤2 cm in greatest dimension.

    e. T2. Tumor >2 cm but ≤5 cm in greatest dimension.

    f. T3. Tumor >5 cm in greatest dimension.

    g. T4. Tumor of any size that invades deep extradermal structures (ie, cartilage, skeletal muscle, or bone).

  2. Lymph node stage

    a. NX. Regional lymph nodes cannot be assessed.

    b. N0. No regional lymph node metastases are present.

    c. N1. Regional lymph node metastases (ipsilateral inguinal lymph nodes) are present.

  3. Metastatic stage

    a. MX. The presence of distant metastases cannot be assessed.

    b. M0. No distant metastases are present.

    c. M1. Distant metastases are present.

  4. Histopathologic grade. The following grading scheme applies to all histologies, except melanoma:

    a. GX. Grade cannot be assessed.

    b. G1. Well differentiated.

    c. G2. Moderately well differentiated.

    d. G3. Poorly differentiated.

    e. G4. Undifferentiated.

  5. Stage groupings

    a. Stage 0. Tis, N0, M0.

    b. Stage I. T1, N0, M0.

    c. Stage II. T2 or 3, N0, M0.

    d. Stage III. T4, N0, M0; or any T, N1, M0.

    e. Stage IV. Any T; any N, M1.

IX. Treatment

  A. Surgery

    1. Primary anal carcinoma

      a. Indications. Formerly, radical surgery was the backbone of treatment for anal malignancies, however, abdominoperineal resection is now indicated **only for locally advanced disease that is unresponsive to combination radiation and chemotherapy**. Conservative surgery is currently indicated in patients with either early superficial disease as the primary treatment or with residual disease after multimodality therapy.

 b. Procedures. For most lesions, the only surgery that is required is wide local excision of the remaining scar/tumor once the patient finishes combination therapy with chemotherapy and radiation therapy. However, other procedures may be necessary as outlined below.

  (1) Excisional biopsy. This minor procedure is frequently performed after completion of chemotherapy and radiotherapy to exclude the presence of persistent tumor in the residual scar tissue.

  (2) Local excision. This limited, sphincter-sparing procedure is commonly used in most anal margin tumors and in small (<2 cm = T1 lesions) anal canal tumors and consists of total excision of the lesion and a small rim of normal tissue. A **split-thickness skin graft** is commonly used to cover the defect if primary closure cannot be performed.

  (3) Inguinal lymphadenectomy. This procedure is only indicated for **metachronous inguinal lymph node metastases** in preparation for chemotherapy, since groin dissection as therapy for synchronous lymph node metastases does not affect the patients disease course or survival.

  (4) Abdominoperineal resection (Miles operation; APR). This procedure requires the creation of a permanent colostomy and is reserved for those **uncommon tumors that cannot be controlled adequately with multimodality therapy**. In addition, **anal melanoma is not an indication for APR** since wide excision with 2 cm margins controls local disease and since APR does not decrease the incidence of distant metastases or improve survival.

 2. Locally advanced and recurrent anal carcinoma

  a. Anal margin tumor. Advanced and recurrent anal margin tumors may only require **local excision**, although **APR may be necessary** in rare instances. In addition, radiation therapy may salvage some tumors that are not amenable to surgical extirpation.

  b. Anal canal tumor. Patients with advanced or recurrent anal canal malignancies not previously exposed to radiation or chemotherapy, should be treated with combined multimodality therapy. Patients previously treated with multimodality therapy can either undergo **APR** or receive **additional chemotherapy and/or radiotherapy if feasible**.

  c. Inguinal nodal involvement. Recommended therapy for locally advanced tumor involving the inguinal nodes includes chemotherapy and radiation therapy to the involved groin. Surgery is reserved for salvage of isolated inguinal recurrences after successful multimodality therapy and for therapeutic groin dissection in patients with metachronous inguinal metastases.

 3. Metastatic anal carcinoma. Surgery plays no role in the therapy of anal carcinoma with distant metastases.

 4. Mortality and morbidity. The complication rate after resection of anal carcinoma remains quite low since limited procedures are favored. If an APR is performed, however, a slightly higher complication rate occurs. Typical problems that may be encountered include the following: wound infection and sepsis, bleeding, donor site infection, failure of the skin graft, incontinence, and recurrent disease.

B. Radiation therapy

 1. Techniques. Prior to the development of megavoltage equipment, interstitial radiation (brachytherapy) with radium needles, ^{192}Ir, and ^{137}Cs was attempted, however, severe complications (necrosis) occurred in up to 25% of patients and poor control was obtained due to inadequate treatment of nodal metastases. Today, megavoltage equipment is used to treat both the primary tumor and regional nodes which are a frequent site of metastatic disease.

 2. Primary anal carcinoma. Most of anal canal tumors are treated with primary radiation therapy. At least 4 studies have demonstrated that a **60–90% local control rate and a 35–75% 5-year survival rate** can be achieved with radiation therapy alone. Doses range from 4500 to 7550 cGy with **severe complications occurring in 5–15%** at the highest doses. When administered together with chemotherapy (ie, multimodality therapy), better response rates are seen.

3. **Adjuvant radiation therapy**
   a. **Preoperative adjuvant radiation therapy.** Anal margin tumors that are not amenable to wide local excision may be responsive to preoperative radiotherapy in an attempt to render them surgically resectable.
   b. **Intraoperative adjuvant radiation therapy.** This modality is not used with anal malignancies
   c. **Postoperative adjuvant radiation therapy.** Postoperative radiotherapy has been used only in those rare patients who are at high risk for recurrence and have undergone **resection of anal melanoma >2.0 mm in depth.**
4. **Locally advanced and metastatic anal cancer.** Radiation therapy, with or without the concomitant administration of chemotherapy, provides good palliation for advanced locoregional tumor. The experience with distant metastases is anecdotal at best and conclusions cannot be drawn.

C. **Chemotherapy**
1. **Primary anal carcinoma.** Agents with activity against anal carcinoma include 5-fluorouracil, mitomycin-C, cisplatin, bleomycin, doxorubicin, and vincristine. The most active regimen and most widely used includes **5-fluorouracil and mitomycin-C. Objective response rates of 50–60%** have been demonstrated with this regimen, although the contribution of mitomycin-C has been questioned recently. Most commonly, this regimen is combined simultaneously or sequentially with radiation therapy.
2. **Adjuvant chemotherapy.** Adjuvant chemotherapy is not used since chemotherapy is an important part of the primary therapy of anal cancers.
3. **Locally advanced and metastatic cancer.** The number of patients in this category is small, and therefore the experience with chemotherapy in the treatment of advanced metastatic disease remains anecdotal. Single agents used in the treatment of primary anal carcinoma (see above) have been tried with only minimal success. Combinations of agents have not proven to be superior to single agents.

D. **Combined modality therapy.** The most common protocol for the treatment of anal carcinoma (excluding anal margin tumors <5 cm) includes combined modality therapy with **5-fluorouracil and mitomycin-C combined with external beam radiation therapy.** The 5-fluorouracil may work both as a cytotoxic agent and as a radiation sensitizer. Chemotherapy and radiotherapy can be administered concomitantly or sequentially (chemotherapy before radiotherapy). Objective response rates approach 100% in 4 of 5 reported clinical trials using this approach. Surgery is then used to excise the remaining scar and/or tumor.

E. **Immunotherapy.** With the success of combined modality therapy, there has been little impetus and few cases to evaluate the possible therapeutic efficacy of different immunotherapeutic protocols in the treatment of anal carcinoma. However, as much as a 30% response rate has been reported with the use of interleukin-2 and either lymphokine-activated killer cells (LAK) or tumor-infiltrating lymphocytes (TILs) in the treatment of **disseminated melanoma**. None of the primary tumors in these trials, however, originated in the anal area.

X. **Prognosis**
A. **Risk of recurrence.** Due to aggressive combined modality therapy, **nearly 75% of all patients remain disease free for at least 5 years**. However, if **recurrences** develop, **85% involve locoregional disease** as the only site. Yet, many of these patients can be salvaged. For instance, **55% of patients** who develop **metachronous inguinal metastases can be cured with inguinal lymphadenectomy**. The most common cause of mortality, however, remains locoregional disease, not distant metastases.

B. **Five-year survival.** The likelihood of surviving 5 years depends on the stage of the primary tumor.
1. **T1 and T2 lesions,** >80%.
2. **T3 and T4 lesions,** <15%.

C. **Adverse prognostic factors.** The following variables are associated with a poor prognosis.
1. **Inguinal lymph node metastases.**
2. **Tumor size >6 cm.**
3. **Small cell histology.**

XI. **Patient follow-up**
A. **General guidelines.** Patients with anal carcinoma should be followed every 3 months for the first 3 years, every 6 months for an additional 2 years, and then annually for evidence of recurrence. The following specific recommendations are suggested:

B. Routine evaluation. The following tests and procedures should be performed with each clinic visit.
   1. **Medical history and physical examination.** A complete interval medical history and a thorough physical examination should be performed with each clinic visit. Careful attention should be paid to those areas outlined in **VI.A.** above.
   2. **Blood tests** (p 1, **IV.A**)
      a. **Complete blood count.**
      b. **Hepatic transaminases.**
      c. **Alkaline phosphatase.**
   3. **Chest x-ray** (see p 3, **IV.C.**)
   4. **Anoscopy** (see p 293, **VI.B.3.a).**
C. Additional evaluation. Other tests which should be obtained at regular intervals include the following examinations.
   1. **Computerized tomography (CT).** The CT test should be obtained every 6–12 months in the routine follow-up evaluation of anal cancer patients (see, also, p 293, **VI.C.2.a**).
   2. **Sigmoidoscopy** (see **VI.B.3.b.** above).
D. Optional evaluation. The following test and procedures may be indicated by previous diagnostic findings or clinical suspicion.
   1. **Blood tests** (see p 293, **IV.A**)
      a. **Nucleotidase.**
      b. **GGTP.**
   2. **Imaging studies** (see p 3, **IV.C**)
      a. **Magnetic resonance imaging.**
      b. **Ultrasound.**
   3. **Intravenous pyelogram** (IVP) (see p 293, **VI.C.2.d**).
   4. **Biopsy.** Local areas near the anus with tissue thickening or clear change from one examination to the next should undergo incisional biopsy. Palpable inguinal lymphadenopathy should be evaluated with either a fine needle aspiration or excisional biopsy to exclude the presence of cancer. Liver and lung lesions should be evaluated with fine needle aspiration cytology, if feasible.

REFERENCES

Cummings BJ: The place of radiation therapy in the treatment of carcinoma of the anal canal. *Cancer Treat Rev* 1982;**9**:125–147.

Gordon PH: Squamous carcinoma of the anal canal. *Surg Clin North Am* 1988;**68**:1391–1399.

Lopez MG et al: Carcinoma of the anal region. *Curr Probl Surg* 1989;**26**:525–600.

Mitchell EP: Carcinoma of the anal region. *Semin Oncol* 1988;**15**:146–153.

Nigro ND, Vaitkeviceus VK, Herskovic AM: Preservation of function in the treatment of cancer of the anus. *Important Adv Oncol* 1989;161–177.

Tiver KW, Langlands AO: Synchronous chemotherapy and radiotherapy for carcinoma of the anal canal—an alternative to abdominoperineal resection. *Aust NZ J Surg* 1984;**54**(2):101–108.

39 Malignancies of the Kidney

Leonard Gomella, MD, and James Stephanelli, MD

I. **Epidemiology.** Renal cell carcinoma accounts for **3% of all adult malignancies**. In 1985, **10.9 cases per 100,000 males and 4.8 cases per 100,000 females** were diagnosed, leading to **4.7 and 2.2 deaths**, respectively. Approximately **27,200 new cases** and **10,900 deaths** are estimated to occur in 1993. Worldwide, the incidence of kidney cancer varies from a high of 11.5 per 100,000 population in Hawaii, Canada, and the Yukon to a low of 1.0 per 100,000 in India. Other areas of high incidence include Northern Europe and those of low incidence include the Far East.

II. **Risk factors**
   A. **Age.** Renal carcinoma occurs in 1.9 per 100,000 children under age 5. After age 5, the incidence remains less than 1 per 100,000 until age 35, when it begins to rise steadily to **42.8 per 100,000 by age 75**.
   B. **Sex.** The risk for **males is 2.3 times greater** than for females.
   C. **Race.** The risk of **whites is 1.1 times greater** than for blacks.
   D. **Genetic factors**
      1. **Family history.** The risk of kidney cancer generally is not increased in first-degree relatives; however, **renal cell carcinoma kindreds** have been reported.
      2. **Familial syndromes. Von Hippel Lindau disease** is an autosomal dominant disorder consisting of angiomas of the cerebellum, pancreas, and retina. **Renal masses** develop in 50–80% of patients. Fifty percent of these patients harbor **renal carcinoma**, whereas the remainder have cystic disease. These tumors tend to be **multiple, bilateral, and localized.**
      3. **Chromosomal abnormalities.** Chromosomal 3;8 translocations and 3p deletions have been implicated in the pathogenesis of kidney cancer.
   E. **Cigarette smoking.** The **risk for smokers is 1.5–2.5 times greater** than for nonsmokers. As many as **30% of all kidney cancers** have been attributed directly to smoking.
   F. **Obesity.** Three studies have implicated obesity as a risk factor in the development of kidney cancer. This may be related to estrogenic stimulation.
   G. **Previous renal pathology**
      1. **Renal failure and chronic dialysis.** About 45% of patients with renal failure who are on chronic dialysis will develop acquired cystic renal disease, and 9% of them **(4% overall)** will develop **renal cell carcinoma—2500 times the incidence in the general population**. Dialysis-associated tumors are more likely to develop after 3 years on dialysis, and they tend to be multiple and bilateral.
      2. **Analgesic nephropathy.** Patients with phenacetin-induced nephropathy have a higher-than-expected incidence of renal cell malignancies.
   H. **Industrial agents.** Certain industries that frequently expose workers to **leather** (tanneries and shoe manufacturers), **asbestos, cadmium, lead acetate** (newspaper printing), and **petroleum products** have been associated with the development of renal cell carcinoma. In addition, the radiologic contrast agent, **Thorotrast**, has been implicated in the genesis of kidney cancer and, consequently, is no longer used.
   I. **Urbanization.** Renal cancer occurs more frequently in urban dwellers and higher income groups than in people in rural areas and in lower income groups. This may be related to exposure to industrial agents.

III. **Clinical presentation**
   A. **Signs and symptoms**
      1. **Local manifestations.** The most common individual presenting symptoms are **hematuria (60%), abdominal mass (45%), and flank pain or discomfort (40%).** The **classic triad** of flank pain, abdominal mass, and hematuria occurs

in only 10–20% of patients (50% of whom have metastatic disease). An **acute varicocele in an adult male,** although present in only 2–5% of patients, strongly suggests renal cell carcinoma.

2. **Systemic manifestations.** Because the kidney is well protected, kidney cancer produces few early signs and symptoms; consequently, **30% of patients present with metastatic disease**. Weight loss (30%), fever and night sweats (20%), anemia (20%), bone pain, and pulmonary nodules are common.

B. **Paraneoplastic syndromes.** Renal cell carcinoma is known as the **"internist's tumor"** because of the multiple paraneoplastic syndromes that have been associated with it.

1. **Amyloidosis.** Secondary amyloidosis is noted in 3% of patients with renal cell carcinoma.
2. **Ectopic ACTH** (see p 90).
3. **Ectopic prolactin.** Galactorrhea from excessive ectopic prolactinlike substances occasionally develops.
4. **Erythrocytosis.** This phenomenon occurs in 3% of patients (see p 77).
5. **Hypercalcemia.** Elevated calcium levels occur in 5% of patients (see p 87).
6. **Hypertension.** Elevated blood pressure occurs in as many as 20–40% of patients and may be the result of **excessive renin production**.
7. **Stauffer's syndrome.** This paraneoplastic syndrome, characterized by reversible hepatosplenomegaly and hepatic dysfunction associated with fever, fatigue, and weight loss, can occur in **10–20% of cases**.
8. **Subacute necrotic myelopathy.** This syndrome, as well as other neuromyopathies, occurs in as many as **3% of patients**.

IV. **Differential diagnosis.** Renal cell carcinoma commonly presents with **hematuria** (see p 313, **IV** for the differential diagnosis of hematuria) and an **abdominal mass**. Only 5–6% of all renal masses identified in asymptomatic patients are malignant. Other diseases that must be considered include **perinephric abscesses, hypertrophied column of Bertin, cysts, and other neoplasms** (angiomyolipoma, oncocytoma, sarcoma, and xanthogranulomatous pyelonephritis).

V. **Screening programs.** Routine urinalysis (to detect hematuria) and a routine physical examination are the most cost-effective means of screening for renal cell carcinoma. High-risk patients (strong family history or history of von Hippel-Lindau disease) should be screened annually with ultrasound or CT examinations (see **VI.C.2** above).

VI. **Diagnostic work-up**

A. **Medical history and physical examination.** A complete medical history and thorough physical examination are essential in the initial evaluation of patients with renal cell carcinoma.

1. **Skin.** Pallor suggesting anemia and jaundice indicating hepatic dysfunction should be noted.
2. **Lymph nodes.** The presence of a signal node (also called **Virchow's or Troisier's node**) should be recorded.
3. **Abdomen.** A palpable mass or hepatomegaly indicating metastatic disease can often be detected, especially in thin patients.
4. **External genitalia.** The presence of a **varicocele**, especially in an older male, may occur from a tumor thrombus obstructing the testicular vein.

B. **Primary tests and procedures.** The following tests and procedures should be performed on all patients with suspected renal cell carcinoma.

1. **Blood tests** (see p 1, **IV.A**)
   a. **Complete blood count.**
   b. **Hepatic transaminases.**
   c. **Alkaline phosphatase.**
   d. **BUN and creatinine.**
2. **Urine tests**
   a. **Urinalysis** (see p 3, **IV.B**).
   b. **Twenty-four-hour creatinine clearance.** Baseline renal function is assessed by calculating the creatinine clearance (urine creatinine x urine volume/serum creatine x 1440 minutes). This is compared with the normal value of 100–125 mL/min in adult males and 85–105 mL/min in adult females.
3. **Imaging studies**
   a. **Chest x-ray** (see p 3, **IV.C.1**).
   b. **Abdominal flat plate.** A plain abdominal x-ray (usually obtained during excretory urography) may demonstrate the position and size of a renal mass. In addition, **calcifications** are present in **10%** of renal cancers. **Punctuate**

        calcifications are associated with a **90% likelihood of malignancy,** whereas **ring-like calcifications** carry only a **20% risk of malignancy.**

    c. **Excretory urography.** An intravenous pyelogram is frequently the primary preliminary imaging study. It can accurately determine the pathologic stage in 70% of cases.

    d. **Computed tomography.** CT scans can differentiate cystic from solid masses because solid masses enhance with contrast administration, whereas cystic lesions do not. CT scans also can identify nodal involvement, perinephric extension, renal vein or caval involvement, and liver metastases.

  C. **Optional tests and procedures.** The following examinations may be indicated by previous diagnostic findings or clinical suspicion.

    1. **Blood tests** (see p 2, **IV.A**)

      a. **Nucleotidase.**

      b. **GGTP.**

    2. **Imaging studies**

      a. **Ultrasound.** The accuracy of ultrasound approaches 100% in differentiating renal cysts from solid masses. Simple **"benign" cysts** have **no internal echoes,** well defined borders, and acoustic enhancement beyond the posterior wall. **Doppler flow ultrasound** can also accurately access the **renal vein for tumor thrombus extension.** (see p 3, **IV.C.3**).

      b. **Magnetic resonance imaging.** MRI can be used in place of CT especially in patients who cannot be given IV contrast. MRI can also be used to evaluate for involvement of the **renal vein or vena cava with tumor thrombus.**

      c. **Angiography.** Angiography, which was used extensively before the development of CT and MRI scans, currently is used only when a **renal parenchymal sparing procedure** (partial nephrectomy) is contemplated.

      d. **Inferior vena cavagram.** As many as 5% of renal cell carcinomas have a **tumor thrombus** that extends into the renal vein and the vena cava. Therefore, a preoperative study of the venous system is usually required. However, the vena cavagram has largely been **replaced by less invasive MRI scans and Doppler flow studies.**

      e. **Renal scan.** This study is especially useful in the diagnosis of renal **"pseudo tumors,"** such as a hypertrophied column of Bertin or lobulations that appear as photodense regions, and renal tumors and cysts that are identified as photodeficient areas on the scan.

      f. **Technetium-99m bone scan** (see p 3, **IV.C.4**).

    3. **Procedures**

      a. **Cyst aspiration.** Cyst aspiration is occasionally helpful when an equivocal cyst does not meet all the criteria noted above. The return of bloody fluid, an irregular outline or **thickened wall** on cystography, **high fat content,** or a **positive cytology** may indicate malignancy.

      b. **Biopsy.** Routine needle biopsy of a renal mass is unreliable because tumor heterogeneity often produces nondiagnostic results. Seeding of the needle tract also may rarely occur. Biopsy of any unusual or unexplained mass remote from the kidney should be performed to exclude the possibility of metastatic disease.

VII. Pathology

  A. **Location.** There is no known variability in the incidence of kidney cancer on the basis of anatomic site.

  B. **Multiplicity. Synchronous or metachronous** renal cell carcinomas occur in 3% of cases. In patients with **von Hippel-Lindau disease,** the incidence is even higher.

  C. **Histology.** Most kidney cancers (> 90%) in adults are **adenocarcinomas** (also called renal cell carcinoma and hypernephroma) originating in the **proximal convoluted tubule.** There are 4 histologic subtypes: **clear, granular, sarcomatoid, and papillary. Sarcomatoid** tumors have a much **poorer prognosis** than do clear and **granular** cell types. **Papillary** renal carcinoma tends to be hypovascular, presents early, and has a **more favorable** 5-year survival rate. In addition, a **cystic variant** of renal cell carcinoma exists in 15% of cases.

  D. **Metastatic spread**

    1. **Modes of spread.** Kidney cancer generally spreads via three mechanisms.

      a. **Direct extension.** Local invasion of contiguous structures occurs in 5% of patients and can involve the **liver and adrenal gland** as well as other adjacent organs. In addition, 5% of patients present with tumor extension into the **renal vein or inferior vena cava.**

        b. Lymphatic metastasis. Regional lymph nodes are involved in 10–25% of patients undergoing radical nephrectomy. The renal lymphatic drainage is highly variable, but it includes the para-aortic, paracaval, and hilar nodes.

        c. Hematogenous metastasis. Tumor cells can travel through systemic blood vessels to distant organs. This occurs in approximately 30% of patients by the time of presentation.

    2. Sites of spread. Renal cell carcinoma can metastasize to the following organs: **lung,** 56–75%; liver, 18–35%; bone, 20–33%; adrenals, 19%; contralateral kidney, 7.5%; soft tissues, 8–36%; and central nervous system, 1–8%.

VIII. Staging. The Robson staging system, which was used for many years, was recently replaced by the TNM classification system devised jointly by the American Joint Committee on Cancer and the Union Internationale Contre le Cancer.

  A. Robson staging system

    1. Stage I. Tumor is completely confined within the kidney.

    2. Stage II. Tumor invades the perinephric fat but is confined within Gerota's fascia.

    3. Stage III. Tumor involves the regional lymph nodes, the renal vein, or the vena cava.

    4. Stage IV. Tumor invades contiguous viscera or distant metastases are present.

  B. TNM staging system

    1. Tumor stage

        a. TX. Primary tumor cannot be assessed.

        b. T0. No evidence of primary tumor.

        c. T1. Tumor is no larger than 2.5 cm in its greatest dimension and limited to the kidney.

        d. T2. Tumor is larger than 2.5 cm in its greatest dimension and is limited to the kidney.

        e. T3. Tumor extends into major veins, adrenal glands, or perinephric tissues but not beyond Gerota's fascia.

          (1) T3a. Tumor invades adrenal gland or perinephric tissue but not beyond Gerota's fascia.

          (2) T3b. Tumor extends into the renal vein or vena cava.

        f. T4. Tumor invades beyond Gerota's fascia.

    2. Lymph node stage

        a. NX. Regional lymph nodes cannot be assessed.

        b. N0. No regional lymph node metastases present.

        c. N1. Metastasis to a single lymph node no larger than 2 cm in its greatest dimension.

        d. N2. Metastasis to a single lymph node larger than 2 but no larger than 5 cm or metastases to multiple lymph nodes no larger than 5.0 cm in their greatest dimension.

        e. N3. Metastasis to a lymph node larger than 5 cm in its greatest dimension.

    3. Metastatic stage

        a. MX. Presence of distant metastases cannot be assessed.

        b. M0. No distant metastases are present.

        c. M1. Distant metastases are present.

    4. Histopathologic grade

        a. GX. Grade cannot be assessed.

        b. G1. Well differentiated.

        c. G2. Moderately well differentiated.

        d. G3–4. Poorly differentiated or undifferentiated.

    5. Stage groupings

        a. Stage I. T1, N0, M0.

        b. Stage II. T2, N0, M0.

        c. Stage III. T1 or 2, N1, M0; T3a or b, N0 or 1, M0.

        d. Stage IV. T4, any N, M0; any T, N2 or 3, M0; any T, any N, M1.

IX. Treatment

  A. Surgery

    1. Primary renal cell carcinoma

        a. Indications. Surgical resection of renal cell carcinoma is generally indicated in all patients **without distant metastases, extensive local tumor invasion,** or both. Resection, however, is contraindicated in patients with poor performance status (see Appendix A).

        b. Approaches. Transabdominal, thoracoabdominal, and extrapleural flank incisions can be used for nephrectomy.

(1) **Transabdominal.** With this approach, a **midline or bilateral subcostal incision** is used most often. This technique affords excellent exposure of the renal vessels and allows intraoperative examination of the contralateral kidney. Like any intra-abdominal operation, transabdominal surgery poses a risk of enterotomy, intra-abdominal abscess, and small bowel obstruction (adhesions).

(2) **Thoracoabdominal.** This approach involves a **midline laparotomy incision that is extended across the costal margin** and into the chest. It is particularly useful with extremely **large lesions,** especially of the **upper pole,** and lesions with an associated **ipsilateral solitary pulmonary nodule.** Like the transabdominal approach, this approach affords excellent exposure of the renal vascular pedicle, but because of the thoracotomy, the **morbidity is greater** than with other approaches.

(3) **Extraperitoneal flank.** This approach uses a **flank incision** and extraperitoneal radical nephrectomy. Although this method is associated with the fewest complications, its use should be limited to situations in which the **lesion is small** and there is **no need to explore the contralateral kidney.** In addition, exposure of the great vessels can be limited.

c. **Procedures.** The cornerstone of therapy for most patients with non-metastatic disease remains radical nephrectomy.

(1) **Radical nephrectomy.** Radical nephrectomy involves initial control of the renal vascular pedicle and en bloc removal of the kidney, surrounding Gerota's fascia, adrenal gland, and upper ureter. The role of extended regional lymphadenectomy remains controversial; however, some local lymphatic tissue should always be included to allow accurate staging. Vena caval involvement occurs in 5% of patients; therefore if a thrombus is present, the vena cava may need to be opened to extract the thrombus. **Aggressive surgical treatment, including cardiopulmonary bypass** to remove thrombus that may extend above the diaphragm and occasionally into the atrium, is recommended because survival rates approaching those of Stage I can be attained, providing that all thrombus is removed.

(2) **Partial Nephrectomy.** Removal of the cancer with a margin of normal renal parenchyma can be utilized in selected cases. Examples include patients with prior renal disease (ie, diabetics) and compromises renal function in whom nephron sparing surgery is desirable.

(3) **Enucleation.** When dealing with very small renal cell carcinomas (< 2–3 cm), simple nucleation with biopsy of the base may be acceptable. Candidates for this are identical to those who are candidates for partial nephrectomy.

(4) **Bilateral Disease.** Surgical therapy for bilateral disease with either bilateral partial nephrectomies or radical nephrectomy coupled with partial nephrectomy is recommended because, stage for stage, survival rates approach those for radical nephrectomy in unilateral disease.

(5) **Embolization.** Rarely angioinfarction is used to devascularize large tumors. Generally, this is performed **immediately preoperatively**.

d. **Morbidity and mortality.** Overall, the **mortality** from radical nephrectomy is **less than 2%.** Difficulties that may be encountered after surgery include the following: pneumothorax, hemorrhage, prolonged ileus, small or large bowel injury or obstruction, pancreatic fistula (left-sided tumors), liver or duodenal injury (right-sided tumors), and splenic injury.

2. **Locally advanced and metastatic renal cell carcinomas.** Metastatic disease occurs in about 30% of patients by the time of diagnosis. Radical nephrectomy is of value only in patients with a **low-grade tumor and a solitary pulmonary metastatic lesion.** When resected, **solitary metastases,** regardless of site, are associated with a **30%–40% 5-year survival.** Nephrectomy with multiple metastases has no effect on survival but occasionally can be used for **palliation** of pain, hemorrhage, hypertension, hypercalcemia, or erythrocytosis or as part of an experimental protocol.

B. **Radiation therapy**

1. **Primary renal cell carcinoma.** Renal cell carcinoma is a relatively radioresistant tumor; therefore, radiation alone is never indicated as the initial treatment of an otherwise resectable lesion.

2. **Adjuvant radiation therapy**
    a. **Preoperative radiotherapy.** Studies using 3000–3600 cGy given before nephrectomy have **failed to demonstrate therapeutic benefit;** however, a high proportion of these patients had early lesions, which would not be expected to profit from preoperative radiation.
    b. **Postoperative radiotherapy.** Although trials of postoperative radiation (5000–5500 cGy over 4 weeks) have been inconclusive because of high complication rates (40–50%), postoperative radiotherapy was recommended at some centers for Stage III and Stage IV lesions without known distant metastases.
3. **Locally advanced and metastatic renal cell carcinoma.** Radiation therapy (4000–5000 cGy over 5–6 weeks) to metastatic lesions can palliate severe pain in 50–67% of patients.
4. **Morbidity and mortality.** The complications that are encountered as a direct result of radiation vary, depending on the location of the lesion, but can include one or more of the following problems: enteritis, pulmonary fibrosis (if the radiation ports extend into the thorax), transverse myelitis, or radiation hepatitis.
C. **Chemotherapy**
    1. **Primary renal cell carcinoma.** Surgical resection of localized renal cell carcinoma is usually preferred; however, chemotherapy may be considered for locally advanced disease.
    2. **Adjuvant chemotherapy.** The few studies of adjuvant chemotherapy that exist fail to demonstrate any benefit to chemotherapy in this setting, however, one trial of **bleomycin and lomustine** suggested a slight survival advantage.
    3. **Locally advanced and metastatic renal cell cancer**
        a. **Single-agent therapy.** The best results have been obtained with **vinblastine** (0.2–0.3 mg/kg weekly) with response rates of 15–30% and improved survival among responders.
        b. **Combination chemotherapy.** No combination chemotherapeutic regimen has been shown to be superior to vinblastine alone, with the possible recent exception of vinblastine, bleomycin, and methotrexate with leucovorin rescue which, in a single report, has demonstrated a 30% response rate.
D. **Hormonal therapy.** Various hormones have been tried in the therapy of renal cell carcinoma, including progestins, androgens, antiestrogens, and corticosteroids. Response rates were only 2–9%, with **megestral acetate** (Megace) demonstrating the best responses. However, this type of therapy has generally been abandoned.
E. **Immunotherapy.** The role of biologic response modifiers in the treatment of advanced renal cell carcinoma is an active area of clinical and basic science research. Because "spontaneous" regression of metastatic disease (0.8%) can occur, immunotherapy may have a major impact on this disease in the future.
    1. **Interleukin-2.** Agents such as interleukin-2, either alone or in combination with lymphokine-activated killer (LAK) cells, have achieved **response rates as high as 30%** and recently have been approved for use in the treatment of renal cell cancer.
    2. **Interferons.** Combination regimens using interferon-alpha or interferon-gamma can result in **overall response rates as high as 28%.** Interferon-alpha has been studied most extensively and has a complete response rate of 14%.
    3. **Cellular therapy.** LAK cells and tumor infiltrating lymphocytes currently are being studied and show some promise.
    4. **Other biologic response modifiers.** Experimental protocols using coumarin and cimetidine have recently been instituted, and objective responses have been reported.
X. **Prognosis**
A. **Risk of recurrence.** The risk of local recurrence is small if surgical margins are adequate. The risk of distant recurrence closely parallels overall survival.
B. **Five-year survival.** Prognosis and 5-year survivals vary with the stage of disease.
    1. **Stage I.** 56–93%.
    2. **Stage II.** 47–75%.
    3. **Stage III.** 34–51%.
    4. **Stage IV.** Less than 10%.
C. **Adverse prognostic factors.** The following factors are associated with a poor outcome: lymph node involvement, positive surgical margins, vena cava invasion, sarcomatoid histology, short disease-free interval, poor performance status, and multiple metastatic sites.

XI. Patient follow-up
   A. General guidelines. Patients with renal cell carcinoma should be followed every 3–4 months for 3 years, every 6 months for an additional 2 years, and then annually. A **long latent period** can precede recurrence, and as many as **11% of patients who survive 10 years subsequently develop recurrence.**
   B. Medical history and physical examination. An interval history and complete physical examination are required during each clinic visit. Particular attention should be focused on the areas discussed under **VI.A.** above.
   C. Routine evaluation. Patients with surgically resected adenocarcinoma should be monitored with the following tests and procedures obtained at the time of each clinic visit.
      1. Blood tests (see p 1, **IV.A**)
         a. Complete blood count
         b. Hepatic transaminases
         c. Alkaline phosphatase
         d. BUN and creatinine
      2. Urinalysis (see p 3, **IV.B**)
      3. Chest x-ray (see p 3, **IV.C.1**)
   D. Additional evaluation. Computed tomography (CT) of the abdomen can be obtained every 6–12 months and is useful in evaluating the retroperitoneum for local recurrence and in assessing the liver, contralateral kidney, and lungs for metastatic disease, especially in patients at high risk for recurrence.
   E. Optional evaluation. The following tests and procedures may be indicated by previous diagnostic findings or clinical suspicion.
      1. Blood tests (see p 2, **IV.A**)
         a. Nucleotidase.
         b. GGTP.
      2. Imaging studies (see p 3, **IV.C**)
         a. Magnetic resonance imaging (MRI).
         b. Technetium-99m bone scan.
      3. Biopsy. Any new or suspicious mass in a patient who is otherwise free of tumor must be subjected to skinny needle, core needle, or open surgical biopsy to document the presence or absence of metastatic disease.

REFERENCES

Breton PN et al: Chronic renal failure: a significant risk factor in the development of renal cysts and renal cell carcinoma. *Cancer* 1986; **57:**1871–1878.

de Kernion JB: Renal tumors. In Campbells Urology, Walsh PC, ed. WB Saunders Co., Philadelphia, volume 2, pp 1294–1338, 1986.

de Malder PN, Gebores AD, Debruyne FM, et al. Recombinant interferon alpha and gamma in the treatment of advanced renal cell carcinoma. Proc Annual Meet. Amer. Soc. Oncology, 7-A506, 1988.

Finney R. The value of radiotherapy in the treatment of hypernephroma: A clinical trial. *Br J Urol* 1973;**45:**258–269.

Horoszewicz JS, Murphy GP. An assessment of the current use of human interferons in the therapy of urologic cancers. *J Urol* 1989;**142:**1173–1180.

Maleh RS et al: Renal cell carcinoma in von Hippel-Lindau syndrome. *Am J Med* 1987;**82:**236–238.

Pritchett TR, Lieskovsky G, Skinner DG: Clinical manifestations and treatment of renal parenchymal tumors In: Skinner DG: *Diagnosis and Management of Genitourinary Cancer.* Philadelphia: WB Saunders: 1988;337–361.

Rosenberg SA, Lotze MT, Yang JC, et al: Experience with the use of high dose interleukin-2 in the treatment of 652 cancer patients. *Ann Surg* 1989;**210:**474–485.

Tanagho EA, McAnich JW. *Smith's General Urology*, 12th ed. Norwalk, Appleton & Lange, 1988.

Vugrin D. Systemic therapy of metastatic renal cell carcinoma. *Sem Nephrol* 1987;**7:**152–162.

Wein AJ, Hanno PM: *A Clinical Manual of Urology.* Norwalk: Appleton-Century Crofts; 1988.

40 Malignancies of the Ureter & Renal Pelvis

Stephen Strup, MD, and Leonard Gomella, MD

I. **Epidemiology.** Carcinoma of the renal pelvis and ureter is **rare,** representing 6% and 1% of all renal malignancies, respectively. Together, these carcinomas account for **1.9% of all genitourinary tumors;** however, the reported incidence of upper-tract tumors is rising. Worldwide, the incidence of renal pelvis and ureteral cancer varies substantially. Balkan countries have a much higher incidence of upper-tract tumors; these neoplasms constitute 40% of all renal cancers.

II. **Risk factors**
   A. **Age.** The incidence of **renal pelvis tumors** peaks between the **ages of 60 and 80,** whereas that of u**reteral carcinoma** increases from less than 1 case per 100,000 before age 55 to **5.7 per 100,000 by age 75.**
   B. **Sex.** The **risk for males is 2–3 times greater** than that for females.
   C. **Diet.** Caffeine ingestion has been implicated in the pathogenesis of urothelial carcinoma.
   D. **Smoking.** Cigarette smoking has been associated with a **2.4-times increased risk** of urothelial tumors.
   E. **Chemicals**
      1. **Phenacetin.** As many as 70% of patients with phenacetin-induced nephropathy develop urothelial cancer of the upper tracts, usually of the **renal pelvis.**
      2. **Thorotrast.** Epidermoid malignancies delayed as long as 19 years have been reported in association with the use of **Thorotrast,** a former radiologic contrast medium.
      3. **Aminophenols.** These chemicals, used in the rubber and dye industry, increase the risk of developing urothelial carcinoma.
   F. **Previous urinary tract pathology**
      1. **Infection.** Both **Danubian endemic familial nephropathy,** which occurs in Balkan countries, and **chronic urinary tract infections** predispose to upper-tract urothelial tumors. Tumors in the former typically are **bilateral** and less aggressive.
      2. **Inflammation.** Chronic inflammation accompanying urolithiasis has been associated with the subsequent development of urothelial malignancies.
      3. **Other urologic neoplasms.** Upper-tract urothelial tumors occur in 2–4% of patients with **previous bladder cancer,** and as many as 30% of patients with **ectopic urothelial tumors** (eg, prostate and urethra) develop upper tract tumors.
      4. **Other factors.** Many factors that predispose to bladder carcinoma also increase the risk of upper-tract urothelial tumors (see p 312, **II**).

III. **Clinical presentation**
   A. **Signs and symptoms.** Approximately 85% of patients present with **nonspecific complaints;** the remaining 15% are asymptomatic.
      1. **Local manifestations.** Patients frequently complain of gross or microscopic **hematuria** (60–75%), **total hematuria** (consistent numbers of red cells throughout urination is more indicative of upper-tract bleeding), flank pain (30–40%), flank mass (< 15%), and bladder irritability (10–15%).
      2. **Systemic manifestations.** Weight loss, anorexia, and fatigue are usually indicative of advanced disease and are present in 10–15% of patients.
   B. **Paraneoplastic syndromes.** No known symptom complexes are associated with upper tract neoplasms.

IV. **Differential diagnosis.** The differential diagnosis for patients presenting with hematuria, flank discomfort, or voiding symptoms is essentially the same as that for bladder cancer (see p 313, **IV**).

V. Screening programs. No useful screening examination is available to detect hematuria other than **routine urinalysis.**

VI. Diagnostic workup

   A. Medical history and physical examination. A meticulous medical history emphasizing common presenting complaints is important, and a careful physical examination is essential.

      1. Skin. Pallor indicating anemia from urologic blood loss, although rare, should be noted.

      2. Lymph nodes. The presence of a signal node (also called **Virchow's or Troisier's node**) must be recorded.

      3. Abdomen. Careful examination may reveal hepatomegaly or an abdominal mass caused by enlarged para-aortic lymph nodes.

      4. Extremities. Edema of the lower extremities from occlusion of the inferior vena cava and abdominal lymphatics should be noted.

   B. Primary tests and procedures. The following diagnostic tests and procedures should be performed in all patients with suspected upper-tract urothelial tumors.

      1. Blood tests

         a. Complete blood count (see p 1, **IV.A.1**).

         b. Hepatic transaminases (see p 1, **IV.A.2**).

         c. Alkaline phosphatase (see p 1, **IV.A.3**).

         d. BUN and creatinine (see p 3, **IV.A.6**).

         e. Tumor markers. No tumor markers are specific for upper tract urothelial tumors, but elevated **carcinoembryonic antigen (CEA), serum gonadotropins, and hypercalcemia** have been reported with these tumors.

      2. Urine tests

         a. Urinalysis

         b. Urine cytology. Cytologic examination of voided urine and bladder or **ureteral washings** (which are more accurate) are highly dependent on the pathologist's expertise. The **false positive rate** resulting from inflammation is **10%,** and the **false negative rate** in low-grade tumors is **as high as 30%,** with an overall **accuracy of 80%.**

      3. Imaging studies

         a. Chest x-ray (see p 3, **IV.C.1**).

         b. Excretory urography. An **abnormal filling defect** is seen on intravenous pyelogram in 50–70% of patients with upper-tract tumors, and another 10% will have **complete obstruction.** Filling defects typically are irregular and occasionally are multiple. Other diseases can produce similar defects (eg, non-opaque calculi, blood clots, sloughed renal papillae, fungus balls, extrinsic compression, hemangioma, or, in rare cases, cholesteatoma).

         c. Retrograde urography. A retrograde pyelogram often visualizes the lesion better, especially with obstruction. It also may differentiate lesions from non-opaque ureteral calculi by demonstrating **poststenotic ureteral dilation** that is characteristic of obstructing urothelial tumors.

      4. Invasive procedures

         a. Cystoscopy. In some cases, cystoscopy can **visualize hemorrhage** from one of the ureteral orifices, and it is essential to exclude associated bladder diseases.

         b. Ureteroscopy. The new flexible ureteroscopes allow **direct visualization and biopsy** of the tumor in as many as 90% of patients.

   C. Optional tests and procedures. The following tests and procedures may be indicated by previous diagnostic findings or clinical suspicion:

      1. Blood tests (see p 2, **IV.A**)

         a. Nucleotidase.

         b. GGTP.

      2. Imaging studies (see p 3, **IV.C**)

         a. Computed tomography. CT scan of the abdomen and pelvis to assess the status of the liver and abdominal lymph nodes is indicated when advanced disease is suspected.

         b. Magnetic resonance imaging (MRI).

         c. Renal ultrasound.

         d. Technetium-99m bone scan.

      3. Invasive procedures. Because of possible tumor seeding, **percutaneous nephroscopy** generally is **discouraged** except in highly selected cases such as that of planned transrenal resection of a malignancy in a solitary kidney.

VII. **Pathology**
   A. **Location.** Ureteral tumors occur most often in the **lower third** of the ureter.
   B. **Multiplicity.** Ureteral and renal pelvis malignancies often are **multifocal,** and 2–4% are **bilateral.** In addition, 21–50% of patients with upper-tract malignancies **develop bladder cancer.**
   C. **Histology**
      1. **Transitional cell carcinoma. Ninety percent** of renal pelvis and ureter cancers are **transitional cell carcinomas.** The transitional cell carcinomas tend to be papillary (85%) rather than sessile (15%).
      2. **Squamous cell carcinoma.** Squamous cell carcinomas account for 7–9% of upper tract neoplasms. These lesions are commonly associated with **chronic inflammation and urolithiasis** and typically are more advanced at presentation.
      3. **Adenocarcinoma.** Adenocarcinomas constitute less than 1% of upper tract tumors. They are **more common in females** and are **associated with urolithiasis, hydronephrosis, and chronic pyelonephritis.** Like squamous cell lesions, they frequently present at an advanced stage.
   D. **Metastatic spread**
      1. **Modes of spread.** Ureteral and renal pelvis cancers can spread by any of the following routes:
         a. **Local extension.** Upper-tract tumors can directly invade contiguous structures such as the small bowel, colon, liver, renal cortex, pancreas, and spleen.
         b. **Lymphatic metastasis.** The principal lymphatic drainage is to the regional lymph nodes, which are the most commonly involved site of metastatic disease. Lymph node metastases present with 22–41% and 37–82% of **ureteral and renal pelvis tumors,** respectively.
         c. **Hematogenous metastasis.** Spread through draining veins results in metastases to distant organs and occurs in approximately 40% of patients.
      2. **Sites of spread.** Ureteral and renal pelvis carcinomas commonly metastasize to the following sites: abdominal and pelvic lymph nodes, lungs, bone, and liver.
VIII. **Staging.** The staging of upper-tract tumors depends on the depth of invasion through the thin muscular wall of the ureter and renal pelvis and the presence or absence of extension into the surrounding structures. The staging is analogous to that of bladder cancer (see p 34, **VIII**), except T2 and T3a cannot be differentiated in the thin muscular wall of the renal pelvis. In 1987 the American Joint Committee on Cancer and the Union Internationale Contre le Cancer jointly adopted a TNM staging system in an attempt to provide a universal staging system.
   A. **Tumor stage**
      1. **TX.** Primary tumor cannot be assessed.
      2. **T0.** No evidence of primary tumor.
      3. **Tis.** Carcinoma in situ.
      4. **Ta.** Noninvasive papillary carcinoma.
      5. **T1.** Tumor invades subepithelial connective tissue.
      6. **T2.** Tumor invades muscularis.
      7. **T3.** Tumor invades beyond muscularis into the periureteric or peripelvic fat or renal parenchyma.
      8. **T4.** Tumor invades adjacent organs or through the kidney into perinephric fat.
   B. **Lymph node stage**
      1. **NX.** Regional lymph nodes cannot be assessed
      2. **N0.** No regional lymph node metastases are present.
      3. **N1.** Metastasis to a single lymph node that is no larger than 2 cm in its greatest dimension.
      4. **N2.** Metastasis to a single lymph node larger than 2 cm but no larger than 5 cm in its greatest dimension or to multiple lymph nodes less than 5 cm in their greatest dimension.
      5. **N3.** Metastasis to a lymph node larger than 5 cm in its greatest dimension.
         Note: Regional lymph nodes include the hilar, abdominal para-aortic, paracaval, and common, internal, and external iliac nodes.
   C. **Metastatic stage**
      1. **MX.** Presence of distant metastasis cannot be assessed.
      2. **M0.** No distant metastases are present.
      3. **M1.** Distant metastases are present.
   D. **Histopathologic grade**
      1. **GX.** Grade cannot be assessed.

2. **G1.** Well differentiated.
3. **G2.** Moderately well differentiated.
4. **G3–4.** Poorly or undifferentiated.
  E. **Stage groupings**
1. **Stage 0.** Ta or Tis, N0, M0 (14% of renal pelvis tumors and 50% of ureteral neoplasms).
2. **Stage I.** T1, N0, M0 (27% and 10% of renal pelvis and ureteral malignancies, respectively).
3. **Stage II.** T2, N0, M0 (together with Stage III tumors: 28% of renal pelvis and 20% of ureteral cancers).
4. **Stage III.** T3, N0, M0 (together with Stage II tumors: 28% of renal pelvis and 20% of ureteral cancers).
5. **Stage IV.** T4, N0, M0; any T, N1–3, M0; any T, any N, M1 (30% of renal pelvis lesions and 15% of ureteral tumors).
IX. **Treatment**
  A. **Surgery**
1. **Primary upper urinary tract carcinoma**
    a. **General considerations**
      (1) **Renal pelvis malignancies.** Because of the multifocal nature of tumors of the renal pelvis, **segmental ureterectomy and nephrectomy** are associated with a 30–60% chance of **recurrent disease** in the ureteral stump.
      (2) **Ureteral malignancies.** Proximal ureteral malignancies typically are **high grade** and are similar to renal pelvis tumors because they often are **multifocal** and carry a 30–75% chance of **recurrence** in the ipsilateral kidney and collecting system after **segmental resection**. Distal ureteral tumors frequently are **low grade and early stage,** with a low likelihood of recurrence. Therefore, they are more amenable to local therapy.
    b. **Indications.** Surgery remains the only potentially curative therapy for cancer of the renal pelvis and ureter and is indicated in all patients with nonmetastatic resectable disease and no medical contraindications to surgery.
    c. **Approaches**
      (1) **Thoracoabdominal incision.** This approach extends a **standard midline abdominal incision through the costal margin and diaphragm.**
      (2) **Combined subcostal and pelvic (Gibson) incisions.** This two-incision approach combines a **subcostal incision with a low pelvic incision.**
    d. **Procedures**
      (1) **Radical nephroureterectomy.** The standard surgical therapy for tumors of the upper urinary tract with a **normal contralateral kidney** is excision of the ipsilateral kidney, renal pelvis, ureter, and a small cuff of bladder surrounding the ureteral orifice. Endoscopic resection or fulguration, followed by intravesical Bacillus Calmette-Guérin (BCG), can be attempted in patients with a single functional kidney and low-grade early stage disease. With a **solitary kidney, nephroureterectomy** and subsequent dialysis would be reserved for those who do not respond to conservative therapy.
      (2) **Partial ureterectomy.** Because of the high rate of recurrence in proximal and high-grade advanced-stage tumors, partial ureterectomy with reimplantation (transureteroureterostomy is **contraindicated in ureteral carcinoma**) should be reserved for patients with a low-grade early tumor of the **distal one-third of the ureter** or for patients with a **single kidney.**
2. **Locally advanced and metastatic urothelial cancer.** Surgery generally is not indicated in the presence of locally advanced or metastatic disease except for palliation of severe symptoms of urinary tract obstruction and bleeding.
3. **Mortality and morbidity.** The mortality and morbidity associated with nephroureterectomy are essentially identical to those associated with radical nephrectomy performed for renal cell carcinoma (see p 303, **IX.A.1.d**). The mortality and morbidity after segmental resection are considerably less and related primarily to the following areas: hemorrhage, infection, urine leak, and ureteral stricture.
  B. **Radiation therapy**
1. **Primary carcinoma of the upper urinary tract.** No data exist to support the

use of radiation therapy in the primary treatment of urothelial malignancies of the upper urinary tract.

2. **Adjuvant radiation therapy.** The incidence of **local recurrence** after surgical resection may be **decreased** from 46% to as low as 1% with postoperative radiotherapy (4500–5000 cGy over 5 weeks). According to a single study, **5-year survival increased** from 17% to 27%, but this remains controversial. Some centers advocate a course of postoperative radiation if the bladder or ureter is opened, if lymph node metastases are present, or if perirenal, peripelvic, or periureteral extension of the tumor is demonstrated.

3. **Locally advanced and metastatic urothelial cancer.** Although radiation therapy has not been shown to be effective in unresectable disease, it may be useful in the palliation of symptomatic metastatic disease.

C. **Chemotherapy**
   1. **Primary carcinoma of the upper urinary tract.** In patients who are not surgical candidates, **thiotepa, mitomycin-C,** and other agents have been shown to be helpful with superficial tumors. In the case of low-grade early stage lesions in a solitary kidney, **thiotepa combined with BCG** has been shown to be effective in a small number of patients.
   2. **Adjuvant chemotherapy.** No studies have been conducted on adjuvant chemotherapy in the treatment of upper-tract urothelial malignancies, and reports of therapeutic benefit remain anecdotal.
   3. **Locally advanced and metastatic urothelial cancer.** Upper-tract urothelial tumors are believed to respond to chemotherapy in a manner identical to the response of bladder tumors. The **M-VAC** (methotrexate, vinblastine, doxorubicin, and cisplatin) regimen has shown promise: the combined complete and partial remission rate **ranges between 50% and 70%.**

D. **Immunotherapy.** Although BCG may have some activity in this disease, no studies have demonstrated definite evidence of therapeutic benefit.

X. **Prognosis**
   A. **Risk of recurrence.** The risk of recurrence and prognosis varies with the grade and stage of the tumor as well as with the type of resection performed. High-grade advanced-stage lesions treated with segmental resection have the highest likelihood of recurrence (64–100%).
   B. **Five-year survival.** The **5-year survival for low- and high-grade tumors** is 80% and 20%, respectively. High-grade tumors do not present with low-stage disease.
      1. **Ureteral carcinoma**
         a. **Stage 0.** 90%.
         b. **Stage I.** 50%.
         c. **Stage II–III.** 15%.
         d. **Stage IV.** Less than 5%.
      2. **Renal pelvis carcinoma**
         a. **Stage 0.** 90–100%.
         b. **Stage I.** 80%.
         c. **Stage II–III.** 75%.
         d. **Stage IV.** 5%.
   C. **Adverse prognostic factors.** The following findings are associated with a particularly poor outlook: high tumor grade and advanced stage.

XI. **Patient follow-up**
   A. **General guidelines.** Patients with ureteral or renal pelvis carcinoma should be evaluated for recurrence every 3 months for 2 years, every 6 months for an additional 3 years, and annually thereafter. The following specific guidelines for tests and procedures are recommended.
   B. **Routine evaluation.** The following examinations should be conducted during each clinic visit.
      1. **History and physical examination.** An interval history and a complete physical examination are mandatory during routine office visits. Special attention should be paid to the areas on p 307, **VI.A.**
      2. **Blood tests** (see p 1, **IV.A**)
         a. **Complete blood count.**
         b. **Hepatic transaminases.**
         c. **Alkaline phosphatase.**
         d. **BUN and creatinine.**
      3. **Urinalysis** (see p 3, **IV.B**)
      4. **Urinary cytology** (see p 307, **VI.C.2**)
      5. **Chest x-ray** (see p 3, **IV.C.1**)

    C. Additional evaluation. Other tests and procedures that should be performed at regular intervals include the following:

        1. Cystoscopy. Patients with upper tract tumors have a 40–50% risk of developing **bladder cancer**. Thus, routine cystoscopy is recommended. Follow-up cystoscopy should be performed every 3 months for 1 year, every 6 months for an additional 4 years, and annually thereafter.

        2. Excretory urography. Close follow-up of the upper tracts is necessary with an **IVP** every 6 months for 2 years and annually thereafter.

    D. Optional evaluation. The following tests may be indicated by previous diagnostic findings or clinical suspicion.

        1. Blood tests (see p 2, **IV.A**)

            a. 5-Nucleotidase.

            b. GGTP.

        2. Imaging studies (see p 3, **IV.C**)

            a. Computerized tomography (CT). If signs or symptoms of liver or lung metastases develop, CT is useful in the evaluation of these organs, however, this test is not universally obtained in the routine follow-up of patients.

            b. Magnetic resonance imaging (MRI).

            c. Technetium-99m bone scan.

REFERENCES

Babaian RJ, Johnson DE. Primary carcinoma of the ureter. *J Urol* 1980;**123**:357–359.

Brookland RK, Richter MP: The postoperative irradiation of transitional cell carcinoma of the renal pelvis and ureter. *J Urol* 1985;**133**:952–955.

Cummings KB. Nephroureterectomy: Rationale in the management of transitional cell carcinoma of the upper urinary tract. *Urol Clin North Am* 1983;**7** (3):569–577.

Droller MJ. Transitional cell cancer: Upper tracts and bladder. In Walsh PC, et al, editors. *Campbell's Urology,* 5th ed., vol. 2. Philadelphia: Saunders; 1986;1408–1440.

Frank IN, Keys HM, McCune CS. Urologic and male genital cancers. In *Clinical Oncology for Medical Students and Physicians,* 6th ed. Atlanta: American Cancer Society; 1983:204–205.

Herr HW. Durable response of a carcinoma in situ of the renal pelvis to topical Bacillus Calmette-Guerin. *J Urol* 1985;**134**:531–532.

Klotz LH: Management of urothelial carcinoma of the upper tracts. *AUA Update,* series 7, lesson 4. American Urological Association; 1988.

McLaughlin JK, et al. Etiology of cancer of the renal pelvis. *JNCI* 1983;**71**:287–291.

Richie JP. Carcinoma of the renal pelvis and ureter. In Skinner D, Lieskowsky G, editors. *Diagnosis and Management of Genitourinary Cancer.* Philadelphia: Saunders; 1988:323–336.

Sternberg CN, Yagoda A, et al. Preliminary results of M-VAC (Methotrexate, Vinblastine, Doxorubicin, and Cisplatin) for transitional cell carcinoma of the urothelium. *J Urol* 1985;**133**:403–407.

Wallace MA, Wallace DM, et al. The late results of conservative surgery for upper tract urothelial carcinomas. *Br J Urol* 1981;**53**:537–541.

Williams WD. Renal, peri-renal, and ureteral neoplasms. In Gillenwater JY, Grayhack JT, Howards SS, Duckett JW, editors. *Adult and Pediatric Urology.* Chicago: Yearbook; 1987:537–554.

41 Malignancies of the Urinary Bladder

Leonard Gomella, MD, and James Stephanelli, MD

I. **Epidemiology.** Bladder carcinoma is the **second most common** urologic **malignancy** in the United States. In 1985, **28.5 cases per 100,000 males** and **7.8 cases per 100,000 females** were reported, leading to 6.0 and 1.7 deaths, respectively. Estimates indicate that **52,300 new cases and 9,900 deaths** occur in 1993. Bladder cancer occurs more commonly in the northeastern United States and in Europe, particularly in Switzerland, where the incidence exceeds 30 cases per 100,000 males annually. Asia, including India, has an exceptionally low incidence: only 2.4 males and 0.5 females per 100,000 develop bladder tumors each year.

II. **Risk factors**
   A. **Age.** The incidence of bladder carcinoma increases from less than 1.0 per 100,000 before age 30 to more than **146 per 100,000 by age 85.** The majority of cases occur between the **fifth and seventh decades.**
   B. **Sex.** The risk for males is **3.6 times greater** than for females.
   C. **Race.** The risk for whites is **1.8 times greater** than for blacks.
   D. **Genetic factors.** There is no evidence that genetic factors play a role in the pathogenesis of bladder carcinoma.
   E. **Diet. Coffee** consumption was once thought to increase the risk of bladder cancer; however, this has not been confirmed by more recent data.
   F. **Cigarette smoking. A 2–3 times increased risk** of bladder malignancies is associated with cigarette smoking; it is estimated that smoking is responsible for **30–40% of all cases.**
   G. **Previous urologic pathology**
      1. **Inflammation.** Patients with chronic inflammation (eg, **indwelling catheters**) are at a slightly higher risk of bladder tumors than the general population.
      2. **Infections.** Chronic infections such as **schistosomiasis or bilharziasis** (infestation with the parasite *Schistosoma haematobium,* commonly found in Egypt) increase the risk of bladder cancer, especially of **squamous cell carcinoma,** by increasing urinary nitrites.
      3. **Congenital anomalies. Bladder exstrophy** is associated with an increased frequency of **adenocarcinoma** of the bladder.
      4. **Other urologic tumors. As many as 40%** of patients with renal pelvis and ureteral tumors will develop bladder cancer.
   H. **Radiation.** Pelvic irradiation increases the incidence of bladder tumors by **2–3 times.**
   I. **Chemicals**
      1. **Industrial chemicals.** Exposure to **arylamine compounds,** common in the dye and rubber industry, increases the risk of developing bladder cancer to **20 times** normal. The latency period varies from **15 to 45 years.**
      2. **Medical compounds. Phenacetin** abuse has been associated with an increased risk of bladder tumors.
      3. **Artificial sweeteners.** Currently, no reliable data is available to link artificial sweeteners **(saccharin, cyclamates)** to bladder cancer in humans.
      4. **Chemotherapeutic agents. A 9-fold** increased risk of carcinoma is present in those who have had prior systemic treatment with **cyclophosphamide.** Tumors usually develop after a **latency period of 5–7 years.** In addition, administration of **chlornaphazine** has been shown to increase the risk of bladder carcinoma.
   J. **Urbanization.** People in certain urban occupations have an elevated risk of bladder cancer, including **painters, printers, metal workers, textile workers, machinists, hairdressers, and truck drivers.** The increased risk in these occupations may be related to exposure to various chemical carcinogens.

III. **Clinical presentation**

A. Signs and symptoms. Although no symptoms or signs are diagnostic of bladder cancer, the following are common presenting complaints and findings:

1. **Local manifestations.** Local signs and symptoms suggesting bladder malignancies include **microscopic or gross painless hematuria (85%)** (the amount of hematuria is not proportional to tumor bulk or invasiveness); urinary **frequency, urgency, and dysuria (30%);** pelvic pain; a **"filling" defect** on intravenous pyelogram or cystogram; rectal mass and obstruction; and lower extremity edema (venous or lymphatic obstruction).

2. **Systemic manifestations.** Patients rarely present with systemic signs and symptoms of bladder cancer, but anorexia, weight loss, and bony or abdominal pain (bone or liver metastases) do occur.

B. Paraneoplastic syndromes. No known paraneoplastic syndromes are associated with bladder cancer.

IV. Differential diagnosis. Many diseases cause **hematuria** and irritative voiding symptoms. Some of them may be confused with bladder carcinoma; these include urinary tract infections, urinary calculi, benign prostatic hypertrophy, trauma, and other urinary tract malignancies.

V. Screening programs. Screening tests are not useful in the general population; however, patients with **microscopic or gross hematuria** must be fully evaluated to exclude urologic malignancies.

VI. Diagnostic workup

A. Medical history and physical examination. A complete medical history emphasizing common presenting symptoms (eg, hematuria, dysuria, frequency) and a thorough physical examination are essential components of a complete examination.

1. **Skin.** Pallor indicating anemia from urologic blood loss, although rare, should be noted.

2. **Lymph nodes.** The presence of a signal node (also called **Virchow's or Troisier's node**) must be recorded.

3. **Abdomen.** Careful examination may reveal hepatomegaly or an abdominal mass caused by enlarged para-aortic lymph nodes.

4. **Pelvis.** All patients with suspected bladder cancer should have a thorough bimanual abdominoperineal examination under anesthesia (at the time of cystoscopy) to determine local extension of the tumor.

5. **Rectum.** Careful palpation of the prostate (in the male) and other pelvic structures may demonstrate distorted anatomy, fixation, or both.

6. **Extremities.** Edema of the lower extremities from occlusion of the iliac vessels and lymphatics should be noted.

B. Primary tests and procedures. The following diagnostic tests and procedures should be obtained in all patients with suspected bladder carcinoma.

1. **Blood tests** (see p 1, **IV.A**)
   a. **Complete blood count.**
   b. **Hepatic transaminases.**
   c. **Alkaline phosphatase.**
   d. **BUN and creatinine.**

2. **Urine tests**
   a. **Urinalysis** (see p 3, **IV.B**).
   b. **Urine cytology.** Cytologic examination of voided urine or bladder washings should be performed and can detect more than **90%** of patients with Grade 3 lesions or carcinoma in situ. However, only **50%** of Grade 1 and Grade 2 lesions are discovered because they resemble normal urothelium on cytologic examination.

3. **Imaging studies**
   a. **Chest x-ray** (see p 3, **IV.C.1**).
   b. **Excretory urography.** Before cystoscopy, **an intravenous pyelogram** should be obtained to assess the upper tracts and to detect abnormalities that may require retrograde pyelography or ureteroscopy. Ureteral obstruction is associated with muscle invasion in 90% of patients. In addition, the primary tumor may appear as an intraluminal filling defect.
   c. **Technetium-99m bone scan** (see p 3, **IV.C.4**).

4. **Invasive procedures. Cystoscopy** is essential in the diagnosis of bladder cancer. Because diffuse urothelial disease (carcinoma in situ) is a possibility, biopsies adjacent to visible tumor as well as **multiple random biopsies** must be obtained. All specimens should include bladder muscle for accurate staging.

C. **Optional tests and procedures.** The following tests and procedures may be indicated by previous diagnostic findings or clinical suspicion:
  1. **Blood tests** (see p 2, **IV.A**)
      a. **Nucleotidase.**
      b. **GGTP.**
  2. **Imaging studies** (see p 3, **IV.C**)
      a. **Computed tomography (CT).** CT scan of the abdomen and pelvis to assess the status of the liver and pelvic lymph nodes is indicated **when muscle invasion is present.** CT scans, however, are less reliable in determining the extent of bladder wall or perivesical tumor involvement, especially after previous transurethral surgical resections.
      b. **Magnetic resonance imaging (MRI).** MRI may be used in patients who cannot receive intravenous contrast agents.
  3. **Invasive procedures. Proctoscopy** to exclude rectal involvement may be indicated for bulky tumors.

VII. **Pathology**
  A. **Location.** Most tumors originate on the **floor** of the bladder; however, **recurrences and adenocarcinomas** are more likely to be found on the **dome.**
  B. **Multiplicity.** Bladder cancer frequently occurs as **multiple lesions** or in association with **carcinoma in situ.**
  C. **Histology.** Most bladder cancers are epithelial in origin; **90% are transitional cell** carcinoma, 7% are squamous cell carcinomas, and 2% are adenocarcinomas. Bladder cancer is graded from 1 to 3, with the higher grade (Grade 3) lesions associated with poor differentiation.
  D. **Metastatic spread**
      1. **Modes of spread.** Bladder cancer can spread by any of the following routes:
          a. **Local extension.** Bladder cancers can directly invade contiguous structures such as the **urethra, rectum, vagina, prostate,** and **small bowel.**
          b. **Lymphatic metastasis.** The principal lymphatic drainage is to the **external iliac, obturator, and hypogastric lymph nodes.** These are the nodes most commonly involved with metastatic disease.
          c. **Hematogenous metastasis.** Spread via the **venous plexus around the bladder** results in metastases to distant organs.
      2. **Sites of spread.** Based on autopsy series, common metastatic sites for bladder carcinoma are the following: **abdominal and pelvic lymph nodes,** 80%; **lungs,** 35%; **liver,** 25%; and **bone,** 25%.

VIII. **Staging.** Traditionally, the **Marshall staging system** has been used to stage bladder cancer. However, in 1987 the American Joint Committee on Cancer and the Union Internationale Contre le Cancer jointly adopted a TNM staging system in an attempt to provide a universal staging system.
  A. **Marshall's staging system**
      1. **Stage 0.** Tumor is limited to the mucosa, including visible papillary carcinoma and carcinoma in situ.
      2. **Stage A.** Tumor invades the lamina propria but not muscle.
      3. **Stage B1.** Tumor penetrates less than halfway through muscle.
      4. **Stage B2.** Tumor penetrates farther than halfway through muscle.
      5. **Stage C.** Tumor invades perivesical fat.
      6. **Stage D1.** Pelvic lymph nodes or contiguous structures are involved.
      7. **Stage D2.** Extrapelvic lymph nodes or distant metastases are present.
  B. **TNM staging system**
      1. **Tumor stage**
          a. **TX.** Primary tumor cannot be assessed.
          b. **T0.** No evidence of primary tumor.
          c. **Tis.** Carcinoma in situ: "flat tumor."
          d. **Ta.** Noninvasive papillary carcinoma.
          e. **T1.** Tumor invades subepithelial connective tissue.
          f. **T2.** Tumor invades superficial muscle (inner half).
          g. **T3.** Tumor invades deep muscle or perivesical fat.
              (1) **T3a.** Tumor invades deep muscle (outer half).
              (2) **T3b.** Tumor invades perivesical fat.
          h. **T4.** Tumor invades any of the following: prostate, uterus, vagina, pelvic wall, abdominal wall.
      2. **Lymph node stage**
          a. **NX.** Regional lymph nodes cannot be assessed.
          b. **N0.** No regional lymph node metastases are present.

  c. **N1.** Metastasis to a single lymph node that is no larger than 2 cm in its greatest dimension.
  d. **N2.** Metastasis to a single lymph node that is larger than 2 cm but no larger than 5 cm in its greatest dimension, or to multiple lymph nodes that are smaller than 5 cm in their greatest dimension.
  e. **N3.** Metastasis to a lymph node that is larger than 5 cm in its greatest dimension

> **Note:** Regional lymph nodes include the hypogastric, obturator, internal and external iliac, perivesical, pelvic, sacral, and presacral nodes. Common iliac nodes metastases are considered distant sites, and metastases to these nodes should be coded as M1.

  3. **Metastatic stage**
     a. **MX.** Presence of distant metastasis cannot be assessed.
     b. **M0.** No distant metastases are present.
     c. **M1.** Distant metastases are present.
  4. **Histopathologic grade**
     a. **GX.** Grade cannot be assessed.
     b. **G1.** Well differentiated.
     c. **G2.** Moderately well differentiated.
     d. **G3–4.** Poorly or undifferentiated.
  5. **Stage groupings**
     a. **Stage 0.** Ta or Tis, N0, M0.
     b. **Stage I.** T1, N0, M0.
     c. **Stage II.** T2, N0, M0.
     d. **Stage III.** T3a or b, N0, M0.
     e. **Stage IV.** T4, N0, M0; any T, N1–3, M0; any T, any N, M1.

IX. Treatment
A. Surgery
  1. **Superficial bladder carcinoma**
     a. **General considerations.** Superficial transitional cell carcinomas consist of **tumors confined to the mucosa** (papillary lesions or carcinoma in situ) and those that involve **only the lamina propria** (< T1). Less than 5% of **low-grade and papillary lesions** progress to invasive disease, whereas 50% of **high-grade lesions** that involve the lamina propria progress to muscle invasion.
     b. **Procedures.** Therapy consists of **cystoscopy and transurethral resection or fulguration of all tumors.** As many as **70%** of superficial bladder tumors will recur. Neodymium yttrium-aluminum-garnet (Nd-YAG) laser fulguration of tumors may result in lower recurrence rates; however, if the laser is used, appropriate biopsies that include muscle should be obtained. Intravesical chemotherapy may be administered subsequently to help prevent recurrence (see p 316, **IX.C.1.a**).
  2. **Invasive bladder cancer**
     a. **General considerations.** Invasive carcinomas **extend into the muscle or perivesical fat** (T2 or greater).
     b. **Procedures**
        (1) **Radical cystectomy.** The most widely accepted therapy remains **bilateral pelvic lymph node dissection and radical cystectomy** (cystoprostatectomy in males). Urethrectomy is indicated when diffuse carcinoma in situ or tumor invasion into the prostatic urethra is present. In females, the bladder and urethra are removed along with the anterior vaginal wall, ureters, cervix, and fallopian tubes (anterior pelvic exenteration), with or without the ovaries (ovaries are generally preserved in patients under 45).
        (2) **Partial cystectomy.** This procedure is rarely performed and is indicated only for low-grade lesions distant from the bladder neck and ureteral orifices.
     c. **Reconstruction.** Urinary diversion is usually accomplished with an **intestinal conduit** (commonly distal ileum) or a **continent catheterizable urinary reservoir** fashioned from small bowel (eg, Koch pouch, Indiana pouch).
     d. **Morbidity and mortality.** Mortality after radical cystectomy is less than **1.5%.** Complications that can occur include the following: **prolonged ureteroileal urine leakage**, 1.9–5.5%; **prolonged ileus/small bowel obstruction**, 3–4%; **infection**, 5–10%; **stomal or ureteral stenosis.**
  3. **Locally advanced and metastatic bladder cancer.** In the face of known met-

astatic disease, **palliative cystectomy** with urinary diversion (ileal conduit) is indicated for **severe pain and intractable bleeding.** Resection of metastases is rarely indicated except in the case of **pelvic lymph nodes,** which, if removed, result in a **10–20% long-term survival.**

B. **Radiation therapy**

1. **Primary bladder carcinoma.** Definitive radiation therapy usually is indicated only for inoperable candidates. Treatment consists of **5000–7000 Cgy administered over 4–6 weeks.** Definitive radiation therapy produces **local control rates of 24–56% and a 5-year survival rate of 15–39%.** Salvage cystectomy after definitive radiation therapy has been advocated at some centers.

2. **Adjuvant radiation therapy**

   a. **Preoperative radiation therapy.** Most recent studies indicate that **1500–5000 cGy** preoperative radiation for muscle invasive lesions does not increase survival (35–52%), although it **may decrease the rate of pelvic recurrence** (88–100%).

   b. **Intraoperative radiation therapy.** Intraoperative treatment with **3250–6500 cGy** by ^{226}Ra or ^{137}Cs implants without resection, or with 2500–3000 cGy by external beam followed by postoperative radiotherapy, has an associated **56–62% overall survival.**

   c. **Postoperative radiation therapy.** Radiotherapy given in the postoperative period, often for positive surgical margins, has yielded mixed results. In one study, a "**sandwich**" technique of **500 cGy preoperatively, followed by 4500 cGy postoperatively,** reportedly resulted in improved disease-free and overall survival, but this has not been confirmed in prospective trials.

3. **Bladder preservation.** Trials combining radiation along with cisplatin-based chemotherapy are currently ongoing to determine the feasibility of bladder preservation.

4. **Morbidity and mortality.** Radiation therapy of primary bladder carcinoma has a **15% rate of major complications.** Difficulties that can develop include **dysuria** (70%), **diarrhea** (70%), **hemorrhagic cystitis,** and **enterovesical and other fistulae.**

C. **Chemotherapy**

1. **Primary bladder carcinoma**

   a. **Intravesical chemotherapy.** Intravesical chemotherapy is used for patients with **recurrent superficial disease or carcinoma in situ.** Patients with multiple mucosal lesions or lamina propria invasion are candidates. Intravesical agents include **thiotepa, doxorubicin, mitomycin-C,** and **BCG** and are generally given weekly for 6–8 weeks with re-evaluation by cystoscopy and biopsy after 3 months. Generally, these agents have **complete response rates of 35–80%.** Currently, **BCG is most widely used** with a **response rate of > 80%.**

   b. **Systemic chemotherapy.** Primary curative chemotherapy is administered as a multidrug regimen. Recently, **MVAC (methotrexate, vinblastine, doxorubicin and cisplatin)** therapy has produced **complete regressions in 30% of patients with transitional cell tumors.** However, its efficacy for existing carcinoma in situ, prevention of future tumors, or for the treatment of nontransitional cell carcinoma has not been proved.

2. **Adjuvant chemotherapy.** Studies examining the efficacy of postoperative adjuvant chemotherapy with **fluorouracil, methotrexate, cisplatin, vinblastine, and mitomycin-C** have failed to demonstrate an impact on survival; however, the number of patients evaluated has been small. Preoperative adjuvant chemotherapy **(neoadjuvant chemotherapy)** with **cisplatin and MVAC combined with radiotherapy** in the treatment of muscle-invasive bladder tumors (Stages II–IV) has been shown by the National Bladder Cancer Group and others to produce **75–77% complete responses and 35–46% overall 5-year survival.** Currently, neoadjuvant therapy is being evaluated to determine whether such therapy will allow more frequent use of bladder-preserving surgical procedures.

3. **Metastatic bladder carcinoma**

   a. **Single agents.** Many chemical agents have been used in the therapy of bladder malignancies with moderate rates of response. **Methotrexate** (40 mg/M^2 IV weekly; 30–45% response rate) and **cisplatin** (70 mg/M^2 IV monthly; 30% response rate) are the most active. Complete responses are rare, however. Others include 10-deazaaminopterin (20%), doxorubicin (17%), vinblastine (16%), fluorouracil (15%), and mitomycin-C (13%).

   b. **Combination regimens.** Although innumerable combination regimens have been used, common combinations include **MVAC, CISCA or CAP** (cyclophosphamide, doxorubicin, and cisplatin), **CM** (cisplatin and methotrexate), **and CMV** (cisplatin, methotrexate, and vinblastine), which have response rates of **55–76%, 41–51%, 38–54%, and 42–70%,** respectively. Despite their increased response rates over single agents, combination regimens have **not increased overall survival.**

D. **Immunotherapy**
1. **Primary bladder carcinoma**
   a. **Intravesical therapy. BCG** response rates are reported by some to be as high as **80–100%** in preventing or treating recurrence, and many consider it to be the most effective intravesical agent. Studies using **intravesical IL-2 and alpha-interferon** have recently been initiated and show early promise.
   b. **Systemic therapy.** Oral BCG has been evaluated without any documented efficacy. Trials using **oral Brompirimine,** an oral biologic response modifier, are underway.
2. **Adjuvant immunotherapy.** No major studies have been done on immunotherapy as an adjuvant treatment for bladder malignancies.
3. **Metastatic bladder carcinoma.** To date, no data support the use of immunotherapy in metastatic bladder cancer.

X. **Prognosis**
A. **Risk of recurrence.** The risk of local recurrence varies with the stage of disease and the type of surgical resection. Risks of recurrence (by Marshall stage) are listed below:
1. **Stage 0/A.** Treated with transurethral resection (TUR), 48–70% (most within 2 years).
2. **Stage B.** Treated with TUR, more than 90%.
3. **Stage B.** Treated with cystectomy, 30%.
4. **Stage C/D.** Higher than 95% regardless of surgical procedure.
B. **Five-year survival.** Five-year survival varies with the stage of disease. The following are typical 5-year survival rates by Marshall stage:
1. **Stage 0/A,** 60–83%.
2. **Stage B1,** 41–70%.
3. **Stage B2/C,** 17–53%.
4. **Stage D,** less than 2%.
C. **Adverse prognostic factors.** The following findings are associated with a particularly poor outcome: **large primary tumor size; advanced stage,** particularly those with positive pelvic lymph nodes; and **high-grade lesion.**

XI. **Patient follow-up**
A. **General guidelines.** Patients with bladder carcinoma should be evaluated for recurrence every 3 months for 2 years, every 6 months for an additional 3 years, then annually thereafter. The following specific guidelines for tests and procedures are recommended.
B. **Routine evaluation.** The following examinations should be obtained with each clinic visit.
1. **History and physical examination.** An interval history and complete physical examination are mandatory during routine office visits. Special attention should be paid to those areas listed under **VI.A.** above
2. **Blood tests** (see p 1, **IV.A**)
   a. **Complete blood count.**
   b. **Hepatic transaminases.**
   c. **Alkaline phosphatase.**
   d. **BUN and creatinine.**
3. **Urinalysis** (see p 3, **IV.B**)
4. **Urinary cytology** (see p 313, **VI.B.2.b**)
5. **Chest x-ray** (see p 3, **IV.C.1**)
C. **Additional evaluation.** Other tests and procedures that should be performed at regular intervals include the following:
1. **Cystoscopy.** In patients with superficial bladder cancer who have not undergone cystectomy, follow-up cystoscopy should be performed every **3 months for 2 years, every 6 months for 2 years, and yearly thereafter.**
2. **Excretory urography.** In patients with urinary diversion, close follow-up of the upper tracts with annual intravenous pyelogram or ultrasound is necessary.
3. **Urethroscopy.** In males who have undergone radical cystectomy without urethrectomy, the urethra should be periodically studied by either urethroscopy or urethral washings for cytology.
D. **Optional evaluation.** The following tests may be indicated by previous diagnostic

findings or clinical suspicion in patients who have undergone cystectomy or received synthetic chemotherapy.

1. **Blood tests** (see p 2, **IV.A**)
   a. **Nucleotidase.**
   b. **GGTP.**
2. **Imaging studies**
   a. **Computerized tomography.** If signs or symptoms of liver or lung metastases develop, CT is useful in the evaluation of these organs. This test is not universally obtained, however, in the routine follow-up of patients.
   b. **Magnetic resonance imaging (MRI).**
   c. **Technetium-99m bone scan.**

REFERENCES

Droller MJ. Transitional cell cancer; upper tracts and bladder. In Walsh PC, editor. *Campbell's Urology*, vol 2. Philadelphia: Saunders; 1986:1343–1440.

Klotz LK. Management of urothelial carcinoma of the upper tracts. *AUA Update* Series 7: Lesson 4, 1988.

Lamm DL, DeHaven JI, Shriver J, et al. A randomized prospective comparison of oral versus intravesical and percutaneous BCG for superficial bladder cancer. *J Urol* 1990:**144:**65–67.

Mohiuddin M, Kramer S, Newall J, et al. Combined preoperative and postoperative radiation therapy for bladder cancer. *Cancer* 1985:**55:**963–966.

Ross RK, Paganine-Hill A, Henderson B. Epidemiology of bladder cancer. In Skinner DG. *Diagnosis and Management of Genitourinary Cancer*. Philadelphia: Saunders; 1988:23–31.

Scher HI, Yagoda A, Herr HW, et al. Neoadjuvant M-VAC (methotrexate, vinblastine, doxorubicin and cisplatin): Effect on the primary bladder lesion. *J Urol* 1988:**139:**470–474.

Skinner DG, Liekovsky G. Management of invasive and high-grade bladder cancer. In Skinner DG, editor. *Diagnosis and Management of Genitourinary Cancer*. Saunders; Philadelphia: 1988:295–312.

Soloway MS. Introduction and overview of intravesical therapy for superficial bladder cancer. *Urology* 1988:**31** (Supl 3):5–16.

Tanagho EA, McAninch JW. *Smith's General Urology*, 12th ed. Norwalk, CT: Appleton & Lange; 1988.

Wein AJ, Hanno PM, editors. *A Clinical Manual of Urology*. Norwalk, CT: Appleton-Century-Crofts; 1988.

42 Malignancies of the Urethra

Michael Grasso, MD, and Leonard Gomella, MD

I. **Epidemiology.** Carcinoma of the urethra is **rare**. Approximately 600 cases in men and 1100 cases in women have been reported in the world literature. Worldwide, the variation in incidence is not precisely known.

II. **Risk factors**
- A. **Age.** The incidence of urethral carcinoma increases between the fifth and eighth decade of life, with **a peak instance at 58 years and 75% occurring in patients older than 50 years.**
- B. **Sex.** The risk for females is **4.6 times** greater than for males.
- C. **Race.** The risk for whites, especially females, is **7 times greater** than for blacks.
- D. **Genetic factors.** The incidence in first-degree relatives is not known to be higher than that of the general population.
- E. **Previous genitourinary pathology**
  1. **Infection**
     - a. **Venereal disease.** As many as **44%** of patients with urethral carcinoma have a history of **sexually transmitted diseases.**
     - b. **Urethritis. Chronic inflammation** of the urethra secondary to bacterial and viral infections has been associated with urethral malignancies.
  2. **Anatomic abnormalities**
     - a. **Urethral strictures.** The presence of urethral strictures closely correlates with the development of urethral tumors. Concomitant strictures and cancer occur in as many as **25–80% of male patients.**
     - b. **Urethral diverticulum.** Urethral cancer occurring in diverticula has been reported. **Urinary stasis and chronic irritation** are two predisposing factors.
  3. **Other neoplasms.** There is a direct correlation between **bladder cancer** and that of **urethral carcinoma.**

III. **Clinical presentation**
- A. **Signs and symptoms**
  1. **Local manifestations.** Common symptoms, such as **urinary frequency, hesitancy, and dysuria,** usually arise from irritation. Other complaints may include urethral discharge, hematuria, fistulae, inguinal masses, and incontinence. In males, **priapism** and penile abnormalities may be the initial presenting symptoms. In females, **vaginal discharge or bleeding** may represent tumor erosion through the vaginal wall. A **palpable mass (39%) and periurethral collections or phlegmon (31%)** also occur.
  2. **Systemic manifestations.** Symptoms of systemic spread rarely occur because of the pronounced local symptoms that precede the development of metastases.
- B. **Paraneoplastic syndromes.** No paraneoplastic syndromes are known to be associated with urethral carcinoma.

IV. **Differential diagnosis.** Voiding symptoms **(frequency, hesitancy,** and **dysuria)** are produced by both benign and malignant diseases. Common conditions that can be confused with urethral carcinoma include **anatomic abnormalities** (urethral stricture and diverticulae), **gynecologic malignancies, prostatic hypertrophy, urethral caruncle, and other urologic neoplasms** (bladder carcinoma).

V. **Screening programs.** Any patient with a chronic inflammatory process within the urethra and male patients who have undergone a cystectomy for bladder malignancies are at a much higher risk for tumor recurrence within the urethra and should be screened with **annual urinary cytologies and a cystoscopic or urethroscopic** examination.

VI. **Diagnostic workup**
- A. **Medical history and physical examination.** A complete medical history emphasizing common presenting complaints and a thorough physical examination are essential in the initial patient evaluation.

319

1. **Lymph nodes.** The presence of a signal node (also called **Virchow's or Troisier's node**) must be recorded.
2. **Abdomen.** Hepatomegaly and abdominal masses may be detected and should be carefully described.
3. **Groin.** Palpable inguinal lymph nodes should be fully described, including their consistency, size, number, and the clinical likelihood of metastatic disease.
4. **Genitalia.** Palpation of the male urethra along the course of the penis and the perineum may show a **periurethral mass**. In the female, bimanual vaginal examination, palpating the urethra between two fingers, may detect a **urethral mass**. Extension into the vagina, rectum, and prostate also should be noted.

B. **Primary tests and procedures.** All patients with suspected urethral carcinoma should undergo the following diagnostic tests and procedures:
  1. **Blood tests** (see p 1, **IV.A**)
    a. **Complete blood count**
    b. **Hepatic transaminases.**
    c. **Alkaline phosphatase.**
  2. **Urine tests**
    a. **Urinalysis** (see p 3, **IV.B**).
    b. **Urine cytology.** Urethral washings and urine cytology can detect **88–100%** of urethral carcinomas.
  3. **Imaging studies**
    a. **Chest x-ray** (see p 3, **IV.C.1**).
    b. **Retrograde urethrogram.** This simple radiologic test may show **irregular strictures, fistulae, or diverticula** with intraluminal filling defects.
    c. **Excretory urography. Intravenous pyelogram (IVP)** is indicated to exclude multifocal transitional cell tumors and upper urinary tract disease.
  4. **Invasive procedures**
    a. **Urethroscopy.** Urethroscopy and biopsy of suspicious areas within the urethra will confirm the diagnosis of malignancy.
    b. **Cystoscopy.** A complete cystoscopic examination is important to exclude a **concurrent bladder malignancy**.

C. **Optional tests and procedures.** The following tests and procedures may be indicated based on previous diagnostic findings or clinical suspicion.
  1. **Blood tests** (see p 2, **IV.A**)
    a. **Nucleotidase.**
    b. **GGTP.**
  2. **Imaging studies**
    a. **Barium enema.** This radiologic test may be indicated if rectal symptoms or masses are discovered.
    b. **Computed tomography (CT).** Abdominal and pelvic CT scans are helpful in determining the local extension of tumor and the status of regional lymph nodes.
    c. **Magnetic resonance imaging (MRI).** (see p 3, **IV.C.2**).
    d. **Technetium-99m bone scan.** (see p 3, **IV.C.4**).
  3. **Invasive procedures**
    a. **Colposcopy.** This procedure should be performed in all females to exclude invasion of the anterior vaginal wall and the existence of gynecologic (vaginal and cervical) neoplasms.
    b. **Proctosigmoidoscopy.** Direct visualization of the distal colon and rectum may be required if evidence or symptoms of rectal invasion are present.

VII. **Pathology**
A. **Location**
  1. **Males.** Most tumors arise in the **bulbomembranous (60%) or penile (35%) urethra,** which are also the most common sites of benign strictures. Malignancies within the **prostatic urethra** constitute only 5% of tumors.
  2. **Females.** The majority of malignancies arise in the **proximal two-thirds** of the urethra.
B. **Multiplicity.** Multiple lesions are rare.
C. **Histology**
  1. **Males. Squamous carcinoma** is the most common malignancy in the **anterior two-thirds** of the urethra (penile and bulbomembranous urethra). In the **penile urethra, 86%** of the tumors are **squamous carcinoma,** whereas 14% are transitional cell. In the **bulbomembranous urethra, 83% are squamous cell tumors,** 8% are transitional cell cancers, and 7% are adenocar-

cinomas. In the **posterior urethra,** the **vast majority are transitional cell carcinomas.**

2. **Females.** As with males, **70% of the tumors in the anterior portion of the urethra are epidermoid lesions.** In one series, 18% of tumors located anteriorly were adenocarcinomas. **Transitional cell neoplasms** constitute **10%** of all lesions and are found **posteriorly.**

D. **Metastatic spread**
1. **Modes of spread.** Urethral tumors spread by 3 mechanisms:
   a. **Direct extension.** Lesions may invade the anterior vaginal wall, the base of the bladder, prostate, and, in advanced cases, the rectum.
   b. **Lymphatic metastasis.**
      (1) **Males.** The lymphatic drainage of the **anterior urethra** is to the **deep inguinal and external iliac lymph nodes.** The **bulbomembranous and prostatic urethral** drainage is to the **internal and external iliac, obturator, and presacral nodes.** When skin is invaded, there also may be spread to the superficial inguinal nodes.
      (2) **Females. Distal urethral** lesions commonly spread to the **superficial and deep inguinal lymph nodes.** The more proximal urethra is drained by both the obturator and external iliac nodes. In females, these rules are not absolute: ie, pelvic nodal metastases have been noted from anterior urethral lesions.
   c. **Hematogenous metastasis.** Tumor cells can gain access to systemic blood vessels, and can spread to distant sites.
2. **Sites of spread.** Common sites involved in the distant spread of urethral carcinoma include the following organs: **lung, liver, and bone.**

VIII. **Staging.** Previously, staging of urethral carcinoma divided tumors into Stages A–D. However, in 1987 the American Joint Committee on Cancer and the Union Internationale Contre le Cancer jointly developed a uniform TNM staging system for use in future reporting.

A. **Traditional staging system**
1. **Stage 0.** Tumor is confined to mucosa only (in situ).
2. **Stage A.** Tumor invades the lamina propria but not beyond.
3. **Stage B.** Tumor invades muscle in the female or invades into but not beyond the substance of the corpus spongiosum or the prostate in males.
4. **Stage C.** Tumor invades periurethral structures: eg, in females, the vagina, bladder, labia and clitoris; in males, direct extension into tissues beyond the corpus spongiosum (surrounding musculature, fat, facia, skin, and beyond the prostate capsule).
5. **Stage D1.** Regional lymph node metastases to inguinal or pelvic lymph nodes.
6. **Stage D2.** Metastases to distant sites or to lymph nodes above the aortic bifurcation.

B. **TNM staging system (male and female)**
1. **Tumor stage**
   a. **TX.** Primary tumor cannot be assessed.
   b. **T0.** No evidence of primary tumor.
   c. **Tis.** Carcinoma in situ.
   d. **Ta.** Noninvasive papillary, polypoid, or verrucous carcinoma.
   e. **T1.** Tumor invades subepithelial connective tissue.
   f. **T2.** Tumor invades the corpus spongiosum, prostate, or periurethral muscle.
   g. **T3.** Tumor invades the corpus cavernosum, beyond prostatic capsule, the anterior vagina, or the bladder neck.
   h. **T4.** Tumor invades other adjacent organs.
2. **Lymph node stage**
   a. **NX.** Regional lymph nodes cannot be assessed.
   b. **N0.** No regional lymph node metastasis.
   c. **N1.** Metastasis in a single lymph node no larger than 2 cm in its greatest dimension.
   d. **N2.** Metastasis in a single lymph node that is larger than 2 cm but no larger than 5 cm in its greatest dimension.
   e. **N3.** Metastasis in a lymph node that is larger than 5 cm in greatest dimension.
3. **Metastatic stage**
   a. **MX.** Presence of distant metastasis cannot be assessed.
   b. **M0.** No distant metastases are present.

        c. M1. Distant metastases are present.
    4. Histopathologic grade
        a. GX. Grade cannot be assessed.
        b. G1. Well differentiated.
        c. G2. Moderately well differentiated.
        d. G3–4. Poorly differentiated or undifferentiated.
    5. Stage groupings
        a. Stage 0. Tis or Ta, N0, M0.
        b. Stage I. T1, N0, M0.
        c. Stage II. T2, N0, M0.
        d. Stage III. T1–2, N1, M0; T3, N0–1, M0.
        e. Stage IV. T4, N0–1, M0; any T, N2–3, M0; any T, any N, M1.
IX. Treatment
  A. Surgery
    1. Primary urethral carcinoma
      a. Indications. Surgical resection is indicated for cure of resectable disease as well as for palliation of locally advanced and metastatic disease.
      b. Procedures
        (1) Male. Anterior urethral tumors can require **transurethral local resection** (small, low-grade lesions), **partial or complete penectomy, or partial or total emasculation**. Posterior urethral lesions involving the bulbomembranous and prostatic urethras necessitate extensive en bloc procedures because of a high local recurrence rate. In addition, **cystoprostatectomy and resection of the public rami and symphysis pubis** may be needed.
        (2) Female. Low-grade, exophytic, distal lesions only require **urethrectomy**, whereas **radical cystectomy with urinary diversion** is necessary for more proximal tumors. Endoscopic resection of low-grade tumors has been described.
        (3) Lymphadenectomy. Regional lymphadenectomy is controversial in patients with urethral carcinoma. Lymphadenectomy in all patients with **anterior** urethral lesions, including those with clinically negative nodes **(prophylactic lymphadenectomy),** and lymphadenectomy in only those patients with clinically positive nodes **(therapeutic lymphadenectomy)** have been advocated. With more **proximal** lesions, however, agreement exists that **staging bilateral pelvic lymphadenectomy** should be performed in all patients along with radical en bloc resection of the primary lesion.
    2. Locally advanced and metastatic urethral cancer. Surgery is rarely indicated for advanced metastatic disease unless severe local symptoms from primary or metastatic deposits demand a palliative resection.
    3. Mortality and morbidity. The nature and rate of complications vary, depending on the location of the primary lesions, and include the following problems: **hemorrhage; infection; urethral stricture; lower extremity edema,** secondary to superficial or deep inguinal lymph node dissection; and **sterility.**
  B. Radiation therapy
    1. Primary urethral carcinoma. In **females,** the highest rate of local control is achieved with **anterior lesions.** Both external-beam and brachytherapy have been used. Radiation therapy is **less valuable** in the treatment of **posterior lesions in females and in all urethral tumors in males**.
    2. Adjuvant radiation therapy. Radiation therapy has been used both pre- and postoperatively with some limited success.
    3. Locally advanced and metastatic urethral cancer. Radiation therapy can be used in an attempt to palliate advanced and metastatic lesions.
    4. Mortality and morbidity. Although mortality from radiation therapy is exceedingly rare, complications are far more common **(42%)** and include the following: **urethral stricture**, vesicovaginal and urethrovaginal **fistulae**, radiation **cystitis**, radiation enteritis and proctitis, **osteonecrosis** of the symphysis pubis, small bowel obstruction.
  C. Chemotherapy
    1. Primary urethral carcinoma. There is no role for treatment of primary lesions in the absence of metastases with systemic chemotherapy.
    2. Adjuvant chemotherapy. Because of the uncommon nature of these lesions,

no studies have been performed to assess the success of adjuvant chemotherapy.

3. **Locally advanced and metastatic urethral cancer**
   a. **Single-agent therapy.** Because of the low incidence of these tumors and the relative success of combination chemotherapy regimens, little is known about the relative effectiveness of single chemical agents.
   b. **Combination chemotherapy.** Chemotherapy with **methotrexate, vincristine, doxorubicin, and cyclophosphamide (MVAC;** see p 317, **IX.C)** may be effective with transitional cell carcinoma.

D. **Immunotherapy.** No data is available on the use of immunotherapy in the treatment of urethral tumors.

X. Prognosis

A. **Risk of recurrence.** Recurrences after potentially curative treatment occur in **45–65%** of patients and most often recur **locally.**

B. **Five-year survival**
   1. **Males. Proximal** lesions present earlier than distal tumors and have a better prognosis. Of patients who refuse treatment, **96% will die within 3 months.** Five-year survival rates depend on the location and stage of the primary lesion.
      a. **Location**
         (1) **Penile urethra,** 50%.
         (2) **Prostatic urethra,** 50%.
         (3) **Bulbomembranous urethra,** 8%.
      b. **Stage**
         (1) **Noninfiltrating lesions,** 50%.
         (2) **Infiltrating lesions,** 8%.
   2. **Females.** The **overall 5-year survival rate is 31%.** As with male cancers, 5-year survival rates vary, depending on location: **anterior urethra,** 47%, and **posterior urethra,** 11%.

C. **Adverse prognostic signs.** Although no correlation exists between survival and patient age, duration of symptoms, or tumor grade or histology, the following factors have been associated with adverse clinical outcomes: size larger than 3 cm and posterior location.

XI. Patient follow-up

A. **General guidelines.** Patients should be followed every 3 months for 2 years, every 6 months for an additional 3 years, then annually thereafter. Local recurrences are common and are potentially curable. The following specific guidelines are recommended.

B. **Routine evaluation.** Each clinic visit should include the following tests and procedures.
   1. **Medical history and physical examination.** An interval history and thorough physical examination should be performed during all routine clinic appointments. Particular attention should be focused on the areas outlined on p 319, **VI.A).**
   2. **Blood tests** (p 1, **IV.A)**
      a. **Complete blood count.**
      b. **Hepatic transaminases.**
      c. **Alkaline phosphatase.**
   3. **Urinalysis** (see p 3, **IV.B)**
   4. **Urine cytology.** Patients who undergo endoscopic resection of low-grade exophytic lesions should be followed by serial cytologies.
   5. **Chest x-ray** (see p 3, **IV.C.1)**
   6. **Urethroscopy.** Patients who undergo endoscopic resection of low-grade exophytic lesions should be followed by serial urethroscopy.

C. **Additional evaluation.** Other tests and procedures that should be obtained at regular intervals include the following examinations.
   1. **Computed tomography (CT).** CT scans of the abdomen and pelvis are performed every 6–12 months to evaluate both regional and distant lymph nodes as well as other visceral metastases.
   2. **Cystourethroscopy.** Direct visualization of the remaining urethra and bladder should be performed every 6 months to exclude recurrence or a new bladder carcinoma.

D. **Optional evaluation.** The following tests and procedures may be indicated based on previous diagnostic findings or clinical suspicion.

1. **Nucleotidase** (see p 2, **IV.A.4**).
2. **GGTP** (see p 2, **IV.A.5**).
3. **Magnetic resonance imaging** (see p 3, **IV.C.2**).

REFERENCES

Prempree T, Amoremarn R, Patanaphan V. Radiation therapy in primary carcinoma of the female urethra. *Cancer* 1984;**54**:729–733.

Sarosdy MF. Urethral Carcinoma. AUA Update VI, Number 13, 1987.

Skinner EC, Skinner DG. Management of carcinoma of the female urethra. In: Skinner DG, Lieskovsky, editors. *Genitourinary Cancer*. Philadelphia: Saunders, 1988.

43 Malignancies of the Prostate

Leonard Gomella, MD, and James Stephanelli, MD

I. **Epidemiology.** Carcinoma of the prostate is the **most common malignancy** in males and the **second leading cause of cancer deaths.** In 1985, **85.5** cases per 100,000 males were diagnosed, leading to **23.5 deaths.** Approximately **165,000 new cases and 35,000 deaths** will occur in 1993. Worldwide, the incidence is high in northwestern Europe and North America and lower in the Orient. Sweden, Norway, and Switzerland report deaths rates of 28.5—32.3 per 100,000, whereas Japan, Hong Kong, and Shanghai experience fewer than 3.6 deaths per 100,000.

II. **Risk factors**
   A. **Age.** Prostate cancer steadily increases from less than 1.0 per 100,000 in males younger than 40 years to **1146 per 100,000 by age 85.** The median age at diagnosis is 70.5 years, and autopsy series indicate that 70% of males older than 90 have at least one focus of prostatic carcinoma.
   B. **Race.** The risk for **blacks** is **1.5 times** greater than for whites, with as many as 125.5 cases per 100,000. In addition, blacks tend to develop cancer at a **younger age.**
   C. **Genetic factors.** The risk for first-degree relatives is slightly higher than for the general population.
   D. **Diet.** High-fat diets have been implicated in the pathogenesis of prostatic carcinoma.
   E. **Previous genitourinary pathology**
      1. **Endocrine factors.** Prostatic carcinoma does not occur in eunuchs. Although **testosterone** is not a direct cause, it may be **permissive** for the development of clinical carcinoma.
      2. **Infections.** A possible **venereal vector** may be responsible for the direct correlation between the incidence of prostate cancer and the frequency of sexual activity; however, this remains unproved.
   F. **Chemical agents. Cadmium** has been implicated in the etiology of prostate cancer, possibly because it is **antagonistic to zinc.**

III. **Clinical presentation**
   A. **Signs and symptoms.** Although early prostatic carcinoma is usually asymptomatic and can be found in as many as **10% of transurethral prostatic resection specimens,** signs and symptoms suggestive of prostate cancer may include the following:
      1. **Local manifestations.** Local tumor growth produces bladder irritation and outlet obstruction with **hesitancy, nocturia, and frequency,** acute urinary retention **(25% of patients with obstruction harbor a malignancy),** hematuria (uncommon), and renal insufficiency from ureteral obstruction (localized disease or metastatic adenopathy).
      2. **Systemic manifestations. Back and hip pain** from bony metastases are the most common complaints, along with pain in the extremities (20–40%) and, occasionally, paralysis (extradural metastases) signifying systemic dissemination. Other systemic symptoms include fatigue, malaise, and weight loss.
   B. **Paraneoplastic syndromes.** No paraneoplastic syndromes are typically associated with prostate cancer.

IV. **Differential diagnosis.** Carcinoma of the prostate is often asymptomatic and is commonly discovered as a **"nodule"** on routine digital rectal examination. Other causes of prostatic nodules include **benign prostatic hypertrophy, granulomatous prostatitis, previous prostatic surgery, and prostatic infarction.**

V. **Screening programs.** Annual digital transrectal examination of the prostate and **serum PSA** is recommended for **all males between age 50 and 70.** Screening is recommended starting at age 40 in patients with a family history of prostate cancer.

VI. Diagnostic workup

A. Medical history and physical examination. A complete medical history emphasizing common presenting symptoms and a thorough physical examination are essential in the evaluation of patients with possible prostatic cancer.

1. **General appearance.** A quick assessment of the patient's functional status should be made.

2. **Lymph nodes.** The presence of a signal node (also called **Virchow's or Troisier's node**) must be recorded.

3. **Abdomen.** Hepatic and intra-abdominal (lymphatic) masses caused by metastases generally are very late manifestations of disease.

4. **Rectum.** The normal prostate is a **rubbery mass slightly larger than a chestnut** (about 3–4 cm). The lateral margins should be distinct (obliteration suggests cancer), and the **seminal vesicles should be nonpalpable** (palpable vesicles are usually cancerous). A hard, nodular, or indurated prostate discovered on routine digital rectal examination may be the first indication of cancer. Approximately **30–50% of prostatic nodules prove to be malignant.**

B. Primary tests and procedures. The following examinations should be performed in all patients with suspected prostate cancer:

1. **Blood tests**
   a. **Complete blood count** (see p 1, **IV.A.1**).
   b. **Hepatic transaminases** (see p 1, **IV.A.2**).
   c. **Alkaline phosphatase** (see p 1, **IV.A.3**).
   d. **BUN and creatinine.** Locally advanced disease or lymphatic metastases can cause ureteral obstruction and renal impairment.
   e. **Prostatic acid phosphatase (PAP).** PAP is elevated in 80% of patients with metastatic disease, 30% of those with local extracapsular extension, and in 4–10% of those with disease contained within the prostate. A normal PAP is 0.8 IU/L. Nonprostatic causes of elevated serum levels include osteogenic sarcoma, osteoporosis, Gaucher's disease, hyperthyroidism, hyperparathyroidism, liver diseases, and erythropoietic disorders. The routine use of PAP is declining.
   f. **Prostatic specific antigen (PSA).** PSA, a protease produced by normal and neoplastic prostatic uroepithelial cells, can be **elevated in carcinoma, benign hypertrophy, and prostatitis.** It may be useful in documenting recurrences following therapy with curative intent. In general, PSA should be less than **0.2 ng/mL after radical prostatectomy, and less than 4 ng/mL in normal males** (monoclonal assay). Values in the range of 4–10 ng/mL may be the result of either cancer or benign enlargement, whereas values **greater than 10 ng/mL most commonly denote carcinoma.** Massively enlarged benign prostate glands occasionally can produce such elevations. **Routine digital rectal exam will not elevate the PSA.** PSA should not be ordered if a patient is experiencing acute prostatitis or for 2–3 weeks after a biopsy of the prostate.

2. **Imaging studies**
   a. **Chest x-ray** (see p 3, **IV.C.1**).
   b. **Excretory urography or ultrasound.** Intravenous pyelogram (IVP) or renal ultrasound may be required to exclude **urinary obstruction** and hydronephrosis.
   c. **Technetium-99m bone scan** (see p 3, **IV.C.4**). Bone scans are used to evaluate for metastatic disease, since bone is a common site of metastasis.

3. **Invasive procedures**
   a. **Prostatic biopsy.** Prostatic biopsy should be performed in all patients. Because carcinoma usually arises from the posterior portion of the prostate, transurethral prostatic biopsy is not optimal. The two most commonly used routes are **transrectal and transperineal.**
      (1) **Fine needle aspiration.** The diagnosis also can be made via fine needle aspiration of the prostate, although well-differentiated carcinomas can be difficult to detect with this technique.
      (2) **Core needle biopsy.** Currently, this is considered the "**gold standard**" in the United States.
         (a) **Transrectal core biopsy.** Although the transrectal route is slightly more accurate than transperineal biopsy, more frequent complications occur, such as acute bacterial prostatitis, septicemia, and bleeding.
         (b) **Transperineal core biopsy.** This technique has fewer complica-

tions than the transrectal approach, although it is slightly less accurate.

    b. Transrectal ultrasound (TRUS). Generally, prostatic cancer appears **"hypoechoic"** on TRUS; however, recent reports suggest that as many as 40% of tumors may be "isoechoic." TRUS does provide accurate information about local capsular penetration and seminal vesical involvement. In addition, it is a useful guide to needle biopsy of the prostate.

C. Optional evaluation. The following tests and procedures may be indicated by prior diagnostic findings or clinical suspicion.

    1. Blood tests (see p 2, **IV.A**)

        a. Nucleotidase.

        b. GGTP.

    2. Imaging studies

        a. Computerized tomography (CT). Abdominal and pelvic CT scan can be useful for determining the extent of local and lymphatic disease. However, microscopic disease is not detected.

        b. Magnetic resonance imaging (MRI). With recent advances (eg, endorectal coil), MRI has become the most accurate imaging method for assessing local tumor spread, however it can still understage many cases.

        c. Pedal lymphangiogram. This uncomfortable examination can provide information about the status of pelvic and intra-abdominal lymph nodes.

        d. Cystoscopy. Although cystoscopy can be performed at the time of biopsy in the operating room, it is not required for the definitive diagnosis of prostate cancer.

VII. Pathology

    A. Location. The **peripheral zone** of the prostate is the most common site for carcinoma, **75% of which occur in the posterior lobe.**

    B. Multiplicity. As many as **85%** of prostate cancers have been shown to be multifocal.

    C. Histology. The majority of prostate malignancies are **acinar adenocarcinomas.** Generally, the malignant acini tend to be closely packed and lined by a single layer of cuboidal epithelium. Although many grading systems exist, most grading is done according to **Gleason's system,** which considers the degree of glandular differentiation and the relationship of the glands to the stroma. Tumors are assigned a total **Gleason score** (ranging from 2 to 10) that represents **the sum of the two most common grades** seen in the tumor (from 1 = well differentiated, 5 = poorly differentiated). Generally, higher scores correlate with a greater likelihood of lymphatic involvement. Rarely, transitional cell carcinomas, lymphomas, and metastatic lesions are found in the prostate.

    D. Metastatic spread

        1. Modes of spread. Prostate cancer can spread by three distinct mechanisms.

            a. Direct extension. Local growth most commonly involves the **seminal vesicles and pelvic side walls. Obstruction of the bladder outlet or ureter** is seen in 35% of cases. Because of the presence of the relatively tough **Denonvillier's fascia,** rectal involvement is rare **(< 10%).**

            b. Lymphatic metastasis. Spread through lymphatic channels to the obturator and iliac lymph nodes occurs frequently. The risk of lymph node metastases by American Urological Association (AUA) state is outlined below:

                (1) A_1, 2%.

                (2) A_2, 23%.

                (3) B_1, 18%.

                (4) B_2, 35%.

                (5) C, 46%.

            c. Hematogenous metastasis. Spread through systemic blood vessels commonly results in distant metastases. **Batson's venous plexus** (vertebral veins), especially, has been implicated in spread to local bony sites, although this mechanism has been questioned.

        2. Sites of spread. The most common sites involved with metastatic prostate carcinoma include the following organs: **bone,** overwhelmingly the most common site and frequently producing **osteoblastic lesions; lung,** 49%; liver, 35%; adrenal, 17%; kidney, 10%.

VIII. Staging. The most common system is the **Whitmore and Jewett staging system** (AUA), but in 1987 the American Joint Committee on Cancer and the Union Internationale Contre le Cancer developed a joint TNM system that has been proposed as a uniform staging system.

A. AUA staging system
    1. Stage A. No palpable lesion.
      a. Stage A_1. Focal disease.
      b. Stage A_2. Diffuse disease.
    2. Stage B. Disease is confined to the prostate.
      a. Stage B_1. A small discrete nodule is present.
      b. Stage B_2. Multiple nodules or a single large nodule is present.
    3. Stage C. Disease localized to the periprostatic area.
      a. Stage C_1. No seminal vesicle involvement and tumor weighs no more than 70 g.
      b. Stage C_2. Seminal vesicles are involved or tumor weighs more than 70 g.
    4. Stage D. Metastatic disease is present.
      a. Stage D_0. Elevated tumor markers alone are present.
      b. Stage D_1. Pelvic lymph node metastases or urethral obstruction causing hydronephrosis are present.
      c. Stage D_2. Metastases to bone, distant organs, soft tissues, or distant lymph nodes are present.
      d. Stage D_3. Tumor is refractory to hormone therapy.
B. TNM staging system
    1. Tumor stage
      a. TX. Primary tumor cannot be assessed.
      b. T0. No evidence of a primary tumor is present.
      c. T1. Tumor is discovered incidentally on histology:
        (1) T1a. Three or fewer less microscopic foci are present.
        (2) T1b. Three microscopic foci are present.
      d. T2. Tumor is clinically or grossly limited to the gland.
        (1) T2a. Tumor is no larger than 1.5 cm in its greatest dimension, with normal tissue present on at least 3 sides.
        (2) T2b. Tumor is no larger than 1.5 cm in its greatest dimension or is present in more than one lobe.
      e. T3. Tumor invades the prostatic apex, the prostatic capsule, the bladder neck, or seminal vesicles but is not fixed.
      f. T4. Tumor is fixed or invades adjacent structures other than those listed under T3.
    2. Lymph node stage
      a. NX. Regional lymph nodes cannot be assessed.
      b. N0. No regional lymph node metastases are present.
      c. N1. Metastases to a single lymph node no larger than 2 cm in its greatest dimension.
      d. N2. Metastases to a single lymph node that are larger than 2 cm but no larger than 5 cm in their greatest dimension, or multiple lymph nodes no larger than 5 cm in their greatest dimension are present.
      e. N3. Metastases to a single lymph node larger than 5 cm in their greatest dimension.
      Note: Regional lymph nodes include periprostatic, pelvic, sacral, iliac, obturator, and hypogastric nodes, whereas aortic, common iliac, inguinal, supraclavicular, cervical, and scalene nodes are considered to be distant metastases.
    3. Metastatic stage
      a. MX. Presence of distant metastases cannot be assessed.
      b. M0. No distant metastases are present.
      c. M1. Distant metastases are present.
    4. Histopathologic grade
      a. GX. Grade cannot be assessed.
      b. G1. Well differentiated, slight anaplasia.
      c. G2. Moderately well differentiated, moderate anaplasia.
      d. G3–4. Poorly differentiated or undifferentiated, marked anaplasia.
    5. Stage groupings
      a. Stage 0. T1–2a, N0, M0, G1.
      b. Stage I. T1–2a, N0, M0, G2–4.
      c. Stage II. T1–2b, N0, M0, any G.
      d. Stage III. T3, N0, M0, any G.
      e. Stage IV. T4, N0, M0, any G; any T, N1–3, M0, any G; any T, any N, M1, any G.

IX. **Treatment**
  A. **Surgery**
    1. **Primary prostate carcinoma**
      a. **Indications.** Patients with **Stage A$_1$** disease can be managed with **observation alone** (periodic rectal examinations and serum tumor markers), although younger patients are probably best served with definitive therapy. **Radial prostatectomy and bilateral pelvic lymphadenectomy** is indicated for clinical **Stages A$_2$, B$_1$, and B$_2$ disease** (TNM Stages I and II) and as an option for young patients with Stage A$_1$ disease. In general, radical prostatectomy is not indicated for Stage C or D disease (TNM Stages III and IV).
      b. **Approaches.** Two main approaches have been used:
        (1) **Perineal approach.** More commonly used in the past, this approach is associated with minimal blood loss and a safe vesicourethral anastomosis. However, it requires a separate incision for lymph node biopsy and **leaves virtually all patients impotent.** With the advent of laparoscopic pelvic lymphadenectomy, however, interest in the perineal approach is increasing.
        (2) **Retropubic approach.** This approach currently is **preferred** by many surgeons because simultaneous resection and lymph node biopsy can be performed and potency may be preserved. It is associated with **greater blood loss** than the perineal approach, however.
      c. **Procedures**
        (1) **Radical prostatectomy.** Radical prostatectomy can be performed through either a transperineal of retropubic approach, although currently the latter is preferred. Initially, a **bilateral pelvic lymphadenectomy is performed,** removing the nodal tissue medial to the external iliac veins and extending to the level of the obturator lymph nodes. Immediate pathologic examination is often performed and, **if tumor cells are identified, the operation is typically terminated.** Otherwise, the radical prostatectomy is completed by **removing the entire prostate and seminal vesicles** and anastomosing the bladder to the membranous urethra. Recently, the **Walsh "nerve-sparing" retropubic approach** has become more popular because **blood loss is reduced, urinary continence is preserved in more than 98% of cases, and potency is preserved in more than 60% of patients.**
        (2) **Transurethral prostatic resection.** This procedure is **rarely** used in the treatment of prostate carcinoma and only if other means of managing bladder outlet obstruction, such as radiation or hormonal therapy, are not successful.
        (3) **Laparoscopic pelvic lymphadenectomy.** This minimally invasive surgical technique may be used as a staging procedure in selected patients.
      d. **Morbidity and mortality.** The **overall mortality** after prostatectomy is **less than 1%;** however, the complication rate depends on the procedure and extent of disease and includes the following potential problems:
        (1) **Hemorrhage,** typically ranging from 1000–2000 mL.
        (2) **Wound infection and pelvic abscess,** which are rare.
        (3) **Impotence.** With the **Walsh technique, as many as 70% of young patients maintain potency,** with an age-dependent decrease to less than 20% by age 70.
        (4) **Urinary incontinence,** usually mild stress incontinence that persists for more than 6 months in 5% of patients.
        (5) **Rectal injury,** 0–7%.
    2. **Locally advanced and metastatic prostate cancer.** In rare cases, radical prostatectomy may be required for palliation of locally advanced prostate cancer. Occasionally, transurethral resection of the prostate may be necessary to relieve obstruction of the bladder outlet. However, radiation therapy and hormonal manipulation generally are preferred to surgical procedures in these patients.
  B. **Radiation therapy**
    1. **Primary prostatic carcinoma.** External-beam radiation therapy **(6000–7000 cGy over 6 weeks)** can be used to treat localized carcinoma of the prostate **(Stages A and B or TNM I and II)** with similar survival to radical surgery. Radi-

ation therapy also has been advocated for Stages C and D_1 (TNM Stages III and IV). Interest in interstitial radiation therapy (primarily ^{125}I seeds) recently has waned because of high recurrence rates and poor dosimetry. New protocols evaluating ultrasonic seed localization and new radioactive agents such as palladium may improve results in the future.

2. **Adjuvant radiation therapy.** After prostatectomy, pelvic radiation can be administered in patients with positive margins, extracapsular extension, and seminal vesicle involvement. External-beam radiation also may be administered to **patients with rising PSA levels** and no evidence of distant metastases after radical surgery. Doses of **4500–6000 cGy** typically are administered, yielding more than **90% long-term disease-free survival** in patients with **Stage C disease** (one study).

3. **Locally advanced and metastatic prostate cancer.** Pain from bony metastases can be significantly palliated with external-beam radiation therapy.

C. **Chemotherapy**

1. **Primary prostatic carcinoma.** Cytotoxic chemotherapy remains a **fourth-line modality** in the treatment of prostate cancer behind surgery, radiation, and hormonal therapy. When used, cytotoxic chemotherapy does not alter survival significantly (see below).

2. **Adjuvant chemotherapy.** There is no indication for adjuvant chemotherapy in the treatment of prostate carcinoma.

3. **Locally advanced and metastatic prostate cancer**

   a. **Single agents.** Multiple agents have been evaluated with minimal response rates, including hydroxyurea (7–50%), fluorouracil (12–29%), cisplatin (2–20%), cyclophosphamide (41%), and doxorubicin (15%). A single randomized study by the National Prostatic Cancer Project involving Stage D patients who failed hormonal therapy demonstrated improved response rates with **both fluorouracil (36%) and cyclophosphamide (41%)** compared with control therapy (19%). Estramustine phosphate (nitrogen mustard bound to estradiol) produces a 17% response rate that is most likely attributable to the hormonal effects of the estradiol. **No prolonged survival has been associated with any agent.**

   b. **Combination regimens.** Several combination regimens have been examined with almost no success. A combination of **cyclophosphamide and doxorubicin** did result in a **31.5% response rate,** but survival was unaffected. Other studies comparing combined hormonal and chemotherapy with hormonal therapy also have demonstrated no additional benefit of chemotherapy. Therefore, chemotherapy currently cannot be recommended in the treatment of prostatic malignancy.

D. **Hormonal therapy.** Hormonal therapy is recommended for **metastatic carcinoma of the prostate**. Therapy has been instituted either before or after the diagnosis of clinically apparent metastases. Recent data suggested that early treatment may prolong survival. The majority of patients with metastatic disease initially respond to **androgen deprivation monotherapy;** however, most disease progresses within 2 years. Many hormonal manipulations produce **gynecomastia**, which can be **prevented in 80% of patients** by irradiating potential breast tissue with 1000 cGy in 3–4 fractions before orchiectomy or any other hormonal therapy. Types of hormonal manipulations that may produce responses include the following:

1. **Orchiectomy.** Transscrotal bilateral orchiectomy, often performed under local anesthesia, is considered the **"gold-standard"** hormonal therapy against which all other therapies are measured.

2. **Diethylstilbesterol (DES) administration.** DES inhibits release of luteinizing hormone from the anterior pituitary gland, resulting in lower testosterone levels. One mg is given orally 3 times daily. **Because of severe side effects, including thromboembolism, cardiovascular complications, and fluid retention**, this agent is not prescribed often.

3. **Luteinizing hormone-releasing hormone (LHRH) agonists.** Agents such as leuprolide (Lupron) and goserelin (Zoladex) disrupt the pulsatile release of LHRH, causing a paradoxical suppression of gonadotropins and testosterone. A "flare reaction" occurs approximately one week after initiation of therapy because of the transient rise in testosterone levels, but "anorchid" levels (2 ng/dL) are reached after 3 weeks. This **"chemical" orchiectomy** is often more acceptable to patients than a "surgical orchiectomy," and new **depot forms** permit monthly administration.

4. **Antiandrogen medications.** Recent data strongly suggest that Flutamide (Eu-

lexin), a nonsteroidal antiandrogen, **combined with LHRH agonists** may increase the long-term survival rate by 25%. These medications, together, attain **"total androgen ablation" because as many as 10% of androgens are made by the adrenal glands.** Protocols combining flutamide with orchiectomy are currently underway.

5. **Other medications.** These agents include **aminoglutethamide, spironolactone, and glucocorticoids** (which produce a "medical adrenalectomy"), **ketoconazole** (a potent inhibitor of both adrenal and gonadal hormone production that can reduce serum levels of testosterone as rapidly as orchiectomy), and **estramustine phosphate.**

E. **Immunotherapy.** The use of biologic response modifiers in this disease requires more study. Currently, early results from clinical trials using **suramin** suggest some activity; however, toxicity is significant unless serum levels are monitored closely.

X. **Prognosis**

A. **Risk of recurrence.** The risk of local or distant recurrence or both varies, depending on stage at presentation:
   1. **Stage A,** less than 10% at 10 years.
   2. **Stage B,** 15–25% at 10 years.
   3. **Stage C,** 20–30% at 5 years.

B. **Five-year survival.** The survival of patients with prostate carcinoma varies with stage:
   1. **Stage A,** 54–80%.
   2. **Stage B,** 54–88%.
   3. **Stage C,** 15%–72%.
   4. **Stage D,** 6–30%.

C. **Adverse prognostic factors.** The following elements are associated with a poor outcome: **hormone unresponsive tumor** (once tumor becomes hormonally unresponsive, median survival is fewer than 12 months); presence of lymph node metastases, seminal vesicle involvement, positive surgical margins, poorly differentiated tumor (Gleason grade > 7).

XI. **Patient follow-up**

A. **General guidelines.** Patients with prostate carcinoma treated with definitive surgery or radiation should be followed every 3–4 months for 3 years, every 6 months for an additional 2 years, and then annually for evidence of recurrence. Patients treated for metastatic disease are generally followed every 3 months.

B. **Routine evaluation.** Patients treated with surgery or radiation should be monitored with the following tests and procedures conducted at the time of each clinic visit:
   1. **Medical history and physical examination.** An interval history and a thorough physical examination are required during every clinic visit. Special attention should be focused on the rectal exam for evidence of recurrent disease. (See p 326, **VI.A**).
   2. **Blood tests**
   3. **Prostatic specific antigen (PSA). PSA has proven to be a sensitive indication of disease progression or recurrence.** It has become the mainstay of routine follow up of all patients with prostate cancer. PAP is no longer routinely followed in most patients.
   4. **Hepatic transaminases and alkaline phosphatase.** These are followed in patients with metastatic disease, to evaluate for any hepatic toxicity that may be related to therapy. Agents such as **flutamide** may cause reversible changes in liver function tests.

C. **Additional evaluation.** Additional tests and procedures that can be used if clinically indicated include:
   1. **Technetium-99m bone scan**
   2. **Computerized tomography (CT).** Local recurrences or nodal metastasis can be detected by this examination.

REFERENCES

Catalona WJ, Scott WW. Carcinoma of the prostate. In: Walsh PC. *Campbell's Urology*, 9th ed., vol. 2. Philadelphia: Saunders: 1986:1763–1834.

Crawford ED, Eisenberger MA, McCleod DG, et. al. A controlled trial of leuprolide with and without flutamide in prostatic carcinoma. *NEJM* 1989;**321**(7):419–424.

Gittes RF. Prostate specific antigen. *NEJM* 1987;**317**(15):954–955.

Labrie F, Belanger A, Simard J, et al. Combination therapy for prostate cancer. Endocrine and biologic basis of its choice as a new standard first line therapy. *Cancer* 1993;**71**(suppl 3):1059–1067.

McCullough DL. Diagnosis and staging of prostatic cancer. In: Skinner DG. *Diagnosis and Management of Genitourinary Cancer*. Philadelphia: Saunders; 1988; 405–416.

Osterling JE. PSA leads the way for detecting and following prostate cancer. *Contemporary Urology*, Feb 1993, 60–81.

Paulson DF. Radiotherapy versus surgery for localized prostatic cancer. *Urol Clin North Am* 1987;**14**(4):675–684.

Resnick MI. Transrectal ultrasound guided versus digitally directed prostatic biopsy: A comparative study. *J Urol* 1988;**139:**754–757.

Tanagho EA, McAninch JW, editors. *Smith's General Urology*, 12th ed. Norwalk, CT: Appleton & Lange; 1988.

Trachtenberg J. Hormonal management of stage D carcinoma of the prostate. *Urol Clin North Am* 1987;**14**(4):685–691.

Walsh PC, Lepor H, Eggleston JC. Radical prostatectomy with preservation of sexual function: Anatomic and pathologic considerations. *Prostate* 1983;**4:**473–485.

Wein AJ, Hanno PM. *A Clinical Manual of Urology*. Norwalk, CT: Appleton & Lange; 1988.

44 Malignancies of the Testis

Leonard Gomella, MD, and Michael Grasso, MD

I. **Epidemiology.** Testicular carcinoma constitutes only **1% of all cancers** in males; however it accounts for **11–13% of all cancer deaths in males ages 15–35.** In 1985, 4.0 cases per 100,000 were diagnosed, resulting in 0.3 deaths. Estimates indicate that **6,600 new cases and 350 deaths** will be reported in the United States in 1993. World-wide, the incidence varies from areas of high risk, such as Switzerland (10.5 per 100,000), to countries of low incidence, such as Cuba (0.3 per 100,000).

II. **Risk factors**

   A. **Age.** Unlike most solid neoplasms, testicular carcinoma is a disease of the **young.** The incidence of testicular cancer increases from less than 1.0 per 100,000 males below age 15 to **a peak of 11.0 per 100,000 between the ages of 25–29;** thereafter, the incidence gradually decreases to less than 1.0 per 100,000 by age 70.

   B. **Race. Whites** are at **4.4 times** greater risk than blacks, and American Indian and Asian males exhibit intermediate risk.

   C. **Genetic factors.** There is an **increased risk** of testicular tumors among first-degree relatives of patients with testicular carcinoma.

   D. **Previous testicular pathology**

   1. **Cryptorchidism.** The lifetime risk of testicular neoplasms in inguinal and abdominal testes is **1.3% and 5%,** respectively. In addition, the incidence of testicular carcinoma in the opposite, normally descended, testis is increased as well.

   2. **Previous testicular cancer.** Patients with a history of testicular cancer are at increased risk of developing a second testicular tumor.

   3. **Infertility.** The incidence of carcinoma in situ ranges from **0.4–1% in patients with oligo- or azoospermia,** and 20–30% of patients with proved carcinoma of the testis will have low sperm counts.

III. **Clinical presentation**

   A. **Signs and symptoms**

   1. **Local manifestations.** Patients may present with a **painless testicular mass,** infertility, and scrotal pain or dull ache (40%). Some are diagnosed during routine **screening after orchiopexy** for an cryptorchid testis.

   2. **Systemic manifestations.** Patients with advanced disease may present with the sequelae of retroperitoneal and pulmonary metastases **(weight loss, lymphedema of the lower extremities, and chronic lower back pain).**

   B. **Paraneoplastic syndromes.** There are no known paraneoplastic syndromes associated with testicular carcinoma.

IV. **Differential diagnosis.** Patients who present with a **scrotal mass** will most often have a benign process, but a malignancy must be considered. The differential diagnosis of a scrotal mass includes **infection** (epididymitis, orchitis, tuberculosis, and genital abscess), **varicocele, hydrocele** (most common), **spermatocele, benign tumors** (epidermoid cyst, adenomatoid tumor, and fibrous pseudotumor of the testicular tunic), **Sertoli and Leydig cell tumors, and other malignancies** and scrotal and spermatic cord sarcomas).

V. **Screening programs.** High school students are now taught testicular self-examination. Patients with a history of a cryptorchidism, atrophic testes, or a previous testicular tumor should be instructed on the importance of a monthly testicular self-examination and should be screened annually with a physical examination and testicular ultrasound. First-degree relatives of patients with testicular tumors also should be examined periodically.

VI. **Diagnostic workup**

   A. **Medical history and physical examination.** A complete medical history and a thorough physical examination are essential to the initial evaluation of patients with suspected testicular tumors.

1. **Lymph nodes.** The presence of a signal node (also called **Virchow's or Troisier's node**) should be noted.
2. **Breasts.** Unilateral or bilateral **gynecomastia** may be present.
3. **Abdomen.** Abdominal and hepatic masses must be described.
4. **Scrotum.** Both testicles should be examined carefully, including the epididy-mis, and spermatic cord and all abnormalities should be noted.
5. **Extremities.** Edema of the lower extremities is an important finding.

B. **Primary tests and procedures.** The following tests and procedures should be per-formed on all patients with suspected testicular carcinoma:
   1. **Blood tests**
      a. **Complete blood count** (see p 1, **IV.A.1**).
      b. **Hepatic transaminases** (see p 1, **IV.A.2**).
      c. **Alkaline phosphatase** (see p 1, **IV.A.3**).
      d. **Tumor markers.** Elevated serum levels of **alpha-fetoprotein (AFP), beta-human chorionic gonadotropin (beta-hCG)**, or both are present in **85% of patients with nonseminomatous germ cell tumors.**
         (1) **Beta-hCG.** This subunit of hCG is produced by the syncytiotrophoblast cells and has a $t_{1/2}$ of 24 hrs. Beta-hCG is **highest in choriocarcinoma** but can be elevated in **67% of embryonal cell carcinomas and 10% of pure seminomas.**
         (2) **Alpha-fetoprotein.** AFP is produced by yolk sac cells with a 7 day $t_{1/2}$. It is **specific for nonseminomatous germ cell** tumors and never ele-vated in pure seminoma.
         (3) **Lactate dehydrogenase (LDH).** LDH is used by some as a relatively "nonspecific" tumor marker.
         (4) **Neuron-specific enolase (NSE).** NSE recently has been shown to be elevated in **73% of patients with seminoma** and may be more widely used as a tumor marker in the future.
   2. **Imaging studies** (see p 3, **IV.C**)
      a. **Chest x-ray.**
      b. **Computed tomography (CT).** Abdominal CT scan is essential to evaluate the retroperitoneum for para-aortic and paracaval lymph node as well as hepatic metastases. **Chest CT** has largely replaced whole lung tomograms for the detection of pulmonary metastases.
      c. **Ultrasound.** Scrotal ultrasonic examination has become the **"gold standard" screening test** for scrotal and testicular masses and is often diagnostic.
   3. **Invasive procedures. Testicular biopsy** of any suspicious testicular mass should be performed using an **inguinal approach**. In most cases, the "biopsy" ultimately requires **a radical orchiectomy** that includes removal of the testis, epididymis, and spermatic cord to the level of the internal inguinal ring, with tourniquet compression on the proximal spermatic cord to help prevent tumor spread. **Transscrotal biopsy of testicular masses is contraindicated** be-cause it may result in scrotal tumor seeding and inguinal nodal metastases. Needle biopsy also is not indicated because of marked tumor heterogeneity and the risk of tumor seeding. Patients with testicular tumors should be evalu-ated for **contralateral overt or in situ carcinoma**.

C. **Optional tests and procedures.** The following tests and procedures may be indi-cated by prior diagnostic findings or clinical suspicion:
   1. **Blood tests** (see p 2, **IV.A**)
      a. **Nucleotidase.**
      b. **GGTP.**
   2. **Imaging studies**
      a. **Magnetic resonance imaging (MRI)** (see p 3, **IV.C.2**).
      b. **Bipedal lymphangiogram.** This test occasionally can be useful in evaluat-ing and following retroperitoneal and pelvic lymph node metastases.

VII. **Pathology**
   A. **Location.** The incidence of testicular tumors is slightly higher on the **right** presum-ably as a result of the higher prevalence of right-sided cryptorchidism.
   B. **Multiplicity.** Multiple **synchronous** tumors occur in **2%** of cases.
   C. **Histology.** Malignant testicular tumors are divided into **non-germ cell tumors and seminomatous and non-seminomatous germ cell lesions.** Although **semi-noma** is the most common germ cell tumor, neoplasms often consist of a mixture of cell types.
      1. **Germ cell tumors.** These malignancies account for **96%** of all malignant testic-ular tumors.

    a. **Seminomas.** Subtypes include classic, spermatocytic (typically seen in older patients), and anaplastic seminoma.

    b. **Nonseminomatous tumors.** These malignancies include embryonal carcinoma, yolk sac carcinoma, choriocarcinoma, teratoma, and teratocarcinoma.

  2. **Non-germ cell tumors**

    a. **Stromal cell tumors.** These tumors account for **3–4%** of all testicular tumors and include **Sertoli cell, Leydig cell, and mixed gonadoblastoma** tumors. Phenotypic changes caused by excess androgen production are often present with these neoplasms.

    b. **Lymphoma.** Testicular lymphoma compromises **less than 5%** of all testicular tumors. However, in males older than **50, it is the most common testicular malignancy.**

    c. **Carcinoma in situ.** This premalignant pattern of intratubular atypical germ cells aggregations is known to precede the development of testicular cancer and occurs particularly in **males with oligospermia and cryptorchism**.

D. **Metastatic spread**

  1. **Modes of spread**

    a. **Direct extension.** Although this is a **rare** mode of spread, the cord or scrotum can become involved from local growth.

    b. **Lymphatic metastasis.** Most often, **right-sided** germ cell tumors will initially spread to the **interaorto-caval nodes and left-sided** tumors to the para-aortic lymph nodes. In **15–25%** of patients without known metastases (Stage A) spread to lymph nodes is found at the time of surgery.

    c. **Hematogenous metastasis.** Although distant metastasis occurs less often than lymphatic metastasis, malignant cells can gain access to the systemic blood vessels and spread to distant organs, especially the **lungs**.

  2. **Sites of spread.** Organs frequently involved with distant spread from testicular tumors include the following: **retroperitoneal lymph nodes, lung, liver, extra-abdominal lymph nodes, and central nervous system.**

VIII. **Staging.** Although testicular carcinoma traditionally has been classified into stages A, B, and C, the American Joint Committee on Cancer and the Union Internationale Contre le Cancer in 1987 developed a joint TNM staging system that has been proposed as a new unifying method of staging testicular carcinoma. Both staging systems are outlined below:

A. **Traditional staging system**

  1. **Stage A.** Tumor is limited to the testis alone.

  2. **Stage B1.** Microscopic metastases to no more than 6 retroperitoneal lymph nodes are present.

  3. **Stage B2.** Microscopic metastases to more than 6 retroperitoneal lymph nodes or gross nodal involvement are present.

  4. **Stage B3.** Bulky retroperitoneal lymph nodes with diameters larger than 6 cm are present.

  5. **Stage C.** Metastases above the diaphragm or to abdominal viscera are present.

B. **TNM staging system**

  1. **Tumor stage**

    a. **TX.** Primary tumor cannot be assessed (in the absence of radical orchiectomy, TX is used).

    b. **T0.** Histologic scar or no evidence of primary tumor.

    c. **TIS.** Intratubular tumor; preinvasive cancer.

    d. **T1.** Tumor is limited to the testis, including rete testis.

    e. **T2.** Tumor invades beyond the tunica albuginea or into the epididymis.

    f. **T3.** Tumor invades the spermatic cord.

    g. **T4.** Tumor invades the scrotum.

  2. **Lymph node stage**

    a. **NX.** Regional lymph nodes cannot be assessed.

    b. **N0.** No regional lymph node metastases are present.

    c. **N1.** Metastases to a single lymph node that is no larger than 2 cm in its greatest dimension.

    d. **N2.** Metastases to a single lymph node that is larger than 2 cm but less than 5 cm in its greatest dimension or metastases to multiple lymph nodes that are no larger than 5 cm in their greatest dimension.

    e. **N3.** Metastases to a lymph node that is larger than 5 cm in its greatest dimension.

  3. **Metastatic stage**

    a. **MX.** Presence of distant metastases cannot be assessed.

       b. M0. No distant metastases are present.

       c. M1. Distant metastases are present.

    4. Histopathologic stage. Testicular carcinomas are not graded.

    5. Stage groupings

       a. Stage 0. TIS, N0, M0.

       b. Stage I. T1–2, N0, M0.

       c. Stage II. T3–4, N0, M0.

       d. Stage III. Any T, N1, M0.

       e. Stage IV. Any T, N2–3, M0, any T, any N, M1.

IX. Treatment. Advances in the therapy of testicular cancer are one of the great success stories in cancer treatment; the **overall survival rate is higher than 90%.**

    A. Surgery

       1. Primary testicular carcinoma

          a. General considerations. Although many patients with testicular cancer have abnormal semen analysis, the option of **semen cryopreservation** for possible future in vitro fertilization should be addressed **before orchiectomy** because surgery, subsequent chemotherapy, or both can produce infertility.

          b. Indications. Radical orchiectomy is indicated in **all patients** with carcinoma in situ, non-germ cell tumors, and both nonseminomatous and seminomatous germ cell cancers. In patients who refuse radical orchiectomy, serial examinations (physical examination, testicular measurements, and chest x-ray every 3 months, ultrasound examination, CT scan, and serum levels of tumor marker every 6 months are indicated. **Limited retroperitoneal lymph node dissection** (RPLND) is commonly used in nonseminomatous germ cell carcinoma with limited local or regional spread (less than T3 or M1 disease). In addition, if a residual mass remains after therapy or if elevated levels of tumor markers persist despite negative x-ray studies, **complete RPLND** is required. In patients explored after chemotherapy, **20% will have residual disease, 40% will have fibrosis, and 40% will have a mature teratoma** (chemotherapy-induced differentiation of the original tumor).

          c. Procedures

             (1) Radical orchiectomy. This operation is performed through an **inguinal incision** (the transscrotal approach is contraindicated). The spermatic cord, is isolated, and divided early unless an immediate pathologic examination is required to confirm a testicular tumor. The testicle is removed with the cord structures up to the level of the internal inguinal ring.

             (2) Retroperitoneal lymph node dissection. RPLND involves transabdominal removal of the remaining spermatic cord structures and retroperitoneal lymph nodes. Previously, "complete" RPLND was associated with a **high incidence of infertility** because resection of sympathetic fibers led to **failure of emission or retrograde ejaculation.** Recent modifications use a **"template" approach** to spare some nerve fibers without compromising the operation. Despite normal preoperative studies, **30% of patients with clinical Stage A testis cancer have nodal disease.** In these patients, RPLND may be curative; however, adjuvant chemotherapy or observation options may be indicated for this group.

       2. Locally advanced and metastatic testicular carcinoma. Surgery is rarely indicated for the palliation of metastatic lesions unless chemotherapy has produced stable resectable lesions that may harbor areas of malignant disease.

       3. Morbidity and mortality. The mortality from radical orchiectomy is essentially 0%, and the mortality from **RPLND is lower than 1%.** Complications after radical orchiectomy are rare (hemorrhage and wound infection), but problems following RPLND are more frequent, especially if chemotherapy was administered before surgery (30%). These problems include the following: **small bowel obstruction, 1–5%; ureteral injury; infertility; lymphocele; and chylous ascites.**

    B. Radiation

       1. Primary testicular carcinoma. There is no role for radiation in the treatment of primary testicular lesions.

       2. Adjuvant radiation therapy

          a. Seminomatous germ cell tumors. Because seminoma is an exquisitely **radiosensitive tumor**, adjuvant radiation to the para-aortic and ipsilateral **pelvic nodes** is recommended to treat the nearly **20% of clinical Stage I**

and Stage II patients who will have **occult nodal disease**. In Stage III and Stage IV disease without metastases above the diaphragm, radiation therapy to the infradiaphragmatic para-aortic, paracaval, and ipsilateral pelvic nodes (and contralateral pelvic nodes if involved) is advocated. **Radiation** above the diaphragm generally is not used because it hinders future chemotherapy.

b. **Nonseminomatous germ cell tumors.** Radiation therapy generally is not used with these tumors because they are not radiosensitive.

3. **Locally advanced and metastatic testicular carcinoma**

a. **Seminomatous germ cell tumors.** In **stages III and IV** without metastases above the diaphragm, **radiation therapy** to the **infradiaphragmatic para-aortic, paracaval, and ipsilateral pelvic nodes (and contralateral pelvic nodes if involved)** is advocated. Radiation above the diaphragm generally is not used because it hinders future chemotherapy.

b. **Nonseminomatous germ cell tumors.** There is no role for radiation therapy in the treatment of these tumors.

4. **Morbidity and mortality.** The complications from retroperitoneal lymph node irradiation are minimal and include **radiation enteritis and small bowel obstruction,** both of which are rare.

C. **Chemotherapy**

1. **Primary testicular carcinoma.** Because of the nature of the testis as a sanctuary site, systemic chemotherapy does not always eradicate primary testicular neoplasms. Therefore, it should never be used in place of radical orchiectomy for therapy of primary lesions.

2. **Adjuvant chemotherapy.** Therapy with **cisplatin-based combination regimens** has been shown to reduce the risk of recurrence in pathologic **Stage II** patients from **48% to less than 2%.** However, it is not clear whether therapy at the time of recurrence will produce identical survival results and simultaneously spare patients who will not recur the morbidity of combination chemotherapy.

3. **Locally advanced and metastatic testicular carcinoma.**

a. **Single agents. Cisplatin** is the **single most active agent** against testicular carcinoma, even against advanced refractory cancer. Other agents with activity include **actinomycin D, mithramycin, vinblastine, and bleomycin (all have a 5–20% complete response rate);** however, because combination regimens are superior, single-agent therapy should never be used as primary therapy.

b. **Combination chemotherapy.** Dramatic advances in the chemotherapy of testicular cancer involve **platinum-based therapy,** as advocated by Einhorn. With the current ability to cure most patients, the development of less toxic regimens now is being emphasized. For example, regimens that exclude bleomycin, which causes pulmonary fibrosis, may be less harmful.

c. **Current regimens.** Some commonly used combinations include those listed below. They generally result in **response rates greater than 90%** and are administered for 3–4 cycles, depending on rapidity of the clinical response:

(1) **PVB.** Cisplatin, vinblastine, bleomycin are administered every 3 weeks.

(2) **VABVI.** Cyclophosphamide, vinblastine, actinomycin-D, bleomycin, and cisplatin are given in monthly cycles.

(3) **BEP.** The combination of bleomycin, etoposide, and cisplatin is delivered every 3 weeks.

(4) **EP.** Etoposide and cisplatin are administered every 3 weeks.

d. **Salvage regimens.** Cisplatin-refractory disease is difficult to control, but trials with **ifosfamide, including the VIP protocol (etoposide [VP-16], ifosfamide and cisplatin)** show promise. Autologous bone marrow transplantation and agents such as carboplatin also are being studied.

D. **Immunotherapy.** This modality has not been adequately studied in the treatment of testicular carcinoma.

E. **Observation.** Patients with **nonseminomatous, nonembryonal testicular carcinoma** with normal tumor markers (alpha-FP, beta-hCG) and radiographic studies (chest x-ray and CT scan) after orchiectomy **(clinical Stage A); no vascular, lymphatic, or cord invasion: and reliable follow-up** can be followed closely for tumor recurrence with monthly tumor marker levels and chest x-rays and CT scans every 3 months. This protocol safely detects patients who manifest distant disease and saves those without distant disease from the morbidity of combination chemotherapy, radical surgery, or both.

X. **Prognosis**

A. **Risk of recurrence.** In the absence of metastatic disease, the risk of recurrence after **orchiectomy alone**, with close surveillance, is about 20%, whereas the risk of recurrence after **orchiectomy and retroperitoneal lymph node dissection** is 10%.

B. **Five-year survival.** Compared with the 50% 5-year survival rate of 20 years ago, the outlook today is markedly improved. Current 5-year survival rates are
   1. **Stage 0,** 100%.
   2. **Stages I and II,** 95–100%.
   3. **Stage III,** 91%.
   4. **Stage IV,** 80%.

XI. **Patient follow-up**
   A. **General guidelines.** Patients with testicular carcinoma should be evaluated every 3 months for 2 years, every 6 months for an additional 3 years, then annually thereafter to exclude the presence of recurrent disease. The following specific guidelines for patient evaluation are recommended.
   B. **Routine evaluation.** The following examinations should be performed during each clinic visit:
      1. **History and physical examination.** An interval medical history and complete physical examination are mandatory during routine office visits. Attention should be focused on those specific areas listed on p 333 **VI.A.**
      2. **Blood tests**
         a. **Complete blood count** (see p 1, **IV.A.1**).
         b. **Hepatic transaminases** (see p 1, **IV.A.2**).
         c. **Alkaline phosphatase** (see p 1, **IV.A.3**).
         d. **Tumor markers** (see p 334, **VI.B.1.d**).
            (1) **Beta-hCG.** Levels of this marker, if originally elevated, can be followed for evidence of recurrence.
            (2) **AFP.** Alpha-fetoprotein, like beta-hCG, can be followed for evidence of recurrence.
            (3) **LDH.**
      3. **Chest x-ray** (see p 3, **IV.C.1**).
   C. **Additional evaluation.** Other tests and procedures that should be performed at regular intervals include the following:
      1. **Computerized tomography (CT).** CT is useful in evaluating retroperitoneal lymph nodes, liver, and lung. **CT scan of the chest, abdomen, and pelvis** should be obtained **every 6–12 months.**
      2. **Ultrasound.** Scrotal ultrasonic examination is required at least **once a year** for adequate periodic evaluation of the **contralateral testis.**
   D. **Optional evaluation.** The following tests may be indicated by prior diagnostic findings or clinical suspicion:
      1. **Blood tests** (see p 2, **IV.A.4**)
         a. **Nucleotidase.**
         b. **GGTP.**
      2. **Biopsy.** Biopsy of any unusual or suspicious mass should be performed to exclude the possibility of recurrent disease.

REFERENCES

Einhorn LH. Chemotherapy of disseminated testicular cancer. In: Skinner DS and Lieskovsky S, editors. *Genitourinary Cancer.* Philadelphia: Saunders; 1988.

Einhorn LH, Crawford ED, Shipley WU, et al. Cancer of the testes. In: DeVita VT, Hellman S, & Rosenberg SA, editors. *Cancer: Principles and Practice of Oncology,* 3rd ed. Philadelphia: Lippincott; 1989:1071–1098.

Frank IN, Keys HM, McCune CS. Urologic and male genital cancers. In: American Cancer Society. *Clinical Oncology for Medical Students and Physicians,* 6th ed. Atlanta: 1983;213–218.

National Cancer Institute. 1987 Annual Cancer Statistics Review. Bethesda, Maryland: National Institutes of Health; 1987.

Loehrer PJ, Lauer R, et al. Salvage therapy in recurrent germ cell cancer: Ifosfamide and cisplatin plus either vinblastine or etoposide. *Ann Int Med* 1988;**109:**540–546.

Peckham MJ, Hamilton CR Horwich A. Surveillance after orchiectomy for stage I seminoma of the testis. *Br J Urol* 1987;**59:**343–347.

Ritchie JP, et al. Management of patients with clinical stage I or II nonseminomatous germ cell tumors of the testis. *Arch Surg* 1987;**122:**1443–1445.

Socinski MA, et al. Stage II nonseminomatous germ cell tumors of the testis: Analysis of treatment options in patients with low volume retroperitoneal disease. *J Urol* 1988;**140:**1437–1441.

45 Malignancies of the Penis

Leonard Gomella, MD, and Michael Grasso, MD

I. **Epidemiology.** In the United States, penile cancer constitutes **less than 4% of all cancers in males and 1% of all cancer deaths.** Worldwide, the incidence varies from areas with high incidence, such as Jamaica and Puerto Rico (5–5.7 per 100,000), to those of low incidence, such as Eastern Europe, Canada, and the United States (0.2–0.7 per 100,000). In South Vietnam, Thailand, and China, penile carcinoma constitutes 12%, 7%, and 20% of all malignances in males, respectively.

II. **Risk factors**
   A. **Age.** Penile carcinoma gradually increases from less than 1.0 per 100,000 in males under 50 years of age to **9.2 per 100,000 by age 85.**
   B. **Race.** There is no difference between blacks and whites, but Asians appear to be at a higher risk.
   C. **Genetic factors.** First-degree relatives are not at greater risk than the general population.
   D. **Previous genital pathology**
      1. **Circumcision.** There has been much debate as to the role of circumcision in preventing penile carcinoma. The **rarity** of this cancer in **Jewish males,** who are routinely circumcised, and the marked difference between **Moslem men,** who are all circumcised at puberty and have a **5% rate** of penile carcinoma, and **Hindu males,** who retain their foreskin into adult life and have a 15–18% incidence of penile carcinoma, support the beneficial effects of circumcision. However, the effect may be related entirely to **hygiene.** Cleansing the foreskin regularly may eliminate the carcinogenic action of bacteria found on the sloughed squamous epithelial surface (smegma).
      2. **Phimosis.** Chronic inflammatory processes of the penile foreskin and glands are associated with a higher incidence of penile carcinoma, and 90% of patients with penile cancer have a **history of phimosis.**
      3. **Venereal disease.** Patients with inadequately treated venereal disease have a higher incidence of penile carcinoma.
   E. **Urbanization.** Penile carcinoma is more prevalent among low socioeconomic groups, probably because of poor hygiene.

III. **Clinical presentation**
   A. **Signs and symptoms**
      1. **Local manifestations.** A variety of lesions may be present. Precancerous lesions may present as **white plaques** (leukoplakia) or **superficial ulcers**. Any diffuse penile lesion, whether exophytic or sessile, may represent carcinoma. Presenting complaints may include **irritative voiding symptoms, penile pain, discharge, and bleeding.**
      2. **Systemic manifestations.** Some patients will present with **painless inguinal lymphadenopathy and weight loss.**
   B. **Paraneoplastic syndromes.** No paraneoplastic syndromes are associated with penile carcinoma.

IV. **Differential diagnosis.** Because a multitude of **exophytic venereal diseases** (syphilis, chancroid, and granuloma inguinale) and **premalignant lesions** (erythroplasia of Querat, Bowen's disease, leukoplakia, Buschke-Lowenstein tumor, and condylomata acuminata) can be confused with penile carcinoma, a **biopsy** should be performed in patients who do not respond to medical therapy. **Balanitis xerotica obliterans** and **trauma** also can mimic penile cancer.

V. **Screening programs.** A biopsy should be performed if penile lesions do not respond to medical therapy; otherwise, no screening programs have been advocated.

VI. **Diagnostic work-up**
   A. **Medical history and physical examination.** A comprehensive medical history,

including a **venereal history**, and a thorough physical examination are essential for a complete evaluation.

  1. **Abdomen.** Any abdominal masses and hepatomegaly should be carefully described.
  2. **Genitalia.** The presence, location, and sensitivity (painless vs painful) of penile lesions should be recorded. The prepuce must be fully retracted (and subsequently reduced) to assure an adequate examination. Squamous carcinoma may appear **exophytic, sessile, or ulcerating**.
  3. **Lymph nodes.** Palpation of the inguinal regions is mandatory. As many as 50% of patients with penile carcinoma have adenopathy. However, most of these are reactive and do not represent metastatic disease. **Antibiotics** (eg, tetracycline) are often administered for 4–6 weeks to differentiate between neoplastic and inflammatory adenopathy.

B. **Primary tests and procedures.** All patients with suspected penile carcinoma should have the following diagnostic tests and procedures performed:
  1. **Blood tests** (see p 1, **IV.A**)
      a. **Complete blood count.**
      b. **Hepatic transaminases.**
      c. **Alkaline phosphatase.**
      d. **BUN and creatinine.**
  2. **Imaging studies** (see p 3, **IV.C**)
      a. **Chest x-ray.**
      b. **Computed tomography (CT).** CT scan of the abdomen and pelvis is useful in evaluating inguinal, pelvic, and para-aortic **lymph nodes** as well as in detecting liver involvement.
  3. **Invasive procedures.** If a presumed infectious lesion fails to respond to antibiotic therapy, an adequate **biopsy** is mandatory. It is important to biopsy the margin of the lesion for an accurate diagnosis.

C. **Optional tests and procedures.** The following tests and procedures may be indicated by prior diagnostic findings or clinical suspicion:
  1. **Blood tests** (see p 2, **IV.A**)
      a. **Nucleotidase.**
      b. **GGTP.**
  2. **Imaging studies**
      a. **Lymphangiogram.** Lymphangiography is an uncomfortable test that is rarely used today to evaluate intra-abdominal adenopathy.
      b. **Magnetic resonance imaging (MRI)** (see p 3, **IV.C.2**).
      c. **Technetium-99m bone scan** (see p 3, **IV.C.4**).

VII. **Pathology**

A. **Location.** Most lesions occur **distally** on the **glans** (48%), the **prepuce** (21%), coronal sulcus (6%), or shaft (< 2%).

B. **Multiplicity.** Approximately 9% of cancers involve more than one area.

C. **Histology. Epidermoid (squamous) carcinoma** is the most common penile neoplasm. Leukoplakia of the penis is a premalignant precursor of squamous carcinoma and is often noted adjacent to frank cancer. Cases of both basal cell and malignant melanoma of the penis have been reported.

D. **Metastatic spread**
  1. **Modes of spread.** Penile cancer spreads by 3 distinct mechanisms:
      a. **Direct extension.** Distal lesions commonly grow into the corporal bodies, which become involved secondarily.
      b. **Lymphatic metastasis.** Lesions of the **prepuce and skin** spread to the **superficial inguinal lymph nodes**. Tumors of the **glands and corpora** spread to the **deep inguinal, external iliac, and pelvic lymph nodes**. The lymphatics cross the midline along the penile shaft, frequently resulting in **bilateral lymphatic involvement**.
      c. **Hematogenous metastasis.** Spread through systemic blood vessels occurs only in the late stages of the disease process.
  2. **Sites of spread.** Common distant organs affected by distant metastases include the following: **lung, liver, bone,** and cutaneous sites.

VIII. **Staging.** The **Jackson staging system** has been the traditional staging system for penile carcinoma. In 1987, however, the American Joint Committee on Cancer and the Union Internationale Contre le Cancer proposed a common TNM staging system to standardize the staging of penile carcinoma:

A. **The Jackson staging system**
  1. **Stage 1.** Lesions confined to the glands or prepuce.

2. **Stage 2.** Lesion extending onto the shaft of the penis.
3. **Stage 3.** Lesions with malignant but operable groin nodes.
4. **Stage 4.** Lesions with a primary tumor extending off the shaft of the penis, those with inoperable groin nodes or distant metastases, or all of these.

B. **TNM staging system**
 1. **Tumor stage**
  a. **TX.** Primary tumor cannot be assessed.
  b. **T0.** No evidence of primary tumor.
  c. **Tis.** Carcinoma in situ.
  d. **Ta.** Noninvasive verrucous carcinoma.
  e. **T1.** Tumor invades subepithelial connective tissue.
  f. **T2.** Tumor invades corpus spongiosum or cavernosum.
  g. **T3.** Tumor invades urethra or prostate.
  h. **T4.** Tumor invades other adjacent structures.
 2. **Lymph node stage**
  a. **NX.** Regional lymph nodes cannot be assessed.
  b. **N0.** No regional lymph node metastasis.
  c. **N1.** Metastasis in a single superficial inguinal lymph node.
  d. **N2.** Metastasis in multiple or bilateral superficial inguinal lymph nodes.
  e. **N3.** Metastasis in deep inguinal or pelvic lymph nodes unilaterally or bilaterally.
 3. **Metastatic stage**
  a. **MX.** Presence of distant metastasis cannot be assessed.
  b. **M0.** No distant metastasis.
  c. **M1.** Distant metastasis.
 4. **Histopathologic stage**
  a. **GX.** Grade cannot be assessed.
  b. **G1.** Well differentiated.
  c. **G2.** Moderately well differentiated.
  d. **G3–4.** Poorly differentiated and undifferentiated.
 5. **Stage groupings**
  a. **Stage 0.** Tis or Ta, N0, M0.
  b. **Stage I.** T1, N0, M0.
  c. **Stage II.** T1, N1, M0; T2, N0–1, M0.
  d. **Stage III.** T1, N2, M0; T2, N2, M0; T3, N0–2, M0.
  e. **Stage IV.** T4, any N, M0; any T, N3, M0; any T, any N, M1.

IX. **Treatment**
A. **Surgery**
 1. **Primary penile carcinoma**
  a. **Indications.** Surgery is the most widely accepted form of therapy for cancer of the penis. Although radiation therapy may be attempted to avoid functional loss, many patients treated with irradiation ultimately require surgery. **Surgery involves both treatment of the local primary tumor and assessment of the metastatic status of the regional lymph nodes.**
  b. **Procedures**
   (1) **Circumcision.** Circumcision as the sole treatment modality should be restricted to those **superficial, noninvasive lesions limited to the foreskin.** However, before instituting radiotherapy, removal of the foreskin always should be performed to avoid significant complications from swelling, desquamation, irritation, and infection.
   (2) **Partial penectomy.** Partial penile amputation is the treatment of choice for **distal lesions. A 2-cm margin** proximal to the lesion is required.
   (3) **Total penectomy with perineal urethrostomy.** In patients with deeply infiltrating or proximal lesions, a total penectomy and perineal urethrostomy is the treatment of choice.
   (4) **Lymphadenectomy.** The role of radical ilioinguinal lymphadenectomy in penile carcinoma is controversial. This procedure involves the **complete removal of superficial and deep inguinal and common iliac lymph nodes to the level of the aorta.** It is associated with significant morbidity, including **wound-healing problems** (flap necrosis) and **lymphedema.** Lymphadenectomy can be performed either in the absence of clinically suspicious lymph nodes **(prophylactic lymphadenectomy)** or once lymph node metastases become apparent **(therapeutic lymphadenectomy).** Recent studies suggest that the 5-

year survival with prophylactic lymphadenectomy is superior to that with therapeutic lymphadenectomy. Some surgeons compromise and perform a **"sentinel" node biopsy,** as described by Cabanas (1977). The sentinel node is located 2 finger breadths lateral and distal to the pubic tubercle at the junction of the superficial epigastric and the saphenous veins. If this node contains metastatic disease, a formal lymphadenectomy is performed. If not, the likelihood of nodal disease is small and an extensive nodal dissection can be avoided.

2. **Locally advanced and metastatic penile cancer.** In metastatic penile carcinoma, surgery is indicated only for palliation of painful, bleeding primary lesions or for symptomatic superficial inguinal masses.

3. **Morbidity and mortality.** The majority of complications following surgery for penile cancer result from previous radiation therapy, lymphadenectomy, and concomitant medical diseases. The following are frequent causes of problems after surgery:

    a. **Penile amputation (partial or complete)**
      (1) **Meatal stenosis,** 0–40%.
      (2) **Wound infection,** 10%.
    b. **Inguinal lymphadenectomy**
      (1) **Lower extremity edema,** 2–40%.
      (2) **Flap necrosis,** mild: 29%; severe: 21%.
      (3) **Hemorrhage,** 18%.
      (4) **Wound infection,** 12%.
      (5) **Thrombophlebitis,** 5%.

B. **Radiation therapy**

1. **Primary penile carcinoma.** Radiation therapy for superficial penile carcinoma produces survival rates that are comparable to those following surgical resection. However, a **10–51% local failure rate** requiring salvage penectomy has been reported, and resection of irradiated tissue is associated with an increased risk of infection and poor wound healing. In cases of **superficial carcinoma, carcinoma in situ, and erythroplasia of Queyrat, 6000 cGy** to the local area **over 5–6 weeks** is successful. To treat more extensive lesions, **6500–7000 cGy of radiation therapy to the entire penis over 5–7 weeks** has been used. This therapy may be indicated in younger patients with superficial disease limited to the prepuce, older patients who are not surgical candidates because of underlying medical diseases, and patients who refuse surgery. Before instituting radiation therapy, the foreskin must be excised in all previously uncircumcised patients to prevent complications from swelling and irritation.

2. **Adjuvant radiotherapy.** Postoperative radiation therapy to the penis, inguinal and pelvic lymph node areas, or both have been used in patients with suspected residual disease (gross or microscopic); **5000–6000 cGy over 6 weeks** is usually delivered.

3. **Locally advanced and metastatic penile cancer.** Palliation from pain, ulceration, and bleeding can be achieved in many patients with locally advanced or metastatic disease with **4000–6000 cGy given over 5–6 weeks.**

4. **Morbidity and mortality.** Complications after radiation therapy to the penis and inguinal/pelvic lymph nodes include the following: **swelling and desquamation of the penis, penile ulceration or necrosis, telangiectasia, urethral (meatal) strictures, and lymphedema.**

C. **Chemotherapy**

1. **Primary penile carcinoma.** Fluorouracil cream is used topically in the treatment of carcinoma in situ in young patients. Those who fail this regimen require surgical resection.

2. **Adjuvant chemotherapy.** Because of the paucity of information and lack of therapeutic benefit, adjuvant chemotherapy currently cannot be recommended.

3. **Locally advanced and metastatic penile cancer**

    a. **Single-agent therapy.** Single agents have been used in the palliation of locally advanced and metastatic disease. Objective responses have been reported with **methotrexate and leucovorin rescue (61%), bleomycin (20–60%), and cisplatin (20%).** In addition, methotrexate has produced rare complete responses.

    b. **Combination therapy.** Although various combinations of the single agents discussed above have been tried, limited data are available regarding the usefulness of combination therapy. Furthermore, many patients are elderly

and have underlying medical problems that preclude the use of most of these agents.
   D. **Immunotherapy.** Immunotherapy has not been used in the treatment of penile carcinoma and remains experimental.
X. **Prognosis**
   A. **Risk of recurrence.** The risk of local recurrence depends on the treatment modality used.
      1. **Surgery. Local** recurrence rates are less than 10% if adequate (> 2 cm) surgical margins are obtained, and risk of **distant** (lymph node) recurrence is 14% within 2 years.
      2. **Radiation.** The local recurrence rate after radiation is 10–50%.
   B. **Five-year survival.** Survival of patients with penile tumors depends on the extent of disease.
      1. **Localized disease limited to the penis,** 65–90%.
      2. **Inguinal node metastases,** 30–50%.
      3. **Iliac node metastases,** less than 20%.
      4. **Distant metastases,** less than 2%.
   C. **Adverse prognostic signs.** The following findings are associated with a more aggressive disease course: **invasion of the corporal bodies and lymph node metastases.**
XI. **Patient follow-up**
   A. **General guidelines.** Patients with penile cancer should be followed every 3 months for 2 years, every 6 months for an additional 3 years, and then annually for evidence of recurrence or metastases. The following specific guidelines are recommended:
   B. **Routine evaluation.** The following examinations should be included with each clinic visit:
      1. **Medical history and physical examination.** An interval medical history and complete physical examination should be performed during routine clinic appointments. Particular emphasis should be placed on the areas outlined on p 339, **VI.A.**
      2. **Blood tests** (p 1, **IV.A**)
         a. **Complete blood count.**
         b. **Hepatic transaminases.**
         c. **Alkaline phosphatase.**
      3. **Chest x-ray** (see p 3, **IV.C.1**)
   C. **Additional evaluation.** Other tests that should be ordered at regular intervals include **computed tomography** (CT). **A CT scan of the abdomen and pelvis** can evaluate the inguinal, pelvic, and para-aortic lymph nodes as well as the liver for the presence of metastatic disease. This test is obtained typically every 6–12 months.
   D. **Optional evaluation.** The following represent additional tests and procedures that may be indicated by prior diagnostic findings or clinical suspicion:
      1. **Blood tests** (see p 2, **IV.A**)
         a. **Nucleotidase.**
         b. **GGTP.**
      2. **Imaging studies** (see p 3, **IV.C**)
         a. **Magnetic resonance imaging (MRI).**
         b. **Technetium-99m bone scan.**
      3. **Biopsy. Biopsy** of any new or unusual mass should be obtained with biopsy forceps (if appropriate), by fine needle aspiration, core needle, or open (incisional or excisional) biopsy to determine the presence or absence of recurrent or metastatic disease.

REFERENCES

Cabanas RM. An approach for the treatment of penile carcinoma. Cancer 1977;**39:**456–466.
Grabstald H, Kelley CD. Radiation therapy of penile cancer: Six to ten year follow-up. *Urology* 1980;**15:**575–576.
Johnson DE: Penile Carcinoma. AUA Update Series, Vol 1, No. 30, 1982.
Johnson DE, Lowe RK. Tumors of the penis, urethra, and scrotum. In: De Kernion J, Paulson D, editors. *Genitourinary Cancer Management.* Philadelphia: Lea and Febiger, 1987.
Mitros FA. Penile neoplasms in genitourinary oncology. In: Culp D, Loening S, editors. Genitourinary Oncology. Philadelphia: Lea and Febiger, 1985.
Sklaroff RB, Yagoda A. Methotrexate in the treatment of penile carcinoma. *Cancer* 1980;**45:**214–216.

46 Malignancies of the Ovary

Laila I. Muderspach, MD

I. **Epidemiology.** In the United States, ovarian carcinoma accounts for **29% of female genital tract tumors** and **3.7% of all malignancies** in females. In addition, it is the leading cause of death from female genital tract tumors (53%) and the fifth most common cause of death from all female malignancies (5.2%) after breast, colon, lung, and pancreas cancer. In 1985, **14.0 cases per 100,000 females** were diagnosed, resulting in 7.7 deaths. Estimates indicate that 22,000 **new cases** and 13,300 **deaths** will occur in 1993. One of every 70 females in the United States (1.4%) will develop ovarian carcinoma, and 1 of every 100 (1%) will die from the disease. Worldwide, the incidence of ovarian carcinoma varies from a high of 17.2 per 100,000 females in Israel to a low of 2.1 per 100,000 in Japan.

II. **Risk factors**
   A. **Age.** Ovarian cancer is predominantly a disease of peri- and postmenopausal females. It gradually increases in frequency from less than 2.0 cases per 100,000 before age 20 to a peak of **55.8 cases per 100,000 by age 70.**
   B. **Race.** The risk in **whites,** particularly upper class females, is **1.5 times** greater than that in blacks.
   C. **Genetic factors**
      1. **Family history. Familial ovarian cancer** is an **autosomal dominant** disease with variable penetrance transmitted by both males and females. First-degree female relatives in the 435 high-risk kindreds identified by the Familial Ovarian Cancer Registry have a **40% risk** of developing ovarian tumors at an early age. In addition, an **increased risk of breast cancer** in these patients also has been reported.
      2. **Familial disease.** Nearly **5%** of females with **Peutz-Jeghers syndrome** (see Chapter 36) develop ovarian **stromal tumors.**
   D. **Diet.** The increased **dietary fat** in western industrialized nations has been implicated in the etiology of ovarian carcinoma, however this requires further confirmation.
   E. **Smoking.** There is no proven association between smoking and ovarian cancer.
   F. **Radiation.** Massive exposure to radiation (atomic bomb survivors) increases the expected number of ovarian cancers by **2 times.**
   G. **History of previous gynecologic abnormalities**
      1. **Infertility.** Continuous gonadotropin stimulation may be important in the pathogenesis of ovarian cancer because **infertility, nulliparity, late child bearing, and delayed menopause increase** the risk of ovarian carcinoma. In contrast, inhibition of gonadotropin release associated with **pregnancy** and **oral contraceptives** reduces the risk of ovarian cancer by **10–50%.**
      2. **Congenital disorders.** Females with **XY gonadal dysgenesis** are predisposed to malignant **germ cell tumors.**
      3. **Previous breast cancer.** Females with breast cancer are at **2 times** greater risk of developing ovarian malignancies than the normal population.
   H. **Urbanization.** For unclear reasons, **western urban populations** are at greater risk for developing ovarian malignancies than are Third World rural populations. One study links **asbestos-contaminated industrial areas** with a heightened risk of ovarian carcinoma.

III. **Clinical presentation**
   A. **Signs and symptoms**
      1. **Local manifestations.** Many patients remain **asymptomatic** until an adnexal mass is discovered on routine pelvic examination or until advanced disease develops; however, nonspecific signs and symptoms may occur at any time, including vague lower abdominal **discomfort (37–57%), endometrial proliferation and vaginal bleeding** from ovarian stromal stimulation **(15–25%); man-**

ifestations of a large pelvic mass with or without ascites, including vaginal/ uterine prolapse, urinary incontinence, and a pressure sensation (35–51%); and gastrointestinal symptoms from rectosigmoid obstruction (10%).

2. **Systemic manifestations.** Patients frequently complain of **dyspepsia, bloating, early satiety, anorexia, "gas pains," and backache** and often are treated initially for an ulcer diathesis, irritable bowel syndrome, or gallbladder disease. **Severe** pain is uncommon. Advanced disease manifests with **weight loss, increased abdominal girth and pressure, ascites, pleural effusions, supraclavicular or inguinal lymphadenopathy, and symptoms of small bowel obstruction.**

B. **Paraneoplastic syndromes.** Like other female genital tract malignancies, ovarian cancer has been associated with various paraneoplastic syndromes.

1. **Thrombophlebitis** (see p 81).
2. **Hypercalcemia** (see p 87).
3. **Hypoglycemia** (see p 88).
4. **Inappropriate ACTH** (see p 90).
5. **Cachexia** (see p 75).
6. **Disseminated intravascular coagulation** (see p 80).

IV. **Differential diagnosis.** Although ovarian cancer may present with evidence of widespread intraperitoneal metastases, an **isolated adnexal or pelvic mass** is often discovered incidentally during a routine pelvic examination. In this setting, true ovarian neoplasms must be distinguished from other **gynecologic processes** such as pregnancy, infection (pelvic inflammatory disease or tuberculosis), and other benign and malignant neoplasms (functional or dermoid ovarian cysts, serous or mucinous cystadenomas, endometriomas, fallopian tube neoplasms, paratubal and para-ovarian cysts, uterine leiomyomata, and endometrial and cervical carcinoma). In addition, these neoplasms must be distinguished from **non-gynecologic diseases** such as infections (appendicitis, diverticulitis, Crohn's disease, and foreign body granuloma), other primary neoplasms (colon, appendiceal, and small bowel adenocarcinoma, retroperitoneal sarcoma, and lymphoma), and metastatic disease (Krukenberg's tumor). Urinary retention, severe constipation, pelvic kidney, sacral meningocele, urachal or omental cysts, and Müllerian anomalies also should be considered.

V. **Screening programs.** As a result of a dearth of specific early symptoms, a poorly defined high-risk population, and inadequate screening tools, routine screening of asymptomatic patients is not recommended. Patients with symptoms, pelvic masses, or significant risk factors should be evaluated by physical examination, serum CA-125 levels, pelvic ultrasound, or CT scan (see below, **VI.B.1.e, VI.B.3.b,** and **VI.B.3.c**).

VI. **Diagnostic workup**

A. **Medical history and physical examination.** A thorough medical history (documenting risk factors) and a complete physical examination should be performed in all patients with suspected ovarian cancer. Particular attention should be directed to the following areas:

1. **General appearance.** An evaluation of the patient's general functional and nutritional status should be included (see, also, p 1, I and III).
2. **Lymph nodes.** The number, consistency, tenderness, and distribution of all cervical, supraclavicular, axillary, and inguinal lymph nodes must be carefully documented.
3. **Chest.** Evidence of pleural effusions and pulmonary metastases (eg, decreased or absent breath sounds, pleural friction rub) should be excluded on pulmonary examination.
4. **Breasts.** Careful breast examination is mandatory to exclude a primary breast lesion.
5. **Abdomen.** Hepatosplenomegaly, ascites, and all masses (intraperitoneal metastases) must be fully described.
6. **Genitalia**
   a. **External genitalia.** The vulva, urethra, vaginal introitus, and anus should be examined for primary or metastatic lesions.
   b. **Vagina.** Visualization and palpation of the entire vagina is necessary to exclude primary or metastatic disease.
   c. **Cervix.** The evaluation includes complete visualization and cytologic (**Papanicolaou smear**) examination as well as bimanual examination.
   d. **Uterus and adnexa.** Initially, the vaginal walls, fornices, and ectocervix should be palpated, and the cervix and uterus should be assessed for position, size, and mobility. In addition, the size of the ovaries must be docu-

mented, and evidence of bladder and rectosigmoid involvement should be noted. Rectovaginal examination is required to evaluate the **cul-de-sac** and **rectovaginal septum.**

  7. **Rectum. Extrinsic compression** and **invasion** of the rectosigmoid must be excluded, and stool should be tested for **occult blood.**

B. **Primary tests and procedures.** The following is a list of diagnostic tests and procedures that should be performed initially on all patients with suspected ovarian carcinoma:
  1. **Blood tests**
    a. **Complete blood count** (see p 1, **IV.A.1**).
    b. **Hepatic enzymes** (see p 1, **IV.A.2**).
    c. **Alkaline phosphatase** (see p 1, **IV.A.3**).
    d. **BUN and creatinine** (see p 3, **IV.A.6**).
    e. **CA-125.** This antigen is detectable in more than 80% of patients with **non-mucinous epithelial ovarian carcinomas,** and levels can be followed as an indicator of disease activity.
    f. **Coagulation times. Prothrombin and partial thromboplastin times** are needed to exclude a coagulopathy.
    g. **Albumin.**
  2. **Urine tests**
    a. **Urinalysis.**
    b. **Beta-human chorionic gonadotropin (beta-hCG).** This test must be obtained to exclude **pregnancy.**
  3. **Imaging studies**
    a. **Chest x-ray.**
    b. **Ultrasound.** A pelvic ultrasound can delineate the uterus, ovaries, and characterize any adnexal pathology. (see p 3, **IV.C.4**).
    c. **Computed tomography (CT).** CT scan of the abdomen and pelvis provide useful information regarding the liver, genitourinary tract, and retroperitoneal lymph nodes as well as peritoneal disease. This is not necessary if an ultrasound diagnosis has been made.

C. **Optional tests and procedures.** The following examinations may be indicated by previous diagnostic findings or clinical suspicion.
  1. **Blood tests**
    a. **Carcinoembryonic antigen.** Serum levels of this antigen are elevated in both **mucinous ovarian tumors** and colorectal carcinoma.
    b. **Alpha-fetoprotein.** Children and young females with endodermal sinus tumors frequently have elevated levels of this tumor marker.
    c. **Arterial blood gas.** Patients with pleural effusions, massive ascites, or borderline pulmonary function require evaluation of arterial oxygenation and gas exchange.
  2. **Imaging studies**
    a. **Barium enema.** Evaluation of the colon should be performed in patients with a change in bowel habits or occult fecal blood to exclude colonic involvement from direct tumor invasion or a primary colon carcinoma.
    b. **Upper gastrointestinal series.** This is necessary if a patient presents with symptoms of upper gastrointestinal disease.
    c. **Intravenous pyelogram (IVP).** IVP should be obtained if ureteral obstruction from tumor invasion is suspected. An **abdominal CT** scan, however, may provide similar information and obviate the need for this test.
    d. **Magnetic resonance imaging (MRI).** (see p 3, **IV.C.3**).
    e. **Technetium-99m bone scan** (see p 3, **IV.C.4**).
  3. **Invasive procedures**
    a. **Fine needle aspiration.** This test can be used to assess suspicious supraclavicular or inguinal lymph nodes as well as lung, liver, and vaginopelvic masses, but it should not be used to evaluate the primary ovarian tumor.
    b. **Endoscopy.** Cystoscopy and proctosigmoidoscopy may be needed in more advanced cases when bladder or rectosigmoid involvement are suspected. Esophagogastroduodenoscopy (EGD) may be necessary if a gastric carcinoma is suspected.
    c. **Paracentesis.** This procedure usually is not done for diagnostic purposes because tumor seeding along the needle tract may occur; however, it may be required to alleviate respiratory distress from massive ascites.
    d. **Thoracentesis.** Significant pleural effusions may require thoracentesis for proper staging (malignant effusions signify Stage IV disease) or for symptomatic relief of respiratory distress.

VII. Pathology

A. Location. There is no predilection for either ovary.

B. Multiplicity. Several **epithelial** tumors may present with bilateral disease, including **serous carcinoma (25%), mucinous malignancies (10–20%), endometrioid tumors (30%),** clear cell neoplasms (rare), and Brenner tumors (rare). However, the only **germ cell** neoplasm with a significant incidence of bilateral disease is **dysgerminoma,** with **10–15% synchronous** and **5–15% metachronous** involvement of the contralateral ovary. In addition, patients with ovarian cancer are at increased risk of **breast, colon, and endometrial** carcinoma.

C. Histology. A continuum of ovarian pathology exists, ranging from benign to frankly malignant disease.

1. **Tumors of low malignant potential (TLMP).** These borderline tumors, which account for **15% of all epithelial ovarian cancers,** have histologic and biologic features of both benign and malignant ovarian neoplasms. The classification of the International Federation of Gynecology and Obstetrics (FIGO) describes TLMP as cystadenomas with nuclear abnormalities, epithelial cell proliferation, but no infiltration.

2. **Epithelial ovarian cancer (85–90%).** Nearly **90%** of ovarian cancers are derived from the **coelomic epithelium.** The most common histologic type is **serous carcinoma (75%).** Less common types are mucinous (20%), endometrioid (2%), clear cell (< 1%), Brenner (< 1%), undifferentiated (< 1%), and a mixture of these types.

3. **Nonepithelial ovarian cancer (10%).** This category includes tumors of germ cell and sex cord-stromal cell origin, sarcomas, lipoid cell tumors, and metastatic carcinomas (see Table 46–1).

D. Metastatic spread

1. **Modes of spread.** The vast majority of ovarian carcinomas (**70–80%**) are metastatic at the time of diagnosis. Ovarian cancers spread by **4 main routes:**

   a. **Direct extension.** After capsular invasion has occurred, direct invasion may involve the **cul-de-sac, sigmoid colon, small intestines, uterus, tubes, and pelvic peritoneum.**

   b. **Lymphatic metastasis.** This mode of spread involves the regional lymphatics in the retroperitoneum of the pelvis and the **para-aorta, supraclavicular, axillary as well as inguinal nodes.** The mediastinal nodes may be affected as a result of diaphragmatic lymphatic drainage.

   c. **Hematogenous metastasis.** In advanced disease, spread through portal and systemic blood vessels leads to distant organs.

   d. **Intraperitoneal exfoliation.** The earliest and most common route of dissemination involves intraperitoneal implantation of exfoliated tumor cells. The distribution of metastases follows the **circulation of peritoneal fluid** and involves the posterior cul-de-sac, paracolic gutters (right to left), the diaphragmatic surfaces (right to left), liver and splenic capsules, the intestinal surfaces and their mesenteries, and the omentum. Large omental cakes that often develop may secrete tremendous amounts of **ascites.**

2. **Sites of metastatic spread.** Distant metastases may involve the following organs: **peritoneum, liver, lung, bone, and central nervous system.**

TABLE 46–1. WHO HISTOLOGIC CLASSIFICATION OF OVARIAN NEOPLASMS

Epithelial tumors	Germ cell tumors
Serous	Dysgerminoma
Mucinous	Teratoma
Endometroid	Immature
Clear cell	Mature (dermoid cyst)
Brenner	Endodermal sinus
Mixed epithelial	Embryonal carcinoma
Undifferentiated	Polyembryoma
Sex-cord stromal tumors	Choriocarcinoma
Granulosa-stromal cell	**Soft-tissue tumors**
Androblastomas	**Unclassified tumors**
Sertoli-Leydig cell	**Metastatic (secondary) tumors**
Gynandroblastoma	

Adapted from the International Histologic Classification of Tumors, No. 9. Geneva: World Health Organization; 1973.

VIII. **Staging.** The **FIGO** and the cancer unit of the World Health Organization have developed staging systems. The TNM staging system is not commonly used in gynecologic cancers, but it correlates with the FIGO stage grouping for ovarian malignancies. Ovarian cancer is a **surgical-histopathologically staged disease.**

   A. **TNM staging system**

   1. **Tumor stage**

   a. **TX.** The primary tumor cannot be assessed.

   b. **T0.** No evidence of a primary tumor exists.

   c. **T1.** Tumor is limited to the ovaries.

   (1) **T1a.** Tumor is limited to one ovary; capsule is intact, no tumor on ovarian surface.

   (2) **T1b.** Tumor is limited to both ovaries; capsules are intact, no tumor on ovarian surface.

   (3) **T1c.** Tumor is limited to one or both ovaries with any of the following: capsule ruptured, tumor on ovarian surface, malignant cells in ascites, or peritoneal washings.

   d. **T2.** Tumor involves one or both ovaries with pelvic extension.

   (1) **T2a.** Extension or implants on the uterus, the tubes, or both.

   (2) **T2b.** Extension to other pelvic tissues.

   (3) **T2c.** Pelvic extension (T2a or T2b) with malignant cells in ascites or peritoneal washing.

   e. **T3.** Tumor involves one or both ovaries with microscopically confirmed peritoneal metastasis outside the pelvis.

   (1) **T3a.** Microscopic peritoneal metastasis beyond the pelvis.

   (2) **T3b.** Macroscopic peritoneal metastasis beyond the pelvis, that is no larger than 2 cm in its greatest dimension.

   (3) **T3c.** Peritoneal metastasis beyond the pelvis, that is larger than 2 cm in its greatest dimension.

   Note: Liver **capsule** metastases are considered T3 disease.

   2. **Lymph node stage**

   a. **NX.** Regional lymph nodes cannot be assessed.

   b. **N0.** No regional lymph node metastases.

   c. **N1.** Regional lymph node metastases are present.

   3. **Metastatic stage**

   a. **MX.** The presence of distant metastasis cannot be assessed.

   b. **M0.** No distant metastases are present.

   c. **MI.** Distant metastasis are present.

   Note: Liver **parenchyma** metastases are considered to be M1 disease.

   4. **Histopathologic grade**

   a. **GX.** Grade cannot be assessed.

   b. **GB.** Borderline malignancy.

   c. **G1.** Well differentiated.

   d. **G2.** Moderately well differentiated.

   e. **G3–4.** Poorly differentiated or undifferentiated.

   5. **Stage groupings**

   a. **Stage IA.** T1a, N0, M0.

   b. **Stage IB.** T1b, N0, M0.

   c. **Stage IC.** T1c, N0, M0.

   d. **Stage IIA.** T2a, N0, M0.

   e. **Stage IIB.** T2b, N0, M0.

   f. **Stage IIC.** T2c, N0, M0.

   g. **Stage IIIA.** T3a, N0, M0.

   h. **Stage IIIB.** T3b, N0, M0.

   i. **Stage IIIC.** T3c, N0, M0; any T, N1, M0.

   j. **Stage IV.** Any T, any N, M1.

   B. **FIGO staging system**

   1. **Stage I.** Growth limited to the ovaries.

   a. **Stage Ia.** Growth limited to one ovary without tumor on the external surface or ruptured capsule and no ascites (T1a, N0, M0).

   b. **Stage Ib.** Growth limited to both ovaries without tumor on the external surface or ruptured capsule and no ascites (T1b, N0, M0).

   c. **Stage Ic.** Tumor either Stage Ia or Stage Ib, but with tumor on the surface of one or both ovaries, ruptured capsule, malignant ascites, or positive peritoneal washings (T1c, N0, M0).

   2. **Stage II.** Growth involving one or both ovaries with pelvic extension.

    a. **Stage IIa.** Extension, metastases, or both to the uterus or tubes (T2a, N0, M0).

    b. **Stage IIb.** Extension to other pelvic tissues (T2b, N0, M0).

    c. **Stage IIc.** Tumor either Stage IIa or Stage IIb, but with tumor on the surface of one or both ovaries, ruptured capsule or capsules, malignant ascites, or positive peritoneal washings (T2c, N0, M0).

3. **Stage III.** Tumor involves one or both ovaries with peritoneal implants outside the pelvis, positive retroperitoneal or inguinal nodes, or all of these.

    a. **Stage IIIa.** Tumor is grossly limited to the true pelvis with negative nodes, but with histologically confirmed microscopic seeding of abdominal peritoneal surfaces (T3a, N0, M0).

    b. **Stage IIIb.** Tumor of one or both ovaries with histologically confirmed abdominal implants no larger than 2 cm in diameter and negative nodes (T3b, N0, M0).

    c. **Stage IIIc.** Abdominal implants larger than 2 cm in diameter and/or positive retroperitoneal or inguinal nodes (T3c, N0, M0; any T, N1, M0).

      Note: liver capsule metastases and tumor limited to the true pelvis, but with histologically proved malignant extension to the small bowel or omentum, are considered Stage III.

4. **Stage IV.** Growth involving one or both ovaries with distant metastases (Any T, any N, M1).

    Note: liver parenchyma metastases are considered to be Stage IV, and malignant ascites and pleural effusions must contain histologically confirmed tumor cells.

IX. Treatment

A. Surgery

1. **Primary ovarian carcinoma**

    a. **Indications.** Except for severely disabled patients with widely metastatic disease, surgery (abdominal exploration with removal of the uterus, fallopian tubes, ovaries, and staging with cytologic washings, omentectomy, and retroperitoneal lymph node biopsy) is indicated in virtually **all patients.**

    b. **Approaches.** Exploratory laparotomy generally is performed through a **low midline incision.** If upper abdominal disease is present, the incision is extended superiorly for optimal exposure and cytoreduction.

    c. **Surgical technique.** Upon entering the peritoneal cavity, surgical staging is performed (see **c.(1)** below). In **young** females with **early unilateral ovarian carcinoma, unilateral salpingo-oophorectomy** is performed, and the contralateral "normal" ovary is biopsied without compromising fertility. Immediate pathologic confirmation (frozen section) may be required. If fertility is not an issue, **total abdominal hysterectomy and bilateral salpingo-oophorectomy** is recommended. Early ovarian carcinoma (Stage I or II) necessitates careful surgical staging (see **c.(1)** below), whereas advanced disease requires meticulous documentation of findings both before and after tumor cytoreduction.

      (1) **Surgical staging.** Initially, **ascites** (if present) is collected for cytologic evaluation. If no ascites is present, washings are obtained from the **pelvic cul-de-sac, bilateral paracolic gutters, and subdiaphragmatic spaces.** Then, the diaphragm, liver, gallbladder, spleen, pancreas, omentum, intestines, and retroperitoneal lymph nodes are thoroughly explored. Any suspicious lesion must be biopsied. In addition, **infracolic omentectomy, appendectomy, retroperitoneal lymph node sampling (pelvic and para-aortic), and random biopsies of the peritoneum overlying the cul-de-sac, paracolic gutters, bladder, and mesentery** are obtained systematically. For patients with low-grade disease limited to the ovaries without a ruptured cyst and positive peritoneal cytology (Stages IA and IB, Grade G1), no further therapy (chemo- or radiotherapy) is required.

      (2) **Cytoreductive surgery.** Prognosis is related to the tumor burden that is present, not only at the time of diagnosis, but also after surgery. Therefore, the goal of surgery in advanced disease (Stages III and IV) is to **remove as much tumor as possible** even if resection of bowel is necessary. **"Optimal" cytoreduction is defined as the removal of all tumor nodules larger than 2.0 cm** in their greatest dimension; however, the best results are obtained when residual tumor implants are smaller than 0.5 cm in their greatest dimension.

2. **Locally advanced and metastatic ovarian cancer**
   a. **Preoperative preparation.** Preoperative orders should include a **mechanical and antibiotic bowel preparation** (see p 277, **IX.A.1.(b)**), and perioperative **total parenteral nutrition** is often beneficial. In addition, the patient and family must be counseled regarding the extent and possible complications of the planned operation.
   b. **Primary cytoreduction.** If feasible, surgical debulking should be attempted. Extensive disease involving the pelvic side wall may require an **en bloc resection of the uterus, fallopian tubes, ovaries, and rectosigmoid.** If small bowel (usually ileum) is involved, a segmental resection should be performed. A large **omental cake must be removed to decrease ascites.** If the spleen is involved, **splenectomy may be necessary** for optimal cytoreduction. Postoperatively, patients receive intensive chemotherapy.
   c. **Secondary cytoreduction.** Removal of recurrent disease can be attempted if no distant metastases are detected. Although secondary cytoreduction does not significantly prolong survival, it is associated with an improved quality of life. However, patients require further postoperative chemotherapy, radiotherapy, or both.
   d. **Second-look surgery.** Following initial chemotherapy, patients without clinical or radiologic manifestation of residual disease undergo a second surgery to determine tumor status. The surgery may be done by laparotomy or laparoscopy. **Multiple strategic biopsies (generally 20–40, including areas of adhesion), washings, and retroperitoneal lymph node biopsies** are performed. Intraperitoneal catheters are placed in selected patients for postoperative intraperitoneal chemotherapy.
3. **Mortality and morbidity.** The mortality and morbidity from surgical staging of early ovarian cancer is low and includes the following problems: **hemorrhage, wound infection, vaginal cuff cellulitis, genital tract fistulae, lymphocele formation, and prolonged ileus.**

B. **Radiation therapy**
   1. **Primary ovarian carcinoma.** Radiation therapy alone is not indicated in the initial treatment of ovarian cancer.
   2. **Adjuvant radiation therapy**
      a. **Preoperative radiotherapy.** This treatment modality has not been successful.
      b. **Intraoperative radiotherapy.** No significant experience with this approach has been reported.
      c. **Postoperative radiotherapy**
         (1) **Whole abdomen and pelvic radiation.** Whole abdomen and pelvic radiation has been used with variable success for residual microscopic disease following cytoreduction surgery (Stage I–IIIA). Generally, the **open-field** rather than moving-strip technique is used, and the entire peritoneal cavity is treated to **2000–3000 cGy in fractions of 100–125 cGy** (shielding only the kidneys). The **pelvis** is boosted in 180 cGy fractions to a total of **5000 cGy.** Following optimal cytoreduction and radiation therapy, the **overall 5-year survival is 43%;** for Stage I–IIIA, although 5-year survival rates as high as **71.5%** have been reported.
         (2) **Intraperitoneal radiocolloids.** Intraperitoneal colloids travel the same route as do malignant cells in ascites (via paracolic gutters to the diaphragm) and, theoretically, are concentrated in the same locations. For this reason, intraperitoneal therapy with the **radiocolloid, ^{32}P,** has been tried in patients with **early ovarian carcinoma (Stage I–IIIA).** The results are identical to those of melphalan, with **5-year survival rates as high as 85%.**
   3. **Locally advanced and metastatic ovarian cancer.** Pain from bony or large soft-tissue metastases may be significantly palliated with external-beam or interstitial therapy.
   4. **Mortality and morbidity.** Postoperative whole abdomen and pelvic radiation produces substantial morbidity **(15–40%).** Complications include all the problems associated with myelosuppression as well as the following difficulties: **diarrhea,** 78%; **bowel obstruction,** 14%; **fistulae** involving the ureters, bladder, small and large intestines, and vagina; **retroperitoneal fibrosis,** causing ureteral obstruction; **proctitis, enteritis, or ileitis; cystitis; hepatitis** (> 2500 cGy); **nephritis** (> 2500 cGy); and **basal pneumonitis.**

C. **Chemotherapy**
  1. **Primary ovarian carcinoma.** Only patients with widely metastatic ovarian cancer, who are **poor surgical candidates,** should be treated initially with combination chemotherapy (see p 349, **IX.C.3**). If a significant response occurs, subsequent surgical intervention then may be beneficial.
  2. **Adjuvant chemotherapy**
      a. **Preoperative chemotherapy.** Because prior pathologic staging and cytoreduction (if necessary) are important for maximum chemotherapeutic response, this approach has not been widely used.
      b. **Postoperative chemotherapy.** Stages IA and IB (Grades G2–4) and Stage IC (all grades) require adjuvant chemotherapy or whole abdomen and pelvic radiotherapy.
          (1) **Single agent therapy.** Until recently, the most widely used single chemotherapeutic agent was **melphalan** (0.2 mg/kg per d for 5 of every 28 days), which yields **5-year survival** as high as **78%**. Other agents (fluorouracil, doxorubicin, hexamethylmelamine, and cisplatin) collectively produce a 34% overall 5-year survival. Because of the side effects of melphalan (10% incidence of **acute nonlymphocytic leukemia** after 12 cycles and 0.3% risk overall) and the development of superior **cisplatin-based combination regimens** (eg, cyclophosphamide and cisplatin = CP; and cyclophosphamide, doxorubicin, and cisplatin = CAP), the use of single agents has been limited.
          (2) **Combination chemotherapy.** Several studies of combination chemotherapy have demonstrated a significant improvement in response rates and survival over those obtained with single agents. Various combinations of cisplatin, carboplatin, cyclophosphamide, doxorubicin, melphalan, and hexamethylmelamine (see Appendix C2) have produced **response rates as high as 84%, compared with 54%** in similar patients treated with single-agent therapy and **4- and 5-year survivals as high as 53% and 34%,** respectively. Currently, **cisplatin or carboplatin and cyclophosphamide** given 3–4 weeks apart for a total of 6–8 cycles are recommended. Carboplatin, which has less gastrointestinal, neural, and nephrotoxicity but greater myelosuppression than cisplatin, can be given as an outpatient since hydration is not necessary.
          (3) **Intraperitoneal chemotherapy.** The usefulness of intraperitoneal chemotherapy is controversial, but currently appears to be limited to patients with **residual disease less than 5 mm** (maximum diameter) and without extensive intra-abdominal adhesions. Like intravenous chemotherapy, **cisplatin** (50–150 mg/m^2 in 2 L every 2–3 weeks for 6–10 cycles) produces the best results: **74% 2-year survival** in nonrandomized trials that evaluated patients with minimal residual disease. Cytosine arabinoside, fluorouracil, doxorubicin, melphalan, and methotrexate also have been infused, but with less success.
  3. **Locally advanced and metastatic ovarian cancer.** Chemotherapy, although usually not curative, often provides significant palliation in patients with locally advanced and metastatic disease. Although one study demonstrated superior results with cyclophosphamide, hexamethylmelamine, doxorubicin, and cisplatin (**CHAP-5;** 19.5 months disease-free and 30.7 months of overall survival) versus cyclophosphamide, fluorouracil, hexamethylmelamine, and methotrexate (**Hexa-CAF;** 6.8 months disease-free and 19.6 months of overall survival), most studies have failed to document improved survival over that obtained with the 2-drug combination of **cyclophosphamide and cisplatin.** Several newer intravenous agents, including etoposide, mitoxantrone, and ifosfamide, as well as oral agents that are less toxic (melphalan, cyclophosphamide, etoposide, and hexamethylmelamine) are being studied. In addition, **taxol** (from the bark of the yew tree) has shown some promising results (approx 20–30% response rate) and is now accepted as part of a second line combination regimen with platinum.
D. **Hormonal therapy. Progestational agents** such as tamoxifen, megestrol, and GnRH analogs produce some responses in the **palliation of endometrioid ovarian carcinomas.** To date, however, no effect on survival has been demonstrated.
E. **Immunology.** Although 2 randomized studies suggested a role for immunotherapy in combination with chemotherapy, the use of biologic response modifiers in the treatment of ovarian carcinoma is currently considered investigational. In-

traperitoneal administration has been used preferentially to systemic delivery in many trials to reduce toxicity. Agents that have been or are currently under study include *Corynebacterium parvum,* interferon, levamisole, interleukin-2, lymphokine-activated killer (LAK) cells, and toxin- or radiolabeled monoclonal antibodies (against cell surface antigens).

X. Prognosis

A. Risk of recurrence. Following a complete pathologic response documented during a second-look laparotomy, **15–20%** of all patients will develop recurrent disease. However, the recurrence rate increases to **nearly 50%** in patients with Grade 2–4 or Stage III–IV tumor.

B. Five-year survival. The 5-year survival is determined by tumor stage and grade and is summarized below:

   1. **Tumor stage**
      a. **Stage I,** 80–100%.
      b. **Stage II or IIIA,** 30–40%.
      c. **Stage IIIB,** 20%.
      d. **Stage IIIC or IV,** 5–10%.
   2. **Tumor grade**
      a. **Grade GB,** more than 95%.
      b. **Grade G1,** 50–60%.
      c. **Grade G2,** 30%.
      d. **Grade G3,** 5–10%.

C. Adverse prognostic factors. The prognosis is related to multiple factors and is adversely affected by the following characteristics:

   1. **Poor performance status.**
   2. **Age older than 50 years** (5-year survival of 15% versus 40% for patients younger than 50 years).
   3. **Residual tumor.** Residual tumor following staging laparotomy and cytoreduction decreases the 5-year survival significantly as outlined below:
      a. **Microscopic disease only,** 50–75%.
      b. **Optimal disease** (< 2 cm maximum residual tumor), 30–40%.
      c. **Nonoptimal disease,** 5%.
   4. **Status at second-look laparotomy.** Residual tumor discovered at second-look laparotomy adversely affects the 5-year survival as follows: **no evidence of disease,** 50–70%; **microscopic disease,** 40–50%; **macroscopic disease,** 5%;

XI. Patient follow-up

A. General guidelines. Patients with ovarian carcinoma should be followed every 3 months for 2 years, every 6 months for 3 additional years, and then annually for evidence of recurrence. Specific guidelines are outlined below.

B. Routine evaluation. Each clinic visit should include the following examinations:

   1. **Medical history and physical examination.** An interval medical history and thorough physical examination should be performed during each office visit. Areas for particular attention are outlined on p 345, **VI.A**).
   2. **Blood tests**
      a. **Complete blood count** (see p 1, **IV.A.1**).
      b. **Hepatic transaminase** (see p 1, **IV.A.2**).
      c. **Alkaline phosphatase** (see p 1, **IV.A.3**).
      d. **BUN and creatinine** (see p 1, **IV.A.6**).
      e. **CA-125** (see p 346, **VI.B.1.e**).
   3. **Urinalysis** (see p 3, **IV.B**).
   4. **Chest x-ray** (see p 3, **IV.C.1**).

C. Additional evaluation. Other tests that should be obtained at regular intervals include the following:

   1. **Computed tomography (CT).** CT scan of the abdomen and pelvis should be obtained **every 6 months for 2 years.**
   2. **Papanicolaou smear (PAP).** This cytologic test should be performed every **6–12 months** in all patients.

D. Optional evaluation. The following tests and procedures may be indicated by previous diagnostic findings or clinical suspicion:

   1. **Blood tests** (see p 2, **IV.A**)
      a. **Nucleotidase.**
      b. **GGTP.**
   2. **Imaging studies** (see p 3, **IV.C**)
      a. **Magnetic resonance imaging (MRI).**

b. **Ultrasound** (see p 3, **IV.C.4**).
c. **Technetium-99m bone scan.**
3. **Biopsy of suspicious lesions.** Any suspicious lesions in the vagina or vaginal cuff should be directly biopsied, and deep masses detected clinically or radiographically should be assessed by fine needle aspiration.

REFERENCES

Berek, JS and Hacker, NF. Staging and second-look operations. In Ovarian Cancer. Albert, PS, Surwit, EA and Hingham, MA, editors. Martinus Nijhoff, Boston: pp. 109–127, 1985.

Berek, JS and Hacker, NF, eds. Practical Gynecologic Oncology. Willams and Wilkins, Baltimore, 1989.

Berek, JS, Hacker, NF, Lichtenstein, A, et al. Intraperitoneal recombinant alpha 2 interferon for salvage immunotherapy in stage III epithelial ovarian cancer: a gynecologic oncology group study. Cancer Res 45:4447–4453, 1985.

Buchsbaum, HJ and Lifshitz, S. Staging and surgical evaluation of ovarian cancer. Semin Oncol 11:227–233, 1984.

Dembo, AJ, Bush, RS, Beale, FA, et al. A randomized clinical trial of moving strip versus open field whole abdominal irradiation in patients with invasive epithelial cancer of the ovary. Int J Radiat Oncol Biol Phys 9(suppl):97–104, 1983.

Griffiths, CT. Surgical resection of tumor bulk in the primary treatment of ovarian carcinoma. NCI Mono 42:101–104, 1975.

Hacker, NF, Berek, JS, Julliard, G, et al. Whole abdominal radiation as salvage therapy for epithelial ovarian cancer. Obstet Gynecol 65:60–66, 1985.

Heintz, AM, Hacker, NF, Berek, JS, et al. Cytoreductive surgery in ovarian carcinoma: feasibility and morbidity. Obstet Gynecol 67:783–788, 1986.

Morkman, M and Howell, SB. Intraperitoneal chemotherapy for ovarian cancer. In Ovarian Cancer. Albert, PS, Surwit, EA and Hingham, MA, editors. Martinus Nijhoff, Boston: pp. 129–212, 1985.

Morrow, C.P., Townsend, D.E., eds. Synopsis of Gynecologic Oncology. Churchill Livingston, New York, 3rd ed., 1987.

Neijt, JP, Ten Bokkel Huinink, WW, Van der Burg, M, et al. Combination chemotherapy with CH4P-5 and CP in advanced ovarian carcinoma: a randomized trial of the Netherlands joint study group for ovarian cancer Proc Am Soc Clin Oncol 4:442–447, 1985.

Piver Steven, M. Ovarian Malignancies: Diagnostic and Therapeutic Advances. Churchill Livingstone, New York, 1987.

Thigren, JT. Single agent chemotherapy in the management of ovarian carcinoma. In Albert, PS, Surwit, EA, and Hingham, MA, editors. Martinus Nijhoff, Boston: pp. 115–146, 1985.

47 Malignancies of the Uterine Corpus

James Heaps, MD

I. **Epidemiology.** Carcinoma of the uterine corpus (endometrial carcinoma) is the **most common** gynecologic cancer and the fourth most common malignancy of any type in females. In the United States, **22 cases per 100,000 females** were diagnosed in 1985, resulting in 3.8 deaths. Estimates indicate that **31,000 new cases** and **5,700 deaths** will occur in 1993. In the early 1970s, with the aggressive administration of **exogenous estrogens** for postmenopausal symptoms, the incidence of endometrial carcinoma abruptly increased to a peak of 32.0 per 100,000 in 1975. When this practice was curtailed, the incidence again declined to the previous stable level. In contrast, the **mortality rates** steadily **decreased 60%** between 1950 and 1985.

Worldwide, the incidence of endometrial cancer varies from 38.5 cases per 100,000 in **Alameda county, California,** to 1.0 per 100,000 in **Japan.** Other countries with a high incidence are Chile, Hungary, and Austria; those with a low incidence include Israel, Australia, and Canada. In addition, epidemiologic data demonstrate that immigrants adopt the risk of the surrounding population.

II. **Risk factors**
   A. **Age.** Endometrial cancer is predominantly a disease of **postmenopausal** females. The incidence steadily increases from less than 1.0 per 100,000 before age 30 to a peak of **116.9 per 100,000** by age 65. The average age at diagnosis is **58 years;** only 2–5% of cases occur in females younger than 40.
   B. **Race.** The risk in whites is **1.6–2.0 times** that in blacks.
   C. **Genetic factors.** A slightly increased risk of endometrial carcinoma has been documented in first-degree relatives of patients with endometrial, breast, ovary, and colon cancer.
   D. **Diet**
      1. **Dietary fat.** Worldwide, the total intake of dietary fat directly parallels the incidence of endometrial cancer.
      2. **Obesity.** Obesity increases the risk of endometrial carcinoma by **3–10 times,** possibly because of increased circulating estrogens.
   E. **Smoking.** The incidence of endometrial carcinoma is **reduced 50%** in smokers, allegedly because of the **antiestrogenic effects of nicotine.**
   F. **History of previous endocrine and medical abnormalities**
      1. **Increased estrogens.** Conditions marked by prolonged exposure to elevated circulating estrogen levels without simultaneous progesterone exposure (conditions with unopposed estrogen) increase the risk of endometrial carcinoma. These conditions include **early menarche, anovulation, nulliparity, polycystic ovarian syndromes, estrogen-secreting neoplasms, and estrogen ingestion.** Unopposed estrogen replacement in postmenopausal females increases the risk of endometrial cancer by **6–8 fold.** In contrast, low-dose progesterone-containing oral contraceptives used by young females have been shown to reduce the risk of subsequent endometrial carcinoma by as much as **50%.**
      2. **Other endocrine disorders.** Other endocrine diseases that have been associated with slightly increased risks of carcinoma of the uterine corpus include **diabetes mellitus, hypothyroidism, and tall stature.**
      3. **Medical disorders.** For unclear reasons, hypertension and arthritis are associated with the development of endometrial carcinoma.
   G. **Ionizing radiation.** Patients with a history of previous pelvic irradiation (often for cervical carcinoma) have an increased risk of both endometrial adenocarcinoma and uterine sarcoma.
   H. **Urbanization.** Urban populations are at greater risk of endometrial carcinoma than are rural residents because of an unknown risk factor.

III. **Presentation**

A. **Signs and symptoms**
   1. **Local manifestations.** More than 90% of patients present with **vaginal bleeding.** Occasionally, a purulent vaginal discharge, pelvic pain, or uterine enlargement is the initial presenting symptom. Abnormal endometrial cells are found on routine cervicovaginal Papanicolaou (Pap) smears in **50%** of patients with endometrial cancer. Conversely, a **25%** incidence of endometrial carcinoma has been associated with abnormal endometrial cells discovered on a routine postmenopausal Pap smear. Even **normal endometrial cells,** however, should not be detected on postmenopausal Pap smear and, if present, increase the risk of endometrial hyperplasia and carcinoma by **6–15%.**
   2. **Systemic manifestations.** Systemic complaints indicating advanced disease include weight loss, bone pain, supraclavicular or inguinal adenopathy, ascites, jaundice, pleural effusions, and hydronephrosis.
B. **Paraneoplastic syndromes.** Like other gynecologic cancers, endometrial carcinoma has been associated with a variety of paraneoplastic syndromes.
   1. **Hypercalcemia** (see p 87, **I**).
   2. **Inappropriate ACTH** (see p 90, **V**).
   3. **Thrombophlebitis** (see p 81, **II**).
IV. **Differential diagnosis.** Endometrial carcinoma typically presents with **irregular postmenopausal vaginal bleeding.** The differential diagnosis of abnormal uterine bleeding includes primary **gynecologic diseases** such as ascending genital tract infections (vaginitis, cervicitis, endometritis, and salpingitis); tuberculosis; foreign body reactions; urinary tract or intestinal fistulae; pregnancy (normal, aborted, ectopic, and trophoblastic); anovulation; and benign neoplasms (endometrial hyperplasia and metaplasia, leiomyoma, polyps, and ovarian hyperthecosis). The differential diagnosis also includes **systemic diseases** such as hypothyroidism, hyperprolactinemia, adrenal dysfunction, liver disease, renal failure (dialysis), factor deficiencies, platelet dysfunction, von Willebrand's disease, idiopathic thrombocytopenia purpura (ITP), aplastic anemia, and leukemia. Other factors include **medications** such as oral contraceptives, estrogen preparations, corticosteroids, androgens, antidepressants, anticoagulants, anticholinergic, and chemotherapeutic agents; **uterine trauma** (abortion, IUD manipulation, and endoscopy); and **metastatic neoplasms** (breast colon, stomach, ovary, fallopian tube, and endocervical carcinoma). In addition, **hematuria and anorectal bleeding** can be confused with vaginal bleeding and must be excluded.
V. **Screening programs.** An ideal mass-screening method has not been developed; however, **obese, hypertensive, diabetic postmenopausal females** as well as those receiving **exogenous estrogens,** those with a strong **family history** of endometrial, colon, breast, or ovarian cancer, and those with **late menopause** (after age 52) or prolonged periods of **anovulation** warrant a screening endometrial biopsy. Others who require a workup to exclude uterine carcinoma include females with **abnormal endometrial cells** on routine Pap smear, **irregular menses,** and irregular **perimenopausal and postmenopausal bleeding.**
VI. **Diagnostic workup**
   A. **Medical history and physical examination.** A complete medical history, emphasizing risk factors (see p 354, **II**) and a thorough physical examination should be performed on all patients with suspected carcinoma of the uterine corpus.
      1. **General appearance.** An assessment of the overall nutritional and functional status of the patient should be made (see p 1, **I** and **III**).
      2. **Lymph nodes.** A thorough survey of the lymphatic system should include the cervical, supraclavicular, axillary, and inguinal regions.
      3. **Chest.** The quality of the breath sounds, presence of wheezing, and evidence of consolidation, pleural effusions, or both are important indications of ongoing pulmonary disease.
      4. **Abdomen.** The abdomen should be examined for hepatomegaly, ascites, and masses suggesting intraperitoneal metastases.
      5. **Genitalia**
         a. **External genitalia.** The vulva, urethra, anus, and vaginal introitus should be examined for evidence of bleeding. Primary and metastatic lesions may involve the external genitalia and are easily biopsied.
         b. **Vagina.** Thorough inspection and palpation are required to exclude metastases.
         c. **Cervix.** Examination is conducted by first obtaining a Pap smear and then by visual and bimanual examination. Endometrial carcinoma can present as either a **gross or a microscopic** cervical lesion.

   d. **Bimanual examination.** Palpation of the vaginal walls and ectocervix may reveal **induration or surface irregularity** that may not be visible with the speculum. Because cancer can cause enlargement, irregularity, and fixation of the uterus, the cervix and uterus should be palpated to assess size, mobility, and symmetry. The remainder of the pelvis must be palpated to exclude ovarian, bladder, and rectosigmoid involvement. A rectovaginal examination is used to assess the **rectovaginal septum** and **cul-de-sac.**
   6. **Rectum.** Stool should be examined for occult blood, and masses must be accurately described.
B. **Primary tests and procedures.** All patients with carcinoma of the uterine corpus should have the following tests and diagnostic procedures performed.
   1. **Blood tests**
      a. **Complete blood count** (see p 1, **IV.A.1**).
      b. **Hepatic transaminases** (see p 1, **IV.A.2**).
      c. **Alkaline phosphatase** (see p 1, **IV.A.3**).
      d. **BUN and creatinine.** These tests may indicate invasion and obstruction of the urinary tract.
      e. **Coagulation times. Prothrombin and partial thromboplastin times** may suggest that vaginal bleeding is caused by a coagulopathy.
      f. **CA-125.** This tumor marker is shed by certain endometrial malignancies and can be followed to evaluate therapeutic responses.
   2. **Urine tests**
      a. **Urinalysis** (see p 3, **IV.B**).
      b. **Beta-human chorionic gonadotropin (beta-hCG). Pregnancy** must be excluded in all females of reproductive age.
   3. **Imaging studies.** Routine radiologic evaluation of a patient with uterine cancer should include **a chest x-ray** (see p 3, **IV.C.1**).
   4. **Invasive procedures.** All patients suspected of having endometrial carcinoma should undergo an **endocervical curettage** and **endometrial biopsy,** which can be done in the office without anesthesia. First, the endocervical canal is scraped up to the internal cervical os using a **Kevorkian curette.** Then, the uterine cavity is measured using a uterine sound, and the depth is recorded (a larger cavity may reflect more extensive uterine involvement). Next, the biopsy device is introduced into the uterus through the cervix and tissue is obtained from all quadrants of the endometrial cavity. The false-negative rate of endometrial biopsies is 10%.
C. **Optional tests and procedures.** The following examinations may be indicated by either previous diagnostic findings or clinical suspicion.
   1. **Blood tests** (see p 2, **IV.A**).
      a. **Nucleotidase.**
      b. **GGTP.**
   2. **Imaging studies**
      a. **Barium enema.** The colon should be evaluated to exclude direct colonic invasion or metastasis as well as a synchronous colon cancer in any patient with occult fecal blood or a change in bowel habits.
      b. **Intravenous pyelogram (IVP).** If renal insufficiency is detected, this test should be done to exclude ureteral obstruction secondary to enlarged lymph nodes or direct tumor infiltration of the urinary tract.
      c. **Computed tomography scan (CT).** When advanced disease is suspected, abdominopelvic CT is the best way to evaluate the extent of the primary uterine tumor. In addition, CT can be substituted for an IVP to determine involvement of the bladder, rectum, uterine adnexa, and ureters as well as retroperitoneal, pelvic, and para-aortic lymph nodes. The possibility of intraperitoneal spread and liver parenchymal metastases also may be assessed.
      d. **Magnetic resonance imaging (MRI).** (see p 3, **IV.C.2**).
      e. **Ultrasound** (see p 3, **IV.C.3**).
      f. **Technetium-99m bone scan** (see p 3, **IV.C.4**).
   3. **Invasive procedures**
      a. **Dilatation and curettage (D & C).** If endometrial biopsy is nondiagnostic, all patients suspected of having endometrial cancer should have a **fractional D & C** under general or regional anesthesia. During this procedure, the cervix is dilated manually to obtain a better sample of the endometrial cavity.
      b. **Hysteroscopy.** This procedure can be used to evaluate patients with uter-

ine bleeding and to help direct endometrial biopsies to improve diagnostic accuracy.

   c. Fine needle aspiration. This technique can be used to assess suspicious retroperitoneal, supraclavicular, or inguinal lymph nodes as well as lung, liver, and vaginopelvic masses.

   d. Endoscopy. In more advanced cases, **cystoscopy** and **proctosigmoidoscopy** are indicated if bladder or rectal invasion is suspected.

VII. Pathology.

  A. Location. The vast majority of endometrial carcinomas arise in the uterine **fundus.** Tumors arising in the lower uterine segment can masquerade as endocervical carcinoma and often involve the cervix secondarily. Uterine sarcomas arise from both the endo- and myometrium.

  B. Multiplicity. Patients with endometrial carcinoma are at an increased risk of concomitant or subsequent **ovarian, breast, and colon carcinomas.**

  C. Histology. The microscopic appearance of endometrial neoplasia and carcinoma is described below:

    1. Endometrial hyperplasia. A variety of terms have been used to describe endometrial hyperplasia, but recent descriptions simplify and standardize the terminology.

      a. Cystic hyperplasia. This term refers to simple or benign hyperplasia that has virtually **no malignant potential** and is characterized by rare mitoses with variations in the size and shape of the endometrial glands.

      b. Adenomatous hyperplasia with and without atypia. The degree of proliferative abnormality (glandular crowding and cellular atypia) in this entity is frequently described as mild, moderate, or severe. **Severe atypia** is associated with as much as a **25%** chance of **malignant progression.**

    2. Endometrial carcinoma. Although many different malignancies—including papillary, serous, mucinous, clear cell, adenosquamous, and squamous cell carcinomas—can arise from the uterine corpus, **adenocarcinoma represents more than 95% of endometrial tumors.** These malignancies often contain areas of benign metaplasia (most commonly squamous) and are given a **grade** of 1 (75%), 2, or 3, depending on the **degree of glandular proliferation.**

    3. Uterine sarcoma. Sarcomas constitute about **3%** of all uterine malignancies and include leiomyosarcomas, endometrial stromal sarcomas, and mixed mesodermal tumors. These mesenchymal tumors can be **pure or mixed** and either **homologous** (tissues usually found in the uterus) or **heterologous** (tissue not normally found in the uterus).

  D. Metastatic spread

    1. Modes of spead. Endometrial cancers spread by 4 distinct routes.

      a. Direct extension. Growth into any of the many contiguous pelvic structures, including the cervix, fallopian tubes, ovaries, vagina, parametria, bladder, ureter, and rectum, occurs through aggressive local invasion.

      b. Transtubal exfoliation. The passage of endometrial cancer cells through the fallopian tubes into the peritoneal cavity may result in peritoneal seeding.

      c. Lymphatic metastasis. Spread through regional lymphatic channels results in parametrial, pelvic, para-aortic, and supraclavicular lymph nodal as well as **vaginal** metastases.

      d. Hematogenous metastasis. Metastases to distant organs occur through a rich supply of pelvic blood vessels.

    2. Sites of metastatic spread. The extent and likelihood of metastatic spread depends on the histology, grade, and depth of myometrial invasion.

      a. Pelvic and para-aortic lymph nodes. Stage 1 (Grade 1) tumors with superficial myometrial invasion have a **0–5%** incidence of nodal spread, whereas tumors with higher grades and deeper penetration exhibit a **10–40%** incidence.

      b. Cervical extension, 15%.

      c. Pelvic extension, 7%.

      d. Liver, less than 3%.

      e. Lung, less than 3%.

      f. Bone, less than 3%.

      g. Central nervous system, less than 3%.

VIII. Staging. The International Federation of Gynecology and Obstetrics (FIGO) recently revised the staging of endometrial carcinoma from a clinical to a **surgical** system that is slowly gaining widespread acceptance. The TMN staging system adopted by the

American Joint Committee on Cancer and the Union Internationale Contre le Cancer, although not commonly used in gynecologic malignancies, was previously modified to correspond to the clinical FIGO classification system. To date, however, it has not been updated to reflect the new surgical FIGO system.

A. **Clinical FIGO staging system**
  1. **Tumor stage**
     a. **Stage 0.** Carcinoma in situ.
     b. **Stage I.** The carcinoma is confined to the corpus.
        (1) **Stage Ia.** The uterine cavity is no longer than 8 cm.
        (2) **Stage Ib.** The uterine cavity is longer than 8 cm.
     c. **Stage II.** The carcinoma has involved the corpus and the cervix but has not extended outside the uterus.
     d. **Stage III.** The carcinoma has extended outside the uterus but not outside the true pelvis.
     e. **Stage IV.** The carcinoma has extended outside the true pelvis or has obviously involved the mucosa of the bladder or rectum. Bullous edema, as such, does not qualify as Stage IV.
        (1) **Stage IVa.** The carcinoma has spread to adjacent organs.
        (2) **Stage IVb.** The carcinoma has spread to distant organs.
  2. **Histopathologic grade.** Stage I cases should be subdivided on the basis of histologic grade.
     a. **Grade 1.** Highly differentiated adenomatous carcinoma.
     b. **Grade 2.** Moderately differentiated adenomatous carcinoma with partly solid areas.
     c. **Grade 3.** Predominantly solid or entirely undifferentiated carcinoma.
B. **TNM staging system**
  1. **Tumor stage**
     a. **TX.** Primary tumor cannot be assessed.
     b. **T0.** No evidence of primary malignancy.
     c. **Tis.** Carcinoma in situ.
     d. **T1.** Tumor is confined to the uterine corpus.
        (1) **T1a.** The uterine cavity is no longer than 8 cm.
        (2) **T1b.** The uterine cavity is longer than 8 cm.
     e. **T2.** Tumor invades the cervix but does not extend beyond the uterus.
     f. **T3.** Tumor extends beyond the uterus but not outside the true pelvis.
     g. **T4.** Tumor invades the bladder or rectal mucosa or extends beyond the true pelvis.
  2. **Lymph node stage**
     a. **NX.** Regional lymph nodes cannot be assessed.
     b. **N0.** No regional lymph node metastases is present.
     c. **N1.** Regional lymph node metastases are present.
  3. **Metastatic stage**
     a. **MX.** Presence of distant metastases cannot be assessed.
     b. **M0.** No distant metastases.
     c. **M1.** Distant metastases are present.
  4. **Histopathologic grade**
     a. **GX.** Grade cannot be assessed.
     b. **G1.** Well differentiated.
     c. **G2.** Moderately well differentiated.
     d. **G3–4.** Poorly differentiated or undifferentiated.
  5. **Stage groups**
     a. **Stage 0.** Tis, N0, M0.
     b. **Stage IA.** T1a, N0, M0.
     c. **Stage IB.** T1b, N0, M0.
     d. **Stage II.** T2, N0, M0.
     e. **Stage III.** T1, N1, M0; T2, N1, M0; or T3, any N, M0.
     f. **Stage IVA.** T4, any N, M0.
     g. **Stage IVB.** any T, any N, M1.
C. **Surgical FIGO staging system**
  1. **Tumor stage**
     a. **Stage IA.** Tumor is limited to endometrium.
     b. **Stage IB.** Tumor invades less than half of the myometrium.
     c. **Stage IC.** Tumor invades more than half of the myometrium.
     d. **Stage IIA.** Tumor involves endocervical glanduls only.
     e. **Stage IIB.** Tumor invades the cervical stroma.

      f. Stage IIIA. Tumor invades the serosa or the adnexa or positive peritoneal cytology.

      g. Stage IIIB. Vaginal metastases.

      h. Stage IIIC. Metastases to pelvic or para-aortic lymph nodes or both.

      i. Stage IVA. Tumor invades the bladder or bowel mucosa or both.

      j. Stage IVB. Distant metastases including intra-abdominal or inguinal lymph nodes or both.

2. **Histopathologic grade.** Tumor grade does not change the stage.

      a. Grade 1. Well differentiated.

      b. Grade 2. Moderately differentiated.

      c. Grade 3. Poorly differentiated.

         Note: Uterine sarcomas generally follow the same staging system, but little information is known about the prognostic significance. All sarcomas with spread outside the uterus have a dismal prognosis.

IX. **Treatment**

   A. **Surgery**

     1. **Primary uterine carcinoma**

       a. Indications. The standard therapy for uterine malignancies of all types is **total abdominal hysterectomy and bilateral salpingo-oophorectomy.** This procedure permits accurate surgical-pathological staging and therefore better tailoring of therapy. Contraindications for immediate surgery include direct extension of the tumor to the pelvic sidewall, a fixed pelvic tumor mass, and metastatic disease in a severely disabled patient.

       b. Approaches. Although laparotomy is generally performed through a **low midline abdominal incision,** it also can be performed through a **transverse Pfannenstiel, Maylard, or Cherney incision** if necessary. In rare instances (eg, morbidly obese, poor medical health), a patient may require a transvaginal hysterectomy and bilateral salpingo-oophorectomy. Even with this approach, surgery with postoperative radiotherapy is superior to radiation alone, especially if it can be accomplished easily as in clinical Stage I disease.

       c. Surgical technique. Upon entering the peritoneal cavity, **cytologic washings** are obtained from the **pelvic cul-de-sac, both pericolic gutters, and subdiaphragmatic spaces,** and any ascites is collected for cytologic examination. Then, thorough *palpation* of the diaphragm, the liver, omentum, intestines, and retroperitoneal lymph node regions is performed. Next, attention is directed to the pelvis. The uterine cornices are each grasped encompassing the round ligaments, ovarian ligaments, and fallopian tubes. The distal ends of the fallopian tubes can be tied or clipped to prevent exfoliation of endometrial cancer cells. The hysterectomy is begun by **dividing the round ligaments** to expose the pararectal and paravesical spaces, the ureter, the paremetria, and the pelvic lymph node chains for inspection and palpation. Enlarged lymph nodes are resected, but, in the absence of obvious nodal involvement, pelvic and para-aortic lymph nodes are sampled to exclude microscopic disease. A standard **extrafascial hysterectomy** is then performed (see p 371, **IX.A.1.c.[2]**). The uterus should be opened in the operating room to assess cervical involvement and the depth of myometrial invasion. Depending on the clinical setting, extension to the cervix can be treated by either radical hysterectomy with pelvic and lower para-aortic lymphadenectomy or pelvic irradiation followed by total hysterectomy and bilateral salpingo-oophorectomy.

     2. **Locally advanced and metastatic uterine cancer**

       a. Locally advanced neoplasm

         (1) Endometrial carcinoma. When feasible, an attempt should always be made to **resect all gross disease,** including enlarged pelvic and para-aortic lymph nodes. Occasionally, patients with localized disease extending into the bladder or rectum should be considered for **pelvic exenteration.** This radical procedure, however, can only be justified if all gross disease is extirpated with adequate margins. In addition, the patient must be willing to **accept reconstruction or diversion** of the urinary or gastrointestinal tract or both.

         (2) Uterine sarcoma. Because of the strong likelihood of distant metastases and poor prognosis associated with extrauterine disease, aggressive surgical procedures generally are not indicated.

       b. Recurrent neoplasm. Isolated local recurrence occurs in as many as **50%**

of patients. Curative surgical resection can be attempted in these cases, but **most require some type of exenteration** procedure, depending on the location of the recurrence and the findings at exploration.

  c. **Metastatic neoplasm.** Although intraperitoneal metastases (usually omental implants), if present, are resected during the initial hysterectomy, **surgery is rarely indicated** for metastatic disease. Although liver and lung metastases are almost always multifocal and unresectable, anecdotal cases of long-term survival after resection of isolated pulmonary metastases have been reported.

3. **Mortality and morbidity.** The mortality and morbidity from hysterectomy is low and includes the following complications: **wound infections, hemorrhage, vaginal cuff cellulitis, genital tract fistulae, urinary tract infection, thrombophlebitis, prolonged ileus, and lymphocele formation.**

B. **Radiation therapy**

1. **Primary uterine carcinoma.** Radiation therapy alone is indicated only in the rare patient whose medical condition precludes surgical intervention.

   a. **Techniques**

      (1) **External beam pelvic irradiation.** Generally, multiple fields are used to deliver **5000 cGy** to the entire pelvis in **180 cGy daily fractions over 5–6 weeks.** If para-aortic disease is present, 4500–5000 cGy is delivered to this area as well.

      (2) **Intracavitary radiation.** Before hysterectomy, radium-226 or cesium-137 can be used via a **Fletcher-Suit afterloading device** to deliver a dose of **6000 cGy** to the uterus and 4000 cGy to the vagina over 48–72 hours. Occasionally, this requires 2 applications.

      (3) **Vaginal vault radiation.** This type of radiation is indicated in postoperative patients with superficially invasive, Grade 2, lesions or in patients who cannot tolerate more extensive therapy. A total surface-vault dose of **5500–6000 cGy** is delivered using a **cylinder or colpostats.**

      (4) **Whole abdominal radiation.** Whole abdominal radiation can be combined with pelvic irradiation and systemic chemotherapy in patients who are at high risk for recurrence and previously had upper-abdominal intraperitoneal metastases removed.

      (5) **Intraperitoneal phosphorus-32.** This method of radiation has been used with some success to prevent recurrences in patients with positive intraperitoneal cytologies but no distant metastases.

      (6) **Interstitial brachytherapy.** Needle implants can be used for vaginal lesions that are unsuitable for a cylinder or colpostats.

2. **Adjuvant radiation therapy**

   a. **Preoperative radiation therapy.** The choice of preoperative (neoadjuvant) versus postoperative adjuvant radiation therapy has been the subject of longstanding debate. Preoperative therapy has been used in the following circumstances:

      (1) **Early disease (Stage 1).** Radiation therapy in early disease is generally limited to a **single radium implant** given before hysterectomy to reduce the incidence of recurrence in the **vaginal cuff and pelvic lymph nodes.**

      (2) **Disease involving the cervix (Stage 2).** Cervical disease can be treated using external-beam pelvic radiation and intracavitary radium-226 or cesium-137, followed in **6 weeks** by **extrafascial radical hysterectomy.** The choice between radical surgery alone versus a combined approach is influenced by the patient's health and the extent of cervical disease. Microscopic disease is more commonly treated with **surgery alone,** and **macroscopic** disease is treated with **combined radiotherapy and surgery.**

      (3) **Advanced disease.** Preoperative irradiation and intracavitary radium-226 or cesium-137 followed by extrafascial hysterectomy, bilateral salpingo-oophorectomy and surgical debulking constitute standard therapy for advanced lesions. Depending on the extent and location of the tumor (eg, pelvic masses, ascites), exploratory laparotomy, hysterectomy, and tumor debulking may be required before radiation therapy. When the bladder, rectum, or both are involved, preoperative radiation may decrease tumor bulk and allow a more complete surgical resection.

    b. **Postoperative radiation therapy.** This procedure is designed to reduce local recurrence in patients with **significant risk factors for recurrence:** eg, high-grade tumors, deep myometrial invasion, large volume tumors, and pelvic, cervical, or adnexal extension. Because standard pelvic radiation generally will not sterilize gross disease (enlarged lymph nodes or metastases), resection must be done before radiotherapy.

3. **Locally advanced and metastatic uterine cancer.** Palliative radiation therapy may improve **pain** associated with **pelvic and bony metastases** as well as **pneumonia** associated with **bronchial obstruction** from pulmonary metastases.

4. **Mortality and morbidity.** Radiation therapy alone or in combination with surgery is generally well tolerated. Major complication rates are **1–2%** with external-beam therapy, but they approach **10%** if **intracavitary therapy** is used. Complications include the following: **gastrointestinal motility disturbances; gastrointestinal obstruction; uretero-, vesico-, or recto-vaginal fistulae; retroperitoneal fibrosis and ureteral obstruction; hemorrhagic cystitis; and proctitis.**

C. **Chemotherapy**

1. **Primary uterine carcinoma.** To date, chemotherapy has no role in the initial therapy of resectable uterine cancer.

2. **Adjuvant chemotherapy.** Adjuvant chemotherapy may play a role in patients at high risk for recurrence—those with adnexal metastases, for example. Clinical trials are currently exploring the possible benefits of ajduvant therapy either alone or in combination with radiotherapy. The agents under study include those used in advanced disease (see below).

3. **Locally advanced and metastatic uterine cancer.** Cytotoxic chemotherapy, although rarely curative, may provide significant palliation for patients with locally advanced and systemic disease.

    a. **Single agents.** Doxorubicin is the most active single agent, with response rates of **30–40%. Cisplatin** has modest activity and usually has been used as a second-line drug; however, as a first-line agent at high doses, response rates (30–40%) approach those of doxorubicin. Other agents with modest cytotoxic activity (10–20%) include **cyclophosphamide and fluorouracil.**

    b. **Combination chemotherapy.** Combination chemotherapeutic regimens, including combinations of doxorubicin and cisplatin, have not improved the **10–40%** response rates seen with single agents. In addition, many of these trials use progestins, thus making the contribution of each agent difficult to assess.

D. **Hormonal therapy.** About **33%** of patients with advanced or recurrent endometrial cancer will respond to progestin therapy. These patients tend to have well-differentiated lesions with **hormone receptors.** Prolonged responses are occasionally reported, and median survival is **24 months** in responders but only **6 months** in nonresponders. The most commonly used progestins include **medroxyprogesterone acetate (Provera), hydroxyprogesterone caproate (Delalutin), and megestrol acetate (Megace).** The antiestrogen agent, **tamoxifen,** also has modest activity in **20–30%** of advanced cases and can be used for palliative therapy. Hormonal therapy, in general, should be continued indefinitely unless tumor progression occurs. Combinations of hormonal agents with other treatment modalities are being investigated.

E. **Immunotherapy.** Immunotherapy of uterine carcinoma has not been studied.

X. **Prognosis**

A. **Risk of recurrence.** Close surveillance for pelvic recurrence is important because the majority of tumors recur within 2 years. Generally, recurrence is either asymptomatic or presents with vaginal bleeding, pelvic pain, or both. In patients with recurrences, the patterns of failure fall into 1 of 3 categories: **pelvic recurrence only,** 50%; **distant recurrence only,** 28%; or **simultaneous local and distant recurrences,** 22%.

B. **Five-year survival.** Generally, endometrial cancer is discovered at an early stage and leads to a favorable prognosis. The overall 5-year survival for all stages is **67%.** The overall 5-year survival of patients with uterine sarcomas with disease limited to the uterus is **50%,** whereas it is less than **20%** with extrauterine spread. Survival by FIGO stage is as follows: **Stage I,** 75%; **Stage II,** 58%; **Stage III,** 30%; and **Stage IV,** 10%.

C. **Prognostic factors.** Within stages, adverse prognostic factors affect the expected outcome significantly and include the following: **poorly differentiated tumors, deep myometrial invasion, and extrauterine spread.**

XI. **Patient follow-up**
   A. **General guidelines.** Patients should be followed closely every 3 months for 2 years, every 6 months for an additional 3 years, and then annually for evidence of pelvic and distant recurrence. Specific guidelines for patient follow-up are detailed below.
   B. **Routine evaluation.** Each clinic visit should include the following tests and procedures.
      1. **Medical history and physical examination.** An interval medical history and a thorough physical examination, including cervical or vaginal cytology (Pap smear), must be performed, paying particular attention to the areas outlined on p 355, **VI.A.**
      2. **Blood tests** (see p 1, **IV.A**)
         a. **Complete blood count.**
         b. **Hepatic transaminases.**
         c. **Alkaline phosphatase.**
         d. **BUN and creatinine.** Pelvic recurrence and **radiation fibrosis** may cause renal failure (see, also, p 356, **VI.B.1.d**).
      3. **Urinalysis** (see p 3, **IV.B**).
      4. **Chest x-ray** (see p 3, **IV.C.1**).
   C. **Optional evaluation.** The following tests may be indicated by previous diagnostic findings or clinical suspicion.
      1. **Blood tests** (see p 2, **IV.A**)
         a. **Nucleotidase.**
         b. **GGTP.**
      2. **Intravenous pyelogram** (see p 356, **VI.C.2.b**)
      3. **Imaging studies** (see p 3, **IV.C**)
         a. **Computed tomography (CT).** CT scan of the abdomen and pelvis is the best radiologic examination for detecting pelvic, intraperitoneal, parenchymal, and retroperitoneal metastases. When recurrence is suspected, this test should be used to establish the diagnosis and define the extent of disease.
         b. **Magnetic resonance imaging (MRI).**
         c. **Technetium-99m bone scan.**
      4. **Fine needle aspiration biopsy.** This simple, low-morbidity technique provides a highly accurate means of demonstrating recurrent tumor in palpable or radiographic masses. A negative result, however, does not exclude the diagnosis of malignancy.

REFERENCES

Berman, ML, Ballon, SC, Lagasse, LD, and Watring, WG. Prognosis and treatment of endometrial cancer. Am J Obstet Gynecol 136: 679–688, 1980.

Creasman, WT, Morrow, CP, Bundy, BN, et al. Surgical pathological spread patterns of endometrial cancer. A Gynecologic Oncology Group study. Cancer 60:2035–2041, 1987.

Grigsby, PW, Perez, CA, Camel, HM, et al. Stage III carcinoma of the endometrium: Results of therapy and prognostic factors. Int J Radiat Oncol Biol Phys 11: 1915–1919, 1985.

Hacker, NF. Endometrial cancer. In Practical Gynecologic Oncology. Berek JS and Hacker, NF, eds. Williams and Wilkins, Baltimore, pp. 285–326, 1989.

Kneale, BLG. Adjunctive and therapeutic progestins in endometrial cancer. Clin Obstet Gynecol 13:789–795, 1986.

Kurman, RJ and Norris, HJ. Endometrial neoplasia. In Hyperplasia and Carcinoma in Pathology of the Female Genital Tract. Blaustein, A., editor. Springer-Verlag, New York, 2nd ed., pp. 311–351, 1982.

Morrow CP, Townsend DE. Synopsis of Gynecologic Oncology. Morrow, CP and Townsend, DE, editors. Churchill Livingston, New York, 3rd ed., pp. 159–205, 1987.

Peters, WA, Anderson, WA, Thornton, WN, and Morley, GW. The selective use of vaginal hysterectomy in the management of adenocarcinoma of the endometrium. Am J Obstet Gynecol 146: 285–291, 1983.

Piver, SM, Yazigi, R, Blumenson, L, and Tsukada, Y. A prospective trial comparing hysterectomy, hysterectomy plus vaginal radium, and uterine radium plus hysterectomy in stage I endometrial carcinoma. Obstet Gynecol 54:85–89, 1979.

Slavik, M, Petty, WM, Blessing, JA, et al. Phase II clinical study of tamoxifen in advanced endometrial adenocarcinoma. A Gynecologic Oncology Group study. Cancer Treat Rep 68:809–811, 1984.

Thigpen, JT, Buchsbaum, HG, Mangan, C, and Blessing, JA. Phase II trial of adriamycin in the treatment of advanced or recurrent endometrial carcinoma: A Gynecologic Oncology Group Study. Cancer Treat Rep 63:21–27, 1979.

Thomas, GM. Radiation therapy. In Practical Gynecologic Oncology. Berek, JS and Hacker, NF, editors. Williams and Wilkins, Baltimore, pp. 37–72, 1989.

48 Malignancies of the Uterine Cervix

Jeffrey Fowler, MD, and F.J. Montz, MD

I. **Epidemiology.** Cancer of the uterine cervix is the third most common gynecologic cancer and the eighth most frequent malignancy of any type in females. In 1985, **8.4 cases per 100,000 females** were diagnosed, leading to **3.1 deaths** per 100,000. Estimates indicate that **13,500 new cases, 4400 deaths, and an additional 55,000 cases of carcinoma** in situ will occur in 1993. Furthermore, 1 in every 770 pregnancies is associated with carcinoma in situ and 1 in 2200 pregnancies is complicated by invasive carcinoma. Since 1940 the incidence of invasive cervical cancer has declined 72% (30 per 100,000 females in 1940), and **overall survival has increased from 47% to 67%** as a result of earlier detection by widespread use of Papanicolaou cervical exfoliative cytology (Pap) smears and frequent pelvic examinations. Worldwide, cervical cancer is the most common gynecologic malignancy.

II. **Risk factors**
   A. **Age.** The incidence of cervical carcinoma rapidly increases from less than 0.3 per 100,000 before age 20 and less than 2.0 per 100,000 before age 25 to 16.6 per 100,000 by age 40, thereafter gradually increasing to **22.4 per 100,000 by age 85**. The **mean age** at diagnosis is **54 years**, with a **bimodal distribution,** peaking at ages 35–39 and 60–64 years.
   B. **Race.** The risk in blacks is **2.0–2.5 times** higher than in white females. At birth the **lifetime probability** of developing cervical cancer is **0.7% in whites vs 1.6% in black females.**
   C. **Genetic factors.** No excess risk has been observed in first-degree relatives of patients with cervical carcinoma, and no genetic factors have been identified.
   D. **Diet.** No dietary factors have been implicated in the pathogenesis of cervical neoplasia.
   E. **Smoking.** Recently, the risk of cervical carcinoma among tobacco smokers was noted to be **4 times** greater than that among nonsmokers.
   F. **Previous gynecologic pathology**
      1. **Sexual behavior.** Major behavioral risk factors include promiscuity, early age at first intercourse, large number of sexual partners, and close temporal relationship between coitarche and menarche.
      2. **Infection.** The epidemiology of cervical carcinoma parallels that of sexually transmitted diseases. **Human papilloma virus (HPV)** now has been linked to all grades of cervical intraepithelial neoplasia (CIN) as well as invasive cancer. **HPV 16 and 18** have been found in more than **90% of invasive squamous cell carcinomas,** and HPV 18 has been isolated from **50% of adenocarcinomas** of the cervix. Possible cofactors in HPV-related neoplasia are genital herpes simplex (HSV–2) infection, other vaginal infections, immunosuppression, and tobacco.
   G. **Urbanization.** Low socioeconomic status is associated with a high risk of cervical neoplasia; however, this may be related to racial and behavioral factors.

III. **Presentation**
   A. **Signs and symptoms.** Nearly **90%** of patients presenting with cervical carcinoma are **symptomatic** with one of the following local or systemic symptoms of the disease.
      1. **Local manifestations. Vaginal bleeding (40%–80%; frequently postcoital)** is the most common presenting complaint. A **watery or purulent vaginal discharge** (10%) is sometimes present and occasionally may be malodorous. Symptoms of advanced local disease include **pain** (pelvic, low back, and leg pain), **edema of the lower extremities, thrombophlebitis, urinary symptoms** (frequency, urgency, hematuria, flank pain), and **rectal complaints** (pain, tenesmus, and bleeding).
      2. **Systemic manifestations.** Systemic signs and symptoms are uncommon, particularly in the absence of local complaints. Occasionally, **adenopathy** (ingui-

nal, para-aortic, and supraclavicular lymph node metastases), **hepatomegaly** (liver metastases), **bone pain** (bone metastases), and **pulmonary nodules** (lung metastases) may occur.

B. **Paraneoplastic syndromes.** In rare cases, cervical cancer presents with one of the following paraneoplastic syndromes as the only manifestation of disease:

1. **Hypercalcemia (see** p 87).
2. **Inappropriate ACTH** (see p 90).
3. **Inappropriate ADH** (see p 89).

IV. **Differential diagnosis.** Many patients with cervical neoplasms present with abnormal **vaginal bleeding,** which can be caused by a myriad of gynecologic diseases (see **Chapter 47**). Once a cervical problem is identified, the differential diagnosis varies with the extent of the disease. **Cervical infections** (condyloma acuminata, chancre, and herpes), **benign neoplasms** (fibroids and nabothian cysts), and **cervical ectropion** may mimic early disease, and **severe pelvic infections** and **other pelvic malignancies** (vagina, uterus, bladder, rectum) may simulate locally advanced disease. Finally, primary lung, breast, endometrial, and gastrointestinal carcinomas as well as lymphoma produce patterns of metastatic disease similar to those of cervical cancer.

V. **Screening programs. Cervical-vaginal exfoliative cytology (Pap smears)** represent one of the most important advances in preventive medicine in the 20th century. The widespread implementation of screening Pap smears precipitated a **40–80% reduction in the incidence and mortality of invasive cervical cancer** through the early diagnosis and treatment of cervical dysplasia and microinvasive cervical carcinoma. Pap smears, however, are limited by a **15% false-negative rate** resulting from cytologic misinterpretation and inadequate sampling and by **patient noncompliance,** particularly in high-risk groups (**60%** of females who die of cervical cancer have never had a Pap smear). In addition, Pap smears **do not reliably detect adenocarcinoma** of the cervix. Currently, the American Cancer Society and the American College of Obstetricians and Gynecologists recommend performing an **annual Pap smear (and pelvic examination) in all sexually active females 18 years old or older.** After 3 **consecutive normal cytologies,** however, this screening can be done less frequently (every 1–3 years) at the physician's discretion.

VI. **Diagnostic workup**

A. **Medical history and physical examination.** In addition to a detailed medical history documenting risk factors and any signs and symptoms of cervical disease, a complete physical examination must be performed, paying particular attention to the following areas:

1. **General appearance.** An evaluation of the patient's nutritional and general functional status should be included (see, also, p 1, **I** and **III**).
2. **Lymph nodes.** Thorough examination of the inguinal, supraclavicular, axillary, and cervical lymph nodes is required.
3. **Chest.** A pulmonary examination may detect pleural effusions and obstructing parenchymal lesions.
4. **Abdomen.** Evidence of ascites, hepatosplenomegaly, and suspicious masses suggesting retroperitoneal lymphadenopathy should be noted.
5. **Genitalia**
   a. **External genitalia.** The vulva, urethra, vaginal introitus, and anus are examined visually and by palpation for primary or metastatic tumor.
   b. **Vagina.** Complete visualization and palpation is mandatory to exclude primary or metastatic lesions.
   c. **Cervix.** A Pap smear should be obtained from the cervix. Visual and bimanual examination also are necessary, noting the size, position, symmetry, and mobility of the cervix. The cervical examination can be **normal in 33% of patients** with cervical cancer. Any abnormality must be biopsied.
   d. **Uterus and adnexa.** The size, position, symmetry, and mobility of the uterus and adnexa must be assessed. In addition, the parametrial, paravaginal, and uterosacral ligaments should be palpated, and any abnormality should be noted. **Cervical fixation,** indicating involvement of the parametrial tissues and pelvic side wall, occurs frequently with large lesions, although central lesions can be extremely large (8–10 cm) without parametrial extension. The remainder of the pelvis should be evaluated for **uterine enlargement (hematometra or pyometra),** vaginal extension and for involvement of the bladder, rectum, or both.
6. **Rectum.** Primary rectal carcinoma must be excluded and stool should be tested for occult blood.

7. **Extremities.** Evidence of lower extremity thrombophlebitis and edema should be noted.

B. **Primary test and procedures.** Except for patients with clinical Stage I disease (see p 367, **VIII**), who do not require IVP, cystourethroscopy, and proctosigmoidoscopy, all patients with suspected cervical carcinoma should have the following diagnostic tests and procedures:

  1. **Blood tests** (see p 1, **IV.A**)
    a. **Complete blood count.**
    b. **Hepatic transaminases.**
    c. **Alkaline phosphatase.**
    d. **BUN and creatinine.**
    e. **Albumin**.

  2. **Urine tests**
    a. **Urinalysis** (see p 3, **IV.B**).
    b. **Beta-human chorionic gonadotropin (beta-hCG). Pregnancy** must be excluded in all females of reproductive age.

  3. **Imaging studies**
    a. **Chest x-ray** (see p 3, **IV.C.1**).
    b. **Intravenous pyelogram.** IVP should be obtained to exclude ureteral obstruction, particularly with **tumors larger than 2 cm** in diameter.

  4. **Invasive procedures**
    a. **Colposcopy.** Direct visualization of the cervix with a colposcope (10–15x) and **green light filter** (to enhance vascular markings) is valuable in the diagnosis of early cervical neoplasms and is recommended in any patient with **a persistently abnormal Pap smear** despite adequate treatment for infection.
    b. **Cystourethroscopy.** Direct visualization of the urethra and bladder should be performed to exclude direct extension of cervical cancer as well as primary bladder carcinoma.
    c. **Proctosigmoidoscopy**. Endoscopic examination of the rectosigmoid colon must be accomplished to dismiss the possibility of secondary rectal involvement and the presence of primary colorectal carcinoma.
    d. **Biopsy. A biopsy** of any suspicious lesion is mandatory and can be obtained by several methods.
      (1) Direct biopsy. A direct biopsy can be obtained with a dermal punch or biopsy forceps with little or no anesthesia.
      (2) Cervical conization. In this procedure, which requires regional or general anesthesia, a conical piece of cervix is removed that includes the transformation zone. This procedure is indicated for patients with high-grade dysplasia (CIN III, CIS) and/or (1) unsatisfactory colposcopy, (2) positive endocervical curettage, (3) no correlation between cytology, colposcopy, and histology, (4) suspicion of invasion on biopsy, and (5) suspicion of adenocarcinoma in situ.

C. **Optional tests and procedures.** The following tests and procedures may be indicated by previous diagnostic findings or clinical suspicion.

  1. **Blood tests**
    a. **Nucleotidase** (see p 2, **IV.A.4**).
    b. **GGTP** (see p 2, **IV.A.5**).
    c. **CA-125.** Associated with **adenocarcinomas,** this serum tumor antigen is not helpful in the initial diagnosis of cervical cancer but may be used to follow patients for tumor regression and recurrence.
    d. **Carcinoembryonic antigen (CEA).** Like CA-125, this serum tumor antigen can be used to monitor patients with cervical carcinoma for tumor regression and recurrence.
    e. **TA-4.** Recent data suggest that serum levels of this multiallele antigen correlate directly with the total volume and stage of cervical carcinoma and in the future may aid in patient evaluation.

  2. **Imaging studies**
    a. **Computed tomography (CT).** CT scan of the pelvis and abdomen provides information regarding the primary tumor, parametrial tissue, liver, retroperitoneal nodes larger than 1–2 cm and the genitourinary tract and **eliminates the need for intravenous pyelography (IVP).** However, a **low sensitivity (50%) and specificity (79%)** as well as a **high false-positive rate of parametrial extension (36%)** precludes its use as a routine imaging study.
    b. **Magnetic resonance imaging (MRI).** (see p 3, **IV.C.2**).

      c. Lymphangiography. Bipedal lymphangiography, in some circumstances, can be helpful in evaluating pelvic lymph nodes for the presence of metastatic disease. The **sensitivity (30–80%) and specificity (50–100%)** of this test, however, are **too low,** and the **false positive (30%) and false negative (12%) rates are too high** for routine use.

      d. Technetium-99m bone scan (see p 3, **IV.C.4**).

   3. Invasive procedures

      a. Pelvic examination under anesthesia. Suboptimal pelvic examination in awake patients necessitates examination under general anesthesia to provide accurate clinical staging. Biopsies can be performed at the same time.

      b. Fine needle aspiration (FNA). Suspicious inguinal, supraclavicular, pelvic, and para-aortic lymph nodes as well as hepatic and pulmonary nodules can be evaluated for metastatic disease by FNA.

VII. Pathology

A. Location. Nearly **90%** of lesions arise in the **transformation zone** or on the ectocervix; **10%** originate in the **endocervical canal.**

B. Multiplicity. Patients with cervical cancer have an increased risk of synchronous and metachronous **vulvar, vaginal, and anal** malignancies, probably the result of common etiologic factors (eg, HPV infection).

C. Histology. As a rule, **ectocervical lesions are exophytic and less extensive** than they first appear, whereas **endocervical lesions are commonly endophytic,** creating a **"barrel-shaped"** expanded cervix, and are **more advanced** than first appreciated.

   1. Squamous cell carcinoma (80–85%). These lesions are commonly **large-cell, keratinizing or non-keratinizing** neoplasms. Variants include a rare, well-differentiated **verrucous variant** that is slow growing, locally invasive, and uniquely radioresistant and a **small-cell variant** that has a poor prognosis and requires electron microscopy to distinguish it from poorly differentiated adenocarcinoma and neuroendocrine tumors.

   2. Adenocarcinoma (15–20%). This histologic type is divided into several subtypes: endocervical, endometrioid, adenoma malignum, colloid producing, adenoid cystic, and adenosquamous and its variant, **glassy cell carcinoma.** Recently, **adenocarcinoma** in situ has been described but can only be diagnosed on cone biopsy. Because endometrial carcinoma may present as a primary cervical lesion, the diagnosis of **endometrioid** cervical cancer warrants a dilation and curettage (D&C) to exclude this possibility before therapy is instituted. Although **adenoma malignum** is well differentiated it has a poor prognosis because of aggressive locoregional spread. Glassy cell carcinomas however spreads to distant as well as locoregional sites.

   3. Carcinoid. Neuroendocrine cell types, such as **carcinoid tumors and small cell variants**, are well-recognized but rare histologic types of cervical cancer. Small cell has a high risk for distant spread, therefore chemotherapy needs to be included in the treatment regimen.

   4. Other cell types. In rare cases, sarcomas, lymphomas, melanomas, and choriocarcinomas originate in the cervix; however, metastatic disease must be excluded in these cases.

D. Metastatic spread

   1. Patterns of spread. Cervical carcinoma spreads via 3 distinct mechanisms.

      a. Direct extension. Growth directly into contiguous structures such as the paracervical tissues and surrounding ligaments (uterosacral, cardinal, pubovesical/cervical) is the most common method of spread. Involvement of the vagina, uterine corpus, bladder, rectum, and parametrial tissue also occurs.

      b. Lymphatic metastasis. Cervical cancer embolizes sequentially to the paracervical, paraurethral, parametrial, pelvic (external iliac, hypogastric, and obturator), common iliac, para-aortic, and supraclavicular lymph nodes. "Skip" metastases are rare. The incidence of pelvic and para-aortic lymph node metastases by stage is outlined in Table 48–1.

      c. Hematogenous metastasis. Spread through vascular channels to distant sites is rare except in advanced cases.

   2. Sites of spread. Once metastatic, cervical cancer may involve the following organs: **lung; bone; liver,** rare, but usually indicates spread from rectosigmoid through the portal vein; **brain,** rare; and **dermis,** rare.

VIII. Staging. In 1987 the **American Joint Committee on Cancer** and the **Union Internationale Contre le Cancer** developed the current uniform **TNM staging system.** This staging system can be used for both clinical and pathologic staging of cervical carci-

TABLE 48–1. FREQUENCY OF LYMPH NODE METASTASES WITH CERVICAL CANCER*

Stage	Pelvic Lymph Nodes (%)	Para-Aortic Lymph Nodes (%)
Ia1	0	0
Ia2 (1–3 mm)	0.6	0
Ia2 (3–5 mm)	4.8	< 1
Ib	16	2.2
IIa	24	11
IIb	31	19
III	45	30
IVa	55	45

*Adapted from Hatch KD: Cervical cancer. In: Berek JS, Hacker NF (editors), Practical Gynecologic Oncology. Baltimore, MD: Williams & Wilkins; 1989: 241–283.

noma and is based on the clinical staging system adopted by the **International Federation of Gynecology and Obstetrics (FIGO).** Staging is established on clinical grounds from inspection, palpation, colposcopy, endocervical curettage, hysteroscopy, cystoscopy, proctoscopy, IVP, chest x-ray, and skeletal radiographs and cannot be changed by pathologic findings. Worldwide, the **frequency of Stages I, II, III, and IV cervical cancer is 32%, 37%, 27%, and 4%,** respectively. In the United States, however, the incidence is slightly different (see below). Although recent studies have demonstrated a poor correlation between clinical and surgical staging, surgical staging is not used universally because of **increased morbidity** (which is reduced with a retroperitoneal approach), **delay in definitive therapy** (in patients normally treated with radiation alone), **high cost,** and the **questionable impact on overall survival.** Possible advantages, however, include **accurate staging** of disease, **resection of bulky (incurable) nodes and adnexa,** and the opportunity for **oophoropexy** to preserve ovarian function in young females. Currently, the routine surgical staging of pelvic and para-aortic lymph nodes is appropriate only as part of an approved investigational treatment protocol.

A. **TNM staging system**
   1. **Tumor stage**
      a. **TX.** The primary tumor cannot be assessed.
      b. **T0.** No evidence of primary tumor exists.
      c. **Tis.** Carcinoma in situ.
      d. **T1.** Tumor is confined to the cervix (extension to the corpus should be disregarded).
         (1) **T1a.** Preclinical invasive carcinoma diagnosed by microscopy only.
            (a) **T1a1.** Tumor with minimal microscopic stromal invasion.
            (b) **T1a2.** Tumor with an invasive component no deeper than 5 mm taken from the base of the epithelium and no more than 7 mm in horizontal spread.
         (2) **T1b.** Tumor is larger than T1a2.
      e. **T2.** Tumor invades beyond the uterus but not to the pelvic wall or to the lower third of the vagina.
         (1) **T2a.** Tumor without parametrial invasion.
         (2) **T2b.** Tumor with parametrial invasion.
      f. **T3.** Tumor extends to the pelvic wall, involves the lower third of the vagina, causes hydronephrosis or a nonfunctioning kidney, or all of these.
         (1) **T3a.** Tumor involves the lower third of the vagina without extension to the pelvic wall.
         (2) **T3b.** Tumor extends to the pelvic wall, causes hydronephrosis or nonfunctioning kidney, or all of these.
      g. **T4.** Tumor invades the mucosa of the bladder or rectum, extends beyond the true pelvis, or both.
         Note: The presence of bullous edema of the bladder is not sufficient to classify a tumor as T4.
   2. **Lymph node stage**

         a. NX. Regional lymph nodes cannot be assessed.
         b. N0. No regional lymph node metastases are present.
         c. N1. Regional lymph node metastases are present.
            Note: Regional lymph nodes include paracervical, parametrial, hypogastric (obturator), presacral, sacral, and common internal and external iliac lymph nodes. **Para-aortic lymph nodes** are considered to be **distant metastases.**

    3. Metastatic stage
        a. MX. The presence of distant metastases cannot be assessed.
        b. M0. No distant metastases are present.
        c. M1. Distant metastases are present.

    4. Histopathologic grade
        a. GX. The grade cannot be assessed.
        b. G1. Well differentiated.
        c. G2. Moderately well differentiated.
        d. G3. Poorly differentiated.
        e. G4. Undifferentiated.

    5. Stage groupings
        a. Stage 0. Tis, N0, M0.
        b. Stage IA. T1a, N0, M0.
        c. Stage IB. T1b, N0, M0.
        d. Stage IIA. T2a, N0, M0.
        e. Stage IIB. T2b, N0, M0.
        f. Stage IIIA. T3a, N01, M0.
        g. Stage IIIB. T1–3a, N1, M0; T3b, any N, M0.
        h. Stage IVA. T4, any N, M0.
        i. Stage IVB. Any T, any N, M1.

B. FIGO clinical staging system
    1. Stage 0. Carcinoma in situ and intraepithelial carcinoma (Tis, N0, M0; TNM Stage 0)
    2. Stage I (55%). Tumor confined to the cervix (extension to the corpus should be disregarded; T1, N0, M0; TNM Stage I).
        a. Stage Ia. Preclinical invasive carcinoma, diagnosed by microscopy only (T1a, N0, M0; TNM Stage IA).
            (1) Stage Ia1. Minimal microscopic stromal invasion (T1a1, N0, M0; TNM Stage IA).
            (2) Stage Ia2: Tumor with invasive component deeper than 5 mm taken from the base of the epithelium (either surface or glandular) from which it originates and no larger than 7 mm in horizontal spread (T1a2, N0, M0; TNM Stage IA).
        b. Stage Ib. Tumor is larger than that of Stage Ia2 whether clinically evident or not (T1b, N0, M0; TNM stage IB).
    3. Stage II (25%). Tumor invades beyond the uterus but not to the pelvic wall or to the lower third of vagina (T2, N0, M0; TNM Stage II).
        a. Stage IIa. Tumor without parametrial invasion (T2a, N0, M0; TNM Stage IIA).
        b. Stage IIb. Tumor with parametrial invasion (T2b, N0, M0; TNM Stage IIB).
    4. Stage III (15%). Tumor extends to the pelvic wall, involves the lower third of the vagina, causes hydronephrosis or nonfunctioning kidney (T3, N0, M0; TNM Stage III), or all of these.
        a. Stage IIIa. Tumor involves the lower third of the vagina without extension to the pelvic wall (T3a, N0, M0; TNM Stage IIIA).
        b. Stage IIIb. Tumor extends to the pelvic wall, causes hydronephrosis or nonfunctioning kidney (T3b, N0, M0; TNM Stage IIIB), or all of these.
    5. Stage IV (5%). Tumor extends beyond the true pelvis, clinically involves the mucosa of the bladder or rectum, distant metastases are present (T4, N0, M0; TNM Stage IV), or all of these.
        a. Stage IVa. Tumor extends beyond the true pelvis and/or clinically involves the mucosa of the bladder or rectum (T4, N0, M0; TNM Stage IVA).
        b. Stage IVb. Distant metastases are present (Any T, Any N, M1; TNM Stage IVB).

IX. Treatment
  A. Surgery
    1. Primary cervical carcinoma
      a. Indications
        (1) General guidelines. Surgery is indicated in all healthy patients with **Stage 0, I, or IIa disease** and without irregular or extensive cervical involvement. Other specific indications for primary surgical therapy are

concomitant pelvic or lower abdominal abscess (eg, inflammatory bowel disease, pelvic inflammatory disease), previous radiation therapy, fear of radiation, pregnancy, and the presence of an adnexal mass.

(2) Carcinoma in situ (Stage 0). Grade 3 cervical intraepithelial neoplasia (CIN-3) or carcinoma in situ requires **conization of the cervix.** In rare cases, simple hysterectomy may be necessary if the margins are involved. **Laser or cryoablation** can be tried in selected **reliable** patients who have **visible lesions** occupying only **one quadrant,** no glandular involvement (**negative endocervical curettage**), a visible transformation zone, and a colposcopic biopsy at least as severe as the cytologic smear.

(3) Microinvasive cervical cancer (Stage Ia). In the United States, microinvasive (squamous cell) carcinoma of the cervix can be diagnosed only by **cone biopsy or hysterectomy** (a punch biopsy is not adequate) and is defined by the **Society of Gynecologic Oncologists** as tumor invading no more than **3 mm in depth from the basement membrane** without vascular space invasion (FIGO considers microinvasive cancer to be tumor that invades no more than **5 mm in depth and no more than 7 mm in width** with or without vascular space involvement). As a rule, local recurrence and pelvic lymph node metastases do not occur and surgery alone (**simple hysterectomy**) serves as definitive therapy.

(4) Invasive cervical cancer (Stage Ib–IV). The standard surgical therapy for Stage Ib and Stage IIa disease is **radical abdominal hysterectomy with pelvic and para-aortic lymphadenectomy** (see below); however, radiation therapy produces equivalent results and the choice of surgery versus radiotherapy is based on the advantages and disadvantages of each (see Table 48–2). Stage Ib and IIa tumors that arise in the cervical stump following supracervical hysterectomy should be treated by a **radical trachelectomy** (resection of the "neck" of the uterus) despite a slightly higher complication rate because brachytherapy is difficult to deliver without an in situ uterus. In more advanced disease (Stages IIb–IV) surgery (pelvic exenteration) is **rarely** indicated.

(5) Residual cervical cancer. Following initial radiation therapy, simple (Type I) hysterectomy (see below) for **bulky or barrel-shaped** cervical lesions larger than **6 cm (10% of Stage I and II** cancers) reduces the **20% central failure rate** (resulting from a large population of hypoxic radio-resistent tumor cells) to **2%.** A significant **risk of severe complications (5–10%)** exists with this procedure, however, because of the previous radiation therapy.

b. **Approaches.** For optimal pelvic exposure, laparotomy is performed through a **low, midline, or transverse (Maylard or Cherney) abdominal incision.**

c. **Procedures**

(1) Conization. A cervical cone biopsy is considered to be the definitive therapy for any female if tumor **invasion is less than 1 mm and the surgical margins are clear** of tumor. This treatment is reserved for women who want to preserve their fertility.

(2) Simple (Type I) hysterectomy. Type I hysterectomy (abdominal or

---

TABLE 48–2. ADVANTAGES OF SURGERY AND RADIOTHERAPY

Surgery	Radiation
Short treatment time	Avoids surgery
Surgical staging available	Given as outpatient
Ovarian preservation	Suitable for poor surgical candidates
Pliable vagina	
Avoids complications of pelvic radiation	

extrafascial hysterectomy) removes the entire uterus. The ureters are retracted laterally while the paracervical tissues are divided. This procedure also can be used with endometrial cancer and carcinoma in situ and with residual cervical cancer after primary radiation therapy (completion hysterectomy). Because the **risk of pelvic lymph node metastases** in this situation is less than **1%, pelvic lymph node dissection is not indicated.**

   (3) **Standard radical (Type III) hysterectomy.** This is the recommended procedure for **Stage Ib (> 5 mm) and IIa disease.** Initially, the entire peritoneal cavity, including the pelvic and para-aortic lymph nodes, is explored to exclude metastatic disease. Next, the **paravesical space** (bordered by the obliterated umbilical artery medially, the obturator internus muscle laterally, the cardinal ligament posteriorly, and the symphysis pubis anteriorly) and the **pararectal space** (bordered by the rectum medially, the cardinal ligament anteriorly, the pelvic vessels laterally, and the sacrum posteriorly) are developed, and the **paravaginal and parametrial tissues are palpated** for evidence of tumor extension. The floor of both spaces is the levator ani muscle. The bladder is then dissected from the lower uterine segment unless anterior tumor extension is present, which makes this difficult, necessitating anterior exenteration (see below). Subsequently, the uterine artery is skeletonized and ligated at its origin and the ureters are isolated as they course medially toward the bladder, allowing for resection of the bladder pillars. This also defines the **cardinal and uterosacral ligaments,** which are completely removed after incising the peritoneum of the posterior cul-de-sac. The rectovaginal septum is developed, then the **upper third of the vagina is removed** to ensure clear margins. A **pelvic and para-aortic lymphadenectomy** is performed either before or after the hysterectomy. **Bilateral salpingo-oophorectomy** is discretionary.

   (4) **Modified radical (Type II) hysterectomy.** This procedure can be used in selected cases of **microinvasive carcinoma and small (< 1 cm) Stage Ib tumors.** The modified radical hysterectomy is less extensive than the standard radical hysterectomy. In the modified radical hysterectomy, only the **medial half** of the cardinal and uterosacral ligaments (rather than all) and the **upper fourth** of the vagina (rather than the upper third) are removed. In addition, the uterine artery is ligated **at the ureter** (not at the origin) and the ureter is **not extensively dissected** to the trigone. A **pelvic and para-aortic lymphadenectomy** is still performed either before or after the hysterectomy, and, again, **bilateral salpingo-oophorectomy** is discretionary.

d. Pelvic exenteration. In rare cases, **Stage IVa** disease is amenable to **anterior** (bladder, uterus, and vagina), **posterior** (uterus, vagina, and rectum), or **total pelvic exenteration** (bladder, uterus, vagina, and rectum). Before undertaking this radical procedure, however, adequate histologic evidence of disease must be present, the patient must be medically and psychologically fit, and no evidence of metastatic disease or pelvic wall extension should exist. Once initial abdominal-pelvic exploration **excludes metastatic disease and pelvic side wall extension,** the appropriate pelvic organs and tumor are removed above or below the levator muscles, depending on the location of the tumor. Next, **a urinary conduit (anterior), neovagina (all), and colostomy or low anterior anastomosis (posterior)** are constructed. Recent technical refinements in this operation include a continent urostomy, low anterior rectal anastomosis without colostomy, omental carpet to close the pelvic floor, vaginal reconstruction with gracilis myocutaneous flaps, rectus abdominus, myocutaneous flaps, or split thickness skin grafts, and improved pre- and postoperative care.

2. Morbidity and mortality. Although morbidity and mortality for simple hysterectomy is low (see p 360, **IX.A.3**), complications following radical hysterectomy are not uncommon despite technical improvements in ureteral dissection (avoiding devascularization) and closed-suction drainage. Pelvic exenteration is associated with a **mortality rate of less than 5%,** a **25–50% incidence of significant morbidity,** and a **15–25% reoperation rate** for fistulae or small bowel obstructions. Frequent problems associated with the radical hysterectomy include the following:

  a. **Wound infection, 1–2%.**
  b. **Hemorrhage,** average blood loss of 600–1200 cc.
  c. **Pelvic cellulitis.**
  d. **Vesicovaginal or ureterovaginal fistulae,** 1–2%.
  e. **Urinary tract infection.**
  f. **Thromboembolism,** 1–2%.
  g. **Small bowel obstruction,** 1–2%.
  h. **Bladder dysfunction,** common with more radical surgery and results from interrupting the autonomic nerves running through the cardinal and utero-sacral ligaments. Full bladder function returns within 2–12 weeks in the majority of patients, although chronic bladder hypertonia may persist in a small number of them.
  i. **Lymphocele,** < 5%.
  j. **Ureteral strictures,** uncommon in the absence of postoperative radiation.
3. **Locally advanced and metastatic cervical cancer.** In this setting, surgery is directed primarily at the **palliation of complications** such as **vesicovaginal and rectovaginal fistulae,** which may require urinary diversion or colostomy, respectively. Diverting colostomy for rectovaginal fistulae should be performed before radiation for optimal perineal hygiene, whereas initial urinary diversion can be established with percutaneous nephrostomy tubes and subsequently be revised to a urinary conduit after radiation therapy. In rare cases, persistent or recurrent disease discovered after primary radiation therapy in the absence of metastatic disease is amenable to surgical resection. **Pelvic exenteration** is recommended and yields **25–50% 5-year survival.** Radical hysterectomy in an irradiated field, however, is associated with high morbidity and mortality rates and should be limited to special situations.

B. **Radiation therapy**
  1. **Primary cervical carcinoma**
     a. **Techniques.** Invasive cervical carcinoma is optimally treated with a combination of external-beam, intracavitary, and frequently interstitial radiation.
        (1) **External beam radiotherapy.** Whole pelvic radiation typically uses 2–4 fields to deliver **180 cGy fractions daily for 5–7 weeks.** The total pelvic dose varies from **4500–7000 cGy,** depending on the location and volume of tumor. The total external-beam dose is directly proportional (whereas the intracavitary dose is inversely proportional) to tumor size. The field includes the pelvic lymph nodes and may be extended to include the para-aortic nodes, if indicated.
        (2) **Intracavitary radiotherapy.** Brachytherapy ([226]radium or [137]cesium) is usually delivered with an afterloading applicator, commonly a **Fletcher-Suit apparatus,** consisting of an intrauterine tandem and two vaginal colpostats. These systems deliver high doses to the tumor but spare the bladder and rectum, and they are initially applied **after 1000–4000 cGy external-beam irradiation,** depending on the tumor geometry. The delivered dose is expressed in terms of point A and B. **Point A,** located 2 cm lateral to the cervical canal and 2 cm superior to the lateral vaginal fornix (corresponding to the **central tumor**), requires **7500–8500 cGy,** whereas **point B,** positioned 3 cm lateral to point A (equivalent to the **pelvic wall**), requires **4500–6500 cGy,** depending on tumor bulk.
        (3) **Vaginal vault radiotherapy.** In selected patients, a total surface dose of **5500–6000 cGy** is given **postoperatively using a vaginal cylinder or two colpostats,** although the dose cannot be accurately calculated with this application and the effective dose is primarily to the surface of the vaginal vault.
        (4) **Interstitial brachytherapy.** In advanced and distorted tumors that are not amenable to therapy with a tandem and a colpostat, interstitial radiotherapy with [226]radium needles or iridium wire can be used. By using a **Syed-Neblett template** to hold the interstitial needles in place, the dosimetry can be **adjusted individually,** according to the geometry of the tumor.
     b. **Indications**
        (1) **Microinvasive disease (Stage Ia or occult Ib).** Appropriately, most patients with microinvasive disease are treated with surgery; however, patients who are poor surgical risks can be adequately treated with **brachytherapy** alone because the risk of lymph node involvement is

extremely low. **External-beam radiotherapy** is reserved for patients with anatomy that is not optimal for intracavitary administration.

   (2) **Early-stage invasive disease (Stages Ib and IIa).** Although surgery often is used for Stages Ib and IIa disease, radiation therapy offers an equivalent alternative with distinct advantages (see Table 48–2). Initially, whole pelvic radiation is given, using multiple fields (box technique) to minimize complications. **Microscopic tumor** deposits in the pelvis are sterilized with **4000–5000 cGy,** whereas **gross tumor** requires more than **6000 cGy** (> 7000 cGy exceeds the normal pelvic tissue tolerance). Although large tumors may not be eradicated completely by external-beam therapy alone, **shrinkage improves the geometry for intracavitary radiation.** In addition, asymmetric cancers can be boosted using smaller external radiation fields. The **pelvic recurrence rate** for early-stage disease is less than **5%** following appropriate radiation therapy.

   (3) **Advanced stage disease (Stages IIb, III, and IV).** Many advanced lesions require large treatment volumes. Interstitial implants are used most often in this setting because they are able to deliver a wider dose distribution. The **pelvic failure rate** for bulky tumors is **40%.** and a substantial risk of pelvic and para-aortic lymph node metastasis as well as distant metastasis exists. Control of pelvic disease using chemotherapy as a radiation sensitizer is currently being investigated. Surgical staging allows for accurate assessment of the para-aortic lymph nodes, and extended field radiation therapy can be delivered to this area if indicated.

2. **Adjuvant radiation therapy**
   a. **Preoperative radiotherapy.** Barrel-shaped and bulky cervical lesions (Stage I and II tumors larger than 5–6 cm in diameter), which constitute less than **10%** of Stage I and Stage II tumors, have a **high incidence of central, pelvic wall, and lymph node recurrence**. The geometry, however, prohibits adequate radiation dosimetry. Therefore, treatment consists of 4000 cGy whole pelvis irradiation followed by an intracavitary implant and, 4–6 weeks later, by a simple (Type I) hysterectomy. Combined surgery and radiation **reduces the central failure rate from 20% with radiation alone to 2%,** although survival is not affected. The individual risk of **recurrence is directly related to the amount of tumor** found in the hysterectomy specimen **and indirectly related to the rate of regression.** Unfortunately, severe complications occur in **5–10%** of patients; these include small bowel **obstruction** as well as genitourinary and gastrointestinal **fistulae.** The addition of radiosensitizing chemotherapeutic agents is currently being investigated.
   b. **Postoperative radiotherapy.** Postoperative whole pelvic radiation therapy **(4500–5000 cGy in 180 cGy daily fractions)** is recommended in **high-risk patients** (ie, those with positive surgical margins or pelvic lymph nodes, large or bulky cervical disease, undifferentiated tumor, deep invasion, parametrial involvement, and lymphatic or vascular invasion). In addition, patients with **undiagnosed invasive cervical carcinoma that is found incidentally** after simple hysterectomy require either external-beam irradiation alone (no residual disease) or external-beam irradiation and a parametrial interstitial implant (gross residual disease). Selected patients who have no gross residual disease, however, can be treated with **radical parametriectomy, upper vaginectomy, and pelvic lymphadenectomy** to complete the staging process and avoid unnecessary radiation.

3. **Locally advanced and metastatic cervical cancer.** The goal of radiotherapy in the presence of locally advanced and metastatic disease is **local tumor control and symptomatic palliation.** For example, if **hemorrhage** occurs, it can be controlled with external-beam pelvic irradiation (a large single fraction or daily 180 cGy fractions) or transvaginal orthovoltage radiation (not included in calculation of total radiation dose). Radiation also can effectively reduce symptoms produced by **recurrent pelvic tumor (after surgery); bone metastases; enlarging supraclavicular, mediastinal, para-aortic, or pelvic lymph nodes; obstructing pulmonary metastases; and brain metastases.** Hyperbaric oxygen, metronidazole, misonidazole, and hyperthermia have been tried as radiation sensitizing agents with increased morbidity but no therapeutic benefit. Thus, at present, the use of these agents cannot be recommended.

4. **Morbidity and mortality.** Acute toxicity results from the adverse effects of radiation on the **rapidly dividing epithelial cells,** whereas chronic toxicity is caused by **obliterative vasculitis and fibrosis.** The risk of a **major** complication depends on the tumor stage and extent of surgical intervention prior to irradiation. Some common problems include the following difficulties: **cystitis; enteritis; proctitis,** 7.1%; **myelosuppression; small bowel obstruction,** 7.1%; **ureteral obstruction,** 2.1–14.3%; and **fistulae,** 2.5–5.0% (rectovaginal, vesicovaginal, ureterovaginal, and small bowel).

C. **Chemotherapy**

1. **Primary cervical carcinoma.** Because of the success of radiation and surgery in the treatment of primary cervical cancer, chemotherapy has not been evaluated in this setting.

2. **Adjuvant chemotherapy.** The adjuvant administration of cytotoxic drugs has not been evaluated extensively because of the lack of effective agents and the overall good response of cervical cancer to radiation and surgery. Cisplatin, hydroxyurea, and fluorouracil, however, have been used as **radiation sensitizing** medications. Several studies of Stage I and II patients suggest that **cisplatin may increase the complete response rate from 20% (radiation alone) to 55% and the disease-free survival from 45% to 54%,** although the results are not consistent. In addition, 2 clinical trials involving patients with Stage II, III, or IV disease (including one randomized prospective trial) demonstrate that **hydroxyurea also increases the complete response rate (48% to 68%) and the 2-year disease-free survival rate (43.5% to 74%).** Unfortunately, in the trials just described, the toxicity observed in the groups receiving radiation sensitizing agents was consistently more severe than in the groups treated with radiation alone. Therefore, although these data are encouraging, more randomized prospective clinical trials are required before this approach is widely endorsed.

3. **Locally advanced and metastatic cervical cancer**
   a. **Single agents. Fluorouracil (1000 mg/m^2 per day continuous IV infusion for 4 days every 21–28 days)** and cisplatin are the most active of the agents that have been adequately studied; **overall response rates are 25–50% and 20–25%, respectively.** The duration of responses, however, is only 4 months, and survival is unaffected. Other agents with activity include ifosfamide (30%), carboplatin (28%), dibromodulcitol (27%), chlorambucil (25%), vincristine (23%), and other platinum derivatives (21%).
   b. **Combination chemotherapy.** Several combination regimens—**doxorubicin and methotrexate, doxorubicin and methyl-CCNU, BVP** (bleomycin, vinblastine, and cisplatin), **BOMP** (bleomycin, vincristine, methotrexate, and cisplatin), and **BOCP** (bleomycin, vincristine, mitomycin-C, and cisplatin)—produce **43–66% overall and 18–29% complete response rates.** The toxicity of these combinations is significant, however, because of myelosuppression, renal insufficiency, and decreased pelvic vascularity from previous radiation, tumor, or both. In addition, no combination has been shown to be superior to single-agent therapy in a prospective trial.
   c. **Intra-arterial chemotherapy.** Although pelvic anatomy is ideal for intra-arterial chemotherapy, infusions of bleomycin, mitomycin-C, and vincristine have produced **disappointing response rates and considerable toxicity.**

4. **Hormonal therapy.** Although hormonal therapy is not effective in the primary or adjuvant treatment of cervical cancer, estrogen replacement often is necessary to keep pelvic tissues well estrogenized. In addition, **no increase in the recurrence rate** has been noted with estrogen administration, even with adenocarcinoma of the cervix.

D. **Immunotherapy.** Limited trials have been conducted using immunomodulatory agents, including *Corynebacterium parvum* and interferon, without success. Currently, **monoclonal antibodies** directed against squamous cell carcinoma are being developed for use in both immunoradiodiagnosis and immunotherapy.

X. **Prognosis**

A. **Risk of recurrence.** Nearly **80%** of recurrences manifest **within 2 years,** and large tumors usually recur earlier than small neoplasms.

B. **Five-year survival.** The 5-year survival by FIGO stage is as follows: **Stage I,** 80–90%; **Stage II,** 50–65%; **Stage III,** 25–35%; and **Stage IV,** 0–15%.

C. **Adverse prognostic factors.** The folowing are independent variables that are associated with a poor prognosis:
   1. **Lymph node involvement.** This extremely important factor reduces 5-year survival from **90% to 65%, 30%, and 25% with unilateral** pelvic node, **bilateral** pelvic node, and **common iliac** node involvement, respectively.
   2. **Large tumor size and volume.** The 5-year survival is **90%, 60%, and 40% for tumors smaller than 2 cm, 2–4 cm, and more than 4 cm** in size, respectively.
   3. **Invasion deeper than 1.5 cm.** This is associated with an **increase** in pelvic lymph node metastases from **2.5% to 44%** and a **decrease** in 5-year survival from **90% to 70%.**
   4. **Parametrial invasion.** This decreases **5-year survival from 95% to 69%** (no lymph node metastases) and 42% (positive lymph node metastases).
   5. **Vascular space invasion (VSI).** Although controversial, VSI is associated with a **4–5 times** increased risk of **pelvic lymph node metastases** and a **30% decrease in 5-year survival.**
   6. **High grade,** with **adenocarcinoma only.** Pelvic lymph node metastases increases from 5% in Grade I to 50% in Grade III.
   7. **Undifferentiated small cell and neuroendocrine histology.**

XI. **Patient follow-up**
   A. **General guidelines.** Patients should be followed closely every 3 months for 1 year, every 4 months for 1 year, every 6 months for an additional 3 years, then annually for evidence of pelvic and distant recurrence. Specific guidelines for patients with cervical cancer are outlined below.
   B. **Routine evaluation.** Each clinic visit should include the following tests and procedures.
      1. **Medical history and physical examination.** An interval medical history and thorough physical examination, including cervical or vaginal cytology (Pap smear), must be completed during each office visit with particular attention paid to the areas summarized above (see p 365, **VI.A**). In addition, the triad of **unilateral leg swelling, pelvic pain, and hydroureter** strongly suggests recurrence in the pelvic wall.
      2. **Blood tests** (see p 1, **IV.A**).
         a. **Complete blood count.**
         b. **Hepatic transaminases.**
         c. **Alkaline phosphatase.**
         d. **BUN and creatinine.**
      3. **Urinalysis** (see p 3, **IV.B**).
      4. **Chest x-ray** (see p 3, **IV.C.1**).
      5. **Colposcopy** (see p 366, **VI.B.4.a**).
   C. **Additional evaluation.** CT scan of the abdomen and pelvis should be obtained **every 6–12 months for 3–5 years** to exclude occult local and distant recurrence.
   D. **Optional evaluation.** The following tests and procedures may be indicated by previous diagnostic findings or clinical suspicion:
      1. **Blood tests**
         a. **5′-nucleotidase** (see p 2, **IV.A.4**).
         b. **GGTP** (see p 2, **IV.A.5**).
         c. **CA-125** (see p 366, **VI.C.1.c**).
         d. **Carcinoembryonic antigen (CEA)** (see p 366, **VI.C.1.d**).
         e. **TA-4** (see p 366, **VI.C.1.e**).
      2. **Imaging studies**
         a. **Intravenous pyelogram** (see p 366, **VI.B.3.b**).
         b. **MRI** (see p 3, **IV.C.2**).
         c. **Ultrasound** (see p 3, **IV.C.3**).
         d. **Technetium-99m bone scan** (see p 3, **IV.C.4**).
         e. **Lymphangiography** (see p 367, **VI.C.2.c**).
      3. **Biopsy.** Because most tumors recur locally, any palpable or radiographic pelvic abnormality must be biopsied by fine needle aspiration, punch biopsy, core needle biopsy, or open biopsy. Occasionally, examination under anesthesia combined with cystoscopy and sigmoidoscopy is required to biopsy suspicious areas. A negative biopsy, however, does not exclude the diagnosis of malignancy.

REFERENCES

Berek, JS, et al. Adenocarcinoma of the cervix: histologic variables associated with lymph node metastasis and survival. Obstet Gynecol 65:46–52, 1985.

Berek, JS, Hacker, NF. Practical Gynecologic Oncology. Williams and Wilkins, Baltimore, 1989, pp. 241–283.

Berman, ML, Walker, JL, and Berek, JS. Cervix. In Cancer Treatment. Haskell, CM, editor. WB Saunders, Philadelphia: 3rd ed. pp. 325–337, 1990.

Boyce, J, et al. Prognostic factors in stage I cancer of the cervix. Gynecol Oncol 12:154–165, 1981.

Copeland, LJ, et al. Gracilis myocutaneous vaginal reconstruction concurrent with total pelvic exenteration. Am J Obstet Gynecol 160:1095–1099, 1989.

Copeland, LJ. Cancer of the Cervix. In Kases Principles and Practice of Clinical Gynecology. Kase, NG, Weingold, AB, and Gershenson, DM., editors. Churchill Livingston, New York: 2nd ed, pp. 763–788, 1990.

Chung, CK, et al. Analysis of factors contributing to the treatment failures in stage Ib and IIa carcinoma of the cervix. Am J Obstet Gynecol 138:550–554, 1988.

Di Saia, PJ, Creasman, WT. Clinical Gynecologic Oncology. CV Mosby, St Louis: 3rd ed, pp. 67–128, 1989.

Gallion, HH, et al. Combined radiation therapy and extrafascial hysterectomy in the treatment of stage Ib barrel-shaped cervical cancer. Cancer 56:262–266, 1985.

Jones, HW. Surgery for advanced or recurrent cervical carcinoma. Cancer 60:2094–2103, 1987.

Krebs, HB, editor. Genital human papilloma virus infection. In Clinical Obstetrics and Gynecology 32:105–214, 1989.

Morely, GW, et al. Pelvic exenteration, University of Michigan: 100 patients at 5 years. Obstet Gynecol 74:934–939, 1989.

Morrow, CP, et al. Panel report: Pelvic radiation in postoperative management of stage Ib squamous cell carcinoma of the cervix with pelvic node metastasis treated by a radical hysterectomy and pelvic lymphadenectomy. Gynecol Oncol 10:105–110, 1980.

Morrow, CP, Townsend, DE. Synopsis of Gynecologic Oncology. Wiley, New York: 3rd ed. pp. 103–158 and 459–520, 1987.

Piver, MS, Barlow, JJ, Vongtama, V, Blumenson, L. Hydroxyurea: A radiation potentiator in carcinoma of the uterine cervix. Am J Obstet Gynecol 147:803–807, 1983.

Potish, RA, et al. Therapeutic implications of the natural history of advanced cervical cancer as defined by pretreatment and surgical staging. Cancer 56:956–960, 1985.

Rubin, SC, et al. Para-aortic nodal metastasis in early cervical carcinoma: long term survival following extended field radiotherapy. Gynecol Oncol 18:213–217, 1984.

Thigpen, JT. Single agent chemotherapy in carcinoma of the cervix. In Cervix Cancer. Surwit EA, Alberts, D.S, editors. Martinus Nijhoff, Boston, MA: pp. 119–136, 1987.

Twiggs, LB, Potish, RA, and McIntyre, S, et al. Concurrent weekly cisplatin and radiotherapy in advanced cervical cancer: a preliminary dose escalating toxicity study. Gynecol Oncol 24:143–148, 1986.

Van Nagel, JR, et al. The significance of vascular space invasion and lymphocytic infiltration invasive cervical cancer. Cancer 41:228–234, 1978.

Van Nagel, JR, et al. Microinvasive carcinoma of the cervix. Am J Obstet Gynecol 145:981–985, 1983.

49 Malignancies of the Vagina

Laila I. Muderspach, M.D.

I. **Epidemiology.** Although secondary involvement of the vagina from other genital tract malignancies (particularly cervical cancer) is relatively frequent, primary cancer of the vagina is uncommon, accounting for only **1–2% of all gynecologic cancers.** The incidence of squamous carcinoma of the vagina is **0.6 per 100,000 females** in the United States.

II. **Risk factors**
   A. **Age.** Vaginal carcinoma increases after age 40 from less than 0.5 per 100,000 to **5.8 per 100,000 by age 85.** The average age at the time of diagnosis is **62 years.**
   B. **Race.** The risk in **black females older than 50** years is **1.5–2 times greater** than in white females of the same age.
   C. **Genetic factors.** The risk of vaginal cancer in first-degree relatives is not increased over that of the general population.
   D. **Diet.** No dietary factors have been associated with the development of vaginal malignancies.
   E. **Smoking.** Tobacco has been implicated in the pathogenesis of squamous cell carcinoma of both the vagina and cervix.
   F. **History of previous genital tract pathology.** Vaginal and cervical squamous cell carcinoma have similar etiologic factors including the following:
      1. **Infection.** A history of frequent sexual activity and sexually transmitted diseases, particularly **human papilloma virus infection,** increases the risk of vaginal tumors.
      2. **Hysterectomy.** For unexplained reasons, **35–59%** of patients with squamous carcinoma of the vagina have had a previous hysterectomy, usually for benign conditions.
      3. **Cervical carcinoma.** Cervical cancer is associated with an increased incidence of vaginal malignancies, and any vaginal carcinoma developing more than 5 years after treatment for cervical cancer should be considered a new primary malignancy.
   G. **Ionizing radiation.** Previous pelvic irradiation (often for cervical carcinoma) increases the risk of vaginal cancer following a latent period of 7–20 years. As many as **20.9% of patients with vaginal malignancies have had pelvic irradiation.**
   H. **Diethylstilbesterol (DES)** exposure. Until its ban in 1971, DES was used to maintain high-risk pregnancies. Subsequently, however, exposure to DES in utero has been reported to cause vaginal adenosis and structural changes in the vagina and cervix in **45%** and 25% of patients, respectively. In addition, **1.4 in 1000 exposed females (0.14%) develop vaginal adenocarcinoma at a mean age of 19 years.**
   I. **Urbanization.** No identifiable risk exists in either rural or urban populations.

III. **Presentation**
   A. **Signs and symptoms**
      1. **Local manifestations.** The most common initial complaint in patients with vaginal malignancies is **abnormal vaginal bleeding,** usually postmenopausal spotting (postcoital and intermenstrual bleeding may occur in younger patients). **Watery malodorous discharge,** vaginal pruritus or pain, urinary complaints, and tenesmus also may be reported, depending on the size of the tumor and its location. **Vesicovaginal and rectovaginal fistulae** as well as pelvic pain (5%) may develop in locally advanced disease, whereas early lesions may be **asymptomatic** and be detected on routine pelvic examination and **Papanicolaou (Pap) smear** (5–10%).
      2. **Systemic manifestations.** Complaints indicating advanced systemic disease include weight loss, supraclavicular or inguinal adenopathy, bone pain, pleural effusions, hydronephrosis, jaundice, and pulmonary symptoms (eg, cough, dyspnea).

   B. **Paraneoplastic syndromes.** Malignancies of the vagina have been associated with the following paraneoplastic conditions, which may be the only manifestation of disease.
      1. **Thrombophlebitis** (see p 81, **II**).
      2. **Hypercalcemia** (see p 87, **I**).

IV. Differential diagnosis. Vaginal carcinoma typically presents with **postmenopausal vaginal bleeding, discharge, a vaginal mass,** or all of these. The differential diagnosis of abnormal vaginal bleeding is extensive (see p 355, **IV**). In addition, other pathologic processes that produce **vaginal masses** and imitate a primary vaginal malignancy include **primary gynecologic diseases** such as the following: endometriosis, infections (herpes simplex, types I and II), autoimmune syndromes (Behçet's disease), trauma (foreign objects, barrier contraceptive devices, and birthing trauma), benign neoplasms (epidermoid inclusion cysts, paramesonephric or Müllerian cysts, mesonephric or Gartner's duct cysts, leiomyomas, and fibromyomas) and malignancies (squamous cell carcinoma of the cervix or vulva, choriocarcinoma, and adenocarcinoma of the uterus and ovary). Finally, **nongynecologic diseases** such as diverticulitis and Crohn's disease and metastases from the breast, colon, kidney, and pancreas can cause vaginal masses and mimic vaginal cancer.

V. Screening programs. Excluding annual pelvic examinations and cervical and vaginal exfoliative cytology, no cost effective method of screening asymptomatic females has been developed.

VI. Diagnostic workup
   A. **Medical history and physical examination.** In addition to a thorough medical history emphasizing risk factors, a complete physical examination directed at the following sites of tumor spread must be documented.
      1. **General appearance.** An evaluation of the patient's nutritional and general functional status should be included (see, also, p 1, **I** and **III**).
      2. **Lymph nodes.** Thorough examination of the inguinal, supraclavicular, axillary, and cervical lymph nodes is required.
      3. **Chest.** Pulmonary examination should detect the presence of pleural effusions.
      4. **Breasts**. The presence of a primary breast lesion must be excluded.
      5. **Abdomen.** Evidence of ascites, hepatosplenomegaly, and suspicious masses suggestive of intraperitoneal spread should be noted.
      6. **Genitalia**
         a. **External genitalia.** The vulva, urethra, vaginal introitus, and anus are examined visually and by palpation for primary or metastatic tumor.
         b. **Vagina.** Complete **visualization and palpation** is mandatory to exclude primary or metastatic lesions. Bimanual examination includes palpation of the vaginal walls, fornices, and ectocervix. Lesions that may be obscured by the speculum are often readily noted as palpable surface irregularities or induration.
         c. **Cervix.** A Pap smear should be obtained from the cervix (or the vaginal cuff if the cervix is absent) and detects **20% of invasive vaginal cancers.** Visual and bimanual examination also is necessary; the size, position, symmetry, and mobility of the cervix should be noted.
         d. **Uterus and adnexa.** The size, position, symmetry, and mobility of the uterus and adnexa must be assessed. The remainder of the pelvis should be evaluated for submucosal extension, paravaginal invasion, and bladder and rectal involvement. Rectovaginal examination is necessary to assess the rectovaginal septum and cul-de-sac.
      7. **Rectum.** Primary rectal carcinoma that directly invades the vagina must be excluded, and stool should be tested for occult blood.
   B. **Primary test and procedures.** All patients with suspected vaginal carcinoma should have the following diagnostic tests and procedures.
      1. **Blood tests** (see p 1, **IV.A**)
         a. **Complete blood count.**
         b. **Hepatic transaminases.**
         c. **Alkaline phosphatase.**
         d. **BUN and creatinine.**
         e. **Albumin.**
      2. **Urine tests**
         a. **Urinalysis** (see p 3, **IV.B**).
         b. **Beta-human chorionic gonadotropin (beta-hCG).** Pregnancy must be excluded in all females of reproductive age. A negative result will exclude choriocarcinoma.

3. **Imaging studies** (see p 3, **IV.C**)
   a. **Chest X-ray**
   b. **Computed tomography (CT).** CT scan of the pelvis and abdomen provides information about the primary tumor, liver, retroperitoneal nodes, and the genitourinary tract and eliminates the need for intravenous pyelography.
4. **Invasive procedures**
   a. **Colposcopy.** Direct visualization of the vaginal mucosa with the aid of **a colposcope** is valuable in the diagnosis of early vaginal neoplasms. Although redundancy of the vaginal mucosa often makes the examination difficult, application of **Lugol's solution** (if the mucosa is well estrogenized) may reveal abnormal areas that **fail to stain brown.**
   b. **Biopsy.** A biopsy of any suspicious lesion is mandatory and can be obtained by direct punch biopsy.
C. **Optional tests and procedures.** The following tests and procedures may be indicated by previous diagnostic findings or clinical suspicion.
   1. **Blood tests**
      a. **Nucleotidase** (see p 2, **IV.A.4**).
      b. **GGTP** (see p 2, **IV.A.5**).
      c. **CA-125.** This monoclonal antibody detects a serum tumor antigen that is associated with adenocarcinomas. Although not helpful in the initial diagnosis of vaginal adenocarcinoma, this test can be used to follow tumor regression and recurrence.
      d. **Carcinoembryonic antigen (CEA).** Although not helpful in the initial diagnosis of vaginal cancer, this serum antigen (if elevated originally) can be used to monitor tumor regression and recurrence.
   2. **Imaging studies**
      a. **Magnetic resonance imaging (MRI)** (see p 3, **IV.C.2**).
      b. **Lymphangiography.** Bipedal lymphangiography, in some circumstances, may be helpful to evaluate pelvic lymph nodes for the presence of metastatic disease.
      c. **Technetium-99m bone scan** (see p 3, **IV.C.4**).
   3. **Invasive procedures**
      a. **Cystourethroscopy.** If involvement of the lower urinary tract is suspected, endoscopic examination of the urethra and bladder must be performed to guide staging and treatment.
      b. **Proctosigmoidoscopy.** Suspicion of rectal involvement requires direct visual inspection of the rectosigmoid colon and anus.
      c. **Fine needle aspiration (FNA).** Suspicious inguinal, supraclavicular, pelvic, and para-aortic lymph nodes as well as hepatic and pulmonary nodules can be evaluated by FNA.
VII. **Pathology**
   A. **Location.** Vaginal carcinoma can be classified according to the **axial** and **circumferential** location of the primary lesion:
      1. **Axial location.** Although as many as **30%** of patients present with disease involving the **entire length** of the vagina, the primary malignancy can be identified as originating from the following areas:
         a. **Upper third,** 50.7% (the most common site with clear cell adenocarcinoma; often confused with cervical carcinoma).
         b. **Middle third,** 18.8%.
         c. **Lower third,** 30.4% (often confused with vulvar cancer).
      2. **Circumferential location**
         a. **Anterior wall,** 26.9% (most common site with clear cell adenocarcinoma).
         b. **Lateral walls,** 15.9%.
         c. **Posterior wall,** 57.2%.
   B. **Multiplicity.** Second primary cancers occur in **3–30%** of patients because of common etiologic factors and predominately include **cervical carcinomas**. Synchronous and metachronous vulvar cancer also may develop.
   C. **Histology.** A continuum of vaginal pathology exists from benign to malignant lesions. Although controversial, **vaginal intraepithelial neoplasia** is considered to be a precursor of vaginal carcinoma and progresses to invasive cancer despite treatment in **3–5%** of females. The histologic types of cancer include **squamous cell carcinoma (85%), adenocarcinoma (8%), sarcoma (3%), melanoma (3%),** small cell carcinoma (< 1%), lymphoma (< 1%), and undifferentiated carcinoma (< 1%). Specific histologic features of the most common types are outlined below:
      1. **Squamous cell carcinoma.** Squamous cell cancers typically are either **ex-**

ophytic or ulcerating tumors that occur in patients older than 50 years of age (76%).

2. **Adenocarcinoma.** Adenocarcinoma of the vagina is most **commonly metastatic**, with **primary tumors** accounting for **6–7%** of vaginal adenocarcinomas. Typically, these patients are younger than patients with squamous cell carcinoma, particularly those exposed to **DES** who develop clear cell carcinoma at a **mean age of 19.**

3. **Sarcoma.** The most common vaginal sarcoma, **sarcoma botryoides (embryonal rhabdomyosarcoma),** occurs in infants, children, and adolescents, with a **peak incidence at age 3.** The Greek term "botrys" means **grapes** and describes the typical presentation of a polypoid mass protruding through the vaginal introitus. This tumor is highly malignant. Fibrosarcomas and leiomyosarcomas are rare, bulky tumors that usually are located in the upper vagina.

4. **Melanoma.** Primary vaginal melanoma accounts for 2.5–3% of all primary vaginal tumors (about 100 reported cases). Most commonly, they are located in the **lower anterior wall** and can be nonpigmented or variegated.

D. **Metastatic spread.** Despite the opportunity for early diagnosis, more than 66% of patients present with disease that has spread beyond the vagina.

  1. **Modes of spread.** Vaginal neoplasms frequently spread via the following 3 routes:

    a. **Direct extension.** Vaginal cancer spreads locally to adjacent paravaginal soft tissue, bladder, rectum, and pelvic bones.

    b. **Lymphatic metastasis.** Spread through the vast vaginal lymphatic network to regional lymph nodes **occurs in 20.8–31.6% of patients.** The lower vagina drains to the **inguinal** and secondarily to the pelvic nodes, whereas the upper vaginal lymphatics drain mainly to the **pelvic** and ultimately the **para-aortic** nodes.

    c. **Hematogenous metastasis.** Spread through systemic blood vessels to distant sites is usually a late finding.

  2. **Sites of spread.** The locations most commonly involved with metastatic vaginal carcinoma include the following sites: **retroperitoneal nodes, lung, liver, and bone**.

VIII. **Staging.** The International Federation of Gynecology and Obstetrics (FIGO) as well as the American Joint Committee on Cancer and the Union Internationale Contre le Cancer have staging systems. The most widely used gynecologic staging system is that of FIGO; however this closely correlates with the TNM system.

A. **TNM staging system**

  1. **Tumor stage**

    a. **TX.** Primary tumor cannot be assessed.

    b. **T0.** No evidence of primary tumor.

    c. **Tis.** Carcinoma in situ.

    d. **T1.** Tumor confined to vagina.

    e. **T2.** Tumor invades paravaginal tissues but not to pelvic wall.

    f. **T3.** Tumor extends to pelvic wall.

    g. **T4.** Tumor invades mucosa of the bladder or rectum, extends beyond the true pelvis, or both.

      Note: Mucosal invasion must be demonstrated to classify a tumor as T4; the presence of bullous edema is not sufficient.

  2. **Lymph node stage**

    a. **NX.** Regional lymph nodes cannot be assessed.

    b. **N0.** No regional lymph node metastases are present.

    c. **N1.** Pelvic lymph node metastases (upper two-thirds of vagina) or unilateral inguinal lymph node metastases (lower one-third of vagina) are present.

    d. **N2 (lower one-third of vagina).** Bilateral inguinal lymph node metastases are present.

  3. **Metastatic stage**

    a. **MX.** Presence of distant metastases cannot be assessed.

    b. **M0.** No distant metastases are present.

    c. **M1.** Distant metastases are present.

  4. **Histopathologic grade**

    a. **GX.** Grade cannot be assessed.

    b. **G1.** Well differentiated.

    c. **G2.** Moderately well differentiated.

    d. **G3.** Poorly differentiated.

  e. **G4.** Undifferentiated.
 5. **Stage groupings**
  a. **Stage 0.** Tis, N0, M0.
  b. **Stage I.** T1, N0, M0.
  c. **Stage II.** T2, N0, M0.
  d. **Stage III.** T3, N0, M0; T1–3, N1, M0.
  e. **Stage IVA.** T1–3, N1, M0; T4, any N, M0.
  f. **Stage IVB.** Any T, any N, M1.
 B. **FIGO staging system.** This staging system is **clinical** and incorporates findings from the physical examination, endoscopy, and imaging studies.
  1. **Stage 0.** Carcinoma in situ, intraepithelial carcinoma (Tis, N0, M0; TNM Stage 0).
  2. **Stage I** (25.6%). Tumor is limited to the vaginal epithelium (T1, N0, M0; TNM Stage I).
  3. **Stage II** (32.5%). Tumor involves the paravaginal tissue but has not extended onto the pelvic wall (T2, N0, M0; TNM Stage II).
  4. **Stage III** (26.1%). Tumor extends to the pelvic wall. (T1–3, N1, M0; T3, N0, M0; TNM Stage III).
  5. **Stage IV** (15.8%). Tumor extends beyond the true pelvis or involves the mucosa of the bladder or rectum.
   a. **Stage IVA.** Tumor invades adjacent organs (T1–3, N2, M0; T4, any N, M0; TNM Stage IVA).
   b. **Stage IVB.** Tumor has spread to distant organs (any T, any N, M1; TNM stage IVB).
IX. Treatment. Careful consideration should be given to the location and size of the lesion and the stage of disease when planning therapy.
 A. **Surgery**
  1. **Primary vaginal carcinoma**
   a. **Indications.** Because of the effectiveness of radiation therapy, initial surgical resection of primary vaginal cancer is indicated only in selected patients with **Stage I disease involving the upper vagina,** patients with **Stage IVA disease and vesico- or rectovaginal fistulae,** and patients with **prior pelvic irradiation.**
   b. **Approaches.** Most surgical procedures are approached through a **lower midline abdominal incision.**
   c. **Procedures**
    (1) **Radical hysterectomy, vaginectomy, and lymphadenectomy. Stage I squamous cell carcinoma of the upper vagina as well as Stage I clear cell carcinoma** can be treated adequately with radical vaginectomy, hysterectomy (if not previously performed), and bilateral pelvic lymphadenectomy.
    (2) **Pelvic exenteration.** Patients with **middle and lower vaginal squamous cell lesions** who are not candidates for radiation therapy (patients with Stage IV disease with vesico- or rectovaginal fistulae and those with prior pelvic irradiation) can be alternately treated with anterior (resection of bladder, urethra, uterus, and vagina), **posterior** (resection of rectum, uterus, and vagina), or **total** (bladder, urethra, uterus, vagina, and rectum) **pelvic exenteration.**
   d. **Reconstruction.** Vaginal reconstruction, usually with **split-thickness skin grafts or myocutaneous grafts,** using the rectus or gracilis muscles, can be performed simultaneously in patients who are sexually active.
  2. **Locally advanced and metastatic vaginal cancer.** Patients with locally advanced tumors (Stage IVA) that are associated with vesico- or rectovaginal fistulae and patients with **central tumor recurrence** following previous surgery or radiation therapy, may be candidates for surgical resection (frequently, **pelvic exenteration**).
  3. **Mortality and morbidity.** The risk of surgery depends on the magnitude of the operation and may include a **10–23% mortality** in radical procedures such as total pelvic exenteration. Common problems include the following: **Wound infection, separation, or both; Hemorrhage; Pelvic cellulitis; Urinary tract infection or fistulae; Thrombophlebitis; Genital tract fistulae; Prolonged ileus; Lymphocele formation; Intestinal fistulae; Perineal hernia; and fecal incontinence.**
 B. **Radiation therapy**

1. **Primary vaginal carcinoma.** Except for **verrucous carcinoma** (which can be transformed by radiotherapy into a more malignant neoplasm) and **melanoma** (which optimally is treated by surgery), most vaginal malignancies are treated best with a **combination of teletherapy and brachytherapy.** External-beam portals include the **entire vagina** to the introitus, the **paravaginal and parametrial tissue, and bilateral pelvic lymph nodes** up to and including the common iliac chains. If the lower third of the vagina is involved, **bilateral inguinal lymph node groups** are included. After 5000–6000 cGy **delivered by external-beam radiotherapy,** intracavitary therapy with **vaginal cylinders** of varying diameter (eg, Bloedorn, Burnett, Delclos) boosts the dose to the **vaginal mucosa to a total of 9000–10,000 cGy.**

2. **Adjuvant radiation therapy**
   a. **Preoperative radiotherapy.** Preoperative radiation therapy followed by radical surgical resection may improve the current **survival and tumor control rates of 25–30%** in selected patients with advanced vaginal cancer **(Stages III and IV).**
   b. **Postoperative radiotherapy.** Patients found to have lymph node metastases at surgery should receive postoperative external-beam irradiation to improve local control.

3. **Mortality and morbidity.** Because of the close proximity of the rectum, bladder, and urethra to the vagina, treatment is difficult and the following complications are possible: **radiation cystitis or proctitis; recto-, entero-, and vesicovaginal fistulae; rectal strictures or ulceration; vaginal necrosis,** with subsequent fibrosis and stenosis; and **vulvar desquamation.**

C. **Chemotherapy**

1. **Primary vaginal carcinoma.** Chemotherapy is not indicated in the initial treatment of vaginal malignancies.

2. **Ajuvant chemotherapy.** No clear role has been demonstrated for chemotherapy in the adjuvant treatment of vaginal cancer.

3. **Locally advanced and metastatic vaginal cancer**
   a. **Single-agent therapy.** Cisplatin (50–100 mg/m^2 every 3 weeks) remains the single most active agent, producing **20–40% overall and 9–13% complete response rates.** The duration of responses, however, is short (4 months). Other agents with some activity include fluorouracil (20%), dibromoducitol (27%), dianhydrogalacticol (17%), ifosfamide (30%), and carboplatin (28%).
   b. **Combination chemotherapy.** Although **CBV** (cisplatin, bleomycin, and vinblastine), **CBOM** (cisplatin, bleomycin, vincristine, and methotrexate), and **MA** (methotrexate and doxorubicin) have achieved **66% overall and 18–22% complete response rates,** combination chemotherapeutic regimens to date have not improved survival over that obtained with single agent (cisplatin) therapy.
   c. **Intra-arterial chemotherapy.** Response rates documented with selective intra-arterial infusion of chemotherapeutic agents such as bleomycin, mitomycin-C, and vincristine have been disappointingly low (8–15%). Therefore, this approach cannot be recommended.

D. **Immunotherapy.** With the possible exception of melanoma (see p 128, **IX.E**), no data currently exist to support the use of immunomodulatory agents in the treatment of vaginal malignancies.

E. **Combined modality therapy**

1. **Combined chemoradiotherapy.** In 2 independent studies, the combination of **hydroxyurea and radiotherapy increased the 2-year survival** from 43.5% and 33% to 74% and 52%, respectively, in patients with Stage IIB or IIIB cervical carcinoma. The beneficial effect of combined chemoradiotherapy also may apply to patients with squamous cell carcinoma of the vagina, although this remains unproved.

2. **Surgery, chemotherapy, and radiation. Survival rates of 46–63%** have been reported for combined treatment of **embryonal rhabdomyosarcoma** with surgery, radiotherapy, and chemotherapy (actinomycin-D, cyclophosphamide, and vincristine). More data is needed, however, before this approach can be recommended.

X. **Prognosis**

A. **Risk of recurrence.** The majority of patients fail locally within 2 years.

B. **Five-year survival.** Survival depends on the extent of disease (stage) at presentation, with **overall 5-year survival reported to be 42%.** The survival by FIGO/TNM stage is summarized below: **Stage I,** 68%; **Stage II,** 47%; **Stage III,** 30%; and **Stage IV,** 17%.

   C. Adverse prognostic factors. The following factors have been variably associated with poor prognosis:

     1. Tumor larger than 2 cm.

     2. High tumor grade (Poorly differentiated tumors).

XI. Patient follow-up

   A. General guidelines. Patients should be evaluated every 3 months for 2 years, every 6 months for an additional 3 years, and then annually for evidence of recurrent disease. Specific guidelines for patients with vaginal cancer are outlined below.

   B. Routine evaluation. Each clinic visit should include the following tests and procedures:

     1. Medical history and physical examination. An interval medical history and a thorough physical examination must be completed during each office visit, paying particular attention to the areas summarized on p 378, **VI.A.**

     2. Blood tests (see p 1, **IV.A**).

       a. Complete blood count.

       b. Hepatic transaminases.

       c. Alkaline phosphatase.

       d. BUN and creatinine.

     3. Urinalysis (see p 3, **IV.B**)

     4. Chest x-ray (see p 3, **IV.C.1**)

     5. Pap smear (see p 379, **VI.B.4.a**) with colposcopy as indicated

   C. Computed tomography (CT). CT scan of the abdomen and pelvis should be obtained **every 6–12 months for 3–5 years** to exclude occult local and distant recurrence.

   D. Optional evaluation. The following tests and procedures may be indicated by previous diagnostic findings or clinical suspicion.

     1. Blood tests

       a. Nucleotidase (see p 2, **IV.A.4**).

       b. GGTP. (see p 2, **IV.A.5**).

       c. CA-125 (see p 379, **VI.C.A.1.c**).

       d. Carcinoembryonic antigen (CEA) (see p 379, **VI.C.1.d**).

     2. Imaging studies

       a. Magnetic resonance imaging (MRI) (see p 3, **IV.C.2**).

       b. Ultrasound (see p 3, **IV.C.3**).

       c. Technetium-99m bone scan (see p 3, **IV.C.4**).

       d. Lymphangiography (see p 79, **VI.C.2.b**).

     3. Biopsy. Because most tumors recur locally, any abnormality of the vagina or vaginal cuff must be biopsied by fine needle aspiration or punch biopsy. Masses detected on clinical or radiographic examination also should be assessed.

REFERENCES

Ball, HG, and Berman, ML. Management of primary vaginal carcinoma. Gynecol Oncol 14:154–163, 1982.

Berek, JS, Hacker, NF, and Lagasse, LD. Vaginal reconstruction performed simultaneously with pelvic exenteration. Obstet Gynecol 63:318–323, 1984.

Dancuart, F, Delclos, L, and Wharton, JT. Primary squamous carcinoma of the vagina treated by radiotherapy: A failures analysis—The M.D. Anderson Hospital Experience 1955–1982. Radiat Oncol Biol Phys 14:745–749, 1983.

Gallup DG, Talledo, OE, and Shah, KJ. Invasive squamous cell carcinoma of the vagina: A 14-year study. Obstet Gynecol 69(5):782–785, 1987.

Hacker, NF. Vaginal cancer. In Practical Gynecologic Oncology. Berek, JS and Hacker, NF. editors. Williams and Wilkins, Baltimore: pp. 425–440, 1989.

Kucera, H, Langer, M, Smekal, G, et al. Radiotherapy of primary carcinoma of the vagina: management and results of different therapy schemes. Gynecol Oncol 21:87–93, 1985.

Manetta, A, Pinto, JL, and Larson, JE. Primary invasive carcinoma of the vagina. Obstet Gynecol 72:77–81, 1988.

Morrow, CP, Townsend, DE, editors. Synopsis of Gynecologic Oncology. Churchill Livingston, New York, 3rd ed., pp. 91–102, 1987.

Perez, CA, Arneson, AN, Dehner, LP, et al. Radiation therapy in carcinoma of the vagina. Obstet Gynecol 44:862–868, 1974.

Pride, GL, Buchler, DA. Carcinoma of vagina 10 or more years following pelvic irradiation therapy. Am J Obstet Gynecol 127:513–519, 1977.

Rutledge, F. Cancer of the vagina. Am J Obstet Gynecol 97:635–636, 1967.

Sulak, P, Barnhill, D, and Heller P. Nonsquamous cancer of the vagina. Gynecologic Oncology 29:309–320, 1988.

Woodruff, JD, Parmley, TH, and Julian, CG. Topical 5-fluorouracil in the treatment of vaginal carcinoma in situ. Gynecol Oncol 3:124–132, 1975.

50 Malignancies of the Vulva

James Heaps, MD

I. **Epidemiology.** Vulvar carcinoma accounts for **3–4% of gynecologic and 1% of all cancers** in females.

II. **Risk factors**
   A. **Age.** The incidence of vulvar carcinoma increases from less than 1.0 per 100,000 before age 45 to **19.1 per 100,000 by age 85.** The mean age of females with **carcinoma in situ, microinvasive, and frankly invasive carcinoma** is 44, 58, and 65 years, respectively.
   B. **Race.** Before age 70, no racial predilection exists; however, **white females older than 80 years** are at **0.25–4.0 times** greater risk than are black females of the same age. In addition, a reduced risk has been documented in **Jewish** females.
   C. **Genetic factors.** No familial predisposition for vulvar malignancies has been identified.
   D. **Previous genital pathology**
      1. **Inflammation.** Although nonspecific and common, **chronic pruritus,** regardless of the underlying pathology, increases the risk of vulvar cancer.
      2. **Infection.** Sexual promiscuity and certain associated **sexually transmitted diseases** increase the risk of vulvar malignancies.
         a. **Viral agents.** Although controversial, both **herpes simplex Type II and human papilloma virus** infection (condyloma acuminata) have been implicated in the pathogenesis of vulvar neoplasia.
         b. **Other agents.** Nearly **5%** of patients have a history or serologic evidence of **syphilis.** Granulomatous venereal diseases (lymphogranuloma venereum and granuloma inguinale) are present in **66% of Jamaican females with vulvar carcinoma** and predispose patients to vulvar cancer, particularly at an early age.
      3. **Premalignant lesions**
         a. **Vulvar intraepithelial neoplasia (VIN).** In 1975, the International Society for the Study of Vulvar Disease classified VIN into 2 types: carcinoma in situ and Paget's disease.
            (1) **Carcinoma in situ (CIS).** Previously termed **Bowen's disease, carcinoma simplex, and erythroplasia of Queyrat,** this entity represents a variety of gross and microscopic appearances. Originally postulated to be a precursor to invasive squamous cell carcinoma of the vulva, CIS now is thought to have a **low (4%) malignant potential.** Most cases occur in females with intense pruritus, immunosuppression, or extreme old age. The **perianal skin,** in particular, is at high risk.
            (2) **Paget's disease.** This **eczematoid** lesion is characterized by large pale epidermal Paget's cells that are associated with a synchronous or metachronous underlying **adenocarcinoma of the adnexal structures,** breast, or Bartholin's glands or squamous cell carcinoma of the cervix in **20–33% of cases.**
         b. **Vulvar dystrophy. Hypertrophic dystrophy with atypia** may predispose to vulvar carcinoma, and **chronic vulvar dermatitis** occurs in more than **50%** of patients with vulvar cancer.
      4. **Other gynecologic malignancies.** As many as **22%** of patients with vulvar cancer harbor a **secondary squamous cell malignancy of the lower genital tract** (primarily the cervix and vagina).
   E. **Medical illnesses.** Although vulvar cancer often occurs in patients with pre-existing **hypertension and diabetes mellitus (18%–25%),** the exact nature of this relationship is unclear.
   F. **Urbanization.** For unknown reasons, females from lower socioeconomic groups often found in urban areas exhibit a higher incidence of vulvar carcinoma.

III. **Presentation**
   A. **Signs and symptoms**
      1. **Local manifestations.** The most common complaint is that of a **palpable vulvar abnormality** (mass or ulceration) often accompanied by **pruritus.** Generally, lesions are raised, red or white, and may weep. Bleeding, pain, and dysuria also are often present, whereas symptomatic inguinal lymphadenopathy develops only occasionally. Although both patient- and physician-related diagnostic delays are common because of the sensitive nature of the involved area, nearly **20% of vulvar cancers are asymptomatic** and are identified on routine pelvic examination.
      2. **Systemic manifestations.** Advanced disease can produce systemic complaints, which include weight loss, anorexia, jaundice (liver metastases), chest pain or dyspnea (lung metastases), renal insufficiency (hydronephrosis from retroperitoneal lymph node metastases), and supraclavicular lymphadenopathy.
   B. **Paraneoplastic syndromes.** Like squamous cell carcinoma at other sites, advanced carcinoma is associated with the following paraneoplastic syndromes:
      1. **Hypercalcemia** (see p 87, **I**).
      2. **Inappropriate ACTH** (see p 90, **V**).
      3. **Inappropriate gonadotropins** (see p 117).

IV. **Differential diagnosis.** Benign and malignant vulvar lesions may present with a **palpable abnormality and pruritus.** It is important to maintain a high index of suspicion and a liberal biopsy policy to avoid unnecessary diagnostic delays. Common benign diseases that can be confused with invasive cancer include **primary gynecologic diseases** such as sexually transmitted diseases (herpes simplex Type II, syphilis, condyloma acuminata, granuloma inguinale, lymphogranuloma venereum, and molluscum contagiosum), other infections (candidiasis, tenia cruris, folliculitis, Crohn's disease, pemphigus, hidradenitis, and tuberculosis), vulvar dystrophies (leukoplakia, lichen sclerosis, sclerotic dermatosis, hyperplastic vulvitis, and kraurosis vulvae), trauma (hematomas, abrasions, and ulcerations), vulvar intraepithelial neoplasia (formerly carcinoma simplex, Bowen's disease, and erythroplasia of Queyrat), Paget's disease (associated with an underlying adenocarcinoma of the cervix, bladder, colon, rectum, and breast in **20–33%** of cases), benign neoplasms (seborrheic keratoses, acanthosis nigricans, syringomas, hidradenomas, epidermal cysts in Fox-Fordyce disease, fibromas, lipomas, neuromas, leiomyomas, neurofibromas, angiomas, freckle-like lesions, lentigo, nevi, inflammatory hyperpigmentation, Bartholin and pilonidal cysts, endometriosis, and canal of Nuck cysts), and other malignancies (urethra, bladder, vagina, and cervix). **Nongynecologic diseases** that can be confused with invasive cancer include inflammatory lesions (Behçet's disease, psoriasis, and eczema) and metastatic neoplasms (breast, colon, cervix, uterus, ovary, and gestational trophoblastic neoplasms).

V. **Screening programs.** No routine screening tests exist for vulvar carcinoma beyond direct visualization and palpation (routine gynecologic examination). **Colposcopy,** although useful to determine the extent of disease once it is diagnosed, is **too time-consuming** for routine screening. Staining of the vulva with toluidine blue to identify suspicious areas is associated with a **20% false-positive rate,** and vulvar Papanicolaou (Pap) smears are not reliable.

VI. **Diagnostic workup**
   A. **Medical history and physical examination.** In addition to a thorough medical history, a complete physical examination directed at the following sites of tumor spread must be documented:
      1. **General appearance.** An evaluation of the patient's nutritional and general functional status should be included (see, also, p 1, **III**).
      2. **Skin.** Signs of systemic infections or diseases that may manifest with vulvar findings should be noted.
      3. **Lymph nodes.** Thorough examination of the inguinal, supraclavicular, axillary, and cervical lymph nodes is required.
      4. **Chest.** Pulmonary examination should detect the presence of pleural effusions and consolidation (eg, diminished breath sounds, dullness to percussion, egophony).
      5. **Breasts.** The presence of a primary breast lesion must be excluded.
      6. **Abdomen.** Evidence of ascites, hepatosplenomegaly, and suspicious masses, suggesting intraperitoneal spread should be noted.
      7. **Genitalia**
         a. **External genitalia.** Using a bright light with the patient in the lithotomy position, the urethra, vaginal introitus, perineum, labia majora and minora, cli-

toris and hood, labial crural folds, and anus are palpated and visually inspected for evidence of primary or metastatic disease. **Acetic acid (5%)** applied to the vulva may help identify existing abnormalities.

b. **Vagina.** Complete visualization and palpation of the vaginal walls, fornices, and ectocervix is mandatory to exclude primary or metastatic lesions.

c. **Cervix.** A Pap smear should be obtained from the cervix (or the vaginal cuff if the cervix is absent). Visual and bimanual examination also is necessary, noting the size, position, symmetry, and mobility of the cervix.

d. **Uterus and adnexa.** The size, position, symmetry, and mobility of the uterus and adnexa must be assessed. The remainder of the pelvis should be evaluated for involvement of the bladder, rectum, or both.

8. **Rectum.** Primary rectal carcinoma must be excluded, and stool should be tested for occult blood.

9. **Extremities.** Evidence of lymphedema (caused by obstructed lymphatics) and thrombophlebitis are important physical findings.

B. **Primary test and procedures.** All patients with suspected vulvar carcinoma should have the following diagnostic tests and procedures:

1. **Blood tests** (see p 1, **IV.A**).
   a. **Complete blood count.**
   b. **Hepatic transaminases.**
   c. **Alkaline phosphatase.**
   d. **BUN and creatinine.**
   e. **Albumin.**

2. **Urine tests**
   a. **Urinalysis. Hematuria** may signify urinary tract involvement, particularly the urethra and bladder.
   b. **Beta-human chorionic gonadotropin (beta-hCG). Pregnancy** must be excluded in all females of reproductive age.

3. **Imaging studies** (see p 2, **IV.C**).
   a. **Chest x-ray.**
   b. **Computed tomography (CT).** CT scan of the pelvis and abdomen provides information about the primary tumor, liver, retroperitoneal nodes, and genitourinary tract and eliminates the need for intravenous pyelography (IVP).

4. **Invasive procedures**
   a. **Colposcopy.** Direct visualization of the vulva with the aid of 5% acetic acid and a colposcope is valuable in the diagnosis of **early** vulvar neoplasms.
   b. **Biopsy.** A biopsy of any suspicious lesion is mandatory and can be obtained **with a Keye's dermal punch** and local anesthesia. An excisional biopsy can be used for lesions smaller than 1 cm. Several sites should be biopsied when multifocal disease is suspected. A handheld magnifying glass or **colposcope with 5% acetic acid staining** may be necessary to guide the biopsy if changes are subtle, such as with vulvar intraepithelial neoplasia. **Stroma** should be obtained to help in determining the **depth of invasion and the type of tumor border** (pushing vs infiltrative).

C. **Optional tests and procedures.** The following tests and procedures may be indicated by previous diagnostic findings or clinical suspicion.

1. **Blood tests**
   a. **Nucleotidase** (see p 2, **IV.A.4**).
   b. **GGTP.** (see p 2, **IV.A.5**).
   c. **VDRL.** If syphilis is suspected, serologies and dark field examination should be performed.
   d. **Herpes titers.** If primary herpes is suspected, serum antibody titers should be measured.
   e. **Genital cultures.** Depending on nature of the lesion, cultures for *Chlamydia, Candida,* and tuberculosis may be indicated. If a primary infectious process is strongly suspected, **empiric therapy can be instituted for a brief period** of time after obtaining cultures and prior to biopsy. **Close follow-up is mandatory,** however, since a delay in the diagnosis of cancer must be avoided.

2. **Imaging studies**
   a. **Magnetic resonance imaging (MRI)** (see p 3, **IV.C.2**).
   b. **Lymphangiography.** Bipedal lymphangiography, in rare circumstances, can be helpful in evaluating pelvic lymph nodes for the presence of metastatic disease.

c. **Technetium-99m bone scan** (see p 3, **IV.C.4**).
d. **Venography.** Venography may be needed to exclude deep vein thrombosis in patients with edematous lower extremities. Noninvasive techniques, however, can be substituted.

3. **Invasive procedures**

a. **Cystourethroscopy.** If involvement of the lower urinary tract is suspected, endoscopic examination of the urethra and bladder must be performed to guide staging and treatment.

b. **Proctosigmoidoscopy.** Suspicion of rectal involvement requires direct visual inspection of the rectosigmoid colon and anus.

c. **Fine needle aspiration (FNA).** Suspicious inguinal, supraclavicular, pelvic, and para-aortic lymph nodes as well as hepatic and pulmonary nodules can be evaluated for metastatic disease by FNA.

VII. Pathology

A. **Location.** Lesions can arise anywhere on the vulva, including the clitoris, urethra, perineum, and anal areas. The **labia majora and minora** are the site of origin in **52% and 18%,** respectively. The **clitoral region** is involved **10–15%** of the time, and the **Bartholin gland area** is involved **in 1–3%.** The remaining tumors are multifocal or too large to determine the exact site of origin.

B. **Multiplicity.** Multifocal disease is identified in **5%** of patients, whereas as many as **22%** are found to have a **second concurrent malignancy** such as cervical, vaginal or anal carcinoma.

C. **Histology.** Because carcinoma may originate within areas of vulvar intraepithelial neoplasia and vulvar dystrophy and may masquerade as condylomas, biopsy of any vulvar lesions is mandatory.

1. **Squamous cell carcinoma.** More than **90%** of vulvar cancers are squamous cell carcinomas and grossly may appear **exophytic, ulcerative, or infiltrative. Verrucous carcinoma** resembling a **giant condyloma of Buschke-Loewenstein** is a locally destructive variant of squamous cell carcinoma that rarely metastasizes.

2. **Melanoma.** Melanoma is the second most common vulvar cancer: it accounts for **5–6%** of cases. Typically, these lesions arise on the labia minora of caucasian women and consist of the **superficial spreading, lentigo maligna, and nodular** types. Staging is identical to melanomas arising on other areas of the body (see p 122, **VIII**).

3. **Adenocarcinoma.** Adenocarcinoma arising in **Bartholin glands** represents **3–5%** of vulvar malignancies. In addition, Bartholin glands also can give rise to **transitional cell, adenoidcystic, adenosquamous, and squamous cell carcinomas.**

4. **Sarcoma.** Sarcomas with a variety of histologies arise in the vulvar area and account for **1–2%** of all vulvar cancers.

5. **Basal cell carcinoma.** Nearly **2%** of vulvar cancers consist of basal cell carcinomas resembling typical lesions that arise on other areas of the body (see Chapter 21).

6. **Paget's disease.** Invasive Paget's disease accounts for less than **1%** of the vulvar malignancies.

D. **Metastatic spread**

1. **Modes of spread.** Vulvar cancer spreads primarily by 3 mechanisms:

a. **Direct extension.** Vulvar carcinoma may enlarge to involve adjacent structures such as the **clitoris, urethra, bladder, vagina, perineum, anus, and rectum.** Invasion deep to the **bony pelvis** and the **ischiorectal fossa** also occurs.

b. **Lymphatic metastasis.** Embolic spread through lymphatic channels initially involves **inguinal lymph nodes and, subsequently, the external and common iliac, obturator, and para-aortic nodes.** Lymphatic spread also may be responsible for vaginal spread, but intervening skin lymphatics are rarely involved unless large fixed inguinal nodes are present. Overall, the **incidence of pelvic node metastases is 5–11%,** most of which occur in the presence of more than 3 involved inguinal nodes. The incidence of inguinal node metastases varies with tumor stage and depth of invasion, as outlined below:

(1) **Tumor stage.** The **overall incidence of inguinal lymph node metastases is 30–40%.** The incidence by tumor stage is as follows: **Stage I,** 10%; **Stage II,** 25%; **Stage III,** 66%; and **Stage IV,** 88%.

(2) **Depth of invasion.** The frequency of inguinal lymph node metastases

varies with the depth of invasion of the primary tumor: less than 1 mm, 0%; **1.1–3.0 mm,** 5–10%; **3.1–5.0 mm,** 20–25%; more than **5.0 mm,** over 35%.

c. **Hematogenous metastasis.** Spread through vascular channels to distant organs occurs as a late phenomenon and is characterized by infiltrative, deeply invasive, large, and advanced local tumors.

2. **Sites of metastatic spread.** Distant metastatic spread most frequently involves the following organs and tissues: **lung,** most common site of distant metastasis; **liver,** <3%; **bone,** <3%; **distant lymph nodes,** para-aortic, mediastinal, and supraclavicular lymph nodes; **central nervous system,** rare.

VIII. **Staging.** The American Joint Committee on Cancer and the Union Internationale Contre le Cancer adopted a uniform TNM **surgical** staging system in 1987. This surgical staging system has been more widely used than the International Federation of Gynecology and Obstetrics (FIGO) **clinical** staging system; however, the FIGO system recently has been revised to a surgical staging system that corresponds to the TNM system.

A. **TNM staging system**
   1. **Tumor stage**
      a. **TX.** Primary tumor cannot be assessed.
      b. **T0.** No evidence of primary tumor exists.
      c. **Tis.** Preinvasive carcinoma (carcinoma in situ).
      d. **T1.** Tumor is confined to the vulva is no larger than 2 cm in its greatest dimension.
      e. **T2.** Tumor is confined to the vulva, and is larger than 2 cm in its greatest dimension.
      f. **T3.** Tumor invades the urethra, vagina, perineum, or anus.
      g. **T4.** Tumor invades the bladder, the rectal mucosa, or the upper part of the urethral mucosa or is fixed to bone.
   2. **Lymph node stage**
      a. **NX.** Regional lymph nodes cannot be assessed.
      b. **N0.** No nodes are palpable.
      c. **N1.** Nodes are palpable in either groin, not enlarged, and mobile (not clinically suspicious for neoplasm).
      d. **N2.** Nodes are palpable in either groin, enlarged, firm, and mobile (clinically suspicious for neoplasm).
      e. **N3.** Fixed or ulcerated nodes are present.
         Note: Regional lymph nodes include the femoral, inguinal, internal and external iliac, and hypogastric nodes.
   3. **Metastatic stage**
      a. **MX.** The presence of distant metastases cannot be assessed.
      b. **M0.** No clinical metastases are present.
      c. **M1a.** Palpable deep pelvic lymph nodes are present.
      d. **M1b.** Other distant metastases are present.
   4. **Histopathologic grade**
      a. **GX.** Grade cannot be assessed.
      b. **G1.** Well differentiated.
      c. **G2.** Moderately well differentiated.
      d. **G3.** Poorly differentiated.
      e. **G4.** Undifferentiated.
   5. **Stage groupings**
      a. **Stage 0.** Tis, N0, M0.
      b. **Stage I.** T1, N0–1, M0.
      c. **Stage II.** T2, N0–1, M0.
      d. **Stage III.** T1–2, N2, M0; T3, N0–2, M0.
      e. **Stage IV.** T4, N0–2, M0; any T, N3, M0; any T, any N, M1a–1b.

B. **Clinical FIGO staging system**
   1. **Stage I.** Tumor is confined to the vulva, it is no larger than 2 cm in its greatest dimension, and no lymph nodes are palpable, or they are palpable in either groin but are not enlarged and mobile (not clinically suspicious of neoplasm) (T1, N0–1, M0).
   2. **Stage II.** Tumor is confined to the vulva, it is larger than 2 cm in its greatest dimension, and no lymph nodes are palpable, or they are palpable in either groin but are not enlarged and mobile (not clinically suspicious of neoplasm) (T2, N0–1, M0).
   3. **Stage III.** Tumor of any size with (1) adjacent spread to the urethra, the vagina,

the perineum, or the anus, (2) palpable lymph nodes in one or both groins that are enlarged, firm, and mobile but not fixed (clinically suspicious of neoplasm) or (3) all these characteristics (T1–2, N2, M0 or T3, N0–2, M0).

4. **Stage IV.** Tumor of any size that (1) infiltrates the bladder mucosa, the rectal mucosa, or the upper part of the urethral mucosa, (2) is fixed to bone or other distant metastases, (3) has fixed or ulcerated nodes in either one or both groins, or (4) has all of these characteristics (T4, N0–2, M0; any T, N3, M0; or any T, any N, M1a–1b).

C. **Surgical FIGO staging system**

1. **Stage I.** Tumor is confined to the vulva or perineum and is no larger than 2 cm in its greatest dimension.

2. **Stage II.** Tumor is confined to vulva or perineum and is larger than 2 cm in its greatest dimension.

3. **Stage III.** Tumor of any size that invades the vagina, rectum, or lower urethra; unilateral regional lymph node metastases are present; or both.

4. **Stage IVa.** Tumor invades the bladder or rectal mucosa, upper urethra, or pelvic bone; bilateral regional lymph node metastases are present; or both.

5. **Stage IVb.** Distant metastases are present.

IX. **Treatment**

A. **Surgery**

1. **Primary vulvar carcinoma**

a. **Indications.** Surgery is the **mainstay of therapy** for vulvar carcinoma. The magnitude of the procedure depends on the stage of the tumor and varies from simple wide local excision to radical vulvectomy, bilateral inguinal-femoral lymphadenectomy, and pelvic exenteration.

b. **Approach.** The **low lithotomy position** is used to prevent excess tension on the vulvar skin and to provide access to the thighs and buttocks for possible skin grafts and flaps. Inguinal-femoral lymphadenectomy and pelvic exenteration for advanced lesions also can be performed using this position. Since its introduction in 1912 by Basset and its promotion by Taussig and Way, en bloc radical vulvectomy with bilateral inguinal-femoral lymphadenectomy has been performed through a **single "butterfly" incision.** Recently, however, a **3-incision approach** (vulvectomy and bilateral groin incisions) in patients without clinically suspicious (N2) lymph nodes has been shown to **decrease wound complication rates** (see p 391, **IX.A.3**) without increasing the risk of local recurrence in the remaining **skin bridges.**

c. **Procedures.** Although extended radical procedures (pelvic exenteration) have been used for advanced lesions and although conservative procedures (hemivulvectomy and ipsilateral inguinal-femoral lymphadenectomy) have been proposed for **superficially invasive vulvar cancer (tumor smaller than 2 cm in diameter with less than 5 mm of stromal invasion),** standard therapy includes **radical vulvectomy and bilateral inguinal-femoral lymphadenectomy with or without pelvic lymphadenectomy.**

(1) **Radical vulvectomy.** En bloc radical vulvectomy removes the entire vulva from the **mons pubis, laterally to the labial crural folds, medially to the vaginal introitus, and posteriorly to include the perineum and perianal skin.** The dissection extends to the deep vulvar fascia. Often, margins encroach on the clitoris, anus, vagina, and urethra, necessitating occasional removal of these structures. The primary tumor should be excised with **2–3 cm margins** in all directions. In rare circumstances, smaller margins are acceptable, but this is controversial. The wound is closed in layers without tension using **rhomboid, tensor fascia lata, and rectus abdominus flaps; Z-plasty incisions; and gracilis myocutaneous grafts** as necessary.

(2) **Inguinal-femoral lymphadenectomy.** Bilateral inguinal and femoral lymph node groups can be removed en bloc with or separately from the vulvectomy specimen. With the 3-incision technique, bilateral incisions are made **1 cm below and parallel to the inguinal ligament.** Skin flaps are raised, and the **superficial inguinal lymph nodes** are removed along with the saphenous vein. The femoral fascia is opened over the cribriform plate, and the **deep femoral lymph nodes** are excised, including the highest femoral node—**Cloquet's node (Jackson's node is the first deep pelvic node located along the external iliac artery).** The origin of the **sartorius muscle** is often

transposed from the anterior superior iliac spine to the pubic tubercle to protect the femoral vessels from exposure in the event of wound breakdown. Femoral nerve injury can be avoided by vertically incising, but not resecting, the cribriform fascia.

   (3) **Pelvic lymphadenectomy.** Previously, the **incidence of pelvic lymph node involvement (2–12% overall)**—particularly in the presence of enlarged, fixed inguinal-femoral lymph nodes—mandated pelvic lymphadenectomy. However, new radiotherapy techniques produce superior results and have reduced the need for this procedure.

2. **Locally advanced and metastatic vulvar cancer.** Local tumor extension may involve the **bladder, vagina, and rectum.** Although distal urethrectomy and partial rectal resection may preserve urinary and fecal continence, these findings usually necessitate a **combined abdominal and perineal approach** with resection of the vagina and bladder **(anterior exenteration)** or vagina and rectum **(posterior exenteration)** in addition to radical vulvectomy and bilateral inguinal-femoral lymphadenectomy. Urinary diversion, vaginal reconstruction (with split-thickness skin graft, omentum, and myocutaneous flap), and permanent colostomy may be required. Following primary therapy, recurrent vulvar disease may be treated successfully with further surgery (although complex plastic surgery may be required. For recurrent nodal and distant metastatic disease, however, surgical therapy has not proved to be beneficial.

3. **Morbidity and mortality.** The frequency and severity of complications is determined by the surgeon's skill, the extent of the resection, and the patient's overall condition. Common postoperative problems include the following:
   a. **Wound breakdown, 80–90%** with single "butterfly" incision; less than **50%** using separate vulvectomy and inguinal incisions (3-incision technique).
   b. **Hemorrhage,** from femoral and vulvar pudendal arteries.
   c. **Lymphedema, lymphangitis, and lymphocele, 10%;** more than 10% if radiation therapy is administered.
   d. **Deep venous thrombosis.** Risk is high because of the patients' advanced age and the presence of postoperative lymphedema.
   e. **Sexual dysfunction.** Alterations in body image and sexual function often lead to clinical depression.
   f. **Urinary or fecal incontinence.**
   g. **Femoral nerve paresthesias or palsy.**
   h. **Femoral and perineal hernia.**
   i. **Osteomyelitis.**

B. **Radiation therapy**
   1. **Primary vulvar carcinoma**
      a. **Indications.** Because of significant associated morbidity, radiation therapy generally plays a limited role in the treatment of primary vulvar cancer and is reserved only for patients who are **not candidates for initial surgical resection.**
      b. **Techniques.** Pelvic radiation portals extend from the **bifurcation of the common iliac arteries (L5–S1),** laterally to encompass the **pelvic and inguinal nodes,** and inferiorly to include the **vulva.** (Anterior-posterior and posterior-anterior (AP-PA) fields are used to deliver a total **midpelvis dose of 5000 cGy and an inguinal nodal dose of 4500–5200 cGy** (the exact dose is tailored to the patient's nodal status). Alternately, the inguinal nodes can be shielded to spare the femoral heads and then boosted with electron beam to a total dose of 5000 cGy. Finally, the **vulva is boosted with an additional 2000 cGy** by either electron beam or interstitial [137]cesium.
   2. **Adjuvant radiation therapy**
      a. **Preoperative radiotherapy.** Patients with extensive disease requiring exenteration or with lesions close to vital structures such as the clitoris, urethra, and anus can be treated with **4500–5500 cGy** preoperatively in anticipation of increasing resectability and decreasing the need for more radical procedures.
      b. **Postoperative radiotherapy.** Following surgery, high-risk patients (those with **large tumors, positive surgical margins, and more than 1 lymph node metastasis)** are appropriate candidates for pelvic, inguinal, and perineal irradiation **(4500–7000 cGy in daily fractions of 175–200 cGy),** depending on the clinical situation. A combination of electrons, cobalt, and photons can be used. In a randomized clinical trial, the Gynecologic Oncology Group demonstrated **improved survival without increased morbid-**

ity with pelvic radiation compared to lymphadenectomy in patients with involved inguinal nodes. Currently, studies are ongoing to evaluate radiotherapy as a substitute for inguinal lymphadenectomy in patients with Stage N0 lymph nodes.

3. **Locally advanced and metastatic vulvar cancer.** Radiotherapy, with or without chemotherapy, can be used to palliate **symptomatic** metastases to the bones, mediastinum, para-aortic or supraclavicular nodes, and lungs.

4. **Morbidity and mortality.** Although all patients experience **vulvar moist desquamation,** which requires a **treatment break of 1 week in 50%** of patients, most ultimately finish therapy. Additional complications include the following: **myelosuppression, cystitis, proctitis, perineal pain, avascular necrosis of the femoral head, pelvic factures, and subcutaneous fibrosis.**

C. **Chemotherapy**

1. **Primary vulvar carcinoma**

a. **Topical chemotherapy.** Topical application of **fluorouracil cream** and contact sensitization induced with **dinitrochlorobenzene (DNCB)** has successfully treated vulvar **intraepithelial neoplasia** and atypical vulvar dystrophy. This approach, however, has not been applied to invasive carcinoma.

b. **Systemic chemotherapy.** Several cycles of systemic chemotherapy with **mitomycin-C (10 mg/m^2 on day 1) and fluorouracil (1000 mg/m^2 continuous infusion on days 1–3)** followed by radiotherapy (days 4–13) has been shown to mediate significant local tumor shrinkage in a small number of patients. In patients with large primary tumors who lack evidence of distant metastases, this approach may reduce primary tumor size enough to permit surgical salvage.

2. **Locally advanced and metastatic vulvar cancer.** Although active agents used in the treatment of squamous cell carcinoma at other sites are **cisplatin, fluorouracil, mitomycin-C, ifosfamide, and hydroxyurea,** little data exist on the effectiveness of these agents to induce significant responses with vulvar cancer, and the experience has been dismal overall.

D. **Hormonal therapy.** To date, no hormonal agents have been shown to be active against squamous cell carcinoma of the vulva.

E. **Immunotherapy.** Immunotherapy for squamous cell carcinoma of the vulva has not been evaluated; however, regimens currently under investigation for head and neck tumors potentially may be used to treat vulvar malignancies. Like melanomas in other locations, vulvovaginal melanomas may respond to several experimental immunomodulatory agents (see p 128, **IX.E**).

X. **Prognosis**

A. **Risk of recurrence.** The risk of local, regional, and distant tumor recurrence correlates closely with the number of involved inguinal lymph nodes. Patients with 3 or more **involved nodes** are at particularly high risk.

1. **Local vulvar recurrence.** With **tumor-free surgical margins of more than 1 cm and fewer than 3 positive inguinal lymph nodes,** the risk of local recurrence is less than 6%. Thirty-three percent to 50% of patients with **margins of less than 1 cm and 3 or more** involved inguinal nodes develop recurrent vulvar disease. Although local recurrences may occur late (commonly after 3 years), they may be amenable to surgical cure.

2. **Regional recurrence.** The risk of lymph node recurrence ranges from **less than 3%** in patients with fewer than **3 involved inguinal lymph nodes** to **33–44%** in those with **3 or more involved inguinal nodes.** Regardless of the therapy used (primarily radiation and chemotherapy), recurrent disease in inguinal and pelvic lymph node areas is difficult to manage and signifies a poor prognosis.

3. **Distant recurrences.** Distant metastases occur in less than **4%** of patients with fewer than **3 involved inguinal lymph nodes** and in more than **65%** of those with **3 or more involved inguinal nodes.** Late metastases are not uncommon.

B. **Five-year survival.** Intensified efforts at early diagnosis have improved survival rates. Currently, the **overall 5-year survival rate is 70%.** The 5-year survival by tumor stage is as follows: **Stage I,** 92%; **Stage II,** 80%; **Stage III,** 54%; and **Stage IV,** 15%.

C. **Adverse prognostic factors.** Several histopathologic findings predict a worse disease course than would be anticipated by the disease stage, and these include the following parameters:

1. **Lymph node status.** This is the most important factor; **overall survival de-**

creases from **92–100% to 46–68%** if involved lymph nodes are present. Less than **20%** of patients with more than **3 involved inguinal lymph nodes** survive more than **2 years.**
  2. **Large primary tumor size.**
  3. **Lymphatic and vascular space invasion.**
  4. **Depth of invasion more than 3 mm.**
  5. **High tumor grade.**
  6. **"Infiltrating" pattern of invasion,** rather than "pushing."
  7. **High mitotic activity.**
  8. **Close or positive surgical margins.**

XI. **Patient follow-up**
  A. **General guidelines.** Patients should be monitored closely every 3 months for the first year and every 6 months thereafter because metachronous primary and recurrent vulvar lesions may arise. Specific guidelines for patients with vulvar cancer are outlined below.
  B. **Routine evaluation.** Each clinic visit should include the following tests and procedures:
    1. **Medical history and physical examination.** An interval medical history and a thorough physical examination must be completed during each office visit, paying particular attention to the areas summarized above (see p 386, **VI.A**).
    2. **Blood tests** (see p 1, **IV.A**).
      a. **Complete blood count.**
      b. **Hepatic transaminases.**
      c. **Alkaline phosphatase.**
      d. **BUN and creatinine.**
    3. **Urinalysis** (see p 3, **VI.B.2.a**).
    4. **Chest x-ray** (see p 3, **IV.C.1**).
    5. **Colposcopy** (see p 387, **VI.B.4.a**).
  C. **Additional evaluation.** CT scan of the abdomen and pelvis should be obtained **every 6–12 months for 3–5 years** to exclude occult local and distant recurrence.
  D. **Optional evaluation.** The following tests and procedures may be indicated by previous diagnostic findings or clinical suspicion:
    1. **Blood tests** (see p 2, **IV.A**).
      a. **Nucleotidase.**
      b. **GGTP.**
    2. **Imaging studies**
      a. **Intravenous pyelogram.** Deteriorating renal function requires IVP (or CT scan with IV contrast) to exclude ureteral obstruction.
      b. **Magnetic resonance imaging (MRI)** (see p 3, **IV.C.2**.)
      c. **Technetium-99m bone scan** (see p 3, **IV.C.4**).
      d. **Ultrasound** (see p 3, **IV.C.3**).
      e. **Lymphangiography** (see p 387, **VI.C.2.b**).
    3. **Biopsy.** Biopsy of vulvar or genital tract lesions can be accomplished easily with **punch biopsy** (see also, p 387 **VI.B.4.b**). In addition, metastatic disease can be diagnosed in suspicious lesions in other locations with extremely low morbidity by **fine needle aspiration.**

REFERENCES

Anderson BL, Hacker NF. Psychological adjustment after vulvar surgery. Obstet Gynecol 62:457–462, 1983.

Berek JS, Heaps JM, Fu YS, et al. Concurrent cisplatin and 5-Fluorouracil chemotherapy and radiation therapy for advanced stage squamous carcinoma of the vulva. Gynecol Oncol 42:197–201, 1991.

Boronow RC. Combined therapy as an alternative to exenteration for locally advanced vulvovaginal cancer. Cancer 49:1085–1091, 1982.

Boyce CR, Mehram AH. Management of vulvar malignancies. Am J Obstet Gynecol 119:48–58, 1974.

DiSaia, PJ. Conservative management of the patient with early gynecologic cancer. CA-A Cancer Journal for Clinicians 39(3):135–154, 1989.

Hacker NF, Berek JS, Juillard GJF, Lagasse LD. Preoperative radiation therapy for locally advanced vulvar cancer. Cancer 54:2056–2061, 1984.

Hacker NF, Leuchter RS, Berek JS, et al. Radical vulvectomy and bilateral inguinal lymphadenopathy through separate groin incisions. Obstet Gynecol 58:574–579, 1981.

Hacker NF, Berek JS, Lagasse LD, et al. The management of regional lymph nodes in vulvar cancer and their influence on prognosis. Obstet Gynecol 61:408–412, 1983.

Hacker NF. Vulvar Cancer. In Practical Gynecologic Oncology. Berek, JS and Hacker, NF, eds. Williams and Wilkins, Baltimore, pp. 391–423, 1989.

Heaps JM, FU YS, Montz FJ, Hacker NF, Berek JS. Surgical-pathologic variables predictive of local recurrence in squamous cell carcinoma of the vulva. Gynecol Oncol 38:309–314, 1990.

Morrow CP, Townsend DE, eds. Synopsis of Gynecologic Oncology. Churchill Livingston, New York, 3rd ed., pp. 57–89, 1987.

Shimizu Y, Hasumi K, Masubuchi K. Effective chemotherapy consisting of bleomycin, vincristine, mitomycin C, and cisplatin (BOMP) for a patient with inoperable vulvar cancer, a case report. Gynecol Oncol 36:423–427, 1990.

Thomas G, Dembo AS, DePetrillo, et al. Concurrent radiation and chemotherapy in vulvar carcinoma. Gynecol Oncol 34:263–267, 1989.

51 Malignancies of the Soft Tissues

Steven Colquhoun, MD

I. **Epidemiology.** Although soft-tissue sarcomas are rare and account for **0.7% of all malignancies in the United States,** the incidence is increasing. In 1985, 2 cases per 100,000 were reported, and estimates indicated that **6000 new cases and 3100 deaths** would occur in 1993. Worldwide, the incidence of soft-tissue tumors varies only slightly.

II. **Risk factors**
   A. **Age.** The incidence of sarcomas in children younger than 5 years of age is 1.4 per 100,000, accounting for **6.5% of all malignancies in childhood** (the fifth most common cause of death in children under the age of 15). After age 5, the incidence falls to less than 1 per 100,000. After age 25, however, the frequency gradually begins to rise, reaching **10.3 per 100,000 by age 85 years.** Approximately **21%** of soft-tissue sarcomas occur in people younger than **40** years, **28%** in those ages **40–60** years, and **52%** in those older than **60** years.
   B. **Sex.** In the United States, the risk for females is **1.1 times** greater than that for males.
   C. **Race.** There are no known racial differences in the incidence of soft tissue sarcomas.
   D. **Genetic factors**
      1. **Family history.** The risk for first-degree relatives of patients with sarcomas is no greater than the risk for the general population. Isolated reports of familial soft-tissue tumors usually involve benign neoplasms.
      2. **Familial syndromes.** The following inherited diseases are associated with increased risk of soft-tissue sarcomas:
         a. **Neurofibromatosis (von Recklinghausen's disease).** Malignant schwannomas occur in **5–15%** of patients with this autosomal dominant disease marked by multiple neurofibromas and characteristic skin lesions **(cafe au lait spots).** An association with **rhabdomyosarcomas** also has been claimed.
         b. **Basal cell nevus syndrome (Gorlin's syndrome).** This hereditary disorder, characterized by multiple basal cell carcinomas, jaw cysts, multiple bony anomalies, and shallow dermal pits of the hands and feet imparts an increased risk of **rhabdomyosarcomas.**
         c. **Tuberous sclerosis (Bourneville's disease).** This autosomal dominant syndrome includes seizures, mental deficiency, and sebaceous adenomas, which pathologically are multiple fibromas occurring on the cheeks and forehead. This disorder is associated with rhabdomyomas and rarely with sarcomas.
         d. **Intestinal polyposis and Gardner's syndrome.** These autosomal dominant diseases are linked to the development of osteomas, fibromas, and lipomas. In rare cases, a true sarcoma occurs.
   E. **Diet.** No dietary factors have been implicated in the etiology of sarcomas.
   F. **Previous soft-tissue pathology**
      1. **Infection.** Oncogenic viruses clearly cause some animal sarcomas and have long been suspected in the pathogenesis of human soft-tissue tumors. To date however, such an association remains unproved, with the possible exception of a correlation between **human immunodeficiency virus (HIV) and Kaposi's sarcoma.**
      2. **Inflammation.** Chronic inflammation and scarring may lead to fibrosarcomas. In addition, inflammation from chronic lymphedema after mastectomy and axillary radiation can induce upper extremity **lymphangiosarcomas (Stewart-Treves Syndrome)** in rare cases.
      3. **Trauma.** Some injury-related lesions, such as **myositis ossificans,** are difficult

to distinguish from true sarcomas, but evidence linking trauma to the formation of sarcomas is anecdotal. In many instances, trauma merely serves to focus attention on a pre-existing occult lesion.

4. **Radiation.** Although osteogenic sarcomas (see Chapter 52), fibrosarcomas, and malignant fibrous histiocytomas occur in irradiated tissue, the actual incidence of irradiation-induced sarcomas is extremely low and the latency period is long (decades).

G. **Environmental toxins.** Carcinogens may be responsible for a small number of sarcomas. **Asbestos** exposure has been linked to the development of **mesotheliomas; polyvinyl chlorides,** to **hepatic angiosarcomas;** and **phenoxybretic acids (herbicides) and chlorophenols (wood preservative),** to a variety of **soft tissue neoplasms.** The last association is controversial.

III. **Clinical presentation**
  A. **Signs and symptoms**
    1. **Local manifestations.** Typically, sarcomas present as **asymptomatic, slow-growing masses.** If signs and symptoms develop, they are often nonspecific and variable, depending on the site of the primary tumor. Occasionally, specific symptoms such as **pain, weakness, paresthesias, and anesthesia** may occur from compression of adjacent nerves or blood vessels. Because benign and malignant lesions are indistinguishable on the basis of clinical presentation, an initial diagnosis of a **"pulled muscle"** or **"organizing hematoma"** is commonly made. Lesions that arise in clinically silent regions such as the retroperitoneum may reach sizeable proportions before detection. The average duration of symptoms before presentation is **4–6 months.**
    2. **Systemic manifestations.** Systemic manifestations of sarcomas include shortness of breath (pulmonary metastases), hepatosplenomegaly (hepatic metastases), and bone pain (bone metastases). Patients also may have vague complaints of weakness, fatigue, and weight loss.
  B. **Paraneoplastic syndromes.** No paraneoplastic syndromes have been described in association with soft-tissue sarcomas.

IV. **Differential diagnosis.** A high index of suspicion is required to diagnose soft-tissue sarcomas. In general, any **enlarging or newly detected mass larger than 2 cm** should be biopsied. A period of observation is appropriate only if a relatively small stable lesion has been present for many years. Other pathologic entities that produce soft-tissue swelling include infections (eg, abscesses, granulomas), inflammation (trauma, hematoma, and myositis ossificans), benign neoplasms (desmoid tumors and dermatofibrosarcomas), and metastases (renal cell carcinoma, melanoma, and lung carcinoma).

V. **Screening programs.** With the exception of a thorough physical examination, no screening tests exist for the detection of soft-tissue sarcomas.

VI. **Diagnostic workup**
  A. **Medical history and physical examination.** A thorough history documenting the duration and progression of signs and symptoms suggesting sarcoma and a complete physical examination are essential during the initial evaluation of patients with suspected soft-tissue tumors. Specific areas that require evaluation during the physical examination are discussed below:
    1. **General appearance.** The patient's functional status (see p 1, I) is important to determine his or her ability to tolerate chemotherapy, be rehabilitated after amputation or limb-sparing operations, and tolerate thoracotomy if pulmonary metastases are detected.
    2. **Lymph nodes.** Although this is uncommon, sarcomas can metastasize to regional lymph nodes.
    3. **Chest.** Evidence for pulmonary metastases (eg, wheezing, decreased breath sounds) may be detected on auscultation in rare cases.
    4. **Abdomen.** The liver and retroperitoneum should be examined for evidence of masses (liver metastases and retroperitoneal sarcomas).
    5. **Extremities.** Any localized soft-tissue mass must be meticulously described, including its **size, depth, position, mobility, and relationship to vital structures.**
  B. **Primary tests and procedures.** All patients with suspected soft-tissue sarcomas should have the following diagnostic tests and procedures performed:
    1. **Blood tests** (see p 1, **IV.A**)
      a. **Complete blood count.**
      b. **Hepatic transaminases.**
      c. **Alkaline phosphatase.**

2. **Imaging studies**
   a. **Chest x-ray** (see p 3, **IV.C.1**).
   b. **Plain x-ray.** Xeroradiography and plain films of a suspected lesion may demonstrate calcifications or fat densities. Calcifications are usually nonspecific, but characteristic patterns sometimes suggest **osteosarcoma (amorphous deposits), chondrosarcoma (ringlet patterns), or synovial cell sarcoma.**
   c. **Computed tomography (CT).** CT scan is the primary method of evaluating soft-tissue masses as well as possible sites of metastatic disease. Because CT scans are **20% more sensitive than plain x-rays** in detecting pulmonary metastases, they have replaced whole-lung tomograms. CT also represents the most accurate means of documenting **vascular bundle invasion, liver or kidney lesions larger than 3–4 mm, and brain lesions larger than 1–3 mm.** Occasionally, the density of the lesion on CT scan suggests a specific particular histologic lesion (eg, fat density = liposarcoma). With extremity masses, it usually is prudent to scan both affected and normal sides for comparison.
3. **Invasive procedures. Soft-tissue biopsy** is essential for the diagnosis and management of soft-tissue sarcomas. Because the diagnosis of soft-tissue neoplasms may be difficult, **a high index of suspicion and an appropriate biopsy are of critical importance.** Several methods of soft-tissue biopsy are discussed below.
   a. **Fine needle aspiration (FNA).** FNA provides **cytologic information** that is generally inadequate for the diagnosis and grading of soft-tissue sarcomas. However, once a diagnosis is made, FNA can be used to confirm residual or recurrent tumor.
   b. **Core needle biopsy.** TRU-CUT needle biopsy provides a **tissue specimen** that often is sufficient for pathologic evaluation. This type of biopsy is particularly useful when the lesion is easily accessible; however, in many instances, an open biopsy (incisional or excisional) may be required.
   c. **Open surgical biopsy.** Frequently, an open biopsy is required to provide satisfactory tissue for the accurate diagnosis of soft-tissue malignancies. Two different techniques are used: **incisional and excisional biopsy.**
      (1) **Incisional biopsy.** In general, an incisional biopsy should be performed if a lesion is larger than **3 cm in diameter.** This enables the surgeon to plan the definitive operation carefully. The incision should be positioned to avoid compromising any future resection. On the extremities, **a longitudinal incision that can be re-excised is made directly over the mass.** A suspected sarcoma should **never** be removed through the pseudocapsule (**"shelled out"**) because of an extremely high local recurrence rate. In addition, hemostasis is crucial because hematomas can spread malignant cells to previously uninvolved areas.
      (2) **Excisional biopsy.** Excisional biopsy can be considered if a lesion is smaller than **3 cm in diameter.** However, if a sarcoma is even remotely suspected, an incisional rather than an excisional biopsy is preferred.
C. **Optional tests and procedures.** The following examinations may be indicated by diagnostic findings or clinical suspicion:
   1. **Blood tests** (see p 2, **IV.A**)
      a. **5′-Nucleotidase.**
      b. **GGTP.**
   2. **Imaging studies**
      a. **Gastrointestinal contrast studies.** In rare cases, **upper gastrointestinal series, small bowel follow-through, and barium enema** may be useful in evaluating patients with soft-tissue sarcomas, especially those of the gastrointestinal tract.
      b. **Excretory urography. Intravenous pyelogram** to evaluate the kidney, ureter, and bladder may be indicated for some retroperitoneal sarcomas.
      c. **Ultrasound** (see p 3, **IV.C.2**).
      d. **Magnetic resonance imaging (MRI).** Although CT scan is currently the preferred radiographic imaging study, MRI ultimately may prove to be superior because of its higher sensitivity, multiplane (transaxial, coronal, and sagittal) imaging abilities, and improved contrast between fascial planes and between malignant and normal tissue. In one study, **MRI accurately pre-**

dicted resectability in 96% of tumors, compared to only 15% with CT scan.

    e. **Angiography.** Before CT, angiograms were used to document tumor neovascularity, vascular encasement (an abrupt change in vessel caliber), and tenting around hypovascular tumors. At present, CT and MRI are more accurate. In certain cases, angiography may be used to demonstrate the vascular supply, the proximity of major vessels before resection, and the feeding vessels for the infusion of intra-arterial neoadjuvant chemotherapy (see p 403, **IX.C.2.a**) or for preoperative embolization.

    f. **Lymphangiography.** Although it is uncommon, some soft tissue tumors may spread through lymphatic channels, blocking normal lymphatic pathways. Suspected pelvic and retroperitoneal lymph node metastases can rarely be documented by lymphangiography.

    g. **Technetium-99m bone scan** (see p 3, **IV.C.5**).

VII. Pathology. The term sarcoma is derived from the Greek word "sarx," meaning **flesh** and the suffix "-oma," meaning **tumor.** Mesenchymal tissues comprise approximately **56%** of the body by weight. Some neuroectodermal tumors are included because their clinical presentation and behavior parallels mesenchymal sarcomas.

    A. Location. Although sarcomas can arise anywhere, they most commonly occur in the extremities; **15% occur in the upper extremities and 40% develop in the lower extremities** (75% of the lesions in the lower extremities are situated at or above the knee). An additional **30% of lesions arise in the trunk** (60% of them involve the abdominal or chest walls and the remaining 40% occur in the retroperitoneum), and another **15% occur in the head and neck region.** Only a small fraction of sarcomas arise from visceral mesenchyma.

    B. Multiplicity. Only **liposarcomas** have been known to present at multiple primary sites.

    C. Histology. Most sarcomas invade locally along fascial planes and along nerves and blood vessels. Expansive growth compresses the surrounding tissues, forming a characteristic **"pseudocapsule."** Originally, histologic classification was based on the appearance of the predominant cell type or the presumed cell of origin (Table 51–1). Currently, histologic classification is based on gross and microscopic appearance, electron microscopy, histochemistry, tissue culture, and clinical history. Because histopathologic classification criteria are not uniform, the reported incidence of each histologic type of sarcoma varies greatly: 1 study found **only 60% agreement in diagnosis among pathologists.** In the distant past, fibrosarcoma was the most common sarcoma; however, in the more recent past, liposarcoma surpassed all other types. Recently, however, **malignant fibrous histiocytoma**

TABLE 51–1. TISSUE ORIGIN OF SELECTED SARCOMAS

Tissue Origin	Tumor
Fibrous tissue	Fibrosarcoma
Muscle, smooth	Leiomyosarcoma
Muscle, skeletal	Rhabdomyosarcoma
Fat	Liposarcoma
Neural tissue	Malignant schwannoma
	Neuroblastoma
	Malignant paraganglioma
	Clear cell tendon sheath
Vascular tissue	Hemangiosarcoma
	Kaposi's sarcoma
	Hemangiopericytoma
	Lymphangiosarcoma
Histiocyte	Malignant fibrous histiocytoma
Synovium	Synovial cell sarcoma
Multipotent	Malignant mesenchymoma
Uncertain	Alveolar soft part
	Epithelioid sarcoma
	Undifferentiated

has become the most frequently diagnosed sarcoma. This evolution in the relative incidence of different sarcomas is the result of multiple revisions of the histopathologic classification criteria rather than of actual changes in the incidence of each histologic type. Some of the more common types of sarcomas are discussed below.

1. **Malignant fibrous histiocytoma (MFH).** MFH arises from tissue histiocytes. Although rarely diagnosed before 1972, MFH is now **the most frequently diagnosed adult soft-tissue sarcoma (> 20%).** Most (40%) occur after age 60, and only 5% develop before age 20. Many tumors, especially pleomorphic rhabdomyosarcomas and undifferentiated fibrosarcomas, are retrospectively being reclassified as MFHs.

2. **Liposarcoma.** Liposarcomas originate in adipose tissue, occur more frequently in males than females (1.5 to 1), and account for **12–33% of adult and 4% of childhood soft-tissue sarcomas.** They can be multicentric and are divided into four subtypes: (1) **well differentiated liposarcomas** that are locally aggressive but rarely metastasize, (2) **myxoid liposarcomas,** (3) **lipoblastic or "round cell" liposarcomas,** which are highly vascular and malignant and have only a 20–30% 5-year survival rate, and (4) **pleomorphic liposarcomas,** which also are highly malignant.

3. **Fibrosarcoma.** Fibrosarcomas arise from fibrous tissue and represent **5.4–43% of all soft-tissue sarcomas.**

4. **Leiomyosarcoma.** The leiomyosarcomas originate from smooth muscle and constitute **2.4–11.4% of adult and 11% of childhood soft-tissue sarcomas.** They are commonly found in the retroperitoneum and often are highly aggressive.

5. **Rhabdomyosarcoma.** Rhabdomyosarcomas arise in skeletal muscle and account for **3–20% of adult and 53% of childhood soft-tissue sarcomas** (see Chapter 69). The incidence of pediatric rhabdomyosarcoma is **bimodal,** with peaks occurring between the ages of 2 and 6 years (genitourinary and head and neck tumors) and during adolescence (genitourinary neoplasms). Rhabdomyosarcomas, especially pediatric genitourinary tract tumors, have a **12% incidence of lymphatic spread.** Three subtypes of rhabdomyosarcomas exist: **pleomorphic, alveolar, and embryonal.** Pleomorphic rhabdomyosarcomas occur more often in adults than in children, commonly involve the extremities, and are usually poorly differentiated. Many are being retrospectively reclassified as MFH. The alveolar and embryonal variants are considered to be juvenile types. The **embryonal subtype is the most common soft-tissue sarcoma of childhood,** whereas the alveolar subtype is somewhat less common and occurs in older children. Alveolar rhabdomyosarcomas frequently involve the genitourinary tract, where a **"botryoid"** (grapelike) appearance is typical, but they also can occur in the nasopharynx and oral cavity.

6. **Synovial cell sarcoma.** Synovial cell sarcomas originate from tendosynovial cells. Despite the cell of origin, these tumors are not commonly associated with joints. They are most common in the lower extremities but can develop anywhere. They usually occur in patients who are 20–40 years old and account for **2.5–19.5% of adult and 5% of childhood soft-tissue sarcomas.** The 5-year survival rate for children varies from 45–70%, which is significantly better than the rate for adults. Synovial cell sarcomas occasionally exhibit characteristic calcifications on plain x-ray films. **There are two subtypes: monophasic and biphasic.** The latter sometimes resembles carcinoma, thus occasionally adding to confusion at the time of diagnosis.

7. **Neurofibrosarcoma.** Neurofibrosarcomas arise from neural sheath cells. These tumors represent **5% of adult and 3% of childhood sarcomas** and include neurogenic sarcomas, malignant schwannomas, or malignant neurilemmomas. They are **associated with von Recklinghausen's disease.** Approximately **10% of patients with neurofibromatosis ultimately develop neurofibrosarcomas.**

8. **Angiosarcomas.** Angiosarcomas originate from blood vessels (hemangiosarcomas) and lymphatics (lymphangiosarcomas). Hemangiosarcomas frequently occur in the skin and superficial soft tissues, in contrast to other soft-tissue sarcomas that occur in deeper tissues. Of those that occur in the skin, **50% develop in the head and neck region** and are exceptionally refractory to therapy. Lymphangiosarcomas are rare **(< 2% of all soft-tissue sarcomas),** uniformly high grade, and associated with chronic lymphedema **(Stewart-Treves syndrome).**

9. **Hemangiopericytoma.** Hemangiopericytomas account for **3% of childhood sarcomas** and arise in **"pericyte" cells** of smooth muscle origin located near small vessels. Both benign and malignant forms exist, creating confusion regarding therapy and survival.

10. **Kaposi's sarcoma.** This tumor arises from **endothelial cells** and often presents as raised pigmented skin lesions. Four subtypes have been described. The **classic form** that was initially described in 1872 occurs in elderly men of Mediterranean or Jewish extraction. This form is extremely rare, generally indolent, and most frequently involves the lower extremities. The **long-term survival exceeds 80%** and is often associated with **second primary malignancies.** The **African form,** which was described in Bantu men in Africa, is more aggressive and has a much worse prognosis. A **third variant** is **associated with renal transplantation and its requisite immunosuppression.** Although this form occurs in only **0.4% of transplant recipients,** this is twice the expected rate. A **fourth form is** extremely aggressive and has been associated with **HIV infection** and AIDS.

11. **Alveolar soft-part sarcoma.** The origin of this tumor is unknown. Alveolar soft-part sarcomas comprise **1.5% of childhood soft-tissue sarcomas.** All are malignant, but they grow slowly and metastasize late. The most commonly involved site is the thigh in adults and in the head and neck region in children.

12. **Epithelioid sarcoma.** The origin of this type also is unknown. Almost all epithelioid sarcomas occur in the extremities and are associated with aponeurotic tissues. This tumor **spreads to regional lymph nodes in 30% of cases.**

D. **Grading.** The original grading system was proposed by Broders at the Mayo Clinic in the 1920s and was used as an estimate of malignant potential and predilection for metastases. Grading remains a more important indicator of biologic behavior than the histopathologic type. **Grade is usually reported as I (low), II (intermediate), or III (high),** depending on microscopic appearance (including mitotic rate and atypia), degree of cellularity and necrosis, nuclear morphology, clinical behavior, and pleomorphism or anaplasia. Because the exact criteria for grading are not uniform, experienced pathologists often disagree, making it difficult to compare results from different institutions. Certain tumors—eg, synovial cell sarcomas and rhabdomyosarcomas—always are considered to be Grade III (high-grade) lesions. The metastatic potential varies with grade. Grade I lesions, although locally aggressive, rarely metastasize, and Grades II and III lesions frequently spread to distant sites.

E. **Metastatic spread**

1. **Modes of spread.** Sarcomas primarily spread by direct extension and hematogenous metastasis; however, certain histologic types can metastasize to regional lymph nodes.

   a. **Direct extension.** Sarcomas commonly spread by direct extension along fascial planes, nerves, and blood vessels.

   b. **Lymphatic metastasis.** Spread to regional lymph nodes occurs in **5% of all sarcomas.** However, this occurs relatively more often in **epithelioid sarcomas (30%), synovial cell sarcomas (17%), rhabdomyosarcoma (12%),** MFH, and clear cell sarcoma.

   c. **Hematogenous metastasis.** The most common route by which soft tissue sarcomas metastasize is through blood vessels.

2. **Sites of spread.** The organs commonly involved with metastatic spread are the following sites: **lung,** most common (34%); **liver,** second most common (25%); **bone,** less frequent (23%); and central nervous system (3%).

VIII. **Staging.** The American Joint Committee on Cancer (AJCC) and the Union Internationale Contre le Cancer have jointly suggested a staging system **based on extent of disease and tumor grade** but not on histologic type. Generally, the AJCC recommendations for the staging of soft-tissue sarcomas are the same for children and adults. The goals of staging are threefold: (1) to establish the probability of distant metastases, (2) to predict the probability of disease control and (3) to accrue information regarding therapeutic success. **Clinical staging** is assessed on the basis of physical examination, imaging studies, laboratory tests, and biopsy results. **Pathologic staging** is determined after resection and pathologic evaluation of the tumor and any metastases (lymph node or distant).

A. **Tumor stage**

1. **TX.** Primary tumor cannot be assessed.
2. **T0.** No evidence of primary tumor exists.
3. **T1.** Tumor is smaller than 5 cm in its greatest dimension.

      4. T2. Tumor is larger than 5 cm in its greatest dimension.
- **B. Lymph node stage**
  1. **NX.** Regional lymph nodes cannot be assessed.
  2. **N0.** No regional lymph node metastases are present.
  3. **N1.** Regional lymph node metastases are present.
- **C. Metastatic stage**
  1. **MX.** Presence of distant metastases cannot be assessed.
  2. **M0.** No distant metastases are present.
  3. **M1.** Distant metastases are present.
- **D. Histopathologic grade**
  1. **GX.** Grade cannot be assessed.
  2. **G1.** Well differentiated.
  3. **G2.** Moderately well differentiated.
  4. **G3–4.** Poorly differentiated and undifferentiated.
- **E. Stage groupings**
  1. **Stage IA.** G1, T1, N0, M0.
  2. **Stage IB.** G1, T2, N0, M0.
  3. **Stage IIA.** G2, T1, N0, M0.
  4. **Stage IIB.** G2, T2, N0, M0.
  5. **Stage IIIA.** G3–4, T1, N0, M0.
  6. **Stage IIIB.** G3–4, T2, N0, M0.
  7. **Stage IVA.** Any G, any T, N1, M0.
  8. **Stage IVB.** Any G, any T, any N, M1.

IX. Treatment
- **A. Surgery**
  1. **Primary soft tissue sarcoma**
     a. **General considerations.** Treatment options depend on several factors, including tumor histology, grade, stage, anatomic location, size, previous therapy administered, and the patient's performance status.
     b. **Indications.** Surgery remains the mainstay of therapy for soft-tissue sarcomas. **Surgery alone is considered adequate for grade I (low-grade) lesions,** but surgery is routinely combined with adjuvant radiation, chemotherapy, or both for Grades II and III (high-grade) neoplasms. **The goal of any surgical resection is to remove the entire tumor with an adequate margin of normal tissue.** Controversy exists, however, regarding the optimal extent of surgical resection. Because of recent advances in adjuvant irradiation and chemotherapy, limb preservation is now preferred, even though, without amputation, some tumor locations may prohibit wide surgical margins. In these situations, limb-sparing procedures combined with adjuvant therapy have produced equal overall survival (compared to amputation) but do have a slightly increased local recurrence rate.
     c. **Procedures.** The extent of surgical resection can be classified into one of several categories.
        (1) **Intracapsular excision.** This procedure removes the bulk of the tumor mass, leaving gross tumor along the pseudocapsule, and is **almost never indicated.**
        (2) **Marginal excision.** This technique, used in **23% of cases,** excises all gross tumor, including the pseudocapsule. These operations leave microscopic tumor and, in the absence of adjuvant therapy, are associated with a **50–93% recurrence rate.** Procedures that **"shell out"** the tumor are classified as marginal resections.
        (3) **Wide excision.** This approach, used in **55% of sarcomas,** includes resection of the tumor with a margin of normal tissue in all directions. With **1–2 cm** margins, the **local recurrence rate is 35–60% without the benefit of adjuvant therapy.**
        (4) **Radical (muscle compartment) excision.** This procedure, used in **14% of resections,** requires the resection of the tumor and all structures within the same anatomic compartment, including all muscles (from origin to insertion) and bone. Retroperitoneal tumors may require the removal of adjacent viscera. The dissection is performed at least 1 tissue plane away in all directions and has an associated **recurrence rate of 7–18% in the absence of further therapy.**
        (5) **Amputation.** Amputation continues to be the only acceptable option in **8% of patients.** The level of amputation should be at least one joint

TABLE 51–2. AMPUTATION LEVEL BY TUMOR SITE

Tumor Location	Amputation Level
Lower extremity	
Foot	Below-knee
Leg	Above-knee
Distal thigh	Hip disarticulation
Proximal thigh	Hemipelvectomy
Buttock	Hemipelvectomy
Upper extremity	
Hand	Below-elbow
Wrist	Below-elbow
Forearm	Above-elbow
Distal arm	Shoulder disarticulation
Proximal arm	Forequarter
Shoulder	Forequarter

above the lesion (see Table 51–2). Without adjuvant chemotherapy or radiation therapy, local recurrence rates after amputation are similar to radical excision **(7–21%).**

2. **Locally advanced and metastatic sarcomas.** Unlike most other malignancies, metastatic sarcoma is often amenable to surgical therapy. The indications for surgery include both local and distant disease.
   a. **Local disease.** Data accumulated from multiple centers also indicate that overall survival is significantly improved with the resection of local recurrences and disease that has metastasized to regional lymph nodes.
   b. **Pulmonary metastases.** The lungs frequently are the first and only site of metastatic spread. Multiple studies have demonstrated that long-term survival is possible after resection of isolated pulmonary metastases. Certain criteria are important when contemplating resection of pulmonary metastases: (1) the primary lesion must be controlled, (2) no other extrapulmonary metastatic disease exists, (3) adequate pulmonary reserve is present, and (4) the lesions are technically resectable. In addition, favorable findings include (1) a small number of lesions (optimally fewer than 4), (2) a tumor doubling time of more than 20 days, and (3) a disease-free interval of more than 12 months (although resection is still recommended if synchronous lesions are found). Because of a high incidence of bilateral disease, **median sternotomy is usually indicated,** although lateral thoracotomy is acceptable if multiple previous sternotomies have been performed or unilateral disease is suspected. Most lesions are peripherally located and can be **locally excised.** In rare cases, lobectomy or pneumonectomy is required.
3. **Mortality and morbidity.** The complications of surgery for sarcomas of the extremities vary with the location of the tumor but include hemorrhage, infection, **nerve and blood vessel injury, functional deficits,** and recurrence. The problems after resection of pulmonary metastases are minimal and include hemorrhage, infection, and bronchopleural fistula.
B. **Radiation therapy.** Radiation therapy has become an extremely important component in the combined modality approach to the treatment of soft-tissue sarcomas. Currently, soft-tissue sarcomas are treated primarily with conventional megavoltage external-beam irradiation. Particle and brachytherapy remain investigational.
   1. **Primary soft-tissue sarcoma.** Radiation therapy as the primary therapy for soft-tissue sarcomas is indicated only in extremely debilitated patients with prohibitive surgical mortality or unresectable lesions.
   2. **Adjuvant radiation therapy.** Radiation can be delivered preoperatively, intraoperatively, or postoperatively, with or without "radiosensitizing" chemotherapeutic agents.
      a. **Preoperative irradiation.** Preoperative irradiation therapy **(1500–5000 cGy)** may be useful because of the limited field, and it may reduce the intraoperative spread of tumor cells.
      b. **Intraoperative irradiation.** Although intraoperative radiation therapy

(2000–3000 cGy) has been used in the treatment of retroperitoneal sarcomas, this modality remains highly experimental.
  c. **Postoperative irradiation.** The entire surgical field, including drain sites, any hematoma, and all tissue planes should be irradiated with **5500–7000 cGy in daily fractions of 150–200 cGy.**
  3. **Locally advanced and metastatic sarcoma.** In some cases, radiation therapy (as much as **8000 cGy**) can be used to convert an otherwise inoperable lesion to one that may be resectable. In addition, painful bone metastases may be significantly palliated with irradiation.
  4. **Mortality and morbidity.** Complications of radiation therapy are more common after preoperative irradiation than after postoperative radiation therapy (**26% versus 8%**) and include the following problems: **fibrosis, delayed wound healing, flap necrosis, osteonecrosis,** and **radiation enteritis.**
C. **Chemotherapy**
  1. **Primary soft-tissue sarcoma.** Currently, primary chemotherapy has no place in the treatment of resectable soft-tissue sarcomas. Patients who are not candidates for surgery or who have unresectable lesions can be treated as if they had metastatic disease (see **IX.C.3**).
  2. **Adjuvant chemotherapy**
    a. **Preoperative (neoadjuvant) chemotherapy.** Limb salvage techniques have given excellent results using preoperative intra-arterial chemotherapy with radiation therapy followed by wide excision. In many cases, this preoperative "neoadjuvant" therapy may convert previously unresectable lesions to those that are resectable. With proper patient selection, limb-sparing protocols have produced **overall survival rates equivalent to those for amputation.** Isolated limb perfusion techniques have not been shown to be significantly better than techniques using systemic chemotherapy. Doxorubicin has been administered intra-arterially with good results; however, significant improvement over systemic therapy has yet to be shown in prospective randomized trials.
    b. **Postoperative chemotherapy.** Although multiple prospective trials of adjuvant postoperative chemotherapy for patients with sarcomas of the extremities have been conducted, only a randomized, prospective trial by the National Cancer Institute with doxorubicin, cyclophosphamide, and methotrexate demonstrated significant benefit in **disease-free (71% vs 46%) and overall (86% vs 51%) survival.** Subsequently, **cyclophosphamide** and lower-dose **doxorubicin** without methotrexate have produced similar results.
  3. **Locally advanced and metastatic sarcoma**
    a. **Single agents.** Many chemotherapeutic agents, including **doxorubicin, cyclophosphamide,** ifosfamide, methotrexate with leucovorin, vincristine, actinomycin-D, and dacarbazine, have been used experimentally in the treatment of the soft-tissue sarcomas. In addition, etoposide has been used for Kaposi's sarcoma. Unfortunately, few agents have significant activity against soft-tissue sarcomas. At present, the most active agent is **doxorubicin,** which has an **overall response rate of 26%** but a 10% rate of significant cardiac toxicity.
    b. **Combination chemotherapy.** Doxorubicin is often used in combination with other agents. Most chemotherapeutic agents are currently used within experimental protocols and, essentially, all are investigational agents.
D. **Immunotherapy.** Interferon has been used for Kaposi's sarcoma with some success.
E. **Combined modality therapy.** Multimodality approaches to the treatment of soft-tissue sarcomas were developed to treat bulky tumors in areas that prohibited adequate surgical resection. Combined approaches use various permutations of surgery, radiation therapy, and chemotherapy and hold the most promise for improving current treatment results.
X. **Prognosis**
  A. **Risk of recurrence.** Patterns of recurrence are influenced by tumor location: eg, retroperitoneal sarcomas disseminate intra-abdominally and chest wall and extremity tumors recur locally. About 80–90% of all recurrences present within 2 years and nearly **100% are evident within 3 years.** Local recurrences are common, and, although most patients do not have metastases at the time of presentation, many develop early hematogenous spread.
  B. **Five-year survival.** Survival at 5 years ranges from a high of 80% for Stage I disease to 67% for Stage II, 47% for Stage III, and 12% for Stage IV.

Note: Survival is not influenced by histologic type.
   C. **Adverse prognostic factors.** Although prognosis is largely determined by tumor stage (including grade), choice of surgical excision, and type of adjuvant therapy, the following factors are associated with a particularly poor outcome: **large size; proximal extremity site** (may be related to larger size); **trunk location,** including retroperitoneum and mediastinum; **head and neck location; lymph node metastases;** and **advanced age.**
XI. **Patient follow-up.** Patients with soft-tissue sarcomas should be followed every 3–4 months for 2 years, every 6 months for an additional 3 years, then annually. The tests and procedures that are indicated depend on the grade and location of the primary tumor and are outlined below.
   A. **Medical history and physical examination.** An interval history and complete physical examination are required during each clinic visit for all patients (Grades I–III). Attention should be directed at the primary site and the areas discussed on p 396, **VI.A**).
   B. **Routine evaluation.** After curative therapy for soft-tissue sarcomas, the following tests and procedures should be monitored during each office visit in all patients with high-grade (Grades II and III) lesions and annually in patients with low-grade (Grade I) tumors:
      1. **Blood tests** (see p 1, **IV.A**).
         a. **Complete blood count.**
         b. **Hepatic transaminases.**
         c. **Alkaline phosphatase.**
         d. **Chest x-ray** (see p 3, **IV.C.1**).
   C. **Additional evaluation.** The following tests and procedures should be obtained at regular intervals in patients with high-grade (Grades II and III) lesions and in some patients with low-grade (Grade I) lesions:
      1. **Electrocardiogram (ECG).** An ECG should be obtained before each dose of chemotherapy in all patients receiving doxorubicin to exclude the development of cardiotoxicity.
      2. **Computerized tomography (CT).** In all retroperitoneal sarcomas (Grades I–III), CT scans of the abdomen and pelvis should be obtained every 6 months for 5 years to exclude local recurrence. With all high-grade (Grades II and III) lesions, CT scan of the chest should be obtained every 6 months for 3 years and then annually for an additional 2 years to detect possible pulmonary metastases.
      3. **Echocardiography.** Cardiac ejection fraction should be quantified and monitored during therapy with doxorubicin.
   D. **Optional evaluation.** The following tests and procedures may be indicated in any patient with Grade I to III lesions by previous diagnostic findings or clinical suspicion:
      1. **Blood tests** (see p 2, **IV.A**).
         a. **5′-Nucleotidase.**
         b. **GGTP.**
      2. **Imaging studies**
         a. **Computerized tomography (CT).** If signs or symptoms of local or distant (liver or lung) recurrences develop, CT should be used to evaluate these sites.
         b. **Magnetic resonance imaging (MRI)** (see p 3, **IV.C.2.d**).
         c. **Technetium-99m bone scan** (see p 3, **IV.C.5**).
         d. **Multiple gated acquisition cardiac scan (MUGA).** MUGA scans may be necessary in patients who have received doxorubicin and subsequently develop signs or symptoms of congestive heart failure or require extensive surgical procedures.

REFERENCES

Antman, KH, Eilber, FR, Shiu, MH. Soft tissue sarcomas: current trends in diagnosis and management. Cur Prob Cancer 13(6):340–367, 1989.

Bramwell, V, Rousesse, J, Santoro, A, et al. European experience of adjuvant chemotherapy for soft tissue sarcoma: a randomized trial comparing CY-VADIC with control. Cancer Treat Symp 3:99–104, 1985.

Chang, A, Kinsella, T, Glatstein, E, et al. Adjuvant chemotherapy for patients with high grade soft tissue sarcoma of the extremity. J Clin Oncol 6:1491–1500, 1988.

Eilber, FR, Morton DL, Sondak VK, and Economou, JS, eds. The Soft Tissue Sarcomas. Grune and Stratton, 1987.

Eilber, FR, Giuliano, AE, Hugh, JF, et al. A randomized prospective trial using postoperative adjuvant chemotherapy (Adriamycin) in high grade extremity soft tissue sarcoma. Am J Clin Oncol 11:39–45, 1988.

Eilber, FR, Guiliano, AE, Huth, J, Mira, J, Morton, DL. High-grade soft tissue sarcomas of the extremity: UCLA experience with limb salvage. Prog Clin Biol Research 201:59–74, 1985.

Elias, AD and Antman, KH. Adjuvant chemotherapy for soft-tissue sarcoma: A critical appraisal. Semin Surg Oncol 4(1):59–65, 1988.

Lawrence, W, Donegan, WL, Natarajan, N, et al. Adult soft tissue sarcomas: A pattern of care survey of the American College of Surgeons. Ann Surg 205:4, 1987.

Lawrence, W. Concepts in limb-sparing treatment of adult soft tissue sarcomas. Sem Surg Oncol 4:73–77, 1988.

Lawrence, W, Neifeld, JP. Soft tissue sarcomas. Cur Prob Surg 26(11):755–827, 1989.

Miser, JS, Pizzo, PA. Soft tissue sarcomas in childhood. Pediatric Clin North Amer, 32(3):779–800, 1985.

Putman, JB, Roth, JA, Wesley, MA, Johnston, MR, Rosenberg, SA. Analysis of prognostic factors in patients undergoing resection of pulmonary metastases from soft tissue sarcomas. J Thor Cardiovas Surg 87(2):260–268, 1984.

Rosenberg, SA. Prospective randomized trials demonstrating the efficacy of adjuvant chemotherapy in adult patients with soft tissue sarcomas. Cancer Treat Report 68(9):1067–1076, 1984.

Shiu, MH, Turnbull, AD, More, D, et al. Control of locally advanced extremity soft tissue sarcoma by function-saving resection and brachy therapy. Cancer 53:1385–1392, 1984.

Suit, H, Mankin, HJ, Wood, WC. Preoperative, intraoperative, and postoperative radiation in the treatment of primary soft tissue sarcomas. Cancer 55:2659–2667, 1985.

52 Malignancies of Bone

Gregory Chow, MD, and Jeffrey Eckardt, MD

I. **Epidemiology.** Bone malignancies are **rare.** Excluding multiple myeloma, which is the most common primary bone malignancy (10 times more frequent than all other types of tumors combined), bone cancer accounts for **0.1% of all new cancer cases and only 0.2% of all cancer deaths.** Estimates indicate that **2000 new cases and 1050 deaths** will occur in 1993. Worldwide, the incidence of bone tumors varies only slightly, although accurate data are not available for many countries.

II. **Risk factors**

A. **Age.** The incidence of bone tumors increases from less than **1 per 100,000 of the population before age 10 years** to an early peak of **1.6 per 100,000 between the ages of 15 and 19 years.** Then, the incidence decreases to **less than 1 per 100,000 until after age 60 years,** when it again increases to **2.2 per 100,000 by age 80.** The age-dependent incidence of bone malignancies varies greatly with histology.

1. **Osteosarcoma.** Although osteosarcoma may occur at any age, nearly **50% of all osteosarcomas arise in adolescents** who are **10 to 20 years of age.**

2. **Chondrosarcoma.** This tumor affects an older age group than does osteosarcoma: patients are usually between **30–60 years of age.**

3. **Fibrosarcoma and malignant fibrous histiocytoma (MFH).** Like osteosarcomas, these tumors can occur at all ages, but they most commonly occur between the **ages of 20 and 30 years.**

4. **Ewing's sarcoma.** Predominantly a disease of children, **85% of all cases** of Ewing's sarcoma are diagnosed **before the age of 20.** This tumor is extremely rare after age 30.

5. **Malignant lymphoma.** Primary lymphoma of bone (previously termed **"reticulum cell sarcoma"**) is generally **a disease of middle-aged and elderly adults;** it is rare in children.

B. **Sex.** Except **fibrosarcoma and MFH,** which have **no sex predilection,** males are at **1.5 times greater risk** than females for bone malignancies.

C. **Race.** With the exception of **Ewing's sarcoma,** which is extremely **rare in blacks,** malignancies of bone affect all races equally.

D. **Genetic factors.** There is no known familial predisposition to bone tumors except as noted below II.F.2.b.

E. **Radiation.** Radiation exposure increases the risk of developing bone tumors, particularly osteosarcomas; however, the incidence is low: less than **0.035% of irradiated patients** develop cancer.

F. **History of previous bone pathology.** The following factors are known to increase the incidence of bone malignancies:

1. **Paget's disease.** An aggressive form of **osteosarcoma** arises in bone affected by Paget's disease.

2. **Benign neoplasms.** The following benign lesions increase the risk of malignancy:

   a. **Enchondromas.** These benign lesions undergo malignant degeneration to **chondrosarcoma in 5% of patients.** Enchondromas in **Ollier's disease (enchondromatosis) and Maffucci's syndrome (enchondromatosis with multiple cavernous hemangiomas)** degenerate at an even faster rate.

   b. **Osteochondromas.** Solitary osteochondromas undergo malignant degeneration to **chondrosarcoma in 1% of patients,** whereas osteochrondromas associated with **hereditary multiple exostoses (osteochondromatosis) degenerate in 10%** of patients.

3. **Polyostotic fibrous dysplasia.** In rare cases, an aggressive form of **fibrosarcoma** arises in patients with polyostotic fibrous dysplasia.

G. **Other factors.** Diet, smoking, and urbanization do not correlate with the incidence of malignant bone tumors.

III. **Clinical presentation**

A. **Signs and symptoms**

1. **Local manifestations.** The most common presenting symptom of bone tumors is **pain**. The pain usually is **localized,** although occasionally radiation occurs from nerve involvement. A **mass or local swelling** may be noted in slender patients, in patients with large tumors, and in patients with tumors in subcutaneous locations (eg, proximal tibia). **Ewing's sarcoma** often presents with **flu-like symptoms, malaise, and low-grade fever.**

2. **Systemic manifestations.** It is extremely uncommon for primary malignancies of bone to present with signs and symptoms of metastatic disease.

B. **Paraneoplastic syndromes.** There are no described cases of primary bone malignancies presenting with paraneoplastic syndromes.

IV. **Differential diagnosis.** Osteosarcoma frequently exhibits a characteristic radiographic appearance. Periodically, however, bone malignancies may be difficult to distinguish from healing **pathologic fractures** (osteosarcoma and fibrosarcoma), **stress fractures** (Ewing's sarcoma), **osteomyelitis** (Ewing's sarcoma and bone lymphoma), **fibrous dysplasia, aneurysmal bone cysts** (telangiectatic osteosarcoma), benign neoplasms of bone (osteoblastoma, giant cell tumors, desmoplastic fibroma, desmoid tumor of bone, and eosinophilic granuloma) and **cartilage** (osteochondroma, enchondroma, chondroblastoma, and chondromyxoid fibroma), and metastatic lesions (neuroblastoma).

V. **Screening programs.** Because of the low incidence of bone malignancies, screening measures are currently impractical.

VI. **Diagnostic workup**

A. **Medical history and physical examination.** In addition to a thorough medical history documenting signs and symptoms of bone disease, a complete physical examination, including an orthopedic examination, should be performed with special attention paid to the following areas:

1. **General appearance.** An assessment of the patient's general functional, nutritional, and ambulatory status should be made (see also, p 1, **I** and **III**).

2. **Chest.** Evidence of pulmonary metastases (eg, wheezing, diminished breath sounds) must be noted.

3. **Abdomen.** Abdominal masses as well as hepatosplenomegaly should be described.

4. **Extremities.** Examination of all 4 extremities should be carefully performed and include detailed descriptions of swelling and masses, evaluation of range of motion of all joints and limitations compared with the contralateral side, tenderness, and neurologic function, including motor strength and sensory function.

B. **Primary tests and procedures.** The following is a list of diagnostic tests and procedures that should be obtained initially in all patients with suspected bone tumors:

1. **Blood tests**

a. **Complete blood count** (see p 1, **IV.A.1**).

b. **Hepatic transaminases** (see p 1, **IV.A.2**).

c. **Alkaline phosphatase.** Serum levels of this enzyme are **elevated in 42%** of patients and have prognostic significance. Nearly **93% of patients** who **survive 10 years had normal preoperative levels,** compared with less than 12% of patients who died (see also, p 1, **IV.A.3**).

d. **Calcium and phosphorus.** With bone destruction, both calcium and phosphorus levels may be elevated.

e. **Erythrocyte sedimentation rate.** Although nonspecific, elevated levels may indicate the presence of **tumor, inflammation, or infection.**

2. **Imaging studies.** These are critical in the diagnostic workup of bone malignancies.

a. **Chest x-ray** (see p 3, **IV.C.1**).

b. **Plain x-rays.** Conventional radiographs (in at least 2 planes) should be obtained. Radiographic findings vary, depending on histology, and are summarized below:

(1) **Osteosarcoma.** A osteoblastic or osteolytic medullary lesion with **periosteal elevation** forming a triangle with the cortex **(Codman's triangle)** is often identified, and cortical bone is frequently eroded and a soft-tissue mass is visible. A **smooth, well-defined mass or spiculated calcifications** adjacent to the cortex without medullary involvement may represent a **parosteal or periosteal osteosarcoma,**

respectively. Generally, radiographic appearances are classified as **sclerotic (32%), osteolytic (22%), and mixed (46%).**

(2) **Chondrosarcoma. Punctate, comma-shaped, and circular calcifications** are characteristic of cartilage-forming tumors. Periosteal reaction and a visible soft-tissue mass also may be present. **Clear-cell chondrosarcoma** produces a distinctive **osteolytic expanding mass** at the end of a long bone.

(3) **Fibrosarcoma.** Although osteolytic destruction of medullary bone and periosteal reaction are sometimes seen, often the only abnormality is **distortion of normal muscle planes.**

(4) **Malignant fibrous histiocytoma.** Typically, a **moth-eaten or permeating osteolytic medullary mass** associated with cortical erosion and soft-tissue ossification is identified. Periosteal reaction is rare.

(5) **Ewing's sarcoma.** This tumor produces a **patchy moth-eaten lesion** associated with a soft-tissue mass and a periosteal reaction characterized as **lamellar or "onion-skin."**

(6) **Lymphoma.** A **mottled mass** eroding into cortical bone, the intramedullary canal, and soft tissue is typical, and **pathologic fractures are common.**

c. **Computerized tomography (CT).** CT scan of the affected bone is the best test to detect tumor-induced abnormalities in cortical structure. **Chest CT** also should be obtained to exclude the presence of **pulmonary metastases.**

d. **Magnetic resonance imaging (MRI).** MRI is the best method to evaluate **medullary involvement, soft-tissue extension, and neurovascular involvement.** However, because it does not demonstrate cortical bone, it should be used to complement, not replace, CT.

3. **Invasive procedures.** Although clinical history and radiographic studies usually can differentiate benign and malignant lesions, tissue examination (biopsy) is essential before a final diagnosis can be made and treatment can be planned.

a. **Fine needle aspiration (FNA).** Rarely, FNA may establish the diagnosis of primary bone malignancy, particularly if a **soft-tissue component** is present and an **experienced cytopathologist** is available.

b. **Percutaneous needle biopsy (PNB).** The role of PNB is controversial. Benefits include (1) a small biopsy tract, (2) a low infection rate, (3) a fast recovery time, and (4) the need for only local anesthesia (outpatient procedure). **Disadvantages** include (1) a small specimen, (2) a potential sampling error with large tumors, (3) the difficult nature of tissue, (4) a frequent requirement for radiologic guidance necessitating coordination between radiologist, surgeon, and pathologist, and (5) pathologists who lack experience in interpreting PNB. With experienced pathologists, the **overall accuracy of PNB is 80–93%.**

c. **Incisional biopsy.** This procedure remains the **"gold"** standard for the diagnosis of bone tumors. To optimize culture results and exclude infection as the cause of a bone lesion, preoperative **antibiotics are not given.** The biopsy must be planned carefully to allow subsequent **en bloc excision of the entire tract with the tumor.** Extremity incisions must be **oriented longitudinally,** and dissection should proceed **directly through muscle tissue** rather than intermuscular planes. **Hemostasis is critical.** Use of a **tourniquet** to reduce hemorrhage and use of a **drain** to reduce hematoma formation are **controversial.** If a tourniquet is used, it must be released and hemostasis must be achieved before the wound is closed, and drain tracts must be placed close to the incision to allow later excision of the tract with the tumor. **Intraoperative radiography and frozen section examination** of the specimen may be needed to confirm that adequate and appropriate tissue was obtained. Ideally, a surgeon experienced in the management of bone malignancies should perform the biopsy and assume the patient's care because poorly planned biopsies may contaminate normal tissues and render limb salvage procedures impossible.

C. **Optional tests and procedures.** The following tests and procedures may be indicated by previous diagnostic findings or clinical suspicion:

1. **Blood tests** (see p 2, **IV.A**)
   a. **5′-Nucleotidase.**
   b. **GGTP.**

2. **Urine tests.** Urinary **catecholamines** that are elevated with metastatic neuroblastoma should be measured to **distinguish Ewing's sarcoma from neuroblastoma.**
3. **Imaging studies**
   a. **Angiography.** Angiography may be useful to **document the vascular supply of the tumor and exclude vascular involvement** before resection (if MRI fails) and to **embolize highly vascular tumors.**
   b. **Technetium-99m bone scan.** Bone scans may be useful for demonstrating **skip lesions** as well as **distant synchronous primary and metastatic lesions.**
4. **Invasive procedures.** In **Ewing's sarcoma and lymphoma,** bone marrow aspiration must be performed to exclude involvement of distant bone marrow.

VII. **Pathology**
A. **Location.** The incidence of bone tumors varies with the histologic type of malignancy.
   1. **Osteosarcoma.** Osteosarcoma occurs most commonly in the **distal femur (50%), proximal tibia (20%),** humerus (10%), proximal femur (5–10%), middle and distal tibia (5–10%), and pelvis (5–10%).
   2. **Chondrosarcoma.** The sites involved with chondrosarcoma most frequently are the **pelvis, femur, and humerus.**
   3. **Fibrosarcoma.** This tumor occurs in the **femur, tibia, and humerus,** whereas involvement of the axial skeleton is rare.
   4. **Malignant fibrous histiocytoma.** MFH usually occurs in the **femur, pelvis,** and **tibia** and rarely in the vertebrae and ribs.
   5. **Ewing's sarcoma.** The most frequent sites involved with Ewing's tumors are the **femur, pelvis, tibia,** and **fibula** and, less commonly, the ribs.
   6. **Lymphoma.** Primary bone lymphomas do not have a predilection for any site and **may occur in any bone.**
B. **Multiplicity.** "**Skip lesions**" **are local hematogenous metastases** that occur in the same bone but are separated by a segment of uninvolved bone. They occur infrequently and can be identified easily on bone scan, CT scan, and MRI.
C. **Histology.** The histologic types of bone sarcomas include **osteosarcoma and its subtypes (30–40%), chondrosarcoma (15–20%), fibrosarcoma and malignant fibrous histiocytoma (10–15%), and small round-cell tumors (Ewing's sarcoma and lymphoma, 5–10%).** The remaining malignancies of bone **(chordoma, adamantimona, angiosarcoma, and malignant giant-cell tumor)** each account for only 1–2% of all bone cancers. The main histologic types of bone sarcomas are discussed below.
   1. **Osteosarcoma.** Although many subtypes exist, the **hallmark of osteosarcoma is the presence of malignant cells that produce osteoid,** which may or may not calcify. Other cell types may be present and even predominant. Table 52–1 summarizes several subtypes of osteosarcoma. Two other subtypes are discussed below.
      a. **Parosteal osteosarcoma.** This **low-grade** (Grade I) tumor arises from the cortex and extends into the soft tissues **without involving the intramedullary cavity.** The tumor usually arises from the **posterior distal femur (80%).** Because this neoplasm does not respond to chemotherapy, surgery represents the only treatment.
      b. **Periosteal osteosarcoma.** This osteosarcoma subtype arises from the cortex **without involving the intramedullary bone.** These tumors almost always exhibit **intermediate aggressiveness (Grade II) and cartilaginous characteristics (chondroblastic).** Adjuvant chemotherapy is indicated for these lesions.

TABLE 52–1. HISTOLOGIC TYPES OF BONE SARCOMAS

Predominate Tissue	Osteosarcoma Subtype
Bone	Osteoblastic
Cartilage	Chondroblastic
Connective tissue	Fibroblastic
Blood vessels	Telangiectatic

2. **Chondrosarcoma.** Because cartilage is relatively **acellular,** the diagnosis of malignancy on the basis of the cellularity and pleomorphism of the chondrocytes may be difficult. If **multicellular lacunae or multinucleated cells** are present, malignancy is likely; however, the histology must always correlate with the clinical and radiographic pictures. Histologic variants of chondrosarcoma exist but are uncommon.

    a. **Juxtacortical (periosteal) chondrosarcoma.** This less aggressive subtype is **devoid of osteoid,** but the distinction between this lesion and the **periosteal osteosarcoma** is unclear.

    b. **Clear-cell chondrosarcoma.** This aggressive lesion represents less than **4%** of all chondrosarcomas and involves **articular cartilage,** particularly around the **femoral neck and intertrochanteric area**.

    c. **Mesenchymal chondrosarcoma.** This rare neoplasm is distinguished by a remarkably cellular component with highly anaplastic small cells that may **resemble Ewing's sarcoma.** The chondroid component is often benign in appearance. Roughly **33% of mesenchymal chondrosarcomas are primary soft-tissue lesions** and do not arise in bone.

    d. **Dedifferentiated chondrosarcoma.** In this extremely malignant tumor, a region undergoes **"dedifferentiation,"** taking on the histologic appearance and **behavior of a fibrosarcoma, osteosarcoma, or MFH.** The transition zone between normal and dedifferentiated tissue is abrupt. Chemotherapy is directed at the metastatic dedifferentiated tumor type.

3. **Fibrosarcoma.** Fibrosarcomas manifest interwoven bundles of spindle cells with narrow tapered nuclei. As with chondrosarcoma, **aggressive behavior is associated with a higher cellularity** and lower proportion of extracellular matrix.

4. **Malignant fibrous histiocytoma.** First recognized as a tumor of soft tissues, primary bone MFH recently has been described. MFH is distinguished by the presence of **spindle cells arranged in a cartwheel or storiform pattern.** Extracellular collagen and anaplastic tumor giant cells also are common.

5. **Ewing's sarcoma.** Grossly, Ewing's tumors are not encapsulated and may be solid or semisolid, **appearing identical to pus** and making it difficult to distinguish from osteomyelitis. Microscopically, numerous small round cells are separated into small compartments by bands of stroma. **Glycogen staining is common** but reticulin staining is not.

6. **Lymphoma.** Primary bone lymphomas exhibit a **mixture of cell types.** The **predominant cell (reticulum cell)** has a prominent nucleus and indistinct cytoplasmic borders and is responsible for the **strong reticulin staining**.

D. **Metastatic spread**

  1. **Modes of spread.** Bone sarcomas can spread by three different routes.

    a. **Direct extension.** Local invasion is a **universal** mode of spread for all bone tumors.

    b. **Lymphatic metastasis.** With the exception of the small round-cell tumors (ie, Ewing's sarcoma and malignant lymphoma), spread to regional lymph nodes is **extremely uncommon.**

    c. **Hematogenous metastasis.** Bone malignancies frequently spread through vascular channels to distant sites, including those within the same bone **("skip" lesions).**

  2. **Sites of spread.** With the rare exception of regional lymph node metastases, distant metastatic sites involved in the spread of bone sarcomas include the following organs: **lung** (50%), **bone** ("skip" or distant metastases), and **liver** (rare).

VIII. **Staging.** The most widely used staging system is that proposed by Enneking in the 1980s and adopted by **The Muscoloskeletal Tumor Society (MSTS).** Recently, however, the American Joint Committee for Cancer and the Union Internationale Contre le Cancer proposed a uniform staging system called TNM. This new system is essentially identical to the MSTS system.

A. **MSTS staging system**

  1. **Tumor stage**

    a. **T1.** Tumor is intracompartmental in location.

    b. **T2.** Tumor is extracompartmental in location.

  2. **Metastatic stage**

    a. **M0.** No metastases are present.

    b. **M1.** Metastases are present.

  3. **Histopathologic grade**

    a. **G1.** Low grade.

    b. G2. High grade.
   4. Stage groupings
    a. Stage I. G1, M0.
     (1) Stage IA. G1, T1, M0.
     (2) Stage IB. G1, T2, M0.
    b. Stage II. G2, M0.
     (1) Stage IIA. G2, T1, M0.
     (2) Stage IIB. G2, T2, M0.
    c. Stage III. Any G, M0.
     (1) Stage IIIA. Any G, T1, M1.
     (2) Stage IIIB. Any G, T2, M1.
 B. TNM staging system
   1. Tumor stage
    a. TX. Primary tumor cannot be assessed.
    b. T0. No evidence of tumor exists.
    c. T1. Tumor is confined within the cortex.
    d. T2. Tumor invades beyond the cortex.
   2. Lymph node stage
    a. NX. Regional lymph nodes cannot be assessed.
    b. N0. No regional lymph node metastases exist.
    c. N1. Regional lymph node metastases are present.
   3. Metastatic stage
    a. MX. Distant metastases cannot be assessed.
    b. M0. No distant metastases exist.
    c. M1. Distant metastases are present.
   4. Histopathologic grade
    a. GX. Grade cannot be assessed.
    b. G1. Well differentiated.
    c. G2. Moderately well differentiated.
    d. G3. Poorly differentiated.
    e. G4. Undifferentiated.
     Note: All Ewing's sarcomas and lymphomas are defined as G4.
   5. Stage groupings
    a. Stage IA. G1–2, T1, N0, M0.
    b. Stage IB. G1–2, T2, N0, M0.
    c. Stage IIA. G3–4, T1, N0, M0.
    d. Stage IIB. G3–4, T2, N0, M0.
    e. Stage III. Not defined.
    f. Stage IVA. Any G, any T, N1, M0.
    g. Stage IVB. Any G, any T, any N, M1.
IX. Treatment
 A. Surgery
   1. Primary bone sarcoma. Surgery remains the mainstay of treatment for nearly
    all types of primary bone malignancies **except lymphoma,** although adjuvant
    radiation and chemotherapy have recently greatly improved survival.
    a. Indications. Except for patients with lymphoma, **surgery is indicated in
     all patients with bone malignancies that are amenable to resection.**
     Neoplasms in surgically **"inaccessible"** locations—eg, the spine or pelvis,
     where a margin of normal tissue cannot be obtained—should be partially
     resected **for palliation** only if the expected benefits outweigh the potential
     morbidity of fracture, paralysis, and so forth.
    b. Approaches. The surgical approach varies tremendously, depending on
     the **location of the primary tumor, the type of tumor present, and the
     procedure planned** (see below). In general, the approach is customized
     for each patient.
    c. Procedures. Although, in the past, amputation was the only surgical option,
     a wider variety of limb-sparing procedures are currently being used with
     equal success.
     (1) Limb-sparing procedures. Recently, limb-sparing surgery **has be-
      come the treatment of choice for bone malignancies because sur-
      vival rates are comparable to amputation.** The extent of resection
      during these procedures is outlined in detail on p 401, **IX.A.1.c.**
      Although **radical (extracompartmental) excision is not manda-
      tory, wide (intracompartmental en bloc) excision is recommended**
      because it safely preserves the maximal amount of normal tissue. Sub-

sequently, several choices exist for reconstruction (see **IX.A.1.d,** below).

   (2) **Amputation.** Amputation may be indicated for patients with extremely **large tumors; debilitating neurovascular involvement; a large, poorly-placed, or contaminated biopsy wound; significant local recurrence following a limb-salvage procedure; and a failure** of limb-salvage because of infection, nonunion, or prosthetic failure. In addition, for **high-grade (Stage IIB) lesions of the distal tibia and foot** functional results are superior with below-the-knee amputations than with limb-salvage procedures.

   d. **Reconstruction.** Types of bone and joint reconstruction that are commonly used in limb-sparing procedures are outlined below. Occasionally, if an expendable bone is involved **(eg, fibula, rib, scapula, distal ulna, or iliac wing),** no reconstruction is required. Lifestyle modifications (ie, avoidance of excessive impact loading activities such as running and jumping) must be made with all types of limb-salvage reconstructions.

   (1) **Arthrodesis.** Fusion of the joint (arthrodesis) following tumor resection may be accomplished with **autologous bone grafts and internal fixation devices.** Although once healed, the extremity is as durable as a normal limb, **loss of motion, a long healing time, and late fractures** complicate this procedure. These problems are increased with postoperative chemotherapy and irradiation.

   (2) **Replacement**
      (a) **Allograft replacement.** Fresh frozen cadaveric bones with or without articulations are inserted and secured by internal fixation. Because bone and cartilage are immunologically privileged, **tissue matching is not required** and rejection does not occur. Grafts must be **matched only for size and side** (right or left). Once healed, these allografts appear and function normally. However, as with arthrodesis, a **long healing time, late fractures, or subchondral collapse** may occur and necessitate total joint replacement. The problem of **disease transmission (eg, hepatitis, AIDS)** also exists. In addition, postoperative chemotherapy and irradiation inhibit allograft healing.
      (b) **Custom endoprosthetic replacement.** Custom endoprostheses are usually made of **titanium, cobalt-chrome,** or both with high-density polyethylene bushings and exterior stops. The prosthesis is either **press-fit or fixed with methylmethacrylate** using techniques similar to those used for conventional joint arthroplasty. This technique **preserves function, cosmesis, and limb length and requires a short healing time that is unaffected by postoperative adjuvant therapy.** Thus, rehabilitation can begin early. However, the **durability of fixation is not known** and the **risk of metal fatigue fracture exists,** although prostheses can be revised without difficulty if problems occur.

2. **Locally advanced and metastatic bone sarcoma.** The 5-year survival after surgical resection of **pulmonary metastases** from osteosarcoma is **nearly 30%.** Wedge resection, segmentectomy, lobectomy, and, in rare cases, pneumonectomy may be performed. Little data exist regarding the treatment of other histologic types and metastatic disease to sites other than the lungs.

3. **Morbidity and mortality.** Although surgical mortality is uncommon (< 1%), complications may be significant and include the following: **hemorrhage,** < 5%; **infection,** 5%; and **prosthetic failure,** uncommon;

B. **Radiation therapy**
   1. **Primary bone malignancies.** Radiotherapy **(4000–5000 cGy over 4–6 weeks) cures more than 90% of patients** with isolated bone **lymphoma.** In addition, radiation therapy **(5000–5500 cGy over 4–6 weeks) results in tumor control in 85% of patients** with localized Ewing's lesions because of their remarkable radiosensitivity. For all other histologic types of bone malignancies, reports of successful radiation therapy are merely anecdotal.

   2. **Adjuvant radiation therapy**
      a. **Preoperative radiation therapy.** The use of preoperative radiation has **not improved the survival** of patients with osteosarcoma, chondrosarcoma, fibrosarcoma, and MFH. In fact, the complications of this treatment (eg, poor wound healing) have discouraged its use.

b. **Intraoperative radiation therapy.** Data about this mode of irradiation are extremely limited and inconclusive.

c. **Postoperative radiation therapy.** Postoperative radiation may kill residual tumor cells that escaped surgical removal. However, it has **not been widely accepted** and should not be substituted for adequate surgery. Radiation therapy also has been used in the treatment of **tumors located in areas that are not amenable to wide excision** (eg, the spine and pelvis) with limited success.

3. **Locally advanced and metastatic bone cancer.** The indications for palliative radiation therapy are limited. This treatment is reserved primarily for **symptomatic local recurrences and bone metastases.**

4. **Morbidity and mortality.** The specific complications of radiation therapy depend on the site of the primary tumor and the extent of irradiation. Common problems include the following: **poor wound healing, growth retardation** (producing limb length discrepancy in children), and **decreased range of motion.**

C. **Chemotherapy**

1. **Primary bone malignancies.** Although primary chemotherapy alone is not curative, **improved survival** with chemotherapy similar to that administered in the adjuvant setting (see **IX.C.2,** below) has been demonstrated for o**steosarcoma and Ewing's sarcoma.**

2. **Adjuvant chemotherapy.** More than 20 studies of various combinations of agents have been reported, with **5-year relapse-free response rates for osteosarcoma ranging from 38–64%.** Currently, therapy is administered both pre- and postoperatively according to the **T10** and **T12** protocols developed at Memorial Sloan-Kettering Cancer Center; these protocols produce **3-year relapse-free survival of 90%** in both favorable and unfavorable responders. **Fibrosarcoma and MFH** are now routinely treated using the same protocol and have shown similar encouraging responses.

a. **Preoperative "neoadjuvant" chemotherapy.** Although the exact combination of drugs and timing of administration are under continued investigation, most patients with osteosarcoma receive **4 (resection or amputation) or 16 (endoprosthetic replacement) weeks** of preoperative therapy with bleomycin, cyclophosphamide, actinomycin-D, doxorubicin, methotrexate (high dose) with leucovorin rescue, and vincristine **(T–10 protocol)** see (Fig. 52–1). Alternately, instead of prolonged postoperative treatment, a single cycle of chemotherapy can be administered to patients with favorable responses (Grade III or IV or > 95% necrosis) with identical results (see T12 protocol, Fig. 52–1).

b. **Postoperative chemotherapy**

   (1) **Osteosarcoma.** According to the T10 protocol, the specimen is examined after surgery for **tumor necrosis,** and, if a **favorable response (> 90% necrosis = grades III and IV)** is observed, the **same drug combination** (bleomycin, cyclophosphamide, actinomycin-D, doxorubicin, methotrexate (high dose) with leucovorin rescue, and vincristine) is continued for three 10-week cycles. If **an unfavorable response (< 90% necrosis = grades I and II)** is noted, the drug combination is **modified** to bleomycin, cisplatin, cyclophosphamide, actinomycin-D, and doxorubicin for three 8-week cycles.

   (2) **Ewing's sarcoma.** Chemotherapy for Ewing's sarcoma relies primarily on varying combinations of **cyclophosphamide, actinomycin-D, doxorubicin, and vincristine.** In addition, **ifosfamide and etoposide** recently have demonstrated solid efficacy against Ewing's sarcoma.

   (3) **Chondrosarcoma.** In general, chemotherapy has **not** been effective against chondrosarcoma; however, chemotherapy directed against the predominant tissue in **dedifferentiated chondrosarcoma** has demonstrated limited success.

3. **Locally advanced and metastatic bone cancer**

a. **Single agents.** Chemotherapy can be used for the **palliation** of bone tumors. The most effective single agents and their response rates are **methotrexate (high dose) with leucovorin rescue (42–82%), cisplatin (33%), ifosfamide (33%), doxorubicin (26%),** cyclophosphamide (15%), and actinomycin-D (15%).

b. **Combination chemotherapy.** Although combinations of chemotherapy agents may produce higher response rates than single agents alone, specific studies are needed.

Week	T10 Protocol[1]	T12 Protocol[2]
0	HDMTX +/– VCR	HDMTX
1	HDMTX +/– VCR	BCD
2	HDMTX +/– VCR	
3	HDMTX	HDMTX
4	Surgery if resection or amputation	HDMTX
5		BCD
6	BCD	
7		HDMTX
8		HDMTX
9	HDMTX	HDMTX
10	HDMTX	Surgery
11	ADR +/– VCR	
12	+/– VCR	
13		
14	HDMTX	
15	HDMTX	
16	Surgery if endoprosthesis	

Week	For grades I/II (< 95% necrosis)	For grades III/IV (> 95% necrosis)	For grades I/II (< 95% necrosis)	For grades III/IV (> 95% necrosis)
0	ADR + CDDP	BCD		
1				
2			HDMTX	BCD
3	ADR + CDDP	HDMTX		
4		HDMTX		HDMTX
5		ADR		HDMTX
6	BCD		Repeat × 6	1 cycle only
7		HDMTX		
8	Repeat × 2	HDMTX		
9				
10		Repeat × 2 (stop MTX after 1–2 cycles)		

[1] High dose (8–12 g/m^2) methotrexate with leucovorin (10–15 mg orally every 6 hours) starting 20 hours after methotrexate (HDMTX); bleomycin (15 mg/m^2/d), cyclophosphamide (600 mg/m^2/d), and dactinomycin (600 μg/m^2/d; BCD); doxorubicin (30 mg/m^2/d; ADR); cisplatin (120 mg/m^2 or 3 mg/kg; CDDP).

[2] Chemotherapeutic agents and doses used are identical to T10 protocol, except bleomycin (20 mg/m^2/d).

FIGURE 52–1. Memorial Sloan–Kettering T10 and T12 chemotherapy protocols.

D. **Immunotherapy.** This relatively new modality has not been widely explored in the treatment of bone tumors.

E. **Other therapies.** Although still in the investigational stage of development, **autologous bone marrow transplantation** may prove to be useful in the treatment of Ewing's sarcoma.

X. **Prognosis**

A. **Risk of recurrence.** The risk of recurrence depends greatly on (1) the histologic type of tumor, (2) the extent of resection and surgical margins attained, and (3) the adjuvant therapy used.

B. **Five-year survival.** The 5-year survival rate varies with the histologic type of malignancy. Overall survival rates are summarized in Table 52–2.

XI. **Patient follow-up**

A. **General guidelines.** Patients with bone malignancies should be examined by the surgeon at 2, 4, 6, and 8 weeks after surgery. Subsequently, patients should be followed **every 3 months for 2 years, every 6 months for an additional 3 years, then annually.** The tests and procedures that are indicated depend on tumor histology, grade and location are outlined below:

B. **Medical history and physical examination.** An interval history and complete physical examination are required during each clinic visit. Attention should be directed toward the areas discussed on p 407, **VI.A,** and orthopedic evaluation must assess **wound problems, tenderness, range of motion, motor strength, gait, and neurovascular status.**

C. **Routine evaluation.** After curative therapy for bone sarcomas, the following tests and procedures should be monitored during each office visit:

1. **Blood tests** (see p 1, **IV.A**)
   a. **Complete blood count.**
   b. **Hepatic transaminases.**
   c. **Alkaline phosphatase.** Serial levels of this enzyme are valuable in detecting locally recurrent or metastatic disease, particularly in **patients who had elevated preoperative levels** that returned to normal after resection.

2. **Imaging studies**
   a. **Chest x-ray** (see p 3, **IV.C.1**).
   b. **Plain x-rays.** Conventional radiographs (in at least 2 planes) demonstrating the entire reconstruction should be obtained. All **internal fixation devices, graft-host junctions, and ends of endoprosthetic devices must be included** to monitor the patient for **graft healing, infection, and loosening and for signs of local tumor recurrence.**

D. **Additional evaluation.** Other tests and procedures that should be obtained at regular intervals include the following:

1. **Computed tomography (CT). Chest CT scan** should be obtained **every 3 months for 2 years, then every 6–12 months.** If signs or symptoms of liver metastases develop, **abdominal CT scan** is useful to evaluate this organ as well, although it should not be obtained routinely.

2. **Technetium-99m bone scan.** This nuclear medicine study must be ordered every **6 months for 2 years** to detect local tumor recurrence (see also, p 3, **IV.C.5**).

E. **Optional evaluation.** The following tests and procedures may be indicated by previous diagnostic findings or clinical suspicion.

TABLE 52–2. FIVE-YEAR SURVIVAL OF PATIENTS WITH BONE MALIGNANCIES

Tumor Histology	5-Year Survival (%)
Osteosarcoma	
Parosteal type	> 80
Other types	> 50
Chondrosarcoma	
Low grade	30–50
High grade	70–80
Fibrosarcoma/MFH	> 50
Ewing's sarcoma	75
Lymphoma	50

1. **Blood tests** (see p 2, **IV.A**)
   a. **5′-Nucleotidase.**
   b. **GGTP.**
2. **Bone marrow aspiration.** This invasive procedure is indicated in the follow-up of patients with **Ewing's sarcoma and lymphoma.**
3. **Biopsy.** All suspicious lesions identified on follow-up examinations must be biopsied. The biopsy techniques are identical to those for primary tumors.

REFERENCES

Aprin, H, Riseborough, EJ, and Hall, JE. Chondrosarcoma in children and adolescents. Clin Orthop 166:226–232, 1982.

Bertoni, F, Boriani, S, Laus, M, and Campanacci, M. Periosteal chondrosarcoma and periosteal osteosarcoma, two distinct entities. J Bone Joint Surg 64B(3):370–376, 1982.

Dahlin, DC, and Unni, KK. Charles C. Bone tumors: general aspects and data on 8,542 cases. Thomas-Publisher, Springfield, Illinois, 1986.

Enneking, WF, ed., Limb salvage in musculoskeletal oncology. Churchill Livingstone, New York, 1987.

Enneking, WF, and Kagan, A. "Skip" metastases in osteosarcoma. Cancer 36:2192–2205, 1975.

Enneking, WF, and Shirley, PD. Resection-arthrodesis for malignant and potentially malignant lesions about the knee using an intramedullary rod and local bone grafts. J Bone Joint Surg 59A(2):223–236, 1977.

Greenspan, A. Tumors of cartilage origin. Orthop Clin North Am 20(3):347–366, 1989.

Heare, TC, Enneking, WF, and Heare, MM. Staging techniques and biopsy of bone tumors. Orthop Clin North Am 20(3):273–285, 1989.

Jaffe, N. Chemotherapy for malignant bone tumors. Orthop Clin North Am 20(3):487–503, 1989.

Kalnicki, S. Radiation therapy in the treatment of bone and soft tissue sarcomas. Orthop Clin North Am 20(3), 487–503, 1989.

Kalnicki, S. Radiation therapy in the treatment of bone and soft tissue sarcomas. Orthop Clin North Am 20(3):505–512, 1989.

Kumar, RV, Mukherjee, G, and Bhargava, MK. Malignant fibrous histiocytoma of bone. J Surg Onc 44:166–170, 1990.

Mankin, HJ, Doppelt, SH, Sullivan, TR, and Tomford, WW. Osteoarticular and intercalary allograft transplantation in the management of malignant tumors of bone. Cancer 50:613–630, 1982.

Marks, KE, and Bauer, TW. Fibrous tumors of bone. Orthop Clin North Am 20(3), 377–393, 1989.

Meyers, PA. Malignant bone tumors in children: osteosarcoma. Hem/Onc Clin North Am 1(4):655–665, 1987.

Meyers, PA. Malignant bone tumors in children: Ewing's sarcoma. Hem/Onc Clin North Am 1(4):667–673, 1987.

Mirra, JM, Picci, P, and Gold, RH, et al. Bone tumors: clinical, radiologic, and pathologic correlations. Lea and Febiger, Malvern, PA, 1989.

Musculoskeletal Tumor Surgery. Enneking, WF, ed. Churchill-Livingstone, New York, 1983.

Pritchard, DJ. Small round cell tumors. Orthop Clin North Am 20(3):367–375, 1989.

Ritts, GD, Pritchard, DJ, Unni, KK, Beabout, JW, and Eckardt, JJ. Periosteal Osteosarcoma. Clin Orthop 219:299–307, 1987.

Rosen, G., Caparros, B, Huvos, AG, et al. Preoperative chemotherapy for osteogenic sarcoma: selection of postoperative adjuvant chemotherapy based on the response of the primary tumor to preoperative chemotherapy. Cancer 49:1221–1230, 1982.

Rosen, G, Murphy, L, Huvos, AG, Gutierrez, M, and Marcove, RC. Chemotherapy, en bloc resection, and prosthetic bone replacement in the treatment of osteogenic sarcoma. Cancer 37:1–11, 1976.

Schajowicz, F. Current trends in the diagnosis and treatment of malignant bone tumors. Clin Orthop 180:220–252, 1983.

Simon, MA. Causes of increased survival of patients with osteosarcoma: current controversies. J Bone Joint Surg 66A(2):306–310, 1984.

Spanos, PK, Payne, WS, Ivins, JC, and Pritchard, DJ. Pulmonary resection for metastatic osteogenic sarcoma. J Bone Joint Surg 58A(5):624–628, 1976.

53 Malignancies of the Breast

Beth Fisher, MD

I. **Epidemiology.** In the United States breast cancer remains the **most common** malignancy and is the second most common cause of cancer mortality in females, accounting for **29%** of all cancers and **18%** of all cancer deaths. In 1985, **102.1** cases per 100,000 females and **0.7** cases per 100,000 males were diagnosed, leading to 27.4 and 0.3 deaths, respectively. Estimates indicate that **183,000 new cases and 46,300 deaths** will occur in females and that 1000 new cases and 300 deaths would occur in males in 1993. The **lifetime risk** (ages 0–110 years) of breast cancer is **7–10%,** and the incidence is increasing rapidly. Worldwide, the incidence of breast cancer varies from areas of low incidence—eg, Japan (8.9 per 100,000) and other Asian, Latin American, and African countries—to areas of high incidence such as the United States (102.1 per 100,000).

II. **Risk factors**
- A. **Age.** Breast cancer gradually increases from less than 1 per 100,000 before age 25 years to **397** per 100,000 by age 80 years. The median age at diagnosis is **57 years.**
- B. **Sex.** The risk in females is **146 times** that in males; male breast cancer accounts for less than 1% of cases.
- C. **Race.** The risk in **white** females is **1.2 times** higher than in black females.
- D. **Genetic factors**
  - 1. **Family history.** Familial risk reflects a combination of genetic and environmental influences that are often difficult to separate.
    - a. **First-degree relatives (mother, sisters, daughters).** The risk varies, depending on several factors such as menopausal status and presence of bilateral disease (see Table 53–1). Although some studies suggest that the risk is directly proportional to the number of family members affected, this is controversial.
    - b. **Second-degree relatives.** Breast cancer in a second-degree relative increases the risk by **1.5 times.**
  - 2. **Familial syndromes**
    - a. **Hereditary breast cancer syndrome.** This uncommon **autosomal dominant** syndrome accounts for **5%** of familial breast cancer cases and is associated with a **50–80%** risk of early **premenopausal bilateral** breast cancer.
    - b. **Li-Fraumeni syndrome.** Leukemia, lung cancer, adrenal cortical neoplasms, breast cancer, and soft tissue sarcomas are characteristic of this rare **autosomal dominant** syndrome.
    - c. **Cowden syndrome.** This rare disease is marked by mucosal and dermal hamartomas as well as a 50% risk of breast cancer.
  - 3. **Genetic abnormalities**
    - a. **Klinefelter's syndrome.** This symptom complex of small testes with hyaline fibrosis and increased gonadotropin levels, azoospermia, and **gynecomastia** is associated with sex chromosomal anomalies (usually XXY) and a **3%** incidence of **male** breast cancer.
    - b. **Oncogenes.** Although the expression of **c-myc, c-erb-2** (HER-2/neu), or both often are increased in breast cancer, their role in the pathogenesis of breast cancer, and their clinical utility, if any, remains unclear.
- E. **History of previous breast pathology**
  - 1. **Atypical ductal hyperplasia (ADH).** Although benign breast pathology (eg, fibrocystic changes) does **not** heighten the risk of breast cancer, ADH with or without a **family history** of breast cancer does increase the risk **11 times** and **5 times,** respectively.

TABLE 53-1. RELATIVE RISK IN FIRST-DEGREE RELATIVES OF PATIENTS WITH BREAST CANCER

Affected Relatives	Unilateral Disease	Bilateral Disease
1 or 2 postmenopause	1	4
1 pre-, 1 postmenopause	1.5	2-3
1 or 2 premenopause	2.5-4.5	7-9

    2. Previous breast cancer. Following unilateral breast cancer, the risk of developing cancer in the contralateral breast is increased **4- or 5-fold.**

    3. Gynecomastia. Conditions associated with **hyperestrogenism and gynecomastia in males,** such as infection with *Schistosoma hematobium* **(bilharziasis)** in Egypt, increase the likelihood of breast cancer **6-fold.**

  F. Endocrine factors. In general, **prolonged estrogen stimulation** increases the risk of breast cancer. Although prolactin and androgens also may increase the risk, the exact role of these hormones remains unclear.

    1. Menarche. Early menarche (particularly before age 12 years) increases the lifetime risk of breast cancer.

    2. Parity. First parity **after age 30** heightens the risk of breast cancer 4–5 times, whereas parity before age 18 lowers it. Although **nulliparity** increases the risk of breast cancer, **first parity after age 35** may be associated with an even greater risk.

    3. Menopause. Late menopause (after age 54) increases the risk of breast cancer **2-fold** compared with natural menopause before age 45. Moreover, early menopause (surgical or natural) lowers the risk.

  G. Exogenous hormones. To date, epidemiologic data **fail to implicate oral contraceptives** in the pathogenesis of breast cancer; however, recent prospective studies demonstrate a dose-dependent correlation between breast cancer and long-term (10–20 years) postmenopausal exogenous estrogen use.

  H. Diet. Obesity, particularly in postmenopausal females, is associated with an increased risk of breast cancer. Experimental evidence incriminates **dietary fat and cholesterol,** although epidemiologic data are inconclusive.

  I. Ethanol. Several studies link alcohol with a dose-related increased risk of breast cancer.

  J. Radiation. Radiation exposure before age 40 from multiple fluoroscopies **(tuberculosis),** radiation therapy **(acne** and postpartum **mastitis),** and atomic bomb blasts may cause breast cancer after a latency period of 10–15 years.

  K. Other malignancies. Ovarian, colorectal, and endometrial carcinoma are associated with a high incidence of breast cancer.

  L. Urbanization. No excessive risk has been reported in either urban or rural populations.

III. Presentation

  A. Signs and symptoms

    1. Local manifestations. Breast cancer most commonly presents with a **painless palpable mass or thickening (74%)** that generally is **larger than 1 cm** and is discovered by the patient or physician on routine physical examination. Increasingly, breast cancers are being discovered as **nonpalpable mammographic abnormalities.** Other presenting local signs and symptoms include pain (6%), nipple discharge (4%), nipple retraction (3%), edema, dimpling, or erythema of the skin, nipple irritation, a mass or pain in the axilla or supraclavicular area, and generalized arm and breast swelling.

    2. Systemic manifestations. Nearly **10%** of patients will have distant metastases at the time of initial presentation manifested by shortness of breath, cough, and pleural effusions **(pulmonary** metastases); bone pain, and pathologic fractures **(bone** metastases); neurologic symptoms (central nervous system [CNS] metastases); and hepatomegaly, abdominal pain, and jaundice **(liver** metastases).

  B. Paraneoplastic syndromes. Breast cancer is often accompanied by one of the following paraneoplastic syndromes, and this may be the only manifestation of disease.

    1. Hypercalcemia (see p 87).

2. **Paget's disease** (see p 108, **X**).
3. **Cowden's disease** (see p 107, **II**).
4. **Erythema gyratum repens** (see p 108).

IV. **Differential diagnosis.** Typically, breast cancer presents as a **breast mass** that is detected during routine self-examination or a physician's examination. Although breast cancer must always be excluded, benign processes also should be considered, including **infection** (bacterial and, rarely, mycobacterial mastitis and abscess), **inflammation** (mammary duct ectasia), **thrombophlebitis** of superficial breast veins (**Mondor's disease**), **trauma** (fat necrosis), **benign neoplasms**, ie, cysts (**45%** of all breast masses), fibroadenoma, intraductal papilloma, sclerosing adenosis, cystosarcoma phylloides.

V. **Screening programs.** The results of 2 large randomized clinical trials demonstrate a 25–30% reduction in breast cancer mortality rates in individuals participating in screening projects.
  A. **Breast self-examination (BSE).** This inexpensive, noninvasive screening method detects **60%** of breast cancers. BSE should be performed at the same time each month, preferably **1 week after menstruation.** Detailed patient instructions on BSE are available from the American Cancer Society (ACS).
  B. **Physician examination.** Annual breast examinations by a physician are inexpensive and important screening tools, but they are not as sensitive as BSE.
  C. **Screening mammography.** This test identifies clinically occult malignancy that manifests as an irregular **spiculated mass,** a cluster of **microcalcifications, asymmetry** in breast density, or distortion of breast architecture. The rapid rise in the incidence of breast cancer noted over the past decade, in part, may be the result of earlier detection of in situ and clinically occult carcinoma.
  D. **Recommendations.** Current screening recommendations endorsed by the American Medical Association, the **ACS,** and the National Cancer Institute are summarized on the inside front cover of this book.

VI. **Diagnostic workup**
  A. **Medical history and physical examination.** In addition to a thorough medical history documenting risk factors as well as signs and symptoms of breast disease (including the site of abnormality, duration of symptoms, and variation of symptoms with menstruation), a complete physical examination should be performed with particular attention paid to the following areas.
    1. **General appearance.** The patient's general functional and nutritional status should be assessed (see p 1, **I** and **III**).
    2. **Breasts.** Performed in both the sitting and supine positions, breast examination must describe (1) **dominant masses** and their size and shape, location (eg, subareolar), texture and consistency (eg, soft, rubbery, hard, cystic), tenderness, and fixation to skin, muscle, or chest wall, (2) **skin changes** such as erythema, edema (**peau d'orange**), dimpling (caused by retraction of Cooper's ligaments), satellite nodules and ulcerations, and (3) **nipple changes and discharge:** eg, asymmetric inversion, retraction, discoloration, thickening, redness (Paget's disease), and erosion.
    3. **Lymph nodes.** The number, size, and location (cervical, supraclavicular, infraclavicular, or axillary) of lymph nodes as well as mobility and any fixation to the chest wall should be documented.
    4. **Chest.** Evidence of pleural effusions and pulmonary metastases (eg, decreased or absent breath sounds, pleural friction rub) should be included in the pulmonary examination.
    5. **Abdomen.** Hepatosplenomegaly (liver metastases), ascites, and all masses (intraperitoneal metastases) must be fully described.
    6. **Rectum.** A stool specimen should be examined for occult blood.
    7. **Nervous system.** A thorough neurologic examination must be carefully documented.
  B. **Primary tests and procedures.** The following diagnostic tests and procedures should be performed initially in all patients with suspected breast cancer:
    1. **Blood tests** (see p 1, **IV.A**)
      a. **Complete blood count.**
      b. **Hepatic transaminases.**
      c. **Alkaline phosphatase.**
    2. **Imaging studies**
      a. **Chest x-ray** (see p 3, **IV.C.1**).
      b. **Mammography.** Bilateral mammography must be performed (by an accredited facility) before biopsy of any suspicious breast mass. The site, size,

and character of the mass and other suspicious **ipsilateral** and **contralateral** occult lesions should be described. The 2 main types of mammograms are conventional **plain films** and **xeromammograms.** Which type is superior is controversial. Although plain films are more widely used, xeromammograms allow greater resolution and better detail in dense breasts. With exposure to radiation of less than 1 cGy, mammography is **90% accurate** in detecting lesions as small as **1 cm** with characteristic calcifications, stellate appearance, and irregular borders. In the presence of a palpable mass, **a normal mammogram does not exclude cancer.**

   3. **Invasive procedures.** A histologic diagnosis of breast cancer is mandatory before treatment and should be established by fine needle aspiration, limited incisional biopsy, or definitive wide local excision.

      a. **Fine needle aspiration (FNA).** FNA is extremely useful for evaluating **both cystic and solid masses.** Cysts can be aspirated and, if no bloody fluid is obtained and the cyst disappears, no further treatment is warranted (cytologic analysis of the cyst fluid is not necessary). If the cyst persists or recurs, or if a solid mass is present, aspirated material (cells and fluid) may be examined for evidence of malignancy and for estrogen and progesterone receptor expression. A 0–4% **false-positive rate** and a 2–10% **false-negative rate** accompanies FNA, depending on the experience of the individual cytologist. The advantage of FNA is that a diagnosis of malignancy allows a definitive single-stage procedure to be planned with the tumor in situ. In some centers, FNA of lesions less than 1 cm in diameter may be possible with stereotactic equipment. However, a negative FNA does not exclude cancer.

      b. **Core needle biopsy.** If FNA is unavailable or inconclusive and the mass is large (> 2.0 cm in diameter), core needle biopsy can rapidly establish the diagnosis. No false-positive results have been reported with this method.

      c. **Open biopsy.** If FNA or core needle biopsy cannot establish the diagnosis, open biopsy under local or general anesthesia provides tissue for histologic analysis with a diagnostic accuracy that approaches **100%.** Tissue must be submitted for measurement of **estrogen and progesterone receptors** as well as **DNA-ploidy level, S-phase evaluation, and mitotic index,** which yield important prognostic information.

         (1) **Excisional biopsy.** Excisional biopsy of small masses should be performed in the manner of a lumpectomy (see p 425, **IX.A.1.d**), thus providing definitive treatment of the breast lesion. Nonpalpable mammographic abnormalities require stereotactic **needle localization** (needle or J-wire placed in the area of the abnormality) by the mammographer and x-ray confirmation that the surgical specimen contains the suspicious area.

         (2) **Incisional biopsy.** In rare cases, a wedge of tissue from a **large** mass may be required if core needle biopsy does not yield a diagnosis.

   4. **Psychosocial evaluation.** Once the diagnosis of breast cancer is established, the patient's psychosocial adaptation skills should be evaluated. A baseline profile may help guide therapy, and skilled intervention and counseling should be available to help the patient with emotional problems that may arise throughout the course of therapy.

C. **Optional tests and procedures.** The following tests and procedures may be indicated by either previous diagnostic findings or clinical suspicion.

   1. **Blood tests**

      a. **5´-Nucleotidase** (see p 2, **IV.A.4**).

      b. **GGTP** (see p 2, **IV.A.5**).

      c. **Calcium** (see p 87).

      d. **Carcinoembryonic antigen (CEA).** This tumor-associated antigen is used to detect recurrence and to monitor response to therapy in advanced disease. It also can be used to screen for hepatic metastases and is **elevated in 70% of patients with metastatic disease.**

      e. **CA 15–3.** This monoclonal antibody to a serum tumor-associated antigen is **more sensitive but less specific than CEA,** and is used to detect recurrence and, with metastatic disease, to detect regression or progression.

      f. **Human chorionic gonadotropin (hCG).** This hormone is **elevated** in 50% of patients **with metastatic disease** and, in rare cases, can be used as a tumor marker.

      g. **Ferritin.** Like CEA, Ca 15–3, and hCG, this serum protein is **elevated** in 67% of patients and can be used in rare instances as a tumor marker.

2. **Imaging studies**
    a. **Computed tomography (CT).** CT scan of the chest is the best imaging technique for evaluating internal mammary nodal and pulmonary metastases, although it offers no advantage over mammography alone for the routine evaluation of the breast. CT scan of the abdomen can be used to assess metastatic involvement of the liver and is obtained routinely in patients with advanced disease (Stages III and IV), whereas CT of the head may be necessary to evaluate neurologic symptoms.
    b. **Magnetic resonance imaging (MRI)** (see p 3, **IV.C.3**).
    c. **Ultrasound** (see p 3, **IV.C.4**).
    d. **Technetium-99m bone scan.** In the presence of advanced disease (Stages III and IV), this test is obtained routinely (see also, p 3, **IV.C.5**).
    e. **Breast thermography.** This imaging study remains experimental without proved clinical usefulness because of its poor sensitivity and specificity.
3. **Invasive procedures.** In addition to its use in evaluating primary breast masses, **fine needle aspiration (FNA)** can be used to assess suspicious supraclavicular or cervical lymph nodes and lung, liver, and subcutaneous masses.
VII. **Pathology**
   A. **Location.** The distribution of carcinomas parallels that of normal breast tissue: **48%** in the **upper outer quadrant,** 15% in the upper inner quadrant, 11% in the lower outer quadrant, and 6% in the lower inner quadrant. The **central area** (within 1 cm of the areola) contains **17%,** and 3% are diffuse.
   B. **Multiplicity**
      1. **Multicentricity.** Distinct and separate microscopic tumor foci located in a quadrant remote from the index cancer have been identified in **4–75%** of mastectomy specimens. The clinical significance of these lesions is controversial and has led to widely disparate treatment approaches.
      2. **Bilaterality.** Asynchronous primary tumors in the contralateral breast are found in **4–17%** of patients.
   C. **Histology**
      1. **Noninvasive neoplasms (minimal breast cancer).** These are primarily small (< 1 cm) adenocarcinomas that are **intraductal** or **intralobular** (do not invade the basement membrane). Nearly **67% of all breast lesions** smaller than 1 cm in diameter are noninvasive neoplasms. The exact nature and malignant potential of these lesions are controversial and a topic of intense research.
         a. **Ductal carcinoma in situ (DCIS).** With screening mammography, the incidence of these intraductal cancers has increased to 20–25% of all cancers detected. DCIS is often **microscopic** (palpable in only 50–65%) and **localized** (axillary nodal metastases are present in only 1%).
         b. **Lobular carcinoma in situ (LCIS).** LCIS is often **multicentric, bilateral,** and an incidental finding on biopsy. Although LCIS itself is not a true premalignant lesion, it increases the risk of **invasive ductal carcinoma** 10-fold.
      2. **Invasive neoplasms.** These ductal or lobular adenocarcinomas invade the surrounding stroma.
         a. **Infiltrating ductal (scirrhous) carcinoma (70–80%).** This histologic type has the poorest prognosis of all ductal cancers.
         b. **Infiltrating lobular carcinoma (5–10%).** The prognosis for the patient with lobular carcinoma is better than that for the patient with ductal cancer.
         c. **Medullary carcinoma (5–7%).** Medullary cancer includes both ductal and lobular structures with a diffuse lymphocytic infiltrate. The prognosis is better than that for ductal carcinoma.
         d. **Mucinous or colloid carcinoma (3%).** This tumor is slow growing.
         e. **Tubular carcinoma (1%).** Tubular cancers carry an intermediate prognosis (better than that for ductal but worse than that for medullary cancer).
      3. **Paget's disease (1–4%).** Typically, Paget's disease presents with **eczematoid** changes of the **nipple and areola** accompanied by itching, burning, oozing, bleeding, or all of these. These findings reflect **epidermal invasion by Paget's cells** (large clear malignant cells with small dark nuclei). **Sixty-seven percent** of these patients have an associated **breast mass** representing either invasive or noninvasive cancer.
      4. **Inflammatory breast cancer (1%).** This advanced lesion is marked by edema **(peau d'orange), erythema,** and warmth of the skin as well as a **poor prognosis.** The sine qua non is histologic demonstration of **dermal lymphatic invasion** by tumor cells.

5. **Cystosarcoma phylloides.** This rare, **"leaf-like"** tumor is the **most common nonepithelial breast neoplasm** and has a peak incidence near menopause. Clinically, it presents as a **large,** infiltrating, yet mobile mass that usually is benign and does not involve axillary lymph nodes but may grow rapidly and metastasize unpredictably.

6. **Other neoplasms.** Metastatic cancer from leukemia, lymphoma, small and non-small-cell lung cancer, melanoma, gastric cancer, and renal cell carcinoma may present as a breast mass.

D. **Metastatic spread.** Traditionally, cancer was thought to spread in an orderly fashion from the breast to regional lymph nodes and, subsequently, to distant organs. This concept of stepwise dissemination has been refuted by laboratory and clinical research. These data suggest that **early systemic spread occurs.**

1. **Modes of spread.** Breast cancer spreads primarily via 3 mechanisms:

   a. **Direct extension.** Direct invasion of the breast **parenchyma, ducts, and lymphatics** may lead to involvement of the pectoralis muscles, chest wall, and, occasionally, the overlying skin. With primary tumors less than 4.0 cm in diameter, microscopic tumor foci are found more than **2.0 cm from the primary tumor in 41% and more than 4.0 cm in 11%.**

   b. **Lymphatic metastasis.** Tumor cells readily embolize through breast lymphatics to **axillary, internal mammary, transpectoral, and supraclavicular lymph nodes.** Previously, these nodes were believed to be barriers to distant metastasis, and the Halsted radical mastectomy was based on this concept. Subsequent studies, however, demonstrated that distant hematogenous spread occurs simultaneously and that regional lymph nodes are a preferred site of spread and are an **indicator** of the risk of developing distant metastases.

      (1) **Axillary lymph nodes.** These nodes are involved in **40–50%** of patients (slightly higher for outer-quadrant and slightly lower for inner-quadrant lesions) and, depending on their relationship to the pectoralis minor muscle, consist of **levels I (inferior), II (beneath), and III (superior) nodes.** Nodes at these levels are involved in 54–58%, 20–22%, and 16–22% of cases, respectively. Physical examination of the axilla is associated with a **25% false-positive and 30–40% false-negative rate.** The incidence of positive nodes is directly proportional to tumor size, and the overall prognosis is directly related to the **total** number of involved nodes.

      (2) **Internal mammary lymph nodes.** These lymph nodes are involved more commonly with **inner-quadrant and central lesions (28%)** than with outer-quadrant tumors (14%) and (with all lesions) less often than axillary metastases (42%). Moreover, they are rarely involved in the absence of axillary nodal metastases (8%). Their prognostic significance is the same as for axillary nodal involvement; however, these nodes are much more difficult to biopsy.

   c. **Hematogenous metastasis.** Spread through blood vessels to distant organs occurs earlier than previously believed and is believed to be responsible for the presence of distant metastases in the absence of regional nodal disease.

2. **Sites of metastatic spread.** The most common sites of metastatic spread (by autopsy studies) are the following organs: **regional lymph nodes,** 40–50%; **lung,** 59–69%; **liver,** 56–65%; **bone,** 44–71%; **pleura,** 23–51%; **adrenal glands,** 31–49%; **central nervous system,** 9–22%; and **skin,** 7–34%.

VIII. **Staging.** In 1987 the Union Internationale Contre le Cancer and the American Joint Committee on Cancer adopted a uniform TNM staging system. **Clinical staging** is based on tissue sampling (biopsy), physical examination, chest x-ray, liver enzymes, alkaline phosphatase, and, in some cases, abdominal CT and a bone scan (to exclude liver and bone metastases). **Pathologic staging** is established by pathologic examination of the primary tumor and at least 6 ipsilateral or at least the lowest level (I) of axillary lymph nodes.

A. **Tumor stage**

1. **TX.** Primary tumor cannot be assessed.

2. **T0.** No evidence of a primary tumor is present.

3. **Tis.** Carcinoma in situ: intraductal carcinoma, lobular carcinoma in situ, or Paget's disease of the nipple with no tumor mass.

4. **T1.** Tumor is no larger than 2.0 cm in its greatest dimension.

   a. **T1a.** Tumor is no larger than 0.5 cm in its greatest dimension.

> **b. T1b.** Tumor is larger than 0.5 cm but no larger than 1.0 cm in its greatest dimension.
>
> **c. T1c.** Tumor is larger than 1 cm but less than 2 cm in its greatest dimension.
>
> **5. T2.** Tumor is larger than 2 cm but no larger than 5 cm in its greatest dimension.
>
> **6. T3.** Tumor is larger than 5 cm in its greatest dimension.
>
> **7. T4.** Tumor of any size with direct extension to chest wall or skin.
>
> > **a. T4a.** Tumor extends to the chest wall.
> >
> > **b. T4b.** Edema (including peau d'orange), ulceration of the skin, or satellite skin nodules confined to the same breast are present.
> >
> > **c. T4c.** Both T4a and T4b.
> >
> > **d. T4d.** Inflammatory carcinoma: diffuse brawny induration of the skin with an erysipeloid edge caused by tumor embolization of dermal lymphatics is present.
> >
> > > ***Note:*** If multiple lesions are present, the size of the largest tumor with the designation of multiple ipsilateral primary carcinomas is recorded. If simultaneous bilateral carcinomas are present, each is staged separately.

B. Lymph node stage (clinical)

1. **NX.** Regional lymph nodes cannot be assessed.
2. **N0.** No regional lymph node metastases are present.
3. **N1.** Metastases to movable ipsilateral axillary lymph nodes are present.
4. **N2.** Metastases to ipsilateral axillary lymph nodes fixed to one another or to other structures are present.
5. **N3.** Metastases to ipsilateral internal mammary lymph nodes are present.

C. Lymph node stage (pathologic)

1. **pNX.** Regional lymph nodes cannot be assessed.
2. **pN0.** No regional lymph node metastases are present.
3. **N1.** Metastases to movable ipsilateral axillary lymph nodes are present.
   - **a. pN1a.** Micrometastases (none larger than 0.2 cm) are present.
   - **b. pN1b.** Metastases to lymph nodes larger than 0.2 cm are present.
     - **(1) pN1bi.** Metastases in 1–3 lymph nodes, at least one larger than 0.2 cm and all smaller than 2 cm in their greatest dimension, are present.
     - **(2) pN1bii.** Metastases to at least 4 lymph nodes, at least one larger than 0.2 cm and all less than 2 cm in their greatest dimension are present.
     - **(3) pN1biii.** Extension of tumor beyond the capsule of a lymph node metastasis smaller than 2 cm in its greatest dimension is present.
     - **(4) pN1biv.** Metastases to lymph nodes larger than 2.0 cm in their greatest dimension are present.
4. **pN2.** Metastases to ipsilateral axillary lymph nodes fixed to one another or to other structures are present.
5. **pN3.** Metastases to ipsilateral internal mammary lymph nodes are present.
   > ***Note:*** Regional lymph nodes include axillary and internal mammary nodes; all others (including supraclavicular nodes) are considered to be distant metastases.

D. Metastatic stage

1. **MX.** Distant metastases cannot be assessed.
2. **M0.** No distant metastases are present.
3. **M1.** Distant metastases are present.

E. Histopathologic grade

1. **GX.** Grade cannot be assessed.
2. **G1.** Well differentiated.
3. **G2.** Moderately well differentiated.
4. **G3.** Poorly differentiated.
5. **G4.** Undifferentiated.

F. Stage groupings

1. **Stage 0.** Tis, N0, M0.
2. **Stage I.** T1, N0, M0.
3. **Stage IIA.** T0–1, N1, M0; T2, N0, M0.
4. **Stage IIB.** T2, N1, M0; T3, N0, M0.
5. **Stage IIIA.** T0–3, N2, M0; T3, N1–2, M0.
6. **Stage IIIB.** T4, any N, M0; any T, N3, M0.
7. **Stage IV.** Any T, any N, M1.

IX. Treatment

A. Surgery

1. **Primary breast carcinoma (Stages I and II).** An algorithm for the surgical approach to patients with breast cancer is presented in Figure 53–1.

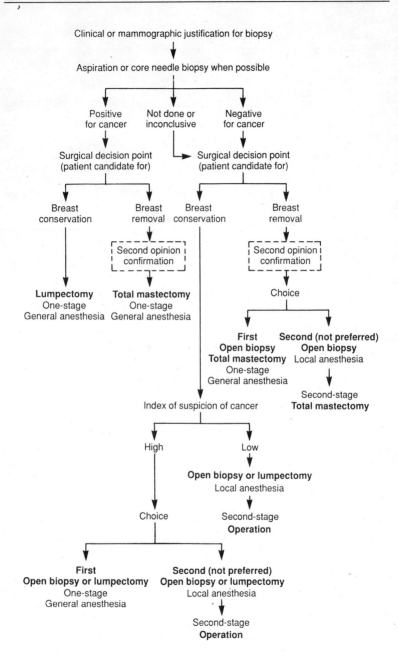

FIGURE 53–1. Summary of the treatment approach for breast abnormalities. *From Fisher B: Reappraisal of breast biopsy prompted by the use of lymphectomy: Surgical strategy. JAMA 253:3586, 1985, with permission.*

a. **General considerations.** In the past 20 years, the surgical approach has changed from radical resection to breast conservation, and the view of breast cancer has simultaneously changed from a local or regional disease to that of a systemic disease. **Trial B04** of the National Surgical Adjuvant Breast Project (NSABP) demonstrated that patient survival with total mastectomy (TM) with axillary dissection (AD) of palpable lymph nodes (TM+AD) was equivalent to radical mastectomy. Subsequently, **NSABP trial B06** established that patient survival with **lumpectomy (L) and axillary dissection followed by regional radiation (RT) (L+AD+RT)** was equivalent to that with TM+AD for **tumors no larger than 4 cm.** Therefore, the 1990 NIH Consensus Conference on Early Stage Breast Cancer recommended breast conservation for Stage I and Stage II disease and endorsed surgical procedures that achieve control of local or regional disease and preserve the breast while offering survival rates equivalent to that of TM+AD.

b. **Indications.** Surgery is indicated as initial therapy for **T0–3, N0–2, M0 lesions (Stages I and II).** In general, **L+AD+RT** is recommended unless (1) the tumor: breast ratio obviates a satisfactory cosmetic result, (2) the patient is unable to obtain or complete postoperative radiation therapy for physical or emotional reasons, (3) multifocal disease is present either by palpation, mammography (diffuse microcalcifications), or biopsy, and (4) the patient prefers a mastectomy. AD is indicated not only to secure regional tumor control but also to obtain important staging and prognostic information. If breast conservation is not possible, **TM+AD** should be performed. Total mastectomy is used for **salvage** in patients with persistent or recurrent disease after L+AD+RT and rarely as **prophylaxis** in high-risk patients. Radical mastectomy is no longer indicated.

c. **Approaches.** For lumpectomy, a **curvilinear incision over the tumor** and parallel with the areola is ideal; however, a **radial incision** may be preferred on the **inferior midbreast** if significant skin and subcutaneous tissue will be resected. Thin skin flaps are not desirable. For axillary dissection, a **transverse axillary incision** that is separate from the lumpectomy incision should be used, even if both incisions are close together. For TM+AD, a **transverse skin incision** is recommended, whereas a **vertical incision** is traditionally used for radical mastectomy.

d. **Procedures.** The following procedures have been used in the local or regional treatment of breast cancer. If previously not obtained, tissue must be submitted during all procedures for measurement of **estrogen and progesterone receptors. DNA-ploidy level, S-phase evaluation, and mitotic index** also should be analyzed and, after further confirmation, may yield important prognostic information.

(1) **Breast conserving operations (lumpectomy, partial or segmental mastectomy, and quadrantectomy).** Lumpectomy consists of wide excision of tumor and enough surrounding normal breast to obtain margins that are grossly and microscopically free of tumor (as determined by the pathologist at the time of surgery). Skin and pectoralis fascia and muscle are **not** included unless they are involved with tumor. For optimal cosmesis, no attempt should be made to **close** or **drain** the dead space. Generally, lumpectomy is accompanied by axillary dissection (see below). **Excisional biopsy** should follow these same technical guidelines because, in this setting, it represents the definitive surgical procedure. **Quadrantectomy** removes an entire breast quadrant along with overlying skin and underlying pectoralis muscle fascia. In a randomized trial survival after quadrantectomy with axillary dissection was shown to be equivalent to that following RM for Stage I disease; however, no advantage over lumpectomy has been documented for this cosmetically inferior procedure.

(2) **Axillary lymphadenectomy.** Axillary dissection is an integral part of surgical staging and includes removal of the axillary contents between the latissimus dorsi muscle posteriorly, the axillary vein superiorly, the medial border of the pectoralis minor muscle anteriorly, the chest wall medially, and the level of the nipple inferiorly. Adequate dissection requires removal of all **Level I and II nodes,** and, in some cases, interpectoral (**Rotter's**) and **Level III** nodes (at least **10 lymph nodes** must be obtained). The nerves to the serratus anterior (**long thoracic** nerve of Bell) and the latissimus dorsi (**thoracodorsal**) muscles should be

identified and preserved. A drain in the axillary bed is recommended for several days.

(3) **Total mastectomy with axillary dissection (modified radical mastectomy).** TM+AD removes the entire breast (including the nipple-areola complex), pectoralis fascia, and axillary contents. The AD generally includes **Level I and Level II lymph nodes.** It also may include dividing or removing the pectoralis minor muscle and excising Level III lymph nodes **(Patey procedure).**

(4) **Total (simple) mastectomy.** In this procedure, the entire breast (including nipple-areola complex) is removed. The **borders** of the dissection are the **clavicle** superiorly, the **sternum** medially, the **rectus** abdominis fascia inferiorly, and the **axilla** laterally.

(5) **Radical mastectomy (Halsted procedure).** This procedure removes the entire breast (including the nipple-areola complex), pectoralis major and minor muscles and fascia, and the ipsilateral axillary contents **(Levels I, II, and III nodes).** The **internal mammary lymph nodes** are excised in an **extended** radical mastectomy.

e. **Breast reconstruction.** The following techniques are used in breast reconstruction following total mastectomy for breast cancer.

(1) **Indications.** Reconstruction should be offered primarily to patients with **Stages I, II, and IIIa** disease who undergo a **total mastectomy.** The primary goal of breast reconstruction is to **restore symmetric breast contour and a nipple-areola complex.** Reconstruction can be performed with **autologous tissue, prosthetic implants, or both,** depending on the presence of adequate skin and soft tissue (eg, pectoralis major muscle), the contour of the contralateral breast, the operative risk, and the patient's preference.

(2) **Procedures with autologous tissue**

(a) **Transverse rectus abdominis myocutaneous (TRAM) flap.** This procedure uses a pedicle flap of **abdominal wall skin, subcutaneous tissue, and underlying rectus abdominis muscle** to reconstruct the breast. This flap provides abundant skin and adipose tissue for reconstruction, and, as an additional benefit, the abdominal wall contour is improved.

(b) **Latissimus dorsi muscle flaps.** Latissimus dorsi muscle or myocutaneous flaps (depending on skin requirements) are useful to recreate bulk lost by removal of the pectoralis major muscle; however, they generally **require an implant** to restore full symmetry.

(c) **Free flaps.** Free rectus abdominis (free TRAM) flaps offer more flexibility than pedicle TRAM flaps. The vascular pedicles are anastomosed to the **thoracodorsal artery and vein.** Although free TRAM flaps are preferred, gluteus maximus and vastus lateralis muscle flaps are acceptable if a TRAM flap is not feasible.

(3) **Prosthetic implants.** Prosthetic implants usually are placed after staged **tissue expansion** to correct the postmastectomy skin deficit. Implants are silicone plastic envelopes filled with silicone gel, saline, or both and generally are placed in a pocket developed **beneath the pectoralis major and serratus anterior muscles.** Implants are particularly well suited for thin or obese patients, who are poor TRAM flap candidates. Other patients who are better suited for implant reconstruction include those with hypertension, diabetes, vascular disease (smokers), and significant abdominal wall scarring from surgery. Because of the recent controversy about the immunologic consequences of silicone gel-filled implants, their use is currently limited and under close surveillance.

(4) **Nipple and areola reconstruction.** The reconstruction of the nipple and areola generally is **delayed,** regardless of the type of breast reconstruction, to correct any breast asymmetry and to determine the optimum location for the nipple-areola complex. The areola may be re-created with full-thickness groin **skin grafts, tattooing,** or areola sharing from the contralateral breast. Nipple reconstruction procedures include use of local **flaps,** contralateral nipple "sharing," or free dermal fat grafts from toe pulp. **"Banking"** of the nipple and areola tissue from

the diseased breast is associated with a **30% recurrence rate** and is not recommended.

(5) **Timing of reconstruction.** The timing of breast reconstruction is flexible. **Immediate reconstruction (33%** of all cases) is becoming increasingly popular because of its psychological and surgical (single operation) advantages. Immediate reconstruction, however, is contraindicated by physiologic instability during surgery, questionable surgical margins, and an ambivalent or unrealistic patient.

f. **Special problems**

(1) **Paget's disease.** Currently, **TM+AD** is indicated for patients with Paget's disease of the nipple, particularly if a palpable mass is present. One study indicated that, in the absence of a palpable mass, total mastectomy alone is sufficient. In addition, limited data from small studies suggest that resection of the nipple-areolar complex and underlying mass, followed by radiation therapy, may be an option, although the latter 2 options are controversial and require confirmation.

(2) **Ductal carcinoma in situ (DCIS).** Formerly, DCIS (intraductal carcinoma) presented with **large, palpable lesions and a high risk (30–70%)** of invasive cancer, requiring a **TM+AD;** however, with the advent of mammography, DCIS lesions are often **small (< 1 cm),** nonpalpable, and amenable to **lumpectomy without axillary dissection.** Recurrences can be treated with a second local procedure (with or without irradiation) or mastectomy with good results. Trials are currently evaluating the value of radiation therapy and systemic therapy.

(3) **Lobular carcinoma in situ (LCIS).** The majority of patients with LCIS do **not** develop invasive carcinoma. Following excisional biopsy with adequate margins, **close follow-up** with breast examination (every 4–6 months) and annual mammography are recommended. Unilateral total mastectomy with contralateral breast biopsy and bilateral total mastectomy are other alternatives. No radiation therapy or systemic treatment is indicated.

(4) **Male breast cancer. TM+AD** is indicated for male patients, although a high incidence of pectoralis muscle invasion frequently necessitates radical mastectomy. Postoperative radiation therapy to the chest wall may improve local control.

2. **Locally advanced breast cancer (Stage III).** Treatment for Stage III breast cancer involves **multimodality therapy** (surgery, radiation, and chemotherapy) because of the high **local-regional recurrence rate (50–67%),** but the optimal regimen is controversial. **TM+AD** with either pre- or postoperative radiation or both and chemotherapy is indicated in locally advanced but **operable** breast cancer **(Stage IIIa).** Locally advanced and **inoperable** breast cancer **(Stage IIIb)** is initially treated with induction chemotherapy and radiation. If a significant response subsequently renders the tumor operable, then **TM+AD** is performed.

3. **Metastatic breast cancer (Stage IV)**

a. **Primary site.** For primary lesions, **lumpectomy,** if possible, is indicated to confirm the diagnosis, achieve local control, and obtain tumor for measurement of **estrogen and progesterone receptors.** Total mastectomy can be used for palliation in patients with bulky local disease and distant metastases. Axillary dissection is appropriate only to control clinically evident nodal disease.

b. **Metastatic sites.** Surgery for metastatic disease is strictly **palliative.** Local recurrences after lumpectomy should be treated by total mastectomy, although local reexcision is being studied. Excisional biopsy (for diagnosis and receptor status) is indicated if a mastectomy was previously performed. Symptomatic metastases may be excised if **technically possible,** and **minimal morbidity** results. Surgical **ablation of endocrine organs**—eg, oophorectomy in premenopausal females, adrenalectomy and hypophysectomy in postmenopausal females, and orchiectomy in males may produce significant palliation in a few cases.

4. **Morbidity and mortality.** The mortality rate of all the procedures just described should be near 0%. The complication rate, however, may be substantial and depends on the type of surgical procedure as well as the type and extent (if any) of perioperative adjuvant therapy. Common problems include the following:

a. **Lumpectomy/mastectomy (all types):** wound infection, hemorrhage or hematoma, seroma, skin necrosis, breast fibrosis, and persistent positive margins.

b. **Axillary dissection (see, also, a above):** lymphedema and nerve injury (thoracodorsal and long thoracic nerves).

c. **Breast reconstruction.** Implant-induced adverse immunologic responses are controversial and are being investigated. Furthermore, reconstruction does not increase the local recurrence rate or make it more difficult to detect recurrent cancer.

(1) **Capsular contraction (prostheses)** occurs in 40–50% of patients and causes loss of natural ptosis, superior migration, and rounding of the breast contour and requires capsulotomy (capsule release).

(2) **Hemorrhage or hematoma; infection, flap ischemia and necrosis, skin necrosis, or prosthesis exposure.**

B. **Radiation therapy**

1. **Primary breast carcinoma (Stages I and II).** Currently, radiation therapy as the initial treatment for **resectable** breast cancer is **not** indicated.

2. **Adjuvant radiation therapy**

a. **Preoperative radiotherapy.** Radiation therapy before resection of early breast cancer (Stages I and II) has not been studied.

b. **Postoperative radiotherapy**

(1) **Indications.** Postoperative adjuvant radiation therapy is used in conjunction with breast conserving surgery (eg, lumpectomy) as part of the primary treatment of early stage disease to destroy microscopic tumor foci and prevent local recurrence. After 9 years of NSABP trial B06, follow-up showed that patients treated with L+AD+RT had a lower recurrence rate (10%) than did those treated with L+AD alone (40%). The third group of patients, treated with TM+AD, also had a 10% local recurrence rate. More important, survival in the 3 groups was equivalent. To date, there is **no indication that radiation therapy increases the risk of secondary neoplasms or contralateral breast cancer.** In contrast, adjuvant radiotherapy is not recommended for patients receiving TM+AD. Although previous studies showed a decrease in the locoregional recurrence rate following TM+AD with radiation therapy, a clear survival advantage was not demonstrated. Some studies actually suggest a decrease in survival for irradiated patients.

(2) **Approach.** The NIH Consensus Conference on Early Stage Breast Cancer in 1990 recommended treatment to the entire breast **in 180–200 cGy daily fractions to a total of 4500–5000 cGy** after lumpectomy. Irradiation of the axilla was not advised, especially if a Level I and II axillary dissection was performed. The Joint Center for Radiation Therapy (JCRT) studied the use of supplemental radiation boost to the primary site, particularly in cases of focal microscopic involvement of the margins or incompletely excised tumors. To date, however, a survival advantage has not been proved.

3. **Locally advanced breast cancer (Stage III).** In conjunction with surgery and chemotherapy, radiotherapy plays a significant role in locally advanced breast cancer. Although the optimum regimen for locally advanced but **operable** breast cancer (Stage IIIa) is unknown, data support the use of **postoperative adjuvant radiation** and chemotherapy following mastectomy to reduce the local recurrence rate. In locally advanced and **inoperable** breast carcinoma (Stage IIIb), nonrandomized retrospective studies using multimodality therapy demonstrate **improved 5-year disease-free survival (40% vs 26%) and overall survival (51% vs 38%).** Two approaches are used: (1) **after induction chemotherapy** and before further systemic therapy, either definitive radiation is administered or a (mastectomy is performed) if the tumor is too large for radiation implantation, the cosmetic appearance is poor, or N2 or N3 nodes were absent initially and (2) **initial** radiation therapy is given at doses higher than 6000 cGy, followed by mastectomy, then chemotherapy. In this setting, the JCRT recommends **4500 cGy in fractions of 180 cGy/d, followed by a 3000 boost** to the primary site. Additional doses to the axilla are required if nodes are clinically involved.

4. **Metastatic disease.** Because breast cancer is a radiosensitive tumor, radiation therapy is used in a palliative fashion to effect local control of disease. Chest wall recurrences treated with radiation therapy will show an initial response of

63–79%; however, 33–66% of patients will have a recurrence. Palliative radiation is indicated for symptomatic **bone** (particularly vertebrae or pelvis), **spine** (to prevent spinal cord compression), and **CNS** metastases.

5. **Morbidity and mortality.** Improved technique has decreased the incidence of the following complications: **fatigue; skin changes** (erythema, desquamation, and hyperpigmentation); **rib fractures; breast and arm edema,** with fibrosis and subsequent nipple or breast retraction or decreased arm mobility; **radiation pneumonitis; radiation pericarditis;** and **peripheral neuropathy,** including brachial plexus disorders.

C. **Hormonal and chemotherapy.** The use of chemotherapy and hormonal therapy (systemic treatment) in conjunction with surgery and radiotherapy (local treatment) stems from the understanding that most patients with breast cancer have disseminated metastases at the time of diagnosis. Numerous clinical trials have been conducted and others are currently ongoing to identify effective agents, the timing and route of administration, the duration of therapy, and the patient subsets most likely to benefit from systemic therapy. At present, therapy varies with stage of disease, nodal involvement, and menopausal status.

1. **Primary breast carcinoma (Stages I and II).** Neither hormonal nor cytotoxic therapy is sufficient initial therapy for primary breast cancer; however, both are used as adjuvant therapy in conjunction with surgery and radiation.

   a. **Node-positive patients.** Adjuvant therapy (administered shortly after surgery) should be considered for all patients with node positive breast cancer because the 10-year relapse rate is 40% or more. The therapeutic approach varies with menopausal status. The NIH Consensus Conference on Adjuvant Therapy in 1985 based the current treatment recommendations on randomized clinical trials.

      (1) **Premenopausal (< 50 years of age)**

         (a) **Chemotherapy.** The NSABP B-05 and Milan CMF trials demonstrated that adjuvant cytotoxic chemotherapy improves disease-free survival and overall survival in premenopausal patients with positive lymph nodes. Patients with **1–3 involved nodes** benefit the most. These findings were confirmed by subsequent trials and led the NIH Consensus Conference to recommend combination chemotherapy for these patients regardless of their hormonal receptor status. The regimen of **cyclophosphamide, methotrexate, and fluorouracil (CMF)** is currently the most widely used one (see Appendix D) and is recommended for these patients. Doxorubicin-based combinations (AC, FAC, and AVCF) also are common. A treatment period of **4–6 months** appears optimal.

         (b) **Hormonal therapy.** No significant survival advantage has been observed with the addition of adjuvant hormonal therapy to the chemotherapy regimen outlined above.

      (2) **Postmenopausal (≥ 50 years of age)**

         (a) **Chemotherapy.** To date, individual trials have not demonstrated an advantage regarding overall survival from the administration of adjuvant chemotherapy in these patients. NSABP trial B-16, however, recently demonstrated prolonged disease-free survival and overall survival in postmenopausal node positive (≥ 4), estrogen receptor positive (ER+) patients treated with short-course cyclophosphamide and doxorubicin and a prolonged course of tamoxifen (compared with tamoxifen alone). This suggests a role for combination chemotherapy in this patient cohort. Until more data is available, however, chemotherapy should be administered to these patients only in the context of a clinical trial.

         (b) **Hormonal therapy.** Randomized trials demonstrate prolonged DFS and OS with adjuvant tamoxifen. The 1990 NIH Consensus Conference recommended **tamoxifen** (20 mg/d for 5 years) as **standard therapy** for postmenopausal, estrogen receptor positive patients.

   b. **Node-negative patients.** Nearly 67% of patients with Stage I or II breast cancer have **no nodal involvement** at the time of axillary dissection, but as many as 30% of these node-negative patients develop a recurrence within 10 years and die of metastatic breast cancer. Until recently, the toxicity of adjuvant treatment was thought to outweigh the benefit in these patients. However, recent data, including a systematic analysis of multiple clinical trials (meta-analysis), demonstrate a role for adjuvant therapy in these patients. Although controversy exists regarding the magnitude of the perceived benefits and toxicities for the individual patient, the results prompted the 1990 NIH Consensus Conference on Early Stage Breast Cancer to recommend that these patients should be encouraged to participate in randomized clinical trials that further evaluate this therapy.

   (a) **Chemotherapy.** Follow-up data (after 4 years) from 3 prospective randomized trials involving more than 2300 pre- and postmenopausal node-negative patients (mostly estrogen receptor negative [ER–]) demonstrate improved disease-free survival and, in some groups, overall survival for patients receiving a combination of cytotoxic drugs compared with control patients treated without systemic therapy (Mansour et al, 1989; Ludwig Breast Cancer Study Group, 1989; and Fisher et al, 1989).

   (b) **Hormonal therapy.** NSABP trial B-14 showed that the disease-free survival of ER+ node-negative patients treated with tamoxifen (10mg twice daily) improved regardless of age (83% vs 77% with placebo; p < 0.00001). Meta-analysis of 30,000 patients by the Early Breast Cancer Trialists Collaborative Group also demonstrated a highly significant reduction in annual recurrence and death rates in patients receiving tamoxifen. In addition, the risk of contralateral breast cancer was reduced by 39%.

2. **Locally advanced breast carcinoma (Stage III)**
   a. **Chemotherapy.** Although the optimum regimen for locally advanced but **operable** breast cancer (Stage IIIa) is evolving, data support the use of **postoperative adjuvant chemotherapy** and radiation following mastectomy to reduce the rate of local recurrence. For locally advanced and **inoperable** breast carcinoma (Stage IIIb), preoperative chemotherapy may reduce the size of the tumor, rendering it resectable. Multiple nonrandomized uncontrolled prospective trials have used induction chemotherapy—eg, **cyclophosphamide, methotrexate, and fluorouracil (CMF);** fluorouracil, doxorubicin, and cyclophosphamide **(FAC);** and thiotepa, methotrexate, fluorouracil, doxorubicin, and vinblastine **(TMFAVs)**—for 4–8 months followed by radiotherapy, surgery, or both. These trials demonstrate **15% complete and up to 90% overall response rates** as well as improved 5-year DFS disease-free survival (28–60%) and overall survival (48–60%) compared with historical controls treated with radiation and surgery alone.
   b. **Hormonal therapy.** To date, the exact role of hormonal therapy in the treatment of Stage III breast cancer has not been completely defined.

3. **Metastatic breast cancer (Stage IV).** Although metastatic breast cancer is incurable, 50–70% of patients will experience significant palliation of disease with hormonal therapy, chemotherapy, or both. The choice of initial therapy often is based on the patient's age (menopausal status), overall performance status, and the aggressiveness of the tumor.
   a. **Chemotherapy.** Chemotherapy in metastatic disease should be reserved for patients who have failed initial hormonal therapy or have aggressive disease: ie, ER– tumor with widespread visceral metastases (particularly lung and liver), a brief disease-free interval, and poor patient-performance status. Previous hormonal therapy does not reduce the likelihood of response to subsequent chemotherapy and vice versa.
      (1) **Single agents.** The most effective single agents and their response rates include **cisplatin (47%), doxorubicin (32–37%),** mechlorethamine (35%), **cyclophosphamide (34%), methotrexate (28–34%), thiotepa (30%), fluorouracil (27%),** ifosfamide (27%), vinca alkaloids (20–22%), mitomycin-C (20–22%), and L-phenylalanine mustard (20%). However, because most studies demonstrate significantly higher complete and overall response rates as well as improved survival with combination chemotherapy, multiple cytotoxic agents are generally administered (see below).
      (2) **Combination chemotherapy.** Combination regimens most frequently used to treat metastatic breast cancer are shown in Appendix D. **Objective response rates of 50–70% with 10–20% complete responses** are common, and the median duration of response and survival is 7–13 months and 12–24 months, respectively. Although the optimal duration of chemotherapy is unknown, **6 months of therapy** in the presence of stable disease is currently recommended. Once pa-

tients fail initial chemotherapy, response rates are only **15–30% and median survival is 4–12 months with salvage regimens** such as vinblastine, doxorubicin, thiotepa, and fluoxymesterone (Halotestin; **VATH**), fluorouracil, and either mitomycin-C **(FMm)** or leucovorin **(FLv)** and methotrexate, mitomycin-C, and teniposide **(MMmTp).** Trials studying dose intensification are in progress. In addition, recent studies using high-dose chemotherapy with either hematopoietic growth factors (G-CSF and GM-CSF) or **autologous bone marrow transplantation** report high rates of **complete response (35–50%);** however, the median disease-free and overall survival are similar to those achieved with conventional chemotherapy.

b. **Hormonal therapy.** Hormonal therapy remains the major source of palliation for patients with advanced breast cancer. The likelihood of response increases with ER+ tumors (see Table 53–2), a **DFI > 2 years, bone and soft tissue** disease, **late premenopausal or postmenopausal** status, and a **previous response** to hormonal therapy. The response time may be long (6–12 weeks). With the exception of androgens and corticosteroids, all hormonal manipulations are **equally effective.** In addition, because combinations are no better than single agents, the choice of therapy should be based on knowledge of the associated toxicities. The following are current recommendations for advanced breast cancer:

(1) **Premenopausal patients** should receive **tamoxifen** or undergo oophorectomy, followed by progestins and subsequently aminoglutethimide (250 mg PO 2–4 times daily) with hydrocortisone (40 mg/d).

(2) **Postmenopausal patients** should be given **tamoxifen,** followed by progestins, aminoglutethimide (with hydrocortisone), and estrogens or androgens. Patients who fail initial hormonal therapy should be given chemotherapy, whereas those who respond can be treated with a different hormonal maneuver on relapse. Specific hormonal maneuvers that can be used include (in order of increasing toxicity):

(a) **Tamoxifen (20 mg/day PO for at least 2 years).** This anti-estrogen agent is the initial hormonal therapy for ER+ patients regardless of menopausal status. Nearly 60% of these patients experience objective regression with a median duration of response of **12 months,** and few toxicities exist.

(b) **Ovarian ablation.** Effective only in **premenopausal** patients (particularly those older than **35**), oophorectomy can be accomplished with either **surgery or irradiation.** This produces a **25–30% response rate** lasting a median of **9–12 months;** however, less than 6% of postmenopausal females respond.

(c) **Progestins.** Either medroxyprogesterone acetate (400 mg PO daily) or megestrol acetate (40 mg PO 4 times daily) have been used as second- or third-line therapy and have **response rates of 20–30%.**

(d) **Aminoglutethimide (250 mg PO 2–4 times daily).** This **aromatase inhibitor** (with 40 mg of hydrocortisone daily) suppresses the adrenal secretion of estrogens. Responses occur in as many as **40–50%** of patients, particularly in those with **bone** metastases, and last a **median of 17 months.** Toxicities include **lethargy,** skin rash, and CNS symptoms. Patients also must receive hydrocortisone (40 mg daily) to replace the suppressed endogenous corticosteroids.

(e) **Luteinizing-hormone-releasing hormone (LHRH) analogs.** Ex-

TABLE 53–2. RESPONSE RATE TO HORMONAL MANIPULATION BY ESTROGEN AND PROGESTERONE (ER/PR) STATUS

Status	Response Rate (%)
ER–, PR–	6–9
ER+, PR–	32–46
ER+, PR+	71–81

perimental LHRH analogs such as **buserelin** and **leuprolide** produce responses in **39–44%** of both pre- and postmenopausal females.

- **(f) Estrogens and androgens.** The most frequently used estrogens are **diethylstilbestrol** (5 mg PO 3 times daily), **ethinyl estradiol** (1 mg PO 3 times daily), and **premarin** (2.5 mg PO 3 times daily). **Fluoxymesterone** (10 mg PO 2–4 times daily) and **testosterone propionate** (100 mg IM 3 times weekly) are common androgens. The mechanism of action is not well understood.
- **(g) Adrenalectomy.** Adrenalectomy is rarely performed today because of numerous side effects.
- **(h) Hypophysectomy.** Like adrenalectomy, hypophysectomy is rarely indicated.
- **(i) Orchiectomy.** Bilateral orchiectomy has been used with some success in the treatment of male breast cancer.

4. **Morbidity and mortality**
   - **a. Chemotherapy.** The complications from combination chemotherapy may be considerable and include the following problems: **nausea and vomiting,** 4–19%; **leukopenia,** 13–28%; **musculoskeletal pain,** 8–29%; **hot flashes,** 3–71%; **neurologic sequelae,** 7–22%; **stomatitis,** 7–11%; **infection,** 1–5%; **thrombophlebitis,** 0.5–4%; and **thrombocytopenia,** 1–10%.
   - **b. Hormonal therapy.** In general, the side effects of hormonal therapy are minimal; however, some complications are distressing and may prompt 10% of patients to discontinue therapy. Side effects include **menopausal symptoms** such as hot flashes and menstrual irregularity, 19–57%; **thromboembolism,** 1–3%; **tumor "flare,"** exacerbation of previous symptoms often in association with hypercalcemia (3–9%); **masculinization** occurs in 50% with androgens; and **fluid retention.**

D. **Immunotherapy.** The use of immunomodulatory agents in the treatment of breast cancer remains anecdotal and should be considered experimental.

X. **Prognosis**

A. **Risk of recurrence.** Nearly **90%** of all recurrences are detected **within 5 years** (38% within 1 year and 60% within 2 years). New evidence indicates that local recurrence should be perceived as a marker of a more aggressive systemic disease as opposed to a failure of local surgical control, necessitating the need for more aggressive systemic therapy. The risk of local and systemic recurrence at 5 and 10 years is related to the number of involved lymph nodes. Once metastatic disease is diagnosed, survival is severely limited.

B. **Five- and 10-year survival. Overall 5-year and 10-year survival** for patients with breast cancer is **64% and 46%,** respectively, and is summarized below by nodal status and TNM stage:

1. **Nodal status**
   - **a. No involved lymph nodes:** 78% and 65%.
   - **b. Only 1–3 involved lymph nodes:** 62% and 38%.
   - **c. Four or more involved lymph nodes:** 32% and 13%.
2. **Pathologic stage**
   - **a. Stage I.** 80% and 65%.
   - **b. Stage IIA.** 75% and 55%.
   - **c. Stage IIB.** 75% and 45%.
   - **d. Stage IIIA.** 55% and 40%.
   - **e. Stage IIIB.** 35% and 20%.
   - **f. Stage IV.** 10% and 5%.

C. **Adverse prognostic factors.** Independent prognostic factors (tumor size and axillary lymph node involvement) and other adverse prognostic influences are summarized below:

1. **Tumor size.** Studies indicate that the larger the tumor, the greater the incidence of lymph node and distant metastases and thus, a poorer prognosis.
2. **Axillary lymph node involvement.** This is the **single most accurate prognostic factor.**
   - **a. No involved lymph nodes.** The 5-year disease-free survival and overall survival are 82% and 78%, respectively.
   - **b. Patients with 1–3 involved lymph nodes.** The 5-year disease-free survival is 50% and the overall survival is 47%.
   - **c. Patients with 4 or more positive nodes.** The 5-year disease-free survival is 21% and the overall survival is **32%.**

3. **Hormone receptor status.** Patients with ER+ and PR+ tumors exhibit a longer disease-free and overall survival than do those with receptor-negative tumors because of a greater likelihood of response to endocrine therapy. Nearly **67%** of all patients are ER+ (postmenopausal > premenopausal), and **50%** of them will respond to endocrine therapy.
4. **Histologic (nuclear) grade.** High nuclear grade (bizarre shapes, tubule formation, hyperchromatism, and frequent mitoses) is designated **Grade 3** (poorly differentiated) and is associated with a poor prognosis.
5. **Histologic types.** Unfavorable histologic types include **inflammatory, undifferentiated, and infiltrating ductal carcinoma.** Tubular, mucinous, papillary, adenoid cystic, secretory, and medullary carcinoma have a more favorable prognosis.
6. **Proliferative rate (S phase).** [3]Thymidine-labeling of cultured tumor cells measures proliferation. Rapid tumor growth (high S phase) is associated with a poor prognosis.
7. **Aneuploidy.** Although still under investigation, aneuploidy may portend an unfavorable outcome.
8. **Oncogene expression.** Preliminary data suggest that high expression of the **c-erbB-2 (HER-2/neu)** oncogene is associated with brief disease-free and overall survival in node-positive patients.
9. **Lymphatic invasion.** Lymphatic emboli occur in **25%** of tumors and predict poor survival.
10. **Vascular invasion.** Vascular invasion is often present in patients with 4 or more positive lymph nodes and portends a poor prognosis.

XI. **Patient follow-up**
  A. **General guidelines.** Patients with breast carcinoma treated with curative intent should be followed every 3 months for 3 years, every 6 months for an additional 2 years, and then annually for evidence of tumor recurrence or second malignancies. Patients with metastatic disease should be followed every 3 months for symptoms requiring palliative measures and for nutritional monitoring. Specific guidelines for following patients with breast cancer are listed below.
  B. **Routine evaluation.** Each clinic visit should include the following examinations:
    1. **Medical history and physical examination.** An interval medical history should be taken and a thorough physical examination should be performed during each office visit. Areas for particular attention are discussed on p 419, **VI.A.**
    2. **Complete blood count** (see p 1, **IV.A.1**).
    3. **Hepatic transaminases** (see p 1, **IV.A.2**).
    4. **Alkaline phosphatase** (see p 1, **IV.A.3**).
    5. **Calcium.** This serum electrolyte may indicate the presence of occult bone disease.
  C. **Additional evaluation.** Other tests that should be obtained at regular intervals include the following examinations.
    1. **Chest x-ray.** A screening chest radiograph is necessary **every 6–12 months** (see p 3, **IV.C.1**).
    2. **Mammography.** An **annual** mammogram should be obtained to exclude metachronous lesions in the ipsilateral (if present) and contralateral breast.
  D. **Optional evaluation.** The following examinations may be indicated depending on previous findings or clinical suspicion.
    1. **Blood tests**
      a. **5′-Nucleotidase** (see p 2, **IV.A.4**).
      b. **GGTP** (see p 2, **IV.A.5**).
      c. **Carcinoembryonic antigen (CEA).** CEA is not useful in early (Stages I and II) breast cancer; however, in **advanced (Stages III and IV)** disease, it is the **most reliable marker** to monitor response to therapy.
    2. **Imaging studies**
      a. **Computed tomography (CT)**
        (1) **Chest CT.** Chest CT scan remains a good method of detecting pulmonary metastases. In patients with no residual tumor, a chest CT scan should be obtained if suspicious findings are identified on chest x-ray.
        (2) **Abdominal CT.** CT scan of the abdomen is the most sensitive test for excluding liver metastases and should be ordered if symptoms or blood tests suggest the possibility of liver disease.
        (3) **Head CT.** CT scan of the head should be obtained if neurologic symptoms occur.
      b. **Magnetic resonance imaging (MRI)** (see p 3, **IV.C.3**).

    c. Technetium-99m bone scan (see p 3, **IV.C.5**).
   3. Invasive diagnostic procedures. In a patient without known residual cancer, a biopsy of any suspicious or abnormal mass detected on physical examination, chest x-ray, or routine blood testing is indicated.

REFERENCES

Bonadonna, G. Valagussa, P, Rossi, A, et al. Ten-year experience with CMF-based adjuvant chemotherapy in resectable breast cancer. Breast Cancer Res Treat 5:95–115, 1985.

Bookman, MA, Goldstein, LJ, and Scheer, RM. Medical management of early-stage breast cancer. Curr Prob Cancer 15(4):161–231, 1991.

Early Breast Cancer Trialists' Collaborative Group. Effects of adjuvant tamoxifen and of cytotoxic therapy on mortality in early breast cancer: an overview of 61 randomized trials among 28,896 women. NEJM 319(26):1681–1692, 1988.

Early Breast Cancer Trialists' Collaborative Group. Systemic treatment of early breast cancer by hormonal, cytotoxic or immune therapy. Lancet 339 no. 8784:1–15 and 8785:71–85, 1992.

Fisher, B. A Biological perspective of breast cancer: contributions of the National Surgical Adjuvant Breast and Bowel Project clinical trials. Ca-A Cancer Journal for Clinicians. 41(2):97–109, 1991.

Fisher, B. Breast Cancer. In Cancer Medicine. Holland, JF and Frei, E., eds. Lea and Febiger, Malvern, PA: 3rd ed., 1991.

Fisher, B. et al. Eight year results of a randomized clinical trial comparing total mastectomy and lumpectomy with or without radiation in the treatment of breast cancer. NEJM 320(13):822–828, 1989a.

Fisher, B, Redmond, C, Dimitrov, NV, et al. A randomized clinical trial evaluating sequential methotrexate and fluorouracil in the treatment of patients with node-negative breast cancer who have estrogen-receptor-negative tumors. NEJM 320(8):473–478, 1989b.

Fisher, B, Costantino, J, Redmond, C, et al. A randomized clinical trial evaluating tamoxifen in the treatment of patients with node-negative breast cancer who have estrogen-receptor-positive tumors. NEJM 320(8):479–484, 1989c.

Fisher, B. Reappraisal of breast biopsy prompted by the use of lumpectomy: surgical strategy. JAMA 253(24):3585–3588, 1985.

Fisher, B, Fisher, ER, Redmond, C, et al. Ten-year results from the National Surgical Adjuvant Breast and Bowel Project (NSABP) clinical trial evaluating the use of 1-phenylalanine mustard (L-PAM) in the management of primary breast cancer. J Clin Oncol 4(6):929–941, 1986.

Fisher, B, Redmond, C, Fisher, ER, et al. Ten-year results of a randomized clinical trial comparing radical mastectomy and total mastectomy with or without radiation. NEJM 312:674–681, 1985.

Fisher, ER, Sass, R, and Fisher, B. Pathologic findings from the National Surgical Adjuvant Project for Breast Cancers (Protocol no. 4): discriminants for tenth year treatment failure. Cancer 53:712, 1984.

Fisher, B, Redmond, C, Brown, A, et al. Influence of tumor estrogen and progesterone receptor levels on the response to tamoxifen and chemotherapy in primary breast cancer. J Clin Oncol 1(2):227–241, 1983.

Fisher, B, Redmond, C, Legault-Poisson, S, et al. Postoperative chemotherapy and tamoxifen compared with tamoxifen alone in the treatment of positive-node breast cancer patients aged 50 years and older with tumors responsive to tamoxifen: results from the National Surgical Adjuvant Breast and Bowel Project B-16. J Clin Oncol 8(6):1005–1018, 1990.

Griem, KL, Henderson, IC, Gelman, R, et al. The 5-year results of a randomized trial of adjuvant radiation therapy after chemotherapy in breast cancer treated with mastectomy. J Clin Oncol 5:1546–1555, 1987.

Lippmann, ME, Lichter, AS, and Danforth D. Diagnosis and Management of Breast Cancer. WB Saunders Co., Philadelphia: 1988.

Ludwig Breast Cancer Study Group. Prolonged disease-free survival after one course of perioperative adjuvant chemotherapy for node-negative breast cancer. NEJM 320(8):491–496, 1989.

Mansour, EG, Gray, R, Shatila, AH, et al. Efficacy of adjuvant chemotherapy in high-risk node-negative breast cancer: an Intergroup study. NEJM 320(8):485–490, 1989.

Margolese, R, Poisson, R, Shibata, H, et al. The technique of segmental mastectomy (lumpectomy) and axillary dissection: a syllabus from the National Surgical Adjuvant Breast Project workshops. Surgery 102(5):828–834, 1987.

Najarian, JS., ed. Progress in Cancer Surgery. Mosby Year Book, Inc., Philadelphia: pp. 51–65, 1991.

National Institutes of Health Consensus Conference. Treatment of early stage breast cancer. JAMA 265(3):391–395, 1991.

National Institutes of Health Consensus Development Panel. Adjuvant chemotherapy and endocrine therapy for breast cancer. JAMA 254:3461–3463, 1985.

Sheldon, T, Hayes, DF, Cady B, et al. Primary radiation therapy for locally advanced breast cancer. Cancer 60:1219–1225, 1987.

Veronesi, U, Zucali, R, and Luini, A. Local control and survival in early breast cancer. The Milan trial. Int J Radiat Oncol Biol Phys 12:717–720, 1986.

54 Malignancies of the Brain

Carl B. Heilman, MD, and Stephen Saris, MD

I. **Epidemiology.** Malignancies of the central nervous system (CNS) are relatively uncommon, constituting only **1.7%** of all cancers. In 1985, **7.5** cases per 100,000 males and **5.1** cases per 100,000 females were diagnosed, leading to **4.9** and **3.3** deaths per 100,000, respectively. Estimates indicate that **17,500 new cases** and **12,100 deaths** will occur in the United States in 1993 from primary brain neoplasms.

II. **Risk factors**
   A. **Age.** Excluding leukemia, malignancies of the CNS are the most common type of cancer in children: **3.1** cases per 100,000 occur each year in **children under 5 years of age.** The incidence then declines to 1.8 cases per 100,000 by the age of 10 and gradually increases thereafter to **20.1** cases per 100,000 over the age of **75.**
   B. **Sex.** American males are **1.47 times** more likely than females to develop a CNS malignancy.
   C. **Race.** Caucasians are **1.5 times** more likely than blacks to develop a CNS malignancy.
   D. **Genetic factors**
      1. **Family history.** First-degree relatives of patients with CNS tumors are not at an increased risk of developing brain malignancies. However, several glioma kindreds have been identified with genetic abnormalities of **chromosomes 17 and 22.**
      2. **Familial syndromes.** Several inherited syndromes have been associated with an increased risk of CNS malignancies.
         a. **Neurofibromatosis.** Gliomas (optic glioma, astrocytoma) have been associated with neurofibromatosis, an autosomal dominant disorder with incomplete penetrance marked by cutaneous pigmented lesions (cafe au lait spots), subcutaneous neurofibromas, bony and mesenchymal abnormalities, and brain tumors.
         b. **Tuberous sclerosis. Subependymal giant-cell astrocytoma and gliomatosis cerebri** are more frequent in patients with tuberous sclerosis, an inherited disorder characterized by **ash-leaf spots,** acneiform skin lesions, angiofibromas, periungual fibromas, epilepsy, periventricular hamartomas, and mental retardation.
         c. **Turcot syndrome.** Familial polyposis of the colon associated with CNS malignancies has been well described.
   E. **History of previous CNS pathology**
      1. **Viral infection.** Although infection with the human immunodeficiency virus (HIV) and the Epstein-Barr virus increase the risk of **primary CNS lymphoma,** no relationship between viral infections and other human nervous system malignancies has been demonstrated.
      2. **Radiation.** Occasional cases of fibrosarcoma or **malignant glioma** have occurred in the radiation field used for pituitary or parasellar tumors. In addition, children with leukemia who received chemotherapy and prophylactic radiation to the CNS have subsequently developed malignant brain tumors. However, proof that an increased risk of CNS malignancies exists after radiation therapy remains anecdotal.
   F. **Urbanization.** Urban dwellers are not at increased risk of developing CNS malignancies. Although industrial workers exposed to **vinyl chloride** were once believed to be at increased risk of gliomas, this has recently been challenged.

III. **Presentation**
   A. **Signs and symptoms**
      1. **Local manifestations.** The presenting signs and symptoms of nervous system malignancies depend on the tumor type and its location.
         a. **Tumors of the cerebral hemispheres.** Supratentorial malignancies usu-

ally present with local irritation of gray matter (ie, **seizures;** 20%), destruction or swelling of the brain (**weakness, sensory changes,** abnormalities of vision, difficulty with speech), or elevated intracranial pressure (**headache, nausea and vomiting,** personality change). Patients with low-grade malignancies (astrocytomas) tend to present with seizures, whereas those with high-grade tumors (glioblastomas) more commonly present with headaches, although seizures and focal neurological deficits also are common. It should be noted that the new onset of focal seizures in an adult should be considered evidence of a brain tumor until proved otherwise.

  b. Tumors of the cerebellum. Patients with infratentorial malignancies often present with **gait disturbance.** If the neoplasm blocks the outflow from the fourth ventricle, however, symptoms of increased intracranial pressure and **hydrocephalus** (headache, nausea, and vomiting) develop. Tumors of the **brainstem** typically produce a combination of **cranial nerve dysfunction** and gait disturbance. If the aqueduct of Sylvius is obstructed, the presenting symptoms, again, are those of increased intracranial pressure and hydrocephalus.

  2. Systemic manifestations. Other than nausea and vomiting, systemic signs and symptoms are uncommon with primary CNS malignancies.

 B. Herniation syndromes. Increased intracranial pressure causing herniation of portions of the brain through various foramina can be life threatening.

  1. Temporal lobe-tentorial herniation. With increasing tumor size and surrounding edema, pressure may cause the temporal lobe to herniate over the edge of the **tentorium.** The earliest sign of transtentorial herniation is a change in the patient's **level of consciousness. Dilation of the ipsilateral pupil** secondary to compression of the third cranial nerve, **ipsilateral hemiplegia** (occasionally contralateral hemiplegia from bilateral compression of cerebral peduncles), homonymous hemianopia, progressive brainstem dysfunction, decorticate and decerebrate posturing, coma, and death follow if the swelling is not rapidly reversed.

  2. Cerebellar-foramen magnum herniation. Although rare, this syndrome is often complicated by hydrocephalus and presents with signs and symptoms that progress from head tilt and stiffness, posturing, and paresthesia of the neck to cerebellar fits (tonic extensor spasms of the limbs), coma, and death. This rapid progression often can be aborted by emergency removal of ventricular fluid and ventricular-peritoneal shunting.

 C. Paraneoplastic syndromes. Paraneoplastic disorders have not been described with primary brain tumors.

IV. Differential diagnosis. The differential diagnosis of a brain tumor depends on the patient's **age** and the tumor's location and appearance on CT or MRI imaging. In **children, infections** (cerebritis and brain abscesses), **vascular abnormalities** (cavernous and venous angiomas, arteriovenous malformations, and capillary telangiectasis), demyelinating disease (multiple sclerosis), and **congenital anomalies** (arachnoid cysts) may mimic primary posterior fossa lesions. In **adults, infections** (brain abscesses), **vascular abnormalities** (arteriovenous malformations and giant aneurysms, and acute cerebral infarcts), **demyelinating disease** (multiple sclerosis), and **metastatic neoplasms** may be confused with primary brain malignancies.

V. Screening programs. Screening programs for primary brain tumors have not been developed because of their low incidence and because early diagnosis has failed to prolong survival.

VI. Diagnostic workup

 A. Medical history and physical examination. In addition to a detailed medical history, a thorough neurologic and general medical examination is important when evaluating patients with CNS neoplasms. The neurologic examination often assists in the anatomic localization of the lesion, and the medical examination may provide evidence suggesting an abscess or metastases to the brain.

  1. Eyes. The optic disc should be examined for evidence of **papilledema,** which indicates elevated intracranial pressure. The presence of hamartomatous elevations of the iris **(Lisch nodules)** suggesting neurofibromatosis must be noted.

  2. Mouth. The state of the patient's dentition should be recorded because poor dentition is associated with the development of brain abscesses.

  3. Breast. The breast should be examined for suspicious masses that could be the source for cerebral metastases.

   4. **Heart.** In the presence of a heart murmur, **bacterial endocarditis**, which can be a source of septic emboli to the brain, must be excluded.
   5. **Rectum.** Rectal and prostate masses should be investigated because malignancies from these organs often metastasize to the brain.
B. **Primary test and procedures.** All patients with suspected CNS malignancies should undergo the following diagnostic tests:
   1. **Blood tests** (see p 1, **IV.A**)
      a. **Complete blood count.**
      b. **Hepatic transaminases.** Elevated levels of these enzymes are associated with alcoholism, which is a risk factor for the development of brain abscesses.
      c. **Alkaline phosphatase.**
   2. **Imaging studies**
      a. **Chest x-ray** (see p 3, **IV.C.1**).
      b. **Computerized tomography.** CT scan of the head with and without IV contrast is the most readily available test to diagnose a CNS neoplasm. In a patient who has had a seizure or has developed a neurologic deficit, a **focal-enhancing abnormality** or one surrounded by edema usually indicates a malignancy.
      c. **Magnetic resonance imaging (MRI).** MRI scan with **gadolinium contrast** is the most accurate test to image lesions in the brain. The anatomic detail is superior and multiplane imaging is available (coronal, sagittal, and axial). Lesions in the **posterior fossa** are characterized much better by MRI than by CT because of the absence of bone artifact. In addition, vascular malformations and aneurysms can be diagnosed by MRI because of the distinctive features (signal void) caused by blood flow.
   3. **Invasive procedures.** In many cases, **stereotactic biopsy** is the simplest method of obtaining a tissue diagnosis, and it usually can be performed under local anesthesia. It is ideal for deep lesions in the cerebral hemisphere and can be done with a complication rate of **< 2%** and a diagnostic accuracy of **96%.** The procedure involves attaching a metal stereotactic device to the patient's head. A contrast CT of the head is performed, and, with the use of a computer and the stereotactic device, three-dimensional coordinates for the lesion are calculated. A small needle is passed into the lesion through a small hole drilled in the skull, and biopsies are sent to the pathologist for histologic diagnosis. This procedure is **contraindicated** if a **vascular lesion** such as an aneurysm or arteriovenous malformation is being considered. In such cases, an arteriogram should be performed first.
C. **Optional tests and procedures.** On the basis of clinical suspicion or previous diagnostic findings, the following tests or procedures may be indicated:
   1. **Blood tests** (see p 2, **IV.A**)
      a. **5′-Nucleotidase.**
      b. **GGTP.**
   2. **Imaging studies**
      a. **Myelography.** Lumbar myelograms are reliable imaging studies to demonstrate drop metastases and also to indicate cord compression.
      b. **Angiography.** In rare cases, cerebral angiography may aid in the diagnosis of intracranial neoplasms by excluding **vascular lesions.** It also can be used before surgery to **embolize** the feeding vessels of some tumors. Careful preoperative embolization of large vascular tumors such as hemangioblastomas, some meningiomas, and metastatic renal cell carcinoma may be indicated to eliminate profuse intraoperative hemorrhage that sometimes can occur with these lesions.
      c. **Technetium-99m bone scan** (see p 3, **IV.C.5**).
   3. **Invasive procedures**
      a. **Lumbar puncture.** When the diagnosis of brain tumor is suspected, lumbar puncture is **contraindicated until a head CT or MRI has been performed.** If a large intracranial mass or noncommunicating hydrocephalus is present, lumbar puncture can cause tentorial herniation and death. However, this procedure is useful for evaluating medulloblastomas or ependymomas in the posterior fossa that are not associated with hydrocephalus or mass effect. The presence of malignant cells indicates dissemination of the tumor in the spinal fluid.
      b. **Open needle biopsy.** Open needle biopsy through a burr hole or small

craniotomy can be performed for diagnosis if stereotactic equipment is not available. This is similar to a CT-guided needle biopsy of a lung mass.

VII. Pathology

A. Location. Neoplasms can arise anywhere in the brain; however, in children **67%** occur below the tentorium, whereas in adults almost **90%** occur above the tentorium and **10–15% occur in the spinal canal.**

B. Multiplicity. Multiple lesions in the brain suggest metastatic disease or infection. In rare cases, patients with **astrocytomas** will develop multiple discrete lesions referred to as **multicentric glioma.**

C. Histology. A wide variation in histology is found between the various CNS malignancies. The cell of origin can be a glial cell, a neuronal cell, a mesenchymal cell (meninges, blood vessel), or a metastatic tumor cell. Most tumors of the brain are of **glial origin**—the "supporting" cells of the nervous system. These include astrocytic neoplasms, oligodendrogliomas, and ependymomas. Tumors of neuronal origin are rare and include neuroblastoma and ganglioneuroma. Medulloblastomas are believed to arise from primitive neuroectodermal cells. Pediatric brain tumors generally include medulloblastoma, astrocytoma, juvenile pilocytic astrocytoma, and ependymoma, whereas astrocytomas, oligodendrogliomas, and ependymomas are common adult tumors.

1. Astrocytic tumors. These tumors constitute approximately **80% of primary brain malignancies.** They typically arise from **white matter** and are most commonly located in the **cerebral hemispheres**, although they occasionally arise in the brainstem or cerebellum. Astrocytic tumors generally are homogeneous but occasionally calcify and form cysts.

2. Juvenile pilocytic astrocytoma. This **benign** tumor usually arises in the **cerebellum of children**, although it also occurs on occasion in the cerebral hemispheres or as an enhancing nodule in a cyst wall. It is characterized by microcysts, microscopic loose and dense areas, and the presence of **Rosenthal fibers.**

3. Oligodendrogliomas. These tumors almost always are found in the **cerebral hemispheres**. The cells typically have a **"fried egg"** appearance with a central nucleus and a poorly staining cytoplasm. **Calcifications** are common.

4. Ependymomas. Usually arising from the floor of the fourth ventricle and often extending through the **foramina of Luschka** into the peripontine cisterns, these malignancies commonly occur in the midline but also may arise in the lateral or third ventricles. These tumors are highly cellular, and they often **calcify** and form **perivascular pseudorosettes** as well as true rosettes.

5. Medulloblastomas. These malignancies of the posterior fossa most commonly are homogeneous **midline tumors** with occasional cysts and calcifications. Histologically, they appear to be highly cellular with hyperchromic nuclei and prominent **pseudorosettes**.

D. Tumor grade. Numerous grading systems are used for gliomas, including the three-tier grading system outlined below.

1. Grade 1. Astrocytoma. This tumor has a mild increase in cellularity, mild nuclear irregularity, and infrequent or absent mitotic cells.

2. Grade 2. Malignant or anaplastic astrocytoma. This tumor has markedly increased cellularity, nuclear pleomorphism, hyperchromasia, occasional giant cell formation, and frequent mitotic figures.

3. Grade 3. Glioblastoma multiforme (GBM). This is the **most malignant** primary brain tumor. It is highly cellular with nuclear pleomorphism, hyperchromasia, and numerous mitotic cells. The hallmarks of GBM are **patches of necrosis and marked endothelial proliferation in blood vessels.**

E. Metastatic spread

1. Modes of spread. Brain tumors can spread by one of several mechanisms.

a. Direct extension. Occasional reports of invasion into the surrounding scalp are almost always associated with and the result of prior surgical excision.

b. Spread through the cerebrospinal fluid (CSF). Tumor cells can be shed into the CSF and **"drop"** down the spinal canal, forming distant metastases. In addition, a medulloblastoma or ependymoma occasionally will spread to the peritoneum through a **ventriculoperitoneal shunt**.

c. Lymphatic metastasis. Because the brain has no lymphatic system, spread to regional lymph nodes does not occur.

d. Hematogenous metastasis. Hematogenous spread through intracranial sinuses and systemic vessels occurs in less than 1% of patients.

2. Sites of spread. At autopsy, few distant organs are likely to be involved in metastatic spread; however, if metastases do develop, the following organs are usually involved: **lung, liver,** and **bone.**

VIII. Staging. Recently, the American Joint Committee on Cancer and the Union Internationale Contre le Cancer developed a TNM staging system for primary CNS cancer. This includes astrocytomas, oligodendrogliomas, ependymomas, glioblastomas, medulloblastomas, meningiomas, malignant neurilemmomas, neurosarcomas, and sarcomas. Although relatively new, it is hoped that this staging system will provide the foundation for accurate comparisons of future therapeutic trials.

   A. Tumor stage
   1. **Supratentorial tumor**
      a. **TX.** The primary tumor cannot be assessed.
      b. **T0.** No evidence of a primary tumor exists.
      c. **T1.** Unilateral tumor smaller than 5 cm in diameter.
      d. **T2.** Unilateral tumor larger than 5 cm in diameter.
      e. **T3.** Tumor invades or encroaches on the ventricular system.
      f. **T4.** tumor crosses the midline, invades the opposite hemisphere, or invades below the tentorium.
   2. **Infratentorial tumor**
      a. **TX.** Primary tumor cannot be assessed.
      b. **T0.** No evidence of a primary tumor exists.
      c. **T1.** Unilateral tumor smaller than 3 cm in diameter.
      d. **T2.** Unilateral tumor larger than 3 cm in diameter.
      e. **T3.** Tumor invades or encroaches on the ventricular system.
      f. **T4.** Tumor crosses the midline, invades the opposite hemisphere, or invades above the tentorium.
   B. Lymph node stage. This category does not apply to this site.
   C. Metastatic stage
   1. **MX.** The presence of distant metastases cannot be assessed.
   2. **M0.** No distant metastases are present.
   3. **M1.** Distant metastases are present.
   D. Histopathologic grade
   1. **GX.** Grade cannot be assessed.
   2. **G1.** Well differentiated.
   3. **G2.** Moderately well differentiated.
   4. **G3.** Poorly differentiated.
   5. **G4.** Undifferentiated.
   E. Stage groupings
   1. **Stage 1A.** G1, T1, M0.
   2. **Stage 1B.** G1, T2 or 3, M0.
   3. **Stage IIA.** G2, T1, M0.
   4. **Stage IIB.** G2, T2 or 3, M0.
   5. **Stage IIIA.** G3, T1, M0.
   6. **Stage IIIB.** G3, T2 or 3, M0.
   7. **Stage IV.** Any G,T4, M0; G4, any T, M0; or any G, any T, M1.

IX. Treatment. In general, the treatment options for malignant gliomas include surgery, radiation, and chemotherapy. Debulking surgery and irradiation are usually offered when the tumor is first diagnosed; at the time of recurrence, chemotherapy or experimental treatments such as immunotherapy and drug-impregnated polymer implants can be considered.

   A. Surgery. Surgery is the most effective means of prolonging survival for malignant brain tumors.
   1. **Primary malignancy of the central nervous system**
      a. **Indications.** Surgery is indicated for purposes of **diagnosis** and **reduction** of **elevated intracranial pressure** and mass effect. Even the most careful preoperative assessment of patients with enhancing intracerebral masses cannot distinguish between primary neoplasms, abscesses, and metastatic tumors. Given the minimal risk of surgery (3% major morbidity and 2–3% mortality rates), a tissue diagnosis should always be obtained. This information is invaluable for treatment planning, avoiding inappropriate radiation therapy of brain abscesses, and patient education. In addition, **debulking** a recurrent tumor to reduce the "tumor load" before chemotherapy or radiation therapy has been shown to be of benefit in controlled clinical studies. Finally, in patients with hydrocephalus, removing an intraventricular tumor may occasionally open up obstructed CSF pathways and obviate the need for a CSF shunt.

b. **Preoperative preparation**

(1) **Anticonvulsants.** All patients with malignant brain tumors should receive anticonvulsants before craniotomy because generalized seizures in the immediate postoperative period can cause intracranial hemorrhage with disastrous results. **Phenytoin** (Dilantin) and **phenobarbital** are preferred perioperatively because they can be administered intravenously. Postoperatively, carbamazepine (Tegretol, Epitol) is an excellent alternative once the patient can tolerate oral medications.

(2) **Steroids.** Corticosteroid should be administered preoperatively to all patients undergoing craniotomy for malignancies. By **decreasing angiogenic edema**, steroids significantly reduce brain swelling. In neurologically intact patients with minimal swelling on imaging studies, **10 mg of dexamethasone** can be started **on the day of surgery**. However, with significant clinical neurologic deficits and mass effect on imaging studies, the steroid dose should be titrated to the patient's clinical status over several days before surgery. Typically, dexamethasone is begun at 4 mg every 6 hours and is increased to as much as 20 mg every 4 hours in severe cases.

c. **Approaches.** The site of a neoplasm dictates the operative approach. Supratentorial lesions are generally approached by a **craniotomy directly over the lesion**, if possible. **Posterior fossa masses** are usually approached by a **midline incision over the occipital bone** with dissection carried through or around the cerebellum. **Third ventricular tumors** are approached through either the **corpus callosum or middle frontal gyrus**.

d. **Procedures.** Craniotomy with complete resection of all gross tumor is the goal of aggressive surgery. However, even though all gross tumor is removed and no residual tumor enhances on postoperative CT or MRI scans, residual tumor is always left behind because of microscopic infiltration of tumor cells. Therefore, if tumor extends into important areas of the brain such as **Broca's area** or the **motor cortex,** tumor is intentionally left behind rather than risk injury to the patient. In the 1930s, hemispherectomies were occasionally performed for these tumors, but because of a remarkable capacity to migrate along white matter pathways to locations distant from the tumor margin, the lesions always recurred within 3 years.

2. **Metastatic CNS malignancy.** Because of the rare occurrence of extracranial metastases and the aggressive nature of the primary lesions, surgical resection of metastatic disease cannot be recommended.

3. **Mortality and morbidity.** Craniotomy for tumor resection, when carefully performed, should carry a **mortality rate of less than 5%.** The most common causes of morbidity after craniotomy include the following: **worsened neurologic deficit, seizures, pneumonia, deep venous thrombosis, pulmonary embolism,** and **wound infection.**

B. **Radiation**

1. **Primary CNS malignancy.** Radiation therapy can be used as the first-line therapy for CNS lesions in patients who are not candidates for surgical debulking. However, a diagnosis must be established first and is frequently obtained by **stereotactic biopsy**.

2. **Adjuvant radiation therapy**

a. **Preoperative radiation therapy.** This modality generally is not used with CNS tumors.

b. **Intraoperative radiation therapy.** No significant experience has been reported with this approach to radiation therapy.

c. **Postoperative adjuvant radiation therapy.** The role of radiation therapy in the management of malignant brain tumors depends on the tumor histology. Previously, patients with gliomas were treated with **4500 cGy whole brain irradiation, followed by a 1500 cGy boost to the tumor**. Currently, however, many centers have abandoned whole brain irradiation and are radiating **only the tumor** and a **3 cm margin** of surrounding brain. Portions of the brain that have no demonstrable tumor on CT or MRI are left unirradiated. The results of postoperative brain irradiation by tumor histology are discussed below:

(1) **Astrocytoma.** The results of retrospective studies evaluating the effect of postoperative radiation therapy vary. Most studies demonstrate either **minimal or no benefit**. A multicenter, prospective, randomized trial designed to answer this question is currently being conducted.

(2) **Anaplastic astrocytoma.** In most studies, whole brain radiation ther-

apy of anaplastic astrocytomas modestly increases the mean patient survival by a few months. In the United States today, **5000–6000 cGy** of external-beam radiation therapy is recommended, and the resulting 5-year survival is approximately **20%.**

(3) **Glioblastoma multiforme.** Radiation therapy has consistently been **beneficial** in the management of glioblastoma multiforme. The median survival after **surgery alone** is approximately **5 months,** and the median survival for glioblastoma multiforme treated by **surgery and postoperative radiation** is approximately **9 months.**

(4) **Oligodendroglioma.** No randomized clinical trial has evaluated the role of radiation therapy for oligodendrogliomas. Retrospective studies have involved small numbers of patients, been uncontrolled, and produced contradictory results. In general, these tumors act like anaplastic astrocytomas and should undergo **5000–6000 cGy** of external-beam radiation therapy after diagnostic or debulking surgery.

(5) **Ependymoma.** Ependymomas are probably the **most radiosensitive** gliomas. Although these tumors are often called benign, they **rarely can be excised completely** because of their location and extension into surrounding brain. Treatment of ependymomas with **surgery alone** has resulted in **5-year survival** rates of approximately **25%. Surgery followed by 4500 cGy** or more has increased **5-year survival rates to 60%.**

(6) **Medulloblastoma.** Before radiation therapy was used, the mean survival of patients following surgery alone ranged from 6 months to a year. Over the past few years, the approach to this tumor has changed. Aggressive debulking surgery followed by a full course of craniospinal radiation is now recommended. The 5-year survival with this approach has improved to **60%.**

3. **Metastatic CNS malignancy.** Because of the rare occurrence of extracranial metastases and the aggressive nature of the primary lesions, radiation therapy is rarely useful.

4. **Morbidity and mortality.** The previously high incidence of acute complications from radiation therapy has been reduced by altered dose-fractionation schedules and concomitant use of steroids. **Daily fractions of 200 cGy,** with a total dose of 5000–6000 cGy, are generally well tolerated. Radiation therapy can lead to the following complications:
   a. **Somnolence and headache** (from increased brain edema).
   b. **Transient worsening of neurologic deficits** (lasts a few weeks).
   c. **Radiation-induced brain necrosis.** This may be delayed for **8–24 months** and may be confused with recurrent tumor (**surgery is required** to distinguish the two).

C. **Chemotherapy**
1. **Primary CNS malignancy.** Chemotherapy has not been tested extensively as an initial therapeutic modality for brain cancer, and it cannot be recommended in place of surgical debulking and postoperative radiation therapy.

2. **Adjuvant chemotherapy**
   a. **Single-agent therapy.** Chemotherapy has been used as adjuvant therapy after surgery and radiation therapy for malignant gliomas. **Carmustine** was first used in the early 1950s for the treatment of malignant gliomas, and still remains the most effective chemotherapeutic agent for this disease. In controlled studies, **survival has been prolonged** by a few months compared with surgery and radiation alone.
   b. **Combination chemotherapy.** The addition of other drugs to carmustine has not increased survival.

3. **Metastatic CNS malignancy.** Because extracranial glioma metastases are rare, information as to the effectiveness of chemotherapy in this setting remains anecdotal.

D. **Immunotherapy.** Despite the attractiveness of this form of therapy, innumerable studies have shown minimal or no efficacy. These include active immunotherapy with BCG, *Corynebacterium parvum,* and glioma cell extract immunization and passive treatment with interferon, peripheral blood lymphocytes, and activated lymphocytes.

X. **Prognosis**
A. **Risk of recurrence.** In general, **all tumors recur**, become progressively more malignant, and result in the demise of the patient.
B. **Five-year survival.** The prognosis for patients with malignant brain tumors de-

pends on the tumor type and grade. In reality, however, the mortality from these diseases is 100%, although some large series have reported a cure rate of 0.4% in young patients with tumors at the edge of the frontal or occipital lobes.

1. **Astrocytoma.** The **5- and 10-year** survival rates for this tumor are **50% and 20%,** respectively.
2. **Anaplastic astrocytoma.** The **5-year** survival rate is approximately **20%.**
3. **Glioblastoma multiforme.** The median survival is 9 months; the **2-year** survival is **15%;** and the **5-year** survival is less than **1%.**
4. **Oligodendroglioma.** The **5- and 10-year** survival rates are **60% and 30%,** respectively.
5. **Ependymoma.** The **5-year** survival rate ranges from **40–87%.**
6. **Medulloblastoma.** The **5-year** survival rate is **60%.**

XI. **Patient follow-up**

A. **General guidelines.** Patients with malignant brain tumors require close careful follow-up. Patients with higher grade tumors should be seen at intervals of **3–4 months** whereas those with low-grade astrocytomas can be seen every 6 months. Specific recommendations are outlined below.

B. **Routine evaluation.** Each clinic visit should include the following tests and procedures:

1. **Medical history and physical examination.** An interim history and complete physical examination, including a neurologic examination, should be performed during each follow-up visit. Particular attention should be focused on the areas highlighted on p 436, **II,** and a **Karnofsky activity rating** (see Appendix A) should be recorded.

2. **Complete blood count.** Patients taking carbamazepine (Tegretol) should have a complete blood count to exclude myelosuppression and aplastic anemia.

3. **Hepatic enzymes.** Patients receiving **valproic acid** (Depakene) should have levels of these enzymes checked to assess possible liver toxicity.

4. **Anticonvulsant levels.** Specific levels of anticonvulsant agents should be checked periodically to avoid subtherapeutic and toxic levels.

5. **Computed tomography (CT).** CT scan is the least expensive test for following patients with malignant supratentorial tumors, and it should be obtained if neurologic deterioration occurs. Patients with **high-grade** tumors should have CT scans every **4 months,** whereas those with **low-grade** lesions can be scanned every **6–12 months.** In routine follow-up, there is little advantage of gadolinium-enhanced MRI over iodine-enhanced CT for supratentorial lesions.

6. **Magnetic resonance imaging (MRI).** This test is ideal for following cerebellar or brain stem tumors or the rare supratentorial lesion that is not seen on CT. In addition, the multiplane images can be indispensable when planning additional surgery.

C. **Additional evaluation.** Other tests that should be obtained at regular intervals include the following:

1. **Chest x-ray.** This simple test should be obtained every **6 months** to exclude the presence of rare pulmonary metastases.

2. **Alkaline phosphatase.** Measurements of this serum enzyme should be obtained every **6 months** to exclude the rare possibility of hepatic (elevation of heat-stable component) or bone (elevation of heat-labile fraction) metastases (see also, p 1, **IV.A.3**).

D. **Optional evaluation.** The following tests and procedures may be indicated by previous diagnostic findings or clinical suspicion:

1. **Blood tests** (see p 2, **IV.A**)
   a. **5'-Nucoeotidase.**
   b. **GGTP.**
2. **Technetium-99m bone scan** (see p 3, **IV.5**)
3. **Biopsy.** Either stereotactic or open biopsy should be performed if recurrent tumor is suspected.

REFERENCES

Kornblith, PL and Walker, M. Chemotherapy for malignant gliomas. *J Neurosurg* 68:1–17, 1988.

Leibel, SA and Sheline, GE. Radiation therapy for neoplasms of the brain. *J Neurosurg* 66:1–22, 1987.

McDonald JD, Dohrmann GJ. Moledular biology of brain tumors. Review Article. Neurosurgery 23(5):537–544, 1988.

Morantz, RA. Radiation therapy in the treatment of cerebral astrocytomas. Neurosurg 20(6):975–982, 1987.

Okazaki, H and Scheithauer, BW. Atlas of Neuropathology. Gower Medical Publishing, New York: 1988.

Piepmeier, JM. Observations on the current treatment of low-grade astrocytic tumors of the cerebral hemispheres. J Neurosurg 67:177–181, 1987.

Rubinstein, LJ. Atlas of tumor pathology. Fascicle 6. Washington DC, Armed Forces Institute of Pathology, 1972.

Shapiro, WR, Green, SB, Burger, PC et al. Randomized trial of three chemotherapy regimens and two radiotherapy regimens in postoperative treatment of malignant glioma. Brain Tumor Cooperative Group Trial 8001. J Neurosurg 71:1–9, 1989.

Shaw EG, Daumas-Duport C, Scheithauer BW et al: Radiation therapy in the management of low-grade supratentorial astrocytomas. J Neurosurg 70:853–861, 1989.

Wallner, KE, Gonzales, M, Sheline, GE. Treatment of oligodendrogliomas with or without postoperative irradiation.J Neurosurg 68:684–688, 1988.

Wilkins, RH and Rengachery, SS. Neurosurgery. McGraw-Hill Book Company, New York: 1985.

55 Malignancies of the Thyroid

Edward Shlasko, MD

I. **Epidemiology.** Although thyroid cancer represents **1–2%** of all malignancies and **90%** of all endocrine cancers, it causes less than **0.2%** of cancer deaths in the United States. The incidence has remained stable for over 10 years, with **2.6** cases per 100,000 males and **6.1** cases per 100,000 females reported in 1985. Estimates indicate that in 1993, **12,700 new cases** will be identified and **1,050 deaths** will occur from thyroid carcinoma. Autopsy series, however, have demonstrated an incidence of **occult carcinoma** as high as **13%**, whereas surgical series have identified carcinoma in as many as **4%** of thyroidectomy specimens obtained for benign disease. Thyroid cancer is much more common in areas of endemic goiter where the local diet is deficient in iodine. Hawaii and China have a high incidence of thyroid cancer: 7.8 per 100,000 males and 17.6 per 100,000 females. India has a low incidence: in males the rate is 0.4 per 100,000, whereas Poland has an incidence in females of only 0.7 per 100,000.

II. **Risk factors**
   A. **Age.** The incidence of thyroid cancer increases from fewer than 3.3 per 100,000 before the age of 20 years to more than **8.0** per 100,000 by the **age of 80** years. **Hurthle cell** tumors usually occur in patients older than **50** years, whereas the incidence of **anaplastic carcinoma** increases greatly after the **age of 60** years. In children, a solitary thyroid nodule, although rare, has a greater than **50%** chance of harboring a malignancy.
   B. **Sex.** The risk in American **females** is **2.3 times** higher than in males, although a solitary thyroid nodule in a male is **3 times** more likely to be malignant than is a nodule in a female.
   C. **Race.** American **blacks** are **1.8 times** more likely than whites to develop thyroid cancer. Worldwide, however, there is no racial difference in the incidence of thyroid carcinoma.
   D. **Genetic factors**
      1. **Family history. Papillary and follicular thyroid carcinoma** have been reported in parent-child pairs and family groupings, often associated with a **B-7, DR-1** HLA haplotype.
      2. **Familial syndromes.** Two familial syndromes are associated with a substantially increased risk for medullary cancer of the thyroid.
         a. **Multiple endocrine neoplasia Type IIa (MEN IIA) or Sipple's syndrome.** This is an autosomal dominant syndrome characterized by **medullary carcinoma of the thyroid, pheochromocytoma, and either parathyroid adenomas or hyperplasia.**
         b. **Multiple endocrine neoplasia Type IIb (MEN IIB).** Similar to MEN IIA, this syndrome is characterized by **medullary carcinoma of the thyroid, pheochromocytoma, multiple mucosal neuromas, a marfanoid habitus, and cafe au lait spots.**
   E. **Diet.** Geographic areas in which **iodine deficiency** and goiter are endemic have an increased incidence of thyroid cancer, and approximately **25%** of thyroid cancers develop in previous multinodular goiters. Normal adults require only **100 mcg/day** of iodine, and iodine supplementation has greatly reduced the risk of goiter in the modern world. It remains to be seen whether this will significantly reduce the risk of developing thyroid cancer.
   F. **History of previous thyroid pathology**
      1. **Multinodular goiter.** Multinodular goiter increases the risk of thyroid carcinoma; approximately **80% of anaplastic tumors and 25% of all thyroid cancers** develop in nodular glands. This finding may reflect the effects of prolonged exposure to thyroid-stimulating hormone (TSH). Similarly, patients who are treated over the long term for hyperthyroidism with antithyroid medications such as propylthiouracil are at an increased risk of developing thyroid cancer.

2. **Inflammatory conditions.** Thyroiditis itself is not associated with a greater-than-normal risk of thyroid cancer. However, **hypothyroidism** that often develops naturally or iatrogenically during the course of the disease may increase the risk of thyroid cancer through the stimulation caused by elevated TSH levels.

3. **Previous radiation exposure.** A **linear relationship** exists between radiation exposure (as high as **2000 cGy**) and the risk of subsequent thyroid cancer. The latency period may be as long as **40 years** but is most commonly 20–30 years after exposure. Japanese survivors of nuclear blasts have an **18%** incidence of thyroid cancer. With extremely high levels of exposure, the risk declines again, reflecting more complete ablation of thyroid tissue. As many as **25%** of **asymptomatic** patients exposed to cervical radiation as children (as therapy for thymic or tonsillar enlargement, cervical adenitis, acne, and tinea capitis) have abnormalities on thyroid screening, and **33%** of them **will have carcinoma**.

G. **Urbanization.** Although urbanization does not affect the incidence of thyroid cancer, the associated widespread iodinization of salt has reduced the prevalence of endemic goiter.

III. **Presentation**

A. **Signs and symptoms**

1. **Local manifestations.** Most patients with well-differentiated thyroid cancer present with **asymptomatic cervical nodules** or masses. Many show cervical lymphadenopathy, which is often their presenting complaint. Hoarseness, dysphagia, choking, dyspnea, laryngeal nerve paralysis, cough, and pain are rare except in patients with **anaplastic** carcinoma.

2. **Systemic manifestations.** Patients with well-differentiated thyroid cancer rarely have systemic symptoms. They may manifest **symptoms of hypothyroidism** (lassitude, intolerance to cold, obesity, constipation, hoarseness, dry skin and hair, myocardial dysfunction, and myxedema), whereas patients with **anaplastic carcinoma** may show significant **weight loss**. Thyrotoxicosis rarely occurs in patients with thyroid cancer because the tumors are usually nonfunctional. As many as **30%** of patients with **medullary** carcinoma complain of **watery diarrhea**, and 10% experience cutaneous flushing.

3. **Paraneoplastic syndromes.** Patients with **medullary** carcinoma of the thyroid may present with a number of systemic symptoms that may represent one of the following paraneoplastic syndromes.

a. **Inappropriate adenocorticotropic hormone (ACTH)** (see p 90).

b. **Hypocalcemia** (see p 84).

IV. **Differential diagnosis.** The differential diagnosis of any cervical mass is extensive, and thyroid malignancies must be distinguished from **inflammatory conditions** (multinodular goiter, focal thyroiditis, Grave's disease, granulomatous disease, colloid cysts, and thyroid abscesses), **congenital abnormalities** (thyroglossal duct cyst, branchial cleft cyst, ectopic thyroid tissue, cystic hygroma, and epidermoid cyst), **other neoplasms** (adenoma, dermoid, teratoma, squamous cell carcinoma, lymphoma, schwannoma of the vagus nerve, chemodectoma, and parathyroid adenoma), and **metastatic disease.**

V. **Screening programs.** Although no cost-effective screening program exists for the general population, the National Cancer Institute recommends the following program for patients exposed to ionizing cervical radiation:

A. **Physical examination.** Careful physical examination every 2 years.

B. **Nodules.** All discrete nodules should be excised regardless of "hot" or "cold" appearance on thyroid scanning. (Nonpalpable scan abnormalities and small [< 1.5 cm] soft nodules should be followed for up to 6 months on T4 suppression therapy).

C. **Goiter.** Diffuse enlargement should be treated with T4 suppression and be followed closely with a careful physical examination every 6 months.

D. **MEN syndromes.** For patients from kindreds with MEN IIA or MEN IIB, frequent careful evaluations are mandatory.

VI. **Diagnostic workup**

A. **Medical history and physical examination.** In addition to a thorough medical history documenting any radiation exposure or significant family history that suggests thyroid disease or other endocrine abnormalities, patients should be examined carefully, paying particular attention to the following areas:

1. **General appearance.** The patient's general functional status and energy level should be carefully assessed.

2. **Skin.** Plaques, papules, and thickening of the skin, especially of the pretibial,

nasal, and oral areas (myxedema) should be excluded as signs of hypothyroidism. **Cafe au lait** spots also should be noted.

3. **Head. Proptosis,** hair texture, and loss of the lateral eyebrow hair should be documented carefully.

4. **Neck.** Size, consistency, number, mobility, fixation, and location of all masses should be recorded.

5. **Pharynx and larynx.** A direct or indirect examination of the vocal cords should be performed in any patient who complains of voice changes, and mucosal neuromas indicative of MEN IIB should be identified.

6. **Lymph nodes.** All lymph node areas must be carefully examined, especially in the cervical, supraclavicular and axillary areas.

7. **Heart.** Any bradycardia consistent with hypothyroidism, or tachyarrhythmias indicating hyperthyroidism, should be noted.

8. **Abdomen.** The size and location of any masses, especially those possibly indicating pheochromocytoma, are carefully documented.

9. **Nervous system.** Deep tendon reflexes are recorded, with specific reference to hypo- or hyperreflexia indicating hypo- or hyperthyroidism, respectively.

B. **Primary test and procedures.** The following tests and diagnostic procedures should be performed initially in all patients with thyroid carcinoma:

1. **Blood tests**
   a. **Complete blood count.** A microcytic, hypochromic sideroblastic anemia may be seen with hypothyroidism.
   b. **Hepatic transaminases** (see p 1, **IV.A.2**).
   c. **Alkaline phosphatase** (see p 1, **IV.A.3**).
   d. **Thyroid function tests.** The total serum **T4** and **T3** are measured using radioimmunoassays, which do not distinguish free from bound thyroid hormone (99% of the circulating hormone is bound to thyroxine binding globulin, thyroxine binding prealbumin, or albumin). The T3 resin uptake test helps to distinguish the amount of biologically available thyroid hormone. **TSH** is obtained to exclude the presence of **hypothyroidism** (elevated TSH levels). However, most patients with thyroid cancer are **euthyroid.** Hypo- or hyperthyroidism usually represents coexisting thyroid diseases.

2. **Imaging studies**
   a. **Chest x-ray.** This simple test often provides important information about thyroid tumors. **Psammoma bodies** (calcific nodules) found with some carcinomas cause a stippled appearance in contrast to the typical **"eggshell"** calcifications that are often present in colloid nodules. Displacement or invasion of the trachea may be apparent, and pulmonary metastases may be recognized (see also, p 3, **IV.C.1**).
   b. **Thyroid scan.** Technetium-99m or ^{123}I are used to document the functional status of thyroid nodules. **"Hot" nodules** (ie, those that are hyperfunctional) **rarely contain carcinoma,** whereas **5–30% of "cold"** (hypofunctional) nodules harbor thyroid cancer.

3. **Invasive procedures**
   a. **Fine needle aspiration.** Cytologists can often diagnose malignant thyroid nodules on the basis of the characteristics of a few cells obtained with a **22–27 gauge needle aspirate;** many series report a false-negative rate of only **0–4%.** Several important caveats must be considered before making treatment decisions based on fine needle aspirate results alone. Because cyst walls may harbor small foci of tumor that are not aspirated into the needle during the procedure, even cases with negative cytology need close follow-up. Cells with large amounts of eosinophilic cytoplasm in Hurthle cell carcinoma may be indistinguishable from inflamed follicular cells in Hashimoto's thyroiditis, so a high level of suspicion must be maintained and **all Hurthle cells should be viewed as malignant.** Finally, because invasion of surrounding structures, not cytologic characteristics, distinguishes follicular carcinoma from adenoma fine needle aspiration **cannot distinguish** follicular adenoma **from follicular thyroid cancer.**
   b. **Core needle biopsy.** Some reports claim that core needle biopsies are more sensitive than fine needle aspiration, but this remains to be confirmed and may be at the expense of increased bleeding.

C. **Optional tests and procedures.** The following tests and procedures may be indicated by previous diagnostic findings or clinical suspicion:

1. **Blood tests**
   a. **5′-Nucleotidase** (see p 2, **IV.A.4**).

      b. GGTP (see p 2, **IV.A.5**).

      c. Carcinoembryonic antigen (CEA). CEA is occasionally elevated in patients with thyroid cancer.

      d. Calcitonin. Elevated serum levels of calcitonin are often found in patients with medullary carcinoma. Calcium and pentagastrin stimulation tests may elicit an abnormally high secretion of calcitonin and can be used to distinguish thyroid from ectopic sources of the hormone.

      e. Adrenocorticotropic hormone (ACTH). Medullary tumors may elaborate other hormones, particularly adrenocorticotrophic hormone, that explain the occasional symptoms of Cushing's syndrome in patients with medullary carcinoma.

  2. Imaging studies

      a. Ultrasound. Ultrasonography often can distinguish solid from cystic lesions, which is important because only 2–3% of purely cystic lesions harbor carcinoma.

      b. Computed tomography. A CT scan of the chest and neck may help define the extent of disease and the involvement of surrounding structures (particularly with anaplastic carcinoma) and provide a clear means of evaluating the presence or absence of pulmonary metastases.

  3. Invasive procedures. Although **esophagoscopy and bronchoscopy** are rarely helpful in evaluating patients with thyroid cancer, they may help define resectability in patients with anaplastic tumors. **Laryngoscopy,** either direct or indirect, may help identify patients with laryngeal nerve involvement preoperatively and should be performed for any complaint of hoarseness.

VII. Pathology

  A. Location. In general, thyroid cancer can develop anywhere in the thyroid gland, including the isthmus, as well as in any ectopic thyroid tissue. However, **medullary carcinoma** is located more commonly within the **lateral and upper two-thirds** of the thyroid gland.

  B. Multiplicity. More than **40% of papillary tumors and 13–16% of follicular tumors** are multifocal. When associated with familial syndromes (MEN IIA and MEN IIB), more than **90% of medullary carcinomas** are multicentric; however, **when sporadic, only 20%** of medullary tumors are multifocal.

  C. Histology. The histologic classification of thyroid cancer is extremely important because it largely determines the patient's prognosis and treatment.

    1. Papillary. The most common type of thyroid cancer, accounting for **60–70%** of all cases, is papillary carcinoma. Commonly associated with previous exposure to **ionizing irradiation**, these tumors usually occur in patients older than 40 years and are multifocal as often as 40% of the time. Microscopic examination shows multiple papillae that are composed of a fibrovascular core surrounded by neoplastic epithelial cells, with occasional follicle formation. **Psammoma bodies** (microcalcifications) are often present, and the tumor cell nuclei show finely dispersed chromatin, which gives them an appearance that has been described as **"Little Orphan Annie" nuclei.** In addition, an inflammatory lymphocytic infiltrate may be present. Tumors with both follicular and papillary elements usually behave like papillary tumors. All papillary tumors must be considered to have malignant potential, and they are classified as **minimal, encapsulated, intrathyroid, or extrathyroid**.

    2. Follicular. Follicular tumors constitute **15–20%** of all thyroid cancers and are **more common in females.** Associated with endemic goiter, they have decreased in incidence since the widespread iodinization of salt. The diagnosis of malignancy in follicular tumors is based, not on cellular morphology, but solely on the presence of **microvascular or capsular invasion.** Pathologists classify these tumors into **minimally or extensively invasive** categories.

    3. Hurthle cell tumors. These tumors are characterized by **large eosinophilic cells**. Although malignancy is diagnosed on the basis of invasion, as many as **85% of these patients eventually die of their disease.** Hurthle cell tumors are notably resistant to irradiation and should always be treated as potentially malignant.

    4. Anaplastic tumors. These extremely aggressive tumors represent **10–15%** of all thyroid cancers. They may be composed of small cells, giant cells, spindle cells, or mixed cellular types and often show areas of hemorrhage and necrosis.

    5. Medullary tumors. Medullary cancer of the thyroid represents only **2–8%** of all thyroid cancers, with no sex predilection. The parafollicular cells that produce calcitonin are the cells of origin, which makes medullary carcinoma a member of the Amine Precursor Uptake and Decarboxylase (APUD) family of cancers. Histologic examination reveals sheets of tumor cells with fibrous septae, Congo red birefringence, vascular invasion, lymphocytic infiltrates, and neurosecretory granules on electron microscopy. Immunohistochemistry may show positive results with staining for calcitonin, somatostatin, CEA, serotonin, histamine, or prostaglandins.

D. Metastatic spread. The pattern of metastatic spread of thyroid cancer depends in large part on the histologic type. Lymphatic spread is more common in papillary tumors, and hematogenous spread is more common with other cell types. Laryngeal nerve paralysis resulting from direct extension may occur with any type of thyroid cancer, although only anaplastic tumors commonly show local invasion of large blood vessels, trachea, and esophagus.

   1. Modes of spread. Thyroid carcinoma can spread by 3 mechanisms.

      a. Direct extension. Although any histologic type of thyroid cancer may extend into the local tissues, **anaplastic thyroid cancer** is associated most often with extensive local invasion.

      b. Lymphatic metastasis. More than **40% of patients with papillary tumors, 10% with follicular cancer, 25% with MEN IIA-associated medullary carcinomas, and 50% with MEN IIB-associated medullary carcinomas** develop cervical or mediastinal lymph node metastases or both during the course of their disease as a result of spread through multiple lymphatic channels to the **Delphian node** overlying the thyroid cartilage and the pretracheal, laterotracheal, jugular, subdigastric, suprahyoid, retropharyngeal, anterior mediastinal, and upper cervical nodes. Only **1–2%** of patients present with disease **outside** the neck.

      c. Hematogenous metastasis. Although only **1–2%** of patients with **papillary cancer** develop distant hematogenous metastases, **75% of follicular tumors** and many **medullary carcinomas** spread to distant sites through blood vessels.

   2. Sites of metastatic spread. The organs often involved with metastatic spread from thyroid cancer include the following: **regional and distant lymph nodes, lung, bone, liver, central nervous system, and pleura and peritoneum.**

VIII. Staging

   A. Clinical staging system. Woolner proposed the clinical staging system described below. This system has not been widely accepted, however.

      1. Clinical Stage I. Intrathyroid disease alone: **unilateral disease** and **multifocal or bilateral disease.**

      2. Clinical Stage II. Cervical lymphadenopathy is present: **unilateral disease** and **bilateral or mediastinal disease.**

      3. Clinical Stage III. Locally invasive disease is detectable.

      4. Clinical Stage IV. Distant metastases are documented.

   B. TNM staging system. After analyzing more than 1000 case protocols, the American Joint Committee on Cancer and the Union Internationale Contre le Cancer proposed the following TNM staging system:

      1. Tumor stage

         a. TX. Primary tumor cannot be assessed.

         b. T0. No evidence of primary tumor.

         c. T1. Tumor is no larger than 1 cm in its greatest dimension and is limited to the thyroid gland.

         d. T2. Tumor is larger than 1 cm but no larger than 4 cm in its greatest dimension and is limited to the thyroid gland.

         e. T3. Tumor is larger than 4 cm in its greatest dimension and is limited to the thyroid gland.

         f. T4. Tumor of any size extends beyond the thyroid capsule.

      2. Lymph node stage

         a. NX. Regional lymph nodes cannot be assessed.

         b. N0. No regional lymph node metastases are present.

         c. N1. Regional lymph node metastases are present.

            (1) N1a. Ipsilateral cervical lymph node metastases are present.

            (2) N1b. Bilateral, midline, or contralateral cervical or mediastinal lymph node metastases are present.

              Note: Submandibular and submental nodes are considered to be distant spread.

3. **Metastatic stage**
   a. **MX.** The presence of metastatic disease cannot be assessed.
   b. **M0.** No distant metastases are present.
   c. **M1.** Distant metastases are present.
4. **Histopathologic grade**
   a. **GX.** Grade cannot be assessed.
   b. **G1.** Well differentiated lesions.
   c. **G2.** Moderately well differentiated lesions.
   d. **G3.** Poorly differentiated lesions.
   e. **G4.** Undifferentiated lesions.
5. **Stage groups**
   a. **Papillary or follicular carcinoma**
      (1) **Under 45 years of age**
          (a) **Stage I.** Any T, any N, M0.
          (b) **Stage II.** Any T, any N, M1.
      (2) **Forty-five years of age or older**
          (a) **Stage 1.** T1, N0, M0.
          (b) **Stage II.** T2 or T3, N0, M0.
          (c) **Stage III.** T4, N0, M0 or any T, N1, M0.
          (d) **Stage IV.** Any T, any N, M1.
   b. **Medullary carcinoma**
      (1) **Stage I.** T1, N0, M0.
      (2) **Stage II.** T2, T3, or T4, N0, M0.
      (3) **Stage III.** Any T, N1, M0.
      (4) **Stage IV.** Any T, any N, M1.
   c. **Undifferentiated carcinoma**
      (1) **Stages I, II, and III.** Do not exist.
      (2) **Stage IV.** Any T, any N, any M.

IX. **Treatment**
   A. **Surgery**
      1. **Primary thyroid carcinoma**
         a. **Indications.** Surgery is the **treatment of choice** for primary lesions in **all cases of localized thyroid cancer** except locally advanced cases of anaplastic carcinoma, when resection is unlikely to increase survival
         b. **Approaches.** Virtually all thyroid cancers are resected using a **transverse cervical incision** placed 2 cm above the level of the clavicles (within the collar area). The platysma muscle is divided; the strap muscles (the sternocleidomastoid, the sternohyoid, the omohyoid, and the sternothyroid) are retracted laterally; and the thyroid gland itself is carefully mobilized. Both **recurrent laryngeal nerves** must be clearly identified and preserved whenever possible (the right nerve may not be recurrent in 1–2% of the population). Similarly, the **parathyroid glands** and their blood supply should be preserved to avoid the difficult management problem of postoperative hypoparathyroidism.
         c. **Procedures.** There are three commonly used procedures for thyroid cancer. The decision about which procedure to use is based on the extent of the primary tumor and on the surgeon's preference.
            (1) **Partial thyroidectomy (lobectomy).** A partial thyroidectomy is often used in **limited unilateral thyroid cancer** and involves removal of the affected lobe with or without the isthmus. However, bilateral and more extensive lesions cannot be treated by this method and require a more radical procedure: either subtotal or total thyroidectomy.
            (2) **Subtotal thyroidectomy.** Subtotal tyroidectomy involves removal of the entire thyroid gland, excluding a small rim of tissue located posteriorly along both lobes near the recurrent nerves and parathyroid glands. Selection of subtotal rather than total thyroidectomy for more extensive or bilateral tumors is based on the following arguments:
                (a) **Nerve damage.** Subtotal thyroidectomy reduces the risk of recurrent laryngeal nerve damage.
                (b) **Multicentricity.** Multicentricity rarely becomes clinically significant.
                (c) **Survival.** Total thyroidectomy has no documented survival advantage.
                (d) **Recurrence.** Repeated resection for local recurrences is safe and technically feasible.

      (e) **Hormonal therapy.** T4 suppression therapy may control residual occult lesions.

      (f) **Residual thyroid tissue.** Postoperative thyroid scanning usually shows residual thyroid tissue even in patients who have undergone total thyroidectomy.

    (3) **Total thyroidectomy.** Total thyroidectomy includes the removal of all thyroid tissue. In the treatment of extensive or bilateral lesions, some surgeons prefer total thyroidectomy over subtotal removal of the gland on the basis of the following information:

      (a) **Nerve damage.** In experienced hands, total thyroidectomy carries only a **minimally increased** risk to the recurrent laryngeal nerve when compared to subtotal thyroidectomy.

      (b) **Parathyroid function.** After total thyroidectomy, less than **2%** of patients develop hypoparathyroidism.

      (c) **Recurrence.** Only 2–11% of patients develop recurrent or persistent cervical disease after subtotal thyroidectomy, and reoperation is technically easier after total thyroidectomy.

      (d) **Evaluation.** Residual thyroid tissue spared by subtotal thyroidectomy complicates the evaluation process for local recurrences.

      (e) **Radiotherapy.** ^{131}I thyroid ablation is rendered simpler by the complete removal of all thyroid tissue, as in total thyroidectomy.

      (f) **Multicentricity.** Because thyroid cancer is often multifocal, total thyroidectomy is required to remove all disease.

    (4) **Cervical lymphadenectomy.** In patients with no clinically suspicious lymphadenopathy, **prophylactic cervical lymphadenectomy** does not result in improved survival. However, clinically suspicious nodes should be removed either individually (ie, in a **"berry picking"** procedure) or, if the clinical situation warrants (ie, in cases of anaplastic carcinoma or marked cervical lymphadenopathy), with a modified radical neck dissection.

  2. Locally advanced and metastatic thyroid cancer. Although surgical resection of distant metastatic foci of thyroid cancer has no proved survival benefit, locally recurrent disease within the neck is an accepted indication for therapeutic or palliative radical neck dissection. Distant metastases rarely produce symptoms that require palliative surgical procedures.

  3. Morbidity and mortality. The mortality rate from thyroid surgery should be less than **1%,** and the morbidity should be minimal as well.

    (a) **Laryngeal nerve paralysis.** Despite even the most diligent attempts to preserve the laryngeal nerves, **1–2% of patients develop laryngeal nerve paralysis.** If the nerve has been clearly identified and remains intact, postoperative swelling or inflammation and intraoperative traction injury may result in **temporary** recurrent laryngeal nerve paralysis that typically resolves within several weeks. In this case, or if the nerve is sacrificed intraoperatively, the resulting paralysis of the ipsilateral vocal cord requires careful postoperative rehabilitation to prevent aspiration during swallowing.

    (b) **Hemorrhage.** In thyroid surgery, as in any surgery involving the neck, bleeding may compromise the airway through direct compression of the trachea. This life-threatening situation must be recognized and treated immediately by **opening the wound** and **evacuating the hematoma.**

    (c) **Wound infection.** Rare.

    (d) **Thromboembolism.** Dislodging plaques or thrombi from the carotid arteries may rarely cause cerebral vascular accidents.

B. Radiation therapy

  1. Primary thyroid carcinoma. Radiation therapy is not an acceptable alternative to surgery in the treatment of primary thyroid carcinoma because these cancers, in general, and Hurthle cell tumors, in particular, are radioresistant. Successful ablative therapy would require doses as high as **30,000 cGy.**

  2. Adjuvant radiation therapy. ^{131}I therapy is commonly used to ablate residual foci of malignancy not identified at the time of surgery. This improves **cure rates** over those observed with surgery alone to as high as **70%** in low-risk patients. ^{131}I ablative therapy also identifies sites of distant disease, improves the identification of recurrences with thyroid scanning, and increases the sensitivity of the thyroglobulin assay in detecting recurrences. ^{131}I therapy and scanning are limited by the efficiency of iodine uptake of the tumor, the location of the tumor, the patient's age, and the amount of ^{131}I uptake in residual normal thyroid tissue.

3. **Locally advanced and metastatic thyroid cancer.** [131]I treatment produces a **45–50% response rate** in patients with widely metastatic disease. Many of these responses are durable, although **lung metastases typically respond better than bony metastases.** External-beam radiation (with 30,000 cGy to primary lesions and **8,000 cGy** to metastases) has been used with limited success in patients who have unresectable anaplastic tumors.
4. **Morbidity and mortality.** The side effects of ^{131}I therapy are usually not severe but may include any or all of the following: **nausea, bone marrow depression, sialoadenitis,** and **leukemia.**

C. **Chemotherapy**
1. **Primary thyroid carcinoma.** Primary thyroid lesions are usually treated with surgery, radiation therapy, or both. There is **no indication** for chemotherapy as a first-line therapy for primary lesions unless the lesion is unresectable and therapy is directed at palliation, as discussed below.
2. **Adjuvant therapy.** Adjuvant chemotherapy has no clear role in patients with thyroid cancer.
3. **Locally advanced and metastatic thyroid cancer.** Metastatic or extensive local disease can be treated with the combination of **doxorubicin, cyclophosphamide, bleomycin, and cisplatin,** which has produced a **50–60% partial response rate.** The combination of **doxorubicin, cisplatin, and streptozotocin** also has been tried, producing a **response rate as high as 50%.** However, no clear survival advantage has been demonstrated with either regimen. Patients with anaplastic tumors are candidates for palliative chemotherapy. Although doxorubicin is often combined with radiation therapy in an attempt to control tumor growth, significant responses are uncommon.

D. **Hormonal therapy.** After subtotal or total thyroidectomy, patients should be treated with exogenous **thyroid hormone to suppress secretion of TSH** and its stimulation of remaining normal and malignant thyroid tissue.

E. **Immunotherapy.** There is no significant experience with immunotherapy in the treatment of patients with thyroid cancer.

X. **Prognosis**
A. **Five-year survival.** The prognosis in thyroid cancer depends more on histology than on tumor stage. However, the recently revised TNM staging system may permit a better correlation between stage and prognosis in the future.
1. **Papillary and papillary-follicular carcinoma.** This histology has the best prognosis: **more than 90%** 5-year survival. Lymph node metastases and multicentricity **do not** influence mortality.
2. **Follicular carcinoma.** Patients with follicular carcinoma have only a **50%** 5-year survival rate because of the development of distant metastases.
3. **Hurthle cell carcinoma.** Approximately **85%** of the patients with this histologic variant **die** of their disease.
4. **Anaplastic carcinoma.** This cancer has a uniformly dismal prognosis: only **7–8%** of patients survive 1 year.
5. **Medullary carcinoma.** Patients with medullary tumors **associated with familial syndromes** generally have a **better prognosis** than do those with sporadic tumors. Although patients with MEN IIB rarely survive beyond age 40 because of intercurrent diseases, as many as **65% of patients with MEN IIA** in some series survive 5 years.

B. **Adverse prognostic factors.** Independent of tumor histology, the likelihood of survival is adversely influenced by the following prognostic factors: **male sex, age older than 45, primary tumor larger than 2.5 cm in diameter, treatment with less radical surgery** (ie, subtotal rather than total thyroidectomy), and **no history of ^{131}I ablation or suppression therapy.**

XI. **Patient follow-up**
A. **General guidelines.** Patients should be followed every 3 months for one year, every 6 months for two years, then annually for evidence of recurrence. Specific recommendations are outlined below.
B. **Routine evaluation.** Every clinic visit should include the following tests and procedures:
1. **Medical history and physical examination.** A complete interval medical history and a thorough physical examination must be performed during each clinic visit. Specific attention should be focused on the areas listed on p 445, **VI.**
2. **Blood tests**
a. **Complete blood count** (see p 1, **VI.B.1.a**).

        b. Thyroglobulin levels. This serum protein serves as a tumor marker, and levels correlate well with the success of ^{131}I therapy.

    3. Chest x-ray (see p 3, **IV.C.1**)

C. Additional evaluation. Other tests that should be ordered at regular intervals include the following:

    1. Thyroid function tests. Serum levels of T4, T3, and TSH should initially be checked every 4–6 months, then annually, to assess the adequacy of thyroid replacement.

    2. [131]I scans. This nuclear medicine scan should be ordered at 6, 12, 36, and 72 months after the completion of treatment or if recurrent disease is suspected.

D. Optional evaluation. The following tests and examinations may be indicated by previous diagnostic findings or clinical suspicion:

    1. Blood tests

        a. Carcinoembryonic antigen (CEA) (see p 447, **VI.C.1.c**).

        b. Calcitonin (see p 447, **VI.C.1.d**).

    2. Imaging studies

        a. Ultrasound. Examination of the neck for local recurrences with ultrasound is occasionally rewarding, especially when surgical scarring makes physical examination difficult (see also, p 3, **IV.C.3**).

        b. Computed tomography (CT). CT scan of the neck and chest is the most sensitive test for detecting local neck recurrences, lymph node metastases, and distant pulmonary metastases.

    3. Magnetic resonance imaging (MRI) (see p 3, **IV.C.3**).

    4. Esophagogastroduodenoscopy. As many as 20% of patients with thyroid cancer develop a peptic ulcer after treatment; therefore, patients should be closely monitored for symptoms of excessive gastric acid. Endoscopic examination is mandatory if symptoms develop, and appropriate treatment should be based on endoscopic findings.

    5. Biopsy. Any abnormal masses in the neck or nodal areas and visceral organs should be subjected to a biopsy to exclude malignancy. The type of biopsy should be appropriate for the location, size, and overall index of suspicion and may include fine needle, needle core, and open biopsies.

REFERENCES

Bell RH. Thyroid carcinoma. Surg Clin North AM, 66(1), 13–30, 1986.

Cance WG and Wells SA. Multiple Endocrine Neoplasia Type IIA. In Ravitch MM et al.: Current Problems in Surgery, Year Book Medical Publishers, Salem, MA, 1985.

Emmertsen, K. Medullary thyroid carcinoma and calcitonin. Dan Med Bull, 32(1), 1–28, 1985.

Gluck WL. Thyroid and parathyroid cancer. Clin Geriatr Med, 3(4), 729–742, 1987.

Lennquist S. The thyroid nodule, diagnosis and surgical treatment. Surg Clin North Am, 67(2), 213–32, 1987.

Mazzaferri EL, de los Santos ET, and Rofagha-Keyrani S. Solitary thyroid nodules, diagnosis and management. Med Clin North Am, 72(5), 1177–1211, 1988.

Ozaki O, Ito K, Kobayashi K, et al. Familial occurrence of differentiated non-medullary thyroid carcinoma. World J Surg, 12: 565–571, 1988.

Van Middlesworth L. Effects of radiation on the thyroid gland. Adv Intern Med, 34, 265–284, 1989.

56 Malignancies of the Adrenal Cortex

Christian Jensen, MD

I. **Epidemiology.** Cancer of the adrenal cortex is **rare;** it represents only **0.05–0.2% of all malignancies.** Estimates indicate that fewer than **400 cases** will occur in 1993 in the United States. The annual incidence is **0.2 per 100,000** of the population. World-wide, the incidence is not known to vary significantly.

II. **Risk factors**
   A. **Age.** The incidence of adrenal cortical carcinoma is **bimodal,** increasing to an early peak **(< 5 years of age)** and again later between the **ages of 35 and 45.**
   B. **Sex.** There is no sex predilection. However, the risk of developing a **functioning** tumor is **2 times** greater in **females,** whereas the risk of developing a **nonfunctioning** cancer is higher in **males**.
   C. **Race.** No racial predilection is known.
   D. **Genetic factors**
      1. **Family history.** The risk in first-degree relatives is not increased.
      2. **Familial syndromes**
         a. **Li-Fraumeni-Lynch syndrome.** An inherited predisposition for **sarcomas** as well as **breast, lung, and adrenal cortical carcinomas** characterizes this syndrome. The pattern of inheritance, however, has not been fully defined.
         b. **Beckwith-Wiedemann syndrome.** This childhood growth disorder—marked by **gigantism, omphalocele, and macroglossia**—is associated with adrenal tumors.
      3. **Genetic abnormalities.** Numerous genetic anomalies, particularly deletions and translocations involving **chromosomes 11p, 13q, 14q, and 17p,** have been identified in patients with adrenal cortical carcinoma.
   E. **Diet.** The importance of dietary factors is unknown.
   F. **Smoking.** Tobacco is not known to increase the risk of developing adrenal carcinoma.
   G. **History of previous adrenal pathology**
      1. **Adrenal hyperplasia.** Adrenal hyperplasia and adenoma do not predispose to carcinoma. However, carcinoma has been reported in patients with hyperplasia.
      2. **Congenital hemihypertrophy.** Adrenal carcinoma has been reported to occur in association with congenital hemihypertrophy.
   H. **Urbanization.** No data are available on the effect of urbanization on the incidence of adrenal tumors.

III. **Presentation**
   A. **Signs and symptoms**
      1. **Local manifestations.** The most common presenting complaints are vague **abdominal pain, weakness, anorexia, and weight loss.** Often, an **abdominal mass** can be appreciated (advanced disease). Direct extension to adjacent structures (kidney, liver, bowel, pancreas, and spleen) may produce symptoms related to these organs. In addition, production of **excess adrenal hormones** leads to numerous additional signs and symptoms, as outlined below:
         a. **Signs and symptoms of excess cortisol.** Many functional tumors secrete cortisol or cortisol-like substances, producing **Cushing's syndrome.** Although both adenomas and carcinomas may produce signs and symptoms of excess cortisol, **carcinomas** generally produce additional signs and symptoms of **excess aldosterone, estrogens, and androgens.** Typical symptoms include **truncal obesity** (88%), **round facies** (75%), **hypertension** (74%), **striae** (66%), **impaired glucose tolerance** (65%), **weakness** (61%), **plethora** (60%), acne (45%), bruising (42%), changes in mental status (42%), osteoporosis (40%), edema (39%), hyperpigmentation (21%),

and hypokalemia (17%). **Females** also may complain of **hirsutism** (65%) and **amenorrhea** (60%).

   b. **Signs and symptoms of excess aldosterone (2%).** Signs and symptoms of pure aldosterone excess **(Conn's syndrome)** are less common with carcinomas than with adenomas and include hypertension, hypokalemia, weakness, muscle cramps, polyuria, and polydipsia.

   c. **Signs and symptoms of excess androgen (10%).** In **prepubertal males and females,** excess androgen leads to increased growth and muscle mass, acne, voice changes, enlargement of the genitalia, and growth of pubic and facial hair. Increased muscle mass, acne, voice changes, hirsutism, amenorrhea, infertility, and temporal balding occur in **adult females.**

   d. **Signs and symptoms of excess estrogen (12%).** Signs and symptoms of excess estrogen are frequently associated with malignancy and include **gynecomastia in prepubertal males; precocious puberty** (vaginal bleeding and breast development) in **prepubertal females;** and **gynecomastia,** decreased libido, impotence, and infertility in **adult males.**

   2. **Systemic manifestations.** Common signs and symptoms of distant metastatic disease include **hepatomegaly** (liver metastases); **lower extremity edema** (lymphatic metastases, tumor mass, or inferior vena cava thrombus); **cervical adenopathy;** and, infrequently, hemoptysis, shortness of breath (pulmonary metastases), bone pain (bone metastases), and changes in mental status (central nervous system [CNS] metastases).

  B. **Paraneoplastic syndromes.** Adrenal carcinoma has no associated paraneoplastic syndromes, other than the syndromes of steroid hormone excess as discussed above.

IV. **Differential diagnosis.** Although some adrenal carcinomas produce hormones and associated syndromes, many do not and instead present as a symptomatic **adrenal mass.** Moreover, expanded use of computed tomography has increased the incidental detection of **asymptomatic adrenal masses** (6 per 1000 scans). The diagnostic possibilities that should be considered (in addition to adrenal cortical carcinoma) include **infections** (tuberculosis, histoplasmosis, and, in rare cases, adrenal or perinephric abscess), **inflammation** (postpartum Waterhouse-Friderichsen syndrome), **congenital cysts, benign neoplasms:** eg, cortical adenomas (generally < 6 cm in diameter), myelolipoma, angioma, and leiomyoma, **other adrenal malignancies** (leiomyosarcoma, malignant lymphoma, plasmacytoma, renal cell carcinoma, pheochromocytoma, and neuroblastoma), and metastatic neoplasms (lung, breast, colorectal, and renal cell carcinoma and melanoma).

V. **Screening programs.** The low incidence of adrenal carcinoma precludes widespread screening.

VI. **Diagnostic workup**

  A. **Medical history and physical examination.** A complete medical history and thorough physical examination are essential in the initial evaluation of patients with suspected adrenal cortical carcinoma. Particular emphasis is placed on the following areas:

   1. **General appearance.** Evidence of peripheral muscle wasting and central obesity should be noted.

   2. **Skin.** Thin atrophic skin, dilated fragile veins, bruising, hyperpigmentation, and jaundice (hepatic dysfunction) must be described.

   3. **Head.** The shape of the face (round facies), plethora, and abnormal facial hair in females (hirsutism) should be indicated.

   4. **Lymph nodes.** The presence of increased dorsal neck fat (buffalo hump) and a signal node (also called **Virchow's or Troisier's node**) should be recorded.

   5. **Abdomen.** Striae, a palpable mass, and hepatomegaly (metastatic disease) may often be detected, especially in thin patients.

   6. **Extremities.** Swelling of the lower extremities (obstruction of the inferior vena cava by tumor thrombus) should be noted.

   7. **Central nervous system.** Changes in mental status from mild depression to florid psychosis may be detected.

  B. **Primary tests and procedures.** The following tests and procedures should be performed on all patients with suspected adrenal cortical carcinoma:

   1. **Blood tests**

     a. **Complete blood count** (see p 1, **IV.A.1**).

     b. **Hepatic transaminases** (see p 1, **IV.A.2**).

     c. **Alkaline phosphatase** (see p 1, **IV.A.3**).

     d. **Electrolytes.** In the absence of diuretic therapy, a serum **potassium** concentration < 3.9 meq/L is suggestive of **hyperaldosteronism.**

   e. **BUN and creatinine** (see p 3, **IV.A.6**).
  2. **Urine tests**
   a. **Urinalysis** (see p 3, **IV.B**).
   b. **24-hour urinary catecholamines.** A 24-hour urine collection demonstrates **elevated epinephrine, norepinephrine, vanillylmandelic acid, and metanephrines in** patients with pheochromocytomas. Alternatively, metanephrine levels can be measured on a spot urine sample. Borderline values require determinations of serum epinephrine and norepinephrine.
   c. **Twenty-four hour urinary 17-hydroxysteroids.** Elevated levels of urinary 17-hydroxysteroids suggest the presence of a **cortisol-producing adrenal tumor,** either an adenoma or carcinoma.
   d. **Twenty-four-hour urinary 17-ketosteroids.** Elevated levels of urinary 17-ketosteroids suggest the presence of an **androgen-secreting adrenal tumor,** either an adenoma or carcinoma.
  3. **Imaging studies**
  4. **Chest x-ray** (see p 3, **IV.C.1**).
   a. **Abdominal flat plate.** A plain abdominal x-ray (usually obtained during excretory urography) may demonstrate the position and size of an adrenal mass. In addition, **fine stippled calcifications** suggest **neuroblastoma.**
   b. **Computed tomography (CT).** CT scan of the abdomen boasts a **95% sensitivity** (although low specificity) in imaging adrenal masses and should be obtained on all patients. Historically, adrenal masses **larger than 6 cm in diameter** are usually **carcinomas,** whereas those smaller than 3.5 cm are adenomas. However, small lesions cannot be ignored because improved imaging techniques (CT and MRI) have increased the incidental detection of small asymptomatic cortical carcinomas and pheochromocytomas, which previously went undiscovered until they had become large (often > 6 cm). Furthermore, CT may identify lymph node, adrenal vein, and caval involvement and liver and lung metastases.
   c. **Magnetic resonance imaging (MRI).** Like CT scans, MRI scans may image adrenal masses as small as 1 cm accurately. Moreover, the **adrenal mass to liver signal ratio on T_2-weighted spin echo scans** may definitely diagnose **pheochromocytomas** (ratio > 3.0) and, in **79%** of cases, help differentiate adrenal **adenomas** (ratio **0.7–1.4,** functioning or nonfunctioning) from **malignancy** (ratio **1.2–2.8,** adrenal carcinoma and metastases from other primary tumors). Adrenal vein and vena cava involvement with tumor thrombus also may be detected.
  5. **Invasive procedures.** No invasive procedures are indicated in the routine workup of adrenal masses. Indeed, they **should be avoided** because of the risk of precipitating an acute hypertensive crisis and death in patients with unsuspected pheochromocytoma.
 C. **Optional tests and procedures.** The following examinations may be indicated by previous diagnostic findings or clinical suspicion.
  1. **Blood tests**
   a. **5′-Nucleotidase** (see p 2, **IV.A.4**).
   b. **GGTP** (see p 2, **IV.A.5**).
   c. **Cortisol.** Although not as sensitive as urinary free cortisol, elevated levels of plasma cortisol **(> 25 mcg/dL) are consistent with the diagnosis of Cushing's syndrome and require evaluation with a low-dose plasma and high-dose (plasma or urinary) dexamethasone suppression test** to determine the cause of the excess cortisol. For the **low-dose plasma test,** dexamethasone (1 mg) is administered at 11 PM, and an 8 AM cortisol level is obtained the following morning. Levels of **less than 5 mcg/dL are normal (3% false-negative rate),** whereas levels greater than 10 mcg/dL should arouse suspicion about Cushing's syndrome, although a **30% false-positive rate** exists with depression, alcoholism, stress, and primary cortical resistance. An abnormal low-dose test then necessitates a high-dose (plasma or urinary) test. For the **high-dose plasma test,** a baseline 8 AM plasma cortisol level is drawn, dexamethasone (8 mg) is given at 11 PM, and an 8 AM plasma cortisol level is obtained the following morning. Suppression to **less than 50% of baseline levels** occurs with **pituitary-dependent Cushing's syndrome** (Cushing's disease) but not with other causes of hypercortisolism such as **adrenal tumors and ectopic ACTH.**
   d. **Adrenocorticotropic hormone (ACTH).** Baseline levels of this hormone will be **elevated in pituitary-dependent Cushing's syndrome** (Cushing's disease), **markedly elevated** in patients with **ectopic ACTH production**

(60% > 300 pg/mL), and **depressed** in adrenal **adenoma and carcinoma** (functioning). Moreover, an alternative test to the dexamethasone suppression test is the corticotropin-releasing hormone (CRH) test. In this test, baseline plasma ACTH and cortisol levels are obtained, CRH (1 mcg/kg) is given, and ACTH and cortisol levels are repeated. An **increased repeat plasma ACTH** (and cortisol) level occurs with **pituitary-dependent Cushing's syndrome** (Cushing's disease) but not with other causes of hypercortisolism such as adrenal tumor and ectopic ACTH.

   e. **Testosterone.** An elevated level of this androgen, particularly if accompanied by **hypercortisolism**, strongly suggests the presence of an **adrenal carcinoma**, even in the presence of normal 17-ketosteroid levels.

   f. **Estrogen.** An elevated level of estrogen, in the presence of an adrenal mass, is usually caused by an adrenal adenoma or carcinoma.

   g. **Aldosterone and renin.** Plasma aldosterone and renin levels should be measured in all patients with **hypertension, hypokalemia,** or symptoms consistent with hyperaldosteronism. Patients must not take **any antihypertensive medication (particularly diuretics and spironolactone) for 1 month** before determination of plasma aldosterone and renin. A plasma **aldosterone to renin ratio of more than 30:1** suggests the presence of an **aldosterone releasing adrenal tumor,** either an adenoma or carcinoma. Alternatively, a **captopril suppression test** can be performed. For this test, captopril (25 mg) is administered in the morning, and 2 hours later, plasma aldosterone and renin measurements are obtained. A plasma **aldosterone level of more than 15ng/dL** and an **aldosterone to renin ratio of more than 50** on this test signify primary aldosteronism and should be followed by a serum 18-hydroxycorticosterone measurement (see below, **VI.C.1.h**).

   h. **18-Hydroxycorticosterone.** In the presence of aldosteronism (see above, **VI.C.1.g**), elevated levels of this steroid metabolite **(> 100 ng/dL)** are found in **adrenal neoplasms,** whereas low levels **(< 90 ng/dL)** are diagnostic of **idiopathic adrenal hyperplasia.**

2. **Urine tests**
   a. **Twenty-four-hour urinary free cortisol.** Elevated levels of urinary free cortisol **(> 100 mg every 24 hours)** require evaluation with a low-dose plasma and high-dose (plasma or urinary) **dexamethasone suppression test** (see p 435, **VI.C.1.c**) to determine the cause of the excess cortisol. For the high-dose urinary dexamethasone suppression test, dexamethasone (2 mg every 6 hours) is given for 48 hrs, and a 72-hour urinary cortisol collection is obtained simultaneously. Suppression to **less than 50% of baseline levels** occurs with **pituitary-dependent Cushing's syndrome** (Cushing's disease) but not with other causes of hypercortisolism such as **adrenal tumors and ectopic ACTH.**

   b. **Twenty-four-hour urinary potassium.** Elevated excretion of urinary potassium **(> 25–30 mEq every 24 hours)** in hypertensive patients who are not taking diuretics is consistent with the diagnosis of primary aldosteronism.

3. **Imaging studies**
   a. **Excretory urography.** An **intravenous pyelogram** frequently demonstrates displacement of the ipsilateral kidney and excludes significant renal pathology. CT, however, obviates the need for the routine use of this study.

   b. **Ultrasound** (see p 3, **IV.C.4**).

   c. **Angiography.** Because of the danger of precipitating a potentially fatal hypertensive crisis with small pheochromocytomas during contrast injection, angiography rarely is indicated in the workup for adrenal masses and must be **preceded** by a **normal biochemical workup** and an MRI that demonstrates an **adrenal mass to liver ratio of less than 1.4.**

   d. **^{131}I-6-beta-iodomethyl-19-norcholesterol (NP–59) scan.** In equivocal cases, NP–59 adrenal scintigraphy may distinguish adrenal hyperplasia and adenoma (**positive** imaging) from cysts, adrenal carcinoma, and metastatic disease (**negative** imaging). However, the **radiation exposure** accompanying this test is considerable, exceeding that of CT.

   e. **^{123}Metaiodobenzylguanidine (MIBG) scan.** Overall, MIBG scans are **87% sensitive** (slightly higher for malignant and familial tumors), **100% specific** in the imaging of pheochromocytomas, and may be helpful in evaluating an adrenal mass with an indeterminate MRI mass to liver ratio.

   f. **Technetium-99m bone scan** (see p 3, **IV.C.5**).

4. **Invasive procedures**
   a. **Bilateral adrenal vein sampling.** For patients with **clinical symptoms** of adrenal hormone excess and a **nonvisualizing tumor** on CT, MRI, and NP–59 scans, the best localizing study (96% sensitivity) is bilateral adrenal vein sampling. Measurement of the appropriate hormone level often localizes the neoplasm to one adrenal gland or the other, which can then be removed.
   b. **Biopsy.** In rare cases, **percutaneous fine needle aspiration (FNA)** may be useful to distinguish a primary adrenal adenoma or carcinoma from a metastatic lesion, but, in general, adrenal adenomas cannot be differentiated from carcinomas. To prevent possible precipitation of a hypertensive crisis in patients with unsuspected pheochromocytoma, patients should have **normal biochemical studies** (eg, urinary catecholamines) and an MRI **adrenal mass to liver ratio of less than 1.4 before FNA.**

VII. **Pathology**
   A. **Location.** Adrenal carcinoma arises in either gland with **equal frequency.** Although it has been reported, extra-adrenal occurrence is rare.
   B. **Multiplicity.** The incidence of bilateral cortical carcinomas is **4%,** but bilateral primary tumors are difficult to distinguish from a unilateral cancer with a contralateral metastasis.
   C. **Histology.** Typically, adrenal carcinomas weigh **100–5000 g** and may be difficult to distinguish from adenomas. The only reliable single discriminating factor is the **presence of metastatic disease;** however, other characteristics may be helpful. With carcinomas, **necrosis** and **hemorrhage** are evident grossly and **pleomorphic cells with large hyperchromatic nuclei and nucleoli** are visible microscopically. **Fibrous bands** are suggestive and **vascular invasion** and **mitoses** are diagnostic of malignancy. With **adenomas, cellular pleomorphism and necrosis** are rare. In addition, adrenal carcinoma may closely resemble renal cell carcinoma and require immunostaining to confirm the diagnosis. For instance, **vimentin** stains strongly in **adrenal tumors** but not in renal cell carcinoma, and **epithelial membrane antigen and cytokeratin** stain well in **renal cell carcinoma.**
   D. **Metastatic spread.** Nearly **25%** of patients with adrenal cancer present with metastatic disease.
      1. **Modes of spread.** Adrenal cancer spreads by 3 distinct mechanisms.
         a. **Direct extension.** Direct growth into contiguous organs and structures is common.
         b. **Lymphatic metastasis.** Embolic spread to regional (celiac and para-aortic) and distant (supraclavicular) lymph nodes occurs in **48%** of patients by the time of presentation.
         c. **Hematogenous metastasis.** Dissemination through vascular channels results in widespread disease.
      2. **Sites of spread.** Large autopsy studies have demonstrated metastatic spread to the following organs: **lung,** 60%; **liver,** 50%; **lymph nodes,** 48%; **bone,** 24%; **pleura and heart,** 10%; and **CNS,** rare.

VIII. **Staging.** Although the American Joint Committee on Cancer and the Union Internationale Contre le Cancer have not adopted an official staging system, Macfarlane proposed the TNM staging system. This was modified by Sullivan and is currently the most widely accepted system, as outlined below:
   A. **Tumor stage**
      1. **T1.** Tumor is no larger than 5 cm without invasion.
      2. **T2.** Tumor is larger than 5 cm without invasion.
      3. **T3.** Any size tumor in periadrenal fat.
      4. **T4.** Tumor invades adjacent organs.
   B. **Lymph node stage**
      1. **N0.** No lymph node metastases are present.
      2. **N1.** Lymph node metastases are present.
   C. **Metastatic stage**
      1. **M0.** No distant metastases are present.
      2. **M1.** Distant metastases are present.
   D. **Stage groupings.** Roughly **30–40%** of patients present with **Stage I or II** disease, whereas, **60–70%** have advanced disease **(Stages III and IV)** at the time of diagnosis.
      1. **Stage I.** T1, N0, M0.
      2. **Stage II.** T2, N0, M0.
      3. **Stage III.** T1–2, N1, M0; T3, N0, M0.
      4. **Stage IV.** T4, N0, M0; T3, N1, M0; any T, any N, M1.

IX. **Treatment**
   A. **Surgery**
      1. **Primary adrenal cortical carcinoma**
         a. **Indications.** Primary therapy for **all** adrenal carcinomas is **complete surgical resection**, whenever feasible, for possible cure as well as for palliation in cases of excess adrenal cortical hormone.
         b. **Preoperative preparation.** Complications from excess secretion of adrenal hormone should be corrected, if possible, preoperatively. For instance, **insulin** therapy controls diabetes associated with hypercortisolism, and **potassium-sparing antihypertensive agents** (spironolactone and amiloride) lower blood pressure and correct hypokalemia in patients with hypercortisolism and aldosteronism. Moreover, in a recent study of patients with aldosteronism, **nifedipine** normalized serum potassium levels and controlled blood pressure in all patients.
         c. **Approaches.** Adrenal tumors can be removed through either anterior or posterior approaches.
            (1) **Anterior approach. Bilateral subcostal, midline, and thoracoabdominal incisions** provide excellent exposure for the excision of **malignant or large (> 6 cm) benign neoplasms.**
            (2) **Posterior approach. Small (< 6 cm) benign neoplasms** can be approached with a posterior **oblique flank incision** with removal of the 12th rib.
         d. **Procedures. Radical adrenalectomy** is the mainstay of surgical therapy for carcinoma of the adrenal cortex. If contiguous organs are involved, **resection of the diaphragm and vena cava, hepatic lobectomy, pancreatectomy, splenectomy, and nephrectomy** (in patients with 2 functioning kidneys) may be necessary for definitive resection.
      2. **Locally advanced and metastatic adrenal cancer.** In the presence of locally advanced (unresectable) and metastatic disease, **tumor debulking** is recommended to decrease the morbidity associated with excess adrenal hormone. Furthermore, reports of long-term survival following resection of pulmonary, hepatic, and intracranial metastases have encouraged an **aggressive approach to the surgical treatment of metastatic disease,** particularly in the light of the known dismal prognosis for widespread disease and the morbidity associated with excess adrenal hormone.
      3. **Morbidity and mortality.** Most of the surgical morbidity occurs because of excess adrenal hormone (hypercortisolism and aldosteronism). Concomitant hypertension, coronary artery disease, diabetes, and obesity greatly increase the risk of medical complications such as **myocardial infarction, stroke, and pneumonia.** In addition, the use of a **thoracoabdominal incision** is associated with a higher rate of complications. Specific problems include **hemorrhage; infection,** subphrenic abscess; **poor wound healing;** and **adrenal insufficiency,** rare.
   B. **Radiation therapy**
      1. **Primary adrenal cortical carcinoma.** Radiation therapy is not indicated in the initial treatment of adrenal carcinoma.
      2. **Adjuvant radiation therapy.** The use of pre-, intra-, and postoperative radiation therapy has not been investigated extensively.
      3. **Locally advanced and metastatic adrenal cancer.** Radiation therapy provides excellent palliation in as many as 67% of patients with locally recurrent and metastatic tumor, particularly lesions associated with **cerebral edema, impending pathologic fracture, spinal cord compression, and severe bone pain.**
      4. **Morbidity and mortality.** Palliative radiation therapy is not associated with significant morbidity.
   C. **Chemotherapy**
      1. **Primary adrenal cortical carcinoma.** The initial and only curative therapy for adrenal carcinoma is surgery. Chemotherapy, as the primary therapy, is indicated only in patients who are poor **surgical risks** or who **refuse surgery.**
      2. **Adjuvant chemotherapy.** Data regarding adjuvant chemotherapy (primarily o,p-DDD or mitotane) for adrenal cortical carcinoma are strictly **anecdotal.** The toxicity of the currently available agents, however, is well known and significant. Therefore, this approach, although promising, cannot be recommended outside of an approved clinical trial.
      3. **Locally advanced and metastatic adrenal cancer.**

        a. **Single agents.** The standard initial chemotherapeutic agent is **o,p-DDD (mitotane),** a derivative of the pesticide DDT. Mitotane (1–12 g/day in 2–3 divided doses) causes necrosis of both normal adrenal gland and large adrenal tumors. With **serum levels greater than 14 mcg/mL, urinary 17-hydroxysteroids and 17-ketosteroids decrease in 67–88%** of patients and a **33% partial response rate** results (0% complete responses). Although patients treated at higher serum levels may respond better, toxicity often becomes dose limiting. Despite this activity, the administration of o,p-DDD has met with disappointing results, and no proof exists that it alters the natural history of this tumor. A **42% partial response rate** has been reported with **suramin.** Additional agents that have been tried as single agents with only rare partial responses are **cisplatin** and **doxorubicin.**

        b. **Combination chemotherapy.** Several multiagent regimens have been tried in limited studies (< 12 patients) with little success. A combination of **cisplatin** (40 mg/m^2 per day) **and etoposide** (100 mg/m^2 per day) for 3 days produced 2 partial responses in 2 patients, and a mixture of **cisplatin** (40 mg/m^2), **etoposide** (100 mg/m^2), **and bleomycin** (30 U) every 4 weeks yielded 1 complete and 2 partial responses in 4 patients. These encouraging results require confirmation in larger trials before definitive recommendations can be formulated.

    4. Morbidity and mortality. The toxicity of o,p-DDD may be considerable, often is dose limiting, and generally occurs with serum levels **greater than 20 mcg/mL. Frequent problems include the following:**

        a. **Gastrointestinal (79–83%).** Anorexia, nausea, vomiting, and diarrhea.

        b. **Neuromuscular (41–50%).** Confusion, weakness, depression, headache, dizziness, and tremors.

        c. **Dermatologic (15%).** Skin rash.

  D. Immunotherapy. No information is available about this therapeutic modality.

X. Prognosis

  A. Risk of recurrence. The risk of recurrence is significant in all patients, but those with disease limited to the adrenal gland (Stages I and II) have the lowest risk.

  B. Mean survival. Although some patients survive long term after surgical resection of small tumors limited to the adrenal gland, most patients die within 2 years. The **mean survival** by tumor stage is outlined below.

    1. Stage I, 25 months.

    2. Stage II, 24 months.

    3. Stage III, 28 months.

    4. Stage IV, 12 months.

  C. Adverse prognostic factors. The following characteristics portend a particularly poor prognosis:

    1. Extra-adrenal spread. Invasion of contiguous structures decreases survival from a mean of **5 years** to a mean of **2.3 years.**

    2. Anaplastic histology. This results in a **mean survival of 5 months,** compared with **40 months** for **differentiated** carcinoma.

    3. Male sex.

    4. Virilizing and nonfunctional tumors.

    5. Vascular invasion.

    6. Tumor cell necrosis.

    7. Fibrous bands on histology.

XI. Patient follow-up

  A. General guidelines. Patients with adrenal cortical carcinoma, whether resected for cure or palliation, should be followed every 3 months for 2 years, every 6 months for an additional 3 years, then annually for evidence of tumor recurrence. Patients with metastatic disease should be followed every 1–2 months for symptoms requiring further palliative measures. Specific guidelines for following patients with adrenal cortical carcinoma are listed below.

  B. Routine evaluation. Each clinic visit should include the following examinations.

    1. Medical history and physical examination. An interval medical history and thorough physical examination should be performed during each office visit. Areas for particular attention are discussed on p 454, **VI.A).**

    2. Blood tests

        a. **Complete blood count** (see p 1, **IV.A.1).**

        b. **Hepatic transaminases** (see p 1, **IV.A.2).**

        c. **Alkaline phosphatase** (see p 1, **IV.A.3).**

        d. **Electrolytes** (see p 454, **VI.B.1.d).**

  e. BUN and creatinine (see p 3, **IV.A.6**).
 3. Urine tests
  a. 24-hour urinary free cortisol. Serum levels of this hormone may confirm (biochemically) the presence of recurrent disease before it may be detected on imaging studies (see also, p 456, **VI.C.2.a**).
  b. Twenty-four-hour urinary 17-hydroxysteroids (see also, p 455, **VI.B.2.c**).
  c. Twenty-four-hour urinary 17-ketosteroids (see also p 455, **VI.B.2.d**).
 4. Chest x-ray (see p 3, **IV.C.1**).
C. Additional evaluation. Other tests that should be obtained at regular intervals **(every 3–4 months)** include a **CT scan of the chest and abdomen** to exclude local recurrence and liver, lung, and distant metastases.
D. Optional evaluation. The following examinations may be indicated, depending on previous findings or clinical suspicion.
 1. Blood tests
  a. 5'-Nucleotidase (see p 2, **IV.A.4**).
  b. GGTP (see p 2, **IV.A.5**).
  c. Testosterone. If virilizing symptoms occur, serum levels of this hormone may confirm (biochemically) the presence of recurrent disease (see also, p 456, **VI.C.1.e**).
  d. Estrogen. If feminizing symptoms arise, serum levels of this hormone may confirm (biochemically) the presence of recurrent disease (see also, p 456, **VI.C.1.f**).
  e. Aldosterone and renin. If hypertension and hypokalemia develop, serum levels of these hormones may confirm (biochemically) the presence of recurrent disease (see also, p 456, **VI.C.1.g**).
 2. Imaging studies
  a. Ultrasound (see p 3, **IV.C.4**).
  b. Magnetic resonance imaging. MRI may detect local recurrences and liver and lymph node metastases (see also, p 456, **VI.B.3.d**).
  c. ^{131}I-6-beta-iodomethyl-19-norcholesterol (NP–59) scan (see also, p 456, **VI.C.3.d**).
  d. Technetium-99m bone scan (see p 3, **IV.C.5**).
 3. Biopsy. A new mass that appears on imaging studies should be biopsied by **FNA** to confirm or exclude the possibility of recurrent or metastatic disease.

REFERENCES

Bergenstal DM, Hertz R, Lipsett MB, and Moy RH. Chemotherapy of adrenocortical cancer with o,p'-DDD. Ann Int Med 53:672–682, 1960.

Bodie B, Novick AC, Pontes JE, et al. The Cleveland Clinic experience with adrenal cortical carcinoma. J Urol 141:257–260, 1989.

Henley DJ, van Heerden JA, Grant CS, et al. Adrenal cortical carcinoma—A continuing challenge. Surgery 94:226–231, 1983.

Jensen JC, Pass HI, Sindelar WF, and Norton JA. Recurrent or metastatic disease in select patients with adrenocortical carcinoma. Arch Surg 126:457–461, 1991.

King DR and Lack EE. Adrenal cortical carcinoma: A clinical and pathologic study of 49 cases. Cancer 44:239–244, 1979.

Macfarlane DA. Cancer of the adrenal cortex. Ann Roy Coll Surg 23:155–186, 1958.

Percarpio B, Knowlton AH. Radiation therapy of adrenal carcinoma. Acta Rad Ther Phys Biol 15:288, 1976.

Petersen RO. Adrenal gland. In Urologic Pathology. Petersen RO, editor. Philadelphia: J.B. Lippincott, pp. 719–751, 1986.

Richie JP and Gittes RF. Carcinoma of the adrenal cortex. Cancer 45:1957–1964, 1980.

Sullivan M, Boileau M, and Hodges CV. Adrenal cortical carcinoma. J Urol 120:660–665, 1978.

Vaughn ED and Carey RM. Adrenal carcinoma. In Adrenal Disorders. Vaughn ED, Carey RM, eds. Thieme Medical Publishers, New York: pp. 231–242, 1989.

Weiss LM, Medeiros LJ, and Vickery AL. Pathologic features of prognostic significance in adrenocortical carcinoma. Am J Surg Pathol 13:202–206, 1989.

57 Malignancies of the Adrenal Medulla

Robert B. Cameron, MD

I. **Epidemiology.** Adrenal medullary tumors (pheochromocytomas; PCCs) are rare. The exact incidence is unknown, but the prevalence estimated from autopsy data is 0.005%, and only 0.1% of hypertensive individuals harbor a PCC.

II. **Risk factors**

   A. **Age.** The incidence of PCC increases from near 0 before age 5 years to a **peak between the ages of 20 and 50 years. Childhood** PCC accounts for **20%** of cases.

   B. **Race.** No racial predilection is known.

   C. **Sex.** Although the overall incidence of PCC is the same in males and females, the risk of **malignant (metastatic) PCC is higher in males** than females.

   D. **Genetic factors**

   1. **Family history.** Although, in general, the risk of PCC is not increased in first-degree relatives, kindreds have been described with hereditary PCC occurring at extra-adrenal locations, often at the same site.

   2. **Familial syndromes**

      a. **Multiple endocrine neoplasia, Type IIa (MEN-IIa).** MEN-IIa **(Sipple's syndrome)** consists of PCC, medullary thyroid carcinoma, and parathyroid hyperplasia and is inherited in an **autosomal dominant** fashion with high penetrance.

      b. **Multiple endocrine neoplasia, Type IIb (MEN-IIb).** MEN-IIb is characterized by PCC, medullary thyroid carcinoma, and characteristic craniofacial abnormalities: ie, prominent lips, mucosal neuromas, prominent jaw, pes cavus, medullated corneal nerves, and occasionally a marfanoid appearance. Like MEN-IIa, this syndrome is inherited as an **autosomal dominant** disease.

      c. **Familial PCC.** This rare syndrome is marked by a genetic predisposition for **bilateral PCC** without other features of MEN syndromes.

      d. **Von Hippel-Lindau's disease.** This **autosomal dominant** disorder includes retinal angiomas, cerebellar hemangioblastoma, renal cell carcinoma, and a **25% risk** of PCC.

      e. **Von Recklinghausen's disease.** Neurofibromatosis is an autosomal dominant disease with variable penetrance that is associated with a **1% risk** of PCC.

      f. **Sturge-Weber syndrome.** In this **phakomatosis,** cavernous hemangiomas of the trigeminal nerve are associated with PCC.

   E. **Smoking.** Tobacco has not been identified as an etiologic agent.

   F. **Diet.** No dietary factors have been implicated in the pathogenesis of PCC.

   G. **Urbanization.** No clear differences exist in the incidence of PCC among urban and rural populations.

III. **Presentation**

   A. **Signs and symptoms**

   1. **Local manifestations.** Classically, patients with PCC complain of **paroxysmal episodes of headache, palpitations, diaphoresis, pallor, and anxiety** that are precipitated by physical and emotional trauma, exercise, alcohol, and increased abdominal pressure (palpation, coughing, sneezing, vomiting, and micturition). Other symptoms include anorexia, nausea, vomiting, nervousness, dizziness, syncope, weakness, flushing, chest pain, and dyspnea. Common physical signs are **hypertension and tachycardia,** whereas weight loss and glucose intolerance are less constant. The hypertension is either **episodic (30–50%) or sustained (50–65%; 90% in children).** Severe attacks may lead to seizures, arrhythmias, myocardial infarction, and death.

      2. Systemic manifestations. Bone pain, hepatomegaly, pulmonary nodules, and soft tissue masses may be signs and symptoms of metastatic disease.

  B. Paraneoplastic syndromes. With the exception of the paroxysmal episodes of hypertension, headache, palpitations, tachycardia, diaphoresis, anxiety, and pallor as well as **hypercalcemia** (see p 87) associated with MEN-IIa, no paraneoplastic syndromes have been associated with PCC.

IV. Differential diagnosis. Although many patients present with diagnostic signs and symptoms of excess catecholamine, a significant number of unsuspected cases are discovered as **adrenal masses** on imaging studies of the abdomen (CT and MRI). The differential diagnosis of an asymptomatic adrenal mass is discussed on p 454, **IV.**

V. Screening programs. The low incidence of PCC precludes widespread screening.

VI. Diagnostic workup

  A. Medical history and physical examination. A complete medical history and a thorough physical examination are essential in the initial evaluation of patients with PCC. Particular emphasis is placed on the following areas:

    1. General appearance. Evidence of weight loss should be noted.

    2. Skin. Cafe au lait spots (neurofibromatosis) and jaundice (hepatic dysfunction) must be described.

    3. Head. The retina should be examined for **arteriole narrowing, hemorrhage, exudates, and papilledema** (chronic hypertension) and **cherry red spots** (von Hippel-Lindau and Sturge-Weber syndromes).

    4. Lymph nodes. The presence of a signal node (also called **Virchow's or Troisier's node**) should be recorded.

    5. Abdomen. A palpable mass and hepatomegaly (metastatic disease) may be detected, especially in thin patients; however the **adrenal mass must not be palpated** because of the risk of precipitating an acute hypertensive crisis.

    6. Extremities. Swelling of the lower extremities (obstruction of the inferior vena cava by tumor thrombus) should be noted.

  B. Primary tests and procedures. The following tests and procedures should be performed on all patients with suspected PCC:

    1. Blood tests (see p 1, **IV.A**)

      a. Complete blood count.

      b. Hepatic transaminases.

      c. Alkaline phosphatase.

      d. BUN and creatinine.

    2. Urine tests

      a. Urinalysis (see p 3, **IV.B**).

      b. Twenty-four-hour urinary catecholamines. A 24-hour urine collection demonstrates **elevated epinephrine, norepinephrine, vanillylmandelic acid, and metanephrines in more than 95%** of patients. Alternately, metanephrine levels may be measured on a spot urine sample. Borderline values require determinations of serum catecholamine.

    3. Imaging studies

      a. Chest x-ray (see p 3, **IV.C.1**).

      b. Computed tomography (CT). CT scan of the abdomen boasts a **98% sensitivity** (although low specificity) in imaging adrenal masses and should be obtained for all patients. Furthermore, CT may identify extra-adrenal primary tumors, lymph node and caval involvement, and liver and lung metastases.

      c. Magnetic resonance imaging (MRI). Like CT scans, MRI scans can accurately image adrenal masses as small as 1 cm. Moreover, the **adrenal mass to liver signal ratio on T_2-weighted spin echo scans** may definitely diagnose **PCCs** (ratio > 3) in **79%** of cases. Lymph node, adrenal vein, and vena cava involvement as well as extra-adrenal primary tumors also may be detected.

      d. Invasive procedures. No invasive procedures are indicated in the routine workup of adrenal masses; indeed, they **should be avoided** because of the risk of precipitating an acute hypertensive crisis and death in patients with unsuspected PCC.

  C. Optional tests and procedures. The following examinations may be indicated by previous diagnostic findings or clinical suspicion:

    1. Blood tests

      a. 5'-Nucleotidase (see p 12, **IV.C.4**).

      b. GGTP (see p 2, **IV.A.5**).

      c. Catecholamines. Serum norepinephrine and epinephrine levels often are elevated, particularly during a hypertensive crisis. However, because of moderately elevated levels (500–2000 pg/mL) in **idiopathic hypertension** and other benign conditions, the specificity of random serum catecholamine levels is low unless **a clonidine suppression test** is performed. For this test, an intravenous catheter is inserted and baseline catecholamine levels are obtained after 30 minutes. Subsequently, 0.3 mg of clonidine is given orally, and repeat catecholamine levels are obtained 3 hours later. Catecholamine levels that do not suppress into the normal range (or at least to **< 50% of baseline levels**) suggest PCC, whereas suppression into the normal range is consistent with idiopathic hypertension and other benign disease. Moreover, patients with normal baseline catecholamine levels may require provocative testing. A **histamine or glucagon stimulation test** may be necessary to confirm the diagnosis of PCC. These tests are performed only with experienced personnel, intensive monitoring, and phentolamine (or nitroprusside) immediately available to abort a hypertensive crisis.

  2. **Imaging studies**
    a. **Excretory urography.** An **intravenous pyelogram** frequently demonstrates displacement of the ipsilateral kidney and excludes significant renal pathology. However, CT obviates the need for the routine use of this study.
    b. **Ultrasound** (see p 3, **IV.C.4**).
    c. **Angiography.** Because of the danger of precipitating a potentially fatal **hypertensive crisis** with small PCCs during contrast injection, angiography is rarely indicated in the workup of adrenal masses.
    d. [123]**Metaiodobenzylguanidine (MIBG) scan.** Overall [123]MIBG scans are **87% sensitive** (slightly higher for malignant and familial tumors) and **100% specific** in the imaging of PCCs and may be helpful in evaluating an adrenal mass with an indeterminate MRI mass to liver ratio and in localizing biochemically evident PCC in patients with normal CT and MRI scans.
    e. **Technetium-99m bone scan** (see p 3, **IV.C.5**).
  3. **Invasive procedures.** For patients with **clinical symptoms** of PCC and a **nonvisualizing tumor** on CT, MRI, and [123]MIBG, the best localizing study (96% sensitivity) is **bilateral adrenal vein sampling.** Measurement of the appropriate hormone level often localizes the neoplasm to one adrenal gland or the other, which then can be removed.

VII. Pathology. The important pathologic aspects of PCC can be summarized by the rule of "tens" (see Table 57–1).
  A. Location. The **adrenal glands** are the site of **87%** of PCC (71% in children) with a slight propensity for the right adrenal gland. Extra-adrenal sites account for 13% of cases (29% in children) and can occur anywhere near the midline, including the **organ of Zuckerkandl** (most common), which is located near the origin of the inferior mesenteric artery, the urinary bladder, the heart, and great vessels (eg, aorta, carotid body).
  B. Multiplicity. In sporadic cases, **8.7%** of adults and 20% of children have **bilateral disease,** whereas the disease in **3.4%** of adults and 16% of children involves **multiple extra-adrenal sites.** In familial cases (eg, MEN-IIa), more than **70%** of PCC is **bilateral.**
  C. Histology. In adults, **9.8–46% of PCC are malignant;** however, it is impossible often to distinguish benign from malignant tumors. All tumors are gray soft masses with cells grouped in cords or in an alveolar pattern. Vascular and capsular invasion and nuclear pleomorphism may be present in both benign and malignant lesions, but numerous **mitoses, extensive necrosis, high nuclear ploidy, and large size**

TABLE 57–1. PCC RULE OF "TENS"

Feature	Proportion of Patients (%)
Bilateral	10
Malignant	10
Extra-adrenal sites	10
Requires provocative test	10

(759 g vs 156 g) favor the diagnosis of **malignancy**. However, the only **absolute criterion for malignancy** is the presence of **metastatic disease**.

D. **Patterns of spread**

   1. **Modes of spread.** Generally, PCC spreads by 3 routes.

      a. **Direct extension.** Direct extension leads to invasion of contiguous structures such as the liver, kidney, spleen, diaphragm, pancreas, and stomach.

      b. **Lymphatic metastasis.** Embolic spread to regional lymph nodes happens occasionally.

      c. **Hematogenous metastasis.** Tumor cells eventually gain access to vascular channels and spread to multiple distant organs and tissues.

   2. **Sites of spread.** Although metastatic PCC may occur virtually anywhere, the following organs are frequent sites of metastatic disease: **liver, lung, bone,** and **lymph nodes.**

VIII. **Staging.** No staging system has been developed for PCC.

IX. **Treatment**

   A. **Surgery**

      1. **Primary PCC**

         a. **Indications.** Because surgical extirpation remains the only curative therapy for PCC, every effort should be made to remove the primary tumor in **all patients.**

         b. **Preoperative preparation.** Chronic vasoconstriction and changes in metabolism caused by excess catecholamines leads to **reduced blood volume and lactic acidosis.** These must be rectified before surgery to reduce perioperative morbidity and mortality. Correction is achieved with the alpha-adrenergic blocking agent **phenoxybenzamine,** starting at 10–20 mg/d and increasing to a maximum of 30–100 mg/d as necessary. After 14 days of adequate alpha blockade, blood volume and lactic acidosis return to normal (normal blood Ph must be documented). Following alpha blockade (never before, because of the risk of worsening hypertension from unopposed vasoconstriction), tachycardia can be treated with **propranolol.** The duration of therapy is controversial. Alpha blockade can be stopped as many as 5 days before surgery or be continued perioperatively, depending on the anesthesiologist's preference. Alternatively, **alpha-methylparatyrosine** (500 mg daily in 2 divided doses, increasing to 4 g/d as needed), which blocks tyrosine hydrolase, can be used to control the effects of excess catecholamines. **Nifedipine** (10–30 mg every 6 hours) in combination with phenoxybenzamine is particularly effective for controlling labile hypertension.

         c. **Perioperative management.** Perioperative monitoring includes a **central venous and arterial catheter** for continuous monitoring of central venous and arterial blood pressures. In patients with cardiac disease, a **Swan-Ganz pulmonary balloon catheter** should be placed. **Light sedation** before placing lines for invasive monitoring is recommended to avoid precipitating a hypertensive crisis. Perioperative blood pressure should be controlled with an intravenous drip of **nitroprusside.**

         d. **Approaches.** Because the entire abdomen must be explored to exclude bilateral adrenal and extra-adrenal disease, a **bilateral subcostal (chevron) or midline incision** is indicated.

         e. **Procedures.** Before **adrenalectomy,** a complete **exploratory laparotomy** must be performed, including Kocherization of the duodenum, exploration of the lesser sac, and examination of the para-aortic area from the celiac axis to Zuckerkandl's organ at the bifurcation of the aorta. Then, resection of all tumor, including unilateral or bilateral adrenalectomy, is accomplished.

      2. **Locally advanced and metastatic PCC.** Although no curative option exists for patients with locally advanced, recurrent, or metastatic PCC, **surgery offers the best palliation** of the symptoms of catecholamine excess. All lesions that are amenable to surgical extirpation should be removed.

      3. **Morbidity and mortality.** Before alpha blocking agents were available, the surgical mortality for PCC was 20%; however, with current monitoring techniques and adequate alpha adrenergic blockade, the mortality rate is lower than 3%. Specific problems that may develop include the following: **uncontrollable hypertension; hemorrhage; infection,** subphrenic abscess; **myocardial infarction;** and **stroke.**

B. Radiation therapy
 1. **Primary PCC.** To date, radiation therapy has **no role** in the initial treatment of PCC.
 2. **Adjuvant radiation therapy.** The data available on adjuvant radiotherapy are not adequate enough to recommend its use.
 3. **Locally advanced and metastatic PCC.** Radiation therapy may successfully control pain associated with **bone metastases.** In addition, [131]MIBG administered in therapeutic quantities yields a low (17–41%) response rate: ie, decreased catecholamine secretion or tumor size.
C. Chemotherapy
 1. **Primary PCC.** Because surgery is effective for the initial management of PCC, chemotherapy has not been used in this setting.
 2. **Adjuvant chemotherapy.** Although no data exist to support the use of adjuvant chemotherapy, new studies showing increased responses in the setting of metastatic disease (see **IX.C.3.b**, below) may provide the rationale for clinical trials of adjuvant chemotherapy in high-risk patients (eg, positive surgical margins).
 3. **Locally advanced and metastatic PCC.** The chemotherapy of locally advanced, recurrent, and metastatic PCC falls into 2 categories: **symptomatic palliation** with alpha and beta blocking agents (see p 464, **IX.1.A.b**) and **cytotoxic therapy.** Various chemotherapeutic agents that have been tried are discussed below:
     a. **Single agents.** On the basis of encouraging results in pancreatic endocrine malignancies, patients with PCC were given **streptozotocin.** However, responses have been anecdotal and inconsistent.
     b. **Combination chemotherapy.** Despite the failure of combinations such as doxorubicin and streptozotocin or carmustine, a regimen often used with neuroblastoma that consists of **cyclophosphamide** (750 mg/m^2 IV on day 1), **vincristine** (1.4 mg/m^2 IV on day 1), and **dacarbazine** (600 mg/m^2 IV daily for 2 days) every 3–4 weeks, produces **overall response rates of 53–79%, complete response rates of 7%,** and improvement in catecholamine levels in as many as 87% of patients. The **median duration** of responses in these studies has been as long as **22 months.** Thus, further experience with this combination in the treatment of PCC is certainly warranted.
D. Immunotherapy. No immunomodulatory agents have been used to treat PCC.
X. Prognosis
A. Risk of recurrence. Tumor recurrence may occur as long as 29 years after original adrenalectomy. The risk for the first 9 years is **5% per year.**
B. Five-year survival. Overall 5-year survival is 36%. All patients die within 3 years after the appearance of metastases.
C. Adverse prognostic factors. Although males develop metastatic PCC more often than do female patients, no specific adverse prognostic factors have been identified.
XI. Patient follow-up
A. General guidelines. Patients with PCC, whether resected for cure or for palliation, should be followed every 3 months for 2 years, every 6 months for an additional 3 years, then annually for evidence of tumor recurrence. Patients with metastatic disease should be followed every 1–2 months for symptoms that require further palliative measures. Specific guidelines for following patients with PCC are listed below.
B. Routine evaluation. Each clinic visit should include the following examinations:
 1. **Medical history and physical examination.** An interval medical history and thorough physical examination should be performed during each office visit. Areas for particular attention are discussed on p 462, **VI.A**).
 2. **Blood tests** (see p 1, **IV.A**)
     a. **Complete blood count.**
     b. **Hepatic transaminases.**
     c. **Alkaline phosphatase.**
 3. **Urine tests**
     a. **Urinalysis** (see p 3, **IV.B**).
     b. **Twenty-four-hour urinary catecholamines.** Serial 24-hour urine collections for catecholamines may be useful for detecting recurrence and following the effects of therapy (see also, p 462, **VI.B.2.b**).
 4. **Chest x-ray** (see p 3, **IV.C.1**)
C. Additional evaluation. Other tests that should be obtained at regular intervals include the following:

1. **Computed tomography (CT).** CT scan of the chest and abdomen should be obtained **every 6 months** to exclude local recurrence as well as liver, lung, and distant metastases.
2. **Magnetic resonance imaging (MRI).** Abdominal MRI should be obtained every 6 months to detect local recurrences and liver and lymph node metastases and may be alternated with CT scans. In addition, suspicious areas on CT scan require MRI to exclude possible recurrent PCC (mass to liver ratio > 3.0 on T_2 image) (see also, p 462, **VI.C.2.c**).
D. **Optional evaluation.** The following examinations may be indicated, depending on previous findings or clinical suspicion.
   1. **Blood tests**
      a. **5'-Nucleotidase** (see p 2, **IV.A.4**).
      b. **GGTP** (see p 2, **IV.A.5**).
      c. **Catecholamines.** Like 24-hour urine catecholamine determinations, serum norepinephrine and epinephrine levels can be followed periodically to detect recurrent disease or to follow the effects of therapy (see also, p 462, **VI.C.1.c**).
   2. **Imaging studies** (see p 3, **IV.C**)
      a. **Ultrasound.**
      b. **Technetium-99m bone scan.**

REFERENCES

Averbuch SD. Malignant pheocromocytoma: Effective treatment with a combination of cyclophosphamide, vinocristine, and dacarbazine. Ann Intern Med 109:267, 1988.

Brennan MF and Keiser HR. Persistent and recurrent PCC: the role of surgery. World J Surg 6:367, 1982.

McEwan A, Shapiro B, Sisson JC, et. al. Radioiodobenzylguanidine for the scintigraphic location and therapy of adrenergic tumors. Semin Nucl Med 15:132, 1985.

Stenstrom G, Haljamae H, Tisell LE. Influence of preoperative treatment with phenoxybenzamine on the incidence of adverse cardiovascular reactions during anaesthesia and surgery for PCC. Acta Anaesthesiol Scand 29:797, 1985.

58 Malignancies of the Endocrine Pancreas

Thomas J. Howard, MD

I. **Epidemiology.** Pancreatic endocrine tumors are **rare**. They include **insulinoma, gastrinoma, glucagonoma, somatostatinoma, pancreatic polypeptide-oma** (PPoma), and **vasoactive intestinal polypeptide-oma** (VIPoma). It is estimated that **250 new cases** of islet cell carcinoma or 0.1 case per 100,000 of the population occur each year in the United States. The relative incidence of each of these tumors is depicted in Table 58–1.

II. **Risk factors**
   A. **Age.** Pancreatic endocrine malignancies are diagnosed most commonly in the **fourth and fifth decades of life;** they occur rarely in the young (< 30 years) and the elderly. Tumors that arise in association with **multiple endocrine neoplasia syndrome Type I (MEN I)** (see **II.D.2** below) develop **10 years earlier** than sporadic tumors.
   B. **Sex.** Although the risk of **gastrinoma is 1.5 times greater in males than in females** and the risk of **somatostatinoma is 1.5 times greater in females than in males,** most pancreatic endocrine tumors (insulinomas, glucagonomas, PPomas, VIPomas) exhibit no sex predilection.
   C. **Race.** No racial preponderance has been identified.
   D. **Genetic factors**
      1. **Family history.** In sporadic cases, the risk in first-degree relatives is not increased.
      2. **Familial syndromes.** MEN I (Wermer's syndrome) is an **autosomal dominant** (variable penetrance) disease characterized by **parathyroid hyperplasia (67%), pituitary adenomas (50%), and pheochromocytomas (33%)** as well as **pancreatic endocrine tumors in 67%.** The incidence of MEN I occurring in association with pancreatic islet cell tumors is outlined in Table 58–2. All patients with MEN I should be evaluated thoroughly for parathyroid, pituitary, pancreatic, and adrenal cortical neoplasms.

III. **Presentation**
   A. **Signs and symptoms**
      1. **Local manifestations.** Local manifestations of pancreatic endocrine tumors occur most often in nonfunctioning islet cell neoplasms and include an **abdominal mass** and **obstruction of the gastrointestinal or biliary tract and pancreatic duct.**
      2. **Systemic manifestations.** Metastatic pancreatic endocrine neoplasms may produce abdominal masses (lymph node metastases), hepatomegaly (hepatic metastases), and pulmonary nodules (lung metastases).
   B. **Paraneoplastic syndromes.** In addition to familial paraneoplastic syndromes, the release of peptide hormones often produces a characteristic and, occasionally, **pathognomonic "paraneoplastic" endocrine syndrome.**
      1. **Insulinoma.** Hypoglycemia from autonomous insulin release causes dysfunction of the central nervous system (92%), producing **confusion, irritability, drowsiness, apathy, visual disturbances, headache, and ultimately seizures (12%) and coma (53%).** Typically, the headaches are mild, persistent, and recurrent but are often not identified as a specific symptom until after surgery, when they no longer occur. A surge in catecholamine and glucagon secretion in response to hypoglycemia also precipitates **palpitations, diaphoresis, tachycardia, and anxiety** in 17% of patients. Patients also may cite vague gastrointestinal complaints (hunger, nausea, vomiting, weight gain). Although symptoms most commonly manifest **2–3 hrs after a meal,** they also are precipitated by fasting or exercise.
      2. **Gastrinoma.** Hypersecretion of gastric acid from excess gastrin production results in symptoms identical to those of peptic ulcer disease: ie, **abdominal pain (95%), dyspepsia, nausea, and vomiting** (these symptoms, in association

TABLE 58–1. RELATIVE INCIDENCE OF PANCREATIC ENDOCRINE NEOPLASMS

Tumor Type	Relative Incidence
Gastrinoma	1000
Insulinoma	100
VIPoma	50
Glucagonoma	10
Somatostatinoma	1
PPoma	< 1

with hypergastrinemia, constitute the **Zollinger-Ellison syndrome**). In addition, excess acid damages small bowel mucosa and inactivates pancreatic enzymes, producing **diarrhea in 28–50% of patients (in 20% as the sole presenting symptom)**. Patients can give a long history of refractory ulcer symptoms (mean time > 32 months) or present with acute catastrophic complications such as **hemorrhage (30–50%) or perforation (10%)**.

3. **Glucagonoma.** Hepatic glycogenolysis and gluconeogenesis from autonomous glucagon secretion produces a wide range of symptoms from **mild glucose intolerance (83%)** to frank **diabetes.** Subsequently, **anemia (85%), stomatitis (34%), anorexia, hypoaminoacidemia, protein-calorie malnutrition, diarrhea (15%), and weight loss (66%)** ensue from the resulting peripheral mobilization of amino acids and a hypercatabolic state. Hypoaminoacidemia produces a characteristic **migratory necrolytic dermatitis (68%)** that is **pathognomonic** and is described as serpiginously spreading, erythematous, scaly patches of the intertriginous areas, mouth, vagina, anus, trunk, thighs, legs, arms, and face that become confluent, raised, vesicular, and necrotic over 2–3 weeks and subsequently heal centrally. The tongue is painful and often appears smooth and erythematous. Superficial spongiosis and necrosis between the stratum corneum and malpighian layers on biopsy is characteristic. Idiopathic, but potentially fatal, **thromboembolism (30%)** also occurs in these patients, necessitating chronic anticoagulation.

4. **Somatostatinoma.** Generalized inhibition of intestinal peptide secretions (eg, insulin), digestive enzyme production, and gallbladder motility from excessive production of somatostatin causes **diabetes mellitus (90%), steatorrhea (20%), and cholelithiasis (25–65%)**. In addition, **abdominal pain (35%), diarrhea (25%), anorexia (13%), weight loss (35%), and anemia** may be present.

5. **PPoma.** Autonomous pancreatic polypeptide secretion can produce numerous symptoms, including **upper abdominal pain, gastrointestinal tract bleeding, weight loss, and diarrhea. An erythematous, pruritic, scaly rash** involving the face, hands, chest, abdomen, and perineum has recently been described.

6. **VIPoma.** Cyclic adenosine monophosphate (cAMP)-dependent stimulation of secretion of small intestinal and pancreatic fluid from autonomous vasoactive intestinal peptide (VIP) production causes a **secretory diarrhea (100%; as much as 5 L per day)** similar to cholera, resulting in **severe dehydration, hypokalemia, weakness, and lethargy (100%)**. In addition, **achlorhydria** from inhibition of gastric acid secretion occurs. Although VIP alone may be re-

TABLE 58–2. INCIDENCE OF MEN I WITH VARIOUS PANCREATIC ENDOCRINE TUMORS

Tumor Type	Frequency of Associated MEN I (%)
Somatostatinoma	28
Gastrinoma	20–40
Insulinoma	5–10
PPoma	4
VIPoma	4
Glucagonoma	Rare

sponsible for this **syndrome of watery diarrhea, hypokalemia and achlorhydria (WDHA syndrome),** similar tumors found in the adrenals and sympathetic nervous system suggest that other polypeptides, such as pancreatic polypeptide, gastric inhibitory peptide, and thyrocalcitonin, may be involved. Additional signs and symptoms of VIPoma include **crampy abdominal pain (62%), hypophosphatemia (60%), hypercalcemia (40%), flushing (20%), glucose intolerance (50%), and kidney stones (5%).**

    7. **Hypercalcemia** (see p 87).

IV. **Differential diagnosis.** The clinical signs and symptoms of pancreatic endocrine tumors, although often characteristic and easily confirmed by radioimmunoassay, occasionally may be confused with inflammatory conditions: ie, peptic ulcer disease (gastrinoma) and pancreatitis (nonfunctioning tumors); neuropsychiatric disorders such as stroke, subdural hematoma, or psychosis (insulinoma); and other neoplasms (pancreatic exocrine tumors and pheochromocytoma).

V. **Screening programs.** The rarity of these tumors precludes large-scale screening programs.

VI. **Diagnostic workup**
  A. **Medical history and physical examination.** A detailed medical history that emphasizes the subtle symptoms of pancreatic endocrine tumors and a complete physical examination are essential to a thorough evaluation.
    1. **General appearance.** A nutritional assessment may reveal mild-to-moderate **weight loss (somatostatinoma and PPoma)** or profound **cachexia (glucagonoma).** Sunken eyes and dry mucous membranes may indicate severe dehydration **(VIPoma)** (see also, p 1, **I** and **III**).
    2. **Skin.** A pretibial and truncal dermatitis is pathognomonic of **necrolytic migratory erythema (glucagonoma).**
    3. **Abdomen.** Hepatomegaly and nodular hepatic masses suggest metastases, whereas **midepigastric masses** are indicative of a large (usually nonfunctioning) primary neoplasm.
    4. **Rectum.** Stool should be examined for **occult blood (gastrinoma or PPoma).**
  B. **Primary tests and procedures.** All patients with suspected pancreatic endocrine neoplasms should have the following diagnostic tests and procedures performed:
    1. **Blood tests**
      a. **Complete blood count.** Anemia **(gastrinoma and PPoma)** resulting from gastrointestinal blood loss may be detected (see also, p 1, **IV.A.1**).
      b. **Hepatic transaminases** (see p 1, **IV.A.2**).
      c. **Alkaline phosphatase** (see p 1, **IV.A.3**).
      d. **Electrolytes.** Potassium, chloride, and bicarbonate levels must be aggressively repleted and closely followed in patients with the **WDHA syndrome (VIPoma).**
      e. **Calcium and phosphate.** Elevated calcium levels accompanied by low phosphate levels may signify the presence of a **concomitant parathyroid neoplasm (MEN I syndrome;** see p 467, **II.D.2**). Isolated hypercalcemia may occur as part of a **paraneoplastic syndrome** (see p 467, **III.B**).
      f. **Polypeptide hormone radioimmunoassay.** The detection of an elevated polypeptide hormone level is the mainstay of diagnosis in patients with pancreatic endocrine malignancies.
        (1) **Gastrin.** An elevated fasting serum **gastrin level (> 500 pg/mL) is diagnostic of gastrinoma;** however, with levels greater than 100 pg/mL but lower than 500 pg/mL, the diagnosis requires confirmation by the secretin stimulation test (see **VI.C.2.a** below). In addition, the diagnosis of insulinoma may necessitate a provocative test (see **VI.C.2.b** below). However, elevated levels of basal plasma polypeptide in association with a pancreatic mass are diagnostic of the following tumors:
        (2) **Glucagon** (> 1000 pg/mL).
        (3) **Somatostatin** (> 150 pg/mL).
        (4) **Vasoactive intestinal peptide** (> 250 pg/mL).
        (5) **Pancreatic polypeptide (PP).** Sensitive but not specific (also elevated in other pancreatic endocrine tumors).
    2. **Imaging studies**
      a. **Chest x-ray** (see p 3, **IV.C.1**).
      b. **Computed tomography (CT).** Abdominal CT scan is the best initial diagnostic test for visualizing **primary pancreatic endocrine neoplasms (> 1.5 cm) and hepatic metastases.** However, because most primary tumors are

smaller than 2 cm in diameter, only **20–40% of malignancies** usually are identified. With new high-resolution CT scanners and the use of bolus intravenous contrast, the sensitivity, particularly for **gastrinomas,** recently has improved to **40–78% with a specificity of 100%.** In contrast, insulinomas are not well visualized by CT and should be evaluated by angiography (see below).

C. **Optional tests and procedures.** The following examinations may be indicated by previous diagnostic findings or clinical suspicion:

1. **Blood tests** (see p 2, **IV.A**)
   a. **5′-Nucleotidase.**
   b. **GGTP.**
2. **Provocative tests**
   a. **Secretin stimulation test.** This test is more than **90% sensitive and 93% specific** and should be performed in all patients with **suspected gastrinoma** and a fasting gastrin level lower than 500 pg/mL. The patient should be **fasting and off all antisecretory medications for 2–3 days.** Initially, intravenous access is established, and 2 baseline serum levels of gastrin are collected. Subsequently, **secretin-kabi (2 mg/kg)** is given by rapid IV infusion, and peripheral blood samples at **2, 5, 10, 15, 20, and 30 minutes** after administration are assayed for gastrin. A marked rise in serum gastrin to more than **200 mcg/mL within 2–5 minutes** is diagnostic.
   b. **Calcium infusion test.** An IV infusion of **calcium (15 mg/kg over 4 hours)** increases gastrin levels in patients with **gastrinoma** but not in normal subjects. Although the **sensitivity is 77% and specificity is 100%,** this test currently is not recommended **because of the cardiac risk** (EKG and symptomatic changes require discontinuation of the infusion in 10% of patients).
   c. **Fasting hypoglycemia.** All patients with suspected insulinoma should be observed in the hospital while fasting for 24–72 hrs. A serum glucose level of less than 50 mg/dL with a simultaneously elevated serum **insulin level of more than 5 mcU/mL** (or an insulin to glucose ratio > 0.3) occurs in 98% and is pathognomonic. Relief of accompanying symptoms characteristically follows intravenous glucose administration. The characteristic central nervous system symptoms (see **III.B.1** above) induced by fasting, a fasting glucose of less than 50 mg/dL and relief of the symptoms with glucose administration constitute **Whipple's triad.** Hypoglycemia occurs within 24 hours in **80% of patients,** whereas failure to develop hypoglycemia during the 72-hour fast and a subsequent 15–30 minute period of strenuous exercise excludes the diagnosis. In rare cases, **calcium infusion** (15 mg/kg over 4 hours), producing hyperinsulinemia and hypoglycemia in 90% of patients with insulinoma, may be required to confirm the diagnosis.
   d. **C-peptide test.** Measurement of serum C-peptide levels (a peptide cleaved from insulin during normal secretion) during hyperinsulinemia may demonstrate the autonomous insulin production associated with **insulinoma** (normal C-peptide levels) instead of the normal feedback inhibition associated with hypoglycemia (suppressed C-peptide levels). However, the accuracy of this test has not been verified.
3. **Imaging studies**
   a. **Angiography.** Angiography remains the single most useful study for the preoperative localization of **insulinomas.** Its accuracy is **60–90% for tumors larger than 0.5 cm in diameter.** Occasionally, selective angiography may be useful to visualize other pancreatic endocrine tumors and hepatic metastases that cannot be documented with CT.
   b. **Ultrasound** (see p 3, **IV.C.4**).
4. **Invasive procedures**
   a. **Esophagogastroduodenoscopy.** EGD should be performed in all patients with gastrinoma to **document the severity of ulcer disease and measure basal gastric acid secretion.** After a 3–6 week course of antisecretory therapy (histamine H_2-receptor antagonists or omeprazole), the EGD and acid secretory studies are repeated. Adequate therapy should reduce acid secretion to **less than 15 meq/h in nonoperated patients** and to **less than 5 meq/h** in patients with **previous ulcer surgery** (vagotomy or antrectomy). Control of acid secretion should be attempted in all patients before exploration because **total gastrectomy** is indicated in patients who are found to have incurable disease and whose acid secretion cannot be controlled successfully with medical therapy.

b. **Endoscopic transduodenal ultrasound.** Recently, small endoscopically placed duodenal ultrasound probes have been used to detect **small tumors located in the head of the pancreas, periduodenal area, and submucosa of the duodenum (gastrinoma and somatostatinoma).** Experience to date has been limited, however.

c. **Percutaneous transhepatic portal venous sampling.** Developed in Sweden, this procedure detects markedly **elevated levels of peptide hormone in the venous effluent draining from specific regions of the pancreas in 50–90% of patients.** Until methods are standardized, however, this procedure should be limited to centers that have the proper equipment and technical personnel to perform the selective catheterization and radioimmunoassays required.

d. **Percutaneous needle biopsy.** CT-guided percutaneous needle aspiration may help differentiate large pancreatic exocrine tumors from nonfunctioning endocrine neoplasms.

VII. **Pathology.** Pancreatic endocrine tumors are a heterogeneous group of pancreatic and peripancreatic tumors that secrete neuroendocrine products (peptide hormones) that resemble those normally produced by islet cells (eg, insulin, glucagon, pancreatic polypeptide, somatostatin) or extrapancreatic tissue (ie, gastrin and vasoactive intestinal peptide). **Corticotropinomas, neurotensinomas, and calcitoninomas** also occur but are extremely rare.

A. **Location.** For most endocrine neoplasms, the relative frequency of tumors in various regions of the pancreas parallels the distribution of the islet cell type (see Table 58–3). However, **gastrinomas** have no related pancreatic endocrine cell, and **90%** are found in the pancreas, duodenum, and lymph nodes within the **gastrinoma triangle.** This area is defined as the confluence of the cystic and common bile duct (superiorly), the second and third portions of the duodenum (inferiorly), and the neck and body of the pancreas (medially).

B. **Multiplicity.** Except for **gastrinoma,** which is multicentric in **30–40% of cases,** multiple primary tumors occur in only **5–10% of sporadic pancreatic endocrine neoplasms.** However, tumors that arise in association with **MEN I** are multiple in **50% of the patients.** In addition, nonfunctioning microadenomas, representing either malignant precursors or benign endocrine cell proliferation, may be present in all such patients.

C. **Histology.** In contrast to the numerous clinical syndromes associated with these tumors, the histopathologic architecture of most pancreatic endocrine neoplasms is strikingly uniform. Cords and nests of well-differentiated homogeneous endocrine cells contain nuclei that are round to oval and deeply chromatic with fine stippling. In addition, diffuse endocrine cell involvement **(nesidioblastosis),** micronodular and macronodular islet cell hyperplasia, or all of these are found throughout the pancreas of patients with MEN I. Although electron and immunofluorescent microscopy may distinguish different tumor types by identifying the peptide hormone contained in secretory granules, distinguishing the biological behavior of these tumors is impossible on the basis of histology alone.

D. **Metastatic spread.** Overall, pancreatic endocrine tumors are indolent. Table 58–4 summarizes the incidence of malignant and metastatic lesions by histologic type of endocrine neoplasm.

1. **Modes of spread**
   a. **Direct extension.** Nonfunctioning tumors and those with ill-defined syn-

TABLE 58–3. LOCATION OF VARIOUS PANCREATIC ENDOCRINE NEOPLASMS

Tumor Type	Head (%)	Body (%)	Tail (%)	Duodenum (%)	Other (%)
Gastrinoma	30	10	30	15	15
Insulinoma	30	35	30	2–3	1–2
Glucagonoma	10	40	50	—	—
Somatostatinoma	50	9	9	19	12
VIPoma	25	37	37	—	—
PPoma	—	—	—	—	—

TABLE 58–4. MALIGNANT POTENTIAL OF VARIOUS PANCREATIC ENDOCRINE NEOPLASMS

Tumor Type	Malignancy Rate (%)	Metastic Rate (%)	Nodal Metastases (%)	Liver Metastases (%)
Gastrinoma	40–60	50–80	20	23
Insulinoma	10–15	30	1	2
Glucagonoma	40–80	50	< 1	33
Somatostatinoma	50–90	75	8	48
VIPoma	50–60	50	10	60
PPoma	45–65	100	28	44

dromes occurring in the body and tail of the pancreas (somatostatinoma, PPoma, glucagon) grow undetected into contiguous structures such as the spleen, stomach, colon, and retroperitoneum.

   b. **Lymphatic metastasis.** Although insulinoma, glucagonoma, VIPoma, and somatostatinoma rarely affect lymph nodes, **gastrinoma and PPoma** exhibit a propensity for periduodenal, common bile duct, and celiac lymph node involvement.

   c. **Hematogenous metastasis.** Because of their vascularity, pancreatic endocrine tumors frequently metastasize through blood vessels.

   2. **Sites of metastatic spread.** The overall incidence of metastases at common sites is outlined in Table 58–4. Other rare sites of metastases include bone and lung.

VIII. **Staging.** Because of their rare nature, no formal staging system has been developed for pancreatic endocrine tumors. In many instances, however, they can be staged in a manner identical to that of pancreatic exocrine malignancies (see p 252, **VIII.B**).

IX. **Treatment**
   A. **Surgery**
      1. **Primary pancreatic endocrine neoplasms**
         a. **General considerations.** Before any surgical intervention, the initial goal of therapy is to control the symptoms of excess hormones. This not only serves as palliation but, in many instances, decreases the morbidity and mortality of subsequent surgical procedures. The agents used for symptomatic control vary with the tumor type and are outlined below.
            (1) **Gastrinoma.** The primary goal of adjuvant therapy in gastrinoma is to control ulcer symptoms and complications. Although **H_2-antagonists** are considered to be first-line medications, followed by **omeprazole, octreotide acetate** has recently been vigorously recommended.
               (a) **Somatostatin analog.** Currently, **octreotide acetate** (Sandostatin; 100–250 mcg sc every 8 hours) is the treatment of choice for symptomatic gastrinoma **because it decreases both acid secretion and hypergastrinemia by 76%.** It also decreases the secretion of secondary peptide hormones and has minimal side effects.
               (b) **H_2-receptor antagonists. Cimetidine** (Tagamet; 300–2500 mg PO every 6 hours, although doses > 2.4 g/d are associated with unacceptable side effects), **ranitidine** (Zantac, 150–2000 mg PO every 8 hours), and **famotidine** (Pepsid, 20–160 mg PO every 6 hours) control symptoms in **more than 66% of patients.** However, unacceptable side effects **(eg, gynecomastia, impotence, decreased libido)** develop at high doses of both cimetidine and, occasionally, of ranitidine. In addition, **tachyphylaxis** leading to **"escape"** and treatment failure occur in **23–50%** of patients with all 3 medications, and the drugs **do not block the trophic effect of gastrin** on the gastric mucosa and, potentially, on the gastrinoma itself.
               (c) **H^+/K^+-ATPase inhibitor.** The benzimidazole **omeprazole** (60–120 mg PO every 8–24 hours) may achieve control of acid secretion in **100%** of patients without blocking the trophic effects of gastrin.

(d) **Anticholinergic agents. Pirenzepine, isopropamide** (5–10 mg PO every 12 hours), and **glycopyrrolate** (1–2 mg PO every 6–8 hours) may reduce the requirements for other medications (eg, H_2-antagonists) but **do not block the trophic effect of gastrin** on the gastric mucosa.

(e) **Antacids.** These agents are only minimally useful for the severe ulcer diathesis seen in patients with gastrinoma.

(2) **Insulinoma.** Because 90% of insulinomas are benign and curable with surgery, the sole purpose of medical therapy is to prevent severe hypoglycemia. Several agents are useful for this task.

(a) **Somatostatin analog.** At present, **octreotide acetate** (Sandostatin; 100–250 mcg SC every 8 hours) may represent the first line of therapy. It normalizes glucose levels in **50–60%** of patients, reduces their serum insulin level by 47%, and blunts the insulin response to provocative stimuli.

(b) **Insulin modulators.** The antihypertensive agent **diazoxide** (100–150 mg PO every 8 hours), suppresses insulin release and controls hyperinsulinemia in the majority of patients.

(c) **Steroids.** Prednisone (5–80 mg PO every day) increases peripheral insulin resistance; however, the side effects generally preclude its widespread use.

(d) **Glucagon.** Because of its short half-life, this gluconeogenic hormone has minimal merit in the treatment of insulinoma.

(e) **Glucose.** In severe cases of insulinoma, **intravenous glucose infusion** is required to prevent life-threatening hypoglycemia before surgery.

(3) **Glucagonoma.** Because most glucagonomas are malignant and unresectable, symptomatic palliation is important. Until recently, no satisfactory agents were available. Now, however, **octreotide acetate** (Sandostatin, 100–250 mcg SC every 8 hours) may reduce the glucagon level by **61%,** blunt provocative responses, relieve symptoms, and promote resolution of the associated dermatitis.

(4) **Somatostatinoma.** At present, the only successful therapy for these tumors is surgery because no agents have been shown to significantly palliate symptoms of somatostatin excess.

(5) **VIPoma.** Following aggressive rehydration, preoperative stabilization includes instituting therapy to decrease the profuse diarrhea with one or more of the agents listed below.

(a) **Somatostatin analog.** The most successful agent is **octreotide acetate** (Sandostatin, 100–250 mcg SC every 8 hours), which controls stool volume and electrolyte losses, decreases serum VIP and calcium levels, and inhibits the secretion of associated gastrointestinal hormones in **70%** of patients.

(b) **Steroids.** Prednisone (60–80 mg PO every day) may aid in the symptomatic management of patients with VIPoma.

(c) **Indomethacin.** Patients with **elevated serum prostaglandin E levels** may respond to indomethacin administration (25 mg PO every 8 hours).

(d) **Lithium carbonate.** This drug (300 mg PO twice daily) **reduces stool volume** through the **inhibition of cAMP.**

(6) **PPoma.** Although the data is limited, **octreotide acetate** (Sandostatin, 100–250 mcg SC every 8 hours) may decrease the secretion of pancreatic polypeptide in as many as **90%** of patients.

b. **Indications**

(1) **Occult disease.** Tumors **smaller than 2 cm in diameter** that radiographically (ie, ultrasound, CT scan, and angiogram) do not localize are termed **"occult"** neoplasms. Because elevated serum peptide hormone levels or provocative tests confirm the presence of these tumors, **meticulous exploration and intraoperative localization** are indicated.

(2) **Resectable local disease.** Surgery represents the **only potentially curative therapy** and is recommended for all patients without extensive metastatic disease.

(3) **Familial disease.** Surgery should **not** be undertaken in patients with **MEN I and occult disease** because exploration in the absence of radiographically localized tumor is almost always fruitless. In addition,

patients with associated hyperparathyroidism must first undergo **parathyroidectomy** because hypercalcemia aggravates both gastric acid secretion **(gastrinoma)** and hypoglycemia **(insulinoma).**

c. **Procedures.** The type of operative procedure is dictated by tumor location, cell type, size, multiplicity, and degree of local invasion. Table 58–5 summarizes the 2 important surgical categories of pancreatic endocrine tumors, ie, those that occur to the **right** of the **superior mesenteric artery (SMA)** more than 50% of the time, which require **subtotal pancreatectomy or pancreaticoduodenectomy,** and those that occur to the **left** of the SMA more than 50% of the time, which require **distal pancreatectomy.**

(1) **Exploratory laparotomy and tumor localization.** This procedure is initiated by a **midline or bilateral subcostal incision.** On entering the abdomen, the liver, stomach, duodenum, pancreas, portal and celiac lymph nodes, small bowel, ovaries, colon, and kidneys must be evaluated. A **Kocher maneuver** is performed to mobilize the duodenum, the head of the pancreas, and the uncinate process and to allow direct palpation of the pancreatic head. The **gastrocolic ligament is divided** and the lesser sac is entered (while the peritoneum over the inferior border of the pancreas is divided) to allow bimanual palpation of the body and tail. The following adjunctive procedures can be used to complement bimanual palpation of the pancreas and peripancreatic tissues:

(a) **Intraoperative ultrasound.** Intraoperative ultrasound, albeit expensive and technically difficult, provides excellent anatomic delineation of the pancreatic duct and portal vein and may discern previously unrecognized intra- or peripancreatic tumors such as **insulinoma and glucagonoma.**

(b) **Intraoperative endoscopic duodenal transillumination.** Intraoperative endoscopic transillumination of the duodenal wall may be useful to identify small **submucosal gastrinomas, somatostatinomas, and PPomas.**

(c) **Duodenotomy with intraluminal palpation.** This risky procedure should be attempted only in patients with **gastrinoma or somatostatinoma** who have no evidence of pancreatic or lymph node disease despite an exhaustive intraoperative search.

(2) **Enucleation.** Solitary, small, well-circumscribed superficial tumors that are located away from the main pancreatic duct (ie, **50% of insulinomas**) are ideal candidates for tumor enucleation.

(3) **Partial pancreatic resection.** Large, poorly-defined lesions close to the pancreatic duct (especially if the issue of malignancy is unresolved) should be removed with a margin of normal surrounding pancreas or a more formal pancreatic resection, as discussed below.

(4) **Distal pancreatectomy.** Removal of the body and tail of the pancreas lying to the left of the SMA is useful in **insulinoma and glucagonoma,** particularly if multiple tumors, pancreatic duct involvement, or a deep location are discovered.

(5) **Subtotal pancreatectomy.** A **90% (subtotal) pancreatic resection** is indicated for lesions located in the head of the pancreas (gastrinoma, somatostatinoma, VIPoma) that are not amenable to local resection. This procedure is preferred over the pancreaticoduodenectomy because of its lower morbidity and mortality rates. In addition, **"blind"** subtotal pancreatectomy may **cure 75% of VIPomas, more than 50% of insulinomas, and 30% of glucagonomas.**

TABLE 58–5. SURGICAL LOCATIONS OF VARIOUS PANCREATIC ENDOCRINE NEOPLASMS

Right of SMA	Left of SMA
Gastrinoma	Insulinoma
Somatostatinoma	Glucagonoma
VIPoma	
PPoma	

(6) **Pancreaticoduodenectomy (Whipple procedure).** Because of the high morbidity and mortality (see below), this procedure can be justified only in the rare and otherwise healthy patient with a large or obstructing malignant lesion located in the head of the pancreas.

(7) **Total pancreatectomy.** This radical procedure is almost never indicated because the resulting **diabetes is extremely brittle** and produces an unacceptably high morbidity rate.

2. **Locally advanced and metastatic disease**

a. **Resectable metastatic disease.** The slow rate of tumor growth and the limited regional as well as extrahepatic distant metastatic potential make extended local resection attractive for patients with metastatic and locally invasive disease. Recent studies suggest that an aggressive surgical approach (ie, major hepatic resection, foregut resection, and orthotopic liver or foregut transplantation) in the face of bulky primary and metastatic gastrinoma may produce a prolonged disease-free survival. However, this strategy cannot be recommended until further confirmation of its efficacy is obtained.

b. **Unresectable metastatic disease.** Although chemotherapy remains the primary therapy for advanced metastatic disease, the following surgical procedures may be indicated in certain circumstances if significant palliation is achieved:

(1) **Tumor debulking.** If complete resection is impossible, subtotal resection of primary and metastatic tumor deposits may provide significant palliation in selected patients with **slow-growing but functionally active pancreatic endocrine tumors.**

(2) **Intestinal bypass.** Large pancreatic endocrine tumors that obstruct the duodenum may necessitate **gastrojejunostomy** for satisfactory palliation.

(3) **Vagotomy and antrectomy.** Combined with H_2-receptor antagonists, this procedure may adequately palliate mild-to-moderate hypergastrinemia; however, the **trophic effects** of the gastrin on the gastric mucosa and the gastrinoma itself is **not inhibited.**

(4) **Total gastrectomy.** Patients with uncontrolled **gastrinoma** and fulminant peptic ulcer disease who are **unresponsive to antisecretory medications** may benefit from total gastrectomy, although this procedure carries a **6–15% mortality rate.**

3. **Morbidity and mortality.** The rates of mortality and complications depend primarily on the surgical procedure performed. The mortality rates by procedure are summarized in Table 58–6. Common problems that develop after pancreatic surgery are **wound infections, subphrenic abscess, pancreatitis, pancreatic fistulae** (9%), **and anastomotic leak or stricture.**

B. **Radiation therapy.** Because of the slow rate of tumor growth and the lack of clinical radiosensitivity, radiation therapy is never indicated for the treatment of pancreatic endocrine malignancies, regardless of histology.

C. **Chemotherapy**

1. **Primary pancreatic endocrine neoplasms.** Chemotherapy as the principal treatment for primary resectable pancreatic endocrine tumors is indicated only in patients who have medical contraindications to surgery. Therapy in these patients is identical to that for locally advanced and metastatic disease (see **C.3** below).

TABLE 58–6. MORBIDITY AND MORTALITY OF VARIOUS PANCREATIC OPERATIONS

Procedure	Mortality (%)	Morbidity (%)
Exploratory laparotomy	< 1	5
Enucleation	< 1	5–10
Partial pancreatectomy	2–5	10
Distal or subtotal pancreatectomy	2–10	10–30
Pancreaticoduodenectomy	2–20	36–60
Total pancreatectomy	2–40	> 50

TABLE 58–7. CHEMOTHERAPY RESPONSE RATES OF PANCREATIC ENDOCRINE NEOPLASMS

Tumor Type	Streptozotocin Alone (%)	Streptozotocin + Fluorouracil (%)
Gastrinoma	20	66
Insulinoma	38–64 (17–25)	86
Glucagonoma	33	—
Somatostatinoma	25	66
VIPoma	50–90	90
PPoma	—	—
Overall	40 (10)	63 (33)

2. **Adjuvant chemotherapy.** No significant data exists for chemotherapy used in this setting.
3. **Locally advanced and metastatic neoplasms**
   a. **Single agents.** Several chemotherapeutic agents, including streptozotocin, dacarbazine, doxorubicin, and fluorouracil, have demonstrated some activity against pancreatic endocrine tumors. **Streptozotocin** has the highest activity of all chemotherapeutic agents: it has a **30–40% overall response rate and a 10% complete response rate** that lasts from **12–17 months.** The response rates by tumor type are tabulated in Table 58–7. Side effects of streptozotocin include **nausea and vomiting** (100%), **renal insufficiency and proteinuria** (65%), **liver dysfunction** (67%), and **leukopenia** (20%). **Chlorozotocin** is a new drug that is similar to streptozotocin but has less nephrotoxicity; however, its efficacy is currently unknown.
   b. **Combination chemotherapy.** The addition of fluorouracil or doxorubicin to streptozotocin nearly **doubles the overall and complete response rates** observed with streptozotocin alone and is recommended in all patients who are able to tolerate such therapy. The known response rates of streptozotocin and fluorouracil are listed in Table 58–7.
   D. **Immunotherapy.** Human **leukocyte interferon (interferon-alpha)** has produced an objective **response rate of 77%** (> 50% reduction in tumor size or marker) in patients with **VIPoma,** but these encouraging results await further confirmation.
X. **Prognosis.** The prognosis for patients with pancreatic endocrine tumors depends on the tumor type and the extent of disease at the time of resection. Although glucagonoma, VIPoma, and PPoma tend to be aggressive, these tumors are generally indolent and patients frequently survive 10 years even with hepatic metastases.
   A. **Risk of recurrence.** The risk of recurrence is directly related to the **extent of surgical resection** and the **incidence of multicentric disease.** Recurrence rates by tumor type are listed in Table 58–8.
   B. **Five-year survival.** The long-term survival rate is highly dependent on the **aggressiveness** of the various histologic tumor types. Although several neoplasms are too rare to accurately predict 5- and 10-year survival statistics, rates for the more common tumors are summarized in Table 58–8.

TABLE 58–8. RECURRENCE AND SURVIVAL RATES FOR PANCREATIC ENDOCRINE NEOPLASMS

Tumor Type	Resectability (%)	Recurrence Rate (%)	5-Year Survival (%)	10-Year Survival (%)
Gastrinoma	21–45	64–88	44–82	40–64
Insulinoma	90	11	> 90	89
Glucagonoma	—	70	—	—
Somatostatinoma	—	25	13	—
VIPoma	—	—	—	—
PPoma	—	—	—	—

C. **Adverse prognostic factors.** Because of the paucity of clinical data, the only significant adverse prognostic factor that can be identified is the **presence of metastatic disease.**

XI. **Patient follow-up**

A. **General guidelines.** Patients with resected and unresected disease should be followed every 3 months for 2 years, every 6 months for an additional 3–7 years, then annually for recurrence and symptoms requiring further palliation. The following specific guidelines are offered for patient follow-up:

B. **Routine evaluation.** Each clinic visit should include the following tests and procedures.

1. **Interval history and physical examination.** An interval history should be obtained and a thorough examination must be performed during all office appointments. Particular attention should be focused on the areas discussed on p 469, **VI.B.**

2. **Blood tests**

a. **Peptide hormone radioimmunoassay.** Serum peptide levels can be used to monitor for tumor recurrence. This is particularly useful in patients whose levels returned to normal following surgical resection.

b. **Complete blood count** (see p 1, **IV.A.1**).

c. **Hepatic transaminases** (see p 1, **IV.A.2**).

d. **Alkaline phosphatase** (see p 1, **IV.A.3**).

e. **Electrolytes** (see p 469, **VI.B.1.d**).

f. **Calcium and phosphate** (see p 469, **VI.B.1.f**).

3. **Chest x-ray** (see p 3, **IV.C.1**).

C. **Additional evaluation.** Other tests that should be obtained at regular intervals include the following examinations:

1. **Computerized tomography.** Rapid-infusion abdominal CT scan with 5 mm slices through the pancreas and liver is an excellent method of detecting **intra-abdominal recurrence and hepatic metastases** and should be obtained **every 6–12 months** in patients resected for cure.

2. **Esophagogastroduodenoscopy.** Periodic **(every 6–12 months)** upper gastrointestinal endoscopy is required in patients with **gastrinoma,** particularly in those with recurrent or metastatic disease who are receiving medical therapy for peptic symptoms.

D. **Optional evaluation.** The following tests and procedures may be indicated by previous diagnostic findings or clinical suspicion:

1. **Blood tests** (see p 2, **IV.A**)

a. **5′-Nucleotidase.**

b. **GGTP.**

2. **Technetium-99m** (see p 3, **IV.C.5**).

3. **Biopsy.** Percutaneous needle or open surgical **biopsy** of any suspicious mass, particularly in the liver, should be performed in any patient who has previously been resected for cure.

REFERENCES

Erikson B, Oberg K, Alm G, et al. Treatment of malignant endocrine pancreatic tumors with human leukocyte interferon. Lancet 2:1307–1309, 1986.

Fraker DL, Norton JA. The role of surgery in the management of islet cell tumors. Gastroenterol Clin N Amer 18:805–829, 1989.

Friesen SR. Tumors of the endocrine pancreas. NEJM 306:580–590, 1982.

Howard TJ, Passaro E, Jr. Gastrinoma; new medical and surgical approaches. Surg Clin N Amer 69:667–681, 1989.

Howard TJ, Stabile BE, Zinner MJ, Chang S, Bhagavan BS, Passaro E, Jr. Pancreatic endocrine tumors: analysis of anatomic distribution. Am J Surg 159:258–264, 1990.

Jaffe BM. Surgery for gut hormone-producing tumors. Am J Med 82(suppl 5B):68–76, 1987.

Modlin IM. Endocrine tumors of the pancreas. Surg Gynecol Obstet 149:751–769, 1979.

Moertel CG, Hanley JA, Johnson LA. Streptozotocin alone compared with streptozocin plus fluoro-uracil in the treatment of advanced islet-cell carcinoma. N Engl J Med 303:1189–1194, 1980.

Mozell E, Stenzel P, Woltering EA, Rosch J, and O'Dorisio TM. Functional endocrine tumors of the pancreas: clinical presentation, diagnosis, and treatment. Curr Prob Surg 27(6):303–386, 1990.

Norton JA, Shawker TH, Doppman JL, et al. Localization and surgical treatment of occult insulinomas. Ann Surg 212:615–620, 1990.

Prinz RA, Badrinath K, Banerji M, Sparagana M, Dorsch T, Lawrence A. Operative and chemotherapeutic management of malignant glucagon-producing tumors. Surgery 90:713–719, 1981.

Roche A, Raisonnier A, Gillon Savouret MC. Pancreatic venous sampling and arteriography in localizing insulinomas and gastrinomas. Procedures and results in 55 cases. Radiology 145;621–
   627, 1982.
Rueckert KF, Klotter HJ, Kummerle F. Intraoperative ultrasonic localization of endocrine tumors of
   the pancreas. Surgery 96:1045–1047, 1984.
Stark DD, Moss AA, Goldberg HI, Deveney CW. CT of pancreatic islet cell tumors. Radiology
   150:491–494, 1984.
van Heerden JA, Smith SL, Miller LJ. Management of the Zollinger-Ellison syndrome in patients
   with multiple endocrine neoplasia Type I. Surgery 100:971–977, 1986.
Welbourn RB, Wood SM, Polak JM, Bloom SR. Pancreatic endocrine tumors. In Gut Hormones.
   Bloom SR, Polak JM, editors. Churchill Livingstone, New York, pp. 547–554, 1981.
Wolfe MM, Jensen RT. Zollinger-Ellison syndrome. NEJM 317:1200–1209, 1987.

59 Carcinoid Malignancies

Alan T. Lefor, MD

I. **Epidemiology.** Carcinoid tumors occur in a variety of sites, but are most common in the **appendix, small bowel, rectum, and bronchus.** Although unusual, carcinoids represent the **most common gastrointestinal APUDoma.** Because they are often asymptomatic, the exact incidence is unknown, but it was estimated that in 1985, **1 case per 100,000** of the population was diagnosed in the United States. In 1993 nearly **2,500 cases** are expected to be identified. The worldwide incidence of carcinoids is not well documented but probably does not vary significantly.

II. **Risk factors**
   A. **Age.** Carcinoid tumors occur equally in all age groups.
   B. **Sex. Females** are at **1.5 times** higher risk of developing carcinoids than are males.
   C. **Race.** There is no known racial bias in the incidence of carcinoid tumors.
   D. **Genetic factors**
      1. **Family history.** A history of carcinoid tumors in a first-degree relative does not affect the risk of carcinoid tumors. However, 6 cases of familial clustering have been reported.
      2. **Familial syndromes.** Two familial diseases are associated with a higher than normal risk of developing carcinoid malignancies.
         a. **Multiple endocrine neoplasia, Type I (MEN I).** This autosomal dominant syndrome, also known as **Wermer's syndrome,** is characterized by pituitary, parathyroid, and pancreatic endocrine tumors and carries an increased risk of **foregut and thymic carcinoids.**
         b. **Von Recklinghausen's disease.** This autosomal dominant disease distinguished by multiple neurofibromas and cafe au lait skin lesions has been correlated with a higher than expected incidence of **ampullary carcinoids.**
   E. **Previous pathology.** Achlorhydric states with accompanying **hypergastrinemia** (achlorhydria; pernicious anemia; retained antrum following gastric surgery; use of H_2 blockers such as cimetidine, ranitidine, and famotidine) are associated particularly with the development of multiple gastric carcinoids.

III. **Presentation**
   A. **Signs and symptoms.** Presenting signs and symptoms vary with the location of the primary lesion and the presence or absence of metastases.
      1. **Local manifestations**
         a. **Stomach.** Most gastric carcinoids are **asymptomatic** and are discovered during routine endoscopy performed for other symptomatic diseases.
         b. **Small bowel.** Most carcinoid tumors occur in the distal small bowel (ileum). Most often, they produce **intermittent abdominal pain (26%) or small bowel obstruction (32%)** as a result of luminal constriction, intussusception, and mesenteric kinking secondary to an aggressive desmoplastic reaction. Small bowel incarceration and strangulation also may happen, but hemorrhage and ulceration rarely occur. Symptoms of the carcinoid syndrome (see p 73) occur in 19% of patients with small bowel carcinoid tumors. Carcinoids of the **stomach and duodenum are asymptomatic** and usually are discovered incidentally at the time of endoscopy. In rare cases, these tumors present with pyelonephritis, renal failure, or both secondary to retroperitoneal fibrosis, and accompanying ureteral obstruction or abdominal pain secondary to retroperitoneal fibrosis and occlusion of the mesenteric vessels.
         c. **Appendix.** Most carcinoid tumors of the appendix are **asymptomatic** and are discovered incidentally during appendectomy for acute appendicitis.
         d. **Rectum.** Rectal lesions are almost always **asymptomatic;** however, obstruction from a large mass may occur. Perforation and hemorrhage are extremely uncommon because of their submucosal location.

   2. **Bronchial tumor.** Bronchial carcinoids may present as **coin lesions** on chest x-ray (43%) or with bronchial obstruction and pneumonia (11%), coughing, wheezing, and hemoptysis (7%), or, less commonly, symptoms of the carcinoid syndrome (6%).
   3. **Thymic tumor.** Thymic carcinoids usually present as **asymptomatic** anterior mediastinal masses.
   4. **Gonadal tumor.** Testicular and ovarian carcinoids frequently present as **mass lesions** detected on physical examination and produce symptoms of **carcinoid syndrome in as many as 50%** of patients.
   5. **Systemic manifestations.** Many carcinoid tumors present with hepatic metastases and advanced disease leading to the development of the carcinoid syndrome (diarrhea, flushing, wheezing, and fibrotic valvular cardiac disease; see p 73) in approximately **35%** of patients. Other complaints include abdominal pain (23%), bone pain from bony metastases (6%), and dorsal angulation of the penis on erection secondary to fibrosis of Buck's fascia producing **Peyronie's disease.**
   B. **Paraneoplastic syndromes.** Several syndromes have been associated with carcinoid tumors, and, although rare (except carcinoid syndrome), these symptoms complexes may be the sole manifestation of disease.
      1. **Carcinoid syndrome** (see p 73).
      2. **Polyneuropathy** (see p 58).
      3. **Inappropriate ACTH** (see p 90).
      4. **Hypercalcemia** (see p 87).
      5. **Hyperglycemia** (see p 89).
IV. **Differential diagnosis.** Carcinoid tumors occur in many sites and must be considered in the differential diagnosis of mass lesions in the chest and abdomen. However, patients may present with **diarrhea alone** (17%), **diarrhea with flushing** (44%), **flushing alone** (6%), or **no carcinoid symptoms at all** (33%). When **diarrhea** with or without flushing suggests the carcinoid syndrome, other diseases should be considered, such as infections (cholera, shigella, and giardiasis), **inflammation** (Crohn's disease), **endocrine disorders** (gastrinomas, medullary carcinoma of the thyroid, and VIP-omas), and **menopause** (flushing), because they may present with identical symptoms. In addition, one cause of diarrhea, **steatorrhea, may falsely elevate the levels of urinary 5-hydroxyindolacetic acid (5-HIAA)** to the intermediate range of 8–30 mg per day.
V. **Screening programs.** Although no screening test is recommended for use in the general population, patients with risk factors or symptoms suggesting carcinoid tumors (ie, chronic flushing, diarrhea, or both) should be screened with a 24-hour urinary 5-HIAA levels and blood, serum, or platelet serotonin levels. **A pentagastrin test** (also used in MEN syndromes) is also a simple provocative test that frequently results in prompt facial flushing that is transient (< 5 minutes) and diagnostic.
VI. **Diagnostic workup**
   A. **Medical history and physical examination.** A complete medical history, with particular emphasis on the frequent symptoms of carcinoid tumors (eg, pain, diarrhea, flushing, wheezing, cough, pneumonia), and a thorough physical examination are mandatory for a complete evaluation.
      1. **Skin.** Evidence of chronic **facial flushing,** such as a permanent cyanotic facial flush, dilated facial veins, telangiectasia, and **deep furrowing of the forehead,** may be noted. An acute facial flush also may be observed.
      2. **Eyes.** Injection of the sclera and evidence of **hyperlacrimation** occurs in some patients with chronic flushing and should be recorded.
      3. **Neck.** Careful palpation of the thyroid and neck for masses must be done to exclude medullary carcinoma of the thyroid, which also is associated in rare cases with the carcinoid syndrome.
      4. **Thorax.** Auscultation of the lungs may reveal **wheezing** or prolonged exhalation as evidence of bronchospasm.
      5. **Heart.** All murmurs should be completely described, and any evidence of valvular disease should be recorded.
      6. **Abdomen.** A thorough palpation of the abdomen may uncover **masses,** particularly in the hepatic or right lower quadrant areas.
      7. **Rectum.** A digital rectal examination is mandatory to exclude the presence of a large rectal carcinoid and to test stool for occult blood.
      8. **Genitalia.** Careful palpation of the testes or ovaries may reveal a carcinoid mass.
      9. **Nervous system.** Evidence of muscle weakness (carcinoid polymyopathy) is important.

B. Primary tests and procedures. All patients with suspected carcinoid malignancies should undergo the following tests and procedures.

1. **Blood tests**
   a. **Complete blood count** (see p 1, **IV.A.1**).
   b. **Hepatic transaminases** (see p 1, **IV.A.2**).
   c. **Alkaline phosphatase** (see p 1, **IV.A.3**).
   d. **BUN and creatinine** (see p 3, **IV.A.6**).
   e. **Blood, serum, or platelet serotonin.** Although not widely available, blood, serum, and platelet levels of serotonin may be valuable in confirming the diagnosis, particularly if the 24-hour urinary 5-HIAA excretion is between 8 and 30 mg.

2. **Urine tests.** The measurement of the 24-hour urinary excretion of serotonin and its metabolites is essential in patients with suspected carcinoid tumors.
   a. **Urinary 5-hydroxyindoleacetic acid.** The "gold standard" test for patients suspected of having metabolically active carcinoid tumors is 24-hour urinary 5-HIAA excretion. **The sensitivity is 73% and the specificity is 100%.** Normal 5-HIAA excretion is 2–8 mg per 24 hours. Levels between 8 and 30 mg per 24 hours suggest carcinoid tumors, whereas those **greater than 30 mg per 24 hours are diagnostic.** However, certain medications (methyldopa, phenothiazines, L-dopa, acetaminophen, salicylates, and the antitussive guaifenesin) and **foods that contain high levels of serotonin** (banana, pineapple, kiwi, avocado, plantain, walnuts, hickory nuts, and pecans) **should be avoided** during the test.
   b. **Urinary serotonin.** Although not always required for the diagnosis, measurement of urinary serotonin may be helpful, especially if the 5-HIAA level falls between 8 and 30 mg per 24 hours.

3. **Imaging studies**
   a. **Chest x-ray.** This is a simple screening test for **"coin" lesions** suggesting bronchial carcinoids as well as pulmonary metastases.
   b. **Computed tomography (CT).** CT scan of the abdomen (and chest if a bronchial carcinoid is suspected) is essential to exclude the presence of **hepatic metastases,** especially if the primary tumor is more than 1 cm in diameter.

C. Optional tests and procedures. The following represent tests and procedures that may be indicated by previous diagnostic findings, clinical suspicion, or the documented presence of carcinoid tumors in various locations.

1. **Blood tests**
   a. **5′-Nucleotidase** (see p 2, **IV.A.4**).
   b. **GGTP** (see p 2, **IV.A.5**).
   c. **Substance P.** Although not widely available, elevated plasma levels of this vasoactive amine are **32% sensitive and 85% specific** for carcinoid tumors.
   d. **Neuropeptide K.** Plasma levels of this amine are elevated in as many as 66% of patients with carcinoid malignancies.
   e. **Pancreatic polypeptide.** As many as **43%** of carcinoid patients have increased plasma levels of this gastrointestinal hormone.

2. **Pulmonary function tests.** Evaluation of the pulmonary function is mandatory in patients with bronchial carcinoids to determine the extent of pulmonary resection that would be tolerated. For instance, a pneumonectomy may be performed safely if the forced expired volume in 1 second (FEV_1) is more than 2.5 L. No resection should be contemplated if the FEV_1 is less than 0.8 L.

3. **Imaging studies**
   a. **Upper gastrointestinal series.** An UGI with small bowel follow-through (UGI + SBFT) is indicated if a foregut carcinoid is suspected, and a SBFT may be helpful to diagnose small intestinal carcinoid tumors.
   b. **Barium enema.** A barium enema may provide evidence of an ileal, appendiceal, or cecal carcinoid (effacement of the cecum) and is essential to exclude the common finding of a synchronous colon carcinoma.
   c. **Ultrasound.** Abdominal ultrasonography may be useful in evaluating the liver for metastatic disease, especially if the CT scan cannot **distinguish between cystic and solid lesions.** In addition, ultrasound examination of the **testes** or **ovaries** may be important.
   d. **Magnetic resonance imaging (MRI)** (see p 3, **IV.C.3**).
   e. **Arteriography.** Occasionally, tumor in the distal ileum, pancreas, liver, and other visceral organs cannot be demonstrated with routine radiographic studies. In these patients, arteriography may be the most sensitive test for localizing the tumor.

    f. Echocardiography. Occasionally, noninvasive evaluation of the cardiac valves is warranted, particularly if a **cardiac murmur** or symptoms of the **carcinoid syndrome** are present.

    g. Technetium-99m bone scan (see p 3, **IV.C.5**).

    h. ^{131}I-metaiodobenzylguanidine. This compound, normally used to image pheochromocytomas (see Chapter 58), is concentrated in carcinoid tumors by a neuronal pump mechanism. It is useful to image lymph node and hepatic metastatic disease (> 1 cm in diameter), and its sensitivity is increased by subtracting the counts from a simultaneous **technetium-99m liver/spleen scan**.

4. Invasive procedures. Numerous procedures may be indicated during the workup of patients with suspected carcinoid malignancies. The indications for each procedure depend on the symptoms and on the location of the primary lesion.

    a. Bronchoscopy. Direct examination of the bronchial tree is indicated in any patient with suspected **bronchial carcinoid or with a "coin" lesion** on chest x-ray. Biopsies of any abnormalities should be taken.

    b. Esophagogastroduodenoscopy. Upper gastrointestinal endoscopy should be performed if a **foregut carcinoid** is suspected, and biopsies should be obtained.

    c. Sigmoidoscopy. A flexible or rigid examination should be performed if a rectal primary tumor is suspected or no primary tumor can be located. Again, biopsy of any abnormalities is mandatory.

    d. Biopsy. Hepatic, testicular, ovarian, and abdominal masses should be biopsied by the most appropriate method. Fine needle aspiration, core needle biopsy, or laparoscopic direct biopsy may be indicated.

    e. Venous sampling. In some instances, the primary tumor cannot be identified. In these cases, selective venous sampling from branches of the **portal, gonadal, and bronchial veins** may reveal the primary site.

5. Provocative tests. Several diagnostic tests that induce the onset of a certain symptom in patients with carcinoid tumors may be necessary to diagnose carcinoid malignancies.

    a. Ethanol. The ingestion of alcohol may cause the release of vasoactive amines from carcinoid tumors, provoking an attack of **flushing and diarrhea**. This will allow the clinician to observe the patient and obtain serum 5-HIAA and serotonin levels. The only other tumor capable of responding in this manner is medullary carcinoma of the thyroid.

    b. Pentagastrin stimulation test. Administration of **pentagastrin** (Pentavlon, 6 mcg/kg SC) causes the immediate release of serotonin **(< 5 minutes),** provoking a **flushing episode** that rapidly resolves and is diagnostic of carcinoid tumors.

    c. Calcium infusion. The infusion of calcium salts intravenously may precipitate the release of serotonin and symptoms of carcinoid syndrome over a period of 23 hours. However, because calcium infusion can be **dangerous,** it requires close monitoring of patients and cannot be recommended for routine use.

    d. Epinephrine infusion. The infusion of epinephrine may induce the release of serotonin and the onset of carcinoid symptoms, but, like calcium, it can be **dangerous** and cannot be recommended.

VII. Pathology

A. Location. Carcinoid lesions may occur throughout the gastrointestinal tract as well as in virtually any other organ of the body.

1. The gastrointestinal tract

    a. The stomach. The stomach is a **rare location** for carcinoid tumors. These tumors are **usually small** (< 1 cm in diameter) and superficial but may become larger and invasive.

    b. The duodenum. The duodenum is a **rare site** for carcinoid tumors. However, when they do occur, they frequently produce other gastrointestinal hormones such as gastrin, causing the Zollinger-Ellison syndrome (see p 72).

    c. The ampulla of Vater. This **rare site** of carcinoid tumors is associated with elevated levels of somatostatin. These tumors are **usually small and present with jaundice.**

    d. Ileum. The ileum is the **second most common site** of carcinoid tumors **(23%).** They are **usually small (< 3 cm in diameter) and multiple (30%).**

Because of their location, they are particularly difficult to diagnose and may be confused with diseases such as Crohn's disease. In addition, carcinoid tumors occurring in **Meckel's diverticula** have been reported.

e. **Appendix.** The appendix is the **most common site** of carcinoids **(38–42%).** Like ileal lesions, they are **usually small (90% are < 1 cm in diameter)** and are discovered incidentally at the time of surgery for appendicitis. It is estimated that 1 of 250 **appendectomies** will reveal carcinoid tumor in the resected specimen. Muscular invasion, lymphatic permeation, and serosal involvement are extremely common. Distant disease is rare when tumors are less than 1 cm in diameter, but 90% of **carcinoids larger than 2 cm** present with simultaneous distant metastases.

f. **Rectum.** The rectum is the **third most common site** of carcinoids (13%). Rectal carcinoids are **usually small** but may grow to become large invasive masses. They are usually located submucosally on the anterior or lateral walls **between 4 and 13 cm from the dentate line** and are discovered incidentally during 1 of every 2500 proctoscopies. The metastatic potential is directly related to the size of the tumor; metastases rarely occur in tumors smaller than 1 cm in diameter.

g. **Pancreas.** Although **extremely rare,** pancreatic carcinoids may be mistaken for nonfunctioning islet cell tumors or pancreatic adenocarcinoma. **Urinary 5-HIAA is normal in 50%** of patients, whereas diarrhea and flushing are unusual. Many tumors still produce **excessive amounts of serotonin,** which may be **detected in the urine.**

h. **Gallbladder.** Carcinoid tumors of the biliary tree are **extremely rare,** but care must be exercised to be certain that a gallbladder carcinoid is not mistaken for symptomatic cholelithiasis.

2. **Bronchus.** Bronchial carcinoids represent the **fourth most common site** of disease **(12%)** but only 16% of all lung cancers. Carcinoids with "typical" features behave less aggressively, and those with **"atypical" features** (high mitotic rate, pleomorphism, lymphatic and vascular invasion) follow a more aggressive pattern. The frequency of lymphatic metastases is directly proportional to the size of these tumors.

3. **Thymus.** Thymic carcinoids are **uncommon.** They often present as asymptomatic masses on chest x-ray; however, they may produce **ectopic parathormone and ACTH**, resulting in hyperparathyroidism and Cushing's disease, respectively. The diagnosis of these carcinoids often requires electron microscopy, and, although radiosensitive, they typically behave **aggressively**.

4. **Breast.** Carcinoid tumors occur in the breast as both primary lesions and metastatic foci. They are exceedingly difficult to distinguish from normal breast cancer.

5. **Ovary.** The ovary may be the site of primary carcinoid tumors as well as metastatic disease. These tumors are **frequently small,** and the ovary often must be **bivalved** to identify them.

6. **Testis.** The testis, like the ovary, is a **rare site** for carcinoid tumors but one that is easily accessible during physical examination.

B. **Multiplicity.** Carcinoid tumors are **multiple in 21–40%** of patients. Multiple tumors most often involve the **small bowel** and specifically the **ileum** (67%). In addition, carcinoid tumors are associated with **other visceral malignancies in 25–50%** of patients. The most common second cancer is **colon carcinoma (30%).**

C. **Histology.** Carcinoid malignancies originate from **Kulschitzsky or enterochromaffin cells,** which are derived from the neural crest and belong to the amine precursor uptake and decarboxylation (APUDoma) system. Grossly, the tumors are typically small **yellow-tan nodules.** The cells are uniform in appearance, contain **electron-dense neurosecretory granules** (the most diagnostic feature) and punctate chromaffin, are acidophilic with rare mitoses, and are organized into insular, trabecular, glandular, or mixed patterns. The glandular and mixed histologies have the worst prognosis, and **insular tumors have a favorable prognosis.** Traditionally, carcinoids also have been grouped according to the following embryologic sites of origin.

1. **Foregut carcinoids.** These include **bronchial, gastric, duodenal, and pancreatic carcinoids.** They do not stain with argentaffin, contain little serotonin, contain small round granules, rarely exhibit insular structure, are associated with types 3 and 4 flushes, may metastasize to bone, and may secrete 5-hydroxytryptophan (5-HTP) or ACTH.

2. **Midgut carcinoids.** This group **(jejunum, ileum, and right colon)** stain positively with argentaffin, contain high levels of serotonin, contain pleomorphic

granules, have an insular structure in 27%, are usually associated with types 1 and 2 flushes, and rarely metastasize to bone or secrete 5-HTP or ACTH.

3. **Hindgut carcinoids.** Carcinoids of the **transverse colon, left colon, and rectum** are argentaffin-negative, rarely contain serotonin, contain large round granules, rarely adopt the insular appearance, are rarely associated with flushing, commonly metastasize to bone, and rarely secrete 5-HTP or ACTH.

D. **Metastatic spread.** The propensity of carcinoid tumors to metastasize is directly related to the **size** of the primary tumor. Tumors smaller than 1 cm in diameter rarely metastasize, whereas more than **90% of those larger than 2 cm present with metastatic disease**. Intermediate sized tumors have intermediate metastatic potential.

1. **Modes of spread.** Carcinoids spread by three distinct mechanisms.

   a. **Direct extension.** The tumor may grow directly into adjacent tissue or organs and may extend along nerves and blood vessels. Local growth may lead to obstruction of structures such as the gastrointestinal tract or the common bile duct.

   b. **Lymphatic metastasis.** Malignant cells may spread through lymphatics to regional and distant lymph nodes.

   c. **Hematogenous metastasis.** Tumor cells may spread through portal and systemic vessels to various distant organs.

2. **Sites of spread.** Although the **liver** is the most common organ involved with metastatic disease, carcinoid tumors also may metastasize to the **bone, lung, brain, or pancreas.**

VIII. **Staging.** No specific staging system for carcinoid tumors exists because the tumors can occur throughout the body. Instead, they are staged in the same way as other tumors that arise in each anatomic location.

IX. **Treatment**

A. **Surgery**

1. **Primary carcinoid tumor**

   a. **Indications.** Carcinoid tumors commonly present with metastatic disease. However, if no metastases can be demonstrated or if the tumor is discovered incidentally, the **lesion should be excised** because surgery is the only potentially curative therapy. Even in the presence of metastatic disease, resection of the primary tumor is indicated for palliation of impending bowel or bronchial obstruction, severe carcinoid symptoms, or for other complications (eg, hemorrhage, pain).

   b. **Approaches.** The surgical approach depends on the location of the neoplasm and usually is identical to that used for other procedures at the particular anatomic site.

   c. **Procedures**

      (1) **Gastric carcinoids.** Because of the **multifocal nature** of gastric carcinoids, either **radical subtotal or total gastrectomy** is commonly required for complete excision. However, if all lesions are less than 1 cm in diameter and urinary serotonin excretion is normal, some surgeons favor annual endoscopic resection of all lesions, avoiding the high morbidity of total gastrectomy. Lesions smaller than 1 cm rarely invade or metastasize.

      (2) **Duodenal carcinoids.** Because most patients with duodenal carcinoids present with metastatic disease, **resection is generally not performed**. However, if discovered early without any evidence of distant metastases, these lesions can be treated with **segmental resection or pancreaticoduodenectomy (Whipple procedure).**

      (3) **Ampulla of Vater carcinoids.** Patients with carcinoids at this site may present with jaundice before metastasis has occurred. If no distant spread is detected, curative **pancreaticoduodenectomy (Whipple procedure)** is indicated.

      (4) **Ileal carcinoids.** Most of these tumors are discovered at laparotomy for bowel obstruction or another intra-abdominal catastrophe. **Segmental resection** is generally indicated for palliation of small bowel obstruction even in the presence of **metastatic disease**. Because these tumors often are multiple, generous margins should be used with **wide excision of the accompanying lymph node-bearing mesentery.**

      (5) **Appendiceal carcinoids.** Appendiceal carcinoids are identified only during routine appendectomy in 70–90% of cases. Because 90% occur

at the tip of the appendix, only 10% are implicated as an inciting factor in the acute appendicitis. **Appendectomy** is adequate therapy in most instances, but **right hemicolectomy should be performed if the tumor is larger than 2 cm in diameter or if vascular invasion or involvement of the mesoappendix is present.**

(6) **Rectal carcinoids.** The surgical procedure of choice depends on the size of the rectal carcinoid. **For tumors less than 1 cm in diameter, sigmoidoscopic resection** is adequate. A more formal **local, trans-anal, full-thickness excision** is indicated with lesions between 1 and 2 cm, whereas those larger than 2 cm demand radical excision—generally—**abdominoperineal resection (Miles operation) or low anterior resection.**

(7) **Pancreatic carcinoids.** These tumors are extremely rare and often present with metastatic disease. **Enucleation or pancreatectomy** may be considered if isolated pancreatic disease is found.

(8) **Biliary carcinoids.** Carcinoids of the gallbladder can be treated with simple **cholecystectomy.** Resection of a wedge of liver may be required if significant invasion exists. Carcinoid tumors of the bile ducts may present with jaundice and, barring distant disease, can be resected in a manner similar to ductal adenocarcinomas (see p 269, **IX.A.1.c**).

(9) **Bronchial carcinoids.** In the absence of distant metastases, patients with bronchial carcinoids can undergo curative resection of their primary disease. If distant spread has occurred, palliative resection for bronchial obstruction can be considered. **Segmental or sleeve resection, lobectomy, and pneumonectomy** can be considered on the basis of the site of the tumor and the patient's pulmonary status.

(10) **Thymic carcinoids.** The primary therapy for these lesions is **thymectomy,** especially because they are aggressive and generally cannot be distinguished from thymomas before surgery.

(11) **Breast carcinoids.** Involvement of the breast with primary or metastatic disease may necessitate **segmental resection, total mastectomy, or modified radical mastectomy,** depending on the size, site, and metastatic status of the tumor.

(12) **Ovarian carcinoids.** Ovarian tumors frequently are small and cannot be identified unless the ovary is bivalved at the time of surgery. If pathology is confirmed, **salpingo-oophorectomy** may be curative. The ovary, however, is also a site of metastatic disease, and more common primary sites should be examined before proceeding with resection.

(13) **Testicular carcinoids.** Testicular masses that suggest carcinoid tumors should be biopsied through a **standard inguinal incision,** and, if pathologic confirmation is obtained, **an orchiectomy** is indicated.

d. **Preoperative preparation.** Patients who do not have symptoms of the carcinoid syndrome require no special preoperative preparation. Those with symptoms require careful cooperation between the anesthesiologist and surgeon. Some recommend preoperative insertion of a pulmonary thermodilution balloon (Swan-Ganz) catheter with alpha-blockade with phentolamine. Exogenous catecholamines and drugs that stimulate endogenous catecholamine release must be avoided. Curare should not be used. Cyproheptadine, somatostatin analogs (Sandostatin), alpha-agonists, and beta-antagonists may be necessary to counteract vasodilation and bronchoconstriction.

2. **Locally advanced and metastatic carcinoid tumor**
   a. **Indications.** Treatment of metastatic disease is more important in patients with carcinoid malignancies than in other tumor types because it not only may improve survival but may also effectively palliate the symptoms of the carcinoid syndrome. In addition, some patients may be cured by definitive surgical resection of metastatic disease.
   b. **Procedures**
      (1) **Hepatic resection.** Localized hepatic metastases may be amenable to surgical resection. This may result in prolonged palliation with a mean survival of 5 years following resection and even **cure in 10%** of patients.
      (2) **Hepatic artery ligation.** Hepatic artery ligation and percutaneous arterial embolization have been used in the presence of multiple diffuse

hepatic metastases with successful palliation of carcinoid symptoms and **partial (> 50%) regression of tumor in 93% of patients.** However, the effects are short-lived, lasting only **5 months** on the average.

- (3) **Hepatic transplantation.** Transplantation has been attempted in patients with disease limited to the liver, but the efficacy of this surgical approach remains anecdotal.

  c. **Mortality and morbidity.** The mortality and morbidity of surgical procedures in patients with carcinoid tumors is similar to that observed in the general population if meticulous pre- and post-operative care is provided by a knowledgeable surgeon and anesthesiologist. Complications that may occur intra- or post-operatively due to the release of vasoactive amines include the following: **bronchospasm, hypotension, hypertension, tachyarrhythmias, altered mental status, facial flushing, and abdominal pain.**

B. **Radiation therapy**
  1. **Primary carcinoid tumor.** No evidence documents a role for radiation therapy in the treatment of primary carcinoid tumors.
  2. **Adjuvant radiation therapy.** Radiation therapy has not been tested extensively in the adjuvant setting because metastatic disease, not local recurrence, determines the level of symptoms and the ultimate survival outcome.
  3. **Locally advanced and metastatic carcinoid tumor.** Although initial successes in the treatment of metastatic disease were reported, subsequent studies have failed to confirm these results. **Thymic carcinoids, however, are especially radiosensitive,** and treatment of recurrence in the chest may be helpful.

C. **Chemotherapy**
  1. **Primary carcinoid.** Chemotherapy has no role in the initial therapy of primary resectable carcinoid tumor.
  2. **Adjuvant chemotherapy.** Chemotherapy in the adjuvant setting has not been adequately studied and remains experimental.
  3. **Locally advanced and metastatic carcinoids.** Chemotherapy has been used to achieve two basic goals: (1) **palliation** of the symptoms caused by the vasoactive substances and (2) **reduction of tumor bulk** to prolong survival. Moreover, intra-arterial (hepatic artery) chemotherapy for hepatic metastases has no advantage over systemic administration. Overall, the results are disappointing, and chemotherapy is currently recommended only for patients with advanced disease, for radiologic documentation of tumor progression, or for patients taking part in clinical trials.
     a. **Single agents.** Agents used only for the relief of carcinoid symptoms are discussed under the heading, "Therapy of the carcinoid syndrome," in Table 13–2. A number of antineoplastic drugs have been evaluated with variable response rates, including **streptozotocin (33%), fluorouracil (26%), cyclophosphamide (23%), doxorubicin (21%),** dacarbazine (13%), actinomycin-D (6%), and cisplatin (6%). In addition, the somatostatin analog **octreotide acetate** (Sandostatin) has a reported response rate of 14%.
     b. **Combination chemotherapy.** Response rates for combination regimens range from 22–40% and have not been superior to single-agent therapy.

D. **Immunotherapy.** The only immunotherapy agent that has been tested in the treatment of metastatic carcinoid tumor is **alpha-interferon.** Preliminary results from two studies indicate that a **partial response may be achieved in 20–47% of cases** (more than 50% reduction of urinary 5-HIAA). Further study of this biologic agent, both alone and in combination with chemotherapy, is warranted.

X. **Prognosis**
  A. **Risk of recurrence.** The prognosis depends entirely on the likelihood of recurrent and metastatic disease. The probability of metastatic disease varies with the site and size of the primary tumor, as outlined in Table 59–1.
  B. **Five-year survival.** Because of the indolent nature of carcinoid tumors, many patients survive 5 years but ultimately succumb to their disease. The rate of 5-year survival depends on the site and metastatic status of the tumor, as indicated in Table 59–1. The **median survival varies from 3.5 to 8.5 years.**
  C. **Adverse prognostic factors.** Although many patients with carcinoid tumors live for long periods, the following characteristics are associated with a shorter than expected rate of survival: **glandular and mixed histology, foregut and hindgut tumors, size larger than 2 cm in diameter, and 5-HIAA excretion of more than 150 mg per day.**

TABLE 59–1. PROGNOSIS OF CARCINOID TUMORS BY SITE AND SIZE

Primary Site & Size	Incidence of Metastases (%)	5-Year Survival		
		No Metastases (%)	*Metastases Present (%)*	*Overall (%)*
Stomach	22	> 90	0–23	52
Ileum	20–35	75	19–59	42–71
< 1 cm	15–18			
1–2 cm	60–80			
> 2 cm	86–95			
Appendix	2–5	95	27–90	92–99
< 1 cm	< 2			
1–2 cm	50			
> 2 cm	33–90			
Rectum	3–15	90	7–44	76–100
< 1 cm	< 20			
1–2 cm				
> 2 cm				
Bronchus	20	95	11–71	87
Overall	23	95	18–64	65–82

XI. **Patient follow-up**
  A. **General guidelines.** Patients should be followed closely for evidence of recurrent or metastatic disease annually for those at low risk (ie, < 1 cm appendiceal lesion), every 4–6 months for those at intermediate risk, and every 2–4 months for those with metastatic disease. The following specific guidelines for patients without evidence of metastatic disease are recommended:
  B. **Routine evaluation.** The following tests and procedures should be performed with each office visit:
    1. **Medical history and physical examination.** An interim medical history and thorough physical examination stressing those areas listed on p 480, **VI,** are mandatory during each visit.
    2. **Blood tests**
      a. **Complete blood count** (see p 1, **IV.A.1**).
      b. **Hepatic transaminases** (see p 1, **IV.A.2**).
      c. **Alkaline phosphatase** (see p 1, **IV.A.3**).
      d. **BUN and creatinine** (see p 3, **IV.A.6**).
      e. **Blood, serum, or platelet serotonin** (see p 481, **VI.B.1.e**).
    3. **Urine tests**
      a. **Urinary 5-HIAA.** Elevated or increasing levels of excretion per 24 hours is a good indication of recurrent, progressive, and metastatic disease.
      b. **Urinary serotonin.** Although not always secreted, measurement of urinary serotonin may be helpful in the follow-up of patients whose tumors originally secreted serotonin (eg, midgut tumors).
    4. **Chest x-ray** (see p 3, **IV.C.1**).
  C. **Additional evaluation.** Other tests that should be obtained at regular intervals include the following:
    1. **Computed tomography (CT).** CT scan of the abdomen to exclude the presence of resectable hepatic metastases should be obtained **every 6–12 months** or if signs or symptoms of liver metastases develop.
    2. **Other examinations.** Various examinations designed to evaluate the site of the primary tumor are indicated at least annually.
  D. **Optional evaluation.** The following tests and procedures may be indicated on the basis of previous diagnostic findings or clinical suspicion:
    1. **Blood tests**
      a. **5′-Nucleotidase** (see p 2, **IV.A.4**).
      b. **GGTP** (see p 2, **IV.A.5**).
      c. **Substance P** (see p 481, **VI.C.1.3**).
      d. **Neuropeptide K** (see p 481, **VI.C.1.4**).

  e. **Pancreatic polypeptide** (see p 481, **VI.C.1.5**).
2. **Imaging studies**
  a. **Magnetic resonance imaging** (see p 3, **IV.A.3**).
  b. **Ultrasound** (see p 3, **IV.C.4**).
  c. **Technetium-99m bone scan** (see p 482, **IV.C.5**).
  d. **Echocardiography** (see p 482, **VI.C.2.f**).
3. **Biopsy.** Any new mass should be biopsied by fine needle aspiration, core needle biopsy, or open wedge incisional biopsy to document the presence or absence of recurrent or metastatic disease.

REFERENCES

Dawes L, Schulte WJ, and Condon RE. Carcinoid tumors. Arch Surg 119:375, 1984.

Elias G. The carcinoid tumors. In Handbook of Surgical Oncology. CRC Press, New York, pp 187–193, 1989.

Engstrom PF, Lavin PT, Folsch E, et. al. Streptozotocin plus fluorouracil versus doxorubicin therapy for metastatic carcinoid tumors. J Clin Oncol 2:1255–1259, 1984.

Feldman JM. Carcinoid tumors and the carcinoid syndrome. Cur Prob Surg 26(12): 831–918, 1989.

Feldman JM and Jones RS. Carcinoid syndrome from gastrointestinal carcinoids without liver metastasis. Ann Surg 196:33–37, 1982.

Godwin JD. Carcinoid tumors: an analysis of 2837 cases. Cancer 36:560, 1975.

Keane TS, Rider WD, Harwood AR, et. al. Whole abdominal radiation in the management of the metastatic gastrointestinal carcinoid tumor. Int J Radiat Oncol Biol Phys 7(11):1519–1521, 1981.

Kvols LK and Buck M. Chemotherapy of the metastatic carcinoid and islet cell tumors: a review. Am J Med 82:77–83, 1987.

Makowka L, Tzakis AG, Mazzaferro V, et. al. Transplantation of the liver for metastatic endocrine tumors of the intestine and pancreas. Surg Gynecol Obstet 168:107–111, 1989.

Martin JK, Moertel CG, Adson MA, and Schutt AJ. Surgical Treatment of functioning metastatic carcinoid tumors. Arch Surg 118: 537–542, 1983.

Oberg K, Norheim I, Lind E, et. al. Treatment of malignant carcinoid tumors with human leukocyte interferon: long-term results. Cancer Treat Rep 70:1297–1304, 1986.

Odurny A and Birch SJ. Hepatic arterial embolization in patients with metastatic carcinoid tumors. Clin Radiol 36:597–602, 1985.

60 Hodgkin's Lymphoma

Mindy S. Bohrer, MD

I. **Epidemiology.** Hodgkin's lymphoma (HL) accounts for less than **25% of all lymphomas and less than 1% of all malignancies,** excluding skin cancer. In 1985, **3.3 cases per 100,000 males** and **2.4 cases per 100,000 females** were diagnosed in the United States, resulting in **0.8 and 0.5 deaths,** respectively. Estimates indicated that **7,900 new cases and 1,500 deaths** would be reported in 1993. Although Albany and Long Island, New York, were initially identified as geographic areas of high incidence, subsequent study has not substantiated this claim. Worldwide, the incidence of HL varies from 4.6 per 100,000 in Switzerland to only 0.4 per 100,000 in Japan.

II. **Risk factors**

A. **Age.** The incidence increases from less than 1 per 100,000 before age 10 to an early **peak of 4.7 per 100,000 between the ages of 20 and 30.** Then the incidence decreases to 2.5 per 100,000 until age 50, when it gradually rises again to a **peak of 4.9 per 100,000 by age 70.** The **median age at the time of diagnosis is 32 years.**

B. **Sex.** Males are at **1.4 times greater risk** than females for HL.

C. **Race.** Whites are at **2.2 times greater risk** of developing HL than are blacks.

D. **Genetic factors.** No hereditary factors have been shown to affect the risk of acquiring HL, although **certain HLA antigens** recently have been implicated. In addition, the risk in first-degree relatives is not increased.

E. **Diet.** No dietary factors have been connected to the pathogenesis of HL.

F. **History of previous pathology. Epstein-Barr virus (EBV) infection** has been incriminated as an etiologic factor in HL. As many as **20% of Hodgkin's patients** harbor the virus, and other human **DNA retroviruses** have recently been investigated. However, conclusive evidence of such relationships is presently lacking.

G. **Socioeconomic status.** HL in children occurs more frequently in families of **low socioeconomic status,** but this finding does not hold true for adults.

H. **Urbanization.** For unknown reasons, **woodworkers are at 2 times greater risk** than the general population.

III. **Clinical presentation**

A. **Signs and symptoms**

1. **Local manifestations. Asymptomatic, superficial, rubbery, matted, discrete lymphadenopathy** represents the most common presentation in HL. Some patients, for unknown reasons, develop transient pain in areas of active disease, especially **after alcohol ingestion.**

2. **Systemic manifestations.** Nearly **40% of patients** present with systemic symptoms of **fever, night sweats, weight loss,** pruritus, noninfiltrating dermal eruptions, papules, skin nodules, pain and weakness (spinal cord compression), uremia (ureteral obstruction from retroperitoneal nodes), and opportunistic infection. **Fever is the most common symptom** and often is characterized by high fever spikes alternating with afebrile periods **(Pel-Ebstein fever). Fever, night sweats, and weight loss,** possibly caused by release of interleukin-1, tumor necrosis factor, or interferon, constitute **"B" symptoms** that are important in staging and prognosis (see p 492, **VIII**).

B. **Paraneoplastic syndromes.** The following paraneoplastic syndromes are rarely associated with HL.

1. **Ophelia syndrome.** This is a rare symptom complex marked by **reversible recent memory loss.**

2. **Progressive multifocal leukoencephalopathy** (see p 58, **IV**).

3. **Subacute cerebellar degeneration** (see p 58, **I**).

4. **Subacute motor neuropathy** (see p 58, **II**).

IV. **Differential diagnosis.** The differential diagnosis of **persistent lymphadenopathy** is extensive and includes (1) **normal variation,** (2) **infection** (ie, EBV, HIV, arbovins

[Dengue fever], tuberculosis **(scrofula),** toxoplasma gondii, syphilis, (3) **inflamma-tory connective tissue disorders** (systemic lupus erythematosus and chronic juve-nile arthritis), (4) granulomatous disease (sarcoidosis), (5) drugs (phenytoin, isoniazid, antithyroid, and antileprosy drugs), and (6) **metastatic neoplasms** (head and neck, skin, lung, and breast neoplasms as well as chronic lymphatic leukemia and non-Hodgkin's lymphoma).

V. **Screening programs.** Because the incidence of HL in the general population is low and the cure rate is high, screening programs are generally not cost-effective and have not been advocated.

VI. **Diagnostic workup**
   A. **Medical history and physical examination.** A thorough medical history should be elicited, and a complete physical examination must be performed in all patients with suspected HL, paying particular attention to the following areas:
      1. **General appearance.** Assessment of the patient's general functional and nutri-tional status should be made, noting evidence of significant **recent weight loss** (see also, p 1, **I** and **III**).
      2. **Skin.** Papules, eruptions, and nodules are recorded and fully described.
      3. **Lymph nodes.** The characteristics (number, size, location, consistency, ten-derness, fluctuancy, mobility) of all lymph nodes must be recorded. This should be done separately for all lymph node areas, including occipital, cervical (ante-rior and posterior), supraclavicular, infraclavicular, axillary, epitrochlear, ingui-nal, and popliteal regions.
      4. **Chest.** Anterior **chest wall tenderness** and certain **auscultation findings** (eg, wheezing, diminished breath sounds) may indicate mediastinal disease, pleural effusions, or both.
      5. **Abdomen.** All abdominal **masses and hepatosplenomegaly** must be com-pletely described.
      6. **Extremities.** Swelling is an important finding that may indicate superior vena cava obstruction from **mediastinal disease** (upper extremity) or inferior vena cava obstruction from **enlarged para-aortic lymph nodes** (lower extremity). In addition, a detailed neurologic examination is crucially important to exclude the possibility of **spinal cord involvement.**
   B. **Primary tests and procedures.** The following diagnostic tests and procedures should be obtained initially in all patients with suspected lymphatic malignancies.
      1. **Blood tests** (see p 1, **IV.A**)
         a. **Complete blood count. Thrombocytopenia** (from hypersplenism, bone marrow involvement, or autoimmunity), normochromic normocytic **anemia** resulting from a **Coombs-positive autoimmune hemolytic anemia (3–10%),** and **eosinophilia (10–20%)** may be noted.
         b. **Hepatic transaminases.**
         c. **Alkaline phosphatase.**
         d. **BUN and creatinine.** Renal impairment may occur from direct infiltration or obstruction of both ureters caused by enlarged para-aortic or pelvic lymph nodes.
      2. **Imaging studies**
         a. **Chest x-ray.** Mediastinal and hilar adenopathy must be excluded (see, also, p 3, **IV.C.1**).
         b. **Computed tomography (CT).** Chest and abdominal CT scan should be obtained for staging purposes. **Abdominal CT is 83% accurate** in detect-ing abdominal lymphadenopathy, particularly in the upper abdomen, but **underestimates splenic involvement** because tumor nodules are often smaller than 1 cm in diameter.
         c. **Bipedal lymphangiogram.** Although inaccurate in the upper abdomen, lymphangiogram boasts a **90–95% positive and 60–80% negative predic-tive value** for retroperitoneal lymphadenopathy. In addition, it may focus attention on suspicious lymph node groups that require biopsy during stag-ing laparotomy.
      3. **Invasive procedures. Excisional lymph node biopsy** is essential to confirm the diagnosis and to determine the histologic subtype of HL that is present (see, also, p 493, **IX.A**). Because superficial lymphadenopathy is present in **90% of patients and 60–80% involve the cervical lymph nodes,** the vast majority of patients undergo **cervical lymph node biopsy.** Axillary and inguinal lymph node biopsies are diagnostic less often and are rarely necessary. Complica-tions following cervical or supraclavicular lymph node biopsy are unusual but include **pneumothorax, cranial nerve injury, infection, and hemorrhage.**

C. **Optional tests and procedures.** The following are examinations that may be indicated by either previous diagnostic findings or clinical suspicion.
1. **Blood tests** (see p 2, **IV.A**)
   a. **5'-Nucleotidase.**
   b. **GGTP.**
2. **Imaging studies**
   a. **Ultrasound.** This test is indicated to exclude obstructive uropathy from enlarged para-aortic nodes if impaired renal function is detected (see also, p 3, **IV.C.4**).
   b. **Gallium scan.** Gallium scans are inaccurate and rarely indicated in documenting the extent of disease but may be helpful in the follow up of large mediastinal masses.
   c. **Technetium-99m bone scan** (see p 3, **IV.C.5**).
3. **Procedures**
   a. **Bone marrow aspiration.** When not obtained at the time of staging laparotomy, bone marrow biopsy **(Jamshidi needle)** is indicated for patients with limited clinical disease (1–2 lymph node areas on one side of the diaphragm) **and suspected bone marrow involvement** (eg, elevated alkaline phosphatase, bone pain, "B" symptoms). Bone marrow involvement in these patients potentially may alter therapy. The likelihood of bone marrow involvement is **1% for clinical Stage I disease, 2% for Stage II, 25% for Stage III, and 45% for Stage IV.** Overall, bone marrow involvement occurs in 6–14% of patients with Hodgkin's lymphoma.
   b. **Staging laparotomy (SL). SL is the "gold standard"** method of staging Hodgkin's patients and includes a systematic exploration of the abdomen, **splenectomy, wedge biopsy of the right lobe of the liver and 3 core needle biopsies of the right and left lobes of the liver, iliac crest bone marrow aspiration, and lymph node sampling.** Lymph nodes from the paraortic, celiac, splenic, mesenteric, portal, iliac, and any suspicious nodal groups noted on lymphangiogram should be biopsied. Oophoropexy may be indicated in females of childbearing age, but it is not routinely performed. Laparotomy findings result in **upstaging 25–35% and downstaging 5–15% of patients,** although it is not clear whether this change has any significant impact on overall survival. Currently, clinical studies designed to evaluate the usefulness of laparotomy as a staging procedure and refine the indications for laparotomy are in progress.
      (1) **Indications.** SL is indicated in patients who otherwise are candidates for radiation therapy because occult abdominal disease in these patients may alter the choice of therapy from radiation to chemotherapy. A general guideline for SL is outlined below:
         (a) **SL is not recommended.** Stage IA lymphocyte predominant (abdominal disease is highly unlikely).
         (b) **SL is indicated.** Stages I, II, and IIIA (III$_{A1}$A) **(therapy is altered in 35–40% of patients).**
         (c) **SL is not indicated.** Stages III$_{A2}$, IIIB, and IV (chemotherapy is indicated).
      (2) **Morbidity and mortality.** Complications following SL, albeit uncommon, include the following problems: **wound infection, hemorrhage, subdiaphragmatic abscess, postsplenectomy sepsis (rare), pancreatitis, and postsplenectomy leukemia or myelodysplasia (controversial).**
   c. **Mediastinoscopy.** In rare cases, this procedure may be indicated in the diagnosis of isolated mediastinal HL (see also, p 194, **VI.C.3.c**).
   d. **Anterior parasternal mediastinotomy (Chamberlain procedure).** Like mediastinoscopy, this surgical procedure may be required in unusual circumstances for the diagnosis of isolated mediastinal HL (see also, p 194, **VI.C.3.d**).
VII. **Pathology.** Hodgkin's disease, a solid tumor of the lymphoreticular system, was first described by Dr. Thomas Hodgkin in 1832.
   A. **Location.** HL typically begins in the cervical lymph nodes, spreading sequentially to contiguous lymph node groups (eg, supraclavicular, axillary, mediastinal, para-aortic), and, finally, to the spleen, liver, and other distant organs.
   B. **Multiplicity.** Multiple areas of involvement separated by normal lymph node regions (ie, cervical and abdominal disease with normal mediastinal nodes) occurs in **15% of patients.**

C. **Histology.** The characteristic, but not pathognomonic, finding in HL is the **Reed-Sternberg (RS) cell,** which—along with the **Hodgkin's cell** (a large monoclonal cell with tetraploid DNA content) and other mononuclear variants—accounts for **0.03–3% of cells** in this lymphoreticular malignancy. The RS cell is a giant polyploid cell with abundant eosinophilic cytoplasm and a bi- or multilobed nucleus that contains **prominent nuclei resembling owl's eyes**. Although its origins are unknown, recent evidence (cell surface markers and immunoglobulin rearrangements) suggests a **B cell origin**. The **Rye modification** of the **Lukes and Butler classification** schema divides the histologic appearances into 4 prognostic groups that are summarized in Table 60–1 and below:

1. **Lymphocyte predominant type.** The **nodular form** is characterized by an **indolent relapsing course,** whereas the **diffuse variety rarely** relapses but is generally fatal. In addition, **10% of patients** with the nodular form develop an **aggressive non-Hodgkin's lymphoma** with or without therapy. This subtype accounts for **5% of HL** and occurs more commonly in **men**.

2. **Nodular sclerosing type.** This type primarily presents with mediastinal and supraclavicular lymphadenopathy and **lacunar cells** (polyploid cells with a halo around the nucleus and less prominent nucleoli). This subtype accounts for **40–60% of HL**, occurs more frequently in **women** and carries an overall **good prognosis**.

3. **Mixed cellularity type.** Frequently presenting at an advanced stage, this type is characterized by a larger number of **RS cells** within a cellular matrix of histiocytes, plasma cells, eosinophils, fibroblasts, and lymphocytes. This subtype accounts for **30% of HL**.

4. **Lymphocyte depleted type.** Scant lymphocytes and a **pleomorphic varient of the RS cell** (a bizarrely shaped, polyploid cell with prominent nucleoli) in a reactive background mark this **aggressive disease**. Like the lymphocyte predominant subtype this subtype of HL occurs in only **5% of patients** and is found more often in the older age groups.

D. **Metastatic spread**
   1. **Modes of spread.** HL can spread by 3 routes:
      a. **Direct extension.** Extension of Hodgkin's cell beyond the capsule of affected lymph nodes is considered to be direct extralymphatic spread and is given the staging designation **"E"**.
      b. **Lymphatic metastasis.** HL is believed to progress in an orderly fashion from its origin in cervical or supraclavicular lymph nodes through contiguous lymph node groups to the abdominal lymph nodes and viscera. The initial lymph node groups involved at the time of diagnosis (in order of frequency) are **cervical or supraclavicular (70%), axillary (20%), and infradiaphragmatic (most commonly inguinal) lymph nodes (5–12%)**.
      c. **Hematogenous metastasis.** Late spread through blood vessels is believed to be responsible for solid organ involvement.
   2. **Sites of spread.** Once Hodgkin's cells have gained access to the circulation, they spread quickly to the following distant organs: **bone marrow,** 2–15%; **liver** (common in the setting of splenic involvement); **spleen,** 35–40% at laparotomy (50% were clinically suspected); and **other extranodal sites,** including renal, gastrointestinal, and neurologic organs.

VIII. **Staging.** The Ann Arbor classification system for HL initially developed in 1970 was adopted by the American Joint Committee on Cancer and the Union Internationale Contre le Cancer in 1983 and is summarized below:
   A. **Histopathologic type**. Lymphocyte predominance, nodular sclerosis, mixed cellularity, lymphocyte depletion, and unclassified.
   B. **Stage groupings**

TABLE 60–1. CHARACTERISTICS OF HISTOLOGIC SUBTYPES IN HODGKIN'S LYMPHOMA

Histology	Incidence (%)	Age	Sex	RS cell	Prognosis
Lymphocyte predominant	5	Young	Male	L and H	Excellent
Nodular sclerosis	40–60	Young	Female	lacunar	Good
Mixed cellularity	30	Young	Male	RS	Fair
Lymphocyte depleted	5	Old	Male	Pleomorphic	Poor

1. **Stage I.** Involvement of **a single lymph node region** with (Stage I$_E$) or without (Stage I) involvement of a single **extralymphatic** organ or site.
2. **Stage II.** Involvement of 2 or more lymph node regions on the **same side of the diaphragm** (Stage II) or localized involvement of a single associated extralymphatic organ or site and its regional lymph nodes, with or without involvement of other lymph node regions on the same side of the diaphragm (Stage II$_E$).
3. **Stage III.** Involvement of lymph node regions on both sides of the diaphragm.
   a. **Stage III.** Involvement of lymph node regions on both sides of the diaphragm, including abdominal disease.
      (1) **Stage III$_{A1}$.** Involvement of lymph node regions on both sides of the diaphragm, including upper abdomen (splenic, celiac, and porta hepatis nodes or the spleen itself).
      (2) **Stage III$_{A2}$.** Involvement of lymph node regions on both sides of the diaphragm, including lower abdomen (para-aortic, iliac, and mesenteric lymph nodes).
   b. **Stage III$_E$.** Involvement of lymph node regions on both sides of the diaphragm accompanied by localized involvement of an associated extralymphatic organ or site.
   c. **Stage III$_S$.** Involvement of lymph node regions on both sides of the diaphragm accompanied by involvement of the spleen.
4. **Stage IV.** Disseminated or multifocal involvement of 1 or more extralymphatic organs with or without associated lymph node involvement or isolated extralymphatic organ involvement with distant (nonregional) nodal involvement.
   Note: Each stage is subdivided into **"A" (asymptomatic) or "B" (patients with unexplained weight loss > 10% of body weight in the last 6 months, unexplained fever > 38° C, and profuse night sweats).** Pruritus is not a consistent "B" symptom. The "E" designation does not alter the prognosis, but pathologic staging is recommended for all cases, especially if therapy would be affected.

IX. **Treatment.** The initial aim of therapy in all Hodgkin's patients is cure. Palliation as a goal in these patients is almost never acceptable.
A. **Surgery**
   1. **Primary Hodgkin's lymphoma**
      a. **General considerations.** Surgery plays a small but crucial role in the **diagnosis and staging of HL and the management of complications,** but surgery has **no direct therapeutic impact.**
      b. **Indications. Excisional lymph node biopsy** must be performed in all patients with suspected HL. In addition, some patients with suspected but unproved infradiaphragmatic disease require SL. In rare cases, patients may require mediastinoscopy or anterior parasternal mediastinotomy for diagnosis or develop complications necessitating surgical palliation (eg, ureteral obstruction from enlarged para-aortic and pelvic nodes and constrictive pericarditis after radiotherapy).
      c. **Procedures.** All procedures in HL are strictly diagnostic and therefore are outlined on pp 490–491, **VI.B.3** and **VI.C.3.**
   2. **Advanced Hodgkin's lymphoma.** As noted above, surgery, in advanced HL, is indicated only for the palliation of disease complications.
   3. **Morbidity and mortality.** The risks of superficial lymph node biopsy and SL are minimal and are discussed on p 490, **VI.C.3.b.**
B. **Radiation therapy**
   1. **Primary Hodgkin's lymphoma**
      a. **Indications.** At present, evidence supports the use of radiotherapy in the treatment of **Stage I (A and B), II (A and B), and III$_{A1}$A** Hodgkin's disease. The use of radiation in Stage III$_{A2}$A and Stage IIIB disease is controversial and is **not indicated** in Stage IV HL. The extent of radiation must be individualized and should include all involved lymph node groups as well as contiguous, presumably normal lymphatic areas.
      b. **Source and doses. Megavoltage** equipment is required to deliver the recommended **4000–4400 cGy to involved areas and 3000–3500 cGy to neighboring ostensibly disease-free nodal groups** at a rate of 150–220 cGy per day for 4–5 weeks (5 d/wk).
      c. **Fields.** Four standard radiation fields have been developed for use in Hodgkin's patients.
         (1) **Local manifestations.** In general, radiation to the local or **"involved"** field (occasionally used in Stage I and Stage II disease) is associated with a **higher relapse rate (as high as 68%)** than is radiation to more

extensive fields, but survival is identical (80%) because of effective salvage chemotherapy.

(2) Mantle. This field includes the **occipital, preauricular, cervical, supraclavicular, axillary, and mediastinal lymph nodes** and is the most common radiation field used (either alone or in conjunction with additional fields) in HL. Extensive high cervical lymphadenopathy may necessitate irradiation of **Waldeyer's ring** (lymphoid tissue of the lingual, pharyngeal, and facial tonsils).

(3) Para-aortic area and spleen. This field includes the **para-aortic nodes** from **T11–12 to the pelvic brim,** the **nodes of the splenic hilum,** and spleen (if not removed during SL). Nodes in the **porta hepatis** are **not** ordinarily irradiated. Although overlap with the mantle field must be limited to minimize the chance of **spinal cord injury,** overlap with pelvic fields is less critical because it occurs below the level of the spinal cord.

(4) Pelvis. Radiation to the **pelvic, inguinal, and femoral nodes** is included in this field while the pelvic bone marrow and testes or ovaries are shielded. In females undergoing SL, the ovaries should be secured above and lateral to the pelvic brim or in front of or behind the uterus for protection. If combined with para-aortic radiation, an **"inverted Y" field** is created. Recently, the need for pelvic irradiation has decreased as a result of improved staging techniques and chemotherapy. Currently, patients with Stage I or Stage II supradiaphragmatic disease do not require pelvic irradiation because of the **low incidence of pelvic disease (3%),** and patients with **Stages III$_{A2}$A, IIIB, or IV** HL usually receive **chemotherapy,** making radiation therapy unnecessary.

2. **Recurrent Hodgkin's lymphoma.** In the setting of recurrent Hodgkin's disease, radiotherapy is **seldom indicated.** Instead, salvage chemotherapy is considered to be the treatment of choice for these patients.

3. **Morbidity and mortality.** The complications that occur as a direct result of radiation therapy may be significant and include the following:

   a. **Myelosuppression. Mantle irradiation** depresses peripheral blood counts to **50% of normal,** whereas **extended fields** typically reduce blood elements by more than **75%.** Concomitant chemotherapy compounds the myelosuppression, but recovery uniformly occurs within several months after therapy is discontinued.

   b. **Gastrointestinal symptoms.** Anorexia, nausea, vomiting, diarrhea, dysphagia, esophagitis, exostomia, and weight loss may occur but generally are **temporary and mild.**

   c. **Radiation-induced pneumonitis.** This problem develops in **5% of patients** receiving mantle irradiation (see, also, p 48 "Radiation-Induced Lung Injury").

   d. **Radiation-induced carditis.** Depending on the amount of myocardium irradiated and the dose used, this complication may occur in **3–50% of patients** undergoing mediastinal radiotherapy (see p 51, "Radiation-Induced Carditis").

   e. **Transverse myelitis.** Although **15%** of patients develop transient numbness, tingling, or "electric" sensations that are aggravated by neck flexion **(Lhermitte's sign),** few sustain permanent neurologic injury.

   f. **Brachial plexopathy** (see p 55, "Lumbar and Brachial Plexopathies").

   g. **Renal insufficiency.** Rarely, irradiation of large para-aortic nodes incorporates the majority of both kidneys and results in renal insufficiency.

   h. **Hypothyroidism.** Although **30%** of patients develop **elevated thyroid-stimulating hormone** levels requiring thyroid hormone replacement, less than **5%** acquire overt **hypothyroidism.**

   i. **Infertility.** Although the testes should be shielded during pelvic irradiation, radiation scatter causes **transitory aspermia.** In females, relocation of the ovaries preserves fertility, but an increased **risk of genetic damage** exists.

   j. **Suppression of bone growth.** Damage to bone (particularly the vertebrae in children) resulting in suppressed growth and scoliosis has not proved to be a significant problem.

   k. **Secondary neoplasms.** The risk of developing a second primary malignancy (eg, myelodysplastic syndrome, acute myelogenous leukemia, non-Hodgkin's lymphoma, osteosarcoma) after completing radiation therapy is small if **radiotherapy is administered alone (0–1%)** and slightly greater if **combined with chemotherapy (6.5%).** Most tumors develop within 10 years.

TABLE 60–2. COMPLETE AND OVERALL RESPONSE RATES IN HODGKIN'S LYMPHOMA

Chemotherapy Agent	Overall Response (%)	Complete Response (%)
Procarbazine	69	38
Vinblastine	68	30
Dacarbazine	68	11
Mechlorethamine	64	13
Chlorambucil	60	16
Prednisone	61	—
Vincristine	58	36
Ifosfamide	55	—
Cyclophosphamide	54	12
CCNU	51	—

C. **Chemotherapy**
 1. **Primary Hodgkin's lymphoma**
  a. **Indications.** Chemotherapy remains the treatment of choice for patients with **Stage III$_{A2}$A, IIIB, or IV disease.** Indications for chemotherapy in Stage IIB (without staging laparotomy) and Stage III$_{A1}$A are controversial. Bulky mediastinal lymphadenopathy is treated best with combined chemoradiotherapy (see p 497, **IX.D**).
  b. **Regimens.** Combination chemotherapy is used almost exclusively in HL, although single agent therapy rarely may be indicated.
   (1) **Single agents.** Because the success of combination regimens, single-agent chemotherapy is indicated **only in elderly or debilitated patients who are unable to tolerate multiple drugs.** Early trials documented activity of many single agents (see Table 60–2).
   (2) **Combination chemotherapy.** Optimal treatment of patients with primary HL usually involves one of **3 regimens:** (1) mechlorethamine, vincristine, procarbazine, and prednisone **(MOPP),** (2) doxorubicin, bleomycin, vinblastine, and dacarbazine **(ABVD),** or (3) an alternating **MOPP and/or hybrid regimen of ABVD.** Although many alternative regimens have been tried (see Table 60–3), none has proven superior to these 3 protocols.
    (a) **MOPP.** MOPP was first used successfully in 1964 to treat patients with advanced-stage Hodgkin's disease. Although the exact dose and administration schedule vary between centers, the protocol is summarized in Appendix D. MOPP is given during 2 out of every 4 weeks for at least 6 courses and produces a **complete response rate higher than 80% and 10-year survival of 66%.** Full doses are administered unless absolutely contraindicated by toxicity, and therapy is discontinued only after **aggressive restaging** fails to document residual disease. If meticulous restaging is performed, **maintenance** chemotherapy has been shown to be **unnecessary.** The **dose-limiting toxicity** of this regimen is **myelosuppression.**
    (b) **ABVD.** Efforts to find a salvage regimen for MOPP-resistant HL, and subsequently for newly diagnosed HL, led to the combination of doxorubicin, bleomycin, vinblastine, and dacarbazine (ABVD). **Acute toxicity** (myelosuppression, gastrointestinal complaints) with ABVD is **diminished,** and the risk of second malignancies associated with alkylating-agent therapy is eliminated. With ABVD, however, chronic irreversible **cardiopulmonary toxicity** is a real hazard. Like MOPP, ABVD is administered during 2 out of every 4 weeks for at least 6 courses and produces a **complete response rate higher than 80%;** however, long-term survival data are not available because few trials have evaluated ABVD alone.
    (c) **Alternating MOPP and/or hybrid ABVD.** In an attempt to improve first-line therapy by adding non-cross-resistant agents to reduce the development of drug-resistant tumor cells **(Goldie-**

TABLE 60–3. ALTERNATIVE COMBINATION CHEMOTHERAPEUTIC REGIMENS IN HODGKIN'S LYMPHOMA

Regimen	MOPP Cross-resistance?	Agents
B-CAVe	No	Bleomycin, CCNU, doxorubicin, vinblastine
B-MOPP	Yes	Bleomycin, nitrogen mustard, vincristine, procarbazine, prednisone
BVCPP	Yes	BCNU, vinblastine, cyclophosphamide, procarbazine, prednisone
BVDS	No	Bleomycin, vinblastine, doxorubicin, prednisone
CABS	No	CCNU, doxorubicin, bleomycin, streptozotocin
CEM	No	CCNU, etoposide, vinblastine, doxorubicin, prednisone
CEP	No	CCNU, etoposide, prednimustine
CVB	No	CCNU, vinblastine, bleomycin
CVPP	Yes	Cyclophosphamide, vinblastine, procarbazine, prednisone
ChlVPP	Yes	Chlorambucil, vinblastine, procarbazine, prednisone
EVAP	No	Etoposide, vinblastine, doxorubicin, prednisone
LOPP	Yes	Chlorambucil, vincristine, procarbazine, prednisone
MOP-BAP	No	Nitrogen mustard, vincristine, bleomycin, doxorubicin, prednisone
MVPP	Yes	Nitrogen mustard, vinblastine, procarbazine, prednisone
MVVPP	Yes	Nitrogen mustard, vincristine, vinblastine, procarbazine, prednisone
VABCD	No	Vinblastine, doxorubicin, bleomycin, CCNU, dacarbazine

Coldman hypothesis), an alternating MOPP-ABVD regimen was developed. This alternative protocol is continued for 6 months and, in at least one randomized clinical trial, produced an **89% complete remission rate and 73% relapse-free survival** compared with 74% and 45%, respectively, for MOPP alone. The MOPP/ABV hybrid combines 7 of the total 8 agents into a single monthly cycle. A recent study comparing MOPP, ABVD and the alternating MOPP and ABVD regimen found ABVD alone or in combination with MOPP to be superior to MOPP alone with regard to complete response rate and overall survival. Further studies are underway in an attempt to identify the ideal regimen for HL.

2. **Recurrent Hodgkin's lymphoma**
   a. **Salvage chemotherapy.** Both patients who fail firstline therapy **(20–30%)** and those who relapse after initial therapy **(20%)** require salvage chemotherapy.
      (1) **Patients who fail more than 12 months after therapy.** These patients should not be assumed a priori to be resistant to the previously administered chemotherapy, and a trial of the same agents should be undertaken. **A complete response** is achieved with retreatment in **93% of patients;** however for patients who do not respond, subsequent therapy with a non-cross-resistant regimen must be pursued.
      (2) **Patients who fail within 12 months after therapy.** These patients require either a non-cross-resistant regimen (either MOPP or ABVD) or a third-line combination. In the case of disease that is resistant to both MOPP and ABVD, **CEVD** (lomustine, etoposide, vindesine, and dexamethasone), **CEP** (CCNU, etoposide, and prednisone), and **MIME** (methyl-gag, ifosfamide, methotrexate, and etoposide) have yielded **44%, 37%, and 24% response rates,** respectively.
   b. **Myeloablative therapy.** High-dose chemotherapy and autologous bone marrow transplantation is a promising but investigational therapy for Hodgkin's patients < 50 years of age who are otherwise in good health and have exhausted all other treatment options (see Chpt 6).
3. **Morbidity and mortality.** A prominent aspect of the acute toxicity of both the

MOPP and ABVD regimen involves **myelosuppression,** and Appendix E outlines suggested dose modifications for ongoing bone marrow toxicity (vincristine and prednisone in MOPP and bleomycin in ABVD do not require dose modification). Administering the **maximum tolerated dose** according to the recommendations is crucial because failure to do so may reduce the chance of cure. Other chemotherapy-related toxicities include the following:

a. **Opportunistic infections** (see Chapter 16).
b. **Anthracycline-induced cardiomyopathy** (see p 451).
c. **Chemotherapy-induced lung injury** (see p 470).
d. **Infertility.** Oligo- and aspermia occur in more than **80% of males** who undergo at least 6 cycles of chemotherapy, whereas only **40–50% of females** (almost all are > 25 years old) experience ovarian dysfunction.
e. **Second malignancies.** Alkylating agents, combination chemotherapy, radiation, advancing age, and splenectomy are factors influencing the **3.3–10% risk of acute myelogenous leukemia and 0–5.9% risk of non-Hodgkin's lymphoma** over the first 10 years following therapy. An increased risk of solid tumors developing 10–15 years after treatment also exists.

D. **Combined modality therapy.** Although not uniformly accepted, Stage IIB (unconfirmed by staging laparotomy), Stage III (particularly III_{A2}), and bulky mediastinal disease may be treated best with combined radiation and chemotherapy.

E. **Immunotherapy.** A multitude of biological response modifiers, including bacille Calmette-Guérin (BCG), interferon-alpha, thymostimulin, tuftsin, and levamisole have been tried without success in the treatment of HL. However, anecdotal responses with interleukin-2 and lymphokine-activated killer cells have been reported in non-Hodgkin's lymphomas and ultimately may lead to application of adoptive immunotherapy to the therapy of HL.

X. **Prognosis**
A. **Risk of recurrence.** The risk of relapse following curative radiotherapy in Stages I to III_{A1} disease is **10–39% (0–11% within the radiation ports).** Subsequent chemotherapy, however, salvages all but 15–50% of these patients. The recurrence rate after complete response to chemotherapy in Stages III_{A2} and IV disease is 20%, and **90%** of these occur **within 2 years** after therapy is discontinued.

B. **Five-year survival.** The 5- and 10-year actuarial survival of patients with HL is depicted in Table 60–4.

C. **Adverse prognostic factors.** A number of factors are associated with a poor outcome.
1. **"B" symptoms.** Patients with "B" symptoms (particularly Stages I to III) experience an **18% worse survival** than asymptomatic patients.
2. **Relapse within 12 months.** Patients recurring within 12 months have a significantly worse 5-year survival than those who relapse after 12 months (**< 20% vs 35%,** respectively).
3. **Advanced age.** Patients who are **older than 40 years** do significantly worse than younger patients.
4. **Advanced stage at diagnosis.**
5. **Histologic subtype.** The actuarial survival varies consistently with the histologic appearance of the disease (see Table 60–5). The lymphocyte predominant subtype has the best 10-year survival at 70%, followed by Nodular sclerosis 65%, mixed celluosity 52% and lymphocyte depleted subtype at less than 20% ten-year survival.

XI. **Patient follow-up**
A. **General guidelines.** Patients with Hodgkin's disease should be followed closely every 3 months for 3 years, every 6 months for an additional 2 years, and annually

TABLE 60–4. FIVE- AND 10-YEAR SURVIVAL IN PATIENTS WITH HODGKIN'S LYMPHOMA

Stage	5–Year Survival (%)	10-Year Survival (%)
I	90	73
II	87	69
III	71	54
IV	45	< 37

TABLE 60–5. FIVE- AND 10-YEAR SURVIVAL BY HISTOLOGIC TUMOR SUBTYPE

Histology	5–Year Survival (%)	10-Year Survival (%)
Lymphoctye predominant	95	70
Nodular sclerosis	84	65
Mixed cellularity	66	52
Lymphocyte depleted	22	< 20

thereafter for evidence of relapse. The following specific guidelines for patient follow-up are offered.

B. Routine evaluation. Patients with HL who have undergone potentially curative therapy require the following routine blood tests and imaging studies:

1. **Medical history and physical examination.** An interval medical history and a complete physical examination should be performed during every clinic visit. Attention is focused on the areas discussed on p 490, **VI.A.**

2. **Blood tests** (see p 1, **IV.A**)
   a. **Complete blood count.**
   b. **Hepatic transaminases**.
   c. **Alkaline phosphatase.**
   d. **BUN and creatinine.**

3. **Chest x-ray** (see p 3, **IV.C.1**)

C. Additional evaluation. Other tests and procedures that should be performed at regular intervals include the following:

1. **Computed tomography (CT).** This radiographic examination should be ordered **every 6–12 months** for at least 5 years (see also, **VI.B.2.b**).

2. **Bipedal lymphangiogram.** This test should be obtained **annually** for 2–5 years (see also, **VIII.B.2.c**).

D. Optional evaluation. The following tests and procedures may be indicated by previous diagnostic findings or clinical suspicion:

1. **Blood tests** (see p 2, **IV.A**)
   a. **5′-Nucleotidase.**
   b. **GGTP.**

2. **Imaging Studies** (see p 3, **IV.C**)
   a. **Ultrasound.**
   b. **Technetium-99m bone scan.**

3. **Biopsy.** Any suspicious or new mass should be surgically biopsied to exclude the possibility of recurrent disease. An aggressive approach may be justified because many patients can be salvaged with additional therapy.

REFERENCES

Anastos J, Bitter MA, and Vordinos JW. The histopathologic diagnosis and subclassification of Hodgkin's disease. Hematol/Oncol Clin N Amer 3(2):187–203, 1987.

Bonadonna G, Santoro A, Vivioni S, and Valagussa P. Treatment strategies for Hodgkin's disease. Sem Hematol 25(2)Suppl:51–77, 1988.

Buzaid AC, Lippman SM, Miller TP. Salvage therapy for advanced Hodgkin's disease. Amer J Med 83:423–532, 1987.

Crnkovich MJ, Leopold K, Hoppe RT, et. al. Stage I to IIB Hodgkin's disease: the combined experience at Stanford University and the Joint Center for Radiation Therapy. J Clin Oncol 5:1041-1049, 1987.

Delaney TF and Glatstein E. The role of staging laparotomy in the management of Hodgkin's disease. Can Updates 1(1):1–14, 1987.

Farch E and Weichselbaum RR. Substaging of Stage III Hodgkin's disease. Hematol/Oncol Clin N Amer 3(2):277–286, 1989.

Jaffe ES. The elusive Reed-Sternberg cell. NEJM 320(8):529- 531, 1989.

Kriterier JG, Porticco CS, and Mach PM. Hodgkin's disease presenting below the diaphragm: a review. J Clin Onc 4(10):1551–1562, 1986.

Longe DL, Young RC, Wesley M, et al. Twenty years of MOPP therapy for Hodgkin's disease. J Clin Oncol 4(9):1295–1306, 1986.

Mauch P, Goffman T, Rosenthal DS, et. al. Stage III Hodgkin's disease: improved survival with combined modality therapy as compared with radiation therapy alone. J Clin Oncol 3:1166–1173, 1985.

Moormeier JA, Williams SF, and Golomb HM. The staging of Hodgkin's disease. Hematol/Oncol Clin N Amer 3(2):1237–1250, 1987.

Portlock CS. Hodgkin's disease. Med Clin N Amer. 68(3):729–740, 1984.

Weiss LM, Morched LA, Worke CA, and Stir J. Detection of Epstein Barr viral cancer in Reed-Sternberg cells of Hodgkin's disease. NEJM 320(8):502–506, 1989.

Wieinik PH. Chemotherapy of Hodgkin's disease. Can Updates 2(3):1–12, 1988.

61 Non-Hodgkin's Lymphoma

Mindy S. Bohrer, MD

I. **Epidemiology.** Non-Hodgkin's lymphomas (NHLs) represent **3.4% of all cancers and 3.6% of all cancer deaths** in the United States. In 1985, **14.7 cases per 100,000 males** and **10.3 cases per 100,000 females** were diagnosed, resulting in **7.0 and 4.6 deaths,** respectively. Estimates indicate that **43,000 new cases** and **20,500 deaths** will occur in 1993. Since 1973 the incidence has **increased 41.8%.** Worldwide, the incidence varies from a low of 1 per 100,000 in Poland to more than 9 per 100,000 in parts of Israel.

II. **Risk factors**
   A. **Age.** In the United States, the incidence of NHL gradually increases from less than 1 per 100,000 before the age of 10 years to **77.9 per 100,000 by age 80.** The **mean age** at presentation is **50 years.**
   B. **Sex.** The risk in **males** is **1.4 times** greater than in females.
   C. **Race.** Whites are at **1.7 times** greater risk than blacks.
   D. **Genetic factors.** In addition to a modest association with **human lymphocyte antigens (HLAs), AW33 and B12,** the following genetic influences have been documented:
      1. **Family history.** Although the risk of NHL in first-degree relatives is slightly greater than in the general population, environmental as well as genetic influences may be responsible.
      2. **Hereditary syndromes.** Certain inherited disorders, including **Klinefelter's syndrome** (47XXY phenotype associated with atrophic testes, azoospermia, gynecomastia, and elevated gonadotropin levels) and **Chédiak-Higashi syndrome or Béguez César disease (**autosomal recessive disease with oculocutaneous albinism, leukocyte inclusions, histiocytic infiltration, and pancytopenia) are associated with an increased risk of NHL (see, also, **II.F.1,** below).
      3. **Chromosomal abnormalities.** Nonrandom clonal chromosomal abnormalities are present in more than **90%** of patients with NHL. **Translocations** such as reciprocal **11q;14q** (diffuse lymphomas), **14q;18q** (85% follicular lymphomas), and **8q;14q** (75–90% Burkitt's lymphoma) may juxtapose oncogenes **bcl-1** (B cell lymphoma or leukemia-1), **bcl-2,** and **c-myc,** respectively, with immunoglobulin enhancers, resulting in clinical lymphoma. Other translocations also occur: eg, 8q;2q (kappa light chain region and 8q;22 (lambda light chain area) in 5–9% and 5–16% of Burkitt's lymphomas, respectively. In addition, **trisomy 11** (partial trisomy) is found in **4%** of patients with NHL.
   E. **Radiation.** Although not definitive, data suggest an **increased incidence** of NHL among atomic bomb survivors and patients irradiated with more than **100 cGy** for ankylosing spondylitis and Hodgkin's disease.
   F. **Previous immunologic pathology.** The diseases discussed below are associated with an increased risk of NHLs:
      1. **Immunodeficiency disease**
         a. **Primary immunodeficiency**
            (1) **Congenital immunodeficiency.** There is a 10,000-fold increased risk of lymphoreticular malignancies, including NHLs, in **ataxia telangiectasia, Louis-Bar's syndrome** (hereditary progressive ataxia associated with oculocutaneous telangiectasia, sinopulmonary disease, and abnormal eye movements), and **Wiscott-Aldrich syndrome** (sex-linked recessive chronic eczema, suppurative otitis media, anemia, and thrombocytopenic purpura).
            (2) **Acquired immunodeficiency**
               (a) **Acquired immunodeficiency (AIDS).** Primary lymphoma of the central nervous system (CNS) and **aggressive high-grade B cell**

lymphoma occur in a high proportion of patients with AIDS and AIDS-related complex (ARC).

(b) Other diseases. Other acquired disorders associated with an increased risk of NHL include **Swiss-type agammaglobulinemia** (autosomal recessive T and B cell disorder), **acquired hypogammaglobulinemia, common variable immunodeficiency,** and autoimmune **collagen vascular diseases** such as rheumatoid arthritis, systemic lupus erythematosus, and Sjögren's syndrome (**10%** develop NHL). **Sarcoid** and **celiac disease** also increase the risk of NHL.

b. Secondary immunodeficiency. Patients undergoing renal and cardiac transplantation are at **40–100 times** greater risk of developing NHLs, especially during the first year following transplant. Discontinuation of the immunosuppressive regimen occasionally reverses the process.

2. Infection

a. Viral infections. Infections with **Epstein-Barr virus** and **human T cell leukemia/lymphoma virus** frequently are implicated in the etiology of African Burkitt's lymphoma and Japanese endemic adult T cell lymphoma, respectively.

b. Parasitic infection. A heightened risk of lymphomas is documented among patients in Brazil who suffer from *Schistosoma mansoni* and **leprosy.**

3. Drugs

a. Cytotoxic drugs. Certain cytotoxic agents (**cyclophosphamide** and **azathioprine**) have been connected with the pathogenesis of NHL and may account for the increased risk observed in patients treated for Hodgkin's lymphoma and in transplant recipients.

b. Other drugs. Chronic administration of **phenytoin** is associated with a lymphoma-like syndrome and a small increased risk of NHL.

G. Diet. No specific dietary habits have been implicated in the pathogenesis of NHL.

H. Urbanization. Although exposure to the **herbicides phenoxyacetic acid and chlorophenol** increases the risk of NHL in rural **farmers** and **veterinarians**, the incidence of NHL is increased among certain urban professions (eg, **chemical workers and anesthesiologists**) for unknown reasons.

III. Clinical presentation

A. Signs and symptoms

1. Local manifestations. The most common clinical manifestation of NHL is **diffuse rubbery, discrete, superficial adenopathy (64–80%)** that is most commonly **painless (90%)**. Symptomatic extranodal disease occurs in **30%** of patients and may produce bone pain (< 5%), spinal cord compression, superior vena cava syndrome and edema (< 5%), gastrointestinal distress (painless mass or painful palpable mass; 67% gastric, 25% small intestine, 8% colon and rectum; rarely bleeding, obstruction, or perforation), pulmonary complaints (< 5%; cough, dyspnea, hemoptysis), skin nodules, anemia, testicular masses, CNS masses, abdominal pain (8%), and nausea and vomiting (8%).

2. Systemic manifestations. Systemic signs and symptoms, including **fever (4%),** malaise (8%), **night sweats (2%), weight loss (9%),** fatigue (10%), and **pruritus,** are less common in NHL than in Hodgkin's disease (20% vs 40%, respectively), and the prognostic significance is less clear.

B. Paraneoplastic syndromes. The following paraneoplastic syndromes rarely are associated with NHL.

1. Progressive multifocal leukoencephalopathy (see p 58, **IV**).

2. Subacute cerebellar degeneration)see p 58, **I**).

3. Subacute motor neuropathy (see p 58, **II**).

4. Myasthenic syndrome (see p 59, **II**).

IV. Differential diagnosis. Most patients with NHL present with localized or diffuse lymphadenopathy. The differential diagnosis of this finding is extensive and is discussed on p 489, **IV.**

V. Screening programs. Because of the low incidence of NHL, the frequency of benign lymphadenopathy, and the lack of a simple diagnostic test, mass screening for NHL is **impractical.**

VI. Diagnostic workup

A. Medical history and physical examination. A thorough medical history should be elicited, and a complete physical examination must be performed in all patients with suspected NHL, paying particular attention to the following areas:

1. General appearance. Assessment of the patient's general functional and nutritional status should be made, noting evidence of significant **recent weight loss.**

2. **Skin.** Papules, eruptions, and nodules are recorded and fully described.
3. **Lymph nodes.** The characteristics (number, size, location, consistency, tenderness, fluctuation, mobility) of all lymph nodes must be recorded. This should be done separately for all lymph node areas, including occipital, cervical (anterior and posterior), supraclavicular, infraclavicular, axillary, epitrochlear, inguinal, and popliteal regions.
4. **Chest. Tenderness** of the anterior **chest wall** and certain **auscultation findings** (eg, wheezing, diminished breath sounds) may indicate mediastinal disease, pleural effusions, or both.
5. **Abdomen.** All abdominal **masses and hepatosplenomegaly,** indicating lymphomatous involvement of the spleen, liver, and intra-abdominal lymph nodes, must be completely described. Nearly **96% of palpable spleens** and **33% of nonpalpable spleens** are involved with lymphoma.
6. **Extremities.** Swelling is an important finding that may indicate obstruction of the superior vena cava from **mediastinal disease** (upper extremity) or obstruction of the inferior vena cava from **enlarged para-aortic lymph nodes** (lower extremity). In addition, a detailed neurologic examination is crucial to exclude the possibility of **spinal cord involvement.**

B. **Primary tests and procedures.** The following diagnostic tests and procedures should be obtained initially in all patients with suspected lymphatic malignancies:
1. **Blood tests** (see p 1, **IV.A**).
   a. **Complete blood count. Thrombocytopenia** (from hypersplenism, bone marrow involvement, or autoimmunity), normochromic normocytic **anemia** resulting from a **Coombs-positive autoimmune hemolytic anemia,** or bone marrow involvement and **abnormal circulating lymphocytes (33%)** may be noted.
   b. **Hepatic transaminases.**
   c. **Alkaline phosphatase.**
   d. **BUN and creatinine.** Renal impairment from direct tumor infiltration or ureteral obstruction may be detected with these tests.
2. **Imaging studies**
   a. **Chest x-ray.** Evidence of mediastinal and hilar **adenopathy (5–25%),** pleural **effusions (8–10%),** and pulmonary parenchymal infiltration (uncommon) should be sought. (see, also, p 3, **IV.C.1**).
   b. **Computed tomography (CT).** Chest and abdominal CT scan should be obtained for staging purposes. **Abdominal CT is 83% accurate** in detecting abdominal lymphadenopathy, particularly in the upper abdomen, but it **underestimates splenic involvement** because tumor nodules are often less than 1 cm in diameter. Because upper abdominal nodes are often enlarged in NHL, CT scans may be particularly useful.
   c. **Bipedal lymphangiogram.** Although inaccurate in the upper abdomen, lymphangiogram boasts a **90–95% positive and 60–80% negative predictive value** for retroperitoneal lymphadenopathy. In addition, it may focus attention on suspicious groups of lymph nodes requiring biopsy during staging laparotomy.
3. **Invasive procedures**
   a. **Lymph node biopsy.** Because 80% of patients present with superficial lymphadenopathy, **excisional lymph node biopsy** is essential to confirm the diagnosis and to determine the histologic type of NHL that is present (see, also, p 506, **IX.A**). The vast majority of patients undergo **cervical lymph node biopsy.** Axillary and inguinal lymph node biopsy is occasionally necessary. Complications after cervical or supraclavicular lymph node biopsy are unusual but include **pneumothorax, cranial nerve injury, infection, and hemorrhage.**
   b. **Bone marrow aspiration.** If not obtained at the time of staging laparotomy, bilateral bone marrow aspirations of the iliac crest and biopsies **(Jamshidi needle)** are indicated in all patients. Overall, bone marrow involvement is identified in **39–45%** of patients **(50–70% with small cell lymphocytic histology)** and results in **upstaging 39–75%** of patients. Only **33%** of patients with bone marrow involvement have **abnormalities on peripheral blood smear.**

C. **Optional tests and procedures.** The following are examinations that may be indicated by either previous diagnostic findings or clinical suspicion:

1. **Blood tests**
   a. **5'Nucleotidase** (see p 2, **IV.A.4**).
   b. **GGTP** (see p 2, **IV.A.5**).
   c. **Lactate dehydrogenase.** The serum level of this enzyme correlates with **tumor burden** and can be monitored to follow response to treatment.
   d. **Uric acid.** Serum levels of this metabolic by-product may be elevated in advanced disease and may cause renal impairment, particularly if **rapid tumor lysis** occurs with chemotherapy (see p 86, "Tumor lysis syndrome").
2. **Imaging studies**
   a. **Upper gastrointestinal series.** This series, with small bowel follow-through, is indicated in patients with gastrointestinal symptoms and lymphoma of **Waldeyer's ring.**
   b. **Barium enema (BE).** A BE should be obtained in patients with symptoms referable to the colon.
   c. **Magnetic resonance imaging (MRI)** (see p 3, **IV.C.3**).
   d. **Ultrasound.** This test is used to exclude **obstructive uropathy** from enlarged para-aortic nodes, if suspected (see also, p 3, **IV.C.4**).
   e. **Gallium scan.** Gallium scans are inaccurate and rarely indicated.
   f. **Technetium-99m bone scan** (see p 3, **IV.C.5**).
3. **Invasive procedures**
   a. **Lumbar puncture. Spinal fluid analysis** reveals meningeal involvement in **8%** of patients with **lymphoblastic lymphoma** and also may be indicated in testicular lymphoma and in diffuse histiocytic lymphoma involving the bone marrow.
   b. **Percutaneous liver biopsy.** Lymphoma is detected in the liver in **20%** of blind needle liver biopsies; however, a **35% false-negative rate** emphasizes that negative results do not exclude this possibility.
   c. **Peritoneoscopy.** Direct visualization of the liver and spleen increases the diagnostic accuracy of needle biopsy, but the results still fall short of open-staging laparotomy.
   d. **Staging laparotomy (SL).** Although **SL is the "gold standard"** method of staging NHL and results in **upstaging 10–20%** of patients (particularly those with follicular histologies), it is useful only in the **rare patients with clinically limited disease** whose therapy may be altered significantly by findings at laparotomy. The technique and complications of SL have been fully discussed previously (see p. 491, **VI,C,3,b**).
   e. **Mediastinoscopy.** In rare cases, this procedure is indicated in the diagnosis of isolated mediastinal NHL (see also, p 491, **VI.C.3.c**).
   f. **Anterior parasternal mediastinotomy (Chamberlain procedure).** Like mediastinoscopy, this surgical procedure may be required in unusual circumstances for the diagnosis of isolated mediastinal NHL (see also, p 491, **VII.C.3.d**).
VII. **Pathology**
   A. **Location**
      1. **Nodal lymphomas.** Superficial lymphadenopathy in NHL frequently is **diffuse (90%)** and **discontinuous** and often involves **cervical (60%),** axillary (14%), mediastinal (20%), intra-abdominal, inguinal (20%), and epitrochlear lymph nodes as well as Waldeyer's ring (15–33%).
      2. **Extranodal lymphomas**
         a. **Head and neck.** Common head and neck locations include the **tonsils (25–35%),** other Waldeyer's ring locations (15–25%), salivary glands, thyroid gland, orbit, and CNS (rare).
         b. **Thorax.** Primary lung and mediastinal (thymic) lymphomas occur occasionally.
         c. **Gastrointestinal tract. Gastric (75%),** small bowel (13%, including Mediterranean lymphoma), colon (6%), and rectum (6%) are common sites. Gastric lymphoma benefits from surgical debulking, whereas resection also may be indicated in small and large bowel lymphoma to prevent hemorrhage, obstruction, and perforation (including that which is treatment related).
         d. **Soft tissue and bone.** Lymphomas limited to the skin, breast, and bone are rare.
         e. **Other sites.** Lymphoma of the testis is well known, whereas isolated disease of the liver, spleen, heart, and kidney are less common.
   B. **Multiplicity.** Multiple areas of discontinuous disease are characteristic of NHL but **do not** represent multiple primary lymphomas.

C. Histology

1. **Classification.** The heterogeneous microscopic appearance of lymphoma has been the basis of 6 independent histologic classification systems worldwide (Rappaport, Lukes and Collins, the World Health Organization, Dorfman, Kiel, and the British National Lymphoma Investigation Group); however, a recent National Cancer Institute study recommended a "Working Formulation" that combined many features of the previous classification systems with data on immunologic phenotype (see Table 61–1). Most systems distinguish between a **follicular** or nodular and a **diffuse** histologic pattern. Furthermore, a second

TABLE 61–1. DIFFERENT HISTOLOGIC CLASSIFICATION SYSTEMS FOR NON-HODGKIN'S LYMPHOMA*

Working Formulation	Lukes and Collins	Modified Rappaport
Low grade	Undefined cell type	**Nodular**
A. Malignant lymphoma, small lymphocytic consistent with CLL plasmacytoid	T cell type, small lymphocytic (A)	Lymphocytic, well differentiated (A)
B. Malignant lymphoma, follicular, predominantly small cleaved cell diffuse areas sclerosis	T cell type, Sezarymycosisfungoides (cerebriform)	Lymphocytic, poorly differentiated (B)
C. Malignant lymphoma, follicular; mixed, small cleaved and large cell diffuse areas sclerosis	T cell type, convoluted lymphocytic (I)	Mixed lymphocytic and histiocytic (C)
	T cell type, immunoblastic sarcoma (T cell) (H)	Histiocytic (D)
Intermediate grade	B cell type, small lymphocytic (A)	**Diffuse**
D. Malignant lymphoma, follicular predominantly large cell	B cell type, plasmacytoid lymphocytic (A)	Lymphocytic, well differentiated (A)
Diffuse areas	Follicular center cell, small cleaved (B-E)	With plasmacytoid features (A)
Sclerosis	Follicular center cell, large cleaved (D-G)	Lymphocytic, poorly differentiated (E)
E. Malignant lymphoma, diffuse small cleaved-cell sclerosis	Follicular center cell, small noncleaved (J)	Lymphoblastic, convoluted (I)
F. Malignant lymphoma, diffuse mixed, small and large cell sclerosis epithelioid cell component	Follicular center cell, large noncleaved (D-G)	Lymphoblastic, nonconvoluted (I)
G. Malignant lymphoma, diffuse:	Immunoblastic sarcoma (B cell)	Mixed, lymphocytic and histiocytic (F)
Large cell	Subtypes of follicular center cell lymphoma (H):	Histiocytic without sclerosis (G)
Cleaved cell	Follicular	Histiocytic with sclerosis (G)
Noncleaved cell	Follicular and diffuse	Burkitt's tumor (J)
Sclerosis	Diffuse	Undifferentiated (J)
High grade	Sclerotic with follicles	**Unclassified**
H. Malignant lymphoma large cell, immunoblastic	Sclerotic without follicles	**Composite**
Plasmacytoid	Histiocytic	
Clear cell	Malignant lymphoma, unclassified	
Polymorphous		
Epithelioid cell component		
I. Malignant lymphoma lymphoblastic:		
Convoluted cell		
Nonconvoluted cell		
J. Malignant lymphoma small non-cleaved cell		
Burkitt's		
Follicular areas		
Miscellaneous		
Composite		
Mycosis fungoides		
Histiocytic		
Extramedullary plasmacytoma		
Unclassifiable		
Other		

*Histologies in the different systems are labeled with letters that corresponding to those of the Working Formulation System of the National Cancer Institute.

Adapted from DeVita VT, Jaffe ES, Mauch P, Longo DL. In DeVita VT, Hellman S, Rosenberg SA, editors. *Lymphocytic Lymphomas in Cancer: Principles and Practice of Oncology.* 4th ed. Philadelphia PA: Lippincott; 1993, with permission.

pathologic feature is the predominant cell type, many classification systems separate a **small cell** (well-differentiated lymphocyte) from a **large cell or histiocyte** (transformed lymphocyte). Lymphomas with **mixed** cell types are regarded as **large-cell** lymphomas unless more than **75%** of the overall cellularity consists of small cells.

2. **Natural history.** Lymphomas can be classified into 2 groups based on natural history: favorable and unfavorable (see Table 61–2).

   a. **Favorable histology.** These lymphomas consist of primarily **follicular small-cell lymphomas and some diffuse small-cell** lymphomas that follow an **indolent clinical course.** Despite protracted and relatively asymptomatic disease, these patients become **increasingly resistant** to cytotoxic agents and, although occasionally cured by radiotherapy, are generally **never cured** by chemotherapy. Conversion to an aggressive cell type often occurs, and the patient ultimately succumbs to widely disseminated disease.

   b. **Unfavorable histology. Diffuse large-cell, some follicular large-cell, and some diffuse small-cell** lymphomas constitute the bulk of these lymphomas, which clinically **behave extremely aggressively.** Paradoxically, **chemotherapy cures 37–60%** of these patients.

D. **Metastatic spread**

   1. **Modes of spread.** NHL spreads via 3 mechanisms:

      a. **Direct extension.** Growth of lymphoma cells through the lymph node **capsule** of involved lymph nodes leads to **extranodal** extension.

      b. **Lymphatic metastasis.** Circulation of lymphatic cells through lymph channels results in diffuse lymphatic involvement marked by areas of apparently discontinuous disease.

      c. **Hematogenous metastasis.** Spread through blood vessels produces involvement in distant organs in **30–33%** patients by the time of diagnosis.

   2. **Sites of spread.** The most common extranodal sites involved at presentation include **bone marrow (30–45%), liver (15–50%),** and **spleen (30–40%).** As with Hodgkin's disease, hepatic involvement invariably is accompanied by splenic involvement. Additional sites are involved in 24% of cases and include the gastrointestinal tract (4.6%; stomach 2.4%; small intestine 1.5%; and colon 0.6%), head and neck (8.7%), bone (4%), scalp (5%), and, in rare cases, lung, kidney, bladder, testes, prostate, ovary, cervix, breast, salivary glands, and CNS.

VIII. **Staging.** The Ann Arbor (AA) classification system for Hodgkin's lymphoma initially developed in 1970, was adopted by the American Joint Committee on Cancer and the Union Internationale Contre le Cancer in 1983 for use in **both** Hodgkin's and non-Hodgkin's lymphoma. The **diffuse** nature of NHL, however, reduces the usefulness of this staging system because **therapeutic strategies rarely are determined by stage.** In addition, this staging system provides little prognostic information because there is no difference in survival between Stage III and Stage IV with histologically favorable lymphoma and between any of the stages with histologically unfavorable lymphoma. Despite these limitations, the AA staging system is still the most widely used one. The **National Cancer Institute (NCI),** however, has proposed a **modified staging system** based on differences in prognosis. The AA staging system for NHL is identical to that outlined for Hodgkin's lymphoma (see p 492, **VIII**), except that the histopathologic

TABLE 61–2. FAVORABLE AND UNFAVORABLE HISTOLOGIES OF NON-HODGKIN'S LYMPHOMA*

Favorable	Unfavorable
Follicular, small cell (B)	Diffuse, large cell (G)
Follicular, mixed (C)	Diffuse, mixed (F)
Diffuse, small cell	Follicular, large cell (D)
Well differentiated (A; small lymphocytic)	Diffuse, large cell immunoblastic (H)
Poorly differentiated (E; diffuse small cleaved cell)	Diffuse, small cell (J; diffuse small non-cleaved cell)
	Diffuse, small cell lymphoblastic (I)

*Histologies are labeled with letters that correspond to those of the Working Formulation System of the National Cancer Institute.

grade is determined by the Working Formulation (see Table 61–1). The NCI's modified staging system is outlined below:

A. Favorable histology (indolent) lymphomas
   1. **Stage I.** Localized disease (AA Stages I and II).
   2. **Stage II.** Disseminated disease (AA Stages III and IV).
B. Histologically unfavorable (aggressive) lymphomas
   1. **Stage I.** Localized nodal or extranodal disease (AA Stages I and I_E).
   2. **Stage II.** Two or more nodal sites of disease or a localized extranodal site plus draining nodes with none of the following poor prognostic features: **performance status of 70 or less, "B" symptoms, any mass larger than 10 cm in diameter (particularly GI), serum lactic dehydrogenase (LHD) higher than 500, or 3 or more extranodal sites of disease.**
   3. **Stage III.** Stage II with any poor prognostic feature.

IX. **Treatment.** Histology and stage of disease are the major factors that need to be defined before any decision is made regarding therapy. By stage, the distinction that must be made is between early Stage I, possibly Stage II, and Stages III and IV disease. It is this distinction that may ultimately affect the choice between radiation and chemotherapy.

A. Surgery
   1. **Primary non-Hodgkin's lymphoma**
      a. **General considerations.** Surgery plays a small but crucial role in the **diagnosis and staging of NHL as well as management of complications,** but surgery has **no direct therapeutic effect.**
      b. **Indications. Excisional lymph node biopsy** must be performed in all patients with suspected NHL. In addition, patients with suspected but unproven infradiaphragmatic disease rarely require SL. A few patients may require mediastinoscopy or anterior parasternal mediastinotomy for diagnosis or may develop complications necessitating surgical palliation (eg, ureteral obstruction from enlarged para-aortic and pelvic nodes, constrictive pericarditis after radiotherapy).
      c. **Procedures.** All procedures in NHL are strictly diagnostic and therefore are outlined under on p 502, **VI.B.3,** and p 503, **VI.C.3.**
   2. **Advanced non-Hodgkin's lymphoma.** As noted in **IX.A.1.b** above, surgery for advanced NHL is indicated only for palliation of disease complications. Patients with gastrointestinal hemorrhage, obstruction, perforation, and intussusception often require surgical intervention. In addition, resection of gastrointestinal lymphomas, particularly gastric lymphomas, may be required to prevent **hemorrhage** and **perforation** induced by thrombocytopenia and tumor lysis associated with intensive chemotherapy.
   3. **Morbidity and mortality.** Although the risk of superficial lymph node biopsy is minimal, the morbidity and mortality following SL may be significant (see p 490, **VI.C.3.b**).
B. Radiation therapy
   1. **Primary non-Hodgkin's lymphoma**
      a. **Localized disease. Radiation therapy (3500–4000 cGy over 4–5 weeks)** is indicated for the **10%** of patients who present with either histologically **favorable or unfavorable NHL limited to one side of the diaphragm** (NCI's indolent Stage I and aggressive Stage I; AA Stage I and I_E and II and II_E). Radiation can be delivered as involved-field, extended-field, total nodal, or total lymphoid (total nodal with whole abdomen) irradiation, although **total lymphoid radiotherapy** generally produces superior results. The 5-year survival following radiation therapy is summarized in Table 61–3. A plateau in the survival curve indicates that **cure** is possible in patients with

TABLE 61-3. FIVE-YEAR SURVIVAL FOLLOWING PRIMARY RADIATION THERAPY

Histology	Stage I/IE*(%)	Stage II/IIE* (%)
Favorable	88	61
Unfavorable	65–100	25
All	50–80	20–60

*Ann Arbor staging system.

both favorable and unfavorable histology. Results improve when **staging** is **rigorous** and when only favorable extranodal sites (intracapsular thyroid, salivary, breast, and lung) are involved. A slightly **worse** outcome is associated with the following features: **unfavorable histology, bulky (> 10 cm)** abdominal disease (unfavorable histology only), **discontinuous or extensive** disease (**> 2 nodal regions** involved), and spread to **unfavorable** extranodal sites, particularly to the **brain, sinus, testis, and small bowel.** Although chemotherapy failed in previous trials to increase the efficacy of radiation therapy because of the use of ineffective cytotoxic combinations, recent studies evaluating **chemotherapy (CVP and CHOP) plus radiation** in the treatment of histologically unfavorable and even histologically favorable NHLs demonstrate **improved** 5-year disease-free survival with the combination compared to radiation alone **(64–88% vs 32–45%)**. Therefore, although radiotherapy continues to be indicated as a potentially curative treatment for localized NHLs, especially those with favorable (indolent) histologies, the administration of chemotherapy in these patients should be seriously considered.

   b. **Diffuse disease.** Palliative **total nodal and total lymphoid** irradiation may yield prolonged survival **(45–50% 5-year and 40% 10-year disease-free survival)** in patients with **Stage III follicular lymphoma.** Moreover, **88% 15-year disease-free survival** has been observed in Stage III patients with no "B" symptoms, fewer than 5 sites of involvement, and a maximum disease diameter of less than 10 cm. However, these results require **staging laparotomy** to exclude patients with occult Stage IV disease. Experimental **total body irradiation** for Stage III and Stage IV disease may induce remission but is less effective than chemotherapy, particularly in patients with acute, bulky, aggressive disease with an unfavorable histology, and is best reserved for **indolent lymphomas** in patients who **cannot tolerate chemotherapy.**

2. **Recurrent non-Hodgkin's lymphoma.** The role of radiation therapy for recurrent NHL is limited to palliation of **symptomatic localized disease in previously nonirradiated fields.**

3. **Morbidity and mortality.** The complications following radiation therapy for early NHL are **minimal** and include salivary dysfunction, transverse myelitis, diarrhea, pneumonitis, nephritis, pericarditis, gastritis, and intestinal obstruction, perforation, and hemorrhage.

C. **Chemotherapy**

1. **Primary non-Hodgkin's lymphoma**

   a. **Single agents.** Active cytotoxic agents in the treatment of NHL include **cyclophosphamide, doxorubicin, mechlorethamine, and vincristine,** which produce **overall and complete response rates of 30–80% and 10–33%, respectively.** Bleomycin, chlorambucil, dacarbazine, procarbazine, vinblastine, and prednisone are only moderately active, with 10–40% overall response rates. The role of cisplatin, high-dose cytosine arabinoside, etoposide, ifosfamide, high-dose methotrexate (with leucovorin rescue), and streptozotocin is unclear. Single chemotherapeutic agents, however, are **rarely** indicated for the treatment of NHL because multiple studies that compared single-agent (or sequential single-agent) treatment (primarily chlorambucil or cyclophosphamide) with combination chemotherapy have demonstrated inferior results with single drugs.

   b. **Combination chemotherapy.** Combination chemotherapeutic regimens have been used extensively in the treatment of NHL. Most combinations include **cyclophosphamide, prednisone, and vincristine.** Although more than 20 years of research have helped to define appropriate therapy for patients with NHL, considerable controversy remains in many areas. In addition, the ideal chemotherapy regimen has not been defined despite studies of numerous cytotoxic regimens (see Table 61–4). General principles of therapy, however, can be deduced from the available data and are based on histology and the extent of disease.

      (1) **Favorable histology**

         (a) **Localized disease (10% of patients).** Previous trials evaluating the addition of chemotherapy to radiation in the treatment of localized disease (NCI's indolent Stage I; AA Stages I and II) generally have used less **intensive** chemotherapy regimens such as **cyclophosphamide, vincristine, and prednisone (CVP),** which

TABLE 61–4. THREE GENERATIONS OF COMBINATION CHEMOTHERAPY REGIMENS

Generation	Change*	CR (%)	Cures (%)	Regimen (variants)
First	—	50	33	MOPP: mechlorethamine, vincristine, procarbazine, prednisone (C-MOPP: cyclophosphamide)
Second	increased number of agents	75	50	CHOP: cyclophosphamide, doxorubicin, vincristine, prednisone (CHOP-bleo, -meth: bleomycin or methotrexate)
				COMLA: cyclophosphamide, vincristine, methotrexate, cytosine arabinoside (ACOMLA: doxorubicin)
				BACOP: bleomycin, doxorubicin, cyclophosphamide, vincristine, prednisone
				M-BACOD: methotrexate, bleomycin, doxorubicin, cyclophosphamide, vincristine, dexamethasone (m-BACOD: lower dose methotrexate)
				COP-BLAM: cylcophosphamide, vincristine, prednisone, bleomycin, doxorubicin, procarbazine
				ProMACE/MOPP: prednisone, methotrexate, leucovorin, doxorubicin, etoposide / mechlorethamine, vincristine, procarbazine, prednisone
Third	increased dose intensity	82	67	COP-BLAM III: cyclophosphamide vincristine (2-day infusion every other cycle), prednisone, bleomycin (5-day infusion every other cycle), doxorubicin, procarbazine
				MACOP-B: methotrexate, doxorubicin, cyclophosphamide, vincristine, prednisone, bleomycin
				ProMACE-CytaBOM: prednisone, methotrexate doxorubicin, cyclophosphamide, etoposide - cytosine arabinoside, bleomycin, vincristine, methotrexate
				F-MACHOP: 5-fluorouracil, methotrexate, cytosine arabinoside, cyclophosphamide, doxorubicin, vincristine, prednisone

*Compared with the previous chemotherapy generation.

have produced poor results. However, a recent study using the potent combination of cyclophosphamide, doxorubicin, vincristine, and prednisone **(CHOP)** documented an **increased 5-year disease-free survival** in patients with follicular lymphomas treated with chemotherapy (+/– radiation) compared with those receiving radiation alone **(64% vs 37%).** Although this study suggests that chemotherapy plus radiation and even chemotherapy alone may yield equivalent or superior results to radiation alone, further data are required to confirm this observation before this approach can be recommended as standard therapy.

   (b) **Diffuse disease (90% of patients).** The exact nature and magnitude of therapy that these diffuse, indolent lymphomas (NCI's indolent Stage II; AA Stages III and IV) require and the actual degree of benefit derived from therapy are **controversial**. Despite **brief (< 2 years) responses** and less than **10% 5-year disease-free survival** in patients previously treated with radiation, chemotherapy, and combined modality therapy, the median survival of these patients, **with** or **without** therapy, approaches **8 years**. Documented cases of **spontaneous regression** and the **indolent** tempo of the disease further complicate the issues. **Asymptomatic patients** with clearly indolent lymphoma by history (chronic waxing and waning lymphadenopathy) can **be observed** without instituting therapy until symptoms develop (median 2–4 years). Delayed therapy **in this setting** does **not** alter the **overall survival,** although this is somewhat controversial and does not apply to symptomatic patients. Furthermore, intensifying the **dose** of chemotherapy **does not have an impact** on long-term results: oral chlorambucil, cyclophosphamide, vincristine, and prednisone (CVP) and high-dose pulse chlorambucil (16 mg/m^2 daily for 5 days per month to reduce irreversible bone marrow damage and risk of secondary leukemia associated with chronic oral therapy) all produce nearly identical 5-year survivals despite a slight initial advantage of combination therapy. Until recently, the most toxic cytotoxic regimen administered in histologically favorable lymphomas was CVP; however, newer, more aggressive (and toxic) combinations— ie, methotrexate, bleomycin, doxorubicin, cyclophosphamide, vincristine, and dexamethasone **(M-BACOD)**; cyclophosphamide, vincristine, procarbazine, and prednisone **(COPP)**; and carmustine, cyclophosphamide, vincristine, melphalan, and prednisone **(M-2)**— are now under investigation. Some protocols include some form of radiation therapy. Preliminary results from a randomized prospective NCI trial with **ProMACE/MOPP** suggests that **improved disease-free** survival (as high as **86% at 4 years**) may be achieved. In addition, **delayed** chemotherapy after an initial period of observation was associated with a **poor (43%) response rate** and **inferior disease-free survival.** The follow-up, however, has been too brief to assess the affect on overall survival. Thus, although observation may be appropriate for **elderly asymptomatic** patients with obvious indolent disease, young, otherwise healthy patients with symptomatic or progressive disease or both may benefit significantly (at least regarding disease-free survival) from immediate aggressive combination chemotherapy. Pulse chlorambucil and CVP remain an option for patients with intermediate disease.

(2) Unfavorable histology

    (a) Localized disease (10% of patients). Although radiation therapy alone may mediate cure in patients with localized disease (NCI's aggressive Stage I; AA Stages I and II), 4 of 6 recent trials (4 involving **intensive** chemotherapy) evaluated involved-field **irradiation plus chemotherapy** versus radiation therapy alone demonstrated a **higher 5-year disease-free survival** with the combination therapy **(76–88% vs 32–45%).** In addition, 1 preliminary study found a **100% and 80% 5-year disease-free survival** following CHOP chemotherapy alone in patients with AA Stage I and II disease, respectively; however, this finding requires independent corroboration. Currently, data clearly indicate that **the combination of (involved-field) radiation and chemotherapy represents the best available therapy.**

    (b) Diffuse disease (90% of patients). Three generations of chemotherapy regimens (see Table 61–4) have been developed to treat diffuse aggressive lymphomas (NCI's aggressive Stages II and III; AA Stages III and IV). Although these malignancies behave aggressively, paradoxically **they are highly curable.** The second and third generation regimens were designed **to either increase the total number of agents used or to increase the dose intensity** of the various agents. Early data suggested higher complete response rates and overall survival with the latter generation regimens. More recent studies suggest that no difference exists in either the rate of complete response or overall survival between CHOP, a first generation regimen and several third generation regimens. In addition fatal toxicities appear to be less with the CHOP regimen.

2. **Recurrent non-Hodgkin's lymphoma.** A particularly ominous prognostic factor in patients with active NHL is a history of prior therapy. Patients who respond poorly to initial chemotherapy or relapse early also respond poorly to salvage regimens. However, high-dose chemoradiotherapy with **autologous bone marrow transplantation (BMT)** recently has produced **40% sustained second remissions.** Thus, **with the possible exception of BMT, the only opportunity to cure these patients is during initial chemotherapy.**

D. **Immunotherapy.** A number of experimental immunomodulatory agents have been tried in NHLs.

1. **Cytokines.** The cytokine that has been studied most extensively is **alpha-interferon** (30×10^6 U/m² daily), which mediates **brief partial responses in 45%** of patients. Anecdotal responses to interleukin-2 (IL-2) have been reported, but tumor necrosis factor has not yielded promising results.

2. **Monoclonal antibodies.** Monoclonal antibodies, particularly **anti-idiotypic antibodies** have produced durable responses (1 complete response for > 5 years) in a small number of patients. Antigenic shedding and modulation as well as human antimouse antibodies have limited the application of this approach.

3. **Adoptive immunotherapy.** Partial responses were reported in 2 of 4 patients given **lymphokine-activated killer cells** with systemic IL-2.

4. **Tumor cell vaccine.** Some experimental data suggests that presentation of tumor antigens on damaged cells may elicit a host antitumor immune response capable of in vivo destruction of tumor cells.

X. **Prognosis**

A. **Risk of recurrence.** The risk of recurrence **after irradiation** is almost always from nodal **regions outside of previously involved areas,** whereas, **after chemotherapy,** relapses occur within **areas of previously documented disease.** The majority of recurrences **manifest within 2 years.**

B. **Five-year survival.** Long-term (5-year and 10-year) survival is related to the histology and extent of disease at presentation.

1. **Favorable histology: localized disease,** 61–90%; **diffuse disease,** 50–70%.
2. **Unfavorable histology: localized disease,** 76–100%; **diffuse disease,** 80–85%.

C. **Adverse prognostic factors.** A number of features are associated with a poor outcome: **poor performance status, abdominal mass larger than 10 cm in diameter, more than 3 extranodal sites, bone marrow involvement, LDH higher than 500 IU/mL, age older than 55 years, advanced stage at diagnosis, and unfavorable histology.**

XI. **Patient follow-up**

A. **General guidelines.** Patients with NHL should be followed closely every 3 months for 3 years, every 6 months for an additional 2 years, and annually thereafter for evidence of relapse. The following specific guidelines for patient follow-up are offered:

B. **Routine evaluation.** Every clinic appointment should include the following tests and procedures:

1. **Medical history and physical examination.** An interval medical history and thorough physical examination should be performed during each office visit. Areas for particular attention are discussed on p 000, **VI.A.**

2. **Blood tests**
   a. **Complete blood count** (see p 1, **IV.A.1**).
   b. **Hepatic transaminases** (see p 1, **IV.A.2**).
   c. **Alkaline phosphatase** (see p 1, **IV.A.3**).
   d. **BUN and creatinine** (see p 3, **VII.B.1.d**).

3. **Chest x-ray** (see p 3, **IV.C.1**).

C. **Additional evaluation.** Other tests and procedures that should be obtained at regular intervals include the following examinations.

1. **Computed tomography (CT).** This radiographic examination should be ordered **every 6–12 months** for at least 5 years. (see also, p 502, **VI.B.2.b**).

2. **Bipedal lymphangiogram.** This test should be obtained annually for 2–5 years (see also, p 502, **VI.B.2.c**).

D. **Optional evaluation.** The following tests and procedures may be indicated by previous diagnostic findings or clinical suspicion:

1. **Blood tests** (see p 2, **IV.A**).

      a. 5'Nucleotidase (see Chp 1, p 2).
      b. GGTP (see Chp 1, p 2).
  2. Imaging studies (see p 3, **IV.C**).
      a. Ultrasound.
      b. Technetium-99m bone scan.
  3. Invasive procedures. Any suspicious or new mass should be surgically biopsied to exclude the possibility of recurrent disease. An aggressive approach may be justified because many patients may be salvaged with additional therapy.

REFERENCES

Berard CW, Greene MH, Jaffe ES, Magrath I, Ziegler J. A multidisciplinary approach to non-Hodgkin's lymphomas. Annalo Int Med 94:218–254, 1981.

DeVita VT. Hematologic malignancies: non-Hodgkin's lymphomas. Hosp Pract 21(9):103–118, 1986.

Ersboll J, Schultz HB. Non-Hodgkin's lymphoma: recent concepts in classification and treatment. Eur J Haematol 42:15–29, 1989.

Glatstein E, Fuks Z, Goffinet DR, et al. Non-Hodgkin's lymphoma of stage III extent. Is total lymphoid irradiation appropriate treatment? Cancer 37:2806–2812, 1976.

Haller DG. Non-Hodgkin's lymphomas. Med Cl 68:741–756, 1984.

List AF. Non-Hodgkin's lymphoma of the gastrointestinal tract an analysis of clinical and pathologic features affecting outcome. J Clin Oncol 6(7):1125–1133, 1988.

Lowder JN, Meeker TC, Campbell M, et al. Studies on B lymphoid tumors treated with monoclonal anti-idiotype antibodies: Correlations with clinical response. Blood 69:199–210, 1987.

Moormeer JA, Williams SF, Golomb HM. The staging of non- Hodgkin's lymphomas. Sem Oncol 17:43–50, 1990.

Paryani SB, Hoppe RT, Cox RS, et al. Analysis of non-Hodgkin's lymphomas with nodular and favorable histologies, stages I and II. Cancer 52:2300–2307, 1983.

Portlock CS. Management of the low-grade non-Hodgkin's lymphomas. Sem Oncol 17:51–59, 1990.

Rosenberg SA, Lotze MT, Muul LM, et al. A progress report on the treatment of 157 patients with advanced cancer using lymphocyte-activated killer cells and interleukin-2 or high-dose interleukin-2 alone. NEJM 316:889–897, 1987.

Urba WJ and Longo DL. Alpha-interferon in the treatment of nodular lymphomas. Semin Oncol 13:40–47, 1980.

Young RC, Largo DL, Glatstein E, Inde DC, Jaffee ES, DeVita VT. The treatment of indolent lymphomas: watchful waiting vs aggressive combined modality treatment. Sem Hematol 25:11–16, 1988.

62 Cutaneous T Cell Lymphoma

Carlin J. McLaughlin, DO

I. **Epidemiology.** Cutaneous T cell lymphomas (CTCLs), including **mycosis fungoides, generalized erythroderma, and Sezary syndrome** as well as **acute T cell leukemia and lymphoma (ATL)** are rare, constituting only **2.2% of all lymphomas**. In 1985, **0.29–0.4 cases per 100,000** of the population **(600–700 cases)** were diagnosed. Worldwide, the incidence of these indolent peripheral T cell lymphomas, particularly ATL, is high in the southwestern provinces of Japan and the Caribbean and southeastern United States.

II. **Risk factors**
   A. **Age.** The incidence of CTCL increases with age, rarely occurring before age 40. The **peak incidence** and mean age at diagnosis occur **between the ages of 50 and 60 for CTCL** and **between the ages of 35 and 55 for ATL.**
   B. **Sex.** The risk in **males** is **slightly greater** than in females for both CTCL and ATL.
   C. **Race.** No clear racial predilection exists.
   D. **Genetic factors.** First-degree relatives are not known to be at increased risk, and no known genetic abnormalities predispose to CTCL.
   E. **Previous immunologic pathology.** Infection with the **human T cell lymphotrophic virus-I (HTLV-I),** a Type C retrovirus, has been causally linked to the development of **ATL,** and **HTLV-V** infection has recently been implicated in the pathogenesis of **CTCL.**
   F. **Diet.** No dietary factors have been identified.
   G. **Urbanization.** The risks in urban and rural populations are identical.

III. **Clinical presentation**
   A. **Signs and symptoms**
      1. **Local manifestations.** Typically, patients present with a long history (4–50 years) of **nonspecific pruritic dermatitis or psoriasiform dermatitis (44%), eczema (10%),** exfoliative erythroderma (7%), dermal nodules or tumors (17%), and other miscellaneous lesions (23%). With progression of the disease, the initial patches evolve into **indurated and erythematous or pigmented, sharply demarcated, irregular plaques.** Early in the disease course **(limited plaque stage),** these lesions cover **less than 10%** of the body surface area and with disease progression grow to cover **more than 10%** of the body surface area **(generalized plaque stage).** In addition, **scaling and fissures** of the palms and soles may occur, and facial involvement may lead to ectropion and the classic **leonine (lion-like) facies.** Peripheral **lymphadenopathy (50%)** also may be present. **Generalized erythroderma (l'homme rogue)** is a common variant accompanied by **intense pruritus, plaques, tumors,** or all of these and **lichenification. Generalized lichenification** (without erythroderma) is a rare variant. The incidence and characteristics of the cutaneous variants are listed in Table 63–1.
      2. **Systemic manifestations.** Abnormal **cerebriform lymphocytes** identified on **peripheral blood smear** are diagnostic of a leukemic variant of CTCL **(Sezary syndrome).** Other systemic findings and symptoms are rare but may include pulmonary infiltrates, hepatomegaly, splenomegaly, and bone symptoms all secondary to tumor infiltration.
   B. **Paraneoplastic syndromes. Hypercalcemia** (see p 87) is a common manifestation of ATL resulting from secretion of an **osteoclast-activating factor** that is difficult to control.

IV. **Differential diagnosis.** The early cutaneous manifestations of CTCL are easily mistaken for **benign dermatologic disorders** (eczema or psoriasis). Nonepidermotrophic T cell lymphomas and T-CLL may also involve the skin but can be distinguished from CTCL by the clinical setting. Dermal involvement with Hodgkin's and non-Hodgkin's lymphoma as well as with **lymphomatoid papulosis** and **lymphoma-**

TABLE 62–1. INCIDENCE AND CHARACTERISTICS OF CUTANEOUS T CELL VARIANTS

Variant	Frequency (%)	Sezary Cells (%)	Lymphadenopathy (%)
Limited plaque	39	0–20	20
Generalized plaque	30	9–30	54
Tumor	16	27–50	84
Generalized erythroderma	12	90–96	81
Generalized lichenification	Rare	—	—

toid granulomatois may have similar appearances but can be reliably distinguished pathologically.

V. **Screening programs.** Because these diseases are rare, no formal screening program has been developed the American Cancer Society recommends a complete annual cutaneous examination to exclude all types of superficial malignancies in all patients over 40 years of age.

VI. **Diagnostic workup**

  A. **Medical history and physical examination.** A complete medical history with reference to common presenting signs and symptoms should be obtained along with a thorough physical examination, including a detailed cutaneous examination with photographs, if necessary.

    1. **General appearance.** An assessment of the patient's functional and nutritional status can be gained simply by observing the patient's appearance (see, also, p 1, **I** and **III**).

    2. **Skin.** Inflammatory lesions (dermatitis) and all neoplastic growths must be accurately described.

    3. **Lymph nodes.** The presence or absence of lymphadenopathy in the cervical, supraclavicular, axillary, epitrochlear, abdominal, inguinal, and popliteal regions should be recorded.

    4. **Thorax.** Auscultation and percussion of the lung fields late in the disease course may reveal evidence of pleural effusions, and parenchymal consolidation.

    5. **Abdomen.** Hepatomegaly, splenomegaly, and other intra-abdominal masses may indicate advanced disease.

  B. **Primary tests and procedures.** The following diagnostic tests and procedures should be performed on all patients with suspected T cell lymphoma.

    1. **Blood tests** (see p 1, **IV.A**).

      a. **Complete blood count.** Leukocyte counts range from 3000 with rare atypical cells to 238,000 with all abnormal cells.

      b. **Hepatic transaminases.**

      c. **Alkaline phosphatase.**

      d. **Lactate dehydrogenase (LDH).** Levels of this serum enzyme may be followed as a prognostic indicator.

      e. **HTLV serology.** Serologic evidence of exposure to HTLV-I aids in the differentiation between endemic and sporadic cases of CTCL and helps define ATL.

      f. **BUN and creatinine.**

    2. **Urine tests** (see p 3, **IV.B**).

    3. **Chest x-ray** (see p 3, **IV.C.1**).

    4. **Invasive procedures**

      a. **Skin biopsy.** Diagnostic skin biopsy is required to confirm the diagnosis of CTCL. A full-thickness specimen is necessary and can be obtained most easily with a **dermal punch** biopsy instrument and local anesthesia. The specimen should be transported to the pathology department in **saline** (not formalin) so that electron microscopic and immunohistochemical studies can be properly performed, providing an accurate immunophenotypic analysis.

      b. **Lymph node biopsy.** Diagnostic **excisional lymph node biopsy** of clinically enlarged lymphadenopathy (if meticulously evaluated with cytogenetics and electron microscopy) may provide definitive evidence of CTCL in as many as **100%** of patients. In addition, the information is essential for accurate staging.

C. **Optional tests and procedures.** The following tests and procedures may be indicated by previous diagnostic findings or clinical suspicion.

1. **Blood tests**
    a. **5'Nucleotidase** (see p 2, **IV.A.4**).
    b. **GGTP** (see p 2, **IV.A.5**).
    c. **Immunoglobulin (Ig) levels.** Generally, serum **IgA** is **increased** in **mycosis** fungoides, whereas **IgE** is **elevated** in **Sezary syndrome**.

2. **Imaging studies** (see p 3, **IV.C**).
    a. **Computed tomography (CT).** A CT scan of the chest, abdomen, and pelvis should be obtained in selected cases if suspicion of visceral involvement is high.
    b. **Magnetic resonance imaging (MRI).**
    c. **Technetium-99m bone scan.** (see Chp 1, p. 3).

3. **Invasive procedures**
    a. **Bone marrow aspiration and biopsy.** This procedure should be considered in patients with evidence of lymphadenopathy or peripheral blood abnormalities; in general, however, the bone marrow is preferentially spared in CTCL.
    b. **Liver biopsy.** The indications for percutaneous liver biopsy are similar to those for bone marrow biopsy. Moreover, liver enzyme abnormalities also should prompt histologic assessment of the liver to exclude malignant infiltration.

VII. **Pathology**

A. **Location.** The initial cutaneous lesions may be localized but quickly become more generalized.

B. **Multiplicity.** As a rule, **CTCL is a systemic disease,** and multiple cutaneous lesions are common.

C. **Histology.** Cutaneous light microscopic characteristics of CTCL—especially of mycosis fungoides—include **patchy mononuclear infiltrates** in the upper dermis and basal epidermis, large hyperchromatic dermal cells **(mycosis cells),** and circumscribed collections of epidermal mononuclear cells **(Pautrier's microabscesses).** Peripheral blood smears and electron microscopic examination of lymph nodes or skin demonstrate **cerebriform (grooved hyperchromatic nuclei) lymphocytes (Sezary cells).** The presence of more than **5%** circulating Sezary cells is pathognomonic of the **Sezary syndrome.** Large T cells suggest the development of a large-cell lymphoma. Immunophenotypic analysis by immunohistochemical staining and fluorescence-activated cell sorting (FACS) reveals **CD4+ (helper) T cells in CTCL** and **CD8+ cells in ATL.**

D. **Metastatic spread**

1. **Modes of spread.** CTCL potentially spreads by 3 different mechanisms.
    a. **Direct extension.** Local growth invariably leads to extensive dermal involvement and may produce tumors several centimeters thick that may ulcerate, bleed, and become infected.
    b. **Lymphatic metastasis.** Embolic spread through lymph channels may be responsible for involvement of draining lymph node groups.
    c. **Hematogenous metastasis.** Spread through blood vessels eventually leads to dissemination to a variety of organs and is generally underestimated by clinical staging methods.

2. **Sites of spread.** Although visceral metastases may not be detected before the cutaneous disease is advanced, widespread involvement is present in **18%** of patients at presentation and is common in advanced disease. Sites frequently affected include the **liver, spleen, lung, bone,** kidneys, pleura, heart, gastrointestinal tract, central nervous system, bone marrow, pancreas, thyroid, and head and neck organs.

VIII. **Staging.** An international standardized staging system has not been developed by the American Joint Committee on Cancer or the Union Internationale Contra le Cancer. The **Mycosis Fungoides Cooperative Group,** however, proposed a TNM staging system that correlates closely with prognosis.

A. **Tumor (skin) stage**

1. **T1.** Limited plaques (< 10% body surface area).
2. **T2.** Generalized plaques (> 10% body surface area).
3. **T3.** Cutaneous tumors.

    4. T4. Generalized erythroderma.
B. Lymph node stage
    1. N0. No adenopathy; histology negative.
    2. N1. Adenopathy present; histology negative.
    3. N2. No adenopathy; histology positive.
    4. N3. Adenopathy present; histology positive.
C. Metastatic (visceral) stage
    1. M0. No visceral involvement.
    2. M1. Visceral involvement is present.
D. Blood stage
    1. B0. No peripheral blood involvement.
    2. B1. Peripheral blood is involved.
E. Stage groupings
    1. Stage I. Plaques are present without adenopathy or histologic involvement of lymph nodes or viscera (T1, N0, M0 or T2, N0, M0).
      a. Stage IA. Limited plaques (T1, N0, M0).
      b. Stage IB. Generalized plaques (T2, N0, M0).
    2. Stage II. Plaques with adenopathy or cutaneous tumors with or without adenopathy but without histologic involvement of lymph nodes or viscera (T1–2, N1, M0 or T3, N0–1, M0).
      a. Stage IIA. Plaques (limited or generalized) with adenopathy and without histologic involvement of lymph nodes or viscera (T1–2, N1, M0).
      b. Stage IIB. Cutaneous tumors with or without adenopathy and no histologic involvement of lymph nodes or viscera (T3, N0–1, M0).
    3. Stage III. Generalized erythroderma with or without adenopathy and without histologic involvement of lymph node or viscera (T4, N0–1, M0).
    4. Stage IV. Histologic involvement of lymph nodes or viscera with any skin lesion and with or without adenopathy (any T, N2–3, M0 or any T, any N, M1).
      a. Stage IVA. Histologic involvement of lymph nodes with any skin lesion and with or without adenopathy (any T, N2–3, M0).
      b. Stage IVB. Histologic involvement of viscera with any skin lesion and with or without adenopathy (any T, any N, M1).
IX. Treatment. Therapy for CTCL has had a limited impact on overall survival; however, treatment may provide substantial palliation from the **disfigurement, pruritus, and infection** associated with this disease. In general, patients with disease limited to the skin are best treated with aggressive topical therapy, while those patients with evidence of visceral/systemic involvement are most appropriate candidates for combined modality therapy.
A. Surgery
    1. Early cutaneous T cell lymphoma
      a. General considerations. Surgery plays a small but crucial role in the **diagnosis and staging of CTCL as well as management of its complications,** but surgery has **no direct therapeutic effect.**
      b. Indications. Excisional lymph node biopsy should be performed in all patients with suspected CTCL for complete staging.
      c. Procedures. All procedures in CTCL are outlined on p 513, **VI.B.3.**
    2. Advanced cutaneous T cell lymphoma. As noted in **A.1.b** above, surgery is indicated for advanced CTCL only for palliation of disease complications (rare).
B. Radiation therapy
    1. Primary cutaneous T cell lymphoma. Cutaneous radiation therapy may be beneficial in patients with **generalized plaque formation** and in those with **limited plaque who have failed topical chemotherapy.** Total skin irradiation with 2–7 MeV **electron** beams are used to deliver **3000–3600 cGy in 100 cGy fractions 4 times per week** using 4–8 fields. With this approach, maximal radiation is deposited **within 5 mm** of the skin surface and almost none penetrates deeper than 2 cm, thus sparing deeper structures (eg, bone marrow). Technically, total body irradiation is challenging because the equipment is designed to deliver radiation to a flat surface. The dose received in areas of **irregular body contour** (eg, hands, feet, face) is highly variable. Moreover, if the eyelids are not involved, **orbital shields** are required, whereas **corneal shields** must be applied with topical anesthesia if the eyelids are to be irradiated. The results of total skin irradiation are similar to topical mechlorethamine, with complete responses in **96%** of patients with **limited plaque (T1),** 87% with **generalized plaque (T2),** and 70% with **tumors (T3)** or **generalized erythroderma (T4) disease.** Duration of response is 4–5 years with limited plaque and 1–2 years

with other lesions. **Fifteen-year disease-free and overall survival** as high as 22% and 32%, respectively, have been reported with this approach. Total skin irradiation also has been combined with total nodal irradiation and total body irradiation, with encouraging results.

2. **Advanced cutaneous T cell lymphoma.** Symptomatic plaques and tumors can often be treated successfully with **"spot"** external beam orthovoltage radiation **(800–1550 cGy in 300–500 cGy fractions).**

3. **Morbidity and mortality.** The primary complication of cutaneous electron-beam irradiation is **sweat gland dysfunction,** with dry skin and an inability to dissipate heat. Furthermore, with doses higher than 3000 cGy, nearly all patients develop erythema.

C. **Chemotherapy**

1. **Early cutaneous T cell lymphoma.** Topical chemotherapy with various compounds, including glucocorticoids, 2,4-dinitrochlorobenzene (DNCB), and cytotoxic agents (eg, nitrogen mustard) has been tried. Topical **mechlorethamine** (nitrogen mustard), is the most useful topical agent. Its antitumor mechanism, however, remains unknown because its alkylating properties disappear after dissolution in water. An aqueous solution **(10 mg per 50–100 mL)** is brushed onto all skin surfaces, taking care to avoid the eyelids and mucosal surfaces (lips, anus, and vagina), **daily for 1 year** and then 3 times per week. Patients with plaque disease respond best: a **complete response rate of 75–80% with T1 or T2** and 54% with T3 disease. Response rates in the presence of adenopathy are lower. The duration of response is brief, however: 87% of patients relapse within 3 years; the median duration of response is 7 months.

2. **Advanced cutaneous T cell lymphoma.** The response of CTCL to systemic chemotherapy is similar to that of low-grade non-Hodgkin's lymphomas. Although **palliative responses are common (70%), cure is rare.**

   a. **Single agents.** Significant **response rates** have been reported in small numbers of patients with **high-dose methotrexate (100%),** etoposide (67%), cyclophosphamide (67%), carmustine (63%), bleomycin (62%), mechlorethamine (64%), doxorubicin (62%), and chlorambucil (57%). In addition, **complete responses** occur in **64% of patients with high dose methotrexate** and 15–25% with etoposide, doxorubicin, bleomycin, and mechlorethamine. A new agent, 2-chlorodeoxy adenosine (2-CDA) can produce **remission rates of approximately 47%** in patients with disease limited to the skin, who have failed prior chemotherapy and radiation therapy. Other experimental medications include deoxycoformycin, retinoic acid (Acutane), cyclosporin, and acyclovir. Anecdotal response rates as high as 50% have been reported with these agents.

   b. **Combination chemotherapy. Response rates are slightly higher** with combinations of cytotoxic drugs than with individual agents, but survival is not improved. Regimens used in non-Hodgkin's lymphomas, such as methotrexate, cyclophosphamide, vincristine, and prednisone **(MCOP);** cyclophosphamide, doxorubicin, vincristine, and prednisone **(CHOP);** and bleomycin, doxorubicin, methotrexate, and topical mechlorethamine **(BAM-M)** produce **80–100% overall and 50–70% complete responses.** In the treatment of ATL, third generation non-Hodgkin's chemotherapy protocols have been minimally effective.

3. **Morbidity and mortality.** Topical mechlorethamine is limited by **intense pruritus and erythematous eruptions** typical of **delayed-type hypersensitivity in 40%** of patients. Desensitization, however, may permit continued therapy.

D. **Photochemotherapy.** Photochemotherapy with **8-methoxypsoralen** (Methoxalen) followed by **ultraviolet A irradiation** (PUVA) may be highly effective in cutaneous disease. Psoralen given orally **(0.4–0.6 mg/kg** 2 hrs before therapy) or topically binds DNA and mediates cell death when exposed to UVA light (1.5–15 J/cm^2). Treatment is given **3 times a week** until skin lesions resolve, then every 2–4 weeks. **Responses** occur in 60–75% of patients, and **long-term control** of cutaneous disease is achieved in **50% of patients** whose disease is limited to cutaneous plaques and eczema. Exposure of leukapheresed blood to UVA light (extracorporeal PUVA) has produced **responses in 64–73%** of patients with **advanced** disease, including Sezary syndrome. However, the ultimate usefulness of this novel approach remains unclear. Complications from PUVA include nausea, pruritus, erythema, and **secondary cutaneous malignancies,** which limit the usefulness of this therapy in patients with a significant life expectancy.

E. **Immunotherapy.** Systemic recombinant **alpha-interferon** is active in **90% of pa-**

tients with **early** plaque and in **50% with advanced** refractory disease, producing as much as **10% complete responses.** Again, responses are **brief** (median of 5.5 months). Preliminary data with intralesional alpha-interferon and systemic gamma-interferon are encouraging. **Monoclonal antibodies** against various T cell antigenic determinants that have been given to patients with ATL have produced some responses; however, those responses are extremely limited and brief.
   F. **Combined modality therapy.** Early results from Phase I trials of combinations of systemic and topical chemotherapy, total skin irradiation and systemic chemotherapy, and systemic alpha-interferon and PUVA suggest that **high response rates (as high as 93%)** may be achieved with multimodality therapy. Until definitive data are available, however, these approaches should be considered experimental.

X. **Prognosis**
   A. **Risk of recurrence.** Despite high response rates and an indolent course, nearly all patients with CTCL relapse and eventually die from their disease. The **15-year survival is less than 20%.** The **prognosis with ATL is dismal:** few patients survive more than a few years.
   B. **Five-year survival.** The 5-year survival depends on the stage of disease at presentation and is summarized below:
      1. **Stage I/IIA (50% of patients).** 90%.
      2. **Stage IIB/III/IVA (40% of patients).** 50%.
      3. **Stage IVB (10% of patients).**
   C. **Adverse prognostic factors.** The following features, independent of stage, are believed to signify a poor outcome: **age older than 50** years, **effaced lymph node architecture,** and presence of **circulating malignant cells** (Sezary cells).

XI. **Patient follow-up**
   A. **General guidelines.** Patients with non-Hodgkin's lymphoma should be followed closely every 3 months for 3 years, every 6 months for an additional 2 years, and annually thereafter for evidence of relapse. The following specific guidelines for patient follow-up are offered.
   B. **Routine evaluation.** Every clinic appointment should include the following tests and procedures:
      1. **Medical history and physical examination.** An interval medical history and a complete physical examination should be performed during every clinic visit. Attention is focused on those areas discussed on p 513, **VI.A.**
      2. **Blood tests** (see p 513, **IV.A**).
         a. **Complete blood count.**
         b. **Hepatic transaminases.**
         c. **Alkaline phosphatase.**
         d. **BUN and creatinine.**
      2. **Chest x-ray** (see p 3, **IV.C.1**).
   C. **Optional evaluation.** The following tests and procedures may be indicated by previous diagnostic findings or clinical suspicion:
      1. **Blood tests** (see p 1, **IV.A**).
         a. **5-Nucleotidase.**
         b. **GGTP.**
      2. **Imaging studies** (see p 3, **IV.C**).
         a. **Ultrasound.**
         b. **Technetium-99m bone scan.**
      3. **Invasive procedures**
         a. **Biopsy.** Any suspicious or new mass should be surgically biopsied to exclude the possibility of recurrent disease. An aggressive approach may be justified since many patients may be salvaged with additional therapy.
         b. **Bone marrow aspiration and biopsy** (see p 514, **VI.C.3.a**).
         c. **Liver biopsy** (see p 514, **VI.C.3.b**).

REFERENCES

Broder S, Bunn PA. Cutaneous T-cell lymphomas. Semin Oncol 7(3):310–311, 1980.

Bunn PA, Foon KA, Ihde DC, et. al. Recombinant leukocyte A interferon: an active agent in advanced cutaneous T-cell lymphomas. Ann Int Med 101:484–487, 1984.

Bunn PA, Ihde DC, Foon KA. The role of recombinant interferon alfa-2a in the therapy of cutaneous T-cell lymphomas. Cancer 57:1689–1695, 1986.

Catovsky D and Matutes E. The classification of T-cell leukemias. In Chronic Lymphocytic Leukemia: Recent Progress and Future Directions. Alan R. Liss, New York: pp. 163–176, 1987.

Edelson R, Berger C, Gasparro F, et. al. Treatment of cutaneous T-cell lymphoma by extracorporeal photochemotherapy. NEJM 316(6):297–303, 1987.

Gallo RC, Kalyanaraman VS, Sarngadharan MG, et. al. Association of the human type C retrovirus with a subset of adult T-cell cancers. Cancer Res 43:3892, 1983.

Hoppe RT, Cox RS, Fuks ZY, et. al. Electron beam therapy in the treatment of mycosis fungoides: the Stanford experience. Cancer Treat Rep 63:691, 1979.

Hoppe RT, Abel EA, Denau DG, et. al. Mycosis fungoides: management with topical nitrogen mustard. J Clin Oncol 5(11):1796–1803, 1987.

Kaplan EH, Rosen ST, Norris DB, et. al. Phase II study of recombinant human interferon gamma for treatment of cutaneous T-cell lymphoma. JNCI 82:208–212, 1990.

Kuzel TM, Gilyon K, Springer E, et. al. Interferon alfa-2a combined with phototherapy in the treatment of cutaneous T-cell lymphoma. JNCI 82:203–207, 1990.

Lutzner M. Cutaneous T-cell lymphomas: the Sezary syndrome, mycosis fungoides, and related disorders. Ann Int Med 83:534–552, 1975.

Micaily B, Vonderheid EC, Brady L et. al. Total electron beam and total nodal irradiation for treatment of patients with cutaneous T cell lymphoma. Int J Radiat Oncol Biol Phys 11:111, 1985.

Sausville EA, Eddy JL, Makuch RW, Fischmann AB, et. al. Histopathologic staging at initial diagnosis of mycosis fungoides and the Sezary syndrome: definition of three distinctive prognostic groups. Ann Int Med 109:372–382, 1988.

Savrn A et. al. 2-Chlorodeoxyadenosine: an active agent in the treatment of cutaneous T-cell lymphoma. Blood 80:587–592, 1992.

Schechter GP, Sausville EA, Fischnhann AB, et. al. Evaluation of circulating malignant cells provides prognostic information in cutaneous T cell lymphoma. Blood 69(3):841–849, 1987.

Shinmoyama M, Ota K, Kikuchyi M, et. al. Major prognostic factors of adult patients with advanced T-cell lymphoma/leukemia. J Clin Oncol 6(7):1088–1097, 1988.

Vonderheid EC, Van Scott EJ, Wallner RE, et. al. A 10 year experience with topical mechlorethamine for mycosis fungoides: comparison with patients treated by total skin electron beam radiation therapy. Cancer Treat Rep 63:681–689, 1979.

63 Acute Leukemia

Carlin J. McLaughlin, DO

I. **Epidemiology.** Acute lymphocytic (ALL) and myelocytic or nonlymphocytic (ANLL) leukemia account for **14.1%** of **hematologic, 43% of leukemic,** and **1.1%** of **all** malignancies in the United States. In 1985, **1.6 cases of ALL and 3.0 cases of ANLL per 100,000 males** and **1.2 and 2.1 per 100,000 females** were diagnosed, leading to 0.7 and 2.3 and to 0.5 and 1.5 deaths, respectively. Estimates indicate that **4300 new cases and 1900 deaths from ALL** and **7600 new cases and 5000 deaths from ANLL** would occur in 1993. Between 1950 and 1975, the incidence of leukemia increased substantially; however, since 1975 it has decreased slightly. Worldwide, the incidence of acute leukemia varies from a high of 5.7 per 100,000 males in **Luxembourg** and 3.7 per 100,000 females in **Kuwait** to a low of 1.1 per 100,000 males and 0.3 per 100,000 females in **Suriname**. Other areas of high incidence include Denmark, Iceland, Hungary, Italy, and Switzerland. Mauritius, Yugoslavia, and Ecuador report a low incidence of new cases.

II. **Risk factors**
   A. **Age.** The incidence of **ALL** reaches an **initial peak of more than 1.1 per 100,000 between ages 5 and 6.** Subsequently, it decreases to less than 0.5 and rises again after **age 50** to **3.0 per 100,000 by age 85.** The incidence of **ANLL** gradually climbs from less than 1.0 per 100,000 before **age 40** to **15.5 per 100,000 by age 85.** Nearly **98% of childhood** but **less than 20% of adult** leukemias are **acute.** Yet **more than 90%** of all cases of acute leukemia occur in **adults.**
   B. **Sex.** The risk of **ALL** in **males** is **1.4 times** greater than in females. The risk of **ANLL** in **males** is **1.5 times** greater than in females.
   C. **Race. Whites** are at **1.2 times** and **1.4 times** greater risk of **ALL** and **ANLL,** respectively, than blacks; however, **black children** may be at slightly higher risk than white children.
   D. **Genetic factors**
      1. **Family history.** A 2–4 fold increase in the risk exists in first-degree relatives of patients with acute leukemia. Moreover, the **concordance rate for identical twins is 17%,** and a number of familial clusters of leukemia have been reported.
      2. **Familial syndromes.** Numerous hereditary disorders are associated with genetic defects and a high incidence of acute leukemia.
         a. **Trisomy 21 (Down's syndrome).** This abnormality of chromosome 21 is associated with a **20-fold** increase in acute leukemia.
         b. **Bloom's syndrome.** This **autosomal recessive** disease includes **dwarfism** and **numerous cutaneous manifestations** (eg, butterfly telangiectatic facial erythema, hypopigmentation, photosensitivity) as well as an association with acute leukemia.
         c. **Fanconi's anemia.** Bone marrow **aplasia** and **melanosis** occur in conjunction with musculoskeletal and genitourinary **anomalies** in this **autosomal recessive** syndrome, which is also associated with a **10% risk** of acute leukemia **(usually ANLL).**
         d. **Wiskott-Aldrich syndrome.** This **sex-linked recessive** symptom complex includes anemia, thrombocytopenia purpura, otitis media and eczema and an increased incidence of acute leukemia.
         e. **Klinefelter's syndrome.** Two X chromosomes (47XXY) in this syndrome result in **atrophic hyalinized testes,** tall stature, elevated urinary gonadotropins, and an increased risk of acute leukemia.
         f. **Other syndromes.** D^1 trisomy, congenital agranulocytosis, celiac disease, Bruton's sex-linked agammaglobulinemia, Ellis-van Creveld syndrome (chondroectodermal dysplasia), and von Recklinghausen's syndrome are rare conditions that may increase the risk of acute leukemia.
   E. **Previous hematologic pathology**

1. **Infection.** The viral RNA-dependent DNA polymerase, **reverse transcriptase,** has been detected in leukemic cells and is indirect evidence of a viral etiology. Recently, human T cell leukemia virus **(HTLV-V),** a type C RNA virus, has been implicated in the pathogenesis of adult T cell leukemia and lymphoma (ATL; see Chapter 62).

2. **Inflammation.** Autoimmune disorders such as systemic lupus erythematosus (SLE), if combined with the administration of alkylating agents, are associated with the development of leukemia.

3. **Neoplasms.** Both **hematologic** (eg, Hodgkin's and non-Hodgkin's lymphomas, multiple myeloma) and **solid** malignancies (eg, breast, ovary) have been linked to a small but definite risk of leukemia, possibly related to **radiation** or chemotherapy with **alkylating** agents.

F. **Radiation.** Studies of patients irradiated for **ankylosing spondylitis;** patients receiving the radioisotope, **thorium dioxide;** radium dial painters; and Japanese **atomic bomb survivors** demonstrate a **10–20 times** greater incidence of leukemia, particularly **ANLL,** occurring after a **latency period of 5–7 years.**

G. **Chemicals.** Acute leukemia (especially ANLL) may develop after exposure to industrial **solvents** (eg, benzene), **alkylating cytotoxic agents** (eg, chlorambucil, melphalan), **radiographic contrast agents** (Thorotrast), and **drugs that cause aplastic anemia** (eg, chloramphenicol, phenylbutazone).

H. **Urbanization.** The risk of leukemia is **higher in urban** populations, most likely because of exposure to industrial chemicals.

III. **Clinical presentation**

A. **Signs and symptoms**

1. **Local manifestations.** Localized infiltrations of leukemic cells and intravascular leukostasis with high peripheral concentrations of blood leukocytes (> 50,000/μL; see, also, Chapter 14) may produce **splenomegaly (ALL 50%; ANLL < 25%), hepatomegaly,** mild adenopathy (ALL, usually cervical), bone or joint pain, hematuria (kidney), testicular enlargement, gingival hypertrophy (monocytic leukemia), neurologic symptoms (headache, nausea, cranial nerve palsies, decreased visual acuity, seizures, and coma), and infections or abscesses (eg, cystitis, pyelonephritis, perirectal abscess, pneumonia; more common in ANLL, 33%).

2. **Systemic manifestations.** Although less than 10% of patients are **asymptomatic,** most present with several weeks (ANLL) to months (ALL) of progressive **fatigue, malaise, bruising and minor hemorrhage (ALL 33%), serious hemorrhage and ecchymosis (ANLL 33%),** as well as weight loss. Fever is not uncommon.

B. **Paraneoplastic syndromes.** The following paraneoplastic syndromes have been described in acute leukemias and may be the sole manifestation of disease.

1. **Progressive multifocal leukoencephalopathy** (see p 58, **IV.**).

2. **Disseminated intravascular coagulation** (see p 80, **I**).

3. **Sweet's syndrome** (see p 109, **II.D**).

4. **Pruritus** (see p 111, **III.G**).

IV. **Differential diagnosis. Peripheral blood leukocytosis** is often discovered on initial evaluation of patients complaining of fatigue and other vague symptoms. Although acute leukemia must always be excluded in these patients, other frequent causes of leukocytosis are **infections** with granulocytosis (meningococcemia, tuberculosis) or lymphocytosis (**mononucleosis,** pertussis, infectious lymphocytosis, herpes zoster, viral hepatitis), functional (sickle-cell anemia, sickle-thal disease, myeloproliferative syndromes) or surgical (ITP, TTP) **splenectomy,** and the following **malignancies:** melanoma, hemangiosarcoma, diffuse histiocytic lymphoma, Hodgkin's disease, glioma, hepatoma, and adenocarcinoma of the stomach, lung, breast, and adrenal cortex. In addition, the **blast phase of chronic myelogenous leukemia** is indistinguishable from AML on morphological grounds.

V. **Screening programs.** Because of their **relatively low incidence,** no widespread screening programs have been instituted for acute leukemias. Peripheral leukocyte counts as a screening tool are unreliable.

VI. **Diagnostic workup**

A. **Medical history and physical examination.** A thorough medical history should be elicited, and a complete physical examination must be performed in all patients with suspected acute leukemia, paying particular attention to the following areas:

1. **General appearance.** Assessment of the patient's general functional and nutritional status should be made, noting evidence of significant weight loss (see, also, p 1, **I,** and **III**).

2. **Skin.** Papules, eruptions, and nodules may reflect cutaneous leukemic infiltration and should be recorded and fully described.
3. **Oral cavity.** The adequacy of dental hygiene should be assessed.
4. **Lymph nodes.** The characteristics (number, size, location, consistency, tenderness, fluctuancy, mobility) of all lymph nodes must be recorded. This should be done separately for all lymph node areas, including occipital, cervical (anterior and posterior), supraclavicular, infraclavicular, axillary, epitrochlear, inguinal, and popliteal regions.
5. **Chest.** Certain auscultation findings (eg, wheezing, diminished breath sounds) may indicate the presence of **pleural effusions.**
6. **Abdomen. Splenomegaly,** hepatomegaly, and all abdominal masses must be completely described.
7. **Rectum.** Evidence of previous or ongoing perianal infections should be noted.
8. **Nervous system.** A detailed neurologic examination is crucially important for assessing the possibility of **central nervous system (CNS) involvement.**

B. **Primary tests and procedures.** The following diagnostic tests and procedures should be obtained initially in all patients with suspected hematologic malignancies:

1. **Blood tests**
   a. **Complete blood count.** This should include a differential white-blood-cell count and evaluation of the peripheral smear. These are the two most important diagnostic tests for acute leukemia.

   (1) **Acute lymphocytic leukemia.** In addition to moderate **thrombocytopenia** (< 50,000 in 33%) and **anemia,** most patients (60%) have normal or slightly elevated leukocyte counts. **Leukopenia (15%) and severe leukocytosis (> 50,000/μL, 25%)** also may occur. **Lymphoblasts** can be identified in essentially all peripheral blood smears; **in 67%, they constitute more than 50% of peripheral white blood cells.**

   (2) **Acute nonlymphocytic leukemia.** Moderate **thrombocytopenia** (< 20,000/μL in many), **anemia** (hematocrit < 35%), and neutropenia (< 1000/μL) are usually present. Furthermore, **leukopenia (33%)** or **leukocytosis (33%)** may be present, but **33%** of patients present with **normal** white cell counts. On examination of the peripheral blood smear, **myeloblasts** may be observed in more than **90%** of patients.

   b. **Hepatic transaminases** (see p 1, **IV.A.2**).
   c. **Alkaline phosphatase** (see p 1, **IV.A.3**).
   d. **BUN and creatinine** (see p 3, **IV.A.6**).
   e. **Lactate dehydrogenase.** The level of this serum enzyme is **usually elevated,** especially in ALL.
   f. **Muramidase.** The serum (and urinary) levels of this lysozyme are **normal or low in ALL** but are **greatly elevated in ANLL.**
   g. **Uric acid.** Serum urate is significantly **increased** in almost **all** patients with ALL and only mildly increased in **50%** of patients with ANLL.
   h. **Coagulation times. Prothrombin and partial thromboplastin** times should be measured to exclude the presence of a coagulopathy induced by a circulating procoagulant or anticoagulant, especially in ANLL.

2. **Imaging studies.** A **chest x-ray** should be obtained in all patients to exclude the presence of pleural effusions as well as pulmonary and mediastinal disease (see p 3, **IV.C.1**).

3. **Invasive procedures**
   a. **Lumbar puncture. All patients with ALL** and certain patients with **ANLL (M4 and M5 monocytic subtypes)** should have a sample of cerebrospinal fluid (CSF) obtained for routine studies and cytologic analysis; however, before lumbar puncture, any existing **coagulopathy must be corrected** and the **platelet count** must be higher than **50,000/μL.** Once a sample is obtained, cells in the CSF are concentrated by **cytocentrifugation or millipore filtration,** stained with **Wright's stain,** and examined for the presence of leukemic cells indicating meningeal involvement.

   b. **Bone marrow aspiration and biopsy. All patients** with acute leukemia should be evaluated with bone marrow aspiration and biopsy. Most commonly, the marrow is obtained from the **posterior iliac crest** with a **Jamshidi needle** after mild sedation, although the **sternum** is an acceptable alternate site (aspiration only). The bone marrow is examined for **cellularity** (increased with obliteration of fat spaces), specific **staining characteristics,** and **leukemia-associated cell surface markers.**

C. **Optional tests and procedures.** The following examinations may be indicated by either previous diagnostic findings or clinical suspicion.
1. **Blood tests** (see p 2, **IV.A**).
   a. **5'-Nucleotidase** (see p 2).
   b. **GGTP.** (see p 2).
2. **Technetium-99m bone scan.** This is rarely indicated in these patients (see p 3, **IV.C.5**).

VII. **Pathology**
A. **Location.** Although leukemia primarily involves the hematopoietic organs **(blood, bone marrow, liver, spleen, and lymph nodes),** it is a hematogenous malignancy, and its location, by definition, is **diffuse.**
B. **Multiplicity.** Although leukemia has been considered a **"clonal" disease** arising from a single progenitor cell, evidence from recent studies of T cell receptor and immunoglobulin gene rearrangements in patients with acute leukemia suggests that multiple stem cells may be involved. In addition, leukemic cells in **33%** of patients with ALL express **myeloid** in addition to lymphoid markers. These findings are more frequent in **adult** patients and appear to have a **worse prognosis.**
C. **Histology.** Important histologic aspects of acute leukemia include morphologic, immunohistochemical, and cytogenetic considerations.
1. **Morphologic and general histochemical properties.** On the basis of multiple histochemical stains and the morphologic appearance of the leukemic cells, a group of **French, American, and British (FAB) hematopathologists proposed the FAB classification system** for acute leukemia. This system distinguishes between lymphocytic and nonlymphocytic malignancies—an important distinction in terms of prognosis and treatment.
   a. **Histochemical stains.** In the FAB system, the following stains are used to determine the **origin** (lymphocytic or nonlymphocytic) of the leukemic cell and to establish subcategories.
      (1) **Myeloperoxidase stain.** This stain selectively reacts with **myeloperoxidase,** an enzyme present only in **nonlymphocytic** (myeloid) cells.
      (2) **Sudan black B stain.** This lipophilic substance specifically stains **primary and specific granules** present in **nonlymphocytic** (myeloid) cells.
      (3) **Esterase stains. Specific naphthol AS-D chloracetate esterase** and **nonspecific alpha naphthyl acetate esterase** selectively bind to granules found in **granulocytes** and **monocytes,** respectively, not to lymphocytic cells.
      (4) **Periodic acid-Schiff (PAS) stain.** Nearly **70% of lymphoblasts** contain coarse granules that stain reddish-brown with PAS stain.
      (5) **Acid phosphatase stain.** Most **T cell lymphoblasts** demonstrate focal acid phosphatase staining.
      (6) **Terminal deoxyribonucleotidyl transferase (TdT) stain.** This stain reacts with the nuclear enzyme TdT, which is present in **95% of lymphoblastic** but fewer than 5% of nonlymphoblastic cells.
   b. **FAB classification of acute lymphocytic leukemia.** Lymphocytic cells fail to react with stains specific for lysosomal granules, such as myeloperoxidase, sudan black B, and esterase stains. PAS and TdT stains, however, are strongly positive in 80% and 95% of patients, respectively. These cells then are further subdivided on the basis of morphology:
      (1) **L1.** These **PAS+ cells** appear as a **uniform** population of small blast cells with a **high nucleus:cytoplasm ratio,** a **single** small inconspicuous **nucleolus,** and a **regular** nuclear contour. This is the most common morphologic type of **childhood ALL** and carries a **favorable prognosis.**
      (2) **L2.** These **PAS+ cells** appear as a **heterogeneous** population of blast cells with a **low nucleus:cytoplasm ratio, multiple** conspicuous **nucleoli,** and an irregular nuclear contour. This is the most common morphologic type in **adult ALL.**
      (3) **L3.** These **PAS− cells** appear as **uniform large cells** with basophilic vacuolated cytoplasm, **multiple** basophilic **nucleoli,** and a **round regular** nuclear contour. Although rare, this occurs **equally in childhood and adult ALL.**
   c. **Acute nonlymphocytic leukemia classification.** In contrast to ALL, these nonlymphocytic cells generally **react strongly** with stains such as

myeloperoxidase, sudan black B, and esterase (monocytic component), which are specific for **lysosomal granules.** PAS and TdT stains are unremarkable in more than 95%. The presence of **Auer rods** (needle-like collections of lysosomal myeloperoxidase) are **pathognomonic** of ANLL. As a prerequisite, the bone marrow aspiration must demonstrate more than **30% myeloblasts** to confirm the diagnosis. These cells are then subdivided further on the basis of morphology and are listed below with their relative incidence:

(1) **M1 (20%).** These **PAS⁻ cells** appear **undifferentiated** with rare cytoplasmic granules (myeloblastic leukemia without maturation).

(2) **M2 (30%).** These **PAS⁻ cells** are **granulated** with occasional **Auer bodies** and monocytoid cells (acute myelocytic leukemia with maturation).

(3) **M3 (10%).** These **PAS⁻ hypergranular cells** contain **large basophilic and eosinophilic granules** and are associated with treatment-induced defibrination (acute promyelocytic leukemia).

(4) **M4 (25%).** These cells may be **PAS⁺** and **include both monocytic (20–80%) and granulocytic (> 20%) precursors.** Serum **lysozyme is elevated** (acute myelomonocytic leukemia).

(5) **M4E.** These cells are the same as M4, except that premature **eosinophils** with small eosinophilic granules and large basophilic granules make up **0.5–30%** of the cells. This type is associated with **16q;22 chromosomal translocation** and a high complete remission rate (acute myelomonocytic leukemia).

(6) **M5A (4%).** These **PAS⁺, nonspecific esterase⁺ cells** are large monoblasts with **basophilic vacuolated cytoplasm.** Tissue infiltration (granulocytic sarcoma or chloroma) and early CNS involvement are common (acute monoblastic leukemia).

(7) **M5B (6%).** These cells are the same as M5A, except the **nucleus is twisted, indented, or folded** with 20% recognizable promonocytes. This type is more common in adults (acute monocytic leukemia).

(8) **M6 (5%).** These **PAS⁺ cells** are associated with **more than 50% megaloblastic and multinucleated red-cell precursors, Howell Jolly bodies, and ringed sideroblasts.** The presence of **30% leukoblasts** is required (erythroleukemia).

(9) **M7.** These cells exhibit a variable morphology with **megakaryoblasts** and intensive **marrow fibrosis** but an absence of the usual cytologic features of chronic myeloproliferative diseases such as myelofibrosis. This type cannot be diagnosed on morphologic grounds alone but requires other data: eg, electron microscopy (acute megakaryocytic leukemia).

2. **Immunohistochemical properties.** Once the importance of cell surface markers was appreciated and a number of **leukemia-associated antigens** were defined, acute leukemias were divided into subgroups on the basis of these markers.

a. **Acute lymphocytic leukemia.** Initially, lymphocytic cells were evaluated for **surface immunoglobulin** and **sheep erythrocyte rosette formation.** The leukemias were then classified into 3 basic categories according to these results.

(1) **B cell acute lymphocytic leukemia (5%).** These leukemias express surface-associated immunoglobulins (SIg), usually of the IgM variety. Most childhood leukemias with FAB L3 morphology are B cell ALL.

(2) **T cell acute lymphocytic leukemia (20%).** These leukemic cells form rosettes with unsensitized sheep erythrocytes (E-rosettes).

(3) **Non-B, non-T cell acute lymphocytic leukemia (75%).** These cells are **SIg⁻ and E-rosette⁻** and require a panel of monoclonal antibodies against **leukemia-associated cell surface antigens** as well as other specific tests to more fully characterize the cell of origin. On the basis of these additional tests, non-B non-T ALL can be classified further into the following 4 categories:

(a) **Common acute lymphoblastic leukemia.** Common acute lymphoblastic leukemia antigen (CALLA) is a 100 kd glycoprotein, encoded on chromosome 3q, that is detected by **rabbit** antiserum. It is present in more than **80% of childhood** and **50% of adult** ALL as well as in **2–6% of normal** bone marrow cells and signifies a **more favorable prognosis.**

- **(b) Pre-B ALL.** Although no SIg is present on these cells, as it is in B cell ALL, cell surface **Class II (Ia) antigens** and intracytoplasmic μ **heavy chains** are detectable.
- **(c) Pre-T ALL.** Although these leukemic cells do not form rosettes with sheep red blood cells, they do have some markers that are characteristic of early T cells and do not express Class II (Ia) antigens.
- **(d) Null cell ALL.** Despite a paucity of cell surface markers, these cells do possess surface **Class II (Ia) antigens** and a marker of early B cells, **BA-2.** Therefore, these cells are mostly likely to represent pre-pre-B cell ALL.

  b. Acute nonlymphocytic leukemia. Myeloid cell lines and markers are more numerous and diverse than the corresponding lymphoid components, and a classification system based on these elements has proved to be more elusive. However, the use of CD antigens and cytogenetic features (see below) may permit the future development of a clinically useful myeloid classification system.

3. **Cluster of differentiation (CD) antigens.** The development of monoclonal antibodies has permitted the characterization of **cell surface antigens (phenotype)** on hematopoietic cells at all levels of differentiation. These antibodies help diagnose and classify the various subsets of acute leukemia. Using several CD antigens, it is now possible to distinguish accurately lymphocytic (both T and B cell) from nonlymphocytic leukemia in more than **95%** of patients. These distinctions can now be used to determine differences in prognosis as well as therapy.

  a. Acute lymphocytic leukemia. A number of CD antigens have been associated with both B and T cells; however, several CD determinants are specific for each lineage. Measurement of these specific CD antigens, along with the demonstration of either **T cell receptor or immunoglobulin gene rearrangement,** represent the most reliable methods of determining cell phenotype.
  - **(1) Acute T cell lymphocytic leukemia.** CD antigens specific for T cells include **CD2, CD3, CD7,** and, for the most part, **CD5.**
  - **(2) Acute B cell lymphocytic leukemia.** Both **CD19** and **CD20** are found exclusively on B cells.

  b. Acute nonlymphocytic leukemia. Antigens present on myeloid elements are numerous, but CD antigens that are specific for the myeloid lineage include **CD11, CD13, CD14, CD15,** and **CD33.**

4. **Cytogenetic properties.** Characteristic chromosomal abnormalities have been demonstrated in **75%** of patients with acute **lymphocytic** leukemia and **50–90%** of patients with acute **nonlymphocytic** leukemia.

  a. Acute lymphocytic leukemia. Genetic abnormalities noted in ALL include anomalies of chromosomal quantity and quality. The modal chromosome number is **greater than 46 (good prognosis) in 30%** and **46 or less with abnormalities (poor prognosis) in another 30%.** The chromosomes most commonly involved include **4, 6, 8, 9, 11, 14, 19,** and **22.** The karyotype may be a more important prognostic factor than age and presenting leukocyte count. Specific abnormalities include the following:
  - **(1) 9;22 translocation.** This **Philadelphia chromosome** anomaly transfers the *abl* **proto-oncogene** on chromosome 9 to chromosome 22 next to the **break-point cluster region (bcr).** Nearly **25% of adults** but only **2–5% of children** with ALL have this translocation, which is associated with a **poor prognosis** and resembles that found in AML in only 50%.
  - **(2) Chromosome 9p deletion.** This abnormality is identified in **10%** of patients and carries a **poor prognosis.**
  - **(3) 4;11 translocation.** Found in **6%** of patients, this anomaly involves the *c-ets-*1 **proto-oncogene** on chromosome 11 and is associated with **biphenotypic** disease (both lymphocytic and myelocytic markers), extremely **high leukocyte counts,** and a **poor prognosis.**
  - **(4) 8;14 translocation.** In this abnormality, the *c-myc* proto-oncogene on chromosome 8 is transferred to the area of the Ig heavy-chain gene on chromosome 14. This change occurs in **5%** of all patients but is the **most common finding in B cell (L3) ALL.**
  - **(5) Chromosome 14 abnormalities.** Translocations (14;11p and 14;10q),

additions, and deletions of chromosome 14—particularly near the gene for the **alpha chain of the T cell receptor** (T cell ALL) and the **Ig heavy chain gene** (B cell ALL)—occur in **5%** of patients and are associated with a **poor prognosis.**

    (6) Chromosome 6q deletion. Arising in only **4%** of acute lymphocytic leukemias, this abnormality has a **favorable** prognostic implication.

    (7) 1;19 translocation. Associated with **pre-B cell ALL** and a **poor prognosis,** this genetic alteration is identified in **4%** of patients.

  b. Acute nonlymphocytic leukemia. Chromosomal anomalies are common and may include multiple abnormalities. Chromosomes **3, 6, 8, 9, 11, 15, 17,** and **22** are most frequently affected.

    (1) 8;21 translocation. This anomaly transfers the *c-myc* proto-oncogene on chromosome 8 to chromosome 21 and, simultaneously, the *c-ets-2* proto-oncogene on chromosome 21 to chromosome 8. This change, found in **5–12%** of all patients with ANLL and **40% of the FAB M2 subtype,** is associated with a **high** initial complete response rate but only **average** survival.

    (2) 15;17 translocation. This cytogenetic abnormality is identified in **5–10%** of all ANLL patients and **90% of the FAB M3 subtype.** It is associated with **trisomy 8** in 33% and carries a **poor prognosis.**

    (3) Chromosome 11q abnormalities. Deletions or translocations involving band q23 are particularly common in ANLL with a prominent **monocytic component.** A **9;11 translocation** juxtaposes the *c-ets-*1 proto-oncogene with the **alpha-interferon** gene in **6%** of all ANLL patients and **10–50% of the FAB M5A subtype.**

    (4) Chromosome 16q abnormalities. Deletions, inversions, and translocations involving band q22 have been linked to **eosinophilia,** the **FAB M4E subtype,** and **trisomy 8.** These alterations occur in **5%** of patients with ANLL and are associated with disruption of the **metallothionin gene** and an increased incidence of **chloromas** of the CNS.

    (5) 9;22 translocation. This **Philadelphia chromosome** anomaly occurs in fewer than **5%** of ANLL patients (predominantly **FAB M1 subtype**) and involves only a small subpopulation of leukemic cells.

    (6) 6;9 translocation. This occurs in **1%** of patients with ANLL and is associated particularly with the **FAB M2 and M4 subtypes.**

    (7) Chromosome 3q inversion. This rare anomaly is observed in the **FAB M7 subtype** as well as other subtypes (particularly M1 and M4) associated with thrombocytosis. It carries a **poor prognosis.**

    (8) Chromosome 5q deletion. This abnormality, especially if accompanied by **trisomy 7,** is associated with chemotherapy-related ANLL, **deletion of M–, GM–, and multi-CSF genes,** and a **poor prognosis.**

D. Metastatic spread

  1. Modes of spread. Unlike solid malignancies, acute leukemia is, by definition, diffuse in nature even at the outset. Therefore, typical mechanisms of spread, including direct extension and lymphatic and hematogenous metastasis do not apply.

  2. Sites of spread. Although acute leukemias diffusely involve all tissues, extensive localized infiltration of various sites such as the liver, spleen, lung, central nervous system, kidney, gastrointestinal tract, and skin may ultimately interfere with organ function.

VIII. Staging. Because acute leukemia is diffuse in all patients at the time of presentation, a staging system has not been developed and is not appropriate.

IX. Treatment

  A. Surgery. Surgery plays essentially no role in the management of acute leukemia.

  B. Radiation therapy. Cranial radiation is indicated in **patients with ALL** following induction chemotherapy to reduce the incidence of **CNS relapse** (see, also, p 526, **IX.C.2.c**). Cranial radiation **(600 cGy in a single dose)** also may be required in **patients with ANLL** and extremely high blast counts to reduce the likelihood of potentially fatal **intracranial hemorrhage** during therapy. Furthermore, males with ALL may require **testicular radiation** because the testes are another **sanctuary site** for leukemic cells. Routine testicular radiation is unnecessary, however, because testicular relapse does not affect survival.

  C. Chemotherapy

    1. Pretreatment preparation. The patient's condition must be optimized to **minimize the complications** and **maximize the therapeutic benefit** of intensive chemotherapy. The substantial risk of **intracranial hemorrhage,** associated with extremely **high peripheral leukocyte (blast) counts,** may be controlled with **cranial irradiation (600 cGy single dose)** and a 2-day course of **hydroxyurea (3 gm/m^2 PO daily). Thrombocytopenia (< 20,000/μL)** also is associated with a high likelihood of hemorrhage and must be corrected with **platelet transfusions** (4–8 units) as needed. **Coagulopathy** secondary to disseminated intravascular coagulation also should be controlled with **heparin** (50 units/kg IV every 6 hours) and **fresh frozen plasma** as required. Evidence of infection (eg, fever) necessitates the prompt institution of **broad-spectrum antibiotics** and amphotericin (if no response occurs in 48–72 hrs). In addition, serious consideration should be given to **prophylactic trimethoprim-sulfamethoxazole and clotrimazole therapy** in patients with ANLL who are undergoing chemotherapy. **Acetazolamide** (Diamox; 500 mg IV or PO every 6 hours) to alkalinize the urine, **allopurinol** (300–400 mg PO 3 times daily) to inhibit xanthine oxidase, and, in extreme cases, **pyrazinamide** (1 g every 8 hours) to inhibit tubular secretion of uric acid may be needed to avoid **urate nephropathy,** particularly if elevated uric acid levels are present before initiation of therapy. If renal failure is already present, dialysis must be started.

2. **Primary acute lymphocytic leukemia.** The treatment of ALL includes 4 separate phases.

a. **Remission induction chemotherapy.** Single-agent chemotherapy with agents such as **prednisone, vincristine,** L-asparaginase, and daunorubicin may induce remission in **40–70% of children** and **10–40% of adults** with ALL. However, combination chemotherapy increases the remission rate and survival with each additional agent, although no clear benefit is obtained from more than **3 drugs** in children. Most combinations include prednisone and vincristine. L-asparaginase or daunorubicin is often added in **"high-risk"** children and in adults (see p 527, **X.C**), but cyclophosphamide, etoposide, and cytarabine also may be included. The optimal treatment regimen, particularly for high-risk patients, is unclear; therefore, **Appendix D** lists several common protocols. Typically, these regimens induce a complete remission in **85–95% of children** and **70–90% of adults** with ALL. If a complete remission is not achieved **within 8 weeks,** an extremely **poor prognosis** should be anticipated.

b. **Consolidation chemotherapy.** Continuing the **same** (or in some cases an alternate) induction chemotherapeutic regimen, often with early **dose intensification,** the consolidation phase **immediately follows induction** and attempts to eradicate the significant, albeit occult, remaining tumor burden. Some protocols make no distinction between induction and consolidation therapy.

c. **Meningeal prophylaxis chemotherapy.** Chemotherapy directed at meningeal leukemia is instituted either just before or immediately after consolidation chemotherapy. This phase consists of **6 weeks** of (1) **intrathecal methotrexate** (12 mg/m^2 weekly) delivered via repeated lumbar puncture or Ommaya reservoir connected to the 3rd ventricle, (2) **intrathecal methotrexate with cranial radiation** (1800 cGy in 180 cGy fractions), (3) combination **intrathecal methotrexate, cytarabine, and hydrocortisone,** or (4) **high-dose systemic methotrexate with leucovorin rescue.** This approach reduces the CNS relapse rate from **33–67% without therapy to 11% in adults and less than 5% in children.** Complications of this therapy include **seizures, transverse myelitis,** chemical arachnoiditis, transient paralysis, somnolence, and **progressive leukoencephalopathy.**

d. **Maintenance chemotherapy.** Long-term chemotherapy is necessary for at least **3–5 years** and usually consists of **oral mercaptopurine** with or without **methotrexate.** Newer regimens that are being developed include multiple additional drugs (cyclophosphamide, L-asparaginase, and vincristine). Early data suggest that these combinations may reduce the relapse rate and increase overall survival. **Bone marrow transplantation** during remission (see, also, Chapter 6) ultimately may improve survival, especially in high-risk children and adults; however, this treatment is currently **experimental.**

3. **Primary acute nonlymphocytic leukemia.** The therapy of ANLL closely parallels that of ALL, with 4 phases of therapy, remission induction, consolidation, meningeal prophylaxis, and maintenance.

a. **Remission induction chemotherapy.** Induction therapy in ANLL is much more toxic than in ALL because ANLL induces more myelosuppression than ALL and the chemotherapeutic agents used are more toxic. Generally, hospitalization is required during this phase of therapy. Primary therapy consists of **cytarabine** (100–200 mg/m^2 per day for 7 days) and an anthracycline such as **daunorubicin** (60–75 mg/m^2 per day for 3 days). Although thioguanine has been advocated as a third agent, additional agents have not proved to be beneficial in most studies (see also Appendix D). As a single agent, cytarabine yields 25% and daunorubicin yields 40–50% complete remission rate, whereas together, the two drugs achieve a **complete remission in more than 65%** of patients within 2 cycles. Remission must be confirmed by bone marrow examination. Failures are the result of tumor resistance in 50% of cases and of leukemia- or treatment-induced complications in the other 50%. The anthracycline **mitoxantrone** is less toxic but as equally effective as is daunorubicin and can be substituted for this drug in the remission induction therapy.

b. **Consolidation chemotherapy.** Chemotherapeutic intensification immediately after remission (usually for **2 cycles**) improves the median duration of response from **8 to 30 months**. The precise choice of cytotoxic agents and their doses remains controversial. Recently, preliminary data indicate that long-term disease-free survival may be improved with **high-dose cytarabine,** but this requires confirmation.

c. **Meningeal prophylaxis chemotherapy.** Unlike the therapy for ALL, specific therapy directed at CNS disease in ANLL is unnecessary.

d. **Maintenance chemotherapy.** Although maintenance therapy with short courses of **cytarabine and thioguanine** or **daunorubicin** for 2–3 years has produced brief prolongations of remissions in 2 trials, including one sponsored by the Cancer and Leukemia Group B, **no effect** of this therapy on **long-term disease-free survival** has been observed. Moreover, the improvement in the duration of remission is no better than are recent results with consolidation therapy. Therefore, maintenance therapy is currently not recommended.

e. **Allogeneic bone marrow transplantation (BMT).** At least 3 prospective trials have documented improved **disease-free survival** with allogeneic BMT in patients younger than **40 years** with compatible donors (HLA identical and MLR negative). Yet, **overall survival rates** were significantly increased in **only 1 study.** In addition, the reported long-term survival of **30–55%** has been nearly equalled recently by high-dose consolidation therapy without BMT.

X. **Prognosis**
A. **Risk of recurrence.** Nearly **30%** of patients with **ALL** (80% with "high-risk" ALL) fail therapy, and more than **40%** of patients with **ANLL** relapse after an initial complete response.

B. **Five-year survival.** The long-term survival rates vary with cell type and the patient's age from a low of 17% in adults with ANLL to 33% for adults with ALL. The corresponding 5-year survival rates for children are 30% for ANLL and 70% for ALL.

C. **Adverse prognostic factors.** Features that are associated with a **poor outcome** vary with the type of malignant cell and include the following factors:
1. **Acute lymphocytic leukemia**
   a. **Childhood acute lymphocytic leukemia: age younger than 3 or older than 10 years, male sex, black race, FAB L2 and L3 subtypes, initial leukocyte count higher than 25,000/μL, Philadelphia chromosome present, CALLA$^-$ phenotype, high nuclear labeling index, and B cell ALL.**
   b. **Adult acute lymphocytic leukemia: age older than 35 years, FAB L3 phenotype, male sex, Philadelphia chromosome present, CNS involvement, high initial leukocyte count, and B cell ALL phenotype.**
2. **Acute nonlymphocytic leukemia: Age older than 70; FAB M5 histologic subtype; 9;11, 9;22, and 4;11 translocations; history of myelodyplastic syndrome; and CNS involvement.**

XI. **Patient follow-up**
A. **General guidelines.** Patients with acute leukemia should be followed closely every 3 months for 3 years, every 6 months for an additional 2 years, and annually thereafter for evidence of relapse. The following are specific guidelines for patient follow-up:

B. **Routine evaluation.** Every clinic appointment should include an interval **medical history;** a thorough **physical examination;** and a **complete blood count,** including a **differential white-blood-cell count, platelet count, and peripheral smear examination** (see, also, p 521, **VI.B.1.a**).

C. **Additional evaluation.** The following tests and procedures should be obtained at regular intervals:

1. **Chest x-ray.** An annual examination is required (see p 3, **IV.C.1**).

2. **Bone marrow aspiration and biopsy.** This test should be obtained serially during induction and consolidation chemotherapy. During maintenance therapy, bone marrow aspiration and biopsy should be performed **every 3–6 months,** depending on the clinical situation. Although positive findings are helpful to confirm relapse, negative findings are a relatively insensitive marker for cure.

D. **Optional evaluation.** The following tests and procedures may be indicated by previous diagnostic findings or clinical suspicion:

1. **Lactate dehydrogenase.** Elevated serum levels of this enzyme may indicate relapse in patients with ALL.

2. **Muramidase.** Elevated serum or urinary levels of this enzyme in patients with ANLL may indicate relapse.

3. **Technetium-99m bone scan** (see p 3, **IV.A.5**).

4. **Lumbar puncture.** This is indicated in the presence of **neurologic symptoms** to exclude CNS relapse (see also p 521, **VI.B.3.a**).

REFERENCES

Arlin, Z, Case, DC, Moore, J, et. al. Randomized multicenter trial of cytosine arabinoside with mitoxantrone or daunorubicin in previously untreated patients with acute nonlymphocytic leukemia (ANLL). Leukemia 4(3):177–183, 1990.

Bennett, JM, Catovsky, D, Daniel, MT, et. al. Criteria for the diagnosis of acute leukemia of megakaryocyte lineage (M7). Ann Int Med 103:450–462, 1985.

Bennett, JM, Catovsky, D, Daniel, MT, et. al. Proposed revised criteria for the classification of acute myeloid leukemia: a report of the French-American-British Cooperative Group. Ann Int Med 103:626–629, 1985.

Bishop, JF, Schiffer, CA, Aisner, J, et. al. Surgery in acute leukemia: a review of 167 operations in thrombocytopenic patients. Am J Hematol 26:147, 1987.

Bloomfield, CD and de la Chapelle, A. Chromosome abnormalities in acute nonlymphocytic leukemia: clinical and biologic significance. Sem Oncol 14:372–383, 1987.

Cassileth, PA, McGlave, P, Harrington, DP, et. al. Comparison of post-remission therapy in AML: maintenance versus intensive consolidation therapy versus allogeneic bone marrow transplantation. Proceed Am Soc Clin Oncol 8:197, 1989.

Chaplin, R, Gajewski, J, Nimer, S, et. al. Post-remission chemotherapy for adults with acute myelogenous leukemia: improved survival with high dose cytarabine and daunorubicin consolidation treatment. J Clin Oncol 8(7):119–126, 1990.

Ortega, JA. J Clin Oncol 5:1646, 1987.

Rai, KR, Holland, JF, Glidewell, OJ, et. al. Treatment of acute myelocytic leukemia: a study by the Cancer and Leukemia Group B. Blood 58:1203, 1981.

Sandler, DP. Epidemiology of acute myelogenous leukemia. Sem Oncol 14:359–364, 1987.

64 Chronic Leukemia

Carlin J. McLaughlin, DO

I. **Epidemiology. Chronic lymphocytic (CLL) and myelogenous (CML) leukemia** account for **13.4% of hematologic,** 41% of leukemic, and 1% of all malignancies in the United States. Two less common chronic leukemias, **hairy cell leukemia (HCL)** and **juvenile CML (JCML)** constitute approximately 2% of adult and childhood leukemias respectively. Estimates indicate that 7400 new cases and 3300 deaths from CLL and 4000 new cases and 2600 deaths from CML will occur in 1993. Since 1950 the relative survival rates have increased from 28% to 69% for CLL and from 6% to 22% for CML. Worldwide, the incidence of chronic leukemia varies from a high of 5.7 per 100,000 males in Luxembourg and 3.7 per 100,000 females in Kuwait to a low of 1.1 per 100,000 males and 0.3 per 100,000 females in Suriname. Other areas of high incidence include Denmark, Iceland, Hungary, Italy, and Switzerland whereas Mauritius, Yugoslavia, and Ecuador report a low incidence of new cases.

II. **Risk factors**
   A. **Age.** The incidence of **CLL** climbs steadily from less than 1 per 100,000 before age 45 to a peak of **36 per 100,000 after age 85,** with more than 90% occurring in patients older than 50. The incidence of **CML** slowly increases from less than 1 per 100,000 before age 20 to **36.7 per 100,000 by age 85.** Furthermore, 95% of patients with **JCML are younger than 4 years old** at presentation, whereas **HCL** presents at a **median age of 52 years.**
   B. **Sex.** The risks of CLL, CML, and HCL in males are 2.1, 2.0, and 4.0 times greater, respectively, than in females.
   C. **Race.** There is no significant racial predisposition, although CLL is rare in Japan and China.
   D. **Genetic factors**
      1. **Family history.** The risk of lymphocytic neoplasms (including CLL) and autoimmune disorders is **slightly higher** in first-degree relatives of patients with CLL than in the general population.
      2. **Genetic abnormalities.** In **CML** a reciprocal translocation between chromosomes 9q and 22q juxtaposes the *c-abl* oncogene from 9q and the *bcr* (breakpoint cluster region) on 22q to produce the **Philadelphia chromosome.** Simultaneously, the *c-sis* oncogene from 22q is transferred to 9q. The Philadelphia chromosome encodes for a novel gene product the **p210 *bcr/abl* protein** that has **tyrosine kinase activity.** In 90% of patients with CML, the Philadelphia chromosome is detectable by routine methods; those patients who are karyotypically Ph negative often have complex translocations which result in the production of the p210 gene product. Those patients who have CML on clinical grounds and do not demonstrate the p210 gene product, have a natural history more in keeping with myelodysplastic syndrome.
   E. **Previous hematologic pathology**
      1. **Infection.** Although viral RNA-dependent DNA polymerase, **reverse transcriptase,** has been detected in some leukemic cells, no direct evidence of a viral etiology exists.
      2. **Inflammation.** The incidence of CLL is increased in families with any one of myriad autoimmune disorders.
   F. **Radiation.** Studies of patients irradiated for ankylosing spondylitis, patients receiving the radioisotope thorium dioxide, radium dial painters, and Japanese atomic bomb survivors have documented a **greater incidence of CML** but not CLL occurring after a latency period of 5–7 years.
   G. **Chemicals.** CML may develop after exposure to industrial solvents (eg, benzene).
   H. **Urbanization.** The risk of leukemia is higher in urban populations most likely because of exposure to industrial chemicals.

III. **Clinical presentation**
   A. **Signs and symptoms**
      1. **Local manifestations. Infiltration of other organs is uncommon** with all of the chronic leukemias. **Hairy cell leukemia** is known to cause **painful lytic lesions of bone** late in the disease, while CLL can cause renal infiltration (hematuria), **testicular infiltration, pulmonary infiltrates,** and **orbital infiltration. Intravascular leukostasis** is not a sign or symptom in three of four chronic leukemias. It is primarily seen in **young patients with CML,** who have high blast counts. Clinical manifestations of this problem are **neurologic symptoms** such as headache, seizures, coma, digital gangrene, and priapism. **Meningeal leukemia (CML)** should be distinguished from intravascular leukostasis. This is only seen with CML in the accelerated or blast phase of the disease and presents with **cranial nerve palsies, decreased mental status, and epidural cord compression. Infections** complicate all of the chronic leukemias; however, patients with CLL have a deficient immunity imparted by hypogammaglobulinemia. **Autoimmune phenomena** are seen in both **NCL** (lupus-like syndrome) and with **CLL** (autoimmune hemolytic anemia, pure red cell aplasia, ITP).
      2. **Systemic manifestations.** Although **25%** of patients are **asymptomatic,** most patients (except those with JCML) present with the insidious onset of progressive **fatigue, malaise, night sweats,** low-grade **fevers, weight loss,** and **bruising or pruritus and urticaria** in **CML** (possibly resulting from histamine release from basophils). However, CML may present in blast phase that is clinically indistinguishable from acute nonlymphoblastic leukemia. Furthermore, CLL may **transform** biologically and clinically to **diffuse large cell lymphoma (Richter's transformation)** or, in rare cases, to **acute lymphocytic leukemia or multiple myeloma.**
   B. **Paraneoplastic syndromes.** The following paraneoplastic syndromes have been described in chronic leukemias and may be the sole manifestation of disease:
      1. **Progressive multifocal leukoencephalopathy** (see p 58, **IV.**).
      2. **Disseminated intravascular coagulation** (see p 80).
      3. **Sweet's syndrome** (see p 109).
      4. **Pruritus** (see p 111).
IV. **Differential diagnosis.** Often, **peripheral blood leukocytosis** is discovered on initial evaluation of asymptomatic patients or patients complaining of vague symptoms. Although leukemia always must be excluded in these patients, other frequent causes of leukocytosis also should be considered (see p 520, **IV**).
V. **Screening programs.** No widespread screening programs for chronic leukemias have been instituted secondary to the relatively low incidence of these illnesses. Screening peripheral leukocyte counts are detecting an increasing number of asymptomatic patients, but they are not cost-effective as a general screening tool.
VI. **Diagnostic workup**
   A. **Medical history and physical examination.** A thorough medical history should be elicited, and a complete physical examination must be performed in all patients with suspected chronic leukemia, paying particular attention to the following areas:
      1. **General appearance.** Assessment of the patient's general functional and nutritional status should be made, noting evidence of significant **weight loss** (see, also, p 1, **I** and **III**).
      2. **Skin.** Papules, eruptions, and nodules may reflect cutaneous leukemic infiltration and should be recorded and fully described. Moreover, **cafe-au-lait spots** and **eczemoid rashes** are associated with **JCML** and should be noted.
      3. **Oral cavity.** The adequacy of dental hygiene should be assessed.
      4. **Lymph nodes.** The characteristics (number, size, location, consistency, tenderness, fluctuancy, mobility) of all lymph nodes must be recorded. This should be done separately for all lymph node areas, including occipital, cervical (anterior and posterior), supraclavicular, infraclavicular, axillary, epitrochlear, inguinal, and popliteal regions.
      5. **Chest.** Certain auscultation findings (eg, wheezing, diminished breath sounds) may indicate the presence of pleural effusions.
      6. **Abdomen. Splenomegaly,** hepatomegaly, and all abdominal masses must be completely described.
      7. **Rectum.** Evidence of previous or ongoing **perianal infections** should be noted.
      8. **Nervous system.** A detailed neurologic examination is critical to assess the

possibility of **central nervous system (CNS) involvement** and **intravascular leukostasis.**

B. **Primary tests and procedures.** The following diagnostic tests and procedures should be performed initially in all patients with suspected hematologic malignancies.

1. **Blood tests**

    a. **Complete blood count.** This test should include a differential white-blood-cell count and evaluation of the **peripheral smear,** which are the single most important diagnostic tests for chronic leukemia.

    (1) **Chronic lymphocytic leukemia.** Sustained **lymphocytosis (> 5,000/mm³),** with mature-appearing lymphoctyes, and numerous "smudge" cells is the diagnostic abnormality of **CLL.** The leukocyte count is characteristically elevated between 15,000 and 200,000/mm³ (70–95% lymphocytes). Other associated findings in this disorder include **thrombocytopenia** (15%) from splenomegaly or bone marrow replacement and **anemia** (15%) resulting from immune hemolysis (10–20%) or marrow failure.

    (2) **Chronic myelogenous leukemia.** A marked, occasionally oscillating, leukocytosis (usually > 200,000/µL in adult CML and < 100,000 in JCML) is typical. White cells demonstrate the ability to terminally differentiate but immature forms such as metamyelocytes (61%), and myelocytes (26%) are seen. **Basophilia** and **eosinophilia** is very common in CML. **Thrombocytosis** (60%), **thrombocytopenia** (10%), or commonly **anemia** (hematocrit 30–35%) may be present at diagnosis.

    (3) **Hairy cell leukemia. Pancytopenia (60%; severe in 20%)** is the most common finding, with **hemoglobin levels** typically **less than 8.5 g/dL** and absolute neutrophil counts < 500/µL. Circulating **"hairy" cells** with cytoplasmic projections that are visible with supravital stains and phase or electron microscopy constitute a variable proportion of the peripheral leukocytes.

    b. **Hepatic transminases** (see p 1, **IV.A.2**).

    c. **Alkaline phosphatase** (see p 1, **IV.A.3**).

    d. **BUN and creatinine** (see p 3, **IV.A.6**).

    e. **Leukocyte alkaline phosphatase (LAP).** The level of this serum enzyme is invariably low in these leukemias, especially in CML, in contrast to **leukemoid reactions,** which are accompanied by **elevated LAP** activity.

    f. **P210 protein.** This product of the ***bcr-abl* fusion gene** is detectable in the serum of patients with CML and soon may be available commercially.

    g. **Uric acid.** Serum urate is significantly **increased** in **all** patients with CML and in some with CLL.

    h. **Coagulation times. Prothrombin and partial thromboplastin times** should be measured to exclude the presence of a coagulopathy induced by a circulating procoagulant or anticoagulant, especially in **CML.**

2. **Chest x-ray.** A **chest x-ray** should be obtained in all patients to exclude the presence of pleural effusions as well as pulmonary and mediastinal disease (see p 3, **IV.C.1**).

3. **Invasive procedures. All patients** with chronic leukemia should be evaluated with **bone marrow aspiration and biopsy.** Most commonly, the marrow is obtained from the **posterior iliac crest** with a **Jamshidi needle** after mild sedation, although the **sternum** is an acceptable alternate site (aspiration only). The bone marrow is examined for cellularity (increased with obliteration of fat spaces), specific **staining characteristics,** and **leukemia-associated cell surface markers.**

    a. **Chronic lymphocytic leukemia.** Bone marrow aspiration reveals more than **30% lymphocytes,** and the biopsy demonstrates one of **4 stages** of disease: (1) **early lymphocytic infiltration without distortion of marrow architecture,** (2) **paratrabecular lymphoid aggregates,** (3) **replacement of marrow fat,** and (4) **diffuse lymphocytic marrow replacement.**

    b. **Chronic myelogenous leukemia. Marked hypercellularity,** particularly with granulocytic precursors and **blasts (10–15%),** is characteristic. The **myeloid:erythroid (M:E) ratio** is strikingly **increased,** and dysmyelopoietic features (eg, giantism, changes in granularity) are prominent. The **reticulin content** is **increased** mildly in the chronic phase and may increase in the blast phase of the disease with secondary myelofibrosis.

    c. **Hairy cell leukemia.** Bone marrow aspiration is difficult and generally unsatisfactory in HCL secondary to **marrow fibrosis.** Biopsy demonstrates **hypercellularity in 60%, hypocellularity in 10%,** and variable patterns of marrow replacement are seen in the remainder. **Panhypoplasia** is seen for normal lineages (particularly granulocytic), whereas a monotonous infiltrate of bland cells with oval nuclei (devoid of nucleoli) and abundant pale-blue cytoplasm replace the normal elements.

- C. **Optional tests and procedures.** The following examinations may be indicated by either previous diagnostic findings or clinical suspicion:
  1. **Blood tests**
     a. **5′Nucleotidase** (see p 2, **IV.A.4**).
     b. **GGTP** (see p 2, **IV.A.5**).
     c. **Lactate dehydrogenase.** The level of this serum enzyme correlates with the size of the leukemic cell mass and can be followed to assess the effects of therapy.
     d. **Serum protein electrophoresis.** Although 95% of patients with CLL have a surface IgM monoclonal immunoglobulin, **hypogammaglobulinemia** is present in **50–75% of patients** and correlates with disease progression. Nearly 5%, however, have a monoclonal gammopathy.
     e. **Coombs test.** In **10–20% of patients** with CLL, a warm-reacting antibody causes a Coombs$^+$ hemolytic anemia.
     f. **Lysozyme.** The serum level of this enzyme is **increased** in JCML.
     g. **Muramidase.** The serum level of this enzyme, like lysozyme, is **elevated** in juvenile CML (JCML).
     h. **Vitamin B$_{12}$ levels.** Serum levels of this vitamin and binding capacity are markedly **elevated** in CML.
  2. **Technetium-99m bone scan.** This is rarely indicated in these patients (see p 3, **IV.C.5**).
  3. **Invasive procedures. All patients with chronic leukemia and neurologic symptoms** should have a sample of cerebrospinal fluid obtained by **lumbar puncture** for routine studies and cytologic analysis; however, prior to lumbar puncture any existing **coagulopathy must be corrected** and the **platelet count must be > 50,000/mm^3.** Once a sample is obtained, cells in the cerebrospinal fluid are concentrated by **cytocentrifugation or millipore filtration,** stained with **Wright's stain,** and examined for the presence of leukemic cells, which indicate meningeal involvement.

VII. **Pathology**
- A. **Location.** Although CLL, CML, JCML, and HCL primarily involve the **hematopoietic organs** (blood, bone marrow, liver, spleen, and lymph nodes), they can infiltrate any site and, by definition, are considered systemic diseases.
- B. **Multiplicity.** These leukemias are **"clonal" diseases** that arise from a single progenitor cell rather than multiple primary cells, as demonstrated by analysis of allelic inactivation of the **X chromosome enzyme G6PD** in CML. In normal tissues with random X chromosome inactivation, 2 alleles for G6PD are expressed, whereas in leukemic cells, a single allele is detected, suggesting a **"clonal" origin.**
- C. **Histology.** Morphologic, immunohistochemical, and cytogenetic aspects of CLL, CML, JCML, and HCL vary in important ways and are discussed below.
  1. **Chronic lymphocytic leukemia**
     a. **Histocytochemical features.** The morphology and histocytochemical appearance of lymphocytic leukemia cells are virtually identical to those of **normal lymphocytes:** ie, small mature cells with scant cytoplasm.
     b. **Immunophenotype** The leukemic cells are **B cells in more than 95% of cases.** The immunophenotype of B-CLL is **CD5, CD19, CD20, CD21, and CD24.** The cells are Ia$^+$ and express **monoclonal Ig (usually IgM)** and a **single light chain** (either kappa or lambda) on the cell surface at levels 10% of normal. Southern blot analysis documents **monoclonal heavy and light chain Ig gene rearrangements.** Rarely (< 5%), T cells with characteristic T cell receptors (CD3, CD4, CD8, and CD56) may present with **T-gamma leukemia,** a **CD8$^+$** indolent leukemia, or **dermatotropic lymphocytic leukemia,** a **CD4$^+$** aggressive leukemia.
     c. **Karyotypic features.** Depending on the stage, **40–70% of patients** with CLL have documented chromosomal abnormalities. **Trisomy 12** is the **most common** finding; however, a **11;14 translocation** is common with advanced disease and juxtaposes the immunoglobulin heavy chain gene with the *bcl*-1 **oncogene.**
  2. **Chronic myelogenous leukemia.**

    a. **Histocytochemical features.** An increase in **basophilic** (and eosinophilic) cells is typical, and **poor staining** with **leukocyte alkaline phosphatase (LAP)** is **pathognomonic of CML.**

    b. **Immunophenotypic features.** Cell surface antigens representative of early myeloid precursors are found on these cells. In the blast phase, however, **33% of patients** will experience **lymphoblastic expansion** with immunoglobulin gene rearrangements and cell surface expression of **terminal deoxynucleotidyl transferase** (TdT) and **common acute lymphoblastic leukemia antigen** (CALLA) suggesting B cell origin.

    c. **Karyotypic features.** The classic **9;22 reciprocal translocation** (see p 000, **II.D.2**) is present in more than 90% of patients. Other chromosomal abnormalities—eg, **duplication of Ph, trisomy 8, and isochromosome 17** (2 long arms and no short arm)—may be identified and indicate a **poor prognosis.**

  3. **Hairy cell leukemia.**

    a. **Histocytochemical features.** Monomorphic cells with abundant light-blue cytoplasm that stain strongly for **tartrate-resistant acid phosphatase** are **highly suggestive** but not pathognomonic of **HCL.**

    b. **Immunophenotypic features.** These leukemic cells are **B cells** with most B cell markers (**CD19 and CD20** but not CD21) and some **plasma-cell antigens (PCA-1).** Furthermore, they all express **CD11c.** Several immunoglobulin heavy chains are generally present on the cell surface. For unclear reasons, hairy cells also express the **TAC antigen (IL-2 receptor),** which is normally only expressed on **T- cells.**

    c. **Karyotypic features.** Southern blot analysis of hairy cells demonstrate monoclonal gene rearrangements for heavy and light immunoglobulin chains.

D. Metastatic spread

  1. **Modes of spread.** Unlike solid malignancies, chronic leukemia is, by definition, a systemic disease. Therefore, typical mechanisms of spread, including direct extension and lymphatic and hematogenous metastasis do not apply.

  2. **Sites of spread.** Although chronic leukemias diffusely involve all tissues, extensive localized infiltration of various sites such as the liver, spleen, lung, CNS, kidney, gastrointestinal tract, and skin may ultimately interfere with organ function.

VIII. Staging. Although no TNM staging system can be applied to these hematologic malignancies, a staging system for CLL based on the extent of disease has been proposed by Rai and modified by Binet. In addition, 3 basic stages of CML have been identified. No staging system has been devised for HCL.

A. Chronic lymphocytic leukemia

  1. **Rai staging system**

    a. **Stage 0.** Blood lymphocytosis more than 15,000/µL and more than 40% bone marrow lymphocytes.

    b. **Stage I. Lymphocytosis with lymphadenopathy.**

    c. **Stage II. Lymphocytosis with splenomegaly or hepatomegaly** (lymphadenopathy is not required).

    d. **Stage III. Lymphocytosis with anemia** caused by hemolysis or decreased production (hemoglobin < 11 g/dL; lymphadenopathy, splenomegaly, and hepatomegaly are not required).

    e. **Stage IV. Lymphocytosis with thrombocytopenia** (platelet count < 100,000/µL; anemia, lymphadenopathy, splenomegaly, and hepatomegaly are not required).

  2. **Binet staging system**

    a. **Stage A.** Lymphocytosis more than 15,000/µL and fewer than three areas of lymph node involvement (liver, spleen, cervical, axillary, and inguinal lymph node regions).

    b. **Stage B.** Lymphocytosis and at least 3 out of 5 areas of leukemic involvement.

    c. **Stage C.** Lymphocytosis and anemia (hemoglobin < 10 g/dL), thrombocytopenia (platelet count < 100,000/µL) or all of these.

B. Chronic myelogenous leukemia

  1. **Chronic phase.** Stable or controllable thrombocytosis.

  2. **Accelerated phase.** Manifested as thrombocytopenia or persistent thrombocytosis, extramedullary disease (chloromas), lymphadenopathy, bone pain, fever, night sweats, progressive weight loss, hypercalcemia, leukocytosis refractory to therapy, and increasing basophilia, eosinophilia, bone marrow pro-

myelocytes and blasts, anemia, karyotype abnormalities, splenomegaly, and myelofibrosis.

    3. **Blast phase.** Detected as a rapid proliferation of **myeloid (67%)** or **lymphoid (33%) blasts** and the decline of other bone marrow elements. Classification of the leukemic cells at this stage follows the FAB system of acute leukemia (see p 522, **VII.**).

IX. Treatment

  A. Surgery. Currently, the only surgical option in patients with chronic leukemia is **splenectomy.** However, it does not alter the disease course and is indicated only for the palliation of symptomatic splenomegaly (eg, pain, hemolytic anemia, immune thrombocytopenia). The response rate to this procedure is not related to the size of the spleen. In **hairy cell leukemia,** the **duration** of response is **longer (19 months)** if the bone marrow **cellularity is less than 85%** than if severe marrow hypercellularity is present (6 months).

  B. Radiation therapy

    1. **Splenic irradiation.** Splenic radiation (1200–1500 cGy in 25–50 cGy fractions over 2–3 weeks) can be substituted for splenectomy in patients who are unable to have surgery (eg, pregnant females, elderly); however, some evidence suggests that this may **adversely affect survival.**

    2. **Total body irradiation.** One study used this approach (400 cGy in 5–10 cGy daily fractions) with CLL and found a **33% complete response rate** and a **57-month median survival;** however, these results have not been replicated.

  C. Chemotherapy

    1. **Chronic lymphocytic leukemia**

      a. Single agents

        (1) Glucocorticoids. Prednisone (0.5–1 mg/kg per day) is indicated for palliation of significant **immune thrombocytopenia or Coombs+ hemolytic anemia.** The lympholytic effect, however, is minimal; in fact, the lymphocyte count usually **rises** during the first 4–6 weeks of therapy. **Splenectomy** should be considered in patients who **fail to respond** and in those who require extended therapy because continued glucocorticoid administration significantly increases the risk of life-threatening infection. However, administration of **intravenous immune globulin (IVIG; 0.4/kg/Q3 weeks)** can be used to lower the frequency of infection substantially in patients with significant **hypogammaglobulinemia.**

        (2) Cytotoxic agents. Chlorambucil has been the mainstay of chemotherapy for CLL. It can be given as a **daily dose** (0.1–0.2 mg/kg), intermittently **every other week** (0.4 mg/kg), or **once a month** (0.4–0.8 mg/kg) until the leukocyte count declines to 20,000/μL. The **response rate is 70–75%. Cyclophosphamide** given daily or intermittently may be useful in lowering the leukocyte counts in chlorambucil-resistant patients. Newer agents include **deoxycoformycin (pentostatin; 4 mg/m^2 every 1–2 weeks),** which inhibits adenosine deaminase and yields a **35–55% overall response rate; fluoro-AMP (fludarabine; 20–30 mg/m^2 per day for 5 days),** which is phosphorylated in vivo and inhibits DNA polymerase, producing **response rates of 45–70%;** and **chlorodeoxyadenosine.**

      b. Combination chemotherapy. Although vincristine is not an effective single agent, several combinations, including vincristine—eg, cyclophosphamide, vincristine, and prednisone (CVP) and vincristine, carmustine, cyclophosphamide, melphalan, and prednisone (**M2 protocol**)—have been administered to CLL patients without significant improvement in response or survival rates. In a French randomized cooperative trial, however, cyclophosphamide, doxorubicin, vincristine, and prednisone (**CHOP**) prolonged the **median survival from 2 to more than 4 years.** Early data from additional studies suggest that CHOP plus cytosine arabinoside (**CHOP-A**) may improve survival as long as **8 years,** although these latest trials require confirmation in additional randomized controlled clinical trials.

    2. **Chronic myelogenous leukemia**

      a. Single agents. The two most commonly used single agents in the treatment of chronic phase CML are **busulfan** (2–6 mg/day PO with allopurinol) and **hydroxyurea** (20–50 mg/kg per day). Both agents have essentially identical efficacy and median duration of response. **Busulfan is the most commonly used alkylating agent.** It produces prolonged and occasionally

unpredictable (10%) leukocyte nadirs and must be discontinued once the leukocyte count is 20,000/µL. **Hydroxyurea** is a **short-acting drug** that requires daily treatment to control the leukocyte count. It is the **drug of choice** for patients who are candidates for **bone marrow transplantation.** Many other single agents have been tried for chronic phase CML without demonstrable therapeutic efficacy over busulfan or hydroxyurea. **Median survival** using single agent therapy is **40–50 months** compared to 31 months without therapy. **Leukapheresis** may be required in **pregnant females** who wish to complete the pregnancy before cytotoxic therapy is instituted.

b. **Combination chemotherapy.** Various combination chemotherapy regimens have been used in patients during the chronic phase without prolongation of the median survival. However, because toxicity is increased substantially, this approach cannot be recommended. During the accelerated and blast phases, combination chemotherapy similar to AML has been used with dismal results. In the 33% of patients with **lymphoid blast crisis,** however, as many as **67% of patients** may attain a **remission lasting 7.5 months** with **vincristine plus prednisone** (VP) or with multiagent chemotherapy regimens.

c. **Bone marrow transplantation (BMT).** Bone marrow transplantation is the **treatment of choice** for CML, provided that the patient is **younger than 50** years of age, has a suitable marrow donor, and is otherwise in satisfactory health. See, also, chapter 6). Preparation for BMT should begin promptly because blast transformation occurs randomly and the long-term relapse-free survival is **60% for BMT during the chronic phase, 30% during the accelerated phase,** and 15% during the blast phase.

3. **Hairy cell leukemia**
   a. **Single agents. Chlorodeoxyadenosine** has recently been released for the initial treatment of hairy cell leukemia. It is associated with **response rates higher than 90%** with a majority being complete responses. **Deoxycoformycin (pentostatin 4–10mg/m² every 2 weeks)** produces **response rates higher than 90%.** Unfortunately, this drug is complicated by a treatment-induced reduction in helper T lymphocytes and occasionally by **opportunistic infections. Chlorambucil is no longer used** for the treatment of HCL secondary to the tremendous success of these two therapies.
   b. **Combination chemotherapy.** Because of unacceptably high therapy-related toxicity (primarily infections) and lack of efficacy, combination chemotherapy has been **abandoned** for this disease.
   c. **Bone marrow transplantation.** BMT, although theoretically useful, is impractical in these patients because nearly all of them are **older than 50 years of age** at presentation, making the morbidity and mortality prohibitively high.

D. **Immunotherapy.** Immunotherapy, primarily interferon therapy, has been explored in the treatment of chronic leukemias with limited success in certain circumstances.
   1. **Chronic lymphocytic leukemia.** Interferon-alpha has been tried in advanced disease without success.
   2. **Chronic myelogenous leukemia.** Administration of **interferon-alpha (5 million units/m² per day)** or **interferon-gamma** is associated with high response rates (80%) and with **complete hematologic remissions in 25–35%** of patients. Complete suppression of the Philadelphia chromosome has been observed. However, the cost and frequent side effects (flu-like symptoms) have limited the acceptance of this promising therapy.
   3. **Hairy cell leukemia.** In large series, therapy with **interferon-alpha-2a** and interferon-alpha-2b has yielded **hematologic improvement** (including immune deficits) in the vast majority of patients **(70–90%)** and **complete remissions in 10–27%.** Therapy must be continued for **1 year,** and repeat treatment may induce a second remission on relapse. The role of maintenance therapy 3 times weekly is controversial.

X. **Prognosis**
   A. **Risk of recurrence.** With the possible exception of BMT, **no therapy for chronic leukemia is curative;** therefore, with time, the risk of recurrence approaches 100%.
   B. **Median survival.** The long-term survival rates vary according to the type of chronic leukemia and the stage of disease at presentation. The median survival by disease and stage is summarized below:
      1. **Chronic lymphocytic leukemia**
         a. **Rai stage**

        (1) Stage 0/I (low risk), 10 years.
        (2) Stage II, 6.5 years.
        (3) Stages III and IV, 1.5 years.
      b. **Binet stage**
        (1) Stage A, 7 years.
        (2) Stage B, 5 years.
        (3) Stage C, 2 years.
  2. **Chronic myelogenous leukemia.** Low-, intermediate-, and high-risk groups have been defined primarily based on **splenomegaly** more than 6 cm below the costal margin and the presence of **more than 1% peripheral blood myeloblasts** as well as multiple other factors (see below). The median survival for these groups is listed below.
    a. **Low-risk group.** Median survival of 5.5 years; 2-year survival is 90%, with a 17–19% annual risk of death.
    b. **Intermediate-risk group.** Median survival of 3 years.
    c. **High-risk group.** Median survival of 2.5 years; 2-year survival of 65–70% with a 30–35% annual risk of death.
  3. **Hairy cell leukemia.** The exact survival with modern therapy is unclear, but it certainly **exceeds the 6–8 year median survival** reported previously. With interferon therapy and **correction of the immune defect,** the risk of infection and death decreases dramatically, and the survival may closely approximate age-matched controls.
  4. **Juvenile chronic myelogenous leukemia.** Prognostic factors are not well established.
C. **Adverse prognostic factors.** Features that are associated with a poor outcome vary according to the type of chronic leukemia and include the following factors:
  1. **Chronic lymphocytic leukemia.** Diffuse bone marrow involvement (vs nodular), karyotypic abnormalities, lymphocytosis greater than 50,000/μL, and high levels of LDH and uric acid.
  2. **Chronic myelogenous leukemia. Age, older than 60; initial leukocyte count** greater than 100,000/μL; **hepatosplenomegaly** more than 6 cm below the costal margin; presence of more than 1% peripheral blood myeloblasts; basophilia and eosinophilia greater than 15%; karyotypic abnormalities; and **platelet count higher than 700,000/μL.**
  3. **Hairy cell leukemia.** The prognostic factors associated with HCL have not been well defined.
  4. **Juvenile chronic myelogenous leukemia.** Prognostic factors are not well established.

XI. **Patient follow-up**
  A. **General guidelines.** Patients with chronic leukemia need individualized follow-up with a frequency dictated by their disease stability, the need for therapeutic intervention or monitoring, and by intercurrent complications of the leukemia such as infectious or hemorrhagic manifestations of their disease.
  B. **Routine evaluation.** Every clinic appointment should include an interval **medical history;** a thorough **physical examination;** and a **complete blood count,** including a **differential white blood cell count, platelet count,** and **peripheral smear examination** (see, also, **VI.B.1.a** above).
  C. **Additional evaluation.** The following tests and procedures should be obtained at regular intervals:
    1. **Chest x-ray.** This should be obtained when signs or symptoms referable to the chest are encountered.
    2. **Bone marrow aspiration and biopsy.** This test should be obtained at regular intervals only if further therapeutic decisions depend on the presence or absence of a pathologic complete remission.
  D. **Optional evaluation.** The following tests and procedures may be indicated by previous diagnostic findings or clinical suspicion:
    1. **Technetium-99m bone scan.** (see p 3, **IV.C.5**).
    2. **Lumbar puncture.** This is indicated in the presence of **neurologic symptoms** to exclude CNS relapse (see, also, p 532, **VI.C.3**).

REFERENCES

Boggs DR, Sofferman SA, Wintrobe MM, et al. Factors influencing the duration of survival of patients with chronic lymphocytic leukemia. Am J Med 40:242–254, 1966.

Brodeur GM, Dow LW, et al. Cytogenetic features of juvenile chronic myelogenous leukemia. Blood 53:812, 1979.

Byhardt RW, Brace KC, Wiernik PH. The role of splenic irradiation in chronic lymphocytic leukemia. Cancer 35:1621, 1975.

del Regato JA. Total body irradiation of chronic lymphocytic leukemia. Am J Roentgenol 120:504, 1974.

French Cooperative Group of Chronic Lymphocytic Leukemia. Prognostic and therapeutic advances in CLL management: The experience of the French Cooperative Group. Sem Hematol 24:275–290, 1987.

Gale RP, Foon KA. Chronic lymphocytic leukemia: Recent advances in biology and treatment. Ann Int Med 103:101, 1985.

Gale RP, Foon KA. Biology of chronic lymphocytic leukemia. Sem Hematol 24:209, 1987.

Golde DW. Therapy of hairy-cell leukemia. NEJM 307:495–496, 1982.

Golomb HM, Fefer A, Golde DW, et al. Sequential evaluation of alpha-2-interferon treatment in 128 patients with hairy cell leukemia. Sem Oncol 11(4 suppl):13–17, 1987.

Golomb HM, Hadad LJ. Infectious complications in 127 patients with hairy cell leukemia. Am J Hematol 16:393, 1984.

Grever MR, Leiby JM, Kraut EH, et al. Low-dose deoxycoformycin in lymphoid malignancy. J Clin Oncol 3:1196–1201, 1985.

Jansen J, Hermans J. Splenectomy in hairy cell leukemia: A retrospective multicenter analysis. Cancer 47:2066,1981.

Keating MJ, Kantarjian H, Talpaz M, et al. Fludarabine: A new agent with major activity against chronic lymphocytic leukemia. Blood 74:19–25, 1989.

Kurzrock R, Blick MD, Tolpaz M, et al. Rearrangement in the breakpoint cluster region and the clinical course in Philadelphia-negative chronic myelogenous leukemia. Ann Int Med 105:673–679, 1986.

Piro LD, Carrera CJ, Beutler E, Carson DA. 1- Chlorodeoxyadenosine: An effective new agent for the treatment of chronic lymphocytic leukemia. Blood 72:1069–1073, 1988.

Quesada JR, Hersh EM, Manning J, et al. Treatment of hairy cell leukemia with recombinant alpha interferon. Blood 68(2):493–497, 1986.

Rubenstein DB, Longo DL. Peripheral destruction of platelets in chronic lymphocytic leukemia: Recognition, prognosis and therapeutic implications. Am J Med 71:729, 1981.

Spiers ASD, Moore D, Cassileth PA, et al. Remissions in hairy-cell leukemia with pentostatin (2'-deoxycoformycin). NEJM 316(14):825–830, 1987.

Talpaz M, Kantarjian H, McCredie K, et al. Chronic myelogenous leukemia: Hematologic remission with alpha interferon. Br J Hematol 64(1):87–95, 1986.

Thomas ED, Clift RA. Indications for marrow transplantation in chronic myelogenous leukemia. Blood 73:861–864, 1989.

Urba WJ, Baseler MW, Koop WC, et al. Deoxycoformycin-induced immunosuppression in patients with hairy cell leukemia. Blood 73(1):38–45, 1989.

65 Malignancies of Plasma Cells

Mindy S. Bohrer, MD

I. **Epidemiology.** Plasma cell neoplasms (PCNs) are uncommon and include **multiple myeloma, essential (Waldenström's) macroglobulinemia, and monoclonal gammopathy** of unknown significance. **Multiple myeloma** is the most important gammopathy and constitutes **14.5% of hematologic malignancies and 1.1% of all malignancies,** excluding skin cancer. In 1985, **4.6 cases per 100,000 males** and **3.1 cases per 100,000 females** were diagnosed, resulting in 3.5 and 2.4 deaths per 100,000 respectively. Estimates indicate that **12,500 new cases and 9,200 deaths** will occur in 1993 in the United States. Worldwide, the incidence of multiple myeloma varies from a high of 8.4 per 100,000 **in black males** living in the San Francisco Bay area to 0.6 per 100,000 in India.

II. **Risk factors**
   A. **Age.** The incidence of multiple myeloma increases from less than 1 per 100,000 before age 45 to a peak of **28.2 per 100,000 by the age of 80.** The **median age** of patients at the time of diagnosis is **68 years.** In addition, nearly **3% of individuals older than 70 years of age** have a **monoclonal spike** on serum protein electrophoresis.
   B. **Sex. Males** are at **1.5 times greater risk** of developing the disease than are females.
   C. **Race. Blacks** are at **1.8 times greater risk** than whites; the incidence among Asian populations is low.
   D. **Genetic factors.** First-degree relatives of patients with multiple myeloma are at **greater risk** of acquiring PCNs because of unknown genetic factors, and familial gammopathy kindred have been reported. Furthermore, genetic abnormalities of **chromosome 14,** the **c-myc oncogene** on chromosome 8, and the **bcl-1 oncogene** on chromosome 11 have been linked to PCNs, as has the **4C group of HLA antigens.**
   E. **History of previous pathology.** Inflammatory diseases that produce chronic antigenic stimulation, such as systemic lupus erythematosus, scleroderma, rheumatoid arthritis, and chronic dermatitis, are associated with an elevated risk of multiple myelomas.
   F. **Radiation.** Radiologists (low dose), radium dial painters (low dose), and atomic bomb survivors (high dose) all are at **4.7 times greater risk** than the general population. The **latency period** for radiation-induced gammopathy is **10–30 years.**
   G. **Urbanization.** For unknown reasons, workers in the **printing, plastics, leather, woodworking, rubber, and petrochemical industries** are at increased risk. In addition, **farmers** and workers exposed to **arsenic, asbestos, or lead** have a high incidence.

III. **Clinical presentation**
   A. **Signs and symptoms.** Although some patients may be asymptomatic and discovered during the workup for an unrelated problem, most patients present with a composite of the following local and systemic signs and symptoms.
      1. **Local manifestations.** Local symptoms arise almost exclusively from **osteolytic bone lesions. Bone pain (60%)** is the most common symptom, but **pathologic fractures (20%)** also occur. Paraspinal extension and spinal compression fractures may produce neurologic symptoms and **spinal cord compression (15%).**
      2. **Systemic manifestations.** Frequent complaints and findings in patients with plasma cell dyscrasias are **anemia (62%)** from marrow replacement, gastrointestinal bleeding, and renal failure; **hypercalcemia (25–33%); fatigue and weakness** (anemia, hypercalcemia, and uremia); **renal insufficiency (20%)** associated with **hypercalcemia** and **Bence Jones proteinuria;** nausea, vomiting and constipation (hypercalcemia); Raynaud's phenomenon (cryoglobu-

linemia); **altered mental status and headache (10%)** caused by hyperviscosity, hypercalcemia, and uremia; **purpura and mucosal bleeding (5% in multiple myeloma, 50% in Waldenström's macroglobulinemia)** from hyperviscosity; fever and encapsulated gram-positive (*Streptococcus pneumoniae, Haemophilus influenzae*) upper respiratory, central nervous system (CNS), or urinary tract **infection** (impaired humoral immunity); granulocytopenia; and thrombocytopenia. A syndrome of glycosuria, aminoaciduria, phosphaturia, acidosis, osteomalacia, and Bence Jones proteinuria **(adult Fanconi syndrome)** also has been reported in patients with multiple myeloma. **Hepatosplenomegaly (40%), lymphadenopathy (30%), coagulopathy, and a mixed sensory-motor peripheral neuropathy (1%)** are associated with Waldenström's macroglobulinemia.

B. **Paraneoplastic syndromes.** The following symptom complexes have been associated with PCNs.

1. **Hypercalcemia.** The frequency and severity of calcium elevations in patients with gammopathies do not correlate with bone involvement. The release of tumor-associated factors (eg, **lymphotoxin, IL-1**) may be responsible.

2. **Erythema annulare centrifugum** (see p 108, **II.F**).

3. **Ichthyosis** (see p 110)

IV. **Differential diagnosis.** Abnormal plasma cell findings and elevated immunoglobulin protein levels do not always imply PCNs. Other possibilities include **reactive plasmacytosis** (viral infections, serum sickness, granulomatous disease, and **autoimmune diseases) primary amyloidosis, benign plasma cell disorders** (benign monoclonal gammopathy and pseudoparaproteinemia), and **other malignancies** (eg, plasma cell leukemia).

V. **Screening programs.** Because of the low incidence of these diseases, routine screening of patients in **not recommended;** however, elderly patients with suggestive symptoms can be screened easily with **serum and urine protein electrophoresis.**

VI. **Diagnostic workup**

A. **Medical history and physical examination.** In addition to a thorough medical history, a complete physical examination is warranted, with particular emphasis on the following areas:

1. **General appearance.** An assessment of the patient's mental, general functional, and nutritional status should be made (see, also, p 1, **I** and **III**).

2. **Skin.** Evidence of **purpura, erythema annulare centrifugum, and ichthyosis** should be sought.

3. **Head.** Palpable bone lesions of the skull should be described.

4. **Lymph nodes.** The extent and size of palpable lymph nodes (infection or WM) must be recorded.

5. **Abdomen.** Hepatic and splenic enlargement suggests the diagnosis of Waldenström's macroglobulinemia.

6. **Skeleton.** Areas of bone pain and tenderness should be accurately cataloged.

7. **Extremities.** Sensation and motor function of all nerves should be assessed to exclude spinal cord compression and the mixed sensory-motor neuropathy associated with Waldenström's macroglobulinemia.

B. **Primary tests and procedures.** The following examinations should be performed initially in all patients with suspected PCNs:

1. **Blood tests**

a. **Complete blood count.** This test may demonstrate **rouleaux formation** if a significant paraproteinemia is present (see, also, p 1, **IV.A.1**).

b. **Hepatic transaminases** (see p 1, **IV.A.2**).

c. **Alkaline phosphatase** (see p 1, **IV.A.3**).

d. **Calcium and phosphate.** Serum levels of these electrolytes are **elevated in 25–33% of patients,** frequently necessitating treatment to prevent nephrolithiasis and pathologic calcification.

e. **BUN and creatinine.** Renal damage from hypercalcemia, hyperuricemia, and Bence Jones protein can be detected with this test.

f. **Electrolytes.** Abnormalities associated with renal insufficiency may be present. In addition, a **decreased anion gap, pseudohyponatremia, and pseudohypoglycemia** may be noted because of a **decreased volume** of distribution and an **increased measurable** chloride and bicarbonate produced by increased concentrations of cationic protein.

g. **Total protein and protein electrophoresis**. This test screens for monoclonal gammopathies and may detect **more than 0.2 g/dL of myeloma pro-**

teins. Total protein is usually elevated with normal albumin levels. Monoclonal spikes usually appear in the **g-b region,** whereas reactive serum proteins migrate to the a-b zone. Peaks should exceed 3.5 g/dL for IgG or 2 g/dL for IgA. **Together with urine protein electrophoresis** (see below), **99% of patients manifest a myeloma protein spike.**

h. **Protein immunoelectrophoresis.** This is the most **sensitive and diagnostic test** for PCNs. It distinguishes polyclonal from monoclonal gammopathies and identifies the class of myeloma protein (ie, g, a, m, d, e and the light chains k, 1).

i. **Quantitative serum immunoglobulin level.** This test measures the amount of specific immunoglobulin by gel immunodiffusion.

j. **Beta-2-microglobulin.** Levels of this serum **protein are elevated in 80–90%** of multiple myeloma patients and correlate with plasma cell mass, renal function, and **prognosis.**

2. **Urine studies**

a. **Sulfosalicylic acid precipitation test.** This is a screening test for urinary protein because "dip" tests for protein do not detect **Bence Jones proteins.**

b. **Urine protein electrophoresis.** Typically, this tests reveals a monoclonal spike in the **g region** as presumptive evidence of light chain disease. If less than **500 mg/dL of protein is present,** the urine must be **concentrated** prior to testing.

c. **Urine protein immunoelectrophoresis.** This test confirms the diagnosis of PCN by demonstrating an **abnormal k to L chain ratio (normal = 2:1).**

d. **Twenty-four hour urine protein.** Quantitation of the 24-hour urinary light chain and total protein excretion is an **important staging criterion** and normally is less than 1 g every 24 hours.

3. **Imaging studies**

a. **Chest x-ray** (see p 3, **IV.C.1**).

b. **Skeletal x-ray survey.** Plain x-rays are obtained of **all long bones, pelvis, sternum, cranium, and spine** to catalog all osteolytic bone lesions.

4. **Invasive procedures. Bone marrow aspiration** should be performed to confirm the presence of myeloma cells in the marrow. **Plasmacytosis (> 10% plasma cells)** in association with **osteolytic lesions,** and **myeloma protein secretion,** is **diagnostic** of PCNs.

C. **Optional tests and procedures.** The following tests and procedures may be indicated by previous diagnostic tests or clinical suspicion.

1. **Blood tests**

a. **5-Nucleotidase** (see p 2, **IV.A.4**).

b. **GGTP** (see p 2, **IV.A.5**).

c. **Cryoglobulin level.** This is determined by isolating the patient's warm serum, cooling it to 4° C for 24–48 hrs, measuring the amount of **cryoprecipitate** with a hematocrit tube, then ascertaining its content by protein immunoelectrophoresis.

d. **Viscosity.** This test measures (with a **Ostwald viscosimeter**) the ratio of the rates of descent past a constriction in a capillary tube of the patient's **serum** (not plasma) and distilled water. **Normal values are less than 2** and symptoms from **hyperviscosity** develop with values **greater than 4.**

e. **Common acute lymphoblastic leukemia antigen (CALLA).** The level of antigen expression on plasma cells correlates with **prognosis** and can be measured to determine response to therapy.

2. **Imaging studies**

a. **Computerized tomography (CT).** If performed after injection of **intrathecal contrast.** CT scan affords an excellent method for evaluating the spinal cord for areas of involvement.

b. **Magnetic resonance imaging (MRI).** Although expensive, this new imaging modality provides the **best detail** of spinal myeloma bone lesions and (with **gadolinium**) epidural extension with impending spinal cord compression (see, also, p 3, **IV.C.3**).

c. **Myelography.** This examination is indicated when neurologic evidence of spinal cord compression exists.

3. **Invasive procedures.** Localized lesions may require **surgical biopsy** to exclude other diseases, including metastatic cancer.

D. **Diagnostic criteria.** The criteria for the diagnosis of myeloma are outlined in Table 65–1.

TABLE 65–1. MAJOR AND MINOR DIAGNOSTIC CRITERIA FOR PLASMA CELL NEOPLASMS*

Multiple myeloma
  Major criteria
    I.   Plasmacytoma on tissue biopsy.
    II. Bone marrow plasmacytosis with > 30% plasma cells.
    III. Monoclonal globulin spike on serum electrophoresis > 3.5 g/dL for IgG peaks or 2.0 g for IgA peaks,
         1.0 g/24 h of kappa or lambda light chain excretion on urine electrophoresis in the absence of
         amyloidosis.

  Minor criteria
    a. Bone marrow plasmacytosis with 10–30% plasma cells.
    b. Monoclonal globulin spike present, but less than the levels defined above.
    c. Lytic bone lesions.
    d. Residual normal IgG < 600 mg/dL, IgA < 100 mg/dL, or IgM < 50 mg/dL

A minimum of 1 major and 1 minor criterion or 3 minor criteria that must include a + b confirm the diagnosis in
symptomatic patients with clearly progressive disease.

Indolent myleoma (same as myeloma except for the following)
    I.   Limited (< 3) bone lesions; no compression fractures.
    II. Myeloma protein levels: IgG < 7 g/dL and IgA < 5 g/dL.
    III. No symptoms or associated disease features, i.e.:
    a. Performance status > 70%.
    b. Hemoglobin > 10 g/dL.
    c. Serum calcium is normal.
    d. Serum creatinine < 2.0 gm/dL.
    e. No infections.

Smoldering myeloma (same as indolent myeloma except for the following)
    I.   No bone lesions.
    II. Bone marrow plasma cells < 30%.

MGUS
    III. Monoclonal gammopathy.
    IV. No symptoms.
    V.   No bone lesions.
    VI. Bone marrow plasma cells < 10%.
    VII. Myeloma protein: IgG < 3.5 g/dL, IgA < 2.0 g/dL, and Bence Jones urinary protein < 1 g/24 hrs.

*Adapted from DeVita V, Rosenberg SA, Hellman S. *Principles and Practice of Oncology.* Philadelphia, PA: JB
Lippincott; 1989: 1863, with permission.

VII. Pathology

A. Variants of plasma cell neoplasms. PCNs represent a spectrum of disease that
includes multiple myeloma and the following rare variants, each accounting for less
than 1% of all PCN patients.

1. **Multiple myeloma variants**
    a. **Osteosclerotic myeloma.** This unusual type of myeloma presents as a
       distinct syndrome, the **POEMS syndrome** (polyneuropathy, organomegaly,
       endocrinopathy, monoclonal gammopathy, and skin changes). This entity
       has been described mainly in the Orient.
    b. **Nonsecretory myeloma.** This variant of multiple myeloma fails to secrete
       a myeloma protein and therefore has no "**M**" **spike** on either serum or urine
       protein electrophoresis.
    c. **"Smoldering" or "indolent" myeloma.** This is probably an early phase
       rather than a true variant of multiple myeloma characterized by slow growth.
       It constitutes **3% of PCNs.**

2. **Essential (Waldenström's) macroglobulinemia.** This is the **second most
    common** PCN and is characterized by more than **2 g/dL of IgM (rather than
    IgG or IgA as in multiple myeloma), uncommon Bence Jones proteinuria
    (10%), hepatosplenomegaly (30%), lymphadenopathy (40%), hypervis-
    cosity syndrome (50%), and peripheral neuropathy (17%)**. Osteolytic bone
    lesions are uncommon with this disease.

3. **Solitary plasmacytoma.** A solitary plasmacytoma consists of a **single local-**

ized **extramedullary or intraosseus bone lesion** that is associated with bone marrow containing less than **5% plasma cells** and a myeloma protein, which, if present (30% of patients), promptly disappears with local therapy.

4. **Monoclonal gammopathy of undetermined significance.** This syndrome is characterized by (1) **less than 3 g/dL** of a stable **myeloma protein,** (2) **less than 10% plasma cells** in the bone marrow, (3) negligible or **absent urinary protein,** and (4) an **absence** of **lytic bone disease,** anemia, azotemia and hypercalcemia. Over a period of 20 years, patients with a monoclonal gammopathy either remain **stable (25%),** develop frank **myeloma (25%),** or **50% die** of unrelated causes.

5. **Heavy chain disease.** On the basis of the type of heavy chain involved (G,A, M or D), diseases involving heavy chains **(Franklin's disease)** can be divided into **g-disease** (presents with fever, weakness, anemia, and lymphadenopathy similar to non-Hodgkin's lymphoma), **a-disease** (presents with gastrointestinal involvement and diarrhea, abdominal pain, and weight loss), **m-disease** (presents in association with chronic lymphocytic leukemia), and **d-disease** (presents with renal failure accompanied by osteolytic bone lesions).

6. **Plasma cell leukemia.** This disease differs from multiple myeloma in that **more than 20% of the peripheral white blood cells are plasma cells,** whereas these cells are rarely identified on peripheral blood smears in patients with multiple myeloma.

B. **Location.** PCNs commonly involve the **cranium, vertebrae,** sternum, pelvis, and long bones.

C. **Multiplicity.** With the exception of a solitary plasmacytoma, these diseases are, by definition, diffuse and multicentric.

D. **Histology.** Plasma cells are **large cells** with abundant bluish-purple (Wright's stain) cytoplasm rich in endoplasmic reticulum. An **eccentric nucleus** is usually present. The cells are characterized further by the subtype of myeloma protein that they secrete. **IgG (54%)** is the most common, followed by **IgA (22%),** light-chain disease alone **(22%),** and, finally, the rare variants of IgD (< 1%) and IgE (< 1%) myeloma.

VIII. **Staging.** The staging of myeloma is based on tumor burden. Although different myeloma staging systems have been proposed, the **Durie-Salmon staging system** is most widely used and is summarized below:

A. **Stage I.** This stage has a low myeloma cell mass (0.6×10^{12} cells/m^2) and meets all of the following criteria:
   1. **Hemoglobin level.** More than 10 g/dL.
   2. **Serum calcium level.** Less than 12 mg/dL.
   3. **Bone x-ray.** Normal bone structure (scale 0) or solitary bone plasmocytoma.
   4. **Myeloma protein.** Low production rate, with IgG less than 5 g/dL; IgA less than 3 g/dL; urine light chain less than 4 g/24 hours.

B. **Stage II.** This stage does not fit the criteria for stage I or III and has an intermediate cell mass ($0.6–1.2 \times 10^{12}$ cells/m^2)

C. **Stage III.** This stage has a high myeloma cell mass ($> 1.2 \times 10^{12}$ cells/m^2) and one or more of the following:
   1. **Hemoglobin level.** Less than 8.5 g/dL.
   2. **Serum calcium level.** More than 12 mg/dL.
   3. **Bone x-ray.** Advanced lytic bone lesions (scale 3).
   4. **Myeloma protein.** High production rates, with IgG more than 7 g/dL, IgA more than 5 g/dL, and urine light chain more than 12 g/24 hours.
      Note: Each stage is subclassified into either A relatively normal renal function (serum creatinine < 2 mg/dL) or B abnormal renal function (serum creatinine >2 mg/dL).

IX. **Treatment.** The therapy for multiple myeloma is directed at both the proliferation of malignant plasma cells and the manifestations and complications of the disease.

A. **Surgery.** Surgical therapy in patients with PCNs (both primary and recurrent) is reserved almost exclusively for the treatment of **orthopedic complications** of osteolytic bone lesions (eg, pathologic fractures, bony instability; see, also, Chapter 17).

B. **Radiation therapy**
   1. **Primary plasma cell neoplasms.** The role of radiation therapy in the treatment of primary PCNs is limited to the following circumstances:
      a. **Solitary plasmacytomas.** Local radiation therapy **(4500–5000 cGy over 4–5 weeks)** directed at solitary plasmacytomas may provide significant palliation and produce **10-year survival rates as high as 80% in the 7% of patients** who present with this entity. Some are resistant to irradiation and

later develop resistance to chemotherapy as well. Myeloma protein levels should decrease during the treatment of the local disease.

   b. **Large osteolytic lesions.** Modest doses of radiation **(2000–2400 cGy over 1–1.5 weeks)** are highly effective in **relieving pain,** arresting localized progression of disease, and restoring functional activity. Higher doses generally deliver no additional benefit. Specific indications include **proptosis or CNS symptoms** from extensive cranial disease and **dental** or **facial symptoms** from involvement of the facial bones.

   c. **Spinal cord compression** (see p 102, **III**).

2. **Recurrent plasma cell neoplasms.** Relapsing PCNs that no longer respond to standard chemotherapy can be treated with the following salvage applications of radiotherapy:

   a. **Hemicorporal radiotherapy.** Sequential irradiation **(750–850 cGy over 5 days)** of the lower and upper body has been attempted initially as **salvage therapy** and subsequently as consolidation therapy after the tumor regresses more than 75% ("complete" response). The results are not encouraging and are inferior to maintenance chemotherapy.

   b. **Bone marrow transplantation (BMT).** Myeloablative therapy in preparation for autologous or allogenic BMT often involves a combination of radiation therapy and chemotherapy.

C. **Chemotherapy**

1. **Primary plasma cell neoplasms**. Most patients with PCNs requiring therapy are treated initially with systemic chemotherapy. Response rates to a variety of agents vary, depending on the aggressiveness of administration and the response criteria used.

   a. **Indications.** Chemotherapy is recommended for all PCNs, except monoclonal gammopathy of unknown significance, stage I multiple myeloma, and "indolent" or "smoldering" myeloma, which often are observed until disease progression occurs. Absolute indications for therapy include **bone pain, hypercalcemia, renal failure, severe myelosuppression, spinal cord compression, and a 2-fold increase in the myeloma protein level in less than 1 year.**

   b. **Induction chemotherapy**

      (1) **Single agents.** As initial therapy, simple regimens consisting of a daily or intermittent alkylating agent such as **melphalan** (16 mg/m^2 IV every 2 weeks × 4, then every 4 weeks; or 8 mg/m^2 PO every 3 weeks) or **cyclophosphamide** (1000 mg/m^2 IV or 250 mg/m^2 PO per day for 4 days every 3 weeks), with or without a glucocorticoid (eg, **prednisone**, 60 mg/m^2 PO per day for 4 days) have been used most often. **Carmustine** (100–150 mg/m^2 IV), and **lomustine** (130 mg/m^2 PO every 4–6 weeks), chlorambucil, procarbazine, azathioprine, doxorubicin, etoposide, cytosine arabinoside, and vincristine also have been tried. Response rates for **melphalan with prednisone (48–72%)** are generally better than those for **melphalan (14–59%)** and for **cyclophosphamide (48%)** alone. However, no regimen is curative, and **median survivals of 18–35 months** are typical.

      (2) **Combination chemotherapy.** Although numerous regimens have been evaluated, the most widely used are the **M2 protocol** developed at Memorial Sloan-Kettering Cancer Center (see Appendix D1),which contain vincristine, BCNU, melphalan, cyclophosphamide, and prednisone **(VMCP);** a combination of vincristine, carmustine, doxorubicin, and prednisone **(VBAP);** and the **Southwest Oncology Group** protocol of **alternating** VMCP and **VBAP.** The M2 protocol has not been proved to be superior to therapy with melphalan and prednisone (MP); however, in randomized clinical trials, the VMCP/VBAP alternating regimen has increased **response rates to 54% (vs 28–32% with MP)** and has prolonged **survival to 42–48 months (vs 23–29 with MP),** particularly in high-risk **Stage III patients.** The observed survival advantage is primarily the result of an increased number of responses in MP-unresponsive patients rather than of prolonged responses in MP-responsive patients.

   c. **Measuring responses.** Responses following cytoreductive therapy are associated with as much as a **90–99% decline in tumor burden** and are measured by the **reduction in myeloma protein,** as outlined below:

      (1) **Responding patients.** Responding patients must satisfy all of the following criteria:

(a) **Myeloma protein synthesis.** The rate of myeloma protein synthesis must decline to **less than 25% of pretreatment levels for at least 4 weeks** (for IgA and IgG3 synthesis, the rates equal the serum concentration; for IgG1, IgG2, and IgG4, the rate must be calculated with a nomogram).

(b) **Bence Jones proteins.** Urinary 24–hour globulin excretion must decrease to **less than 10% of pretreatment levels and less than 0.2 g per 24 hours for at least 4 weeks.**

(c) **Osteolytic bone lesions.** All osteolytic skull lesions must **not increase in size or number.**

(d) **Serum calcium.** This electrolyte must remain **normal.**

(e) **Hematocrit.** Myeloma-induced anemia must correct to a **hematocrit** of more than **27%.**

(f) **Serum albumin.** Myeloma-induced hypoalbuminemia must correct to a **albumin concentration** of **more than 3 g/dL.**

(g) **Additional data.** In nonsecretors and in patients with equivocal or incomplete data, additional evidence of response **includes recalcification** of osteolytic skull lesions and **normalization of** depressed nonmyelomatous immunoglobulin levels (IgG of > 4000 mg/dL; IgA of > 400 mg/dL; and IgM of > 200 mg/dL).

(2) **Improved patients.** Synthesis of myeloma protein declines in these patients to **less than 50% but to more than 25%** of pretreatment values.

(3) **Nonresponding patients.** These patients do not satisfy the criteria for either responding or improved status.

d. **Maintenance chemotherapy.** Despite several large cooperative studies of continued therapy with MP, **no efficacy** has been demonstrated for maintenance chemotherapy; thus, this form of treatment cannot be recommended at present.

2. **Recurrent plasma cell neoplasms.** Nearly **30–50%** of patients either (1) **do not respond** to first-line therapy or they relapse while receiving treatment (**refractory patients**) or (2) **relapse** after undergoing treatment (**relapsing patients**). Retreatment with the same drugs reinduces remission (> 50% reduction in myeloma protein) in **50–80%** of patients who **relapse after more than 6 months of remission,** although these second remissions only **last 8–11 months.** Refractory patients and those who relapse **within 6 months** of initial remission have a **poor prognosis.** The following therapeutic maneuvers may be helpful in salvaging these patients:

a. **High-dose glucocorticoids.** Alternate-day or pulse high-dose prednisone or **dexamethasone** produces consistent, albeit brief, responses in **40% of refractory patients.** This therapy is often combined with additional chemotherapy (VAD).

b. **Chemotherapy.** The combination of **vincristine** and **doxorubicin** with dexamethasone (VAD; see Appendix D1) may induce responses in **73% of patients** who **relapse** during or **within 6 months** following therapy and **43%** of previously **unresponsive patients.** All patients on this regimen also must receive H_2**-antagonists** and **trimethoprim-sulfamethoxazole** for prophylaxis of **ulcer and infection,** respectively.

c. **Hemicorporal radiotherapy.** Hemibody irradiation has been used for patients who are resistant to salvage chemotherapy (VAD) and have significant bone pain, but responses are uncommon (see p 543, **IX.B.2.a**).

d. **Bone marrow transplantation.** Autologous BMT (and allogeneic BMT in the rare patient with myeloma who is younger than 40 years of age) can be considered. However, this form of therapy is considered to be purely investigational and should not be attempted in any but experienced centers with approved clinical trials.

3. **Complications of plasma cell neoplasms.** Specific therapy directed at the complications of PCNs frequently reduces the morbidity and mortality of these diseases.

a. **Hypercalcemia.** High levels of **osteoclast activating factor** and cyclic adenosine monophosphate produce significant **hypercalcemia (> 11.5 mg/dL) in 25–33% of patients,** leading to nausea, vomiting, constipation, polyuria, dehydration, renal failure, changes in mental status, and, ultimately, to coma and death. Aggressive therapy is required to avert these complications and is outlined on p 87).

b. **Hyperviscosity.** This syndrome occurs in **5% of patients with multiple myeloma and 50% of those with Waldenström's macroglobulinemia.** Symptoms develop because of sludging and oncotic expansion of the plasma volume with **viscosities greater than 4.0** (normal < 2.0) and include **hematologic manifestations** (bruising, purpura, recurrent mucosal and retinal hemorrhage), **congestive heart failure,** and **neurologic problems** (fatigue, weakness, vertigo, papilledema, headache, confusion, transient paralysis, and coma). **Plasmapheresis (2–3 L/d for 4–5 days or until serum viscosity is < 4.0)** is an effective method of palliation until the primary PCN can be brought under control with chemotherapy. For patients who have an inadequate response to therapy, intermittent plasmapheresis may be required.

c. **Infection.** Because of impaired humoral immunity, neutropenia, and deficient bacterial opsonization, infection with encapsulated organisms (*Haemophilus influenzae and Streptococcus pneumoniae*) as well as *Staphylococcus aureus* and gram-negative organisms is a frequent problem in patients with PCNs. The **most common sites** of infection are the **upper respiratory and urinary tracts.** Oral (amoxicillin-clavulanate or cefaclor) or intravenous (vancomycin and ceftazidime) antibiotics may be necessary, depending on the severity of infection; however, **aminoglycosides should be avoided** because of the risk of renal impairment. Gamma globulin and pneumococcal vaccine have not proved to be useful.

d. **Renal insufficiency.** Renal disease occurs in **50% of patients** with PCNs and may manifest as (1) **acute renal failure,** (2) **proximal tubular defects** (renal tubular acidosis or the Fanconi syndrome), (3) **distal tubular defects** (renal tubular acidosis), or (4) **the nephrotic syndrome.** Factors that contribute to the development of renal insufficiency are **Bence Jones proteinuria, dehydration, hypercalcemia (nephrocalcinosis), hyperviscosity syndrome,** hyperuricemia, amyloidosis, renal plasma cell infiltration, pyelonephritis (*Escherichia coli* and *Proteus mirabilis*), and bladder atony. In addition to treatment of the underlying PCN, therapy includes **hydration (3 L/d),** allopurinol (during the first few courses of chemotherapy in Stage III patients), and prompt treatment of infections and hypercalcemia. **Plasmapheresis** for Bence Jones proteinuria and for hyperviscosity may reverse the azotemia.

e. **Coagulopathy.** Myeloma proteins may bind to coagulation factors II, V, VII, VIII, and X and act either directly as an **inhibitor** or indirectly to precipitate large quantities of coagulation proteins, leading to **purpura, ecchymosis, and mucosal (particularly epistaxis) and retinal hemorrhage.** Binding to **fibrinogen** and **platelets** also occurs to some extent.

f. **Myelosuppression.** Bone marrow replacement leads to **thrombocytopenia (15%), leukopenia (15%), and anemia (60%)** that may be mild or severe, causing symptoms of fatigue, weakness, abnormal bleeding, and an increased incidence of infection. Increased plasma volume in Waldenström's macroglobulinemia aggravates the anemia. Primary therapy involves treatment of the underlying PCN; however, supportive care with **transfusions, androgens** (testosterone enanthate 600 mg IM every 6 weeks or fluoxymesterone 15–30 mg PO daily), and **recombinant erythropoietin** (epoietin-a or Epogen; 150 U/kg IV or SC 3 times/wk) for anemia may be necessary. In addition, recombinant granulocyte colony-stimulating factor (G-CSF); filgrastim or Neupogen; 5–115 mcg/kg per day SC or IV) or granulocyte-macrophage colony-stimulating factor (GM-CSF); sarcogrammastim or Leukine) may be useful for treatment of febrile neutropenia.

g. **Cryoglobulinemia.** Cryoglobulins are usually **IgG or IgM myeloma proteins** that agglutinate in exposed areas of the body and cause acrocyanosis and Raynaud's phenomenon. The only known therapy is that directed at the underlying malignancy.

h. **Amyloidosis.** Fibrillar **"L-chain"** proteins are deposited in a wide range of tissues, generating symptoms such as **weakness, congestive heart failure, nephrotic syndrome,** hepatomegaly, paresthesias, carpal tunnel syndrome, macroglossia, periorbital purpura **("raccoon eyes")** with dependent head positions, and syncope in **15–20% of patients.** An **apple-green birefringence after Congo red staining** of a **rectal biopsy or abdominal fat aspiration** (19-gauge needle) specimen establishes the diagnosis in **60–85%** of patients. Although **colchicine** may be of some benefit, therapy aimed at the underlying neoplasm remains the only proved method of arresting progression of the disease.

    i. Neurologic complications. Spinal cord compression (10–15%), neoplastic meningitis, and a motor polyneuropathy associated with the POEMS syndrome may arise. Treatment of spinal cord compression and neoplastic meningitis is discussed on p 54. Furthermore, **carpal tunnel syndrome** and **sensorimotor polyneuropathy** secondary to amyloidosis occur.

  4. Morbidity and mortality. Several potential problems accompany the administration of alkylating agents and glucocorticoids to patients with PCNs.

    a. Second malignancies. Patients treated with alkylating agents are at a **93–230 times greater** risk of developing **myelodysplastic syndrome** or **acute myelocytic leukemia**. The risk is estimated to be **3% at 5 years, 10% at 8 years, and 11.2% at 10 years**. The risk is highest with **melphalan**.

    b. Myelosuppression. Although therapy for PCNs may aggravate a preexisting pancytopenia, bone marrow depression secondary to the PCN may diminish with therapy, thereby improving overall bone marrow function. Consequently, myelosuppression from PCNs is **not** a contraindication to chemotherapy.

D. Immunotherapy. Limited data (almost exclusively involving **interferon-alpha-2**) are available for this modality. Clearly, much research is needed before the usefulness of biologic modifiers in this disease will be known.

  1. Primary plasma cell neoplasms

    a. Induction immunotherapy. After initial reports of **50–69% response rates** in previously untreated patients given **interferon-alpha-2**, randomized trials demonstrated a **response rate of only 14%**.

    b. Maintenance immunotherapy. Interferon-alpha-2 (3×10^6 IU/m^2 SC 3 times per wk) after induction chemotherapy maintained a significantly greater number of responses than no therapy **(76% vs 41%)** at 27 months.

  2. Recurrent plasma cell neoplasms. Interferon as salvage therapy for patients with PCNs has not been fully evaluated, but early results are not encouraging: response rates of only **11–21%** have been achieved.

X. Prognosis

A. Risk of recurrence. Excluding the 20% of patients who do not respond to initial therapy, the risk of recurrence (disease-free survival) is only slightly better than overall survival. Nearly **90%** of all recurrences occur **within 2 years,** and all patients ultimately recur.

B. Five-year survival. The chance of 5-year survival depends on multiple factors. In general, patients with multiple myeloma achieve a **5-year survival of 21–32%** and a 10-year survival of less than 20%. Those with **medullary plasmacytoma** attain a **79% 5-year survival** and 51% are alive at 10 years, whereas **88% of those with extramedullary plasmacytoma live for 5 years** and 82% survive for 10 years.

C. Adverse prognostic factors. The following variables are associated with a poor response to therapy, brief periods of remission, and brief survival: **renal failure, serum beta-2-microglobulin higher than 5 mg/mL, serum albumin lower than 3.0 g/dL, serum LDH higher than 200 μ/L, aneuploidy greater than 75%, tritiated thymidine labeling index greater than 3%, low cytoplasmic RNA, myeloma cell mass greater than 1.2×10^{12}, lambda light chains** (rather than kappa), **IgD immunoglobulin** (rather than IgG or IgA), **and elevated CALLA titers** (common acute lymphoblastic leukemia antigen).

XI. Patient follow-up

A. General guidelines. High-risk patients and those receiving chemotherapy should be examined monthly for 1–2 years, every 3 months for an additional 3 years, then annually for evidence of relapsing disease.

B. Routine evaluation. Every clinic visit should include the following tests and procedures:

  1. Medical history and physical examination. An interval medical history and a thorough physical examination should be performed during each office visit. Areas for particular attention are on p 539, **VI.A.**

  2. Blood tests

    a. Complete blood count (see p 1, **IV.A.1**).

    b. Hepatic transaminases (see p 1, **IV.A.2**).

    c. Alkaline phosphatase (see p 1, **IV.A.3**).

    d. Calcium and phosphate (see p 539, **VI.B.1.d**).

    e. BUN and creatinine (see p 3, **VI.B.1.e**).

    f. Serum electrolytes (see p 539, **VI.B.1.f**).

    g. **Serum total protein and protein electrophoresis.** (see p 539, **VI.B.1.g**).

    h. **Twenty-four hour urine protein** (see p 540, **VI.B.2.d**).

    i. **Chest x-ray** (see p 3, **IV.C.1**).

C. Additional evaluation. Other tests and procedures that should be obtained at regular intervals (every 6–12 months) include the following:

    1. **Quantitative serum immunoglobulin level** (see p 540, **VI.B.1.i**).

    2. **Beta-2-microglobulin** (see p 540, **VI.B.1.j**).

    3. **Skeletal x-ray survey** (see p 540, **VI.B.3.b**).

    4. **Bone marrow aspiration** (see p 540, **VI.B.4.a**).

D. Optional evaluation. The following examinations may be indicated by previous diagnostic findings or clinical suspicion:

    1. **Blood tests**

        a. **5′Nucleotidase** (see p 2, **IV.A.4**).

        b. **GGTP** (see p 2, **IV.A.5**).

        c. **Protein immune electrophoresis** (see p 540, **VI.B.1.h**).

        d. **Cryoglobulin level** (see p 540, **IV.C.1.c**).

        e. **Serum viscosity** (see p 540, **VI.C.1.d**).

        f. **CALLA** (see p 540, **VI.C.1.e**).

        g. **UPEP** (see p 540, **VI.B.2.b**).

        h. **UPIEP** (see p 540, **VI.B.2.c**).

        i. **Computed tomography (CT).** (see p 540, **VI.C.2.a**).

    2. **Imaging studies**

        a. **Magnetic resonance imaging (MRI)** (see p 540, **VI.C.2.b**).

        b. **Myelography** (see p 540, **VI.C.2.c**).

    3. **Invasive procedures** (see p 540, **VI.C.3**).

REFERENCES

Barlogie B, Epstein J, Selvenayagan P, Alexanion R: plasma cell myeloma—new biologic insights and advances in therapy. Blood 73(4):865–879, 1989.

Chak, LY, Cox, S, Bostwick, DG, et. al. Solitary plasmacytomas of bone: treatment, progression, and survival. J Clin Oncol 5:1811–1815, 1987.

Dune BGM. Staging and kinetics of multiple myeloma. Sem Oncol 13(3):300–309, 1986.

Dune BGPI, Buzaid AC. Management of refractory myeloma. A Review. J Clin Oncol 6(5):889–905, 1988.

Kyle RA, Lust JA. Monoclonal gammopathies of undetermined significance. Sem Hematol 26(3):176–200, 1989.

Mandell, F, Tribalto, M, Cantonetti, M, et. al. Recombinant alpha 2_b interferon as maintenance therapy in responding multiple myeloma patients. Blood 70(suppl 1):247a, 1987.

Martinez-Maldonado M, Yiun J, Suki WN, Eknoyon G. Renal complications in multiple myeloma: Pathophysiology and some aspects of clinical management. J Chron Dis 24:221–237, 1971.

Oker MO. Multiple myeloma. Med Clin N Amer 68(3):757–787, 1984.

Sporn JR, McIntyre OR. Chemotherapy of previously untreated multiple myeloma patients. An analysis of recent treatment results. Sem Oncol 13(3):318–325, 1986.

Tobias, JS, Richards, JDM, Blackman, GM, et. al. Hemibody irradiation in multiple myeloma. *Radiother Oncol* **3**:11–16, 1985.

Yang JL, Perry CL, Asire AJ. Surveillance, epidemiology, and end results incidence and mortality data, 1973–1977. NCI Monograph 81–2300, 1981.

Zucchelli P, Pasquali S, Cognoli L, Ferrai G: Controlled plasma exchange trial in acute renal failure due to multiple myeloma. Kidney International 33:1175–1180, 1988.

66 Malignancies of Undetermined Primary Site

Robert B. Cameron, MD

I. **Epidemiology.** Malignancies of undetermined primary site (occult malignancies) constitute **0.5–9.0% of all cancers** and include all neoplasms with pathologically confirmed metastases but a primary site that cannot be determined by **medical history, physical examination (including stool guiaic), complete blood count, urinalysis, chest x-ray, and meticulous histologic evaluation.**

II. **Risk factors.** Although risk factors depend on the primary site of the tumor (whether known or occult), data support the following generalizations:
   A. **Age.** The **median age** at presentation is **56–60 years** of age.
   B. **Sex.** There is no apparent sex predilection.
   C. **Race.** There is no racial preponderance.
   D. **Genetic factors.** No genetic predisposition has been identified, and first-degree relatives are not at increased risk.
   E. **Previous pathology.** A previous diagnosis of **cancer** is present in **10% of patients.**
   F. **Diet.** No dietary factors have been recognized.
   G. **Tobacco.** Tobacco is associated with the development of squamous cell carcinoma of the head and neck region that may present as cervical metastases of unknown origin (see Chapter 26).
   H. **Urbanization.** There is no propensity for occult malignancies in either urban or rural populations.

III. **Presentation**
   A. **Signs and symptoms.** Although **1–3% of patients** with occult cancer are **asymptomatic,** the vast majority (> 95%) present with signs and symptoms from specific metastases.
      1. **Local manifestations.** Patients often complain of **jaundice, abdominal distention, and abdominal masses (26–47%);** hemptysis, dyspnea, and chest x-ray abnormalities (18–27%); lymphadenopathy (11–26%), bone pain or fracture (6–26%); seizures and other neurologic symptoms (0–17%); and dermal abnormalities (0–2%).
      2. **Systemic manifestations.** Fatigue, malaise, anorexia, **weight loss,** and cachexia are common findings in patients with advanced (metastatic) cancer.
   B. **Paraneoplastic syndromes.** Although any paraneoplastic syndrome may occur in patients with occult cancer, the following symptom complexes are particularly associated with occult malignancies and may be the sole manifestation of disease.
      1. **Fever of unknown origin** (see p 99).
      2. **Migratory thrombophlebitis** (see p 81).

IV. **Differential diagnosis.** The differential diagnosis of **a mass lesion** depends on its size, consistency, and location and on the patient's age. Because malignancies with undetermined primary sites can arise essentially anywhere in the body, the diagnostic possibilities are practically limitless and cannot be elaborated easily.

V. **Screening programs.** Other than annual physical examinations, screening programs are impractical.

VI. **Diagnostic workup**
   A. **Medical history and physical examination.** A complete medical history (emphasizing common presenting symptoms) and a thorough physical examination are essential components of a complete assessment.
      1. **General appearance.** An assessment of the patient's functional and nutritional status should be made.
      2. **Skin.** Pallor (indicating anemia), suspicious **nevi** or lesions, and other characteristic findings of underlying malignancy (see Chapter 18) should be noted.

    3. **Head and neck.** A thorough head and neck examination, including direct palpation of the entire oral cavity and thyroid gland as well as laryngoscopy are required, especially in patients with palpable **cervical adenopathy.**

    4. **Lymph nodes.** Significant cervical, supraclavicular, axillary, epitrochlear, and inguinal adenopathy must be described, particularly the presence of an isolated left supraclavicular **(signal, Virchow's, or Troisier's node)** or axillary lymph node (such as **Irish's node; see p 233, VI.A.3**) that may signify a visceral or breast cancer.

    5. **Breasts.** A complete breast examination may reveal a **breast mass,** nipple discharge, or other skin or nipple changes that suggest a primary breast malignancy.

    6. **Chest.** Meticulous auscultation and percussion of the lungs may disclose evidence of pleural effusions, pulmonary consolidation, atelectasis, and other pulmonary pathology.

    7. **Abdomen.** Careful examination may reveal hepatomegaly, splenomegaly, or an abdominal mass caused by primary tumor or lymphadenopathy.

    8. **Pelvis.** All female patients should have a thorough speculum and bimanual pelvic examination, including Papanicolou cervicovaginal cytology to exclude gynecologic neoplasms.

    9. **Rectum.** Careful palpation of the prostate (male) and pelvic reproductive organs (female) is essential. Furthermore, rectal masses and occult fecal blood are important findings.

   10. **Extremities.** Edema from venous or lymphatic obstruction, soft tissue or bone masses, and thrombophlebitis may provide diagnostic clues about the site of occult cancer.

   11. **Nerves.** The nature and extent of neurologic deficits should be documented and are crucial in the diagnosis and management of patients with malignancies of undetermined origin.

B. Primary tests and procedures. In general, the following diagnostic tests and procedures must be obtained in all patients before designating the malignancy as one of an undetermined primary site (occult neoplasm); in practice, however, the exact diagnostic needs must be balanced with consideration of the expense and therapeutic implications of the individual studies.

    1. **Blood tests** (see p 1, **IV.A**)
       a. **Complete blood count.**
       b. **Hepatic transaminases.**
       c. **Alkaline phosphatase.**
       d. **BUN and creatinine.**

    2. **Urine tests.** Routine **urinalysis** may detect **hematuria** (see, also, p 3, **IV.B**).

    3. **Imaging studies.** A **chest x-ray** should be obtained (see p 3, **IV.C.1**).

    4. **Invasive procedures. Biopsy** of any abnormal mass identified on physical or radiologic examination must be performed and carefully reviewed to exclude a recognizable primary source of tumor.

C. Optional tests and procedures. The extent of the diagnostic workup should be dictated by the patient's **age, social situation, performance level, and extent of disease** as well as previous diagnostic findings, clinical suspicion, and the possible **therapeutic implications** of the various tests and procedures.

    1. **Blood tests**
       a. **5′Nucleotidase** (see p 2, **IV.A.4**).
       b. **GGTP** (see p 2, **IV.A.5**).
       c. **Calcium.** Because of overwhelming bone disease or parathormonelike substances, the serum level of this electrolyte may be significantly elevated and require therapeutic intervention (see p 87).
       d. **Uric acid.** Neoplasms with rapid cell proliferation (and destruction) often raise the serum level of uric acid and threaten **renal function,** necessitating treatment (see p 84).

    2. **Imaging studies**
       a. **Computed tomography.** As a single screening test, a CT scan of the chest and abdomen may provide the most information about the etiology of malignancies of undetermined primary site.
       b. **Magnetic resonance imaging (MRI)** (see p 3, **IV.C.3**).
       c. **Technetium-99m bone scan** (see p 3, **IV.C.5**).
       d. **Upper gastrointestinal (UGI) series.** Although frequently ordered, this radiologic study, in the absence of significant and specific symptoms, yields a diagnosis in **less than 10% of patients.**

      e. Barium enema. Like UGI series, this common test is fruitless in the vast majority of patients in the absence of specific symptoms.

      f. Intravenous pyelogram (IVP). Substantial **hematuria** is a valid indication for IVP, although **abdominal CT scan** may be preferred because it affords superior resolution.

      g. Mammography. Unless isolated axillary lymph node metastases are present in females, **mammography generally is not indicated.**

VII. Pathology

A. Location. Although **only 10–15% of primary tumor locations are ultimately identified,** certain generalizations exist regarding occult malignancies that manifest with the following sites of disease:

1. **Head and neck.** The majority (> 80%) of malignant cervical masses, particularly in the **upper anterior triangle,** signify local metastatic spread from primary head and neck tumors, 5–10% of which remain occult even after extensive evaluation (see Chapter 26). Histologically, **50%** of tumors exhibit features of **squamous cell carcinoma,** whereas **25% are undifferentiated** and 25% appear to be **adenocarcinoma.** However, **supraclavicular and low cervical masses,** are most likely to represent distant metastases derived from distant **lung,** breast, and prostate (right side) or **lung,** breast, and intra-abdominal (left side) primary sites. In addition, **multiple posterior** neck masses often indicate **lymphoma** or, occasionally, **melanoma.**

2. **Axilla.** In females, **solitary** axillary lymph node metastases from an otherwise occult primary neoplasm most often represent **breast cancer (70%),** even with a normal breast examination. **Estrogen and progesterone receptors** are important diagnostic and therapeutic findings in these patients. Furthermore, **gastric carcinoma** may present with a metastatic left axillary lymph node **(Irish's node),** and **melanoma** regularly produces axillary adenopathy that stains strongly for **S-100** protein.

3. **Thorax.** The most likely cancer to present with pulmonary nodules is **lung cancer,** particularly if microscopic examination reveals **squamous cell** histology. However, adenocarcinoma may represent metastatic pancreatic, breast, gastric, colorectal, renal cell, and hepatocellular carcinoma. Furthermore, **50% of pleural effusions** in adults are malignant and **20%** have no identifiable primary site.

4. **Abdomen.** Metastatic adenocarcinoma involving the liver is a common manifestation of a wide variety of malignancies (pancreas, stomach, colon rectum, lung, and breast) and may be accompanied by **ascites** in cancer of the ovary, pancreas, stomach, and colon. Occult fecal blood suggests a gastrointestinal source, but CT may demonstrate a pancreatic, renal, or ovarian primary lesion.

5. **Groin.** Although metastatic disease occasionally occurs in groin nodes and may represent neoplasm of the reproductive tract (40%), dermis (32%), anrectum (6%), bladder (3%), or other sites (20%), **occult** malignancies are rare and usually signify **lymphoma** or **melanoma.**

6. **Bone.** Prostate and ovarian carcinoma, carcinoid tumors, Hodgkin's lymphomas, and, in rare cases, small-cell lung cancer may produce **osteoblastic** bony lesions. In contrast, **mixed** osteoblastic and osteolytic lesions are typical of breast, kidney, lung, and gastrointestinal cancers, and multiple myeloma produces osteolytic lesions.

7. **Effusions.** Malignant **pleural** effusions as the sole manifestation of disease, although uncommon, may arise from lung, breast, pancreatic, and ovarian cancer. In addition, **ascites** may represent ovarian, pancreatic, gastric, or colon carcinoma. **Pericardial** effusion as the only evidence of lung cancer is extremely rare.

B. Multiplicity. The incidence of multiple lesions is unknown but is related to the site of origin.

C. Histology. The microscopic appearance and staining characteristics of occult cancers may provide invaluable evidence as to the location of the primary tumor. To optimize the available diagnostic information, however, the biopsy specimen must be submitted **fresh** for pathologic examination so that appropriate preparations can be made, including glutaraldehyde preservation (or Karnofsky fixative) for electron microscopy, liquid nitrogen freezing for immunohistochemistry, B5 fixative for immune peroxidase stains, and formaldehyde for routine permanent (hematoxylin and eosin) stains.

1. **Adenocarcinoma.** Representing **35–45%** of occult malignancies, this cell type may contain **signet rings** (suggesting a primary gastrointestinal, ovarian, or

breast lesion), **psammoma bodies** (implying a thyroid, breast, or ovarian origin), **estrogen receptors** (characteristic of breast, ovarian, and endometrial cancers as well as melanoma), **diastase-resistant periodic acid-Schiff-positive cells** (indicating gastric cancer), **mucin** (excluding renal cell carcinoma), and, occasionally, **cellular architecture** pathognomonic of well-differentiated colon, breast, renal cell, and thyroid carcinoma.

2. **Squamous cell carcinoma (SCC).** SCC constitutes **10–15%** of occult neoplasms and histologically appears to be similar, regardless of the primary tumor site. Metastatic cervical disease is most likely to originate from head and neck, lung, or esophageal neoplasms, whereas inguinal metastases arise most often from the cervix, anorectum, or penis.

3. **Undifferentiated carcinoma.** Accounting for **35–45%** of occult cancer, these malignancies can be classified as either large cell or small cell.

   a. **Large-cell undifferentiated cancer.** These tumors can represent numerous neoplasms, including adenocarcinoma, lymphoma, and melanoma. Furthermore, **germ-cell tumors** should be suspected in patients with large-cell **midline malignancies in patients 20–50 years of age,** especially if serum beta-human chorionic gonadotropin or alpha-fetoprotein levels are elevated.

   b. **Small-cell undifferentiated cancer.** These malignancies include **small-cell carcinoma**—which can originate in almost any organ but, most prominently, in the **lung**—as well as lymphoma, plasmacytoma, Ewing's sarcoma, amelanotic melanoma, and seminoma.

4. **Melanoma.** As many as **5%** of melanomas present with metastatic disease and no detectable primary lesion, and they represent **2–5%** of occult cancers. In many instances, the original lesion undergoes **regression** and is never identified.

D. **Metastatic spread.** The characteristics of tumor spread are directly related to the unknown primary tumor site and therefore are difficult to predict.

   1. **Modes of spread.** Occult neoplasms can spread by 3 routes.

      a. **Lymphatic metastasis.** Embolization through lymphatic channels leads to regional and distant nodal metastases.

      b. **Hematogenous metastasis.** Spread through blood vessels is a common sequela in patients with occult malignancies.

      c. **Direct implantation.** Malignant effusions (pleural, pericardial, and peritoneal) spread tumor cells throughout the body cavity and may lead to surface implantation.

   2. **Sites of spread.** Once metastases are detected, subsequent sites of disease often include the lung, liver, bone, and brain.

VIII. **Staging.** Because patients with malignancies of undetermined primary site present with metastatic disease from a variety of locations, a staging system would theoretically be difficult to devise and in practice would be of little prognostic significance.

IX. **Treatment**

A. **Surgery.** In general, surgery is not indicated in the treatment of occult malignancies except for peripheral lymph node metastases from occult squamous cell carcinoma of the **head and neck** (see Chapter 26) and **melanoma,** which may produce **25–50% 5-year survival.** Furthermore, metastatic adenocarcinoma that is isolated to the axillary lymph nodes of females (presumed **breast cancer**) necessitates upper outer quadrantectomy (not total mastectomy, as recommended previously) because this limited procedure detects nearly all identifiable breast lesions and yields a **20–25%** long-term survival. In addition, symptomatic distant metastases may be palliated successfully with simple excision in selected cases.

B. **Radiation therapy.** In addition to empiric radiation to **suspected primary sites** in metastatic squamous cell carcinoma of the head and neck, palliative radiotherapy may be indicated for many painful bone and soft tissue metastases.

C. **Chemotherapy.** If breast, ovarian, prostate, germ cell, or lymphoid malignancies are identified, appropriate chemotherapy should be instituted. However, cytotoxic agents do not improve the survival of patients who have other neoplasms (eg, adenocarcinoma, poorly differentiated carcinoma) and should not be administered routinely.

   1. **Single agents.** Numerous chemotherapeutic drugs, including **doxorubicin, fluorouracil, cyclophosphamide, methotrexate, mitomycin-C,** vincristine, and others have been given with reported response rates of **6–16%.** No impact on survival has been noted, however.

   2. **Combination chemotherapy.** Despite 3 randomized prospective trials of vari-

ous combination chemotherapy regimens, no consensus has been reached regarding the optimal cytotoxic management of patients with occult malignancies. Most combinations consist of doxorubicin, fluorouracil, mitomycin-C, or cyclophosphamide, or all of these. Initial **response rates of 40–70%** are common, but survival is unaffected. Furthermore, **toxicity may be substantial** and must be balanced against the likelihood of clinical benefit.

X. Prognosis

A. **Risk of recurrence.** Except for patients with melanoma, breast carcinoma, and head and neck cancer, more than **97%** of all patients recur **within 5 years.**

B. **Five-year survival.** Within the first year, **75–80%** of all patients with occult malignancies die, and the **5-year survival is less than 10%.**

C. **Adverse prognostic factors.** Although identification of the primary tumor site does **not** affect the overall prognosis, the following presenting features do imply a particularly poor outcome:

1. **Advanced age** (older than 60 years).
2. **Extralymphatic site of disease.**
3. **Poor performance status.** Patients with no symptoms or mild or severe symptoms (good, intermediate, and poor performance status) have reported response rates to chemotherapy of 75%, 19–42%, and 11%, respectively.

XI. Patient follow-up

A. **General guidelines.** Patients with occult malignancies should be examined monthly for 1 year, every 3 months for 2 years, every 6 months for an additional 2 years, then annually thereafter. The following specific guidelines for tests and procedures are recommended:

B. **Routine evaluation.** An interval history and a complete physical examination are mandatory during routine office visits. Special attention should be paid to the areas listed on p 548, **VI.A.** Because of extremely low yield, however, no laboratory tests, imaging studies, or invasive procedures should be performed on a routine basis.

C. **Optional evaluation.** The following tests may be indicated by previous diagnostic findings, clinical suspicion, or symptoms that are amenable to therapeutic intervention:

1. **Blood tests** (see p 1, **IV.A**)
   a. **Complete blood count.**
   b. **Hepatic transaminases.**
   c. **Alkaline phosphatase.**
   d. **5′Nucleotidase.**
   e. **GGTP.**
   f. **BUN and creatinine.**
2. **Urinalysis** (see p 3, **IV.B**).
3. **Chest x-ray** (see p 3, **IV.C.1**).

REFERENCES

Guarischi, A, Keane, TJ, Elhakim, T. Metastatic inguinal nodes from an unknown primary neoplasm: a review of 56 cases. Cancer 59:572–577, 1987.

Klausner, JM, Gutman, M, Inbar, M, et. al. Unknown primary melanoma. J Surg Oncol 24:129–131, 1983.

Lopez, R, Holyoke, ED, Moore, RH, et. al. Malignant melanoma with unknown primary site. J Surg Oncol 19:151–154, 1982.

Walach, N and Horn, Y. Combination chemotherapy in the treatment of adenocarcinoma of unknown primary origin. Cancer Treat Rep 71:605–607, 1987.

Wood, RL, Rox, RM, Tattersall, MHN, et. al. Metastatic adenocarcinoma of unknown primary site: a randomized trial of two combination chemotherapy regimens. NEJM 303:87–89, 1980.

67 Malignancies of the Liver

Cynthia A. Corpron, MD

I. **Epidemiology. Hepatoblastoma (HB)** and **hepatocellular carcinoma (HCC)** are uncommon, representing only **0.5–2%** of all pediatric neoplasms (the **10th** most common malignancy in children). Each year **0.16 cases per 100,000 children** are diagnosed. Estimates indicate that **120 new cases** will occur in 1993. Worldwide, HBs are more common in the **Far East** than in western countries.

II. **Risk factors**
   A. **Age.** The median ages at diagnosis of **HB and HCC** are **1 year and 12 years of age,** respectively. The majority of cases of HB occur in the first 18 months of life, whereas the age range for HCC is much wider.
   B. **Sex.** The risks of HB and HCC in **males** are **1.7 and 1.4 times** greater, respectively, than in females.
   C. **Race.** HB and HCC are **2.4 and more than 7 times,** respectively, more common in **whites** than in blacks.
   D. **Genetic factors**
      1. **Family history.** The risks of HB and HCC are not increased in first-degree relatives.
      2. **Familial syndromes.** An increased incidence of **HCC** has been reported with hereditary tyrosinemia, progressive familial cholestatic cirrhosis, glucose-6-phosphatase deficiency, and alpha-1-antitrypsin deficiency. Moreover, neurofibromatosis, telangiectasia, and familial polyposis also may predispose to **HCC,** whereas the **Beckwith-Wiedemann syndrome** is associated with **HB.**
   E. **History of previous hepatic pathology**
      1. **Infection.** HCC is strongly associated with **hepatitis B virus infection.**
      2. **Congenital anomalies. Extrahepatic biliary atresia** and **biliary cirrhosis** predispose to HCC.
   F. **Chemicals. Anabolic steroids** as well as maternal **alcohol** and **hormone** use may cause HCC. Furthermore, the chemotherapeutic agent, **methotrexate,** may induce the disease.

III. **Presentation**
   A. **Signs and symptoms**
      1. **Local manifestations.** HB and HCC most often presents as an **asymptomatic abdominal mass** (10% are noted on routine physical examination). Abdominal pain and associated nausea, vomiting, anorexia, and jaundice are more common with **HCC (50%).** Other findings include hemihypertrophy and tumor rupture precipitating an acute abdominal crisis.
      2. **Systemic manifestations.** Less common systemic symptoms include anorexia, weight loss (< 25%), and bone pain (metastases).
   B. **Paraneoplastic syndromes.** The following paraneoplastic symptom complexes may be the sole manifestation of disease.
      1. **Inappropriate gonadotropins.** This syndrome usually develops with HB (see p 117.
      2. **Erythrocytosis.** This may occur with HCC (see p 77, **I**).

IV. **Differential diagnosis.** HB and HCC usually present as an **asymptomatic abdominal mass.** The differential diagnosis includes diseases found in both children and adults as well as those that are specific to pediatric patients (see p 259, **IV**).

V. **Screening programs.** Because of the rare nature of HCC and HB, no screening programs (other than routine physical examination) have been developed.

VI. **Diagnostic workup**
   A. **Medical history and physical examination.** A thorough medical history should be obtained and a complete physical examination should be performed in all patients

with suspected HB or HCC. Particular attention should be directed at the following areas:

1. **Head and neck.** Scleral icterus should be noted.
2. **Lymph nodes.** The number, consistency, tenderness, and distribution of all cervical, supraclavicular, axillary, and inguinal lymph nodes must be carefully documented.
3. **Chest.** Decreased breath sounds, wheezing, and pleural rubs on pulmonary examination should be recorded.
4. **Abdomen.** Hepatosplenomegaly and all masses must be fully characterized.
5. **Rectum.** Stool should be tested for occult blood, and any rectal masses must be carefully described.
6. **Nervous system.** A thorough neurologic examination must be carefully documented.

B. **Primary tests and procedures.** The following diagnostic tests and procedures should be performed initially on all patients with suspected hepatoblastoma:
   1. **Blood tests**
      a. **Complete blood count** (see p 1, **IV.A.1**).
      b. **Hepatic transaminases** (see p 1, **IV.A.2**).
      c. **Alkaline phosphatase** (see p 1, **IV.A.3**).
      d. **Bilirubin.** This is elevated in **5% and 25%** of patients with **HB and HCC,** respectively.
      e. **BUN and creatinine** (see p 3, **IV.A.6**).
      f. **Alpha fetoprotein.** Although nonspecific, serum levels of this tumor marker are elevated in **40% and 67%** of patients with **HCC and HB**, respectively.
   2. **Imaging studies** (see p 3, **IV.C**)
      a. **Chest x-ray.**
      b. **Computed tomography (CT).** CT scan of the chest and abdomen is indicated to assess the primary tumor and to assess the lungs for metastatic disease. The functional status of the kidneys also may be evaluated.
   3. **Invasive procedures.** Any suspicious lesion, particularly in high-risk patients, should be biopsied (see, also, p 260, **VI.B.3**).

C. **Optional tests and procedures.** The following examinations may be indicated by previous diagnostic findings or clinical suspicion:
   1. **Blood tests**
      a. **5'-Nucleotidase** (see p 2, **IV.A.4**).
      b. **GGTP** (see p 2, **IV.A.5**).
      c. **Vitamin B_{12} binding protein.** This serum protein is elevated in the **fibrolamellar variant** of HCC.
      d. **Hepatitis screen.** HB_sAg, HB_sAb and HB_cAb should be obtained in patients with suspected HCC.
      e. **Beta-human chorionic gonadotropin (beta-hCG).** Serum levels of this hormone may be elevated in **3% of HB,** particularly if **sexual precocity** is present.
   2. **Imaging studies**
      a. **Magnetic resonance imaging (MRI)** (see p 3, **IV.C.3**).
      b. **Angiography.** Visceral angiography is important to **define the vascular anatomy** before surgery, particularly the origin of the **right hepatic artery** (from the proper hepatic or superior mesenteric artery).
      c. **Ultrasound** (see p 3, **IV.C.4**).
      d. **Technetium-99m bone scan** (see p 3, **IV.C.5**).
   3. **Invasive procedures**
      a. **Fine needle aspiration.** FNA may be used to assess suspicious supraclavicular or inguinal lymph nodes as well as lung, liver, and pelvic masses.

VII. **Pathology**
   A. **Location.** The **right** lobe of the liver is affected more often, probably because of its **greater size (70% of liver parenchyma).**
   B. **Multiplicity.** HB is almost always **unifocal,** whereas often HCC is **multicentric.**
   C. **Histology**
      1. **Hepatoblastoma.** Two types of HB exist: (1) a pure **epithelial type** containing fetal or embryonal cells, and (2) a **mixed hepatoblastoma type** consisting of epithelial and mesenchymal elements.
      2. **Hepatocellular carcinoma.** HCC is characterized by large pleomorphic cells. The **fibrolamellar variant** is characterized by **eosinophilic** hepatocytes, fibrous stroma, a **younger age** at presentation (mean age of **25 years**), and a **favorable prognosis.**

    D. Metastatic spread. The spread of HB and HCC is identical to that of HCC in adults (see p 261, **VII.D**).

VIII. Staging. Although no widely accepted staging system exists, pediatric HB and HCC can be staged according to the adult HCC TNM staging system (see p 261, **VIII**) or according to the clinical staging system proposed by the Children's Cancer Study Group, which is based on surgical resectability and is outlined below:

    A. Group I. Tumor is initially treated with complete resection by wedge resection, lobectomy, or extended lobectomy.

    B. Group IIA. Tumor is initially treated with irradiation, chemotherapy, or both and is rendered completely resectable.

    C. Group IIB. Residual disease confined to 1 lobe is present.

    D. Group III. Tumor involves both lobes of the liver.

    E. Group IIIB. Regional lymph nodes are involved.

    F. Group IV. Distant metastases are present (regardless of the extent of liver involvement).

IX. Treatment

    A. Surgery

        1. Primary hepatic cancer

            a. Indications. Complete surgical resection is the **treatment of choice** for both resectable HB and HCC (ie, tumor is confined to 1 lobe of the liver or involves both lobes but spares the left lateral segment and is free of extension into the hepatic vein and porta hepatis). Only **50% of HB** and **33% of HCC** are resectable by the time of presentation.

            b. Approaches. Tumors can be resected through a **bilateral subcostal** (chevron) incision or a **thoracoabdominal** incision.

            c. Procedures

                (1) Hepatic lobectomy. This procedure removes part or all of one hepatic lobe. In addition, **trisegmentectomy** removes the entire right lobe and the medial segment of the left lobe. Initially, the **liver is mobilized** and **control of the vena cava** is achieved. Next, the **porta hepatis is dissected** and the hepatic artery, portal vein, and bile duct to the diseased lobe are ligated. Then the liver capsule is divided and the substance is **dissected bluntly** (preferably with an ultrasonic surgical aspirator or "CUSA"). Blood vessels and bile ducts are ligated or clipped as necessary. Following resection, **hemostasis is obtained, drains are placed,** and the incision is closed. Modifications using hypothermia, generalized or isolated hepatic circulatory arrest, and hemodilution have not gained wide acceptance.

                (2) Liver transplantation. Although transplantation can be considered for otherwise unresectable HBs and HCCs, its use in resectable tumor has not yet been defined.

        2. Locally advanced and unresectable liver cancer. Resection of pulmonary metastasis with long-term survival has been described; however, because the true effect on survival is unclear, this approach cannot be recommended at present.

        3. Mortality and morbidity. The perioperative **mortality** for lobectomy ranges from **10–25%.** Frequent complications include **hemorrhage,** hypoglycemia, **coagulopathy,** hemobilia, **subphrenic abscess or biloma,** pleural effusions, and prolonged ileus.

    B. Radiation therapy

        1. Primary hepatic cancer. Radiation is not indicated as initial therapy for hepatic malignancies.

        2. Adjuvant radiation therapy

            a. Preoperative radiotherapy. In unresectable tumors, preoperative therapy **(1200–2000 cGy)** may increase the resectability rate. However, impact on survival has not been demonstrated.

            b. Postoperative radiotherapy. Following surgery, radiotherapy may decrease the incidence of local recurrence in the remaining liver parenchyma, particularly with HCC.

        3. Locally advanced and metastatic hepatic cancer. Radiation rarely provides palliation of symptoms from metastatic disease.

        4. Morbidity and mortality. If given preoperatively, radiotherapy may cause **failure of hepatic regeneration.** Moreover, radiation doses are limited by **radiation hepatitis.**

    C. Chemotherapy

1. **Primary hepatic cancer.** As the initial therapy in otherwise resectable hepatic cancer, chemotherapy is not widely advocated.
2. **Adjuvant chemotherapy**
   a. **Preoperative chemotherapy. Cisplatin** and **doxorubicin** may reduce tumor size and allow resection of initially **unresectable HB.** In addition, doxorubicin, etoposide, and fluorouracil may increase the resectability rate in **HCC,** but this has not been as extensively studied.
   b. **Postoperative chemotherapy.** In uncontrolled trials, alternating **VAC** (vincristine, doxorubicin, and cyclophosphamide) and **FAC** (fluorouracil, doxorubicin, and vincristine) **reduced** the historical **metastatic rate of HB from 64% to 6%.** A combination of cisplatin and doxorubicin also has been beneficial and is currently recommended for **HB.** For **HCC** a regimen of **doxorubicin, etoposide, and fluorouracil** may improve the results obtained with surgery alone.
3. **Locally advanced and metastatic hepatic cancer**
   a. **Single agents.** The following agents have proved to be active in the therapy of malignant hepatic tumors: actinomycin-D, **cisplatin,** cyclophosphamide, dacarbazine, **doxorubicin,** fluorouracil, and vincristine. However, because of the increased efficacy of combination regimen, drugs are rarely administered as single agents.
   b. **Combination chemotherapy.** Currently, most chemotherapeutic regimens are based on **cisplatin** or **doxorubicin.** Therapy with a combination of **cisplatin and doxorubicin** for **HB** and a regimen of **doxorubicin, etoposide, and fluorouracil** for **HCC** produces tumor regression in some patients with metastatic disease. Long-term survival, however, remains elusive.

D. **Immunotherapy.** The role of immunotherapy in hepatic neoplasms remains unknown.

X. **Prognosis**
   A. **Risk of recurrence.** Nearly all patients who fail therapy recur **within 1–2 years.**
   B. **Five-year survival.** Following complete surgical resection, 5-year survival rates for **HB and HCC are 60% and 33%,** respectively. The **fibrolamellar variant** of HCC, however, is more favorable, with a **62% 5-year survival.**
   C. **Adverse prognostic factors.** The following features portend a poor prognosis: **multicentric tumor and local recurrence.**

XI. **Patient follow-up**
   A. **General guidelines.** Patients with hepatic malignancies should be followed monthly for 1 year, every 2 months for the second year, every 6 months for an additional 3 years, then annually for evidence of tumor recurrence. Specific guidelines are listed below.
   B. **Routine evaluation.** Each clinic visit should include the following examinations:
   1. **Medical history and physical examination.** An interval medical history and thorough physical examination should be performed during each office visit. Areas for particular attention are discussed on p 553, **VI.A.**
   2. **Blood tests**
      a. **Complete blood count** (see p 1, **IV.A.1**).
      b. **Hepatic transaminases** (see p 1, **IV.A.2**).
      c. **Alkaline phosphatase** (see p 1, **IV.A.3**).
      d. **BUN and creatinine** (see p 3, **IV.A.6**).
      e. **Alpha fetoprotein.** This tumor marker can be followed for evidence of disease activity (see, also, p 554, **VI.B.1.f**).
   3. **Chest x-ray** (see p 3, **IV.C.1**).
   C. **Additional evaluation.** Other tests that should be performed at regular intervals **(every 3–4 months)** in patients resected for cure include a **computed tomography scan of the chest and abdomen** to exclude local recurrence and lung metastases.
   D. **Optional evaluation.** The following examinations may be indicated, depending on previous diagnostic findings or clinical suspicion:
   1. **Blood tests** (see p 2, **IV.A**)
      a. **5′-Nucleotidase** (see p 2).
      b. **GGTP.**
   2. **Imaging studies** (see p 3, **IV.C**)
      a. **Magnetic resonance imaging (MRI).** MRI may detect local recurrences as well as liver and lymph node metastases (see, also, p 3, **VI.B.3.d**).
      b. **Technetium-99m bone scan.** (see p 3 **IV.C.5**)
   3. **Biopsy.** A new mass that appears on imaging studies should be biopsied by

fine needle aspiration to confirm or exclude the possibility of recurrent or metastatic disease.

REFERENCES

Evans, AE, Land, VJ, Newton, WA, et. al. Combination chemotherapy in the treatment of children with malignant hepatoma. Cancer 50:821–826, 1982.

Exelby, PR, Filler, RM, and Grosfeld, JL. Liver tumors in children in the particular reference to hepatoblastoma and hepatocellular carcinoma. American Academy of Pediatric Surgical Section Survey, 1974. J Pediat Surg 10:329–337, 1975.

Giancomantonio, M, Ein, SH, Mancer, K, and Stephens, CA. Thirty years of experience with pediatric primary malignant liver tumors. J Pediat Surg 19:523–526, 1984.

Koneru, B, et. al. Liver transplantation of hepatoblastoma, the American experience. Ann Surg 213(2):118–121, 1991.

Ohaki, Y, Misugi, K, Sasakki, Y, and Tsunoda, A. Hepatitis B surface antigen positive hepatocellular carcinoma in children. Report of a case and review of the literature. Cancer 51:822–828, 1983.

Sitzman, J, Order, S, and Klein, J. Conversion by new treatment modalities of nonresectable to resectable hepatocellular cancer. J Clin Oncol 5:1566, 1987.

68 Malignancies of Bone

Joe K. McIntosh, MD, and Robert B. Cameron, MD

I. **Epidemiology. Ewing's sarcoma** is the **second** most common primary pediatric bone tumor after osteosarcoma (see Chapter 52). Annually, less than **0.2 cases per 100,000** children are diagnosed, and estimates indicate that **160 new cases** will occur in 1993. Worldwide, the incidence varies from regions of high incidence (United States and Europe) to areas of low incidence (Africa and China).

II. **Risk factors**
   A. **Age.** The incidence of Ewing's sarcoma rapidly increases from nearly 0 before age 5 years to a **peak** between the **ages of 10 and 18** years. After age 20, the incidence decreases again to nearly 0 by age 30.
   B. **Sex.** The risk in **males** is **slightly** higher than in females but **only after age 13.**
   C. **Race.** Ewing's sarcoma is particularly **rare** in **blacks** (both African and American) and in the **Chinese.**
   D. **Genetic factors**
      1. **Family history.** The risk in first-degree siblings is **not** increased over that of the other children, and no familial syndromes are associated with Ewing's sarcoma.
      2. **Genetic anomalies.** Anomalies of chromosome 22—eg, **(11;22) transloca-tion or deletion**—have been documented in **85%** of Ewing's sarcomas.
   E. **Previous bone pathology.** Certain congenital anomalies of the skeleton (**aneu-rysmal bone cysts** and **enchondroma)** increase the risk of Ewing's sarcoma (genitourinary anomalies such as hypospadias and duplication also are associated).

III. **Clinical presentation**
   A. **Signs and symptoms**
      1. **Local manifestations.** Most patients complain of **pain** and **swelling** in the area of the **femur or pelvis**, although any bone can be affected. A bony and soft tissue **mass** often can be appreciated and may be fluctuant and erythematous from **intratumoral hemorrhage.**
      2. **Systemic manifestations.** Fatigue, malaise, weight loss, and fever sometimes occur, and pulmonary masses (metastases) may be detected.
   B. **Paraneoplastic syndromes.** No paraneoplastic symptom complexes have been described in association with Ewing's sarcoma.

IV. **Differential diagnosis.** The differential diagnosis is that of a **bone mass** and is discussed with osteosarcoma (see p 407, **IV**).

V. **Screening programs.** No screening tests or procedures have been developed for this rare malignancy.

VI. **Diagnostic workup**
   A. **Medical history and physical examination.** A thorough medical history and a complete physical examination should be performed in all patients with suspected Ewing's sarcoma. Particular attention should be directed at the following areas:
      1. **General appearance.** An evaluation of the patient's general functional and nutritional status should be included (see, also, p 1, **I** and **III**).
      2. **Lymph nodes.** The number, consistency, tenderness, and distribution of all cervical, supraclavicular, axillary, and inguinal lymph nodes must be carefully documented.
      3. **Chest.** Evidence of pleural effusions and pulmonary metastases (eg, decreased or absent breath sounds, pleural friction rub) should be excluded on pulmonary examination.
      4. **Abdomen.** Hepatosplenomegaly, ascites, and all masses must be fully described.
      5. **Pelvis.** Palpation of as much of the pelvis as possible is mandatory, noting **masses, areas of tenderness**, and so forth.

6. **Extremities.** A thorough skeletal examination, including range of motion testing, is imperative.
7. **Nervous system.** A thorough neurologic examination must be carefully documented.

B. **Primary tests and procedures.** The following diagnostic tests and procedures should be performed initially on all patients with suspected Ewing's sarcoma.

1. **Blood tests**
   a. **Complete blood count** (see p 1, **IV.A.1**).
   b. **Hepatic transaminases** (see p 1, **IV.A.2**).
   c. **Alkaline phosphatase** (see p 1, **IV.A.3**).
   d. **Lactate dehydrogenase.** Elevated serum levels of this enzyme correlate with the presence and extent of metastatic disease.

2. **Imaging studies**
   a. **Chest x-ray** (see p 3, **IV.C.1**).
   b. **Computed tomography (CT).** CT scan of the area of the suspected neoplasm (eg, pelvis, extremity, head) and the chest is vital to document the size and location of the mass, its relationship to neighboring structures, and the presence of metastatic disease (pulmonary). In the presence of neurologic symptoms, a head CT also is indicated.
   c. **Technetium-99m bone scan** (see p 3, **IV.C.5**).

3. **Invasive procedures**
   a. **Bone marrow aspiration and biopsy.** Aspiration and biopsy of a sample of bone marrow at a site distant from the tumor is mandatory to exclude metastatic disease.
   b. **Biopsy.** An incisional or needle biopsy of the tumor mass is critical for the diagnosis of Ewing's sarcoma. If a **soft tissue** component is present, biopsy of this area is generally more reliable (see, also, **IX.A.1.c.[1]**).

C. **Optional tests and procedures.** The following examinations may be indicated by previous diagnostic findings or clinical suspicion:

1. **Blood tests** (see p 2, **IV.A**)
   a. **5′-Nucleotidase.**
   b. **GGTP.**

2. **Magnetic resonance imaging (MRI)** (see p 3, **IV.C.3**).

3. **Invasive procedures. Fine needle aspiration** can be used to assess suspicious supraclavicular or inguinal lymph nodes as well as lung, liver, and pelvic masses.

VII. **Pathology**

A. **Location.** The most common sites of Ewing's sarcoma are **pelvis (21%), femur (21%), fibula (12%), tibia (11%), humerus (11%)**, ribs (7%), vertebrae (5%), scapula (4%), skull (3%), and all other sites (< 2% each).

B. **Multiplicity.** Ewing's sarcoma is **rarely multicentric**.

C. **Histology.** The diagnosis of Ewing's sarcoma is one of **exclusion**. Other small round-cell neoplasms (small-cell osteosarcoma, rhabdomyosarcoma, neuroblastoma, and lymphoma) must be eliminated. A **striking vascularity, necrosis, and a biphasic population of large clear and small dark cells are characteristic**. These periodic acid-Schiff stain positive cells also exhibit stippled nuclei, faint nucleoli, and absent cytoplasmic organelles.

D. **Metastatic spread**

1. **Modes of spread**
   a. **Direct extension.** Ewing's sarcoma may directly invade contiguous structures and soft tissue.
   b. **Lymphatic metastasis.** Occasionally, Ewing's sarcoma may metastasize to regional lymph nodes.
   c. **Hematogenous metastasis.** Ewing's sarcoma typically has spread through vascular channels to distant sites in **50%** of patients by the time of presentation.

2. **Sites of spread.** Distant sites commonly involved with metastatic Ewing's sarcoma consist of **lung,** bone (including bone marrow), and central nervous system (1–5%).

VIII. **Staging.** No widely accepted staging system has been developed for Ewing's sarcoma.

IX. **Treatment.** All patients with Ewing's sarcoma, even those with distant metastases, should be treated with curative intent.

A. **Surgery**

1. **Primary Ewing's sarcoma**
   a. **Indications.** Advances in radiation therapy and a recent emphasis on func-

tional preservation as well as tumor control have reduced the role of surgery in the treatment of Ewing's sarcoma. Currently, primary surgical resection (usually after preoperative adjuvant chemotherapy) is advocated in patients with **pelvic** lesions and tumors of **expendable bone:** eg, fibula, rib, and tarsal bones. Furthermore, **amputation** is required for **pathologic fractures** and **infrageniculate primary tumors** that cannot be locally managed with irradiation.

   b. Approaches. The surgical approach varies tremendously, depending on the size, **location,** and extent of the primary tumor.

   c. Procedures

      (1) Biopsy. The technique for performing a biopsy on bone tumors is identical to that for osteosarcoma (see p 397, **VI.B.3.c**).

      (2) Radical resection. If surgery is indicated, removal of tumor with a margin of normal tissue is pursued **unless the functional deficit is excessive**. For example, primary **amputation** and sacrifice of peripheral nerves (eg, peroneal) should be **avoided** in Ewing's sarcoma of the extremities.

  2. Locally advanced and metastatic Ewing's sarcoma. Occasionally, isolated **pulmonary metastases** are amenable to surgical resection with improved long-term survival.

  3. Morbidity and mortality. The nature and severity of the complications hinges on the location and extent of the surgical procedure and include virtually any surgical problem.

B. Radiation therapy

  1. Primary Ewing's sarcoma. Ewing's sarcoma is especially **radiosensitive,** and radiation represents the preferred therapeutic modality for most lesions. Doses of **4000–5500 cGy in daily fractions of 200 cGy** alone may locally control **44–86%** of tumors. **If appropriate chemotherapy is added, local control** is achieved in more than **90% of the distal** and **60–80% of proximal** lesions (overall, 80–85%).

  2. Adjuvant radiation therapy

   a. Preoperative radiotherapy. Because of the high rate of local control with irradiation (alone and with chemotherapy), this modality has not been widely used.

   b. Postoperative radiation therapy. Following appropriate surgical resection of Ewing's sarcoma, irradiation is indicated only if **gross or significant microscopic residual disease remains**.

  3. Locally advanced and metastatic Ewing's sarcoma. Radiation therapy is often used in the treatment of distant metastases, particularly after systemic chemotherapy. **Prophylactic bilateral pulmonary irradiation** has been attempted but is **inferior** to systemic chemotherapy in preventing pulmonary metastases.

  4. Morbidity and mortality. Complications following radiation therapy are common and vary with the primary tumor site. If doses do not exceed 5000 cGy, severe **functional deficits** and **secondary malignancies** occur in less than **18%** of patients.

C. Chemotherapy

  1. Primary Ewing's sarcoma. Currently, **3–5 cycles** of chemotherapy are administered before treatment of the primary site with irradiation or surgery. This allows accurate assessment of the response to the chemotherapy. The regimens used are discussed below (see **IX.C.3**).

  2. Adjuvant chemotherapy

   a. Preoperative chemotherapy. Initial chemotherapy (3–5 cycles) is now **standard** in patients with surgical indications. Appropriate regimens are outlined below (see **IX.C.3**).

   b. Postoperative chemotherapy. Additional chemotherapy can be combined with radiation therapy if complete resection cannot be accomplished.

  3. Locally advanced and metastatic Ewing's sarcoma

   a. Single agents. Numerous chemotherapeutic agents are active in Ewing's sarcoma, producing the following overall response rates: **cyclophosphamide (50%); doxorubicin (40%);** and actinomycin-D, carmustine, etoposide, fluorouracil, and ifosfamide (30%).

   b. Combination chemotherapy. Combination therapy has been shown by multiple studies (Intergroup Ewing's Sarcoma Study, National Cancer Institute, and St. Jude Children's Research Hospital) to be highly effective. The most common regimens include **AC** (doxorubicin and cyclophosphamide), **VAC** (vincristine, actinomycin-D, and cyclophosphamide), and **VACA** (VAC plus doxorubicin). Typically, chemotherapy is followed by radiation to the primary tumor as well as to metastatic sites. Although the initial **rates of complete and overall response** are relatively high **(83–97%)**, only **25–79%** of patients remain **disease-free for more than 3 years.** Currently, new chemotherapeutic regimens for recurrent Ewing's sarcoma, such as ifosfámide and etoposide, are being investigated.

    D. Immunotherapy. No significant experience with this modality has been reported.

X. Prognosis

    A. Risk of recurrence. Although most recurrences manifest within 2–3 years, patients may continue to relapse as long as **15 years** after treatment.

    B. Three-year survival. The overall survival for all patients depends on the presence of metastatic disease and the site of the primary tumor.

        1. Localized tumor. Overall, more than **60%** of patients survive 3 years.

            a. Skull and spine, more than 95%.

            b. Ribs, tibia, and fibula, 60–70%.

            c. Femur and humerus, 50%.

            d. Pelvis, less than 40%.

        2. Metastatic tumor. Overall survival is less than **40%.**

    C. Adverse prognostic factors. In the absence of distant metastases, the following pathologic features portend a particularly poor prognosis.

        1. The tumor is situated in the proximal skeleton.

        2. The tumor is large (> 8 cm) and situated in the extremities. This reduces **5-year disease-free survival** from **72% to 22%** and increases **local** recurrence from **10% to 30%.** Pelvic lesions larger than **5 cm** diminish the **local control rate** from **92% to 83%.**

        3. Extraosseous extension decreases survival from **87% to 20%.**

        4. Serum lactate dehydrogenase is elevated.

        5. Filigree histology is present.

        6. The tumor responded poorly to initial chemotherapy.

XI. Patient follow-up

    A. General guidelines. Patients with Ewing's sarcoma should be followed every 3 months for 3 years, every 6 months for an additional 2 years, then annually for evidence of tumor recurrence. Specific guidelines are listed below:

    B. Routine evaluation. Each clinic visit should include the following examinations:

        1. Medical history and physical examination. An interval medical history should be obtained and a thorough physical examination should be performed during each office visit. Areas for particular attention are discussed on p 558, (**VI.A**).

        2. Blood tests

            a. Complete blood count (see p 1, **IV.A.1**).

            b. Hepatic transaminases (see p 1, **IV.A.2**).

            c. Alkaline phosphatase (see p 1, **IV.A.3**).

            d. Lactate dehydrogenase (LDH) (see p 559, **VI.B.1.d**).

        3. Chest x-ray (see p 3, **IV.C.1**).

    C. Additional evaluation. Other tests and procedures that should be obtained periodically (every 6 months) include the following:

        1. Technetium 99-m bone scan (see p 3, **IV.C.5**).

        2. Computed tomography (CT) (see **VI.B.2.b**).

    D. Optional evaluation. The following tests and procedures may be indicated by previous diagnostic findings or clinical suspicion:

        1. Blood tests (see p 2, **IV.A**)

            a. 5-Nucleotidase.

            b. GGTP.

        2. Magnetic resonance imaging (MRI) (see p 3, **IV.C.3**).

        3. Biopsy. In patients without known residual cancer, **biopsy** of any suspicious or abnormal mass detected on physical examination, chest x-ray, or routine blood testing is indicated.

REFERENCES

Enneking WF, editor. Limb Salvage in Musculoskeletal Oncology. Churchill Livingstone, New York, 1987.

Heare TC, Enneking WF, and Heare MM. Staging techniques and biopsy of bone tumors. Orthop Clin North Amer 20(3):273–285, 1989.

Kissane JM, Askin FB, Foulkes M, et. al. Ewing's sarcoma of bone: clinicopathological aspects of 303 cases from the Intergroup Ewing's Sarcoma Study. Hum Pathol 14:773–779, 1983.

Miser JS, Kinsella TJ, Triche TJ, et. al. Ifosfamide with MESNA uroprotection and etoposide: an effective regimen in the treatment of recurrent sarcomas and other tumors of children and young adults. J Clin Oncol 8:1171–1198, 1987.

Razek A, Perez CA, Tefft M, et. al. Intergroup Ewing's Sarcoma Study. Local control related to radiation dose, volume, and site of primary lesion in Ewing's sarcoma. Cancer 46:516–521, 1980.

69 Malignancies of the Soft Tissues

Joe K. McIntosh, MD, and Robert B. Cameron, MD

I. **Epidemiology.** The primary sarcoma of childhood, **rhabdomyosarcoma (RMS),** accounts for **5–10%** of all solid pediatric malignancies. Every year, **0.4 cases per 100,000** children are diagnosed, and estimates indicate that **275 new cases** will occur in 1993. Worldwide, the incidence of RMS does not vary substantially.

II. **Risk factors**
   A. **Age.** The incidence of RMS is **bimodal,** peaking at **2–6 years** of age (genitourinary and head and neck tumors) and again at **14–18 years** (particularly alveolar RMS).
   B. **Sex.** The risk in **males** is **1.2 times** greater than in females.
   C. **Race.** The incidence in **blacks** is **slightly** higher than in whites.
   D. **Genetic factors**
      1. **Family history.** The risk of RMS in first-degree relatives is not increased, although siblings with brain and adrenal cortical cancers may be at higher risk than are normal children.
      2. **Familial syndromes.** Some inherited disorders are associated with an excessive risk of RMS, including **basal cell nevus syndrome** and **neurofibromatosis.**
      3. **Chromosomal anomalies.** Abnormalities of chromosome **3p, t(2;13) translocation,** and the **N-*ras* oncogene** have been implicated in the pathogenesis of RMS.
   E. **Previous soft-tissue pathology.** Although trauma and chronic inflammation have been suggested as inciting factors in soft-tissue malignancies, no proof of this exists.

III. **Clinical presentation**
   A. **Signs and symptoms**
      1. **Local manifestations.** Most often, RMS presents as a **mass** with symptoms that vary with the location of the lesion, such as proptosis (orbit); ear pain or discharge, chronic otitis media, sinusitis, epistaxis, dysphagia, airway obstruction, and cranial nerve deficits (head and neck); pain suggesting cholecystitis or appendicitis and hyperbilirubinemia (abdomen); hematuria, urinary frequency, urgency, and retention and a scrotal or vaginal mass (genitourinary tract); and a soft-tissue mass (extremity).
      2. **Systemic manifestations. Dyspnea** and **pulmonary masses** (pulmonary metastases), **hepatomegaly** and **abdominal masses** (hepatic and abdominal lymph node metastases), and **bone pain** (bone metastases) may be present. Malaise, fatigue, weight loss, and fever also may occur.
   B. **Paraneoplastic syndromes.** No paraneoplastic symptom complexes have been described in association with RMS.

IV. **Differential diagnosis.** Diagnostic considerations vary with the location of the primary tumor and include disorders that produce masses in the **head and neck, genitourinary tract, abdomen, or extremities.**

V. **Screening programs.** No screening tests or procedures have been developed for this rare malignancy.

VI. **Diagnostic workup**
   A. **Medical history and physical examination.** A thorough medical history should be obtained and a complete physical examination should be performed in all patients with suspected RMS. Particular attention should be paid to the following areas:
      1. **General appearance.** An evaluation of the patient's general functional and nutritional status should be included (see also, p 1, I and III).
      2. **Eyes.** Both eyes should be examined for evidence of RMS of the orbit.
      3. **Lymph nodes.** The number, consistency, tenderness, and distribution of all cervical, supraclavicular, axillary, and inguinal lymph nodes must be carefully documented.
      4. **Chest.** Evidence for pleural effusions and pulmonary metastases (eg, decreased or absent breath sounds, pleural friction rub) should be excluded on pulmonary examination.

5. **Abdomen.** Hepatosplenomegaly, ascites, and all masses must be fully described.
6. **Genitalia.** A speculum and bimanual examination may reveal vaginal, scrotal, or bladder masses.
7. **Rectum.** Stool should be tested for occult blood, and perineal and rectal masses excluded.
8. **Nervous system.** A thorough neurologic examination must be carefully documented.

B. **Primary tests and procedures.** The following diagnostic tests and procedures should be performed initially on all patients with suspected rhabdomyosarcoma:
   1. **Blood tests** (see p 1, **IV.A**)
      a. **Complete blood count.**
      b. **Hepatic transaminases.**
      c. **Alkaline phosphatase.**
      d. **BUN and creatinine.**
   2. **Urine tests.** Routine **urinalysis** is indicated (see, also, p 3, **IV.B**).
   3. **Imaging studies** (see p 3, **IV.C**)
      a. **Chest x-ray.**
      b. **Computed tomography (CT).** CT scan of the area of the suspected neoplasm (ie, head, neck, thorax, abdomen, pelvis, or extremity) is vital to document the size and location of the mass, its relationship to neighboring structures, and the presence of metastatic disease (chest CT).
   4. **Invasive procedures.** Any suspicious lesion should be **biopsied** to exclude the possibility of RMS (see, also, **IX.A.1.c**).

C. **Optional tests and procedures.** The following examinations may be indicated by previous diagnostic findings or clinical suspicion:
   1. **Blood tests** (see p 2, **IV.A**)
      a. **5′-Nucleotidase.**
      b. **GGTP.**
   2. **Imaging studies** (see p 3, **IV.C**)
      a. **Magnetic resonance imaging (MRI).**
      b. **Technetium-99m bone scan.**
   3. **Invasive procedures. Fine needle aspiration** can be used to assess suspicious supraclavicular or inguinal lymph nodes as well as lung, liver, and pelvic masses.

VII. **Pathology**
A. **Location.** The most common sites of RMS are the **head and neck (38%), genitourinary tract (21%), extremities (18%),** thorax (7%), and abdomen and retroperitoneum (7%).
B. **Multiplicity.** RMS is rarely multicentric.
C. **Histology.** RMS can be classified according to either its histologic appearance or prognostic features.
   1. **Histologic classification.** On the basis of histologic appearance, **3 types** of RMS exist.
      a. **Embryonal rhabdomyosarcoma (60%).** Characterized by large acidophilic and undifferentiated round and spindle-shaped cells, this type includes the **botryoides variant** diagnosed by the pathognomonic **cambium layer of Nicholoson** (submucosal spindle-cell band).
      b. **Alveolar rhabdomyosarcoma (35%).** This type arises most often in the perineum and extremities and forms alveoli containing multinucleated giant cells similar to pulmonary alveoli.
      c. **Pleomorphic rhabdomyosarcoma (< 5%).** This type contains spindle and multinucleated giant cells.
   2. **Prognostic classification.** The **Intergroup Rhabdomyosarcoma Study (IRS)** categorizes RMS as favorable or unfavorable depending on histologic features.
      a. **Favorable rhabdomyosarcoma (82%).** Tumors that fail to fulfill the criteria of unfavorable RMS are considered "favorable."
      b. **Unfavorable rhabdomyosarcoma (18%).** This group of tumors includes an **anaplastic** variety (bizarre mitotic figures and diffuse nuclear hyperchromatism) and a **monomorphous** (uniform round cells) variety.
D. **Metastatic spread**
   1. **Modes of spread**
      a. **Direct extension.** RMS may directly invade contiguous structures and is surrounded by a **pseudocapsule.**
      b. **Lymphatic metastasis.** Overall, RMS, particularly **alveolar** RMS, metasta-

sizes to regional lymph nodes in **12%** of patients. The rate of lymph node metastasis also depends on the primary site: **scrotum (26%), genitourinary (20%), perineum (17%),** and extremities (10%).
- c. **Hematogenous metastasis.** In advanced disease, RMS typically spreads through vascular channels.
2. **Sites of spread.** Distant sites commonly involved with metastatic RMS are lung, liver, and bone (including marrow).

VIII. **Staging.** The IRS developed a clinical grouping system that ignores local tumor size and other characteristics that are incorporated into the TNM staging system adopted jointly by the American Joint Committee on Cancer and the Union Internationale Contre le Cancer. Both systems are outlined below.

A. **IRS staging system**
 1. **Group I.** Localized disease that is completely resected.
   a. **Group Ia.** Tumor is confined to the muscle or organ of origin.
   b. **Group Ib.** Tumor involves contiguous structures outside the muscle or organ of origin, such as through fascial planes.
 2. **Group II.** Regional disease is present.
   a. **Group IIa.** Tumor is resected without gross residual disease and regional lymph node involvement but **with microscopic** residual disease.
   b. **Group IIb.** Regional lymph node metastases are present but are completely resected **without microscopic** residual disease.
   c. **Group IIc.** Regional lymph node metastases are present and are completely resected but **with microscopic** residual disease.
 3. **Group III.** Tumor is **incompletely** resected, or biopsy is performed **with gross** residual disease.
 4. **Group IV.** Distant metastases are present.

B. **TNM staging system**
 1. **Tumor stage**
   a. **Clinical tumor stage**
     (1) **TX.** The primary tumor cannot be assessed.
     (2) **T0.** No evidence of a primary tumor exists.
     (3) **T1.** Tumor is limited to the organ or tissue of origin.
     (4) **T2.** Tumor invades contiguous organs or tissues, adjacent malignant effusion is present, or both.
     Note: T1 and T2 are subdivided into "a" and "b" for primary tumors no larger than 5 cm and larger than 5 cm in their greatest diameter, respectively.
   b. **Pathologic tumor stage**
     (1) **TX.** The primary tumor cannot be assessed.
     (2) **T0.** No evidence of a primary tumor exists.
     (3) **T1.** Tumor is limited to the organ or tissue of origin and is completely excised with histologically tumor-free margins.
     (4) **T2.** Tumor invades beyond the organ or tissue of origin and is completely excised with histologically tumor-free margins.
     (5) **T3.** Tumor invades beyond the organ or tissues of origin and is incompletely excised.
       (a) **T3a.** Microscopic residual tumor is present.
       (b) **T3b.** Macroscopic residual tumor or adjacent malignant effusion is present.
       (c) **T3c.** Surgical exploration only was performed; tumor was not resected.
 2. **Lymph node stage**
   a. **Clinical lymph node stage**
     (1) **NX.** Regional lymph node metastases cannot be assessed.
     (2) **N0.** No regional lymph node metastases exist.
     (3) **N1.** Regional lymph node metastases are present.
   b. **Pathologic lymph node stage**
     (1) **NX.** Regional lymph node metastases cannot be assessed.
     (2) **N0.** No regional lymph node metastases exist.
     (3) **N1.** Regional lymph node metastases are present.
       (a) **N1a.** Regional lymph node metastases are completely resected.
       (b) **N1b.** Regional lymph node metastases are incompletely resected.
 3. **Metastatic stage**
   a. **MX.** The presence of distant metastases cannot be assessed.
   b. **M0.** No distant metastases exist.

        c. M1. Distant metastases are present.
    4. Histopathologic grade
        a. GX. Grade cannot be assessed.
        b. G1. Well differentiated.
        c. G2. Moderately well differentiated.
        d. G3. Poorly differentiated.
        e. G4. Undifferentiated.
    5. Stage groupings
        a. Clinical stage groupings
           (1) Stage I. T1a–b, N0, M0.
           (2) Stage II. T2a–b, N0, M0.
           (3) Stage III. Any T, N1, M0.
           (4) Stage IV. Any T, any N, M1.
               Note: Each stage can be subdivided by tumor size, and NX should be considered N0 for Stages I and II.
        b. Pathologic stage groupings
           (1) Stage I. T1, N0, M0.
           (2) Stage II. T1, N1a, M0; T2, N0–1a, M0.
           (3) Stage IIIA. T3a, N0–1a, M0.
           (4) Stage IIIB. T3b–c, any N, M0; any T, N1b, M0.
           (5) Stage IV. Any T, any N, M1.

IX. Treatment
  A. Surgery
    1. Primary rhabdomyosarcoma
        a. Indications. Although radical surgery previously offered the only hope of cure, more conservative surgery is currently appropriate. In general, surgical excision is indicated in patients with RMS if resection **does not create a major functional** deficit, and it **decreases or eliminates the need for radiation therapy.**
        b. Approaches. The surgical approach varies tremendously, depending on the size, **location,** and extent of the primary tumor.
        c. Procedures
           (1) Biopsy. If complete tumor removal is impossible, **incisional biopsy and regional node sampling** (except in Stage IV disease) followed by chemotherapy, radiation therapy, or both is advocated.
           (2) Radical resection. Removal of the tumor with a margin of normal tissue is the preferred treatment for RMS particularly if no functional deficit results. Primary **amputation** currently is **avoided** for RMS of the extremities, although secondary amputation for extensive local recurrence after limb-sparing procedures may be necessary. Furthermore, orbital RMS responds well to biopsy followed by chemotherapy and radiation therapy and **rarely** requires orbital **exenteration.**
           (3) Regional lymphadenectomy. Meticulous dissection of the draining regional lymph nodes, including retroperitoneal lymphadenectomy for pelvic and genitourinary RMS, is **not indicated.** However, lymph node **sampling** is required to guide radiation therapy.
    2. Locally advanced and metastatic rhabdomyosarcoma. Occasionally, isolated **pulmonary metastases** may be amenable to surgical resection, with improved long-term survival.
    3. Morbidity and mortality. The nature and severity of the complications hinge on the location and extent of the surgical procedure and include virtually any surgical problem.
  B. Radiation therapy
    1. Primary rhabdomyosarcoma. Treatment of primary RMS with radiation (and chemotherapy) is indicated if complete surgical **resection is impossible** or would produce an **unacceptable functional deficit.** Radiation therapy, however, is not required for tumors that are completely resected (Group I). Doses of **5500–6500 cGy in 150–180 cGy fractions** covering wide fields (with appropriate chemotherapy) may control **75–90%** of primary RMS (90% of orbital RMS).
    2. Adjuvant radiation therapy
        a. Preoperative radiotherapy. Preoperative radiation (with chemotherapy) may improve the rate of resection as well as the functional results.
        b. Postoperative radiotherapy. Radiation doses of **4000 cGy** control more than 95% of **microscopic** (Group II) disease, whereas **5000–6500 cGy** in

150–180 cGy daily fractions yields local control in **75–90%** of patients with **gross** residual tumor. Moreover, **central nervous system tumor extension** in patients with parameningeal RMS may be reduced **from 15% to less than 5%.**

3. **Locally advanced and metastatic rhabdomyosarcoma.** Radiation therapy may be useful in the palliation of systemic disease, particularly painful **bone** metastases.

4. **Morbidity and mortality.** Complications after radiation therapy are common and vary with the primary tumor site. Specific problems following **orbital irradiation** include enophthalmus, keratoconjunctivitis, lacrimal duct stenosis, cataract formation, and photophobia. These require corrective surgery in **33%** of patients and **enucleation in 8%. Irradiation** of the **extremity** may cause limb length discrepancy, edema, lymphedema, skin necrosis, and functional limitations. **Head and neck irradiation** produces numerous facial, dental, and endocrine abnormalities.

C. **Chemotherapy**

1. **Primary rhabdomyosarcoma.** Chemotherapy as the initial therapy for resectable RMS is limited to specific circumstances (eg, orbital RMS), which have **high response rates** (> 90%) with chemotherapy (with or without radiation therapy) and **high morbidity (or failure) rates** with surgery. The regimens used are similar to those used with metastatic disease (see **IX.C.3** below).

2. **Adjuvant chemotherapy.**
   a. **Preoperative chemotherapy.** Chemotherapy before surgery may increase the resectability rate of borderline lesions and reduce any associated functional deficit. Chemotherapy regimens that are used are outlined below (see **IX.C.3**).
   b. **Postoperative chemotherapy. AC** (actinomycin-D and vincristine) and **VAC** (vincristine, actinomycin-D, and cyclophosphamide) are equally effective **(83–87% 2-year disease-free survival)** in patients without gross residual tumor **(Groups I and II)** and eliminate the need for adjuvant radiation therapy in Group I patients. Grade III and IV patients derive less benefit. The advantage of additional drugs (eg, doxorubicin) is controversial.

3. **Locally advanced and metastatic rhabdomyosarcoma**
   a. **Single agents.** Numerous chemotherapeutic agents that are active in RMS produce the following overall response rates: **methotrexate (50%); actinomycin-D and cyclophosphamide (40–45%); doxorubicin and vincristine (30–35%);** and cisplatin, dacarbazine, and etoposide (20–25%).
   b. **Combination chemotherapy.** Combination therapy has been shown to be superior to single agents. The most common regimens include **VAC** (National Cancer Institute), **VACA** (VAC plus actinomycin-D; IRS), and **VACAD** (VACA plus dacarbazine; St. Jude Children's Research Hospital).

D. **Immunotherapy.** No significant experience with this modality has been reported.

X. **Prognosis**

A. **Risk of recurrence.** After curative resection, the risk of recurrence is **43%** in patients with **unfavorable** or **embryonal** histology and **15%** in patients with **favorable** histology. Nearly all patients who recur do so within 2 years.

B. **Five-year survival.** Survival is largely determined by histology and stage.
   1. **Histology**
      a. **Favorable histology,** 89%.
      b. **Unfavorable histology,** 72%.
   2. **Stage**
      a. **Group I.** 80–95%.
      b. **Group II.** 70–85%.
      c. **Group III.** 40–70%.
      d. **Group IV.** 20–30%.

C. **Adverse prognostic factors.** The following pathologic features portend an especially poor prognosis: **alveolar histology, truncal and retroperitoneal location,** and **invasion of the central nervous system** (head and neck tumors).

XI. **Patient follow-up**

A. **General guidelines.** Patients with RMS should be followed every 3 months for 2 years, every 6 months for an additional 3 years, then annually for evidence of tumor recurrence. Specific guidelines are listed below.

B. **Routine evaluation.** Each clinic visit should include the following examinations:
   1. **Medical history and physical examination.** An interval medical history should be obtained and a thorough physical examination should be performed

during each office visit. Areas for particular attention are discussed on p 563, **VI.A**.
2. **Blood tests** (see p 1, **IV.A**)
   a. **Complete blood count.**
   b. **Hepatic transaminases.**
   c. **Alkaline phosphatase.**
   d. **BUN and creatinine.**
3. **Urine tests** (see p 3, **VI.B.2**).
4. **Chest x-ray** (see p 3, **IV.C.1**).
C. **Optional evaluation.** The following tests and procedures may be indicated by previous diagnostic findings or clinical suspicion:
   1. **Blood tests** (see p 2, **IV.A**)
      a. **5'-Nucleotidase.**
      b. **GGTP.**
   2. **Imaging studies**
      a. **Computed tomography** (see p 3, **VI.B.3.b**).
      b. **Magnetic resonance imaging** (see p 3, **IV.C**).
      c. **Technetium-99m bone scan** (see p 3, **IV.C.5**).
   3. **Invasive procedures.** In a patient without known residual cancer, **biopsy** of any suspicious or abnormal mass detected on physical examination, chest x-ray, or routine blood testing is indicated.

REFERENCES

Halperin EC. Pediatric radiation oncology. Invest Radiol 21(5):429–436, 1986.

Leonard AS, Alyono D, Fischel RJ, et. al. Role of the surgeon in the treatment of children's cancer. Surg Clin North Am 65(6):1387–1422, 1985.

Maurer HM, Beltangady, M, Gehan EA, et. al. The Intergroup Rhabdomyosarcoma Study-I. A final report. Cancer 61:209–220, 1988.

70 Neuroblastoma

Joe K. McIntosh, MD, and Robert B. Cameron, MD

I. **Epidemiology.** Neuroblastoma is the **fourth most common childhood malignancy,** accounting for **8–10%** of all pediatric tumors. Every year, **1 case per 100,000** children is diagnosed, and estimates indicate that **590 new cases** will occur in 1993. Worldwide, the incidence of neuroblastoma varies from countries with a relatively high incidence (eg, the United States) to regions with a correspondingly low incidence (eg, African countries).

II. **Risk factors**

   A. **Age.** The incidence of neuroblastoma peaks at **2 years** of age. Nearly **50%** of all malignancies in neonates **less than 1 month old** are NBs.

   B. **Sex.** The risk in **males** is **1.4 times** greater than in females.

   C. **Race.** The incidence in **whites** is **1.6 times** higher than in blacks. Moreover, **American blacks** are at substantially greater risk than African blacks.

   D. **Genetic factors**

   1. **Family history.** The risk of neuroblastoma in first-degree relatives is **slightly** increased.

   2. **Familial syndromes. Familial neuroblastoma** is a rare **autosomal dominant** disorder associated with multiple primary neoplasms and early presentation. Other inherited diseases that are associated with an increased risk of neuroblastoma include **Beckwith-Wiedemann syndrome** (hypoglycemia, macroglossia, omphalocele, and hyperplasia of the adrenal cortex, kidney, pancreas, and Leydig cells), **nisidioblastosis,** and **neurofibromatosis.**

   3. **Chromosomal anomalies.** In addition to trisomy 18, chromosomal abnormalities documented in neuroblastoma patients include **1p22 deletion,** chromosome 17 anomalies, hypo- and hyperdiploidy, **N-*myc* oncogene amplification (30%),** and N-*ras* and c-*src* oncogene expression. A **"2-hit" hypothesis** has been proposed to explain the behavior of neuroblastoma with both pre- and postzygotic chromosomal mutations.

   E. **Previous adrenal pathology. Neuroblastoma in situ** is present in all 20-week fetal adrenal glands and in many neonates and may predispose to the development of frankly invasive disease.

   F. **Chemicals.** Maternal ingestion of hair coloring **dyes,** some **medicines,** and even **alcohol** has been implicated in the pathogenesis of neuroblastoma.

III. **Clinical presentation**

   A. **Signs and symptoms**

   1. **Local manifestations.** Most often, neuroblastoma presents as a **large irregular abdominal or flank mass** that extends across the midline, a pelvic or posterior mediastinal mass producing respiratory or urinary symptoms, or a cervical mass often confused with lymphadenopathy but associated with **heterochromia irides** and **Horner's syndrome.** Neuroblastoma also may produce **sinusitis** (olfactory or **esthesioneuroblastoma**) and neurologic symptoms (cerebral neuroblastoma).

   2. **Systemic manifestations.** Skin lesions, hepatomegaly, ecchymosis, and proptosis may indicate metastatic disease.

   B. **Paraneoplastic syndromes.** The following symptom complexes have been described in association with neuroblastoma:

   1. **Blueberry muffin syndrome.** Neonates may develop firm **blue-tinged subcutaneous nodules** resembling blueberry muffins.

   2. **Opsoclonus-polymyoclonus syndrome.** Associated with a favorable prognosis, this syndrome includes acute cerebellar and truncal **ataxia** as well as **"dancing" eyes.**

   3. **Watery diarrhea, hypokalemia, achlorhydria (WDHA syndrome)** (see p 468, **III.B.6**).

IV. Differential diagnosis. Diagnostic considerations vary with the location of the primary tumor and include disorders that produce **head and neck, mediastinal, abdominal, and pelvic masses,** including Ewing's sarcoma, rhabdomyosarcoma, neuroepithelioma, and lymphoma.

V. Screening programs. No screening tests or procedures have been developed for this rare malignancy.

VI. Diagnostic workup

   A. Medical history and physical examination. A thorough medical history should be obtained and a complete physical examination should be performed in all patients with suspected neuroblastoma. Particular attention should be paid to the following areas:

   1. **General appearance.** An evaluation of the patient's general functional and nutritional status should be included (see, also, p 1, **I** and **III**).

   2. **Eyes.** Both eyes should be examined for evidence of periorbital neuroblastoma metastases.

   3. **Lymph nodes.** The number, consistency, tenderness, and distribution of all cervical, supraclavicular, axillary, and inguinal lymph nodes must be carefully documented. The association of **Horner's syndrome** and a **cervical "lymph node"** is **suggestive of neuroblastoma**.

   4. **Chest.** Evidence for pleural effusions and pulmonary metastases (eg, decreased or absent breath sounds, pleural friction rub) should be excluded on pulmonary examination.

   5. **Abdomen.** Hepatosplenomegaly, ascites, and all masses must be fully described.

   6. **Nervous system.** A thorough neurologic examination must be carefully documented.

   B. Primary tests and procedures. The following diagnostic tests and procedures that should be performed initially on all patients with neuroblastoma.

   1. **Blood tests** (see p 1, **IV.A**)
       a. **Complete blood count.**
       b. **Hepatic transaminases.**
       c. **Alkaline phosphatase.**
       d. **BUN and creatinine.**

   2. **Imaging studies** (see p 3, **IV.C**)
       a. **Chest x-ray.**
       b. **Computed tomography.** CT scan of the area of the suspected neoplasm (ie, head, neck, thorax, abdomen, pelvis, or extremity) is vital to document the size and location of the mass, its relationship to neighboring structures, and the presence of metastatic disease. Abdominal CT is extremely reliable for abdominal neuroblastoma with **calcifications** documented in **more than 85%** of patients.
       c. **Technetium-99m bone scan.**

   3. **Invasive procedures**
       a. **Biopsy.** Any suspicious lesion should be biopsied to exclude the possibility of neuroblastoma.
       b. **Bone marrow aspiration and biopsy.** Bone marrow should be aspirated and biopsied from both iliac crests to exclude the presence of bone marrow metastases.

   C. Optional tests and procedures. The following examinations may be indicated by previous diagnostic findings or clinical suspicion:

   1. **Blood tests**
       a. **5′-Nucleotidase** (see p 2, **IV.A.4**).
       b. **GGTP** (see p 2, **IV.A.5**).
       c. **Coagulation times.** The prothrombin and partial thromboplastin times, along with fibrinogen and D-dimer levels, should be ascertained in patients with advanced disease to determine if **disseminated intravascular coagulation (DIC)** is present.

   2. **Urine tests**
       a. **Vanillylmandelic (VMA) and homovanillic acid (HVA).** VMA and HVA together are elevated in > **90%** of patients.
       b. **Cystathionine.** This substance is increased in **more than 50%** of patients with neuroblastoma.

   3. **Imaging studies**
       a. **Magnetic resonance imaging (MRI)** (see p 3, **IV.C.3**).
       b. **[123]Metaiodobenzylguanidine (MIBG) scan.** This nuclear medicine scan images most NBs (see, also, p 463, **VI.C.2.d**).

   4. **Invasive procedures. Fine needle aspiration** can be used to assess suspicious supraclavicular or inguinal lymph nodes as well as lung, liver, and pelvic masses.
VII. **Pathology**
   A. **Location.** The most common sites of neuroblastoma are the **adrenal gland (40%), abdominal paraspinal ganglia (25%)**, thorax (15%; more common in children < 1 year of age), pelvis (5%; **organ of Zuckerkandl**), nasal cavity (**esthesioneuroblastoma**), and cerebrum.
   B. **Multiplicity.** Occasionally, multiple primary neuroblastomas arise.
   C. **Histology.** Derived from **neural crest cells,** neuroblastoma is made up of small round cells with abundant blue granules, Homer-Wright rosettes, calcifications, necrosis, and hemorrhage. Antibodies to cell surface antigens such as glycosphingolipid diganglioside (GD_2), CE7, KP-NAC8, 5G3, 6–19, Neurofilament, synaptophysin, NSE and UJ13A also may aid in the diagnosis. The histologic grading system proposed by Shimida is the most widely accepted, and correlates the presence or absence of stroma, the degree of differentiation, the mitotic index, and patient age with clinical outcome.
   D. **Metastatic spread**
      1. **Modes of spread**
         a. **Direct extension.** Neuroblastoma may directly invade contiguous structures.
         b. **Lymphatic metastasis.** Neuroblastoma may metastasize to regional lymph nodes.
         c. **Hematogenous metastasis.** Neuroblastoma typically spreads through vascular channels to distant sites in **50% of infants** and **75%** of older **children** by the time of diagnosis.
      2. **Sites of spread.** Distant sites commonly involved with metastatic neuroblastoma consist of bone (particularly **periorbital bone,** producing proptosis and ecchymosis), bone marrow, liver, soft tissues, and, in rare cases, lung.
VIII. **Staging.** Although the Evans and Pediatric Oncology Group (POG) staging systems have been most widely used, a TNM staging system adopted jointly by the American Joint Committee on Cancer and the Union Internationale Contre le Cancer attempts to unify the staging of neuroblastoma. All 3 systems are outlined below.
   A. **Evans staging system**
      1. **Stage I.** Tumor is confined to the organ of origin.
      2. **Stage II.** Tumor extends in continuity beyond the organ of origin but does not cross the midline with or without ipsilateral regional lymph node involvement.
      3. **Stage III.** Tumor extends in continuity beyond the midline with or without ipsilateral and contralateral lymph node involvement.
      4. **Stage IV.** Distant metastases involving the skeleton, soft tissues, distant lymph nodes, or all of these are present.
      5. **Stage IV-S.** Local Stage I or II tumor with distant metastases confined to the liver, skin, and bone marrow but without radiographic evidence of bone metastases.
   B. **POG surgical staging system**
      1. **Stage A.** Tumor that, grossly, is completely resected (negative or positive microscopic margins) with excised but histologically uninvolved intracavitary lymph nodes and normal liver (abdominal and pelvic tumor).
      2. **Stage B.** Tumor that, grossly, is incompletely resected but with lymph nodes and liver that are histologically uninvolved.
      3. **Stage C.** Tumor that, grossly, is completely or incompletely resected but with involved intracavitary lymph nodes and normal liver.
      4. **Stage D.** Distant metastases beyond the intracavitary lymph nodes (ie, bone, bone marrow, liver, skin, and distant lymph nodes or body cavities).
   C. **TNM staging system**
      1. **Tumor stage**
         a. **Clinical tumor stage**
            (1) **TX.** Primary tumor cannot be assessed.
            (2) **T0.** No evidence of a primary tumor exists.
            (3) **T1.** Single tumor no larger than 5 cm in its greatest dimension.
            (4) **T2.** Single tumor larger than 5 cm but no larger than 10 cm in its greatest dimension.
            (5) **T3.** Single tumor larger than 10 cm in its greatest dimension.
            (6) **T4.** Synchronous multicentric tumor.
         b. **Pathologic tumor stage**

(1) **TX.** Primary tumor cannot be assessed.
(2) **T0.** No evidence of a primary tumor exists.
(3) **T1.** Tumor excision is complete with histologically free margins.
(4) **T2.** This category does not apply to neuroblastoma.
(5) **T3.** Residual tumor exists.
    (a) **T3a.** Microscopic residual tumor.
    (b) **T3b.** Macroscopic residual tumor or grossly incomplete resection.
    (c) **T3c.** Surgical exploration alone was performed without tumor resection.
(6) **T4.** Multicentric tumor is present.

2. **Lymph node stage**
  a. **Clinical lymph node stage**
    (1) **NX.** Regional lymph node metastases cannot be assessed.
    (2) **N0.** No regional lymph node metastases exist.
    (3) **N1.** Regional lymph node metastases are present.
  b. **Pathologic lymph node stage**
    (1) **NX.** Regional lymph node metastases cannot be assessed.
    (2) **N0.** No regional lymph node metastases exist.
    (3) **N1.** Regional lymph node metastases are present.
      (a) **N1a.** Regional lymph node metastases are completely resected.
      (b) **N1b.** Regional lymph node metastases are incompletely resected.

3. **Metastatic stage**
  a. **MX.** The presence of distant metastases cannot be assessed.
  b. **M0.** No distant metastases exist.
  c. **M1.** Distant metastases are present.

4. **Histopathologic grade**
  a. **GX.** Grade cannot be assessed.
  b. **G1.** Well differentiated.
  c. **G2.** Moderately well differentiated.
  d. **G3.** Poorly differentiated.
  e. **G4.** Undifferentiated.

5. **Stage groupings**
  a. **Clinical stage groupings**
    (1) **Stage I.** T1, N0, M0.
    (2) **Stage II.** T2, N0, M0.
    (3) **Stage III.** T1–2, N1, M0; T3, any N, M0.
    (4) **Stage IVA.** T1–3, any N, M1.
    (5) **Stage IVB.** T4, any N, any M.
  b. **Pathologic stage groupings**
    (1) **Stage I.** T1, N0, M0.
    (2) **Stage II.** T1, N1a, M0.
    (3) **Stage IIIA.** T3a, N0–1a, M0.
    (4) **Stage IIIB.** T1–3a, N1b, M0; T3b–c, any N, M0.
    (5) **Stage IVA.** T1–3c, any N, M1.
    (6) **Stage IVB.** T4, any N, any M.

IX. **Treatment**
  A. **Surgery**
    1. **Primary neuroblastoma**
      a. **Indications.** Surgical excision is indicated in all patients with resectable cervical, mediastinal, and pelvic neuroblastoma. Abdominal disease, however, is usually not resectable because of encasement of major blood vessels and requires initial chemotherapy.
      b. **Approaches.** The surgical approach varies tremendously, depending on the size, **location,** and extent of the primary tumor.
      c. **Procedures**
        (1) **Biopsy.** If complete tumor removal is not possible (common with abdominal neoplasms), **incisional biopsy** followed by chemotherapy, radiation therapy, or both is advocated.
        (2) **Radical resection.** Removal of the tumor with a margin of normal tissue is the preferred treatment for neuroblastoma. This goal should be vigorously pursued unless encasement of blood vessels is present.
    2. **Locally advanced and metastatic neuroblastoma.** Resection of the primary tumor may prolong survival in patients whose metastatic disease is initially controlled with chemotherapy. In addition, **long-term survival of 75–80%** has

been achieved with secondary surgical resection of initially unresectable tumor following chemotherapy.

3. **Morbidity and mortality.** The nature and severity of the complications depends on the location and extent of the surgical procedure. The **mortality rate** associated with resection, however, should be **less than 10%.**

B. **Radiation therapy**
 1. **Primary neuroblastoma.** Radiation therapy has no defined role in the initial treatment of neuroblastoma.
 2. **Adjuvant radiation therapy**
   a. **Preoperative radiation therapy.** Preoperative irradiation (with chemotherapy) may improve the rate of resection as well as the functional results, although no data exist to support this belief.
   b. **Postoperative radiation therapy.** Radiotherapy **(2000–4000 cGy)** for residual local disease that does not involve regional lymph nodes is controversial; however, with lymph node metastases (Evans Stage III or POG Stage C), irradiation may improve **overall survival** from **33% to 84%.**
 3. **Locally advanced and metastatic neuroblastoma.** Radiation therapy may be useful in the palliation of systemic disease, particularly painful **bony** metastases.
 4. **Morbidity and mortality.** Complications following radiation therapy are common and vary widely with the tumor site.

C. **Chemotherapy**
 1. **Primary neuroblastoma.** Chemotherapy is indicated only in patients with **unresectable** primary lesions. **Surgery** remains the primary therapeutic modality for resectable localized disease.
 2. **Adjuvant chemotherapy**
   a. **Preoperative chemotherapy.** Chemotherapy before surgery may increase the resectability rate of borderline lesions, particularly abdominal and pelvic neoplasms and produce **long-term survival rates of 75–80%.** Chemotherapy regimens that are used are outlined below (see **IX.C.3**).
   b. **Postoperative chemotherapy. AC** (actinomycin-D and vincristine) and **VAC** (vincristine, actinomycin-D, and cyclophosphamide) are equally effective **(83–87% 2-year disease-free survival)** in patients without gross residual tumor **(Groups I and II)** and eliminate the need for adjuvant radiation therapy in Group I patients. Grade III and Grade IV patients derive less benefit. The advantage of additional drugs (eg, doxorubicin) is controversial.
 3. **Locally advanced and metastatic neuroblastoma**
   a. **Single agents.** Numerous chemotherapeutic agents are active in neuroblastoma, producing the following overall response rates: **cyclophosphamide (60%); cisplatin (45%);** ifosfamide, melphalan, and vincristine (20–25%); and dacarbazine (15%).
   b. **Combination chemotherapy.** Combination therapy has been shown to be superior to single agents. The most common regimens include **AC** (cyclophosphamide and doxorubicin) and **cisplatin plus VM-26** (St. Jude Children's Research Hospital), which produce as much as **70% overall and 50% complete response rates.** A **short interval (1–2 weeks)** between cycles is believed to be important for successful therapy because of the rapid growth of NB.

D. **Immunotherapy.** Although the administration of **bacillus Calmette-Guérin (BCG)** extract has not proven efficacious, radioactive **monoclonal antibodies** to neuroblastoma cell surface antigens (see p 571, **VII.C**) have produced some responses in patients with metastatic disease. This approach, however, remains experimental and cannot be recommended at present.

X. **Prognosis**
 A. **Risk of recurrence.** Most recurrences occur within 2 years. In addition, **2%** of patients younger than 2 years of age experience a **spontaneous regression or maturation** of the tumor.
 B. **Five-year survival.** Survival varies significantly with stage and age.
   1. **Age**
     a. **Age younger than 1 year,** 70–88%.
     b. **Age older than 1 year,** 30%.
   2. **Tumor stage.** The 3-year survival by POG stage is summarized below:
     a. **Stage A,** > 90%.
     b. **Stage B,** 80–85%.
     c. **Stage C,** 50–65%.

      d. Stage D, 30–48%.
- **C. Adverse prognostic factors.** The following pathologic features portend an especially poor prognosis:
  1. **Age older than 1 year.**
  2. **N-*myc* oncogene amplification.**
  3. **Diploidy.**
  4. **VMA:HVA ratio less than 1.5.**
  5. **High tumor marker levels.** Elevated levels of **serum neuron-specific enolase** and **ferritin** and increased **urine** levels of **cystathionine** portend a poor prognosis.
  6. **Abdominal tumor site.**
  7. **Bone metastases.**

XI. Patient follow-up
- **A. General guidelines.** Patients with neuroblastoma should be followed every 3 months for 2 years, every 6 months for an additional 3 years, then annually for evidence of tumor recurrence. Specific guidelines are listed below.
- **B. Routine evaluation.** Each clinic visit should include the following examinations:
  1. **Medical history and physical examination.** An interval medical history should be obtained and a thorough physical examination should be performed during each office visit. Areas for particular attention are discussed on p 570, **VI.A.**
  2. **Blood tests** (see p 1, **IV.A**)
     - a. **Complete blood count.**
     - b. **Hepatic transaminases.**
     - c. **Alkaline phosphatase.**
     - d. **BUN and creatinine.**
  3. **Chest x-ray** (see p 3, **IV.C.1**)
- **C. Additional evaluation.** Other tests and procedures that should be obtained at regular intervals include computed tomography scans (see p 570, **VI.B.2.b**).
- **D. Optional evaluation.** The following tests and procedures may be indicated by previous diagnostic findings or clinical suspicion:
  1. **Blood tests** (see p 2, **IV.A**)
     - a. **5′-Nucleotidase.**
     - b. **GGTP.**
  2. **Imaging studies** (see p 3, **IV.C**)
     - a. **Magnetic resonance imaging (MRI).**
     - b. **Technetium-99m bone scan.**
  3. **Invasive procedures.** In a patient without known residual cancer, **biopsy** of any suspicious or abnormal mass detected on physical examination, chest x-ray, or routine blood testing is indicated.

REFERENCES

Kretschmar CS, Frantz CN, Rosen EM, et. al. Improved prognosis for infants with stage IV neuroblastoma. J Clin Oncol 2:799–803, 1984.

Kushner BH and Helson LH. Coordinated use of sequential escalated cyclophosphamide and cell-cycle-specific chemotherapy (N4SE protocol) for advanced neuroblastoma: experience with 100 patients. J Clin Oncol 5:1746–1751, 1987.

Leonard AS, Alyono D, Fischel RJ, et. al. Role of the surgeon in the treatment of children's cancer. Surg Clin North Am 65(6):1387–1422, 1985.

Rosen E, Cassady JR, Frantz C, et. al. Neuroblastoma: the Joint Center for Radiation Therapy/Dana Farber Cancer Institute/Children's Hospital experience. J Clin Oncol 2:719–732, 1984.

71 Malignancies of the Eye

Joe K. McIntosh, MD, and Robert B. Cameron, MD

I. **Epidemiology. Retinoblastoma** is the most common ocular malignancy in children, accounting for **1–3% of all pediatric neoplasms**. In the United States, **0.3 cases per 100,000 children** are diagnosed each year, and estimates indicate that **225 new cases** will occur in 1993. Worldwide, the incidence of RB is not known to vary significantly.

II. **Risk factors**
   A. **Age.** The incidence of RB rises rapidly to a peak at **17 months,** and **90%** of cases occur in children **younger than 5 years.**
   B. **Sex.** The risk in **females** is **slightly higher** than in males.
   C. **Race.** The incidence in **blacks** is **slightly higher** than in whites.
   D. **Genetic factors**
      1. **Family history.** In sporadic RB, the risk in first-degree relatives is not increased.
      2. **Familial syndromes**
         a. **Hereditary retinoblastoma.** Hereditary RB is an **autosomal dominant** disorder with high penetrance that constitutes **40% of all cases.** Offspring of patients with hereditary RB (nearly all **bilateral cases** and 12% of unilateral cases) are at a **50% risk** of developing RB.
         b. **Other syndromes.** A rare syndrome of microcephaly, skeletal abnormalities, dysmorphic features, and mental retardation is associated in some cases with chromosome 13 anomalies and RB.
      3. **Chromosomal anomalies. Deletion** of the specific **RB locus, Rb-1, on chromosome 13q** has been identified in a small number of patients.
   E. **Previous central nervous system (CNS) pathology.** Bilateral RB is unusually common in some patients with **pineoblastoma (trilateral retinoblastoma)** because of a genetic defect in photoreceptors.

III. **Clinical presentation**
   A. **Signs and symptoms**
      1. **Local manifestations.** Because most children do not complain of pain or poor vision, the most common signs include **strabismus, leukocoria ("cat's eye" reflex), retinal detachment,** and **vitreous seeds.** Less commonly, proptosis and ocular inflammation may be present. In patients with a known family history, the diagnosis is often made during a screening examination.
      2. **Systemic manifestations.** Cervical adenopathy and other evidence of distant metastases are often present.
   B. **Paraneoplastic syndromes.** No paraneoplastic symptom complexes have been described in association with RB.

IV. **Differential diagnosis.** Diagnostic considerations include **retrolental fibroplasia, persistent hyperplastic vitreous, Coats' disease** (chronic progressive exudative retinopathy), **visceral larva migrans** (toxocara granuloma), and other ocular neoplasms (see p 145, **IV**).

V. **Screening programs.** With the exception of routine funduscopic examination, no screening tests or procedures have been developed for this rare malignancy. Genetic screening is not yet available on a routine basis.

VI. **Diagnostic workup**
   A. **Medical history and physical examination.** A thorough medical history should be obtained and a complete physical examination, including meticulous ocular examination, should be performed in all patients with suspected RB. Particular attention should be paid to the following areas:
      1. **General appearance.** An evaluation of the patient's general functional and nutritional status should be included (see also, p 1, **I** and **III**).

2. **Eyes.** Both eyes, including the entire fundus, should be examined by direct and indirect ophthalmoscopy. General anesthesia is occasionally required.

3. **Lymph nodes.** The number, consistency, tenderness, and distribution of all cervical, supraclavicular, axillary, and inguinal lymph nodes must be carefully documented.

4. **Chest.** Evidence for pleural effusions and pulmonary metastases (eg, decreased or absent breath sounds, pleural friction rub) should be excluded on pulmonary examination.

5. **Abdomen.** Hepatosplenomegaly, ascites, and all masses must be fully described.

6. **Nervous system.** A thorough neurologic examination must be carefully performed.

B. **Primary tests and procedures.** The following diagnostic tests and procedures should be performed initially on all patients with suspected retinoblastoma:

1. **Blood tests** (see p 1, **IV.A**)
   a. **Complete blood count.**
   b. **Hepatic transaminases.**
   c. **Alkaline phosphatase.**

2. **Imaging studies**
   a. **Chest x-ray** (see p 3, **IV.C.1**).
   b. **Computed tomography (CT).** CT scan of the orbit that demonstrates **calcifications** in **80%** of patients is virtually **diagnostic** of RB in patients **younger than 3 years** of age. CT also is imperative to document **orbital and intracranial extension.**

3. **Invasive procedures**
   a. **Biopsy.** All suspicious lesions should be biopsied to exclude the possibility of RB.
   b. **Lumbar puncture.** Cytologic examination of cells found in the cerebrospinal fluid may detect involvement of the central nervous system.
   c. **Bone marrow aspiration and biopsy.** Distant metastases to bone marrow can be documented by aspiration and biopsy of one or both iliac crests.

C. **Optional tests and procedures.** The following examinations may be indicated by previous diagnostic findings or clinical suspicion:

1. **Blood tests** (see p 2, **IV.A**)
   a. **5′-Nucleotidase.**
   b. **GGTP.**

2. **Imaging studies** (see p 3, **IV.C**)
   a. **Magnetic resonance imaging (MRI).**
   b. **Ultrasound.**
   c. **Technetium-99m bone scan.**

3. **Invasive procedures. Fine needle aspiration** can be used to assess suspicious cervical lymph nodes and lung and other masses.

VII. **Pathology**

A. **Location.** RB arises in the **outer retinal layer** and occurs with equal frequency in the right and left eyes.

B. **Multiplicity.** RB is **bilateral** in **75%** of patients with **hereditary** RB and **in fewer than 5%** of patients with **sporadic** RB. Moreover, **tumors often are multifocal; 4–5 discrete lesions** are present in **84%** of patients. **Second primary malignancies** such as osteo-, fibro-, and Ewing's sarcomas and Wilms' tumor arise in **15–20%** of patients with **bilateral** RB up to 40 years after diagnosis.

C. **Histology.** Small round cells with abundant dark chromatin and scant cytoplasm characterize RB. **Calcification, necrosis, perivascular infiltration, and Flexner-Winterstainer rosettes** also may be present.

D. **Metastatic spread**

1. **Modes of spread**
   a. **Direct extension.** RB may directly invade the **vitreous cavity (endophytic** growth) and produce vitreous seeding, the **subretinal space (exophytic** growth) causing retinal detachment and, occasionally, glaucoma, the **lamina cribrosa,** or both resulting in **meningeal** involvement.
   b. **Lymphatic metastasis.** Cervical lymph nodes are involved in advanced disease.
   c. **Hematogenous metastasis.** RB typically spreads through vascular channels.

      2. **Sites of spread.** Distant metastases may be detected in nearly **50%** of patients and may include bone (including marrow) and lungs (uncommon).

VIII. Staging. The American Joint Committee on Cancer and the Union Internationale Contre le Cancer adopted a joint TNM staging system that includes clinical and pathologic components. In addition, several other staging systems have been proposed, including the **Reese-Ellsworth** and **St. Jude's staging systems**.

    A. Reese-Ellsworth clinical grouping system
        1. **Group I (very favorable).** One or more tumors no larger than 4 disc diameters (6.4 mm) in size at or behind the equator.
        2. **Group II (favorable).** One or more tumors 4–10 disc diameters (6.4–16 mm) in size at or behind the equator.
        3. **Group III (doubtful).** Solitary tumor larger than 10 disc diameter (16 mm) behind the equator or any tumor anterior to the equator.
        4. **Group IV (unfavorable).** Multiple tumors, at least 1 larger than 10 disc diameters (16 mm), or any tumor extending to the ora serrata.
        5. **Group V (very unfavorable).** Massive tumor involving more than 50% of the retina or tumor with vitreous seeding.

    B. St. Jude's staging system
        1. **Stage I.** Tumor (uni- or multifocal) is confined to the retina.
          a. **Stage IA.** Tumor occupies no more than 1 quadrant.
          b. **Stage IB.** Tumor occupies less than 2 quadrants.
          c. **Stage IC.** Tumor occupies **more than 50%** of the retinal surface.
        2. **Stage II.** Tumor (uni- or multifocal) is confined to the globe.
          a. **Stage IIA.** Vitreous seeding is present.
          b. **Stage IIB.** Tumor extends to the optic nerve head.
          c. **Stage IIC.** Tumor extends to the choroid.
          d. **Stage IID.** Tumor extends to the choroid and optic nerve head.
          e. **Stage IIE.** Tumor extends to the emissary veins.
        3. **Stage III.** Tumor (regional) with extraocular extension.
          a. **Stage IIIA.** Tumor extends beyond the cut end of the optic nerve (including subarachnoid extension).
          b. **Stage IIIB.** Tumor extends through the sclera into orbital contents.
          c. **Stage IIIC.** Tumor extends to the choroid and beyond the cut end of the optic nerve (including subarachnoid extension).
          d. **Stage IIID.** Tumor extends through the sclera into orbital contents and beyond the cut end of the optic nerve (including subarachnoid extension).
        4. **Stage IV.** Distant metastases.
          a. **Stage IVA.** Tumor extends through the optic nerve to the brain.
          b. **Stage IVB.** Soft tissue and bone metastases (hematogenous) are present.
          c. **Stage IVC.** Bone marrow metastases are present.

    C. TNM staging system
        1. **Tumor stage**
          a. **TX.** Primary tumor cannot be assessed.
          b. **T0.** No evidence of primary tumor exists.
          c. **T1.** Tumor is limited to no more than 25% of the retina.
          d. **T2.** Tumor involves more than 25% but no more than 50% of the retina.
          e. **T3.** Tumor involves more than 50% of the retina, invades beyond the retina but remains intraocular, or both.
            (1) **T3a.** Tumor involves more than 50% of the retina, tumor cells are present in the vitreous, or both.
            (2) **cT3b.** Tumor involves the optic disc.
            (3) **pT3b.** Tumor invades the optic nerve as far as the lamina cribrosa.
            (4) **cT3c.** Tumor involves the anterior chamber, uvea, or both.
            (5) **pT3c.** Tumor is present in the anterior chamber, uvea, or intrascleral invasion is present, or all of these.
          f. **T4.** Tumor with extraocular invasion.
            (1) **cT4a.** Tumor invades the retrobulbar optic nerve.
            (2) **pT4a.** Intraneural tumor goes beyond the lamina cribrosa but not at the line of resection.
            (3) **cT4b.** Extraocular extension is present other than invasion of the optic nerve.
            (4) **pT4b.** Tumor is present at the line of resection, or other extraocular extension has occurred.

Note: "M" indicates multiple tumors; "f" labels cases with known family history; and "d" signifies diffuse retinal involvement without formation of discrete masses.

2. **Lymph node stage**
   a. **NX.** The regional lymph nodes cannot be assessed.
   b. **N0.** No regional lymph node metastases are present.
   c. **N1.** Regional lymph node metastases are present.
3. **Metastatic stage**
   a. **MX.** The presence of distant metastases cannot be assessed.
   b. **M0.** No distant metastases exist.
   c. **M1.** Distant metastases are present.
4. **Stage groupings**
   a. **Stage IA.** T1, N0, M0.
   b. **Stage IB.** T2, N0, M0.
   c. **Stage IIA.** T3a, N0, M0.
   d. **Stage IIB.** T3b, N0, M0.
   e. **Stage IIC.** T3c, N0, M0.
   f. **Stage IIIA.** T4a, N0, M0.
   g. **Stage IIIB.** T4b, N0, M0.
   h. **Stage IV.** Any T, N1, M0; any T, any N, M1.

IX. **Treatment**
   A. **Surgery**
      1. **Primary retinoblastoma**
         a. **Indications. Enucleation** is indicated for patients with advanced **unilateral** disease and either **glaucoma** or **optic nerve head involvement.** In addition, **radiation failure** (because of progression of the tumor or complications) necessitates surgery in **50%** of patients with **advanced** and **bilateral** disease.
         b. **Approaches.** A **transorbital approach** is universal.
         c. **Procedures.** Although conservative surgery may be possible in some patients, particularly after radiation therapy, radical resection (enucleation) is more common.
            (1) **Cryotherapy.** During this procedure, a small conjunctival incision is made and a probe is advanced under ophthalmoscopic guidance to the area of the tumor. The tumor is then observed to blanch as it is frozen. Clinical cure is attained in **95%** and **88%** of patients who have **small** primary tumors **(fewer than 4 disk diameters that are 6.4 mm) or have failed irradiation,** respectively. Vitreous seeding is not amenable to this form of treatment.
            (2) **Enucleation.** Enucleation includes removal of the entire **globe,** some of the **orbital contents,** and at least **10 mm of the optic nerve.**
         d. **Reconstruction.** An **ocular prosthesis** can be worn after **6 weeks.**
      2. **Locally advanced and metastatic retinoblastoma.** Surgical resection of distant metastases is indicated only in rare cases.
      3. **Morbidity and mortality.** In addition to hemorrhage and infection, complications are limited to the cosmetic and functional deficits (visual) associated with the loss of an eye.
   B. **Radiation therapy**
      1. **Primary retinoblastoma.** Radiation is often the preferred therapeutic modality because it usually both controls local disease and **preserves vision.** Typically, **3500–3600 cGy** is delivered over 4–5 weeks to the **entire retina,** including the **ora serrata** via lateral fields (avoids exophthalmia and cataract). Because of radiation failure or complications, however, **50% of patients ultimately need enucleation**.
      2. **Adjuvant radiation therapy**
         a. **Preoperative radiotherapy.** Because irradiation often results in cure, it is used more as definitive therapy than as preoperative "neoadjuvant" therapy. In rare advanced cases, the combination of preoperative radiation therapy and cryotherapy may produce long-term survival without compromising vision.
         b. **Postoperative radiation therapy.** Residual orbital or optic nerve tumor after enucleation is a candidate for postoperative radiation **(5000–5500 cGy over 5–6 weeks).**
      3. **Locally advanced and metastatic retinoblastoma.** Extension of intracranial

or **dural tumor necessitates full cranial irradiation**. In rare cases, radiation therapy also may be useful in the palliation of distant metastases.
  4. **Morbidity and mortality.** Specific problems following **orbital irradiation** include **enophthalmus, keratoconjunctivitis, lacrimal duct stenosis (xerophthalmia), cataract formation**, and **photophobia**. These require corrective surgery in **33% of patients** and **enucleation** in **8%**.
C. **Chemotherapy**
  1. **Primary retinoblastoma.** Because of the effectiveness of surgery and radiation, the role of chemotherapy as the initial therapy for resectable RB is limited.
  2. **Adjuvant chemotherapy.**
    a. **Preoperative chemotherapy.** Chemotherapy in the preoperative "neoadjuvant" setting has not been evaluated extensively.
    b. **Postoperative chemotherapy.** Chemotherapy has no role in the treatment of patients who are completely resected.
  3. **Locally advanced and metastatic retinoblastoma**
    a. **Single agents.** Numerous chemotherapeutic agents are active in RB, including cyclophosphamide, doxorubicin, methotrexate, triethanolamine, and vincristine. Cisplatin and ifosfamide are less effective. **Triethanolamine** is almost always given as **regional therapy (carotid infusion)**. Intracranial disease may require **intrathecal** chemotherapy (primarily methotrexate).
    b. **Combination chemotherapy.** Common regimens include **cyclophosphamide plus either actinomycin-D or doxorubicin** and **cisplatin plus VM–26**. These combinations are reserved for patients with **choroidal** or **optic nerve involvement**, regional or distant **metastases**, or both. Unfortunately, responses have only been partial or mixed.
D. **Immunotherapy.** No significant experience with this modality has been reported.
X. **Prognosis**
  A. **Risk of recurrence.** The greatest risk of recurrence occurs in the first 6–12 months after treatment.
  B. **Five-year survival.** Recent data indicate that, with improved radiation therapy, local disease control is attained in **more than 80%** of patients and that **5-year survival exceeds 88%,** even in patients with Reese-Ellsworth Group IV or V disease.
  C. **Adverse prognostic factors.** The following pathologic features portend an especially poor prognosis: **meningeal invasion,** usually along the optic nerve; **scleral involvement;** and **choroidal involvement.**
XI. **Patient follow-up**
  A. **General guidelines.** Patients with RB should be followed every 3 months for 3 years, every 6 months for an additional 2 years, then annually for evidence of tumor recurrence. Specific guidelines are listed below.
  B. **Routine evaluation.** Each clinic visit should include the following examinations:
    1. **Medical history and physical examination.** An interval medical history and thorough physical examination should be performed during each office visit. Areas for particular attention are discussed on p 576, **VI.A.**
    2. **Blood tests** (see p 1, **VI.A**).
      a. **Complete blood count.**
      b. **Hepatic transaminases.**
      c. **Alkaline phosphatase.**
    3. **Chest x-ray** (see p 3, **IV.C.1**).
  C. **Optional evaluation.** The following tests and procedures may be indicated by previous diagnostic findings or clinical suspicion.
    1. **Blood tests**
      a. **5′-Nucleotidase** (see p 2, **IV.A.4**).
      b. **GGTP** (see p 2, **IV.A.5**).
    2. **Imaging studies** (see p 3, **IV.C**)
      a. **Computed tomography.**
      b. **Magnetic resonance imaging (MRI).**
      c. **Technetium-99m bone scan.**
    3. **Invasive procedures.** In a patient without known residual cancer, **biopsy of** any suspicious or abnormal mass detected on physical examination, chest x-ray, or routine blood testing is indicated.

REFERENCES

Harnett AN. Ocular radiotherapy: a review of current management. Br J Radiol 22(suppl):122–132, 1988.

Leonard AS, Alyono D, Fischel RJ, et. al. Role of the surgeon in the treatment of children's cancer. Surg Clin North Am 65(6):1387–1422, 1985.

Maurer HM, Beltangady M, Gehan EA, et. al. The Intergroup Rhabdomyosarcoma Study-I. A final report. Cancer 61:209–220, 1988.

72 Childhood Leukemia

Victor Santana, MD

I. **Epidemiology.** Leukemia is the **most common pediatric malignancy** in the United States and is the second leading cause of death in children younger than 15 years. Childhood leukemias include **acute lymphoblastic (ALL), acute non-lymphocytic leukemia (ANLL), and chronic myelogenous leukemia (CML).** Each year, **4 cases per 100,000** children are diagnosed. Estimates indicate that **1820 new cases of ALL and 370 of ANLL** will occur in 1993. Worldwide, the incidence of acute leukemia varies substantially from areas of low incidence (North Africa, the Middle East, India, and China) to regions of high incidence (United States, Great Britain, and Japan).

II. **Risk factors**

A. **Age.** The incidence of **ALL** increases after birth, **peaks** by **3–5 years** of age, then declines again. However, **T cell ALL** occurs primarily in **older** children and **pre-B cell ALL** commonly arises in children younger than **7 years.** The incidence of **ANLL** remains **constant** throughout childhood, whereas **juvenile CML** occurs in **young** children (median age=2 years) and **Philadelphia chromosome-positive CML** develops predominantly in **older** children.

B. **Sex.** Except in infants (< 1 year of age), the **risk of ALL in males is considerably greater** than in females. Overall, **no sex predominance exists** in ANLL and CML, although the incidence of **ANLL** is **slightly higher among females younger than 5 years and males older than 15 years.**

C. **Race.** In the United States, the risk of **ALL** in **whites** is **greater** than in blacks, but ANLL and CML occur with equal frequency in both races.

D. **Genetic factors**

a. **Family history.** The risk of leukemia in siblings of children with **ALL or ANLL** is **4 times** higher than in the general population. Moreover, the risk in **identical twins** is **20 times higher.**

b. **Genetic abnormalities.** A high incidence of **acute leukemia** is associated with certain genetic disorders such as **Down's (ALL), Bloom's (ANLL), Klinefelter's and Wiskott-Aldrich syndromes** as well as **ataxia-telangiectasia (ALL), trisomy G, Fanconi's anemia, congenital agammaglobulinemia,** and **neurofibromatosis.**

E. **Previous hematologic abnormalities**

1. **Immunosuppression.** Children with **immunodeficiency syndromes** (eg, Wiskott-Aldrich, congenital agammaglobulinemia) and those on **chronic immunosuppressive agents** exhibit a higher incidence of leukemia than does the general population.

2. **Infection.** Viral infection has been implicated in the pathogenesis of leukemia although, with the exception of **human T cell lymphoma-leukemia infection,** this remains unproved.

F. **Radiation.** Evidence from atomic bomb survivors; children irradiated for thymic enlargement, ankylosing spondylitis, and tinea capitis; and children exposed to radiation in utero (first trimester) indicate that ionizing **irradiation increases the risk of leukemia.**

G. **Chemicals**

1. **Chemotherapeutic agents.** Treatment of childhood malignancies with **alkylating agents** increases the probability of subsequently developing acute leukemia (**especially ANLL**), particularly if radiation therapy also has been administered.

2. **Industrial chemicals.** Exposure to environmental carcinogens such as **benzene** has been implicated in the development of acute leukemia.

H. **Urbanization.** The incidence in **industrialized** countries with large urban populations is significantly higher than in nonindustrialized rural nations.

III. **Clinical presentation**
  A. **Signs and symptoms.** Childhood leukemia most commonly presents as a **subacute illness** with symptoms developing over weeks to months.
    1. **Local manifestations.** Common presenting complaints and findings include **fever, malaise, pallor, hemorrhage, coagulopathy, lymphadenopathy, hepatosplenomegaly, pain (bone, joint, or abdominal),** and **anorexia.** The frequency of presenting signs and symptoms is outlined in Table 72–1.
    2. **Systemic manifestations.**
      a. **Central nervous system (CNS). Headache, nausea, vomiting, visual disturbances,** and **cranial nerve deficits** (most frequently the sixth) are among presenting complaints in **less than 10%** of patients.
      b. **Kidney. Oliguria, hyperuricemia, hypokalemia,** and **renal failure** occur secondary to renal infiltration or metabolic damage.
      c. **Skin. Nodules** and **"chloromas"** (common in infants and patients with monocytic leukemia) develop in some children.
      d. **Lung. Cough** and **tachypnea** may be associated with mediastinal adenopathy or **hyperleukocytosis** (see p 79).
      e. **Gingival infiltration.** Typically, this develops in **5–10%** of patients with **monocytic** or **myelomonocytic** leukemia.
  B. **Paraneoplastic syndromes.** No specific paraneoplastic syndromes are associated with pediatric leukemia.
IV. **Differential diagnosis.** Conditions that may produce signs and symptoms which may be confused with acute leukemia include **infections** (mononucleosis, pertussis, parapertussis, and infectious lymphocytosis), **inflammation** (juvenile rheumatoid arthritis), **idiopathic thrombocytopenic purpura, aplastic anemia,** and **other malignancies** (lymphoma, neuroblastoma, rhabdomyosarcoma, and retinoblastoma).
V. **Screening programs.** No cost-effective methods of mass screening are available.
VI. **Diagnostic workup**
  A. **Medical history and physical examination.** A complete history and a thorough physical examination are essential when evaluating a child with suspected leukemia. Particular attention should be paid to the following areas:
    1. **General appearance.** Patients may have pallor secondary to anemia (bleeding or marrow failure), fever from infection, or general malaise.
    2. **Skin.** Petechiae, hemorrhage, and ecchymoses (thrombocytopenia) should be noted, as should minor skin abrasions with cellulitis and **gingival infiltration.** Patients with ANLL as well as infants with ALL may have **skin nodules.**
    3. **Lymph nodes.** All lymph node areas should be systematically examined and enlargement or tenderness should be noted. **Tonsillar hypertrophy** may be prominent.
    4. **Abdomen.** Hepatosplenomegaly may be a prominent feature at presentation.
    5. **Nervous system.** A full examination of sensorium as well as cranial and peripheral nerves may identify **cranial nerve paresis** or **retinal hemorrhages** indicating leukemic CNS infiltration, hemorrhage, or infection.
  B. **Primary tests and procedures.** All children with suspected leukemia should have the following diagnostic tests and procedures.
    1. **Blood tests**
      a. **Complete blood count.** A complete blood count and a peripheral blood

TABLE 72–1. FREQUENT PRESENTING SIGNS AND SYMPTOMS IN ALL AND ANLL

Sign or Symptom	ALL	ANLL
Fever	50%	30%
Hemorrhage	42%	30%
Coagulopathy	Uncommon	Common
Lymphadenopathy	Common	Uncommon
Hepatosplenomegaly	Common	Uncommon
Pain		
Bone or joint	10–20%	18%
Abdominal	Common	Uncommon

smear are essential and almost always suggest the diagnosis. Multiple abnormalities are common in acute leukemia (eg, anemia and thrombocytopenia; anemia and lymphocytosis; leukemic blast cells, neutropenia and thrombocytopenia). Furthermore, in **ANLL**, typical morphologic changes such as **Auer rods, hypo- or hypersegmentation** (neutrophils), and **abnormal granulation** (neutrophils) generally are present.

   b. **BUN and creatinine** (see p 3, **IV.A.6**).
   c. **Uric acid.** High levels of uric acid, particularly during therapy, are associated with the **tumor lysis syndrome** (see p 86) and **renal dysfunction**.
   d. **Electrolytes.** Serum levels of **potassium, magnesium**, and **calcium** may be abnormal and require correction.
   e. **Lactate dehydrogenase.** The serum level of this enzyme closely correlates with **total tumor burden** and can be followed as an indication of the extent of disease.
   f. **Coagulation times.** Prolonged prothrombin and partial thromboplastin times as well as elevated fibrin degradation products and low fibrinogen levels suggest **tumor-associated disseminated intravascular coagulation** (see p 80) in children with hyperleukocytosis, T cell ALL, and promyelocytic leukemia.

2. **Imaging studies. Chest x-ray** may detect a **mediastinal mass or pleural effusion** (common in T cell ALL) and other pathologic processes (see, also, p 3, **IV.C.1**).

3. **Invasive procedures**
   a. **Bone marrow aspiration and biopsy.** A definitive diagnosis **requires careful examination of a bone marrow aspirate** and biopsy specimen for morphology, cytochemistry, cytogenetics, and immunophenotype.
   b. **Lumbar puncture.** Cytologic examination of cerebrospinal fluid for malignant cells is indicated in all children.

C. **Optional tests and procedures.** The following tests and procedures may be indicated by previous diagnostic findings or clinical suspicion:

1. **Blood tests**
   a. **Quantitative immunoglobulin.** Serum levels of immunoglobulin are **depressed in 30%** of patients with **ALL,** indicating immunosuppression.
   b. **Hepatic transaminases.** Elevation of these enzymes suggests leukemic infiltration of the liver (see p 1, **IV.A.2**).
   c. **Alkaline phosphatase** (see p 1, **IV.A.3**).
   d. **5′-Nucleotidase** (see p 2, **IV.A.4**).
   e. **GGTP** (see p 2, **IV.A.5**).

2. **Urine tests.** Lysozyme levels may be elevated.

3. **Imaging studies**
   a. **Computed tomography (CT).** In rare cases, CT scan of the head and abdomen may demonstrate leukemic infiltration of the brain, liver, spleen, and other organs.
   b. **Technetium-99m bone scan** (see p 3, **IV.C.5**).

VII. **Pathology**

A. **Location.** Because leukemia is a diffuse hematologic neoplasm, it involves not only hematopoietic organs (blood, bone marrow, liver, and spleen) but potentially all organs.

B. **Multiplicity.** Leukemia is considered a **"clonal"** disease arising from a single progenitor cell, although evidence of multiple clones may be present in rare cases.

C. **Histology**

1. **Classification.** The classification of childhood leukemia is based mainly on the morphologic criteria of the **French-American-British (FAB) Cooperative Group** (see p 522, **VII.C**). Additional studies are needed to distinguish between the different biologic types of ALL and ANLL. Cytochemical stains, biochemical markers, immunophenotyping, and cytogenetic analysis are used in the subclassification of the acute leukemias. The same classification system is used for childhood and adult leukemia (see p 522, **VII.C.**) with the following distinctions:
   a. **Morphology.** The frequency distribution of FAB classes of acute leukemia is different than adults and is summarized in Table 71–2. Overall, **ALL** accounts for **75%** of childhood leukemia, whereas **acute myelogenous and acute myelomonocytic leukemia** constitute only **12.5–17.5%** and **5–10%**, respectively.
   b. **Immunohistochemical properties**

TABLE 72–2. FREQUENCY OF FAB CLASSES

Morphology	Frequency
ALL	
L1	85–90%
L2	5–15%
L3	< 1%
ANLL	
M0	< 1%
M1	17–25%
M2	25%
M3	5–10%
M4–M5	40%
M6	< 1%
M7	< 1%

(1) **Acute lymphoblastic leukemia.** In most children with ALL, leukemic cells arise from **early pre-B (60–68%) or pre-B cells (20%)** and express the **common ALL antigen (CALLA) in 90–94%** of cases (but in only 50% of infants). Pre-B ALL often presents with a high leukocyte count and is more frequent among **blacks.** In **adolescents,** however, **T cell** immunophenotypes are more common **(23%),** particularly in **males.** Typically, **T cell ALL** presents with a **high leukocyte count, frequent CNS disease,** and often a **mediastinal mass.**

(2) **Acute nonlymphocytic leukemia.** Although a variety of cell surface antigens have been used to refine the classification of ANLL, the immunologic marker system is not well established in this disease.

c. **Cluster of differentiation antigens (CD).** No significant differences exist between adult and childhood leukemias.

d. **Cytogenetic properties.** Chromosomal abnormalities—eg, number (ploidy) and structure—may be detected in **90%** of patients with **ALL** and in **50%** with **ANLL** and may alter the prognosis. A **modal chromosome number larger than 51** (DNA index of ≥ 1.16) is found in **22%** of patients with **ALL** and confers an **excellent prognosis.** Common structural alterations are discussed on p 522, **VII.C.4,** and are listed in Table 72–3.

VIII. **Staging.** Because childhood leukemia is a diffuse disease, a TNM staging system would not be useful and has not been developed.

IX. **Treatment**

A. **Surgery.** Except for establishing long-term venous access for chemotherapy, surgery plays **no role** in the management of childhood leukemia.

B. **Radiation therapy**

1. **Primary childhood leukemia**

a. **Acute lymphoblastic leukemia. Prevention of CNS relapse** is crucial to maintain remission. In addition to intrathecal chemotherapy, cranial irradiation is often used. Because of a high incidence of neurologic and intellectual impairment following radiation with 2400 cGy, however, the **standard dose** is now **1800 cGy,** which is combined with intrathecal chemotherapy (see **C** below).

b. **Acute nonlymphocytic leukemia.** Cranial irradiation is recommended only for **infants with hyperleukocytosis, patients with monocytic ANLL, and cases of documented CNS leukemia.**

2. **Recurrent childhood leukemia.** Radiation therapy is rarely useful for extracranial recurrent leukemia.

3. **Morbidity and mortality. Postirradiation somnolence syndrome,** characterized by anorexia, somnolence, and lassitude, commonly develops **6 weeks** after treatment.

C. **Chemotherapy**

1. **Primary childhood leukemia.** Chemotherapy remains the **cornerstone of therapy** for childhood leukemias. The **3 main components** of therapy are **remission induction** (4–6 weeks), **CNS prophylaxis,** and **remission maintenance** (2–3 years).

TABLE 72–3. CHROMOSOME ABNORMALITIES IN CHILDHOOD LEUKEMIA

Disease	Karyotype	Characteristics
ALL	t(1;19)(q23p13.3)	Pre-B cell; clg+
	t(9;22)(q34q11)	B-lineage; high leukocyte count
	dic(9;12)(p11p12)	B-lineage
	t(12;v)(p12;v)	B-lineage
	t(8;14)(q24q32)	B-cell ⎫
	t(8;22)(q24q11)	B-cell ⎬ Burkitt's leukemia or lymphoma
	t(2;8)(p12q24)	B-cell ⎭
	t(11;14)(p13q11-q13)	T-lineage
	t(8;14)(q24q11)	T-lineage
	t(10;14)(q24q11)	T-lineage
	t(1;14)(p32q11)	T-lineage
	inv(14)(q11q32)	T-lineage
ANLL	t(8;21)(q22q22)	FAB-M2
	t(15;17)(q22q12)	FAB-M3
	inv16(p13q22)/del (16)(q22)	FAB-M4Eo (M2)
	t(9;22)(q34q11)	FAB-M1 (M2)
	t(9;11)(p21–p22q23)	FAB-M5 (M4)
	inv(3)(q21q26)	FAB-M1 (M2, M4, M7)
	-7/7q-	FAB-M1-M5
	5q-	FAB-M1-M5
	t(3;5)(q25.1q34)	preleukemia, M2, M6

   a. **Pretreatment preparation. Anemia** should be corrected with **packed red blood cells** (10 cc/kg increases the hemoglobin 1 g/dL, and **platelet transfusions (3–4 units/m^2)** are recommended to maintain platelet counts higher than 20,000/μL. Moreover, prophylactic oral **trimethoprim-sulfamethoxazole** dramatically reduces the morbidity and mortality of *Pneumocystis carinii* pneumonia. Febrile neutropenia also may represent other opportunistic infections (see Chapter 16). In addition, **allopurinol,** vigorous intravenous **hydration** (3–4 L/m^2 per day), **alkalinization** of the urine, and blood products are essential to avoid the complications caused by rapid destruction of leukemic cells (**hyperuricemia, hypocalcemia, hyperphosphatemia,** and **renal failure**) and disseminated intravascular coagulation (DIC). This **tumor lysis syndrome** (see p 86) occurs more frequently in patients with **hyperleukocytosis** and **T cell ALL,** whereas DIC develops more commonly in **promyelocytic (M3) ANLL** and **T cell ALL.**

   b. **Acute lymphoblastic leukemia**

      (1) **Remission induction. The combination of vincristine, prednisone, L-asparaginase, and daunorubicin** is the combination most commonly used for induction of remission, and it yields a **90–95% remission rate.** Furthermore, recent data suggest that the addition of **cytarabine** and the **epipodophyllotoxin (VM–26)** or **etoposide (VP–16)** may increase the initial complete response rate to **95–97%.**

      (2) **Central nervous system prophylaxis.** Prevention of CNS relapse is crucial to maintain remission. In addition to cranial irradiation, **intrathecal** (methotrexate, cytarabine, hydrocortisone) and **high-dose systemic** chemotherapy (methotrexate, cytarabine) have been used. Currently, a **combination of irradiation and intrathecal chemotherapy** is preferred.

      (3) **Remission maintenance.** Combination chemotherapy with agents such as methotrexate, 6-mercaptopurine, etoposide, cyclophosphamide, vincristine, and prednisone must be continued for **2–3 years** to eradicate or at least suppress residual leukemic cells.

      (4) **Bone marrow transplantation (BMT).** BMT is **not** indicated for the initial management of ALL.

   c. **Acute nonlymphocytic leukemia.** Chemotherapy for ANLL, like ALL, can be divided into **3 elements.**

      (1) Remission induction. Clinical remission may be induced in **75–87%** of patients by a combination of **cytarabine and daunomycin.** In addition, **6-thioguanine** is often administered.

      (2) Central nervous system prophylaxis. Despite a low incidence of CNS involvement (< 5%), **intrathecal chemotherapy for CNS prophylaxis is considered routine.**

      (3) Remission maintenance. Although the value of maintenance chemotherapy is controversial, **6–24 months** of therapy with various combinations of 5-azacytidine, etoposide, cyclophosphamide, m-AMSA, cytarabine, doxorubicin, 6-thioguanine, 6-mercaptopurine, methotrexate, and vincristine are widely used.

      (4) Bone marrow transplantation. BMT during the first remission is under investigation. Early data indicates that **disease-free survival** following BMT is **40–50%;** however, patients often develop complications caused by **acute or chronic graft-versus-host disease** (see Chapter 6).

    2. Recurrent leukemia. Some patients with **recurrent ALL** may be salvaged with intensive chemotherapy or BMT. The prognosis is significantly better if relapse occurs after the completion of initial therapy and outside of the bone marrow. Patients with **recurrent ANLL** rarely achieve a prolonged second remission unless BMT is attempted.

    3. Morbidity and mortality. Chemotherapeutic agents may adversely affect the liver (methotrexate and 6-mercaptopurine), heart (doxorubicin), gonads (cyclophosphamide), urinary bladder (cyclophosphamide), bone (prednisone), brain (high-dose methotrexate and cytarabine), and the endocrine glands (prednisone). Furthermore, **3–10%** of patients develop chemotherapy-related **second malignancies** (brain and bone tumors, lymphomas, or ANLL) following successful therapy.

X. Prognosis

  A. Risk of recurrence. The rate of relapse depends on the anatomic site.

    1. Bone marrow. Bone marrow is the **most common** site of treatment failure. It accounts for **12% and 39%** of failures (with or without CNS involvement) in **ALL and ANLL,** respectively.

    2. Central nervous system. Primary CNS relapse occurs in **5%** of patients with acute leukemia, although the incidence is higher in infants and in **T cell ALL.**

    3. Gonads. Because of intensive chemotherapy, testicular and ovarian relapses are **rare (< 10%).**

  B. Five-year survival. The 5-year **disease-free** survival for children with **ALL and ANLL ranges** from **58–74% and 20–30%,** respectively. With recurrent disease, cure rates for patients with **bone marrow relapse** are **30–50%,** whereas for patients with **extramedullary relapse alone,** the rate may be as high as **70–80%.**

  C. Adverse prognostic factors. Many features influence the prognosis in acute childhood leukemia. With improved therapy, however, the prognostic significance of these factors has diminished.

    1. Acute lymphoblastic leukemia

      a. Age younger than 1 year.

      b. Leukocyte count greater or equal to 50,000/μL.

      c. Ploidy of no more than 51 chromosomes (DNA index ≤ 1.16).

      d. Translocations, particularly t(4;11), t(1;19), and t(9;22).

      e. Black race.

      f. Serum LDH more than 300 U/L.

      g. T cell immunophenotype.

    2. Acute nonlymphocytic leukemia. Because of the poor overall prognosis, few factors impact on the prognosis.

XI. Patient follow-up

  A. General guidelines. Patients with childhood **leukemia** should be followed every 1–2 weeks during therapy, every 3–4 months for the first 2 years after completion of therapy, every 6 months for an additional 3 years, then annually for evidence of tumor recurrence and treatment-related toxicity. Specific guidelines are listed below.

  B. Routine evaluation. The following examinations should be included with each clinic visit:

    1. Medical history and physical examination. An interval medical history and a thorough physical examination is essential during every office visit. Particular attention should be directed to the areas outlined on p 582, **VI.A.**

   2. **Blood tests**
      a. **Complete blood count** (see p 582, **VI.B.1.a**).
      b. **BUN and creatinine** (see p 3, **IV.A.6**).
      c. **Uric acid** (see p. 583, **VI.B.1.c**).
      d. **Electrolytes** (see p 583, **VI.B.1.d**).
      e. **Lactate dehydrogenase** (see p 583, **VI.B.1.d**).
   3. **Chest x-ray** (see p 583, **VI.B.2**).
C. **Additional evaluation.** Other tests and procedures that should be obtained at regular intervals include the following:
   1. **Bone marrow aspiration and biopsy** (see p 583, **VI.B.3.a**).
   2. **Lumbar puncture** (see p 583, **VI.B.3.b**).
D. **Optional evaluation.** The following tests and procedures may be indicated by previous diagnostic findings or clinical suspicion:
   1. **Blood tests**
      a. **Hepatic transaminases** (see p 583, **VI.C.1.b**).
      b. **Alkaline phosphatase** (see p 1, **IV.A.3**).
      c. **5'-Nucleotidase** (see p 2, **IV.A.4**).
      d. **GGTP** (see p 2, **IV.A.5**).
      e. **Thyroid function studies.** Serum TSH, free T_4, and free T_3 may indicate therapy-related hypothyroidism.
   2. **Imaging studies**
      a. **Computed tomography (CT).** (see p 583, **VI.C.3.a**).
      b. **Technetium-99m bone scan** (see p 3, **IV.C.5**).
      c. **Echocardiogram.** This cardiac imaging study, along with the electrocardiogram, is indicated in patients receiving large cumulative doses of doxorubicin (> 300 mg/m^2).
   3. **Psychosocial testing.** The psychological and social impact of the disease and therapy on the patient (including school attendance) should be closely monitored.

REFERENCES

Bennett, JJ, Catovsky, D, Daniel, MT, et. al. Proposals for the classifications of acute leukemias. Br J Haematol 33:451–458, 1976.

Bleyer, WA. Central nervous system leukemia. Ped Clin NA 35:789–814, 1988.

Buckley, JD, Chard, RL, Baehner, RL, etl. al. Improvement in outcome for children with acute non-lymphocytic leukemia. A report from the Children's Cancer Study Group. Cancer 63:1457–1465, 1989.

Hustu, HO, Aur, RJA, Verzosa, MS, et al. Prevention of central nervous system leukemia by irradiation. Cancer 32:585–597, 1973.

Kalwinsky, D, Mirro, J, Schell, M, et. al. Early intensification of chemotherapy for childhood acute nonlymphoblastic leukemia: improved remission induction with a five-drug regimen including etoposide. J Clin Oncol 6:1134–1143, 1988.

Krischer, JP, Steuber, CP, Vietti, TJ, et. al. Long-term results in the treatment of acute non-lymphocytic leukemia. A Pediatric Oncology Group Study. Med Pediatr Oncol 17:401–408, 1989.

Lampkin, BC, Lange, B, Bernstein, J, et. al. Biologic characteristics and treatment of acute non-lymphocytic leukemia in children. Ped Clin North Amer 35:743–764, 1988.

Nesbit, ME, Sather, HN, Robison, LL, et. al. Presymptomatic control nervous system therapy in previously untreated childhood acute lymphoblastic leukemia: comparison of 1800 rad and 2400 rad. A report for the Children's Cancer Study Group. Lancet 1:461–466, 1981.

Ochs, J, Mulhern, RK. Late effects of antileukemic treatment. Ped Clin North Amer 35:815, 1988.

Rivera, GK. Therapeutic options for children with acute lymphocytic leukemia who fail on contemporary protocols. In Current Controversies in Bone Marrow Transplantation. Robert P. Gale and Richard E. Champlin, eds. New York: Alan Liss, Inc. pp. 31–45, 1989.

Rivera, GK and Pui, C-H. Acute lymphoblastic leukemia. In Rudolph, AM, ed. Pediatrics. Norwalk, CT: Appleton & Lange 1987:1186–1189.

Rivera, GK, Raimondi, SC, Hancock, ML, et. al. Improved outcome in childhood acute lymphoblastic leukemia with reinforced early treatment and rotational chemotherapy. Lancet 337:61–66, 1991.

Weinstein, HJ, Mayer, RJ, Rosenthal, DS, et. al. Treatment of acute myelogenous leukemia in children and adults. NEJM 303:473–478, 1980.

73 Childhood Lymphoma

Victor Santana, MD

I. **Epidemiology.** In the United States, Hodgkin's (HL) and non-Hodgkin's lymphoma (NHL) each account for **4–10%** of all pediatric malignancies; however, children younger than 16 years account for only **5–15%** and **3%** of all patients with **HL and NHL,** respectively. Each year **0.9 and 0.75 cases of NHL and HL per 100,000 children** are diagnosed, and estimates indicate that **690 and 550 new cases,** respectively, will occur in 1993. Worldwide, NHL represents the third most common childhood malignancy after leukemia and brain cancer in developed countries, and childhood HL, although rare in some areas (Japan), is relatively common in other regions (the Middle East and South America).

II. **Risk factors**
   - A. **Age.** In children, both HL and NHL are **rare before age 3,** but the incidence increases gradually after this age, **peaking at 9–10 years** of age. The incidence of HL steadily increases throughout the pediatric age range.
   - B. **Sex.** The risk of **NHL** for **males** is **2.5 times greater** than for females. The risk of HL in **prepubertal males** is **3 times greater** than in females but only **1.5 times** greater after puberty.
   - C. **Race.** The risk of **NHL** in **whites** is **1.4 times** higher than in blacks. The risk of **HL** also is **higher** in **white** children.
   - D. **Genetic factors**
      1. **Family history.** The risk of **NHL** in first-degree relatives is not known to be **substantially higher** than in the general population.
      2. **Hereditary syndromes.** NHL occurs with increased frequency in patients with certain genetic immunodeficiency disorders (see **F.1.a** below).
      3. **Chromosomal abnormalities.** Translocations and other anomalies of **chromosome 14** are associated with B cell malignancies.
   - E. **Radiation.** Evidence from atomic bomb survivors suggests that ionizing irradiation **(> 100 cGy)** may cause NHL.
   - F. **Previous immunologic pathology**
      1. **Immunodeficiency disease**
         - a. **Primary immunodeficiency.** An increased incidence of NHL is associated with **primary immunodeficiency syndromes** such as the Wiskott-Aldrich syndrome, ataxia-telangiectasia, Chédiak-Higashi disease, common variable immunodeficiency, Swiss-type agammaglobulinemia, and X-linked lymphoproliferative disorder.
         - b. **Secondary immunodeficiency.** Immunosuppression related to solid organ **transplantation** increases the risk of NHL.
      2. **Infection.** Viral infection with **Epstein-Barr virus (EBV)** has been implicated in the pathogenesis of **African Burkitt's lymphoma** and HL, whereas **human immunodeficiency virus (HIV)** may cause high grade B cell lymphomas. Patients with African Burkitt's lymphoma also have a high incidence of **malaria.** Both EBV and *Plasmodium malariae* (malaria) are known B cell mitogens.
   - G. **Diet.** No dietary factors have been identified.
   - H. **Socioeconomic status. HL** in chldren occurs more frequently in families of **high** socioeconomic status.
   - I. **Urbanization.** Other than African Burkitt's lymphoma, which occurs in rural Africa, no differences have been observed between rural and urban populations.

III. **Clinical presentation**
   - A. **Signs and symptoms**
      1. **Local manifestations. Abdominal complaints** (pain, distention, nausea, vomiting, and altered bowel habits) are common in childhood lymphomas. Thoracic symptoms lead to the discovery of **a mediastinal mass in 25% of NHL patients and 50% of HL patients** and may be accompanied by a pleural effusion, dyspnea, dysphagia, upper extremity and facial edema (superior vena

cava syndrome), or all of these. HL and, less frequently, NHL may present as **painless rubbery peripheral lymphadenopathy (15%),** which is most often cervical. Painless **swelling of the jaw** and **neurologic problems** from central nervous system (CNS) involvement or spinal cord compression (10–15%) also occur, particularly with Burkitt's lymphoma.

2. **Systemic manifestations.** Fever, night sweats, and weight loss are common (< 50% of HL patients) and constitute "B" symptoms (see p 590, VIII). Pruritus and dermal eruptions, papules, and nodules also may develop, particularly in HL, but are **less common** than in adults.

B. **Paraneoplastic syndromes.** Although paraneoplastic syndromes have not been associated with childhood NHLs, rare syndromes have been described with HL (see p 489, **III.B**).

IV. **Differential diagnosis.** The differential diagnosis varies with the site of localized disease. Abdominal disease may present as an **abdominal mass** and mimic **infections** (abscess) and **other neoplasms** (Wilms' tumor and neuroblastoma). **Thoracic disease** (mediastinal mass) can be confused with numerous disease entities (see p 214, **IV**). Finally, localized or **generalized lymphadenopathy** is associated with numerous pathologic processes (see p 489, **IV**).

V. **Screening programs.** Because of the low incidence of lymphoma compared to the high frequency of benign lymphadenopathy, screening is not feasible.

VI. **Diagnostic workup.** The appropriate tests and procedures required for the workup of HL and NHL are essentially identical to those used in adults (see p 490, **VI,** and p 501, **VI**) with the following exceptions and additions:

A. **Complete blood count. Coombs' autoimmune hemolytic anemia** is present in **less than 1%** of patients.

B. **Erythrocyte sedimentation rate.** This is a useful parameter of disease activity.

C. **Lactate dehydrogenase.** The serum level of this enzyme correlates with **tumor burden** and can be monitored to follow response to treatment.

D. **Computed tomography (CT).** Chest CT detects thoracic (primarily **mediastinal**) disease in **60% of patients** compared with only 50% by chest x-ray; however, abdominal CT **fails** to detect **splenic** involvement in **60%** of patients.

E. **Lymphangiogram.** This test is contraindicated in children with pulmonary or mediastinal disease.

F. **Staging laparotomy (SL).** The most common sites of HL identified by SL in children are the **spleen (39%)** and the splenic hilar (28%), celiac (17%), periportal (15%), and periaortic (15%) lymph nodes. Although proposed as a splenic-preserving procedure, hemisplenectomy is not recommended.

VII. **Pathology**

A. **Location.** Childhood **NHL** frequently arises in the **abdomen (31%), head and neck region (29%),** and **mediastinum (26%).** Uncommon sites include skin, bone, and the epidural space. HL typically begins in **cervical lymph nodes** and **mediastinum.**

B. **Multiplicity.** Because most childhood NHLs are diffuse, multiple areas of disease are common; however, these separate areas **do not** represent individual primary lymphomas.

C. **Histology.** The histology of childhood lymphomas is similar to that of adult HL and NHL (see p 491, **VII.C,** and p 504, **VII.C**), with the following caveats:

1. **Hodgkin's lymphoma.** The 4 classifications of HL—**lymphocyte predominant, nodular sclerosis, mixed cellularity,** and **lymphocyte depletion**—occur in **8–15%, 40–60%, 20–40%,** and **1–8% of patients,** respectively. The **lymphocyte predominant** type arises primarily in children under **10 years of age,** and **nodular sclerosis** is the most common type to develop in **adolescents.**

2. **Non-Hodgkin's lymphoma.** The current "Working Formulation" for classifying NHL is outlined in Table 61–1. The 3 major pediatric NHL histologies are **small noncleaved cell** (SNCC, including Burkitt's and non-Burkitt's NHL; 39%), **lymphoblastic** (28%), and **diffuse large cell** (LC, 26%). Burkitt's lymphoma consists of 2 distinct disease entities: the **sporadic type** that occurs worldwide, and the **EBV-associated type** that is endemic to equatorial Africa and New Guinea. Nearly all childhood NHLs are **diffuse high-grade** lymphomas; follicular lymphomas are rare.

a. **Immunophenotype. SNCC** lymphomas typically express **B cell** antigens (CD19, CD20, CD22) and surface immunoglobulin (SIg), whereas **lymphoblastic** lymphomas generally manifest **T cell** markers (eg, CD3, glycoprotein gp40). However, **common acute lymphoblastic leukemia antigen (CALLA)** may be present regardless of histology.

        b. Cytogenetics. SNCC lymphomas may exhibit one of 3 characteristic chromosomal translocations: t(8;14) (85% of cases), t(8;22), and t(2;8), which juxtapose the *c-myc* proto-oncogene on chromosome 8 and an immunoglobulin gene on the other chromosome. **Lymphoblastic** lymphomas may reveal chromosomal translocations involving breakpoints within the **T cell receptor (TCR) genes:** 14q11-q13 (TCR-alpha locus) and 7q32-q36 (TCR-beta locus).

  D. Metastatic spread

    1. Modes of spread. Childhood lymphomas spread in a manner similar to adult lymphomas.

    2. Sites of spread. The major sites of metastatic disease include the CNS, bones, eyes, testicles, and ovaries. In addition, bone marrow is often involved in children with NHLs, particularly **Burkitt's lymphoma (20%)** and **lymphoblastic lymphoma (25–30%).**

VIII. Staging

  A. Hodgkin's lymphoma. The staging of Hodgkin's disease is outlined on p 492, **VIII.**

  B. Non-Hodgkin's lymphoma. The Murphy staging system (St. Jude Children's Research Hospital) uses the following criteria for assessing the extent of pediatric NHL; however, many centers have abandoned all staging systems, because childhood NHLs are **disseminated** in essentially all patients:

    1. Stage I. Tumor is limited to a **single extranodal site or lymph node region**, excluding the mediastinum and abdomen.

    2. Stage II. Tumor involves a single extranodal site with regional lymph node involvement; **no more than 2 lymph node regions are on the same side of the diaphragm;** 2 extranodal sites are on the same side of the diaphragm, with or without regional lymph node involvement; or primary gastrointestinal lymphoma (usually ileocecal) is present, with or without mesenteric lymph node involvement (grossly completely resected).

    3. Stage III. Tumor involves 2 or more lymph node regions or extranodal sites **above and below the diaphragm**; primary intrathoracic lymphoma (mediastinal, pleural, thymic) is present; extensive primary intra-abdominal disease (unresectable) is present; or paraspinal or epidural lymphoma is present regardless of other involved sites.

    4. Stage IV. Tumor involves the **CNS, bone marrow,** or both.

IX. Treatment

  A. Surgery

    1. Primary childhood lymphoma

      a. Indications. The major role of surgery in pediatric lymphoma is to confirm the diagnosis by tissue biopsy. Resection of lymphomas generally is not indicated, although Stage III abdominal Burkitt's lymphoma may benefit from debulking procedures to lower the patient's stage.

      b. Procedures. Excisional lymph node biopsy or occasionally exploratory laparotomy usually is required to obtain diagnostic material. However, because of the exquisite chemosensitivity, major surgical procedures should be avoided. Children with HL occasionally require **staging laparotomy** (see p 491, **VI.C.3.b**).

    2. Advanced childhood lymphoma. Surgery is necessary only for **acute surgical complications** of advanced lymphoma (eg, gastrointestinal obstruction, perforation, hemorrhage).

    3. Morbidity and mortality. Complications following diagnostic procedures are unusual (see p 491, **VI.C.3.b.[2]**) and generally are limited to bleeding and infection, although therapy-induced myelosuppression may aggravate simple problems.

  B. Radiation therapy

    1. Primary non-Hodgkin's lymphoma. Radiation therapy plays a **minor role** in the initial therapy of childhood lymphoma and is indicated only for **respiratory compromise** from mediastinal disease, neurologic symptoms caused by **spinal cord compression,** symptomatic **superior vena cava compression, cranial nerve palsy, orbital proptosis,** and **persistent localized disease** after initial chemotherapy. Doses are usually low (eg, **1200 cGy** over 5–10 days). Although cranial irradiation has been used in the past to prevent CNS relapse, intrathecal chemotherapy alone is now believed to be adequate.

    2. Primary Hodgkin's lymphoma. Because of the risk of **infraclavicular narrowing, shortened sitting height, decreased mandibular growth and neck size,** and **atrophy of soft tissue and muscle,** full adult doses are not recommended. Instead, low-dose radiation therapy (**1500–2000 cGy**) to involved areas and intermediate-dose therapy (2500 cGy) to sites of bulky disease (**> 6 cm** in diameter or mediastinal disease **> 33% of the thoracic diameter**), combined with chemotherapy, is used for patients with **Stage I-IIIA disease.**

3. **Advanced childhood lymphoma.** In rare cases, radiation therapy is recommended for **palliation** in patients with advanced HL or NHL and **localized symptomatic disease.**

4. **Morbidity and mortality.** In children, numerous problems may develop following significant irradiation, including suppression of bone growth, pneumonitis, gastrointestinal complaints (eg, stomatitis, diarrhea), and myelosuppression (see, also, p 494, **IX.B.3**).

C. **Chemotherapy**
1. **Primary childhood lymphoma.** Chemotherapy is recommended for nearly all patients with childhood lymphoma.
   a. **Pretreatment preparation.** Steps should be taken to avert complications from **rapid tumor cell lysis** (see, also, p 494, **IX.C.1**).
   b. **Single-agent chemotherapy.** Doxorubicin, prednisone, vincristine, methotrexate, cyclophosphamide, 6-mercaptopurine, asparaginase, cytosine arabinoside, and teniposide are active agents. However, because of the success of combination chemotherapy, chemotherapeutic drugs generally are not used as single agents.
   c. **Combination chemotherapy**
      (1) **Hodgkin's lymphoma.** Combination chemotherapy for HL in children is essentially identical to that given in adults (see p 494, **IX.C**). In addition, a reduced number of cycles of multiagent chemotherapy (MOPP and ABVD) and **low-dose (2000 cGy) involved-field irradiation** is being investigated at several centers in the United States and Europe. Preliminary data indicate that **2-year disease-free survival is more than 95%** with this approach; however, side effects, including acute leukemia, azoospermia, and pulmonary fibrosis, have been encountered. Further study of this promising approach is warranted.
      (2) **Non-Hodgkin's lymphoma.** Combination chemotherapy is the principal treatment for childhood lymphomas, although the optimal treatment strategy remains unknown. **APO** (doxorubicin, prednisone, vincristine, methotrexate, asparaginase, 6-mercaptopurine) and **ACOP+** (doxorubicin, prednisone, vincristine, methotrexate, and cyclophosphamide) are used to treat advanced (Stage III and IV) large-cell lymphoma with some success (eg, 3-year disease-free survival of 83% and 65%, respectively). The preliminary data with **MACOP-B** predict a **cure rate of 55%** with this brief **12-week regimen.**
   d. **Central nervous system prophylaxis.** The administration of intrathecal chemotherapy (methotrexate and cytosine arabinoside) has eliminated the need for cranial irradiation and decreased the incidence of CNS relapse from **20% to 2%** in NHL.
2. **Recurrent childhood lymphoma.** Local recurrent disease outside original radiation treatment portals may be treated simply by using additional irradiation. Systemic recurrence, however, is more difficult to control (particularly with remissions lasting < 12 months) and requires salvage chemotherapy, which may control the disease in **20–30%** of patients.

X. **Prognosis**
A. **Risk of recurrence.** Nearly all relapses occur less than **2 years** after therapy is completed.
B. **Five-year survival**
1. **Hodgkin's lymphoma.** Overall, the complete remission rate and long-term survival with HL is **excellent (80–90%).** The 5-year disease-free survival by stage is **Stage I–IIIA,** more than 75–80%; **Stage IIIB–IV,** 40–60%.
2. **Non-Hodgkin's lymphoma.** The long-term survival of patients with NHL varies with stage and histology. Overall 2-year disease-free survival (DFS) by stage is as follows: **limited stage (I and II),** 90%; **Stage III,** 81%; and **Stage IV,** 20%.
C. **Adverse risk factors.** The following disease features are associated with a particularly poor prognosis: **high lactate dehydrogenase level** (NHL) and **relapse within 12 months.**

XI. **Patient follow-up.** Patients with childhood lymphoma should be followed closely every month during treatment, every 3 months for the first 3 years following therapy, every 6 months for an additional 2 years, then annually for evidence of relapse. Specific guidelines for patient follow-up are outlined on p 498, **XI.B–D,** and p 510, **XI.B–D,** with the following additions:

A. Blood tests
   1. **Lactate dehydrogenase** (see p 589, **VI.C**).
   2. **Erythrocyte sedimentation rate.**
B. Echocardiography. This noninvasive test evaluates cardiac function.
C. Pulmonary function tests (PFTs). Some regimens include bleomycin, which may cause pulmonary fibrosis that can be detected with serial PFTs.
D. Other tests. Specific testing should include evaluation of **skeletal growth** and **fertility.**

REFERENCES

Cramer, P and Andrieu, JM. Hodgkin's disease in childhood and adolescence: results of chemotherapy-radiotherapy in clinical stage IA-IIB. J Clin Oncol 3:1495–1502.

Dahl, GV, Rivera, G, Pui, C-H, et. al. A novel treatment of childhood lymphoblastic non-Hodgkin lymphoma: early and intermittent use of teniposide plus cytarabine. Blood 66:1110–1114, 1985.

Donaldson, SS, Glatstein, E, and Kaplan, HS. Pediatric Hodgkin's disease: II. Results of therapy. Cancer 37:2436–2447, 1976.

Donaldson, SS and Link, MP. Combined modality treatment with low-dose radiation and MOPP chemotherapy for children with Hodgkin's disease. J Clin Oncol 5:742–749, 1987.

Donaldson, SS, Link, MP, McDougall, IR, Parker, BR, and Shochat, SJ. Clinical investigations of children with Hodgkin's disease at Stanford University Medical Center: a preliminary overview of pediatric Hodgkin's disease protocol using low-dose irradiation and alternating ABVD/MOPP chemotherapy. In *Hodgkin's Disease in Children*. Kamps, WA, Poppema, S, and Humphrey, GB, eds. Kluwer Academic Publishers, Boston pp. 307–315, 1988.

Fleming, ID, Turk, PS, Murphy, SB, et. al. Surgical implications of primary gastrointestinal lymphoma of childhood. Arch Surg 125:252–256, 1990.

Hvizdala, E, Berard, C, Callihan, T, et. al. Lymphoblastic lymphoma in children—a randomized trial comparing LSA_2L_2 with the A-COP+ therapeutic regimen: a Pediatric Oncology Group study. J Clin Oncol 6:26–33, 1988.

Kaplan, HS. Hodgkin's Disease. Harvard University Press, Boston: 2nd ed., 1980.

Lange, B and Littman, P. Management of Hodgkin's disease in children and adolescents. Cancer 51:1371–1377, 1983.

Magrath, IT, Lwanga, S, Carswell, W, et. al. Surgical reduction of tumor bulk in management of abdominal Burkitt's lymphoma. Brit Med J 2:308–312, 1974.

Murphy, SB. Classification, strategy, and end results of treatment of childhood non-Hodgkin's lymphoma. Semin Oncol 7:332–339, 1980.

Murphy, S, Bowman, WP, Abromowitch, M, et. al. Results of treatment of advanced stage Burkitt's lymphoma and B-cell (sIg^+) acute lymphoblastic leukemia with high-dose fractionated cyclophosphamide and coordinated high-dose methotrexate and cytarabine. J Clin Oncol 4:1732–1739, 1986.

Murphy, SB, Fairclough, D, Hutchison, RE, et. al. Non-Hodgkin's lymphomas of childhood: an analysis of the histology, staging and response to treatment of 338 cases at a single institution. J Clin Oncol 7:186–193, 1989.

Murphy, SB and Hustu, HO. A randomized trial of combined modality therapy of childhood non-Hodgkin's lymphoma. Cancer 45:630–637, 1980.

Patte, C, Philip, T, Rodary, C, et. al. Improved survival rate in children with stage III and IV B cell non-Hodgkin's lymphoma and leukemia using multi-agent chemotherapy: results of a study of 114 children from the French Pediatric Oncology Society. J Clin Oncol 4:1219–1226, 1986.

Weinstein, HJ, Cassady, JR, and Levey, R. Long-term results of the APO protocol (vincristine, doxorubicin, and prednisone) for treatment of mediastinal lymphoblastic lymphoma. J Clin Oncol 1:537–541, 1983.

Wollner, N, Burchenal, JH, and Lieberman, PH. Non-Hodgkin's lymphoma in children: a comparative study of two modalities of therapy. Cancer 37:123–134, 1976.

74 Wilms' Tumor

Richard G. Nord, MD, and R. Bruce Filmer, MD

I. **Epidemiology.** Wilms' tumor (renal embryoma, nephroblastoma) is the **most common genitourinary malignancy** and the fifth most common solid tumor in children, accounting for **8%** of all pediatric malignancies. The incidence in the United States has remained constant at **0.8 cases per 100,000** children younger than 15 years of age. Estimates indicate that **510 new cases** will be diagnosed in 1993. Worldwide, there is little variation in the incidence of Wilms' tumor.

II. **Risk factors**
   A. **Age.** Wilms' tumor has a bimodal age distribution: **hereditary** and **sporadic** cases present at a **median age** of **2.5** and **3.5** years, respectively, and **90%** of patients are younger than **7 years.**
   B. **Genetic factors**
      1. **Family history.** First-degree relatives of patients with the sporadic form of Wilms' tumor are not at increased risk; however, an **autosomal dominant** form of Wilms' tumor (with variable penetrance) accounts for **1% of all cases.**
      2. **Hereditary syndromes. Aniridia** is associated with **11p chromosomal deletion** and a **33%** chance of developing Wilms' tumor. In addition, the incidence of **hemihypertrophy** among children with Wilms' tumor is **2.4%.** Other genetic disorders with a high incidence of Wilms' tumor include **neurofibromatosis** and the **Beckwith-Wiedemann, Drash,** and **Perlman syndromes.**
   C. **Previous genitourinary pathology.** Congenital genitourinary malformations such as **hypospadias, renal anomalies** (horseshoe, ectopic, and hypoplastic kidneys), **ureteral duplication,** and **cryptorchidism** occur in **4.4%** of patients with Wilms' tumors.

III. **Clinical presentation**
   A. **Signs and symptoms**
      1. **Local manifestations.** Most children present with an **asymptomatic abdominal or flank mass (69%), whereas 31%** complain of vague abdominal **pain.** Hematuria (26%; gross or microscopic) is less common.
      2. **Systemic manifestations.** Symptoms such as fever (18%), malaise, and anorexia (14%) may be present. Hypertension (25%) caused by elevated renin levels also may occur.
   B. **Paraneoplastic syndromes.** No known paraneoplastic symptom complexes are associated with Wilms' tumor.

IV. **Differential diagnosis.** Most patients present with an **asymptomatic abdominal mass,** which, in a child, also may be the result of **congenital abnormalities** (mesoblastic nephroma), **infections** (paranephric and intra-abdominal abscesses), **cysts** (multilocular cysts, multi- and polycystic kidneys, and mesenteric cysts), **obstructive uropathy** (hydronephrosis), and **other neoplasms** (neuroblastoma and lymphoma).

V. **Screening programs.** Because of the rare nature of Wilms' tumors, screening (other than a careful physical examination) is not warranted.

VI. **Diagnostic workup**
   A. **Medical history and physical examination.** A complete medical history and a thorough physical examination are essential for the initial evaluation of patients with suspected Wilms' tumor. Particular emphasis is placed on the following areas:
      1. **Chest.** Abnormal breath sounds may be the first clue to lung metastases.
      2. **Abdomen.** A smooth palpable mass and hepatomegaly (metastatic disease) may be detected.
      3. **Extremities.** Swelling of the lower extremities (obstruction of the inferior vena cava) should be noted.
      4. **Nervous system.** Neurologic findings may indicate brain metastases.
   B. **Primary tests and procedures.** The following tests and procedures should be performed on all patients with suspected Wilms' tumor:

1. **Blood tests** (see p 1, **IV.A**)
   a. **Complete blood count.**
   b. **Hepatic transaminases.**
   c. **Alkaline phosphatase.**
   d. **BUN and creatinine.**
2. **Urine tests**
   a. **Urinalysis** (see p 3, **IV.B**).
   b. **Twenty-four-hour urinary catecholamines.** Pheochromocytoma must be excluded (see p 462, **VI.B.2.b**).
3. **Imaging studies**
   a. **Chest x-ray** (see p 3, **IV.C.1**).
   b. **Abdominal flat plate.** Plain abdominal x-ray (usually obtained during excretory urography) demonstrates the presence of a renal mass with displacement of abdominal gas. Although unusual, **peripheral** calcium deposits may be noted. **Central, finely stippled calcifications suggest neuroblastoma.**
   c. **Intravenous pyelography (IVP).** This imaging test not only demonstrates an **intrarenal mass with calyceal distortion** but evaluates the function and possible involvement of the **contralateral** kidney.
   d. **Computed tomography (CT). Abdominal CT** is an extremely accurate method of assessing the extent of the primary tumor and the presence of lymph node and hepatic metastases. In addition, **head CT** is appropriate for patients with neurologic symptoms. Routine **chest CT**, however, is **not** indicated.
4. **Invasive procedures. Fine needle aspiration** or open surgical **biopsy** (through a retroperitoneal approach) is indicated, particularly if preoperative therapy (radiation therapy, chemotherapy, or both) is contemplated.
C. **Optional tests and procedures.** The following examinations may be indicated by previous diagnostic findings or clinical suspicion:
   1. **Blood tests**
      a. **5′-Nucleotidase** (see p 2, **IV.A.4**).
      b. **GGTP** (see p 2, **IV.A.5**).
      c. **Cortisol** (see p 455, **VI.C.1.c**).
      d. **Adrenocorticotropic hormone** (see p 455, **VI.C.1.d**).
      e. **Aldosterone and renin** (see p 456, **VI.C.1.g**).
   2. **Urine tests** (see p 455, **VI.B.2**, and p 456, **VI.C.2**)
      a. **Twenty-four-hour urinary 17-hydroxysteroids**
      b. **Twenty-four-hour urinary 17-ketosteroids**
      c. **Twenty-four-hour urinary free cortisol**
   3. **Imaging studies**
      a. **Magnetic resonance imaging (MRI).** MRI is particularly useful for detecting renal vein and vena cava **tumor thrombus.**
      b. **Ultrasound** (see p 3, **IV.C.4**).
      c. **Angiography** (see p 456, **VI.C.3.c**).
      d. **Technetium-99m bone scan** (see p 3, **IV.C.5**).
      e. **Inferior vena cavography.** Although almost entirely replaced by MRI and ultrasound, this test may be necessary to exclude **tumor thrombus**.
   4. **Invasive procedures. Cystoscopy with retrograde pyelography** occasionally may document involvement of the upper collecting system that requires en bloc nephroureterectomy.
VII. **Pathology**
   A. **Location.** Wilms' tumors occur in either kidney with equal frequency and, in **rare** cases, arise in **extrarenal locations** (retroperitoneum and pelvis).
   B. **Multiplicity.** Wilms' tumors are multicentric (most commonly **bilateral**) in **12%** of patients. Bilateral Wilms' tumors usually occur **synchronously (metachronous** lesions are uncommon, arising in less than **3%** of patients).
   C. **Gross pathology.** Characteristically, tumors develop an inflammatory **pseudocapsule** with adhesions to adjacent structures. Focal **hemorrhage, necrosis, cavitation,** and **invasion of the collecting system** may occur.
   D. **Histology.** Wilms' tumor consists of a mixture of blastemal, stromal, and epithelial cells. **Nephroblastomatosis** refers to the presence of **multiple or diffuse nephrogenic rests** (persistent metanephric blastema beyond 36 weeks of gestation). These lesions may be **bilateral,** cause massive renal enlargement, and progress to Wilms' tumor (nephroblastomatosis has been demonstrated in **44%** of Wilms' tumors and **100%** of bilateral Wilms' tumors). With the exception of **anaplasia (unfa-**

vorable histology), which increases with the patient's age and is present in **11%** of all cases, histologic features do **not** affect prognosis. Previously, unfavorable histological patterns included **clear cell sarcoma** and **malignant rhabdoid tumor;** however, these are now considered to be distinct entities rather than variants of Wilms' tumor.

E. **Metastatic spread**
1. **Modes of spread.** Wilms' tumor generally spreads by three mechanisms.
    a. **Direct extension.** Local invasion of contiguous structures commonly occurs and may involve the **liver and adrenal gland** as well as other adjacent organs. In addition, **10%** of patients present with tumor extension into the **renal vein, inferior vena cava, or right atrium.**
    b. **Lymphatic metastasis.** Regional lymph nodes are involved in **20%** of patients. The renal lymphatic drainage is highly variable but includes the **paraaortic, paracaval, and hilar nodes.**
    c. **Hematogenous metastasis.** In **15%** of patients, tumor cells may travel through **systemic blood vessels** to distant organs by the time of presentation.
2. **Sites of spread.** The following organs may be involved with metastatic Wilms' tumor: **lung, 85%, liver, 15%, bone; and CNS**.

VIII. **Staging.** The **National Wilms' Tumor Study (NWTS)** defined a staging system based on the extent of the primary tumor and the presence of lymph node and distant metastases. The American Joint Committee on Cancer and the Union Internationale Contre le Cancer adopted a unified **TNM staging system** according to the recommendations of the Societe Internationale d'Oncologie Pediatrique, that includes both clinical and pathologic components. Both systems are discussed below.

A. **NWTS staging system**
1. **Stage I.** Tumor is limited to the kidney and is completely excised. The surface of the renal capsule must be intact (tumor was not ruptured before or during removal). Furthermore, no residual tumor is apparent beyond the margins of resection.
2. **Stage II.** Tumor extends beyond the kidney but is completely removed—ie, there is regional extension of the tumor (penetration through the outer surface of the renal capsule into perirenal soft tissues)—or vessels outside the kidney substance are infiltrated or contain tumor thrombus. Alternately, the tumor may have been biopsied or spillage of tumor is confined to the flank. Furthermore, no residual tumor is apparent at or beyond the margins of excision.
3. **Stage III.** Residual nonhematogenous tumor is confined to the abdomen with one or more of the following:
    a **Lymph nodes** on biopsy are found to be involved in hilus, the periaortic chains, or beyond.
    b. **Diffuse peritoneal contamination** has occurred: eg, tumor spillage has occurred beyond the flank before or during surgery or tumor growth has penetrated through the peritoneal surface.
    c. **Peritoneal implants** are found.
    d. **Tumor extends beyond the surgical margins** either microscopically or grossly.
    e. **Tumor is not completely resected** because of local infiltration of vital structures.
4. **Stage IV.** Hematogenous metastases or deposits beyond Stage III: eg, lung, liver, bone, and brain metastases are present.
5. **Stage V.** Bilateral renal involvement is present at diagnosis. An attempt should be made to stage each side according to the above criteria on the basis of the extent of disease before biopsy.

B. **TNM staging system**
1. **Tumor stage**
    a. **Clinical tumor stage**
        (1) **TX.** Primary tumor cannot be assessed.
        (2) **T0.** No evidence of a primary tumor exists.
        (3) **T1.** Unilateral tumor no larger than 80 cm^2 (including the kidney) exists.
        (4) **T2.** Unilateral tumor larger than 80 cm^2 (including the kidney) exists.
        (5) **T3.** Unilateral tumor is present that ruptures before treatment.
        (6) **T4.** Bilateral tumors exist.
    b. **Pathologic tumor stage**
        (1) **pTX.** Primary tumor cannot be assessed.
        (2) **pT0.** No evidence of a primary tumor exists.

      (3) pT1. Tumor is intrarenal and completely encapsulated; excision is complete and margins are histologically free.

      (4) pT2. Tumor invades beyond the capsule or renal parenchyma; excision is complete.

      (5) pT3. Tumor invades beyond the capsule or renal parenchyma; excision is incomplete or tumor undergoes preoperative or operative rupture.

         (a) pT3a. Microscopic residual tumor is limited to the tumor bed.

         (b) pT3b. Macroscopic residual tumor, spillage, or malignant ascites is present.

         (c) pT3c. Surgical exploration only; tumor is not resected.

      (6) pT4. Bilateral tumors.

         Note: Tumor invasion beyond the capsule or renal parenchyma includes breach of the renal capsule or tumor seen microscopically outside the capsule; tumor adhesions microscopically confirmed; infiltrations of, or tumor thrombus within, the renal vessels outside the kidney; infiltration of the renal pelvis or ureter or parapelvic and pericaliceal fat.

  2. Lymph node stage

    a. Clinical lymph node stage

      (1) NX. Regional lymph nodes cannot be assessed.

      (2) N0. No regional lymph node metastases exist.

      (3) N1. Regional lymph node metastases are present.

    b. Pathologic lymph node stage

      (1) pNX. Regional lymph nodes cannot be assessed.

      (2) pN0. No regional lymph nodes are involved.

      (3) pN1. Regional lymph node metastases are present.

         (a) pN1a. Regional lymph node metastases are completely resected.

         (b) PN1b. Regional lymph node metastases are incompletely resected.

  3. Metastatic stage

    a. MX. Distant metastases cannot be assessed.

    b. M0. No distant metastases exist.

    c. M1. Distant metastases are present.

  4. Stage groupings

    a. Clinical stage groupings

      (1) Stage I. T1, N0, M0.

      (2) Stage II. T2, N0, M0.

      (3) Stage III. T1–2, N1, M0; T3, any N, M0.

      (4) Stage IVA. T1–3, any N, M1.

      (5) Stage IVB. T4, any N, any M.

    b. Pathologic stage groupings

      (1) Stage I. T1, N0, M0.

      (2) Stage II. T1, N1a, M0; T2, N0–1a, M0.

      (3) Stage IIIA. T3a, N0–1a, M0.

      (4) Stage IIIB. T1–3a, N1b, M0; T3b–3c, any N, M0.

      (5) Stage IVA. T1–3c, any N, M1.

      (6) Stage IVB. T4, any N, any M.

IX. Treatment. The treatment of Wilms' tumor involves a combination of surgery, irradiation, and chemotherapy.

  A. Surgery

    1. Primary Wilms' tumor

      a. Indications. Surgery remains the cornerstone of treatment for Wilms' tumor and is **indicated in all patients** (even in the presence of metastases) except the **5–15%** whose malignancies that are too large for safe resection (ie, those that cross the midline or are fixed to adjacent structures).

      b. Approaches. A **transverse** or **midline abdominal** incision is used, as for a transperitoneal approach. A **thoracoabdominal** incision is preferred for large upper-pole tumors and for excision of ipsilateral pulmonary metastases.

      c. Procedures

         (1) Radical nephrectomy. Before surgery, the status of the vena cava and renal pelvis also should be ascertained. Following initial abdominal exploration, **radical nephrectomy** is generally required to remove the tumor (see p 303, **IX.A.1.c**). Contiguous structures that are involved can be excised en bloc. Subsequently, Gerota's fascia of the contralateral kidney should be opened and the contralateral kidney should be gently explored to exclude bilateral disease. In addition, suspicious lymph nodes are excised and perihilar, pericaval, and periaortic lymph nodes are sampled. Any unresectable tumor is marked by surgical clips to facilitate postoperative radiation therapy. Special care should be taken to avoid intraoperative **tumor spillage (occurs in 16% of** cases) because this adversely affects tumor stage and **doubles the rate of abdominal recurrence.**

(2) **Partial nephrectomy.** If **bilateral** disease is discovered, exploration with **lymph node sampling** and bilateral incisional or excisional (if ≥ 67% of the renal parenchyma can be salvaged) renal **biopsy** is indicated. Postoperative chemotherapy is given according to the stage of the more advanced lesion. A **second-look procedure** is performed within 6 months, and partial nephrectomy, excisional biopsy, or both are performed, if possible. Subsequently, chemotherapy is continued (radiation therapy may be added) and a **third-look operation** is performed after another 6 months. During treatment, tumor size is carefully monitored by CT because the tumor may grow rapidly. **Survival** after **bilateral nephrectomy** and renal transplantation **remains poor.**

2. **Locally advanced and metastatic Wilms' tumor.** Excluding lesions that are too large for safe resection, surgical extirpation of the primary tumor is indicated even in patients with distant metastases. In addition, resection of **pulmonary metastases** and, in rare cases, other distant sites of disease may be beneficial.

3. **Morbidity and mortality.** Complications are identical to those occurring after nephrectomy for renal cell carinoma (see p 303, **IX.A.1.d**).

B. **Radiation therapy**
1. **Primary Wilms' tumor.** Radiation as the initial definitive therapeutic modality is not widely accepted.
2. **Adjuvant radiation therapy**
   a. **Preoperative radiation therapy.** Although preoperative radiation improves the rate of resectability and disease-free survival in patients with large tumors, it is no longer used because of the **success of preoperative chemotherapy.**
   b. **Postoperative radiation therapy.** NWTS cooperative studies have established that radiation therapy (**2000–27900 cGy** in 150 cGy fractions) after surgery **may eliminate abdominal recurrence** and is **indicated in patients** with **Stage III and Stage IV favorable** histology and in **all** patients with **unfavorable** histology; however, NWTS 2 established that postoperative radiation in patients with Stage 1 tumors (favorable histology) did not improve the results obtained with vincristine and actinomycin-D chemotherapy.
3. **Locally advanced and metastatic Wilms' tumor.** In rare cases, radiation therapy may improve control of locally advanced and metastatic Wilms' lesions.
4. **Morbidity and mortality.** The long-term side effects of therapy include radiation nephritis, musculoskeletal damage, and hepatic and enteric injury.

C. **Chemotherapy**
1. **Primary Wilms' tumor.** Chemotherapy remains necessary for all patients with Wilms' tumors. As the sole means of initial tumor control, however, it does not represent adequate therapy.
2. **Adjuvant chemotherapy**
   a. **Preoperative chemotherapy.** Large locally advanced Wilms' tumors may shrink with preoperative chemotherapy, **increasing the rate of resection** and reducing the recurrence and morbidity associated with surgery.
   b. **Postoperative chemotherapy**
      (1) **Single agents.** Studies on the effectiveness of **actinomycin-D, doxorubicin, vincristine,** cyclophosphamide, and cisplatin have demonstrated **response rates of 58%, 63%, 60%,** 27%, and 16%, respectively.
      (2) **Combination chemotherapy.** NWTS 1 documented that combination chemotherapy with **vincristine** and **actinomycin-D** is superior to either agent alone. NWTS 3 demonstrated that **less aggressive chemotherapy regimens** produce comparable results to more intensive schedules for children with all stages and favorable histology. The aim of NWTS 4 is to shorten and simplify chemotherapy for patients with favorable histology and to improve the results with Stage IV disease and tumors of unfavorable histology that account for the majority of treatment failures.
3. **Locally advanced and metastatic Wilms' tumor.** Intensive combination che-

motherapy remains the only systemic therapy available for these patients. Wilms' tumor has a **high rate of cure** even in the face of metastatic disease.

X. **Prognosis**

    A. **Risk of recurrence.** Most recurrences manifest **within 4 years.**

    B. **Two- and 5-year survival.** Overall, the 2-year survival rates for patients with **favorable** histology versus **unfavorable** histology are **90%** and **54%**, respectively. The 2-year relapse-free survival rates for **Stages I, II, III, and IV** are **95%, 90%, 84%, and 54%,** respectively. With **bilateral disease**, 3-year survival is estimated to be **76%.**

    C. **Adverse prognostic factors.** The following disease features are associated with an unusually poor outcome:

        1. **Anaplasia (unfavorable histology).** The single most important histologic indicator of adverse prognosis is the presence of anaplasia, particularly if diffuse.

        2. **Lymph node involvement.** A significant adverse prognostic sign is nodal metastasis.

XI. **Patient follow-up**

    A. **General guidelines.** Patients with Wilms' tumor should be followed every 3 months for 2 years, every 6 months for an additional 3 years, then annually for evidence of tumor recurrence. Specific guidelines are listed below.

    B. **Routine evaluation.** Each clinic visit should include the following examinations:

        1. **Medical history and physical examination.** An interval medical history and thorough physical examination should be performed during each office visit. Areas for particular attention are discussed on p 593, **VI.A**)

        2. **Blood tests**

            a. **Complete blood count** (see p 1, **IV.A.1**).

            b. **Hepatic transaminases** (see p 1, **IV.A.2**).

            c. **Alkaline phosphatase** (see p 1, **IV.A.3**).

            d. **Electrolytes** (see p 454, **VI.B.1.d**).

            e. **BUN and creatinine** (see p 2, **IV.A.6**).

        3. **Chest x-ray** (see p 3, **IV.C.1**).

    C. **Additional evaluation.** Other tests that should be obtained at regular intervals (**every 3–4 months**) include **computed tomography scans of the chest and abdomen** to exclude local recurrence and metastases to the liver, lung, and distant areas.

    D. **Optional evaluation.** The following tests and procedures may be indicated by previous diagnostic findings or clinical suspicion:

        1. **Blood tests** (see p 2, **IV.A**)

            a. **5′-Nucleotidase.**

            b. **GGTP.**

        2. **Imaging studies**

            a. **Magnetic resonance imaging (MRI).** MRI may detect local recurrences and liver and lymph node metastases (see, also, **VI.C.3.a**).

            b. **Technetium-99m bone scan** (see p 3, **IV.C.5**).

        3. **Biopsy.** A new mass that appears on imaging studies should be biopsied by **fine needle aspiration** to confirm or exclude the possibility of recurrent or metastatic disease.

REFERENCES

Beckwith, JB, et. al. Nephrogenic rests, nephroblastomatosis, and the pathogenesis of Wilms' tumor. Pediat Pathol 10:1–36, 1990.

Broecker, BH and Klein, FA. Pediatric Tumors of the Genitourinary Tract. Allen R. Liss, New York: pp. 25–86, 1988.

D'Angio, GJ et. al. Treatment of Wilms' tumor: Results of the Third National Wilms' Tumor Study. Cancer 64:349–360, 1989.

D'Angio, GJ, Duckett, JW, and Belasco, JB. Upper urinary tract tumors. In Clinical Pediatric Urology, Kelalis, PP and King, LR, eds. WB Saunders, Philadelphia: 2nd ed, pp. 1157–1183, 1985.

Halperin, EC. Pediatric radiation oncology. Invest Radiol 21(5):429–436, 1986.

Kramer, SA and Kelalis, PP. Wilms' Tumor 1984. AUA Update Series 3(lesson 18), 1984.

Leonard, AS, Alyono, D, Fischel, RJ, et. al. Role of the surgeon in the treatment of children's cancer. Surg Clin North Am 65(6):1387–1422, 1985.

Mesrobian, HG, Wilms' Tumor: Past, Present, Future. J Urol 140(2):231–238, 1988.

Tefft, M, D'Angio, GJ, and Grant, W. Postoperative radiation therapy for residual Wilms' tumor. Review of Group III patients in the National Wilms' Tumor Study. Cancer 37(6):2768–2772, 1976.

75 Malignancies of the Germ Cell

Cynthia A. Corporan, MD

I. **Epidemiology.** Germ cell neoplasms (choriocarcinoma, embryonal carcinoma, germinoma, gonadoblastoma, polyembryoma, teratoma, and yolk sac tumor) represent **3% of all childhood tumors.** Nearly **0.1 cases per 100,000** children are diagnosed each year. Estimates indicate that **215 new cases** will occur in 1993.

II. **Risk factors**
   A. **Age.** A **bimodal** age distribution characterizes germ cell tumors; **extragonadal** teratomas and testicular **yolk sac** neoplasms present **before age 3** years and **other gonadal tumors** (particularly ovarian teratomas and dysgerminomas) arise **after the age of 10 years.**
   B. **Sex.** The risk of germ cell neoplasms and, in parlticular, **sacrococcygeal teratomas in females** is **2–3 times** greater than in males.
   C. **Race. Testicular** neoplasms are **rare** in **black** children.
   D. **Genetic factors**
      1. **Family history.** In general, first-degree siblings are **not** known to be at increased risk of germ cell cancers.
      2. **Familial syndromes.** A rare familial syndrome of **presacral teratomas,** sacral defects, and anal stenosis has been reported.
      3. **Chromosomal anomalies.** Duplication and loss of **chromosome 1p** and the **c-myc oncogene** have been implicated in the pathogenesis of germ cell neoplasms.
   E. **Previous germ cell pathology.** Previous congenital and acquired germ cell disorders do not predispose to germ cell tumors; however, an association with **hematologic malignancies** exists.

III. **Presentation**
   A. **Signs and symptoms**
      1. **Local manifestations.** Signs and symptoms vary with site of the tumor.
         a. **Sacrococcygeal tumor.** Neurologic involvement of the bladder, rectum (constipation), and lower extremities (weakness) may be present. A **presacral mass diagnosed within 2 months of birth** is typical of sacrococcygeal teratoma, although abdominal and buttock masses also occur.
         b. **Gonadal tumor. Females** may present with **abdominal pain,** distention, nausea, vomiting, constipation, frequency, urgency, and an abdominal or pelvic mass, whereas a **painless testicular mass** usually occurs in **males. Vaginal germ cell tumors** present with a **bloody vaginal discharge.**
         c. **Intracranial tumor. Headache** is the most common symptom, but **cranial nerve paralysis** (upward gaze) may arise.
         d. **Mediastinal tumor.** Although **often asymptomatic,** mediastinal germ cell neoplasms may present with **chest pain, coughing,** wheezing, dyspnea, hemoptysis, and a **mediastinal mass.**
         e. **Abdominal** germ cell tumors present with symptoms identical to ovarian teratomas (see **III.A.1.b** above).
         f. **Head and neck tumor.** Germ cell tumors of the head and neck often produce **dyspnea,** wheezing, stridor, **dysphagia,** and a **palpable mass.**
      2. **Systemic manifestations.** Fever, malaise, anorexia, weight loss are rare, but **pulmonary and hepatic masses** (metastases) are not unusual.
   B. **Paraneoplastic syndromes.** Syndromes related to overproduction of beta-human chorionic gonadotropin (beta-hCG) and sex hormones are identical to syndromes of gonadotropin excess (see p 117).

IV. **Differential diagnosis.** Most germ cell neoplasms present with a **mass;** however, the differential diagnosis varies with the site of the tumor. Sacrococcygeal teratomas produce **sacral masses** similar to other disorders (perirectal and pilonidal abscesses, meningocele, lipomeningocele, rectal duplication, vestigial tail, hemangiomas, lipomas, epidermal cyst, chondromas, chordomas, lymphomas, ependymomas, neuroblastomas, mucinoid carcinomas, and gliomas). Similarly, the list of diagnostic possibilities for **abdominal, pelvic, and mediastinal masses** is extensive (see p 284, **IV;** p 345, **IV;** p 593, **IV;** and p 214, **VI;** respectively). In rare cases, germ cell neoplasms must be considered in the differential diagnosis of **intracranial** (see p 436, **IV**) and **genital** (see p 333, **IV,** and p 378, **IV**) **masses.**

V. **Diagnostic workup**
  A. **Medical history and physical examination.** A thorough medical history and a complete physical examination should be performed in all patients with suspected germ cell neoplasms. Particular attention should be paid to the following areas:
    1. **Head and neck. Tracheal deviation**, stridor, and neck masses should be noted.
    2. **Lymph nodes.** The number, consistency, tenderness, and distribution of all cervical, supraclavicular, axillary, and inguinal lymph nodes must be carefully documented.
    3. **Chest.** Cyanosis, tachypnea, muffled heart tones, and improved breathing while the patient is prone should be excluded on pulmonary examination.
    4. **Abdomen.** Hepatosplenomegaly and all masses must be fully described.
    5. **Genitalia.** Pelvic (ovarian), testicular, and polypoid vaginal masses should raise the suspicion of germ cell tumors.
    6. **Rectum.** A **presacral mass**, with or without extension to the buttocks, pelvis, and abdomen, strongly suggests sacrococcygeal teratoma.
    7. **Nervous system.** A thorough neurologic examination, including the presence of **upward gaze paralysis** and incoordination, must be carefully documented.
  B. **Primary tests and procedures.** The following diagnostic tests and procedures should be performed initially on all patients with suspected germ cell tumors:
    1. **Blood tests**
       a. **Complete blood count** (see p 1, **IV.A.1**).
       b. **Hepatic transaminases** (see p 1, **IV.A.2**).
       c. **Alkaline phosphatase** (see p 1, **IV.A.3**).
       d. **BUN and creatinine** (see p 3, **IV.A.6**).
       e. **Alpha fetoprotein (AFP).** This tumor marker is produced by **embryonal carcinoma, yolk sac tumors** (sacrococcygeal teratoma), and **polyembryomas.**
       f. **Beta-human chorionic gonadotropin (beta-hCG).** Embryonal carcinoma, choriocarcinoma, and polyembryoma produce this hormone.
    2. **Urine tests**
       a. **Urinalysis** (see p 3, **IV.B**).
       b. **24-hour urinary catecholamines.** A neuroblastoma may be excluded by this test (see, also, **VI.B.2.b**).
    3. **Imaging studies** (see p 3, **IV.C**)
       a. **Chest x-ray.**
       b. **Computed tomography (CT).** CT scan of the **head** (cranial teratoma), **chest** (mediastinal germ cell tumors), and **abdomen** and **pelvis** (ovarian, testicular, and sacrococcygeal teratoma) are indicated to assess the primary tumor and the liver and lung for metastatic disease. The urinary system also should be evaluated.
    4. **Invasive procedures.** A biopsy should be performed for any suspicious lesion, particularly in high-risk patients.
  C. **Optional tests and procedures.** The following examinations may be indicated by previous diagnostic findings or clinical suspicion:
    1. **Blood tests** (see p 12, **IV.A**)
       a. **5′-Nucleotidase.**
       b. **GGTP.**
    2. **Imaging studies**
       a. **Plain radiographs.** Lateral x-ray of the pelvis may show **anterior** displacement of the rectum by sacrococcygeal teratomas.
       b. **Barium enema.** In rare cases, this imaging study may be necessary to evaluate the rectum and anus.
       c. **Intravenous pyelogram (IVP).** In the absence of a CT scan demonstrating the anatomy and functional status of the urinary tract, an IVP is required.
       d. **Magnetic resonance imaging (MRI)** (see p 3, **IV.C.3**).
       e. **Ultrasound** (see p 3, **IV.C.3**).
       f. **Technetium-99m bone scan** (see p 3, **IV.C.5**).

3. **Invasive procedures**
   a. **Fine needle aspiration (FNA).** FNA can be used to assess suspicious supraclavicular or inguinal lymph nodes as well as lung, liver, and pelvic masses.
   b. **Lumbar puncture.** With intracranial germ cell tumors, cerebrospinal fluid may contain AFP, beta-hCG, or both.

VI. Pathology
A. **Location.** Only **one-third of germ cell tumors** arise in **gonadal tissue** (ovary 29%, testes 7%), whereas nearly two-thirds occur at extragonadal sites: **sacrum or coccyx 41%, mediastinum 6%,** cranium 6%, abdomen 5%, head and neck 4%, and vagina 1%.
B. **Multiplicity.** Multiple primary germ cell neoplasms are **rare.**
C. **Histology.** By histology, germ cell tumors are classified into 7 **types:**
   1. **Germinoma.** Marked by large, monotonous, round cells with vesicular nuclei and clear eosinophilic cytoplasm, these tumors occur in the **ovary, anterior mediastinum, pineal gland,** and **undescended testes.**
   2. **Embryonal carcinoma.** These **anaplastic** neoplasms arise in the **testes** and display a solid or glandular pattern, often with necrosis.
   3. **Endodermal sinus (yolk sac) tumor.** Characterized by a papillary, reticular, or solid pattern and **Schiller-Duval bodies** (perivascular papillary projections), these malignancies begin in the **testes, ovaries,** and **sacrococcygeal region.**
   4. **Choriocarcinoma.** Large round cells with clear cytoplasm and vesicular nuclei (**cytotrophoblasts**), syncytia (**syncytiotrophoblasts**), hemorrhage, and necrosis distinguish these cancers, which are found in the **ovary, mediastinum,** and **pineal gland.**
   5. **Teratoma.** These tumors contain cells from all 3 embryonic layers (ectoderm, mesoderm, and endoderm) and usually arise in midline structures (eg, **mediastinum, sacrococcygeal region**). Only **18–25%** of sacrococcygeal teratomas are frankly **malignant.**
   6. **Polyembryoma.** These embryoid bodies with amniotic cavity, yolk sac, and embryonic disc may occur in the **ovary** and **mediastinum.**
   7. **Gonadoblastoma.** Large germ cells, small Sertoli cells, calcium, and hyaline bodies may be identified in these **gonadal tumors,** which are associated with **germinomas** in **33% of patients.**
D. **Metastatic spread.** The modes and sites of metastatic spread are similar to those of tumors arising in adult germ cells (see p 335, **VII.D,** and p 347, **VII.D**).

VII. Staging.
Testicular and ovarian germ cell tumors can be staged in a manner similar to that with adult tumors (see p 335, **VIII,** and p 348, **VIII**); otherwise, no widely accepted staging system has been developed for pediatric germ cell neoplasms.

VIII. Treatment
A. **Surgery**
   1. **Primary germ cell cancer**
      a. **Indications.** The initial treatment of germ cell neoplasms in all patients is surgical resection.
      b. **Approaches.** The surgical approach depends on the site of the primary germ cell neoplasm.
         (1) **Cranium.** Craniotomy is indicated.
         (2) **Head and neck.** Numerous neck incisions can be used.
         (3) **Mediastinum.** Tumors can be approached through a **posterolateral thoracotomy** or a **median sternotomy.**
         (4) **Abdomen.** A **transverse abdominal** or **midline laparotomy** incision is used.
         (5) **Sacrococcygeal region. A 1-stage posterior approach** to remove the coccyx and lower sacrum is preferred. However, for **lesions that extend into the pelvis,** a **2-stage transabdominal and posterior approach** (v-shaped incision) is required.
      c. **Procedures.** In general, wide excision is performed, but the exact procedure depends on the site of the primary tumor. Special considerations exist when tumor is in the following sites:
         (1) **Ovarian tumor.** The procedures for pediatric and adult ovarian neoplasms are identical (see p 349, **IX.A**). **Initial staging** is followed by **ipsilateral salpingo-oophorectomy** (tumors > 5 cm) and by contralateral salpingo-oophorectomy if bivalve examination of the opposite ovary reveals suspicious nodularity.

(2) **Testicular tumor.** Like adult testicular malignancies (see p 336, **IX.A**), these neoplasms require **transinguinal radical orchiectomy** and, in some cases, **unilateral retroperitoneal lymphadenectomy** (controversial).

(3) **Sacrococcygeal teratoma.** With abdominal or pelvic extension, the superior extent of the tumor is defined **transperitoneally.** Subsequently, the sacrum is divided and the mass is removed **posteriorly.**

2. **Locally advanced and metastatic germ cell cancer.** With the rare exception of symptomatic metastases that are amenable to palliation by simple excision, surgery is **not** indicated for metastatic lesions.

3. **Morbidity and mortality.** The type of postoperative complications vary with the site of the primary tumor and are identical to those that occur with surgery for other malignancies in similar locations (see Chapters 26, 29, 37, 44, 46, and 54).

B. **Radiation therapy**

1. **Primary germ cell cancer.** Although **germinomas** can be treated successfully with **2500–3500 cGy,** radiation therapy is **not** indicated as the initial therapy for common germ cell neoplasms such as **embryonal carcinomas** and **malignant extragonadal teratomas**. In the rare patient who is not a surgical candidate, local control of sacrococcygeal teratoma has been reported with 4000–4500 cGy.

2. **Adjuvant radiation therapy.** Although radiation has been used in patients failing surgery and chemotherapy, no reliable data supports the use of adjuvant radiotherapy.

3. **Locally advanced and metastatic germ cell cancer.** Palliative radiation therapy may be indicated for certain patients.

4. **Morbidity and mortality.** As with surgery, the specific complications of radiation therapy vary with the site of the lesion treated and run the gamut from mucositis to severe myelosuppression.

C. **Chemotherapy**

1. **Primary germ cell cancer.** Chemotherapy plays no role in the initial management of localized germ cell neoplasms.

2. **Adjuvant chemotherapy.** Because of their high malignant potential, **embryonal carcinoma, yolk sac tumors,** and certain advanced **dysgerminomas** and **teratomas** require postoperative chemotherapy even if completely resected. Recommended chemotherapy is discussed below.

3. **Locally advanced and metastatic germ cell cancer**

a. **Single agents. Methotrexate,** actinomycin-D, bleomycin, cisplatin, cyclophosphamide, doxorubicin, etoposide, vinblastine, and vincristine have produced **response rates as high as 47%,** whereas epipodophyllotoxin and ifosfamide have been tried as salvage therapy.

b. **Combination chemotherapy.** Combination chemotherapy, most commonly **VAC** (vincristine, actinomycin-D, and cyclophosphamide), **VAB** (vincristine, actinomycin-D, and bleomycin), or **PVB** (cisplatin, vinblastine, and bleomycin), has proved to be superior to single agents and is similar to therapy used in adults (see p 337, **IX.C.3**, and p 351, **IX.C.3**), producing **complete response rates of 70%.** Patients with **poor-risk** germ cell tumors (39% with metastatic disease) treated with **actinomycin-D, bleomycin, cisplatin, cyclophosphamide, doxorubicin, and vinblastine** (Children Cancer Group study) demonstrated a **69% complete and 27% partial response rate** and a **45% 4-year survival.**

D. **Immunotherapy.** The role of immunotherapy in the treatment of germ cell tumors has not been explored.

IX. **Prognosis**

A. **Risk of recurrence.** The vast majority of patients who fail therapy recur **within 2 years.**

B. **Five-year survival.** The long-term survival of patients with germ cell tumors depends on the histology of the malignancy. In general, the 5-year survival of patients with **extragonadal germ cell tumors** is 60–90%.

1. **Teratomas.** The 1-year survival for **sacrococcygeal tumors** is 60%.

2. **Testicular nonseminomatous germ cell tumors.** The 5-year survival is 45–55%.

3. **Ovarian teratomas.** Survival varies with **stage** and **histologic grade** and ranges from **33–100%** (85–100% with Stage I or II and 20% with Stage IV tumors).

C. **Adverse prognostic factors.** Patients with sacrococcygeal teratomas and the following features face a poor prognosis: **tumor diagnosed after age 2** and **tumor extending into the pelvis or abdomen.**

X. **Patient follow-up**
  A. **General guidelines.** Patients with germ cell tumors should be followed every 1–2 months for 3 years, every 4–6 months for an additional 2 years, then annually for evidence of tumor recurrence. Specific guidelines are listed below.
  B. **Routine evaluation.** Each clinic visit should include the following examinations:
  1. **Medical history and physical examination.** An interval medical history should be obtained and a thorough physical examination should be performed during each office visit. Areas for particular attention are discussed on p 599, **VI.A**.
  2. **Blood tests**
    a. **Complete blood count** (see p 1, **IV.A.1**).
    b. **Hepatic transaminases** (see p 1, **IV.A.2**).
    c. **Alkaline phosphatase** (see p 1, **IV.A.3**).
    d. **BUN and creatinine** (see p 3, **IV.A.6**).
    e. **Alpha fetoprotein (AFP).** This tumor marker may be used to monitor for recurrence and progression (see, also, **VI.B.1.e** above).
    f. **Beta-human chorionic gonadotropin (beta-hCg).** Like AFP, beta-hCG can be used to monitor for disease recurrence and progression (see, also, **VI,B.1.f**).
    g. **Chest x-ray**
  C. **Additional evaluation.** A **computed tomography scan** of the area of the primary tumor as well as the lungs and liver should be obtained **every 3 months** for 2 years and then every 6–12 months depending on the clinical setting.
  D. **Optional evaluation.** The following examinations may be indicated depending on previous findings or clinical suspicion.
  1. **Blood tests** (se p 2, **IV.A**)
    a. **5′-Nucleotidase.**
    b. **GGTP.**
  2. **Imaging studies** (see p 3, **IV.C**)
    a. **Magnetic resonance imaging (MRI).**
    b. **Ultrasound.**
    c. **Technetium-99m bone scan.**
  3. **Invasive diagnostic procedures.** In a patient without known residual cancer, a biopsy of any suspicious or abnormal mass detected on physical examination, chest x-ray, or routine blood testing is indicated.

REFERENCES

Bilmore, DF and Grosfeld, JL, Teratomas in childhood: analysis of 142 cases. J Pediat Surg 21(6):548–551, 1986.

Ein, SH, Mancer, K, and Adeyemi, SD. Malignant sacrococcygeal teratomas-endodermal sinus yolk sac tumors in infants and children: a 32 year review. J Pediat Surg 20:473–477, 1985.

Peckham, MJ, Hamilton, CR Horwich, A. Surveillance after orchiectomy for stage I seminoma of the testis. Br J Urol 59:343–347, 1987.

Perlin, E, Engler, JE, Edson, M, et al. The value of serial measurements of both human chorionic gonadotropin and alpha-fetoprotein for monitoring germ cell tumors. Cancer 37:215–219, 1976.

Socinski, MA, et al. Stage II nonseminomatous germ cell tumors of the testis: Analysis of treatment options in patients with low volume retroperitoneal disease. J Urol 140:1437–1441, 1988.

Taylor, MH, Depetrillo, AO, and Turner, RA. Vinblastine, bleomycin and cisplatin in malignant germ cell tumors of the ovary. Cancer 56:1341–1349, 1985.

Thomas, WJ, Kellcher, JF, and Duval/Arnuld, B. Successful treatment of metastatic extragonadal endodermal sinus (yolk sac) tumors in childhood. Cancer 48:2371–2374, 1981.

Appendix A: Performance Status Scales

APPENDIX A. PERFORMANCE STATUS SCALES

Karnofsky		ECOG		AJCC	
Functional Status	**% Normal Status**	**Activity Level**	**Grade**	**Activity Level**	**Grade**	**Activity**

Karnofsky Functional Status	% Normal Status	Activity Level	ECOG Grade	ECOG Activity Level	AJCC Grade	AJCC Activity
Able to carry on normal activity; no special care is needed	100	Normal; no complaints; no evidence of disease	0	Normal activity	H0	Normal activity
	90	Able to carry on normal activity; minor signs or symptoms of disease				
	80	Normal activity with effort; some signs or symptoms of disease	1	Symptoms but ambulatory	H1	Symptomatic and ambulatory; cares for self
Unable to work; able to live at home; cares for most personal needs; a varying amount of assistance is needed	70	Cares for self; unable to carry on normal activity or do active work				
	60	Requires occasional assistance but is able to care for most of his or her needs	2	In bed < 50% of time	H2	Ambulatory more than 50% of time; occasionally needs assistance
	50	Requires considerable assistance and frequent medical care				
Unable to care for self; requires equivalent of institutional or hospital care; disease may be progressing rapidly	40	Disabled; requires special care and assistance	3	In bed > 50% of time	H3	Ambulatory 50% or less of time; nursing care needed
	30	Severely disabled; hospitalization is indicated though death not imminent				
	20	Very sick; hospitalization is necessary	4	100% bedridden	H4	Bedridden; may need hospitalization
	10	Moribund; fatal processes progressing rapidly				
	0	Dead				

ECOG, Eastern Cooperative Oncology Group; AJCC, American Joint Committee on Cancer

Appendix B: Chemotherapeutic Agents

Name	Class	Mechanism	Cell Cycle Specificity	Indications	Form	Dosage/Administration
Asparaginase (L-asparaginase; Elspar)	Miscellaneous	Hydrolyzes asparaginase into aspartic acid and ammonia	G1 phase specific	Pediatric acute lymphocytic leukemia	Powder for injection (10,000 units/vial): Reconstitute in 5 mL sterile water or NS (2 mL NS for IM injection); Use reconstituted solution within 8 h and only if clear	Pediatric or adult single agent dose: 200 units/kg/day IV for 28 days (perform skin test prior to initial dose and if 1 or more weeks have passed since the last dose) IV infusion: give over at least 30 min through side port of a running NS or D_5W infusion IM: Inject no more than 2 mL per injection site
Bleomycin sulfate (BLM; Blenoxane)	Antibiotic	Inhibits DNA, RNA, and protein synthesis	G2 and M-phase	Squamous cell carcinoma of the head and neck, penis, cervix, and vulva; Hodgkin's disease; reticulum cell sarcoma, lymphosarcoma; nonseminomatous testicular carcinoma	Powder for injection (150 units/vial; Reconstitute in 1–5 mL sterile water, D_5W, or NS for IM/SC injection and in D_5W or NS for IV infusion; Stable for 24 h in D_5W, D_5W with heparin (100 or 1000 units/mL), or NS at room temperature (1 unit = 1 mg of Bleomycin A2)	Dose: 0.25–0.50 units/kg (10–20 units/M2) given IV, IM, or SC 1–2 times/wk (maximum dose = 400 units due to pulmonary toxicity) Note: anaphylactoid reactions occur; treat lymphoma patients with 1–2 units/dose for 2 doses, and if no acute reactions occur, follow with regular dose Hodgkin's disease: begin maintenance dose of 1 unit/day or 5 units/week IV or IM after >50% induction response IV: dilution to 50–100 mL is preferred
Busulfan (Myleran)	Alkylating agent	Alkylates DNA, forming covalent cross-links, and inhibits DNA, RNA, and protein synthesis	Nonspecific	Chronic myelocytic leukemia (less effective in Ph chromosome negative patients; no benefit in blast phase)	2 mg tablets	Induction: 4–8 mg/day until total leukocyte count is < 15,000/mm³ Maintenance: repeat induction dose when total leukocyte count is > 50,000/ mm³; give 1–3 mg/d continuously to prevent relapse if remissions are shorter than 3 months Pediatric dose: 0.06–0.12 mg/kg/d or 1.8–4.6 mg/m²/d until total leukocyte count is < 20,000/mm³

(continued)

CHEMOTHERAPEUTIC AGENTS (cont.)

Name	Class	Mechanism	Cell Cycle Specificity	Indications	Form	Dosage/Administration
Carboplatin (Paraplatin)	Alkylating agent	Alkylates DNA, forming covalent cross-links, and inhibits DNA, RNA, and protein synthesis	Nonspecific	Resistent ovarian carcinoma	Powder for injection (50, 150, and 450 mg/vial with mannitol); Reconstitute in D_5W or NS to a concentration of 10 mg/mL (may further dilute to 0.5 mg/mL); Protect from light; store unopened vial at room temperature; use diluted solution within 8 h	Dose: 360 mg/m² IV q 4 wk (Avoid aluminum containing equipment because it can cause precipitation and loss of potency)
Carmustine (BCNU, BiCNU)	Alkylating agent	Alkylates DNA, forming covalent cross-links, and inhibits DNA, RNA, and protein synthesis	Nonspecific	Gliomas, multiple myeloma, and refractory Hodgkin's and non-Hodgkin's lymphomas	Powder for injection (100 mg/vial); Reconstitute in supplied diluent and 27 mL sterile water giving 3.3 mg/mL (may further dilute to 500 mL with NS or D_5W); Stable for 24 h at 4°C and 8 h at room temperature when reconstituted in ethanol; Stable for 48 h at 4°C and 8 h at room temperature when diluted in 500 mL NS or D_5W	Single agent: 150–200 mg/m² IV on day 1 or 75–100 mg/m² IV days 1 and 2 every 6 weeks Note: use only glass containers and administer IV over 1–2 h; adjust dose in patients with marrow suppression and when given in combination with other myelosuppressive agents; avoid skin contact
Chlorambucil (Leukeran)	Alkylating agent	Alkylates DNA, forming covalent cross-links, and inhibits DNA, RNA, and protein synthesis	Nonspecific	Chronic lymphocytic leukemia and Hodgkin's and non-Hodgkin's lymphomas	2 mg tablets	Initial dose: 0.1–0.2 mg/kg/d for 3–6 weeks (may be given as a single dose not to exceed 0.1 mg/kg/d if bone marrow is hypoplastic or infiltrated with tumor) Hodgkin's lymphoma: 0.2 mg/kg/d for 3–6 weeks

Drug	Classification	Mechanism of Action	Cell Cycle	Uses	Preparation	Dosage/Administration
						Non-Hodgkin's lymphoma or CLL: 0.1 mg/kg/day Chronic lymphocytic leukemia (alternate therapy): initial dose of 0.4 mg/kg increasing by 0.1 mg/kg given in biweekly or monthly doses until maximum effect or toxicity is reached. Subsequent dosage is titrated to produce mild hematologic toxicity (1000–2000 granulocytes/mm³; 50,000–75,000 platelets/mm³; and 8–10 mg hemoglobin/dL) Maintenance: 0.03–0.1 mg/kg/d until maximal control achieved
Cisplatin (CDDP, DDP, CisDDP, Platinol, PlatinolAQ)	Alkylating agent	Alkylates DNA, forming covalent cross-links, and inhibits DNA, RNA, and protein synthesis	Nonspecific	Testicular, lung, ovarian, and bladder carcinoma	Powder for injection (10 and 50 mg/vial); solution for injection (1 mg/mL; 50 and 100 mL/vial) Reconstitute in sterile water to a concentration of 1 mg/mL; stable for 20 h at room temperature; do not refrigerate reconstituted solution; further dilute in 2L of D_5W with 1/2 or 1/3 NS and 37.5 g of mannitol	Bladder carcinoma: 50 –70 mg/m² IV q 3–4 wk depending on previous chemotherapy or radiation-induced bone marrow suppression Metastatic testicular carcinoma: 20 mg/m² IV on days 1–5 of 3 week cycle for 3 courses in combination with bleomycin and vinblastine (see Appendix D2 for combination therapy suggestions for testicular and ovarian cancer) Do not repeat courses until serum creatinine is <1.5 mg/dL, BUN is < 25 mg/dL, and platelet count, WBC count, and auditory acuity are normal Hydration: Infuse 1–2 L of fluid over 8–12 h prior to dose; use solutions containing chloride ions. Infuse dose over 6–8 h; maintain hydration and urinary output over the next 24 h; avoid aluminum containing equipment which can cause precipitation and loss of potency

(continued)

CHEMOTHERAPEUTIC AGENTS (cont.)

Name	Class	Mechanism	Cell Cycle Specificity	Indications	Form	Dosage/Administration
Cyclophosphamide (CPM, CTX, CYT, Cytoxan, Cytoxan, lyophilized, Neosar)	Alkylating agent	Alkylates DNA, forming covalent cross-links, and inhibits DNA, RNA, and protein synthesis	Nonspecific	Hodgkin's lymphoma, non-Hodgkin's lymphoma, multiple myeloma, acute lymphocytic leukemia, chronic lymphocytic leukemia, acute myelocytic leukemia, Neuroblastoma, ovarian carcinoma, breast carcinoma, mycosis fungoides, retinoblastoma sarcomas	Powder for injection (0.1, 0.2, 0.5, 1, and 2 g/vial); 25 and 50 mg tablets; Reconstitute in sterile or bacteriostatic water to a concentration of 20 mg/mL; solution stable for 24 h at room temperature, 6 days at 4°C; may be given IV bolus or infusion (in D_5W, D_5NS, D_5LR, LR), IM, or intracavitary	Induction: 40–50 mg/kg IV in divided doses over 2–5 days (1/3–1/2 reduction in patients with depressed bone marrow) or 1–5 mg/kg/d PO Maintenance: 10–15 mg/kg IV q 7–10 days, 3–5 mg/kg IV twice weekly, or 1–5 mg/kg PO daily Give maximum tolerated maintenance dose (ie. to leukocyte count between 2000–3500/mm³)
Cytarabine (ARA-C, Cytosine arabinoside, Cytosar-U)	Antimetabolite	Inhibits DNA polymerase	S-phase specific	Acute lymphocytic leukemia, acute myelocytic leukemia, chronic myelocytic leukemia, erythroleukemia, meningeal leukemia, childhood non-Hodgkin's lymphoma	Powder for injection (100 and 500 mg/vial) Reconstitute in bacteriostatic water (preservative-free NS for IT administration) to a concentration of 20 mg/mL; stable for 48 h When diluted to 500 mg/L, stability in D_5W and NS is 94–96% at 192 h; discard hazy solution	Acute myelocytic leukemia: Adult single agent induction: 200 mg/m²/d continuous infusion for 5 days to a total dose of 1000 mg/m² over 2 weeks; modify dosage according to hematologic parameters Adult combination therapy for induction: (see appendix C2); For persistent leukemia administer additional complete or modified courses Adult maintenance therapy: schedule is similar to induction therapy Children induction and maintenance: calculate dose based on age, body weight, or body surface area Acute lymphocytic leukemia: Dose schedules are similar to those used in acute myelocytic leukemia

Drug	Classification	Mechanism	Uses	Preparation	Dosage
Dacarbazine (DTIC, Imidazole carboxamide, DTIC-Dome)	Alkylating agent	Alkylates DNA, forming covalent cross-links, and inhibits DNA, RNA, and protein synthesis	Metastatic malignant, melanoma, Hodgkin's lymphoma (in combination with other agents as second line therapy)	Powder for injection (100, 200, and 500 mg/vial) Reconstitute in sterile water to a concentration of 10 mg/mL; stable for 72 h (24 h after further dilution) at 4°C; 8 h at room temperature Change in color from pale yellow to pink or red is a sign of decomposition	Malignant melanoma: 2–4.5 mg/kg/day IV for 10 days every 4 weeks or 250 mg/m²/d IV for 5 days q 3 wk Hodgkin's lymphoma: 150 mg/m²/day for 5 days q 4 wk or 375 mg/m² on day 1 every 15 days in combination with other agents Protect from light IV infusion: further dilute with D_5W or NS
Dactinomycin (Actinomycin-D, ACT, Cosmegen)	Antibiotic	Intercalates between DNA base pairs and inhibits messenger RNA synthesis	Wilm's tumor, rhabdomyosarcoma, choriocarcinoma, nonseminomatous testicular carcinoma, Ewing's sarcoma, sarcoma botryoides	Powder for injection (0.5 mg with 20 mg mannitol/vial) Reconstitute with 1.1 mL preservative-free sterile water; discard within a few hours	IV: Individualize dose, calculate using BSA; do not exceed 15 µg/kg or 400–600 µg/m² IV every day for 5 days; give IV infusion over 10–15 min Adults: 0.5 mg/d IV to a maximum of 5 days; administer second course after 3 weeks provided all signs of toxicity have disappeared Children: 0.015 mg/kg/d IV for 5 days or 2.5 mg/m² over 1 week; administer second course after 3 weeks provided all signs of toxicity have disappeared Isolation–perfusion: 0.05 mg/kg for lower extremities or pelvis; 0.035 mg/kg for upper extremities (lower doses in obese patients or when previous therapy has been employed) "Two needle technique" should be used if given directly into vein; reconstitute and withdraw dose with one needle, use another for injection

Meningeal leukemia: ARA-C 5–75 mg/m² IT every day for 4 days or once every 4 days; most common dose is 30 mg/m² every 4 days until CSF findings are normal, and then give one additional course

(continued)

CHEMOTHERAPEUTIC AGENTS (cont.)

Name	Class	Mechanism	Cell Cycle Specificity	Indications	Form	Dosage/Administration
Daunorubicin (DNR, Cerubidine)	Antibiotic	Intercalates between DNA base pairs and inhibits nucleic acid synthesis	Nonspecific	Acute myelocytic leukemia, acute lymphocytic leukemia (adults and children)	Powder for injection (20 mg with 100 mg mannitol/vial) Reconstitute with 4 mL of sterile water for injection for a total of 5 mg/mL; For IV use only; color change from red to purple is a sign of decomposition	Induction: Acute myelocytic leukemia: Adult < 60 years: see ARA-C + DNR in Appendix D2 for suggested doses Acute lymphocytic leukemia: Adult dose: see Appendix D2 for VP + L-asparaginase + DNR Pediatric dose: see Appendix D2 for VP + DNR Administration: withdraw dose into syringe with 10–15 mL of normal saline; inject into tubing or sidearm of a rapidly flowing infusion of D₅W or NS over 2–3 min; do not mix with other drugs or heparin; protect from light
Doxorubicin HCL (ADR, Adriamycin RDF, Adriamycin PFS)	Antibiotic	Intercalates between DNA base pairs and inhibits nucleic acid synthesis	Nonspecific	Acute lymphocytic leukemia, acute myelocytic leukemia, breast carcinoma, Wilm's tumor, neuroblastoma, soft tissue and bone sarcomas, ovarian carcinoma, transitional cell carcinoma, thyroid carcinoma, Hodgkin's and non-Hodgkin's lymphoma, bronchogenic carcinoma	Powder for injection with lactose (10, 20, 50, and 150 mg/vial); preservative-free solution for injection (2 mg/mL); IV use only Reconstitute in D₅W, NS or sterile water to 2 mg/mL; stable at 4°C for 48 h and 24 h at room temperature Color changes from red to purple indicates decomposition	Dose: 60–75 mg/m² IV as a single dose q 3 wk, 30 mg/m² IV for 3 days q 4 wk, or 20 mg/m² IV weekly (may produce a lower incidence of congestive heart failure) IV push: Administer over no less than 3–5 min into tubing of a freely running infusion of normal saline or D₅W Attach the tubing to a butterfly needle inserted into a large vein; avoid veins over joints or extremities with compromised venous or lymphatic drainage Local erythematous streaking along vein and facial flushing may indicate too rapid administration; protect from light.

Etoposide (VP-16-213, Vepesid)	Mitotic inhibitor	Inhibits DNA synthesis	G2 phase specific	Testicular carcinoma (in combination therapy), small cell lung cancer (in combination therapy)	50 mg capsules; ampules for injection (100 mg/5 mL) Dilute with either D_5W or NS to a concentration of 0.2–0.4 mg/mL; store capsules in refrigerator; stability at 0.2 mg/mL for 96 h and 0.4 mg/mL for 48 h at room temperature	Testicular carcinoma: 50–100 mg/m²/day IV for 5 days or 100 mg/m²/d IV on days 1, 3, and 5 Small cell lung cancer: 35–50 mg/m²/d IV for 4–5 days or twice the IV dose rounded to the nearest 50 mg IV Give courses q 3–4 wk; administer IV over 30–60 minutes; do not give rapid IV injection
Floxuridine (FUdR)	Antimetabolite	Inhibits thymidylate synthetase and DNA synthesis	S phase specific	Gastrointestinal adenocarcinoma	Powder for injection (500 mg/vial); preservative-free injection (500 mg/ampule) Reconstitute in 5 mL sterile water and dilute in D_5W or NS to an appropriate volume for infusion	Dose: 0.1–0.6 mg/kg/d continuous arterial infusion (administer the higher dose range 0.4–0.6 mg/kg/d with hepatic artery infusion because it is metabolized by the liver reducing potential for systemic toxicity) Administer until adverse reactions occur, hold drug and resume when subsided; maintain as long as response continues Use arterial pump to overcome arterial pressure in large arteries, ensuring constant infusion rate
Fluorouracil (5-fluorouracil, 5-FU, Adrucil)	Antimetabolite	Inhibits thymidylate synthesis and DNA synthesis	S phase specific	Colon, rectum, breast, stomach, and pancreatic carcinoma	Ampules for injection (500 mg and 5 g/vial at 50 mg/mL) Store at room temperature; protect from light	Initial dose: 12 mg/kg IV daily for 4 days (max daily dose is 800 mg) and 6 mg/kg on days 6, 8, 10, and 12 unless toxicity occurs Poor risk patients or those with poor nutrition: 6 mg/kg IV daily for 3 days (max daily dose is 400 mg/kg), and if no toxicity is observed, give 3 mg/kg IV on days 5, 7, and 9; discontinue drug promptly if toxicities appear Maintenance: repeat dosages of first course every 30 days after the last day of previous therapy or 10–15 mg/kg/wk as a single dose (max dose is 1 g/wk); use reduced doses for poor risk patients;

(continued)

CHEMOTHERAPEUTIC AGENTS (cont.)

Name	Class	Mechanism	Cell Cycle Specificity	Indications	Form	Dosage/Administration
Hydroxyurea (Hydrea)	Miscellaneous	Inhibits thymidine incorporation and DNA synthesis	S phase specific	Melanoma, resistant chronic myelocytic leukemia, recurrent metastatic or unresectable ovarian carcinoma, squamous cell carcinoma of the head and neck excluding lip	500 mg capsules	Base dose on actual or ideal weight, whichever is less; give therapy for 6 weeks; continue therapy until disease progresses, monitoring white blood count and platelet count. Solid tumors: Intermittent therapy: 80 mg/kg single dose every third day. Continuous therapy: 20–30 mg/kg as a single dose every day. Carcinoma of the head and neck (with irradiation): 80 mg/kg as a single dose every third day starting 1 week prior to radiation therapy and continuing indefinitely. Resistant chronic myelocytic leukemia: 20–30 mg/kg as a single dose every day
Ifosfamide (Ifex)	Alkylating agent	Alkylates DNA, forming covalent cross-links, and inhibits DNA, RNA, and protein synthesis	Nonspecific	Germ cell testicular carcinoma	Powder for injection (1 g/vial). Reconstitute in 20 mL of sterile water (50 mg/mL) and dilute in D_5W, NS, or LR to a concentration of 0.6–20 mg/mL; stable for 7 days at room temperature and 3 weeks at 4°C; if reconstituted without bacteriostatic water, refrigerate and use within 6 h	Dose: 1.2 g/m²/d IV for 5 days every 3 weeks or after recovery from hematologic toxicity; give with slow IV infusion over at least 30 min; give with a prophylactic agent for hemorrhagic cystitis, such as mesna; hydrate with at least 2 L of fluid PO or IV per day

| Interferon α-2a (rIFN-a, 1FLrA, Roferon-a) | Immunomodulatory | Antiproliferative and immunostimulatory agent | Unknown | Hairy cell leukemia (adults), AIDS-related Kaposi's sarcoma (adults) | Powder for injection (18 million IU/vial); Solution for injection (3 and 18 million IU/ampule) Reconstitute with provided diluent to a concentration of 6 million IU/mL; do not freeze or shake; use reconstituted powder within 30 days | Administration: give SC or IM. SC administration is suggested for thrombocytopenic patients Hairy cell leukemia: Induction: 3 million units IM or SC every day for 16–24 weeks Maintenance: 3 million units IM or SC 3 times/wk, decrease dose by 1/2 or hold for severe adverse reactions; treat for 6 months, then evaluate for continuation AIDS-related Kaposi's sarcoma: Induction: 36 million units IM or SC daily for 10–12 weeks Maintenance: 36 million units IM or SC 3 times/wk, decrease dose by 1/2 or hold for severe adverse reactions or use an escalating schedule of 3, 9, and 18 million units/d for 3 days followed by 36 million units/d for the remainder of the 10–12 weeks (this may decrease toxicity); continue until no further evidence of tumor or severe opportunistic infection or adverse reactions requiring discontinuation |

(continued)

CHEMOTHERAPEUTIC AGENTS (cont.)

Name	Class	Mechanism	Cell Cycle Specificity	Indications	Form	Dosage/Administration
Interferon α-2b (IFN-a 2, rIFN-a 2, a-2-interferon, Intron a)	Immuno-modulatory	Antiproliferative and immunostimulatory agent	Unknown	Hairy cell leukemia (adults), AIDS-related Kaposi's sarcoma, condylomata acuminata (intralesional) refractory to other forms of therapy	Powder for injection (3, 5, 10, 25, and 50 million IU/vial) Reconstitute in supplied diluent to a concentration of 3–5 million IU/mL (10 million IU/mL for treatment of condylomata and 50 million IU/mL for treatment of Kaposi's sarcoma); stable for one month after reconstitution at 4°C.	Hairy cell leukemia: 2 million units/m² IM or SC 3 times/wk for > 6 months; patients may self-administer dose at bedtime AIDS-related Kaposi's sarcoma: 30 million units/m² IM or SC 3 times/wk; if severe adverse reactions occur, modify dosage or hold drug; continue until no further evidence of tumor or severe adverse reactions occur Condylomata acuminata: 1 million units/lesion 3 times/wk for 3 weeks intralesionally; use only 10 million unit vial; reconstitute with 1 mL of diluent, use 25-gauge needle, and take care not to inject too deeply or superficially; give in evenings with acetaminophen to alleviate side effects Maximum response in 4–8 weeks; one more course may be given after 12–16 weeks; patients with > 10 condylomata may require additional courses
Leucovorin calcium (Wellcovorin, Citrovorum Factor, 5-formyl tetrahydrofolate)	Unclassified	Converts readily to tetrahydrofolic acid derivatives	None	Antidote for folic acid antagonists (methotrexate) and in combination with 5-FU for colorectal cancer	5, 10, 15, and 25 mg tablets; powder for oral solution (60 mg); powder for injection (25, 50, 100, and 350 mg/vial); solution for injection (3, 5, and 25 g/ampule) Reconstitute oral powder with 60 mL for a concentration of 1 mg/mL; reconstitute powder for injection in sterile water containing preservatives (benzyl alcohol) to a concentration of 10 mg/mL (except 350 mg vial should be reconstituted in 17 mL for 20 mg/mL); stable for 7 days	See methotrexate under dose modifications of Appendix E for leucovorin rescue

Levamisole (Ergamisol, 1-tetramisole hydrochloride)	Immuno-modulator	Restores depressed immune factors	None	In combination with 5-FU as adjuvant chemotherapy for Duke's C colon cancer	50 mg tablets	Give 50 mg PO 3 times daily after surgery and with 5-FU 21–34 days after surgery; For more information call the Drug Management and Authorization Section (DMAS) of the National Cancer Institute at (301) 496–5725, 9AM–4PM EST, Mon–Fri
Lomustine (CCNU, CeeNu)	Alkylating agent	Alkylates DNA, forming covalent cross-links, and inhibits DNA, RNA, and protein synthesis	Nonspecific	Hodgkin's lymphoma, glial tumors	10, 40, and 100 mg capsules	Adults and children: 130 mg/m² PO as a single dose q 6 wk Patients with myelosuppression: 100 mg/m² q 6 wk Monitor blood counts weekly and do not repeat courses until counts are at acceptable levels
Mechlorethamine HCL (Nitrogen mustard, HN2, Mustargen)	Alkylating agent	Alkylates DNA, forming covalent cross-links, and inhibits DNA, RNA, and protein synthesis	Nonspecific	Hodgkin's lymphoma (stage III, IV), polycythemia vera, lymphosarcoma, chronic lymphocytic leukemia, chronic myelocytic leukemia, mycosis fungoides, bronchogenic carcinoma, malignant pleural effusions, pericardial effusions, and ascites	Powder for injection (10 mg/vial) Reconstitute in 10 mL sterile water or NS for a concentration of 1 mg/mL; prepare solution immediately before each use because it will decompose on standing	IV: 0.4 mg/kg as a single dose or in 2–4 divided doses/d based on ideal body weight; administer at night in case sedation required for side effects; repeat courses after hematologic recovery (about 3–6 weeks) Administer through rubber or plastic tubing of a running IV infusion set Intracavitary administration: consult label

(continued)

CHEMOTHERAPEUTIC AGENTS (cont.)

Name	Class	Mechanism	Cell Cycle Specificity	Indications	Form	Dosage/Administration
Melphalan (L-PAM, L-Phenylalanine mustard, L-Sarcolysin, Alkeran)	Alkylating agent	Alkylates DNA, forming covalent cross-links, and inhibits DNA, RNA, and protein synthesis	Nonspecific	Multiple myeloma, ovarian carcinoma	2 mg tablets	Multiple myeloma: 6 mg/d PO for 2–3 weeks monitoring blood counts and adjusting dose, then hold drug for up to 4 weeks (monitoring blood counts); when WBC and platelet counts begin to rise start maintenance dose of 2 mg/d; may carefully increase the dose until myelosuppression develops to assure therapeutic levels; maintain leukocytes between 2000–3500/mm³ Alternate regimens: 1. 10 mg/d for 7–10 days and wait for marrow recovery (WBC > 4000/mm³ and platelets > 100,000/mm³; about 4–8 weeks), and then begin maintenance dose of 2 mg/d (adjust dose between 1–3 mg/d based on hematologic response) 2. 0.15 mg/kg/d for 7 days then hold for 2–6 weeks and begin maintenance dose of 0.05 mg/kg/d when WBC and platelet counts are rising; adjust according to blood counts Ovarian carcinoma: 0.2 mg/kg/d for 5 days every 4–5 weeks
Mercaptopurine (6-Mercaptopurine, 6-MP, Purinethol)	Antimetabolite	Inhibits purine synthesis	S phase specific	Acute lymphocytic leukemia, acute myelocytic leukemia	50 mg tablets	Induction: 2.5 mg/kg/d until improvement or up to 4 weeks; if no improvement, increase the dose to 5 mg/kg/d (in multiples of 25 mg); monitor leukocyte counts and hold drug for abnormally large or rapid falls, and resume after 2–3 days if counts remain stable or rise Maintenance: begin if complete remission obtained; 1.5–2.5 mg/kg/d (use in combination with other agents)

Drug	Classification	Cell cycle specificity	Indications	Mechanism	Preparation/Stability	Administration/Dosage
Mesna (Mesnex)	Detoxifier	None	Inhibition of ifosfamide-induced hemorrhagic cystitis	Reduced thiol form neutralizes toxic ifosfamide metabolites (acrolein and 4-hydroxyifosfamide) in the kidney	Solution for injection (200, 400, and 1000 mg/ampule) Dilute in D₅W, D₅NS, NS or LR to a concentration of 20 mg/mL; stable for 24 h at 24°C; refrigerate and use within 6 h; store ampules at room temperature	Give 20% of ifosfamide (W/W) dose as IV bolus at the time of ifosfamide administration and again after 4 and 8 h (total mesna dose is 60% of ifosfamide dose)
Methotrexate (Amethopterin, MTX, Folex, Folex PFS, Mexate, Mexate AQ, Methotrexate LPF, Abitrexate, Rhematrex dose pack)	Antimetabolite	S phase specific	Acute lymphocytic leukemia, breast cancer, gestational choriocarcinoma, chorioadenoma destruens, hydatidiform mole, lung carcinoma, mycosis fungoides, squamous cell carcinoma of the head and neck, meningeal leukemia, non-Hodgkin's lymphoma, osteosarcoma	Inhibits dihydrofolate reductase, conversion of dihydrofolate to tetrahydrofolate, and DNA synthesis	25 mg tablets, powder for injection (20, 25, 50, 100, 250, and 1000 mg/vial), solution for injection (5, 50, 100, 200, and 250 mg/vial at 2.5 mg/mL), preservative-free injection (50, 100, 200, and 250 g/vial at 25 mg/mL) Stable for 1 week at room temperature; preservative-free preparations may be given IM, IV, or IT; for intrathecal (IT) use, dissolve in preservative-free diluent to a concentration of 1 mg/mL immediately prior to use; stable for 8 h; protect from light	**Administration:** may be given PO, IM, IV, IT, or intra-arterially; PO is preferred. **Choriocarcinoma and trophoblastic disease:** 15–30 mg PO or IM daily for 5 days, then hold until toxicity resolves (1 or more weeks); repeat course 3–5 times measuring human chorionic gonadotropin (hCG); continue 1–2 courses after hCG is normalized. **Leukemia:** Induction: 3.3 mg/m² daily for 4–6 weeks (with prednisone 60 mg/m² daily for 4–6 weeks) Maintenance: 30 mg/m²/wk PO or IM in 2 doses/week or 2.5 mg/kg IV every 2 weeks (repeat induction if relapse occurs) Meningeal leukemia: 12 mg/m² IT or an empirical dose of 15 mg IT every 2–5 days until CSF normal, then give one additional dose; suggested dose guidelines for IT administration (based on BSA):

Age (years)	Dose (mg)
<1	6
1	8
2	10
>2	12
elderly	adjust individually

(continued)

CHEMOTHERAPEUTIC AGENTS (cont.)

Name	Class	Mechanism	Cell Cycle Specificity	Indications	Form	Dosage/Administration
Methotrexate (continued)						Lymphomas: Burkitt's stage I and II: 10–25 mg/day PO for 4–8 days, then hold for 7–10 days Burkitt's stage III: same dose with other agents Lymphosarcoma stage IV: 0.625–2.5 mg/kg/day with other agents Mycosis fungoides: 2.5–10 mg PO daily, 50 mg IM weekly, or 25 mg IM twice weekly Osteosarcoma: 12 mg/m² IV infusion over 4 h on weeks 4–7, 11–12, 15–16, 29–30, 44, and 45 after surgery; dose may be increased to 15 mg/m² if peak serum concentration is below 1000 μ molar at end of infusion Leucovorin rescue: 15 mg PO q 6 h for 10 doses starting 24 h after the start of methotrexate infusion; if patient unable to tolerate PO, give IV at same dose and schedule; monitor using leucovorin suggested guidelines Hydration: infuse 1 L/m² over 6 h, starting 6 h prior to methotrexate infusion and continue hydration at 125 mL/m²/h (3 L/m²/d) during methotrexate infusion and for 2 days following completion of infusion Alkalinization: give sodium bicarbonate PO or IV to maintain urine pH > 7.0 during methotrexate and leucovorin infusion

Drug	Classification	Mechanism	Specificity	Indication	Preparation	Dose/Administration
Mitomycin (mitomycin-C, MTC, mutamycin)	Antibiotic	Inhibits DNA, RNA, and protein synthesis	Nonspecific	Gastric carcinoma, pancreatic carcinoma	Powder for injection with mannitol (5 and 20 mg/vial). Reconstitute in sterile water to a concentration of 0.5 mg/mL; stable for 14 days at 4°C and 7 days at room temperature	Dose: 20 mg/m² IV as a single dose q 6–8 wk, and monitor hematologic parameters after each course of therapy and adjust therapy based on response
Mitotane (o, p'-DDD, Lysodren)	Miscellaneous	Inhibits adrenal function	Nonspecific	Adrenocortical carcinoma	500 mg tablets	Dose: 2–6 g/d in 3–4 divided doses; increase incrementally to 9–10 g/day For severe side effects reduce to a maximum tolerated dose; if patient can tolerate higher doses and improvement of clinical response is possible, increase dose until adverse reactions interfere; continue treatment as long as there is clinical response; stop treatment if no clinical response after 3 months at maximum dose
Mitoxantrone HCL (Novantrone)	Antibiotic	DNA reactive agent	Nonspecific	Acute myelocytic leukemia	Solution for injection (20, 25, and 30 mg/vial at 2 mg/mL) Dilute to at least 50 mL in D₅W or NS	Induction and consolidation: see Appendix D2 for Mitoxantrone with ARA-C combination therapy doses; infuse slowly over 3 min or more into tubing of a running IV line of NS or D₅W

(continued)

CHEMOTHERAPEUTIC AGENTS (cont.)

Name	Class	Mechanism	Cell Cycle Specificity	Indications	Form	Dosage/Administration
Pipobroman (Vercyte)	Alkylating agent	Alkylates DNA, forming covalent cross-links, and inhibits DNA, RNA, and protein synthesis	Nonspecific	Polycythemia vera, chronic myelocytic leukemia refractory to busulfan	25 mg tablets	Polycythemia vera: Induction: 1 mg/kg/d in divided doses; if no improvement after 30 days, increase dose to 1.5–3.0 mg/kg/d Maintenance: 0.1–0.2 mg/kg/d in divided doses; begin when hematocrit reduced to 50–55% and continue as long as needed for clinical response Chronic myelocytic leukemia: Induction: 1.5–2.5 mg/kg/d in divided doses; continue until maximum clinical or hematologic response and hold drug if leukocyte count falls too rapidly Maintenance: 50 mg/week–175 mg/d in divided doses; initiate as leukocyte count approaches 10,000/mm^3; if leukocyte count doubles in 70 days use continuous treatment; if count doubles in greater than 70 days, use intermittent therapy
Plicamycin (Mithramycin, Mithracin)	Antibiotic	Inhibits DNA-dependent RNA synthesis	Nonspecific	Testicular carcinoma, hypercalcemia of malignancy	Powder for injection (2.5 mg with 100 mg mannitol/vial) Reconstitute in 4.9 mL sterile water for a concentration of 0.5 mg/mL; dilute dose in 1 L D$_5$W or NS; discard unused portion	Testicular carcinoma: 25–30 µg/kg/d IV for 8–10 days every month (base on IBW), do not exceed 30 µg/kg/d or give for more than 10 days Hypercalcemia/hypercalciuria: 25µg/d IV for 3–4 days repeating at 1 week intervals until desired calcium level reached, then maintain with 1–3 weekly doses Administer over 4–6 h; prepare fresh solution daily

Procarbazine HCL (N-methylhydrazine, MIH, Matulane)	Miscellaneous	Damages DNA, causes aberrant transmethylation of tRNA, oxidation of sulfhydryl groups on DNA bound protein	Nonspecific	Hodgkin's lymphoma	50 mg capsules	See MOPP in Appendix D2. Adults: base dose on IBW; to minimize nausea and vomiting give in single or divided doses of 2–4 mg/kg/d for the first week; maintain at 4–6 mg/kg/d until WBC < 4,000/mm^3 or platelets < 100,000/mm^3 or maximum response. Hold drug for hematologic toxicity and resume at 1–2 mg/kg/d when recovered; when maximum response is obtained, maintain at 1–2 mg/kg/d. Children: Monitor carefully and give 50 mg/m^2 daily the first week; maintain at 100 mg/m^2 daily until leukopenia or maximum response occurs and when maximum response is reached, maintain at 50 mg/m^2 daily
Streptozocin (Zanosar)	Alkylating agent	Alkylates DNA, forming covalent cross-links, and inhibits DNA, RNA, and protein synthesis	Nonspecific	Pancreatic islet cell carcinoma	Powder for injection (1 g/vial) Reconstitute in 9.5 mL D$_5$W or NS for a concentration of 100 mg/mL; use reconstituted solution within 12 h	Daily schedule: 500 mg/m^2 IV for 5 days every 6 weeks until maximum response or limiting toxicity. Weekly schedule: 1 g/m^2 IV weekly for 2 weeks; increase subsequent doses up to 1500 mg/m^2 in patients not achieving therapeutic response and who have not experienced significant toxicity; do not exceed 1500 mg/m^2 BSA, as this may cause azotemia
Thioguanine (TG, 6-thioguanine)	Antimetabolite	Inhibits purine synthesis	S phase specific	Acute and chronic myelocytic leukemia	40 mg tablets	Initial dose: 2 mg/kg/d PO for 4 weeks, then increase cautiously to 3 mg/kg/d if no improvement or no leukocyte or platelet depression

(continued)

CHEMOTHERAPEUTIC AGENTS (cont.)

Name	Class	Mechanism	Cell Cycle Specificity	Indications	Form	Dosage/Administration
Thiotepa (Triethylenethiophosphoramide, TSPA, TESPA)	Alkylating agent	Alkylates DNA, forming covalent cross-links, and inhibits DNA, RNA, and protein synthesis	Nonspecific	Breast carcinoma, ovarian carcinoma, bladder carcinoma, malignant pleural, pericardial, and peritoneal effusions	Powder for injection (15 mg/vial) Reconstitute in 1.5 mL of sterile water for a concentration of 10 mg/mL; dilute further in NS, D_5W, D_5NS, or LR	IV: 0.3–0.4 mg/kg every 1–4 wk by rapid administration (in converting from mg/kg to mg/m² a ratio of 1:30 is a good guideline) Intralesional administration: Initial dose: 0.6–0.8 mg/kg (for local use into sites, dilute in sterile water to 10 mg/mL); may mix with 2% procaine HCL, 1:1000 epinephrine or both, or inject the local anesthetic first, remove the syringe, and inject the drug through the same needle Maintenance: 0.07–0.8 mg/kg q 1–4 wk Intracavitary: 0.6–0.8 mg/kg through same tube used to remove cavity fluid Intravesical: for papillary carcinoma dehydrate patient 8–12 h, then instill into bladder by catheter 60 mg in 30–60 mL of distilled water; retain for 2 h (reduce volume to 30 mL if patient cannot retain volume of 60 mL for 2 h) and reposition patient every 15 min for maximum area contact Give weekly for 4 weeks; repeat 1–2 times cautiously monitoring bone marrow
Uracil mustard	Alkylating agent	Alkylates DNA, forming covalent cross-links, and inhibits DNA, RNA, and protein synthesis	Nonspecific	Chronic lymphocytic leukemia, chronic myelocytic leukemia, non-Hodgkin's lymphoma, polycythemia vera, mycosis fungoides	1 mg capsules	Administration: Give 2–3 weeks after maximum effect of previous radiation or cytotoxic drug therapy on bone marrow has been obtained, best determined by increase in WBC count Adults: 0.15 mg/kg/wk as single dose for 4 wk Children: 0.3 mg/kg/wk as single dose for 4 wk Continue until relapse if responding

| Vinblastine sulfate (VLB, Velban, Velsar, Alkaban-AQ) | Mitotic inhibitor | Inhibits nucleic acid synthesis, citric acid cycle, urea cycle, and energy production required for mitosis | M phase specific | Hodgkin's lymphoma, lymphocytic and histiocytic lymphoma, mycosis fungoides, testicular carcinoma, Kaposi's sarcoma, Letterer-Siwe disease, choriocarcinoma, breast carcinoma, lung carcinoma | Powder for injection (10 mg/vial), solution for injection (10 mg/vial). Reconstitute in 10 mL of NS with preservative (phenol or benzyl alcohol) for a concentration of 1 mg/mL; refrigerate |

Administration: Give IV only. Suggested weekly incremental doses:

Dose #	Adult dose mg/m^2	Pediatric mg/m^2
1	3.7	2.5
2	5.5	3.75
3	7.4	5.0
4	9.25	6.25
5	11.1	7.5
Max dose	18.5	12.4

Do not increase dose after WBC count reduced to about $3000/mm^3$
Maintenance: after WBC > $3999/mm^3$ begin with a dose 1 increment smaller weekly, waiting until WBC count has returned to $4000/mm^3$ before the next dose
Give in a running IV infusion or directly into vein over 1 min; if giving directly into vein, rinse syringe and needle with venous blood before withdrawing needle to reduce extravasation; do not dilute dose in large volumes of diluent (ie, 100–250 mL) or give over prolonged times (ie, 30–60 min), these irritate veins; do not inject into extremities where circulation is impaired due to possibility of thrombosis

(continued)

CHEMOTHERAPEUTIC AGENTS (cont.)

Name	Class	Mechanism	Cell Cycle Specificity	Indications	Form	Dosage/Administration
Vincristine sulfate (VCR, LCR, Oncovin, Vincasar PFS)	Mitotic inhibitor (metaphase)	Interferes reversibly with tubulin function and arrests cell division in metaphase	M phase specific	Acute lymphocytic and myelocytic leukemia, Hodgkin's lymphoma, non-Hodgkin's lymphoma, lymphosarcoma, reticulum cell sarcoma, rhabdomyosarcoma, Wilm's tumor, neuroblastoma, lung carcinoma	Solution for injection (1, 2, and 5 mg with 100 mg mannitol/vial) Refrigerate	Adults: 1.4 mg/m^2 IV weekly Children: 2 mg/m^2 IV weekly Children < 10 kg or < 1 m^2: give 0.05 mg/kg IV weekly Impaired hepatic function: 0.05–1.0 mg/m^2, increase to maximum tolerated dose Inject into vein or tubing over 1 min

Appendix C:
Side Effects of Chemotherapeutic Agents

APPENDIX C. SIDE EFFECTS OF CHEMOTHERAPEUTIC AGENTS

Drug	Local	Skin	Hematologic	Gastrointestinal	Hepatic
Asparaginase			Hypofibrinogenemia, fibrinolysis, decreased factor V, VII, VIII, and IX, leukopenia, thrombocytopenia, bleeding, consumptive coagulopathy	Nausea, vomiting, weight loss, abdominal pain, anorexia, pancreatitis, hyperglycemia	Elevated transaminases, alkaline phosphatase, gamma-globulin, ammonia, bilirubin; decreased albumin, cholesterol, fibrinogen
Bleomycin sulfate	Phlebitis	Erythema, rash, striae, vesiculation, hyperpigmentation, tenderness, alopecia, stomatitis		Nausea, vomiting, anorexia, weight loss	
Busulfan		Hyperpigmentation, urticaria, erythema multiforme, erythema nodosum, porphyria, cutanea tarda, dryness, fragility, anhidrosis, cheilosis, alopecia	Myelosuppression, agranulocytosis (rare; usually due to overdose; may progress to aplastic anemia)	Epigastric distress	
Carmustine	Burning, venospasm	Flushing	Myelosuppression	Nausea, vomiting, diarrhea, anorexia, esophagitis, dysphagia	Elevated transaminases, alkaline phosphatase, bilirubin
Chlorambucil		Dermatitis, pruritus, occurrence or exacerbation of herpes zoster, oral ulceration	Myelosuppression, irreversible bone marrow toxicity with doses approaching 6.5 mg/kg	Nausea, vomiting, diarrhea, anorexia, abdominal pain, epigastric discomfort	Elevated transaminases (rare), alkaline phosphatase (rare), bilirubin
Cisplatin		Mild alopecia	Myelosuppression, Coombs' hemolytic anemia (rare)	Nausea, severe vomiting, anorexia	Elevated transaminases (rare)

APPENDIX C: SIDE EFFECTS OF CHEMOTHERAPEUTIC AGENTS

Renal	Pulmonary	Cardiovascular	Neurologic	Reproductive	Misc.
Azotemia, acute and chronic renal insufficiency			Fatigue, somnolence, confusion, agitation, hallucination, headache, irritability, depression, Parkinson-like syndrome, coma		Fatal hyperthermia, fatal anaphylaxis, hypersensitivity, fever, chills
	Pneumonitis, fibrosis				Idiosyncratic reactions similar to anaphylaxis (hypotension, confusion, fever, chills, wheezing) in lymphoma patients
	Bronchopulmonary dysplasia with fibrosis (Busulfan lung)			Ovarian supression, amenorrhea, menopausal symptoms, azoospermia, testicular atrophy, sterility	Syndrome resembling adrenal insufficiency (weakness, severe fatigue, anorexia, weight loss, nausea, vomiting, melanoderma) after prolonged therapy
Renal insufficiency, decreased kidney size	Fibrosis		Optic nerve fiber infarcts, retinal hemorrhage		Conjunctival suffusion with rapid IV infusion
Sterile cystitis	Fibrosis, dysplasia, interstitial pneumonitis		Peripheral neuropathy, seizures	Amenorrhea, azoospermia, sterility	Drug fever, keratitis
Renal tubular damage, hyperuricemia, dose-dependent cumulative renal insufficiency			Peripheral neuropathy, seizures, loss of taste, Lhermitte's sign, autonomic neuropathy, optic neuritis (rare), cerebral blindness (rare), high frequency hearing loss, tinnitus, papilledema		Tetany, vestibular toxicity, altered vision and color perception, anaphylactoid reactions (facial edema, wheezing, tachycardia, hypotension), hypomagnesemia, hypocalcemia, hyponatremia, hypokalemia, hypophosphatemia

APPENDIX C. SIDE EFFECTS OF CHEMOTHERAPEUTIC AGENTS (cont.)

Drug	Local	Skin	Hematologic	Gastrointestinal	Hepatic
Carboplatin		Alopecia	Myelosuppression, bleeding	Nausea, severe vomiting, diarrhea, constipation	Elevated transaminases, alkaline phosphatase, bilirubin
Cyclophosphamide		Alopecia, darkening of the skin and fingernails, dermatitis, oral ulcerations, stomatitis	Leukopenia, anemia (rare), thrombocytopenia (rare)	Nausea, vomiting, anorexia, diarrhea, hemorrhagic colitis, hypokalemia	Elevated transaminases, alkaline phosphatase, bilirubin
Cytarabine	Pain, inflammation, thrombophlebitis, cellulitis	Rash, ulcerations, freckling, pruritus, conjunctivitis	Myelosuppression, bleeding	Nausea, vomiting, diarrhea, anorexia; oral esophageal, and anal inflammation and ulceration; bowel necrosis; abdominal pain	Elevated transaminases, alkaline phosphatase, bilirubin
Dacarbazine	Pain, burning, irritation; extravasation may produce tissue necrosis, severe pain	Erythematous or urticarial rash, photosensitivity, alopecia	Leukopenia, thrombocytopenia	Nausea, vomiting, anorexia	
Dactinomycin	Pain, erythema, extravasation may produce cellulitis, phlebitis, inflammation, necrosis, and tissue damage	Alopecia, eruptions, acne, exacerbation of radiation-induced erythema and hyperpigmentation, ulcerative stomatitis, cheilitis	Myelosuppression	Nausea, vomiting, diarrhea, anorexia, pharyngitis, dysphagia, esophagitis, abdominal pain, ulceration, proctitis	
Daunorubicin HCL	Extravasation may produce painful induration, thrombophlebitis, severe cellulitis, tissue necrosis	Alopecia, rash, pruritus, radiation-recall dermatitis, stomatitis, hyperpigmentation	Myelosuppression	Nausea, vomiting, diarrhea, anorexia, abdominal pain, constipation, dysphagia	

Renal	Pulmonary	Cardiovascular	Neurologic	Reproductive	Misc.
Renal insufficiency			Peripheral neuropathy, paresthesias, ototoxicity, visual disturbances, loss of taste, asthenia		Hypersensitivity reactions (rash, urticaria, pruritus, wheezing, hypotension), pain, hypomagnesemia, hypocalcemia, hypokalemia, hyponatremia
Hemorrhagic and non-hemorrhagic cystitis, bladder fibrosis, renal insufficiency, renal pelvis hemorrhage, SIADH with doses > 50 mg/kg, hyperuricemia	Interstitial fibrosis, (with prolonged high doses)	With massive doses: hemorrhagic cardiac necrosis, transmural hemorrhage, coronary vasculitis		Amenorrhea, azoospermia	Type 1 hypersensitivity reactions, increased B cell activity and IgE, anaphylaxis, secondary neoplasia
Urinary retention, renal insufficiency	Pneumonia, shortness of breath		Dizziness, headache, neuritis		Cytarabine syndrome (fever, myalgias, bone pain, occasional chest pain, maculopapular rash, conjunctivitis, malaise), fever, sepsis, pharyngitis, chest pain, anaphylaxis, allergic edema Facial flushing and paresthesias, flu-like syndrome (fever, myalgias, malaise) Malaise, fatigue, lethargy, fevers, myalgia, hypocalcemia
Hyperuricemia, red urine color		CHF with cumulative doses > 550 mg/m^2, non–dose-related pericarditis/myocarditis (rare)			Fever, chills

(continued)

APPENDIX C. SIDE EFFECTS OF CHEMOTHERAPEUTIC AGENTS (cont.)

Drug	Local	Skin	Hematologic	Gastrointesti- nal	Hepatic
Doxorubicin HCL	Pain, indura- tion, lymphan- gitis, cellulitis, thrombophle- bitis, vesica- tion; extravasa- tion may pro- duce tissue ne- crosis	Alopecia, nail and dermal crease hyperpigmenta- tion, stomati- tis, conjunctivi- tis, lacrima- tion, radiation- recall dermati- tis	Myelosuppres- sion	Nausea, vomit- ing, diarrhea, anorexia, esophagitis, colonic ulcer- ation and ne- crosis	
Etoposide	Local pain, phlebitis	Alopecia, rash, mucos- itis	Myelosuppres- sion	Nausea, vomit- ing, diarrhea	
Floxuridine		Alopecia, ery- thema, derma- titis, pruritus, rash, ulcer- ation, excoria- tion, macera- tion, glossitis, stomatitis	Myelosuppres- sion	Nausea, vomit- ing, diarrhea, anorexia, crampy ab- dominal pain, enteritis, duo- denal ulcer- ation, duoden- itis, gastritis, pharyngitis	Elevated trans- aminases, al- kaline phos- phatase, LDH, bilirubin; he- patic arterial infusion is as- sociated with intra- and extra-hepatic biliary sclero- sis, acalculus cholecystitis, and abnormal BSP excretion
Fluorouracil		Alopecia, nail loss, dermati- tis (maculo- papular ex- tremity rash), dryness, fis- suring, scal- ing, erythema, hyperpigmenta- tion, stomatitis	Myelosuppres- sion	Nausea, vomit- ing, diarrhea, anorexia, esophagitis, proctitis, phar- yngitis, ulcer- ation and bleeding	Elevated trans- aminases, al- kaline phos- phatase, LDH, bilirubin
Hydroxyurea		Maculopapu- lar rash, facial edema, alope- cia (rare), sto- matitis	Myelosuppres- sion	Nausea, vomit- ing, diarrhea, anorexia, con- stipation	Elevated trans- aminases, al- kaline phos- phatase, LDH, bilirubin, ab- normal BSP excretion
Ifosfamide	Phlebitis	Dermatitis, sal- ivation, stoma- titis, alopecia	Leukopenia, thrombocyto- penia	Nausea, vomit- ing, diarrhea, anorexia, con- stipation	Elevated trans- aminases, al- kaline phos- phatase, LDH, bilirubin

Renal	Pulmonary	Cardiovascular	Neurologic	Reproductive	Misc.
Hyperuricemia, red urine color		Acute LV failure (rare); acute life-threatening arrhythmias; cardiomyopathy, CHF, and cardiorespiratory decompensation with cumulative doses > 550 mg/m^2			Facial flushing with rapid IV infusion, hypersensitivity (fever, chills, urticaria, anaphylaxis), cross-sensitivity to lincomycin
		Transient hypotension after rapid IV infusion, hypertension	Peripheral neurotoxicity, altered taste, transient cortical blindness, headache		Anaphylactic reaction (hypotension, fever, chills, tachycardia, dyspnea, wheezing)
		Myocardial ischemia	Lethargy, malaise, weakness, euphoria, acute cerebellar syndromes		Photophobia, fever, decreased visual acuity, nystagmus, diplopia, epistaxis, intra-arterial infusion complications (ischemia, aneurysms, thrombosis, bleeding, malfunctioning catheter, embolism, fibromyositis, abscesses, thrombophlebitis)
		Myocardial ischemia, angina	Lethargy, malaise, weakness, euphoria, acute cerebellar syndromes		Photophobia, fever, decreased visual acuity, nystagmus, diplopia, epistaxis
Increased uric acid, dysuria (rare), temporary renal tubular insufficiency					Fever, chills, malaise
Hemorrhagic cystitis, dysuria, urinary frequency, renal toxicity, hematuria, transient renal insufficiency	Pulmonary symptoms	Cardiomyopathy, hypertension, hypotension	Polyneuropathy, somnolence, confusion, depressive psychosis, hallucinations, dizziness, disorientation, cranial nerve dysfunction, seizures, coma		Fever, allergic reactions, fatigue, malaise

(continued)

APPENDIX C. SIDE EFFECTS OF CHEMOTHERAPEUTIC AGENTS (cont.)

Drug	Local	Skin	Hematologic	Gastrointestinal	Hepatic
Interferon α–2a	Erythema, pruritus	Partial alopecia, rash, dryness, inflammation, pruritus, urticaria, flushing, rhinorrhea, rhinitis, sinusitis, conjunctivitis, salivation, eye irritation	Myelosuppresssion	Nausea, vomiting, diarrhea, anorexia, constipation, abdominal pain, hypermotility, epigastric distress, weight loss	Elevated transaminases, alkaline phosphatase, LDH, bilirubin; hepatitis
Interferon α-2b	Erythema, pruritus	Alopecia, nasal congestion, dry mouth, rash, rhinitis, sinusitis, dryness, pruritus, dermatitis, urticaria, monilia, stomatitis, gingivitis	Myelosuppression	Nausea, vomiting, diarrhea, anorexia, constipation, eructation, pharyngitis, abdominal pain	Elevated transaminases, alkaline phosphatase
Levamisole		Dermatitis	Myelosuppression (rare), Leukopenia	Nausea, vomiting, diarrhea	
Lomustine			Myelosuppression	Nausea, vomiting	Elevated transaminases, alkaline phosphatase, bilirubin
Mechlorethamine HCL	Thrombophlebitis; extravasation may produce painful inflammation and induration	Maculopapular rash, erythema multiforme, herpes zoster	Myelosuppression, bleeding, petechiae, subcutaneous hemorrhages	Severe nausea, vomiting, anorexia	

Renal	Pulmonary	Cardiovascular	Neurologic	Reproductive	Misc.
	Coughing, dyspnea	Hypotension, edema, hypertension, chest pain, congestion, palpitations, hot flashes, syncope, arrhythmias, stroke, TIAs, CHF, myocardial infarction, Raynaud's phenomenon	Dizziness, confusion, paresthesias, numbness, lethargy, coma, apathy, depression, decreased mental status, visual disturbances, diaphoresis, vertigo, nervousness, forgetfulness, gait disturbances, hallucination, seizures, stroke, encephalopathy, dysarthria, psychomotor retardation, aphasia, aphonia, dysphasia, amnesia, sedation, emotional lability, anxiety, irritability, hyperactivity, weakness, involuntary movements, claustrophobia, loss of libido, transient impotence, neuropathy, tremor, altered taste		Flu-like symptoms (fever, fatigue, arthralgias, myalgias, headache, chills), reactivation of herpes labialis, night sweats, muscle contractions, earache, cyanosis
	Coughing, dyspnea	Tachycardia, hypotension, arrythmia with doses 2 million IU/m^2 IV	Dizziness, paresthesias, depression, anxiety, agitation, confusion, hypesthesia, weakness, amnesia, impaired concentration, altered taste, vision disorder, hearing disorder, insomnia, migraine, somnolence, diaphoresis, decreased libido, hypertonia, asthenia		Flu-like symptoms (fever, fatigue, chills, headache, myalgias, arthralgias, rigors), leg cramps, arthrosis, back pain, malaise, gynecomastia, stye, flushing, chest pain; condylomata acuminata patients (tremor, vertigo, emotional lability, epistaxis, nervousness, acne, eye pain, herpes simplex, lymphadenopathy)
			Headache, blurred vision, drowsiness, malaise, irritability, metallic taste		Fever, arm pain
Azotemia, renal insufficiency, decreased kidney size	Fibrosis, infiltrates				Secondary malignancies (long-term use)
			Vertigo, tinnitus, weakness, headache, convulsions, cerebral degeneration, progressive muscle paralysis, death	Delayed menses, oligo- or amenorrhea, impaired spermatogenesis, azoospermia	

(continued)

APPENDIX C. SIDE EFFECTS OF CHEMOTHERAPEUTIC AGENTS (cont.)

Drug	Local	Skin	Hematologic	Gastrointestinal	Hepatic
Melphalan		Alopecia, hypersensitivity, ulcerations	Myelosuppression, Coombs' hemolytic anemia	Nausea, vomiting, diarrhea	
6-Mercaptopurine		Rash, hyperpigmentation, thrush, mucositis	Myelosuppression	Nausea, vomiting, diarrhea, anorexia, ulceration	Elevated transaminases, alkaline phosphatase, bilirubin; intrahepatic cholestasis, hepatic necrosis, ascites, hepatic encephalopathy
Methotrexate		Erythematous rash, pruritus, urticaria, photosensitivity, pigment changes, ecchymosis, telangiectasia, acne, furunculosis, alopecia, ulcerative stomatitis, gingivitis	Myelosuppression, hemorrhage	Nausea, vomiting, diarrhea, anorexia, pharyngitis, ulceration, hemorrhage, enteritis, epigastric distress	Elevated transaminases, alkaline phosphatase, LDH; cirrhosis, fibrosis
Mitomycin	Pain, induration, thrombophlebitis, cellulitis; extravasation may produce necrosis and tissue sloughing	Alopecia, stomatitis, rash (rare)	Leukopenia, thrombocytopenia, microangiopathic hemolytic anemia	Nausea, vomiting anorexia	
Mitotane		Transient rash		Nausea, vomiting, diarrhea, anorexia	
Mitoxantrone HCL	Phlebitis; extravasation may produce necrosis	Alopecia, conjunctivitis, mucositis, stomatitis	Myelosuppression, petechia, ecchymosis, hemorrhage	Nausea, vomiting, diarrhea, abdominal pain	Elevated bilirubin
Pipobroman		Rash	Myelosuppression	Nausea, vomiting, diarrhea, abdominal pain	

Renal	Pulmonary	Cardiovascular	Neurologic	Reproductive	Misc.
	Interstitial pneumonitis	Vasculitis			Allergic reactions
Hyperuricemia					Fever (rare)
Cystitis, hematuria, azotemia, renal insufficiency	Interstitial pneumonitis, fibrosis		Headache, drowsiness, blurred vision, aphasia, hemiparesis, convulsions; IT administration: arachnoiditis (headache, back pain, nuchal rigidity, fever), paresis (paraplegia involving spinal nerve roots), leukoencephalopathy (confusion, irritability, somnolence, ataxia, dementia, seizures)	Amenorrhea, anovulation, azoospermia or oligospermia, infertility, abortion, congenital defects, vaginal discharge	Fever, chills, malaise, fatigue, immunosuppression
Renal insufficiency	Dyspnea, cough, infiltrates				Fever; syndrome of hypertension, microangiopathic hemolytic anemia, thrombocytopenia, and renal insufficiency
Proteinuria, hematuria, hemorrhagic cystitis		Hypertension, orthostatic hypotension, flushing	Depression, lethargy, somnolence, diplopia, vertigo, blurred vision, dizziness		Fever, myalgias, arthralgias, toxic retinopathy, lens opacification, adrenocortical insufficiency
Renal insufficiency	Dyspnea, cough, pneumonia	Tachycardia, ECG changes, chest pain, congestive heart failure, decreased LV ejection fraction, cardiomyopathy	Seizures, headache		Fever, allergic reactions, fungal infections, sepsis

(*continued*)

APPENDIX C. SIDE EFFECTS OF CHEMOTHERAPEUTIC AGENTS (cont.)

Drug	Local	Skin	Hematologic	Gastrointestinal	Hepatic
Plicamycin	Phlebitis; extravasation may produce irritation, cellulitis	Rash, facial flushing, stomatitis	Myelosuppression, coagulopathy (elevated prothrombin, bleeding times), hemorrhagic diathesis	Nausea, vomiting, diarrhea, anorexia	Elevated transaminases, alkaline phosphatase, LDH, bilirubin, ornithine carbamyl transferase, isocitric dehydrogenase; poor BSP excretion
Procarbazine HCL		Rash, pruritus, urticaria, hyperpigmentation, flushing, alopecia, photosensitivity, dermatitis, stomatitis, dryness, herpes	Myelosuppression, anisocytosis, hemolysis, poikilocytosis, eosinophilia, erythrocyte Heinz-Erlich inclusion bodies, petechiae, purpura, epistaxis	Nausea, vomiting, diarrhea, anorexia, constipation, hemorrhage, abdominal pain	Elevated bilirubin
Streptozotocin	Burning; extravasation may produce necrosis		Myelosuppression, severe and potentially fatal leukopenia, thrombocytopenia	Nausea, vomiting, diarrhea	
Thioguanine		Stomatitis	Myelosuppression	Nausea, vomiting, anorexia, necrosis, perforation	Elevated transaminases, alkaline phosphatase, bilirubin, right upper quadrant pain, hepatomegaly, toxic hepatitis
Thiotepa	Pain	Rash, urticaria, alopecia	Myelosuppression	Nausea, vomiting, anorexia	
Uracil mustard		Pruritus, alopecia, dermatitis, hyperpigmentation	Myelosuppression	Nausea, vomiting, diarrhea	Elevated bilirubin and glycogen infiltration (rare)

Renal	Pulmonary	Cardiovascular	Neurologic	Reproductive	Misc.
Proteinuria, renal insufficiency			Drowsiness, headache, depression		Fever, malaise, lethargy, weakness, hypokalemia, hypocalcemia, hypophosphatemia
Hematuria, frequency, nocturia	Cough, hemoptysis, pneumonitis, effusions	Hypotension, tachycardia, syncope	Dysphasia, paresthesias, neuropathy, headache, dizziness, depression, apprehension, nervousness, insomnia, nightmares, hallucinations, lethargy, fatigue, drowsiness, ataxia, foot drop, decreased reflexes, tremors, nystagmus, photophobia, blurred vision, diplopia, papilledema, hearing loss, slurred speech, confusion, seizures, coma		Gynecomastia, pain, myalgias, arthralgias, fever, diaphoresis, chills, immunosuppression, edema, hoarseness, retinal hemorrhage, allergic reactions, secondary malignancies
Proteinuria, glycosuria, renal tubular acidosis, azotemia, anuria, renal insufficiency			Confusion, lethargy, depression		
Hyperuricemia					
Hemorrhagic cystitis			Dizziness, headache	Amenorrhea, oligospermia, azoospermia	Febrile reactions, allergic reactions (rare)
			Nervousness, depression, irritability	Amenorrhea, azoospermia	

(*continued*)

APPENDIX C. SIDE EFFECTS OF CHEMOTHERAPEUTIC AGENTS (cont.)

Drug	Local	Skin	Hematologic	Gastrointestinal	Hepatic
Vinblastine sulfate	Phlebitis; extravasation may produce pain, cellulitis, necrosis	Alopecia, dermatitis, photosensitivity, vesiculation	Myelosuppression	Nausea, vomiting, diarrhea, anorexia, pharyngitis, ileus, constipation, hemorrhage, abdominal pain, enterocolitis	
Vincristine sulfate	Phlebitis; extravasation may produce pain, cellulitis, necrosis	Rash, alopecia, ulcerations	Myelosuppression	Nausea, vomiting, diarrhea, anorexia, constipation, weight loss, paralytic ileus mimicking a "surgical abdomen," abdominal pain, impaction, necrosis, perforation	

Renal	Pulmonary	Cardiovascular	Neurologic	Reproductive	Misc.
SIADH	Acute shortness of breath, bronchospasm	Hypertension, myocardial infarction, cerebral vascular accident in combination with bleomycin, cisplatin	Numbness, paresthesias, peripheral neuritis, depression, malaise, fatigue, weakness, loss of deep tendon reflexes, headache, dizziness, seizures		Pain in jaw, bones, and at tumor site
Polyuria, dysuria, bladder atony, urinary retention, SIADH	Acute shortness of breath, bronchospasm	Hypertension, hypotension	Headache, loss of deep tendon reflexes, foot drop, cortical blindness, diplopia, photophobia, ptosis, optic atrophy, ataxia, paralysis, seizures; sequence: first sensory impairment, then pain, and finally motor difficulties		Fever

REFERENCES

General

American Hospital Formulary Service. Bethesda, MD: American Society of Hospital Pharmacists, 1989.

Carter SK, Glatstein E, Livingston RB. Principles of Cancer Treatment. New York: McGraw-Hill, 1982.

Clinical Oncology, 6th ed. American Cancer Society, 1983.

Dorr RT. Antineoplastic Agents. In Knoben JE, Anderson PO, eds. Handbook of Clinical Drug Data. Drug Intelligence Publications, Hamilton: 6th ed., pp. 397–429, 1988.

Dorr RT, Fritz WL, COMPS. Cancer Chemotherapy Handbook. New York: Elsevier, 1980.

Drug Facts and Comparisons. St. Louis: Lippincott; 1988; pp. 642–689.

Morra ME. Cancer Chemotherapy Treatment and Care. Boston: Hall Medical Publishers, 1981.

Trissel LA. Handbook on Injectable Drugs, 5th ed. Bethesda, MD: American Society of Hospital Pharmacists, 1988.

Specific

Alexander M, Glatstein EJ, Gordon DS, et al. Combined modality treatment for oat cell carcinoma of the lung: A randomized trial. Cancer Treat Rep 61:1–6, 1977.

Barlogie B, Smith L, Alexanin R. Effective treatment of advanced multiple myeloma refractory to alkylating agents. New Engl J Med 310:1353–1356, 1984.

Butler TP, MacDonald MC, Smith FP, et al. 5-Flurouracil, adriamycin, and mitomycin-C (FAM) chemotherapy for adenocarcinoma of the lung. Can 43:1183–1188, 1979.

Cooper RG. Combination chemotherapy in hormone resistant breast cancer. Proc Am Assoc Cancer Res 10:15, 1969.

DeLorenzo L, Stewart JA. Levamisole toxicity. J Clin Oncol 8:365, 1990.

Einhorn LH, Donohue J. Cis-diamminedichloroplatinum, vinblastine, and bleomycin combination chemotherapy in disseminated testicular cancer. Ann Int Med 87:293–298, 1977.

Knospe WH, Loeb V, Huguley CM. Bi-weekly chlorambucil treatment of chronic lymphocytic leukemia. Can 33:555–562, 1974.

Konits PH, Aisner J, Van Echo DA, et al. Mitomycin C and vinblastine chemotherapy for advanced breast cancer. Can 48:1295–1298, 1981.

Laufman LR, Krzeczowski KA, Roach R, et al. Leucovorin plus 5-fluorouracil: an effective treatment for metastatic colon cancer. J Clin Oncol 5:1394–1400, 1987.

Livingston RB, Moore TN, Heilbrun L, et al. Small cell carcinoma of the lung: combination chemotherapy and radiation. Ann Int Med 88:194–199, 1978.

Logothetis CJ, Samuels ML, Selig DE, et al. Cyclic chemotherapy with cyclophosphamide, doxorubicin, and cisplatin plus vinblastine and bleomycin in advanced germinal tumors. Am J Med 81:219–228, 1986.

MacDonald JS, Woolley PV, Smythe T, et al. 5-Fluorouracil, adriamycin, and mitomycin-C (FAM) combination chemotherapy in the treatment of advanced gastric cancer. Can 44:42–47, 1979.

Moertel CG, Fleming TR, MacDonald JS, et al. Levamisole and fluorouracil for adjuvant therapy of resected colon carcinoma. New Engl J Med 322:352–358, 1990.

Rosen G, Caparros B, Mosende C, et al. Curability of Ewings sarcoma and considerations for future therapeutic trials. Can 41:888–899, 1978.

Sawitsky A, Rai KR, Glidwell O, et al. Comparison of daily versus intermittent chlorambucil and prednisone therapy in the treatment of patients with chronic leukemia. Blood 50:1049–1059, 1977.

Stevenson, H (Senior Investigator). Levamisole plus 5-fluorouracil as an adjuvant to surgery for resectable adenocarcinoma of the colon. Group C/Treatment protocol NCI #189–0017. Bethesda, Maryland: Division of Cancer Treatment, National Cancer Institute, 20892, 1989.

Appendix D1: Combination Chemotherapeutic Regimens

Abbreviation	Use	Regimen	Frequency
ABDIC	Hodgkin's disease (MOPP resistant)	Doxorubicin 45 mg/m² IV day 1 Bleomycin 5 units/m² IV days 1, 5 Dacarbazine 200 mg/m²/day IV days 1–5 CCNU 50 mg/m² PO days 1–5 Prednisone 40 mg/m²/d PO days 1–5	Every 4 weeks
ABVD	Hodgkin's disease (MOPP resistant, induction)	Doxorubicin 25 mg/m²/d IV days 1, 14 Bleomycin 10 units/m²/d IV days 1, 14 Vinblastine 6 mg/m²/d IV days 1, 14 Dacarbazine 375 mg/m²/d IV days 1, 14	Twice monthly until remission, then continue 2 more cycles
ACE	Lung cancer (small cell)	Doxorubicin 45 mg/m² IV day 1 Cyclophosphamide 1 mg/m² IV day 1 Etoposide 50 mg/m²/d IV days 1–5	Every 3 weeks
ACe	Breast cancer (metastatic or recurrent)	Doxorubicin 40 mg/m² IV day 1 Cyclophosphamide 200 mg/m²/d PO days 3–6	Every 3–4 weeks
	Ovarian cancer (advanced)	Doxorubicin 40 mg/m² IV day 1 Cyclophosphamide 500 mg/m² IV day 1	Every 3–4 weeks
AP	Ovarian cancer (advanced)	Doxorubicin 50 mg/m² IV day 1 Cisplatin 50 mg/m² IV day 1	Every 3 weeks
A-COPP	Hodgkin's disease (Children, induction)	Doxorubicin 60 mg/m² IV day 1 Cyclophosphamide 300 mg/m²/d IV days 14, 20 Vincristine 1.5 mg/m²/d IV days 14, 20 (2 mg maximum dose) Procarbazine 100 mg/m²/d PO days 14–28 Prednisone 40 mg/m²/d PO days 1–27 (1st and 4th cycles only) Prednisone 40 mg/m²/d PO days 14–27 (2nd, 3rd, 5th and 6th cycles)	Every 6 weeks for 6 cycles
ADR + BCNU	Multiple myeloma (alkylator resistant)	Doxorubicin 30 mg/m² IV day 1 Carmustine 30 mg/m² IV day 1	Every 3–4 weeks
ARA-C + ADR	Acute myelocytic leukemia (induction)	Cytarabine 100 mg/m²/d continuous 24 h IV infusion times 7–10 days Doxorubicin 30 mg/m²/d IV over 30 min times 3 days	Every 2–4 weeks
ARA-C + ADR + VCR + Prednisolone	Acute myelocytic leukemia (induction)	Cytarabine 100 mg/m²/d continuous 24 h IV infusion days 1–7 Doxorubicin 30 mg/m²/d IV days 1–3 Vincristine 1.5 mg/m²/d IV infusion days 1, 5 Prednisolone 40 mg/m²/d IV infusion q 12 h days 1–5	Every 2–4 weeks

(*continued*)

APPENDIX D1. COMBINATION CHEMOTHERAPEUTIC REGIMENS (cont.)

Abbreviation	Use	Regimen	Frequency
ARA-C + 6-TG	Acute myelocytic leukemia	*Induction* Cytarabine 100 mg/m^2/q 12 h IV times 10 days Thioguanine 100 mg/m^2/q 12 h PO times 10 days	Every month until remission
		Maintenance Cytarabine 100 mg/m^2/q 12 h IV times 5 days Thioguanine 100 mg/m^2/q 12 h PO times 5 days	Every month
ARA-C + 6-TG + DNR	Acute myelocytic leukemia (induction)	Cytarabine 100 mg/m^2/d q 12 h IV infusion days 1–7 Thioguanine 100 mg/m^2 q 12 h PO days 1–7 Daunorubicin 60 mg/m^2/d IV infusion days 5–7	Every 2–4 weeks
ARA-C + DNR	Acute lymphocytic leukemia (induction)	Cytarabine 100 mg/m^2/d IV infusion times 7 days during 1st course and 5 days on subsequent courses Daunorubicin 45 mg/m^2/d IV days 1, 2, 3, 1st course and days 1, 2 on subsequent courses	Every 2–4 weeks
ARA-C + DNR + 6-TG + VCR + Pred	Acute lymphocytic leukemia (induction)	Cytarabine 100 mg/m^2/d q 12 h IV infusion days 1–7 Daunorubicin 70 mg/m^2 IV infusion days 1–3 Thioguanine 100 mg/m^2/d q 12 h PO days 1–7 Vincristine 1 mg/m^2/d IV infusion days 1, 7 Prednisone 40 mg/m^2/d PO days 1–7	Every 2–4 weeks
ARA-C + DNR + MP + Pred	Acute myelocytic leukemia (children)	*Induction* Cytarabine 80 mg/m^2/d IV times 3 days Daunorubicin 25 mg/m^2/d IV times 1 day Mercaptopurine 100 mg/m^2 PO daily Prednisone 40 mg/m^2 PO daily *Maintenance* Same dosage	Every week until remission
BACOP	Non-Hodgkin's lymphomas (unfavorable histology)	Bleomycin 5 units/m^2 IV days 15, 22 Doxorubicin 25 mg/m^2 IV days 1, 8 Cyclophosphamide 650 mg/m^2 IV days 1, 8 Vincristine 1.4 mg/m^2 IV days 1, 8 Prednisone 60 mg/m^2 PO days 15–28	Every 4 weeks for 6 or more cycles
B-CAVe	Hodgkin's disease, advanced (resistant to MOPP)	Bleomycin 5 units/m^2 IV days 1, 28, 35 CCNU 100 mg/m^2 PO day 1 Doxorubicin 60 mg/m^2 IV day 1 Vinblastine 5 mg/m^2 IV day 1	Continue until patient receives the maximum tolerated dose of doxorubicin
BCVPP	Hodgkin's disease (induction)	Carmustine 100 mg/m^2 IV day 1 Cyclophosphamide 600 mg/m^2 IV day 1 Vinblastine 5 mg/m^2 IV day 1 Procarbazine 50 mg/m^2/d PO day 1 Procarbazine 100 mg/m^2/d PO days 2–10 Prednisone 60 mg/m^2/d PO days 1–10	Every 4 weeks for 6 cycles

(*continued*)

APPENDIX D1. COMBINATION CHEMOTHERAPEUTIC REGIMENS (cont.)

Abbreviation	Use	Regimen	Frequency
CAF	Breast cancer (meta-static)	Cyclophosphamide 100 mg/m^2/d PO days 1–14 Doxorubicin 30 mg/m^2/d IV days 1, 8 Fluorouracil 500 mg/m^2/d IV days 1, 8	Every 4 weeks until 450 mg/m^2 of doxorubicin then start methotrexate 40 mg/m^2 IV and increase 5-FU to 600 mg/m^2 IV
CAMP	Lung cancer (non-small cell)	Cyclophosphamide 300 mg/m^2/d IV days 1, 8 Doxorubicin 20 mg/m^2/d IV days 1, 8 Methotrexate 15 mg/m^2/d IV days 1, 8 Procarbazine 100 mg/m^2/d PO days 1–10	Every 4 weeks
CAP	Lung cancer (non-small cell)	Cyclophosphamide 400 mg/m^2 IV day 1 Doxorubicin 40 mg/m^2 IV day 1 Cisplatin 40 mg/m^2 IV day 1	Every 4 weeks
	Ovarian cancer (advanced)	Cyclophosphamide 300 mg/m^2 IV day 1 Doxorubicin 30 mg/m^2 IV day 1 Cisplatin 50 mg/m^2 IV day 1	Every 4 weeks
CAV	Lung cancer (small cell, induction)	Cyclophosphamide 750 mg/m^2 IV Doxorubicin 50 mg/m^2 IV Vincristine 2 mg IV	Every 3 weeks
CAVe	Hodgkin's disease (resistant to MOPP, induction)	Lomustine 100 mg/m^2 PO day 1 Doxorubicin 60 mg/m^2 IV day 1 Vinblastine 5 mg/m^2 IV day 1	Every 6 weeks for 9 cycles
CHL + Pred	Chronic lymphocytic leukemia	Chlorambucil 0.4 mg/kg PO day 1 Prednisone 100 mg/d PO times 2 days adjust dosage to blood counts q 2 wk prior to therapy. Increase initial dose of 0.4 mg/kg by increments of 0.1 mg/kg q 2 wk until toxicity or disease control reached	Every other week
CHOP	Non-Hodgkin's lymphomas (unfavorable histology)	Cyclophosphamide 750 mg/m^2 IV day 1 Doxorubicin 50 mg/m^2 IV day 1 Vincristine 1.4 mg/m^2 IV (max dose 2 mg) Prednisone 60 mg/d PO days 1–5	Every 3–4 weeks for 6 cycles
CHOR	Lung cancer (small cell)	Cyclophosphamide 750 mg/m^2/d IV days 1, 22 Doxorubicin 50 mg/m^2/d IV days 1, 22 Vincristine 1 mg/d IV days 1, 8, 15, 22 Radiation total dose 3000 cGy, 10 daily fractions over a 2-week period beginning on day 36	Every 3–4 weeks for 6 cycles
CISCA	Urinary tract (metastatic)	Cyclophosphamide 650 mg/m^2 IV day 1 Doxorubicin 50 mg/m^2 IV day 1 Cisplatin 100 mg/m^2 IV infusion over 2 h day 2 Discontinue doxorubicin when total dose of 450 mg/m^2 is reached and increase cyclophosphamide to 1000 mg/m^2 IV	Every 3 weeks for 9 cycles
CISCA-II/VB-IV	Germ cell tumors (advanced)	Cyclophosphamide 500 mg/m^2/d IV days 1, 2 Doxorubicin 40–45 mg/m^2/d IV days 1, 2 Cisplatin 100–120 mg/m^2 IV day 3 *Alternate with* Vinblastine 3 mg/m^2 continuous IV infusion for 5 days Bleomycin 30 mg/d continuous IV infusion for 5 days	Every 3–4 weeks for 6 cycles or 2 cycles beyond a complete response

(*continued*)

APPENDIX D1. COMBINATION CHEMOTHERAPEUTIC REGIMENS (cont.)

Abbreviation	Use	Regimen	Frequency
CMC-High Dose	Lung cancer (small cell, induction)	Cyclophosphamide 1000 mg/m²/d IV days 1, 29 Methotrexate 15 mg/m²/d IV twice weekly times 6 wk Lomustine 100 mg/m² PO day 1	One cycle only
CMF	Breast cancer (metastatic or recurrent and adjuvant therapy)	Cyclophosphamide 100 mg/m²/d PO days 1–14 Methotrexate 40–60 mg/m²/d IV days 1, 8 Fluorouracil 600 mg/m²/d IV days 1, 8	Every 4 weeks
CMFP	Breast cancer (metastatic)	Cyclophosphamide 100 mg/m²/d PO days 1–14 Methotrexate 60 mg/m²/d IV days 1, 8 Fluorouracil 700 mg/m²/d IV days 1, 8 Prednisone 400 mg/m²/d PO days 1–14	Every 4 weeks
CMFVP (Cooper's regimen)	Breast cancer (metastatic or recurrent)	Cyclophosphamide 2.5 mg/kg PO daily Methotrexate 25–50 mg IV weekly Fluorouracil 12 mg/kg/d IV days 1–4, then 500 mg IV weekly Vincristine 0.035 mg/kg IV weekly (max dose 2 mg) Prednisone 0.75 mg/kg PO daily	Every week for 8 weeks followed by reduced therapy for maintenance
COMLA	Non-Hodgkin's lymphomas (unfavorable histology)	Cyclophosphamide 1.5 g/m² IV day 1 Vincristine 1.4 mg/m²/d IV days 1, 8, 15 Cytarabine 300 mg/m²/d IV days 22, 29, 36, 43, 50, 57, 64, 71 Methotrexate 120 mg/m²/d IV days 22, 29, 36, 43, 50, 57, 64, 71 Leucovorin 25 mg/m² PO q 6 h times 4, start 24 h after methotrexate	Every 12 weeks for 3 cycles
COP	Non-Hodgkin's lymphomas (favorable histology)	Cyclophosphamide 800–1000 mg/m² IV day 1 Vincristine 1.4 mg/m² IV day 1 (max dose 2 mg) Prednisone 60 mg/m²/d PO days 1–5	Every 3 weeks for 6 cycles
COP-BLAM	Non-Hodgkin's lymphomas (advanced histiocytic, stage III or IV)	Cyclophosphamide 400 mg/m² IV day 1 Vincristine 1 mg/m² IV day 1 Prednisone 40 mg/m²/d PO days 1–10 Bleomycin 15 mg IV day 14 Doxorubicin 40 mg/m² IV day 1 Procarbazine 100 mg/m²/d PO days 1–10	Every 3 weeks for 8 cycles
COPP or "C" MOPP	Non-Hodgkin's lymphomas (favorable, unfavorable histology), Hodgkin's disease	Cyclophosphamide 650 mg/m²/d IV days 1,8 Vincristine 1 4 mg/m²/d IV days 1, 8 (max dose 2 mg) Procarbazine 100 mg/m²/d PO days 1–14 Prednisone 40 mg/m²/d PO days 1–14	Every 4 weeks for 6 cycles
CVP	Non-Hodgkin's lymphomas (favorable histology)	Cyclophosphamide 400 mg/m²/d PO days 2–6 Vincristine 1.4 mg/m² IV day 1 (max dose 2 mg) Prednisone 100 mg/m²/d PO days 2–6	Every 3 weeks for 6 cycles
CVAD	Soft tissue sarcomas (adult)	Cyclophosphamide 500 mg/m² IV day 1 Vincristine 1.4 mg/m²/d IV days 1, 5 (max dose 2 mg) Doxorubicin 50 mg/m² IV day 1 Dacarbazine 250 mg/m²/d IV days 1–5	Every 3 weeks

(continued)

APPENDIX D1. COMBINATION CHEMOTHERAPEUTIC REGIMENS (cont.)

Abbreviation	Use	Regimen	Frequency
5-FU + leucovorin	Colon cancer	5-FU 400 mg/m^2/d IV days 1–3 of first cycle and then day 1 only thereafter Leucovorin 80–500 mg/m^2 IV over 20 h prior to 5-FU dose(s)	Every week until toxicity or tumor progression occurs
5-FU + levamisole	Colon cancer	*Cycle 1:* Levamisole 50 mg PO 3 times daily days 1–3 *Cycle 2:* 5-FU 450 mg/m^2/d IV days 1–5 then 450 mg/m^2 IV weekly beginning on day 28 Levamisole 50 mg PO 3 times daily days 1–3	Every 2 weeks for 1 year
FAC	Breast cancer (metastatic)	Fluorouracil 500 mg/m^2/d IV days 1, 8 Doxorubicin 50 mg/m^2 IV day 1 Cyclophosphamide 500 mg/m^2 IV day 1	Every 3 weeks
FAM	Lung cancer (non-small cell), gastric carcinoma (advanced)	Fluorouracil 600 mg/m^2/d IV days 1, 8, 29, 36 Doxorubicin 30 mg/m^2/d IV days 1, 29 Mitomycin 10 mg/m^2 IV day 1	Every 8 weeks
	Pancreatic carcinoma	Fluorouracil 600 mg/m^2/wk IV weeks 1, 2, 5, 6, 9 Doxorubicin 30 mg/m^2/wk IV weeks 1, 5, 9 Mitomycin 10 mg/m^2/wk weeks 1, 9	Every 8 weeks
FOMi	Lung cancer (non-small cell)	Fluorouracil 300 mg/m^2/d IV days 1–4 Vincristine 2 mg IV day 1 Mitomycin 10 mg/m^2 IV day 1	Every 3 weeks for 3 cycles then every 6 weeks
M-2 Protocol	Multiple myeloma	Vincristine 0.03 mg/kg IV day 1 (max dose 2 mg) Carmustine 0.5 mg/kg IV day 1 Cyclophosphamide 10 mg/kg IV day 1 Melphalan 0.25 mg/kg/d PO days 1–4 Prednisone 1.0 mg/kg/d PO days 1–7 then taper to 21	Every 3–4 weeks and continue treatment through remission until disease progresses
MAC	Ovarian cancer (advanced)	Mitomycin 7 mg/m^2 IV Doxorubicin 45 mg/m^2 IV Cyclophosphamide 450 mg/m^2 IV	Every 3 weeks
MACC	Lung cancer (non-small cell)	Methotrexate 40 mg/m^2 IV Doxorubicin 40 mg/m^2 IV Cyclophosphamide 400 mg/m^2 IV Lomustine 30 mg/m^2 PO	Every 3 weeks
MAP	Multiple myeloma	Melphalan 6 mg/m^2/d PO days 1–4 Doxorubicin 25 mg/m^2 PO day 1 Prednisone 60 mg/m^2/d PO days 1–4	Every 4 weeks for 22 cycles
Mitoxantrone + Ara-C	Acute myelocytic leukemia	*Induction* Mitoxantrone 12 mg/m^2/d IV infusion days 1–3 Cytarabine 100 mg/m^2/d continuous 24-h IV infusion days 1–7 *Consolidation* Mitoxantrone 12 mg/m^2/d IV days 1, 2 Cytarabine 100 mg/m^2/d continuous 24-h IV infusion days 1–5	Repeat doses for incomplete induction giving mitoxanthrone for 2 days and cytarabine for 5 days Give first course about 6 weeks after final induction and second course after an additional 4 weeks

(continued)

APPENDIX D1. COMBINATION CHEMOTHERAPEUTIC REGIMENS (cont.)

Abbreviation	Use	Regimen	Frequency
MOPP	Hodgkin's disease (induction)	Mechlorethamine 6 mg/m^2/d IV days 1, 8 Vincristine 2 mg/m^2/d IV days 1, 8 (max dose 2 mg) Procarbazine 50 mg/m^2/d PO day 1 Procarbazine 100 mg/m^2/d PO days 2–14 Prednisone 40 mg/m^2/d PO days 1–14	Every 4 weeks for 6 cycles

MOPP/ABVD	Hodgkin's disease (advanced)	Mechlorethamine 6 mg/m^2/d IV days 1, 8
		Vincristine 1.4 mg/m^2/d IV days 1, 8
		Procarbazine 100 mg/m^2/d PO days 1–14
		Prednisone 40 mg/m^2/d PO days 1–14
		Alternate with
		  Doxorubicin 25 mg/m^2/d IV days 1, 15
		  Bleomycin 10 mg/m^2/d IV days 1, 15
		  Vinblastine 6 mg/m^2/d IV days 1, 15
		  Dacarbazine 375 mg/m^2/d IV days 1, 15
			Every other month
			
			Every other month

MOPP-LO BLEO	Hodgkin's disease (induction)	Mechlorethamine 6 mg/m^2/d IV days 1, 8 Vincristine 1.5 mg/m^2/d IV days 1, 8 (max dose 2 mg) Procarbazine 100 mg/m^2/d PO days 2–7, 9–12 Prednisone 40 mg/m^2/d PO in divided doses days 2–7, 9–12 Bleomycin 2 units/m^2/d IV days 1, 8	Every 4 weeks for 6 cycles
MPL + Pred(MP)	Multiple myeloma	Melphalan 8 mg/m^2/d PO days 1–14 Prednisone 75 mg/m^2/d PO days 1–7	Every 4 weeks for 6 cycles
MTX + MP	Acute lymphocytic leukemia (maintenance)	Methotrexate 20 mg/m^2/wk IV Mercaptopurine 50 mg/m^2/d PO	Continue until relapse or 3 years of remission
MTX + MP + CTX	Acute lymphocytic leukemia (maintenance)	Methotrexate 20 mg/m^2/wk IV Mercaptopurine 50 mg/m^2/d PO Cyclophosphamide 200 mg/m^2/wk IV	Continue until relapse or 3 years of remission
M-VAC	Bladder cancer (transitional cell)	Methotrexate 30 mg/m^2 IV day 1 Vinblastine 3 mg/m^2/d IV days 2, 15, 22 Doxorubicin 30 mg/m^2/d IV days 2, 15, 22 Cisplatin 70 mg/m^2 IV day 2	Every 4 weeks for 6 cycles
MV1b	Breast cancer (metastatic or recurrent)	Mitomycin 15–20 mg/m^2 IV day 1 Vinblastine 6 mg/m^2 IV/d days 1, 21	Every 6–8 weeks
POCC	Lung cancer (small cell)	Procarbazine 100 mg/m^2/d PO days 1–14 Vincristine 2 mg/d IV days 1, 8 Cyclophosphamide 600 mg/m^2/d IV day 1, 8 Lomustine 60 mg/m^2 PO day 1	Every 4 weeks
PVB	Testicular carcinoma	Cisplatin 20 mg/m^2/d IV days 1–5 Vinblastine 0.2–0.4 mg/kg IV day 1 Bleomycin 30 units/d IV days 1, 8, 15	Every 3 weeks for 4 cycles

T-2 Protocol	Ewing's sarcoma	*Cycle 1:*
		  Month 1
		    Dactinomycin 0.45 mg/m^2/d IV days 1–5
		    Doxorubicin 20 mg/m^2/d IV days 20–22
		    Radiation days 1–21 then 2 weeks rest period
		  Month 2
		    Doxorubicin 20 mg/m^2/d IV days 8–10
		    Vincristine 1.5–2 mg/m^2 IV day 24 (max dose 2 mg)
		    Cyclophosphamide 1200 mg/m^2 IV day 24
		    Radiation days 8–28
			Every 12 months for 2 cycles

(continued)

APPENDIX D1. COMBINATION CHEMOTHERAPEUTIC REGIMENS (cont.)

Abbreviation	Use	Regimen	Frequency
		Month 3	
		Vincristine 1.5–2 mg/m²/d IV days 3, 9, 15 (max dose 2 mg)	
		Cyclophosphamide 1200 mg/m² IV day 9	
		Cycle 2: Repeat cycle 1 without radiation	
		Cycle 3:	
		Month 1	
		Dactinomycin 0.45 mg/m²/d IV days 1–5	
		Doxorubicin 20 mg/m²/d IV days 20–22	
		Month 2	
		Vincristine 1.5–2 mg/m²/d IV days 8, 15, 22, 28 (max dose 2 mg)	
		Cyclophosphamide 1200 mg/m²/d IV days 8, 22	
		Month 3	
		No drug for 28 days	
		Cycle 4: Repeat cycle #3	
VAB-6	Testicular carcinoma	*Induction*	Every 3–4 weeks for 2 cycles
		Cyclophosphamide 600 mg/m² IV day 1	
		Dactinomycin 1 mg/m² IV day 1	
		Vinblastine 4 mg/m² IV day 1	
		Bleomycin 30 mg IV day 1	
		Bleomycin 20 mg/m²/d continuous 24-h IV infusion days 1–3	
		Cisplatin 120 mg/m² IV day 4	
		Maintenance	Every 3 weeks for 12 months
		Vinblastine 6 mg/m² IV	
		Dactinomycin 1 mg/m² IV	
VAC Pulse	Soft tissue sarcomas (rhabdomyosarcoma pediatric)	Vincristine 2 mg/m²/wk IV (max dose 2 mg)	Every 3 months for 5–6 courses
		Dactinomycin 0.015 mg/kg/d IV days 1–5 (max dose 0.5 mg/d)	
		Cyclophosphamide 10 mg/kg/d IV or PO days 1–7 and 43–49	
VAC Standard	Soft tissue sarcomas (rhabdomyosarcoma and undifferentiated sarcomas)	Vincristine 2 mg/m²/wk IV (max dose 2 mg)	Every 3 months for 5–6 cycles
		Dactinomycin 0.015 mg/kg/d IV days 1–5 (max dose 0.5 mg/d)	
		Cyclophosphamide 2.5 mg/kg/d PO daily for 2 years	
VAD	Multiple myeloma (refractory)	Vincristine 0.4 mg/d continuous IV infusion days 1–4	Every 25 days for 12 cycles
		Doxorubicin 9 mg/m²/d continuous IV infusion days 1–4	
		Dexamethasone 40 mg/d PO days 1–4, 9–12, and 17–20	
VBAP	Multiple myeloma	Vincristine 1.0 mg IV day 1	Every 3 weeks for 5 cycles then continue vinblastine 0.3 mg/kg IV every 3 weeks
		Carmustine 30 mg/m² IV day 1	
		Doxorubicin 30 mg/m² IV day 1	
		Prednisone 60 mg/m²/d PO days 1–4	
VBP	Testicular cancer (disseminated)	Vinblastine 0.2 mg/kg/d IV days 1, 2	Every 4 weeks for 2 years
		Cisplatin 20 mg/m²/d IV infusion over 15 min on days 1–5	
		Bleomycin 30 units/wk IV to a total cumulative dose of 360 units (4 cycles)	

(continued)

APPENDIX D1. COMBINATION CHEMOTHERAPEUTIC REGIMENS (cont.)

Abbreviation	Use	Regimen	Frequency
VMCP	Multiple myeloma	Vincristine 1 mg IV day 1 Melphalan 6 mg/m^2/d PO days 1–4 Cyclophosphamide 125 mg/m^2/d PO days 1–4 Prednisone 60 mg/m^2/d PO days 1–4	Every 3 weeks
VP	Acute lymphocytic leukemia (induction)	Vincristine 2 mg/m^2/wk IV times 4–6 weeks (max dose 2 mg) Prednisone 60 mg/m^2/d PO in divided doses times 4 weeks then taper weeks 5–7	One cycle only
VP + DNR	Acute lymphocytic leukemia (children, induction)	Daunorubicin 25 mg/m^2 IV day 1 Vincristine 1.5 mg/m^2 IV day 1 Prednisone 40 mg/m^2/d PO (for children < 2 years or < 0.5 m^2 calculate dose based on mg/kg)	Every week for 4–6 cycles
VP-L-as-paraginase	Acute lymphocytic leukemia (induction)	Vincristine 2 mg/m^2/wk IV for 4–6 weeks (max dose 2 mg) Prednisone 60 mg/m^2/d PO for 4–6 weeks then taper L-asparaginase 10,000 units/m^2/d IV days 1–14	One 4–6 week cycle only
	Acute lymphocytic leukemia (children, induction)	Vincristine 2 mg/m^2/d IV days 1, 8, 15 (max dose 2 mg) Prednisone 40 mg/m^2/d PO in 3 divided doses days 1–15, then taper: 20 mg/m^2 days 16–17, 10 mg/m^2 days 18–19, 5 mg/m^2 days 20–21, 2.5 mg/m^2 days 22–23 L-asparaginase 1000 units/kg/d IV days 22–31 **Or**	One 4–6 week cycle only
		Vincristine 1.5 mg/m^2/d IV days 1, 8, 15, 22 (max dose 2 mg) Prednisone 40 mg/m^2/d PO in 3 divided doses for 28 days (round to nearest 2.5 mg) gradually discontinue over 14 days L-asparaginase 6000 units/m^2/d IM on days 4, 7, 10, 13, 16, 19, 22, 25, 28	One 4–6 week cycle only
VP + L-as-paraginase + DNR	Acute lymphocytic leukemia (induction)	Daunorubicin 45 mg/m^2/d IV days 1, 2, 3 Vincristine 2 mg/d IV days 1, 8, 15 Prednisone 40 mg/m^2/d PO days 1–22, taper days 22–29 L-asparaginase 500 units/kg/d IV days 22–32	One 4–6 week cycle only

This listing of representative combination chemotherapy regimens is not all inclusive and some combinations may be reported in the literature with variations. Modifications may be required for dose-limiting toxicities.

Appendix D2: Combination Chemotherapeutic Regimens

Cancer	Suggested Combination Regimens*
Acute lymphocytic leukemia (adult, induction)	VP
	VP + DNR
	VP + L-asparaginase
	VP + L-asparaginase + DNR
Acute lymphocytic leukemia (pediatric, induction)	VP + L-asparaginase
	VP + DNR
Acute lymphocytic leukemia (maintenance)	MTX + MP
	MTX + MP + CTX
Acute myelocytic leukemia (adult, induction)	ARA-C + ADR
	ARA-C + ADR + VCR + Prednisolone
	ARA-C + 6-TG
	ARA-C + 6-TG + DNR
	ARA-C + DNR
	ARA-C + DNR + 6-TG + VCR + Pred
	Mitoxantrone + ARA-C
Acute myelocytic leukemia (adult, maintenance)	ARA-C + 6-TG
	Mitoxantrone + ARA-C
Acute myelocytic leukemia (pediatric)	ARA-C + DNR + MP + Pred
Bladder cancer (transitional cell)	M-VAC
Breast cancer (metastatic or recurrent)	CAF
	CMFP
	FAC
	ACe
	CMF
	CMFVP (Cooper's regimen)
	MV1b
Chronic lymphocytic leukemia	CHL + Pred
Colon cancer	5-FU + leucovorin
	5-FU + levamisole
Ewing's sarcoma	T-2 Protocol
Gastric carcinoma	FAM
Germ cell tumors	CISCA-II/VB-IV
Hodgkin's lymphoma (adult, induction)	BCVPP
	MOPP
	MOPP-LO BLEO
Hodgkin's lymphoma (pediatric, induction)	A-COPP
Hodgkin's lymphoma (MOPP resistant, induction)	ABVD
	CAVe
Hodgkin's lymphoma (MOPP resistant)	ABDIC
Hodgkin's lymphoma (advanced)	MOPP/ABVD
Hodgkin's lymphoma (advanced, MOPP-resistant)	B-CAVe

(continued)

APPENDIX D2. COMBINATION CHEMOTHERAPEUTIC REGIMENS (cont.)

Cancer	Suggested Combination Regimens
Lung cancer (non-small cell)	CAMP
	FAM
	MACC
	CAP
	FOMi
Lung cancer (small cell, induction)	CAV
	CMC-high dose
Lung cancer (small cell)	ACE
	CHOR
	POCC
Multiple myeloma	M-2 Protocol
	MPL + Pred (MP)
	MAP
	VMCP
Multiple myeloma (alkylator resistant)	ADR + BCNU
Multiple myeloma (refractory)	VAD
Non-Hodgkin's lymphoma (favorable histology)	COP
	COPP or "C" MOPP
	CVP
Non-Hodgkin's lymphoma (unfavorable histology)	BACOP
	CHOP
	COMLA
	COPP or "C" MOPP
Non-Hodgkin's lymphoma (with Hodgkin's disease)	COPP or "C" MOPP
Non-Hodgkin's lymphoma (advanced histiocytic, stage III or IV)	COP-BLAM
Ovarian cancer	ACe
	AP
	CAP
	MAC
Pancreatic cancer	FAM
Soft Tissue sarcomas (adult)	CVAD
Soft Tissue sarcomas (pediatric rhabdomyosarcoma)	VAC Pulse
Soft Tissue sarcomas (rhabdomyosarcoma and undifferentiated)	VAC Standard
Testicular carcinoma (nonseminomatous)	VBP
	VAB-6
Urinary tract cancer	CISCA

*This list of representative combination chemotherapies is not all inclusive and some combinations may be reported in the literature with several variations. Modifications are required for dose-limiting toxicities.

Drug	Dose-Limiting Toxicity	Dose Modifications
Asparaginase	Hypersensitivity reactions that are frequent and may occur during the primary course of therapy and are not completely predictable by skin test; there is an increased risk of hypersensitivity with retreatment	Perform intradermal skin test with 2 IU in 0.1 mL prior to initial administration and when it is given after one or more weeks between doses. Observe site for at least 1 hour for wheal or erythema; a negative test does not preclude possible hypersensitivity reactions; Administer only after successful desensitization in patients found hypersenstitive by skin test and any patient previously treated with asparaginase; one suggested method of desensitization is to begin with 1 IU IV and double the dose every 10 minutes if no reaction has occurred until the planned daily dose has been administered:

Injection #	Dose (IU)	Cumulative Dose (IU)
1	1	1
2	2	3
3	4	7
4	8	15
5	16	31
	Until cumulative dose equals planned dose	

Drug	Dose-Limiting Toxicity	Dose Modifications
		Alternatively, endotoxin-free Erwinia asparaginase (not derived from E Coli) is available from the National Cancer Institute for special circumstances
	Pancreatitis (monitor serum amylase)	Discontinue drug if pancreatitis develops
	Hepatopathy	Improves if drug is stopped; treat with IV fluids and insulin
Bleomycin sulfate	Pulmonary fibrosis (earliest signs and symptoms include fine rales and dyspnea)	Fibrosis is dose related; give total doses over 400 IU with caution (if given with other agents, toxicity may occur at lower doses); discontinue drug if forced vital capacity (FVC) decreases rapidly
	Anaphylactoid reaction (occurs in lymphoma patients)	Treat with 2 IU or less for first 2 doses, and if no acute reactions occur, then start regular dose schedule
	Mucocutaneous toxicity	If severe, may need to discontinue therapy
Busulfan	Myelosuppression (monitor CBC weekly)	Withdraw drug if leukocyte count declines to < 15,000/mm^3
	Pulmonary fibrosis or "busulfan lung" (earliest signs and symptoms include fine rales, dyspnea, cough, and fever)	Stop drug

(continued)

APPENDIX E. DOSE MODIFICATIONS FOR CHEMOTHERAPEUTIC AGENTS (cont.)

Drug	Dose-Limiting Toxicity	Dose Modifications
Carbopla-tin	Myelosuppression (monitor CBC)	Do not repeat dose until neutrophil count > 2000/mm³ and platelet count is > 100,000/mm³; suggested dose modification based on nadir values is outlined below:

Platelets/mm³	Neutrophils/mm³	% Prior Dose
> 100,000	> 2000	125
50,000–100,000	500–2000	100R
< 50,000	< 500	75

| | Nephropathy (monitor creatinine clearance) | Suggested dose modification based on creatinine clearance: |

Baseline Creatinine Clearance (mL/min)	Recommended Dose on Day 1 (mg/m²)
41–59	250
16–40	200

| Carmus-tine | Myelosuppression (monitor CBC for at least 6 weeks after therapy due to delayed cumulative toxicity; do not repeat dose within 6 weeks) | Suggested dose modification based on nadir counts from previous dose: |

Nadir Counts		
Leukocytes/mm³	*Platelets/mm³*	% Prior Dose
> 4000	> 100,000	100
3000–3999	75,000–99,999	100
2000–2999	25,000–74,999	70
< 2000	< 25,000	50

Do not repeat dose until circulating blood elements are at acceptable levels (platelet count > 100,000/mm³ leukocyte count > 4000/mm³, and adequate neutrophils)

Drug	Dose-Limiting Toxicity	Dose Modifications
Chloram-bucil	Myelosuppression (monitor CBC twice weekly for first 3–6 weeks of therapy)	Decrease dose if leukocyte or platelet count fall below normal values or there is an abrupt drop in the leukocyte count; Discontinue if more severe depression occurs
	Bone marrow infiltration (persistently low neutrophils, platelets, and peripheral lymphocytosis)	Do not exceed a daily dose of 0.1 mg/kg
	Radiation or chemotherapy (in past)	Do not give at full dose within 4 weeks of a full course of radiation or chemotherapy
Cisplatin	Nephropathy (monitor BUN, creatinine, creatinine clearance, magnesium, calcium, and potassium)	Administration of cisplatin over 6–8 hours with IV hydration and mannitol has been used to reduce nephrotoxicity; do not give repeat doses unless serum creatinine < 1.5 mg/dL and BUN < 25 mg/dL; electrolyte disturbances can be corrected by electrolyte supplements and discontinuing therapy
	Auditory impairment manifested by tinnitus or high frequency hearing loss (4000–8000 Hz); may be unilateral or bilateral; perform audiometry before starting therapy and prior to each dose	Do not give repeat doses unless audiometric analysis shows normal auditory acuity
	Neuropathy (examine weekly)	Discontinue at first sign of neurotoxicity

(continued)

APPENDIX E. DOSE MODIFICATIONS FOR CHEMOTHERAPEUTIC AGENTS (cont.)

Drug	Dose-Limiting Toxicity	Dose Modifications
	Myelosuppression (monitor CBC weekly)	Do not repeat dose until circulating blood elements are at acceptable levels (platelet count > 100,000/mm^3, leukocyte count > 4000/mm^3, and adequate neutrophils)
	Gastrointestinal symptoms	Severe nausea and vomiting may necessitate discontinuation of therapy; high dose metaclopramide may be used as prophylaxis
Cyclophosphamide	Hepatopathy (monitor bilirubin and SGOT)	Dose modifications recommended based on bilirubin level include the following:

Bilirubin (mg/dL)	SGOT (IU/dL)	% Prior Dose
3.1–5.0	> 180	25
> 5.0		0

Drug	Dose-Limiting Toxicity	Dose Modifications
	Nephropathy (monitor creatinine)	Decrease dose by 50% for a glomerular filtration rate of < 10 mL/min
	Hemorrhagic cystitis (monitor for hematuria)	Hold therapy for cystitis; hydration should be used as prophylaxis; SIADH may occur with IV doses > 50 mg/kg; it is both a limitation to and a consequence of fluid loading
	Myelosuppression (monitor CBC, especially in patients with previous radio- and chemotherapy)	Reduce dose by 33–50% of the initial loading dose
Cytarabine	Myelosuppression (monitor CBC daily; manufacturer recommends frequent bone marrow examinations in acute leukemia after blast cells have disappeared from the peripheral blood)	Hold or modify dose if platelets decrease to < 50,000/mm^3 or neutrophil counts fall below 1000/mm^3
	Hepatopathy (monitor bilirubin)	Decrease dose in patients with poor hepatic function
Dacarbazine	Myelosuppression (monitor CBC)	Recommended dose modifications based on nadir leukocyte and platelet counts are summarized below (when used in combination therapies, such as ABVD):

Leukocytes/mm^3	Platelets/mm^3	% Prior Dose
> 4000	> 130,000	100
3000–3999	100,000–129,999	100
2000–2999	80,000–99,999	50
1500–1999	50,000–79,999	25
< 1500	< 50,000	0

Drug	Dose-Limiting Toxicity	Dose Modifications
Dactinomycin HCL	Myelosuppression (monitor CBC daily)	Hold drug until recovery for markedly decreased platelet or leukocyte counts
	Gastrointestinal symptoms (monitor for stomatitis and severe diarrhea)	In multi-agent therapy, discontinue therapy until patient has recovered
Daunorubicin HCL	Cardiomyopathy (monitor ECG, systolic ejection fraction, and cumulative dose)	Occurs with cumulative doses exceeding 550 mg/m^2 in adults, 400 mg/m^2 in patients with prior chest irradiation, 300 mg/m^2 in children ≥ 2 years old, and 10 mg/kg in children < 2 years old (if toxicity should occur, risk and benefits of continued therapy must be weighed before continuing therapy)
	Myelosuppression (monitor CBC at frequent intervals)	Use primarily as a treatment guide; bone marrow suppression will always occur

(continued)

APPENDIX E. DOSE MODIFICATIONS FOR CHEMOTHERAPEUTIC AGENTS (cont.)

Drug	Dose-Limiting Toxicity	Dose Modifications
	Nephropathy (monitor creatinine) Hepatopathy (monitor bilirubin)	Suggested dose modifications inlcude the following:

Bilirubin (mg/dL)	Creatinine (mg/dL)	% Prior Dose
1.2–3.0		75
> 3.0	> 3.0	50

Drug	Dose-Limiting Toxicity	Dose Modifications
Doxorubicin HCL	Cardiomyopathy (monitor ECG, ejection fraction, and cumulative dose)	For a cumulative dose > 550 mg/m^2 (400 mg/m^2 in patients with previous chest irradiation or chemotherapy), risk and benefits should be weighed before continuing therapy
	Hepatopathy (monitor bilirubin)	Suggested dose modification:

Bilirubin (mg/dL)	% Prior Dose
1.2–3.0	50
> 3.0	25

Drug	Dose-Limiting Toxicity	Dose Modifications
	Myelosuppression (monitor CBC)	Recommended dose modifications based on nadir leukocyte and platelet counts are summarized below (when used in combination therapies, such as ABVD):

Leukocytes/mm^3	Platelets/mm^3	% Prior Dose
> 4000	> 130,000	100
3000–3999	100,000–129,999	50
2000–2999	80,000–99,999	25
1500–1999	50,000–79,999	0
< 1500	< 50,000	0

Drug	Dose-Limiting Toxicity	Dose Modifications
Etoposide	Myelosuppression (monitor CBC before and twice weekly after each dose)	Hold dose until hematologic recovery occurs if platelet count is < 50,000/mm^3 or absolute neutrophil count is < 500/mm^3
	Hypotension (monitor BP)	Administer slowly over 30–60 minutes to avoid hypotension; if hypotension occurs, stop administration, give fluids and other supportive agents, and restart infusion at a slower rate
Floxuridine/	Hepatopathy (monitor bilirubin)	For bilirubin > 5.0, stop fluorouracil
Fluorouracil	Severe adverse reactions (monitor for stomatitis, esophagopharyngitis, intractable vomiting, diarrhea, GI ulceration, GI bleeding, rapidly falling WBC, leukopenia < 3500/ mm^3 WBC, thrombocytopenia < 100,000/mm^3, and hemorrhage)	Discontinue therapy
Hydroxyurea	Myelosuppression (monitor CBC weekly)	For WBC < 2500/mm^3 or platelet count < 100,000/mm^3 hold therapy and recheck counts every 3 days; resume treatment when counts are normal; hold any concomitant radiation if hematologic rebound is not prompt

(continued)

APPENDIX E. DOSE MODIFICATIONS FOR CHEMOTHERAPEUTIC AGENTS (cont.)

Drug	Dose-Limiting Toxicity	Dose Modifications
Ifosfamide	Myelosuppression (monitor CBC prior to each dose and at appropriate intervals)	Do not administer therapy if WBC < 2000/mm^3 or platelet count < 50,000/mm^3
	Hemorrhagic cystitis (monitor for hematuria prior to each dose)	Prevent by dose fractionation, vigorous hydration, and using mesna; hold therapy if microscopic hematuria occurs (> 10 RBCs/high power field)
	Neuropathy (monitor for somnolence, confusion, hallucinations, and coma)	Discontinue therapy
Interferon α-2a	Severe adverse reactions	Reduce dose by 50% or hold treatment until reaction abates
	Neuropathy (monitor for somnolence, confusion, hallucinations, and coma)	Hold drug
	Myelosuppression (monitor for thrombocytopenia and bleeding)	For platelet counts < 50,000/mm^3, give SC not IM
Interferon α-2b	Severe adverse reactions	Reduce dose by 50% or hold drug until reaction abates
	Neuropathy (monitor for somnolence, confusion, hallucinations, and coma)	Hold drug
	Hypersensitivity reactions	Discontinue treatment and start appropriate medical therapy
	Cardiovascular effects (monitor for hypotension, arrhythmias and ischemia)	Modify or decrease dose
	Myelosuppression (monitor for thrombocytopenia and bleeding)	For platelet counts < 50,000/mm^3, give SC not IM
Levamisole	Myelosuppression (monitor CBC)	Discontinue drug if persistent leukopenia develops
	Dermatitis	Discontinue drug
Lomustine	Myelosuppression (monitor CBC weekly for at least 6 weeks; toxicity is cumulative and delayed)	Suggested doses based on prior nadir leukocyte counts are the following:

Leukocytes/mm^3	Platelets/mm^3	% Prior Dose
> 4000	> 100,000	100
3000–3999	75,000–99,999	100
2000–2999	25,000–74,999	70
< 2000	< 25,000	50

With compromised bone marrow function, reduce dose to 100 mg/M^2 q 6 wk; do not repeat dose until circulating blood elements are at acceptable levels (platelet count > 100,000/mm^3, leukocyte count > 4000/mm^3, and adequate neutrophils)

Mechlorethamine — Myelosuppression (monitor CBC) — Hold therapy until complete hematologic recovery; recommended dose modification (when used in combination therapies, such as MOPP) based on nadir leukocyte and platelet counts is summarized below:

Leukocytes/mm^3	Platelets/mm^3	% Prior Dose
> 4000	> 100,000	100
3000–3999		75
1000–2999	50,000–100,000	50
< 1000	< 50,000	0

(*continued*)

APPENDIX E. DOSE MODIFICATIONS FOR CHEMOTHERAPEUTIC AGENTS (cont.)

Drug	Dose-Limiting Toxicity	Dose Modifications
	Gastrointestinal symptoms (monitor for severe vomiting 1–3 hours after dose; may precipitate intracranial bleeding due to severe emesis)	Premedicate with antiemetics and sedatives
Melphalan	Myelosuppression (monitor CBC weekly)	Decrease or stop therapy until hematologic recovery if leukocytes fall to < 3000/mm³ or platelet count is < 100,000/mm³
Mercapto-purine	Myelosuppression (monitor CBC weekly and bone marrow if status is uncertain)	Continue, modify, or stop therapy based on absolute blood cell counts, rate of fall, indications for therapy, as well as the availability of supportive facilities
	Hepatopathy (monitor bilirubin; jaundice, hepatomegaly, anorexia, right upper quadrant pain, toxic hepatitis, and biliary stasis can occur with doses > 2.5 mg/kg/d)	Discontinue therapy and investigate etiology
Metho-trexate	Myelosuppression (monitor CBC weekly)	Hold therapy if blood counts fall rapidly and restart only if benefit outweighs the risk of severe myelosuppression
	Hepatopathy (monitor bilirubin, transaminases, and albumin prior to each dose)	Modify dose as indicated below:

Bilirubin (mg/dL)	SGOT (IU/dL)	% Prior Dose
3.0–5.0	> 180	25
> 5.0		0

	Pulmonary fibrosis (monitor for dyspnea, nonproductive cough, hypoxemia, fever, and pulmonary infiltrates	Stop the drug and evaluate etiology
	Gastrointestinal symptoms (monitor for severe diarrhea, vomiting, ulcerative stomatitis, hemorrhagic enteritis, and intestinal perforation)	Hold drug until recovery
	Nephropathy (monitor creatinine and creatinine clearance prior to each dose)	Discontinue therapy until improvement
	Leucovorin rescue	Suggested leucovorin guidelines:

Methotrexate Elimination	Lab Findings	Leukovorin
Normal	Serum MTX approx. 10 µM at 24 h, 1µM at 48 h, and < 0.2 µM at 72 h	15 mg PO or IV q 6 h for 60 h (10 doses starting 24 h after start of MTX infusion)
Delayed	Serum MTX remains above 0.2 µM at 72 h, and > 0.05 µM at 96 h	Continue 15 mg PO or IV q 6 h until MTX level is < 0.05 µM
Delayed early or acute renal injury	Serum MTX > 50 µM at 24 h, > 5 µM at 48 h; or > 2 times increase in serum creatinine levels at 24 h	150 mg IV q 3 h until MTX level is < 1 µM, then 15 mg IV q 3 h until MTX level is < 0.05 µM

Delay methotrexate until recovery for the following:
1. WBC < 1500/mm³
2. Neutrophils < 200/mm³
3. Platelets < 75,000/mm³
4. Serum bilirubin > 1.2 mg/dL
5. SGPT > 450 U/dL
6. Mucositis present
7. Persistent pleural effusions present

(continue

APPENDIX E. DOSE MODIFICATIONS FOR CHEMOTHERAPEUTIC AGENTS (cont.)

Methotrexate Elimination (cont.)

Adequate renal function must be documented with normal serum creatinine and creatinine clearance >60 ml/min before starting therapy; if serum creatinine levels increase by > 50%, creatinine clearance must be documented to be > 60 mL/min even if the serum creatinine level is within normal levels

Drug	Dose-Limiting Toxicity	Dose Modifications
Mitomycin	Myelosuppression (monitor CBC weekly and for 8 weeks after therapy)	Suggested dose modification based on nadir leukocyte and platelet counts of prior dose:

Leukocytes/mm^3	Platelets/mm^3	% Prior Dose
> 4000	> 100,000	100
3000–3999	75,000–99,999	100
2000–2999	25,000–74,999	70
< 2000	< 25,000	50

Do not repeat dose until the leukocyte count is > 3000/mm^3 and the platelet count is > 75,000/mm^3

Drug	Dose-Limiting Toxicity	Dose Modifications
	Nephropathy (monitor creatinine)	Hold drug if serum creatinine > 1.7 mg/dL
	Pulmonary fibrosis (monitor for dyspnea, nonproductive cough, and infiltrates)	Discontinue therapy if other etiologies are eliminated
Mitotane	Severe adverse reactions	Reduce dose to maximum tolerated levels
Mitoxantrone HCL	Severe adverse reactions (monitor during first induction course)	Hold second induction course until toxicities abate
	Myelosuppression, severe (monitor CBC frequently)	Continue treatment only if benefits outweigh risks of severe myelosuppression
Pipobroman	Myelosuppression (monitor CBC every other day and bone marrow prior to therapy and at maximal response)	Stop therapy if leukocytes are < 3000/mm^3 or if platelets are < 150,000/mm^3; discontinue for rapid fall in hemoglobin, rise in bilirubin and reticulocyte count (hemolysis)
Plicamycin	Thrombocytopenia, severe with hemorrhagic tendencies (monitor for epistaxis and hematemesis; monitor platelets, prothrombin and bleeding time frequently)	Discontinue treatment if thrombocytopenia or prolongation of prothrombin or bleeding times occurs
Procarbazine HCL	Myelosuppression (monitor CBC and reticulocyte count twice weekly)	Recommended dose modifications based on nadir leukocyte and platelet counts are summarized below (when used in combination therapies, such as MOPP):

Leukocytes/mm^3	Platelets/mm^3	% Prior Dose
> 4000	> 100,000	100
3000–3999	> 100,000	75
2000–2999	50,000–100,000	50
1000–1999	50,000–100,000	25
< 1000	< 50,000	0

Drug	Dose-Limiting Toxicity	Dose Modifications
	Neuropathy (monitor for somnolence, confusion, hallucinations, and coma)	Hold drug until reaction abates
	Hypersensitivity reactions	Hold drug until reaction abates
	Gastrointestinal symptoms (monitor for stomatitis and diarrhea)	Hold drug until reaction abates
	Hemorrhagic tendencies (monitor for epistaxis and hematemesis)	Hold drug until reaction abates

(continued)

APPENDIX E. DOSE MODIFICATIONS FOR CHEMOTHERAPEUTIC AGENTS (cont.)

Drug	Dose-Limiting Toxicity	Dose Modifications
Thiogua-nine	Myelosuppression (monitor CBC)	Modify or discontinue drug based on absolute value and rate of change in hematologic parameters
	Hepatopathy (monitor bilirubin, transaminases, and alkaline phosphatase weekly at first and then monthly; monitor for toxic hepatitis, biliary stasis, jaundice, hepatomegaly, anorexia, and right upper quadrant pain)	Stop drug and determine etiology
Thiotepa	Myelosuppression (monitor CBC weekly and for at least 3 weeks after therapy)	Stop drug if WBC falls to < 3000/mm^3 or platelet count decreases to < 150,000/mm^3 or a rapid fall occurs
Streptozo-tocin	Myelosuppression (monitor CBC weekly)	Stop drug if WBC falls to < 3000/mm^3 or platelet count decreases to < 150,000/mm^3 or a rapid fall occurs
	Hepatopathy (monitor bilirubin, transaminases, alkaline phosphatase weekly)	Decrease or discontinue drug
	Nephropathy (monitor creatinine, BUN, electrolytes, urinalysis, and creatinine clearance prior to, weekly during, and weekly for 4 weeks after drug administration)	Decrease or discontinue drug
Uracil mustard	Myelosuppression (monitor CBC twice weekly and for permanent bone marrow damage)	Decrease or discontinue drug for severe toxicity
Vinblas-tine sul-fate	Myelosuppression (monitor CBC weekly)	Recommended dose modifications based on nadir leukocyte and platelet counts are summarized below (when used in combination therapies, such as ABVD):

Leukocytes/mm^3	Platelets/mm^3	% Prior Dose
> 4000	> 130,000	100
3000–3999	100,000–129,999	50
2000–2999	80,000–99,999	25
1500–1999	50,000–79,999	0
< 1500	< 50,000	0

Drug	Dose-Limiting Toxicity	Dose Modifications
	Hepatopathy (monitor direct bilirubin)	With serum bilirubin > 3.0 mg/dL, decrease dose to 50%
Vincris-tine sul-fate	Neuropathy (monitor for reversible loss of deep tendon reflexes, sensory impairment, paresthesias, neuritic pain, and motor difficulties)	Toxicity is dose-dependent and cumulative; stop drug after 30–50 mg
	Gastrointestinal symptoms (monitor for paralytic ileus)	Hold drug until resolution; provide symptomatic relief
	Hepatopathy (monitor bilirubin and SGOT)	Dose modification guidelines are the following:

Bilirubin (mg/dL)	SGOT IU/dL	% Prior Dose
1.5–3.0		50
> 3.1	> 180	0

Appendix F: WHO Grading for Therapy-Induced Toxicity

Toxicity	Grade 0	Grade 1	Grade 2	Grade 3	Grade 4
Cardiac Function	None	Abnormal but asymptomatic	Transient symptoms, no therapy required	Symptomatic, responsive to therapy	Symptomatic, unresponsive to therapy
Pericarditis	None	Asymptomatic effusion	Symptomatic, no therapy required	Tamponade requiring pericardiocentesis	Tamponade requiring surgery
Rhythm	None	Sinus tachycardia > 110	Unifocal PVC atrial arrhythmia	Multifocal PVCs	Ventricular tachycardia
Dermal	None	Erythema	Dry desquamation, vesiculation, pruritus	Moist desquamation, ulceration	Exfoliative dermatitis, necrosis requiring surgery
Drug allergy	None	Edema	Bronchospasm, no parenteral therapy required	Bronchospasm requiring parenteral therapy	Anaphylaxis
Drug fever	None	Fever < 38°C	Fever 38–40°C	Fever > 40°C	Fever with hypotension
Gastrointestinal Nausea/emesis	None	Nausea	Transient vomiting	Vomiting requiring therapy	Vomiting unresponsive to therapy (intractable)
Diarrhea	None	Transient < 2 days	> 2 days but tolerable	Intolerable diarrhea requiring therapy	Hemorrhagic dehydration
Oral	None	Soreness/erythema	Erythema and ulcers but can eat solids	Ulceration requiring liquid diet	Alimentation not possible
Bilirubin	$\leq 1.25 \times nl$	$1.26–2.5 \times nl$	$2.6–5.0 \times nl$	$5.1–10.0 \times nl$	$> 10 \times nl$
Alkaline phosphatase	$\leq 1.25 \times nl$	$1.26–2.5 \times nl$	$2.6–5.0 \times nl$	$5.1–10.0 \times nl$	$> 10 \times nl$
SGOT/SGPT	$\leq 1.25 \times nl$	$1.26–2.5 \times nl$	$2.6–5.0 \times nl$	$5.1 \times 10.0 \times nl$	$> 10 \times nl$
Hematologic Hemoglobin (g/dL)	≥ 11.0	9.5–10.9	8.0–9.4	6.5–7.9	< 6.5
Leukocytes ($\times 10^3/mm^3$)	≥ 4.0	3.0–3.9	2.0–2.9	1.0–1.9	< 1.0

(continued)

APPENDIX F. WHO GRADING FOR THERAPY-INDUCED TOXICITY (cont.)

Toxicity	Grade 0	Grade 1	Grade 2	Grade 3	Grade 4
Hematologic (cont.)					
Granulocytes ($\times 10^3/mm^3$)	≥ 2.0	1.5–1.9	1.0–1.4	0.5–0.9	< 0.5
Platelets ($\times 10^4/mm^3$)	≥ 10.0	7.5–9.9	5.0–7.4	2.5–4.9	< 2.5
Hemorrhage	None	Petechiae	Mild hemorrhage	Gross hemmorrhage	Debilitating hemorrhage
Neurologic					
Consciousness	Alert	Transient lethargy	Somnolent < 50% of waking hrs	Somnolent > 50% of waking hours	Comatose
Constipation	None	Mild	Moderate	Abdominal distention	Distention/vomiting
Peripheral neuropathy	None	Paresthesias/decreased deep tendon reflexes	Severe paresthesias/mild weakness	Intolerable paresthesias/marked motor loss	Paralysis
Pain	None	Mild	Moderate	Severe	Intractable
Pulmonary	None	Mild symptoms	Exertional dyspnea	Dyspnea at rest	Total bed rest required
Urologic					
Blood urea nitrogen (BUN)	$<1.25 \times nl$	$1.26–2.5 \times nl$	$2.6–5.0 \times nl$	$5–10 \times nl$	$> 10 \times nl$
Creatinine	$\leq 1.25 \times nl$	$1.26–2.5 \times nl$	$2.6–5.0 \times nl$	$5–10 \times nl$	$> 10 \times nl$
Hematuria	None	Microscopic	Gross	Clots present	Obstructive uropathy
Proteinuria	None	< 0.3 g/dL (1+)	0.3–1.0 g/dL (2–3+)	> 1.0 g/dL (4+)	Nephrotic syndrome

General References

American Cancer Society. *Cancer Facts and Figures*. Atlanta, GA: American Cancer Society; 1989.

Beahrs OH, editor. *Manual for Staging of Cancer*, 4th ed. Philadelphia, PA: JB Lippincott; 1992.

Boring CC, Squires TS, Tong T. Cancer statistics, 1993. *CA—A Cancer J for Clinicians* 1993;**43**:7.

DeVita VT, Hellman S, Rosenberg SA, editors. *Cancer: Principles and Practice of Oncology,* 4th ed. Philadelphia, PA: JB Lippincott; 1993.

Haskell CM, editor. *Cancer Treatment,* 3rd ed. Philadelphia, PA: WB Saunders; 1990.

Holleb AI, Fink DJ, Murphy GP, editors. *American Cancer Society Textbook of Clinical Oncology.* Atlanta, GA: American Cancer Society; 1991.

National Cancer Institute. *1987 Annual Cancer Statistics Review.* Bethesda, MD: National Institutes of Health; 1987.

Wilson J, et al, editors. *Harrison's Principles of Internal Medicine,* 12th ed. New York: McGraw-Hill; 1990.

Index

Page numbers followed by *t* and *f* indicate tables and figures, respectively.

665